TURNBULL'S OBSTETRICS

For Harcourt Brace

Publisher: Miranda Bromage
Project Editor: Tim Kimber

Freelancers

Project Manager: Nora Naughton
Copy-editor: Ruth Swan
Indexer: Nina Boyd

TURNBULL'S OBSTETRICS

Third edition

Edited by

Geoffrey Chamberlain
RD MD FRCS FRCOG FACOG (Hons)

Emeritus Professor,
St George's Hospital Medical School
London, UK

Philip J Steer
BSc MD FRCOG

Professor, Imperial College School of Medicine
Chelsca and Westminster Hospital
London, UK

Associate Editors

Gérard Bréart MD
Professor, Epidemiological
Research Unit on Women and Children,
Paris, France

Allan Chang MBBS PhD FRCOG FRACOG
Professor, Chinese University, Hong Kong

Mark Johnson PhD MRCP MRCOG
Senior Lecturer, Imperial College School of Medicine
Chelsea and Westminster Hospital
London, UK

James Purdie Neilson BSc MB ChB MRCOG MD FRCOG
Professor, University of Liverpool
Liverpool, UK

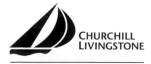
CHURCHILL
LIVINGSTONE

LONDON   EDINBURGH   NEW YORK   PHILADELPHIA   ST LOUIS   SYDNEY   TORONTO 2001

CHURCHILL LIVINGSTONE

An imprint of Harcourt Publishers Limited

ISBN 0 443 063 656

British Library Cataloguing in Publication Data
A catalogue record for this book is available from the British Library.

Library of Congress Cataloging in Publication Data
A catalog record for this book is available from the Library of Congress.

Note
Medical knowledge is constantly changing. As new information becomes
available, changes in treatment, procedures, equipment and the use of
drugs become necessary. The editors and contributors and the publishers
have, as far as it is possible, taken care to ensure that the information
given in this text is accurate and up to date. However, readers are
strongly advised to confirm that the information, especially with regard
to drug usage, complies with current legislation and standards of
practice.

The publishers have made every effort to trace holders of copyright of
original material and to seek permission for its use. Should this have
proved impossible, then copyright holders are asked to contact the
publishers so that suitable acknowledgement can be made at the first
opportunity.

During the production of this book, there was an international
agreement to change the names Lignocaine to Lidocaine, Thiopentone to
Thiopental and Suxamethonium to Succinyldioline. This edition uses the
older names more familiar to contemporary obstetricians but will change
by the next edition.

Printed and bound in China

Contents

Section 4

Normal Labour

Section 5

Abnormal Labour

Section 6

The Puerperium

Section 7

The Baby

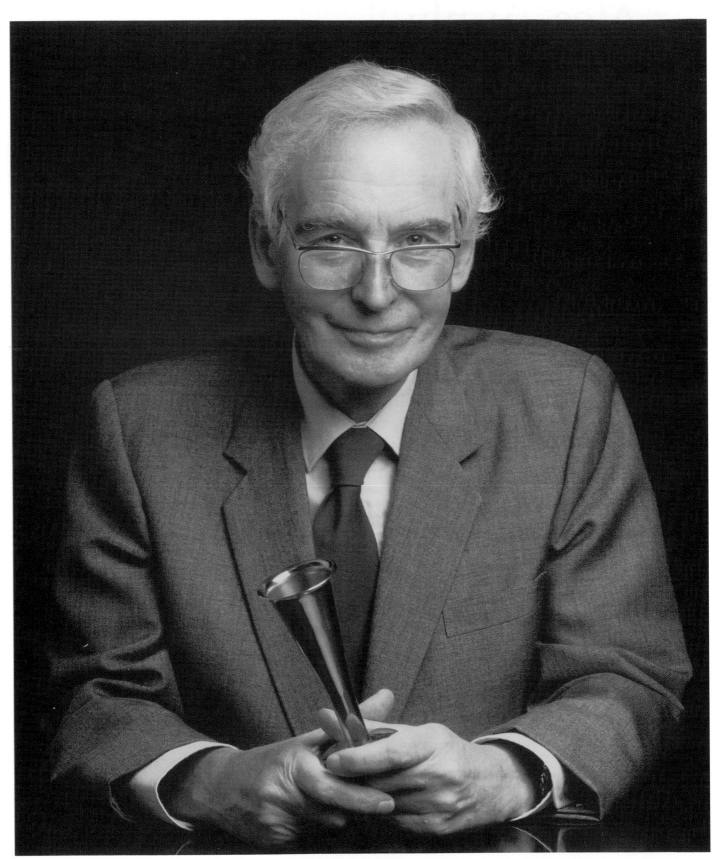

Sir Alec Turnbull 1925–90

Sir Alec Turnbull

The architects of the first edition of *Obstetrics*, Professors Turnbull and Chamberlain, laid their opening plans in a garden at Chandigar in the Punjab in 1984. They were lecturing at the Postgraduate Medical Centre of India as a part of a British Council course and one evening were sitting and talking about the future of postgraduate medical education in the United Kingdom. They both realized that a big definitive postgraduate book, an account of the best in British obstetrics, was required and agreed that evening to co-edit such a volume. In the foothills of the Himalayas, the first discussions took place and a provisional list of authors was considered. This was modified several times and, as soon as they returned to Britain, invitations went out.

At the time, the editors were both Vice-President of the Royal College of Obstetricians and Gynaecologists. The book, therefore, had an emphasis from that educational establishment, and had a commonwealth flavor. During the course of the next two or three years, unfortunately Professor Turnbull developed a recurrence of his previous malignancy. He still, however, worked hard at the planning and editing of the first edition. The publication of Obstetrics in 1989 corresponded with one of the last appearances of Alec Turnbull on the international scene at the XXV British Congress of Obstetrics and Gynaecology in London.

A few years went by and the science of obstetrics has advanced, in 1994 a new edition of the 1989 volume was required. With the permission of Lady Elsie Turnbull, we decided to turn the title into Turnbull's Obstetrics, thus creating a memorial for a man who was probably the greatest British obstetrician of his generation. Professor Chamberlain, the remaining editor who was by then serving as President RCOG was happy to edit this new edition as a memorial to Alec Turnbull who did so much for his college. Now in 2000 comes a third edition, the last to be piloted by Geoffrey Chamberlain. The now senior editor is glad to invite Professor Philip Steer to help make this edition up to date and accurate.

Alec was born in Aberdeen in 1925. He went to school and medical school there, qualifying in 1947. With the exception of a period with Professor James Walker at Dundee, he stayed in the Aberdeen school under the aegis of Sir Dugald Baird until 1966. Whilst there, he meet Elsie noted clinical scientist herself, and they married. She was his staunch companion for the rest of his life.

From Aberdeen, Alec Turnbull moved to Cardiff as Professor and then on to Oxford. In all these changes his colleague, Anne Anderson, with whom he made a strong team, examining much of the physiology of labour and control of uterine contractions, accompanied him. Anne unfortunately died in 1983 and Alec continued in his department at Oxford with other workers. As well as his grasp of science, Sir Alec Turnbull was a great humanitarian, looking at each woman as an individual and caring for all those who consulted him. Alec was the ideal obstetrician, and in 1984 The Observer honoured him, with the title of *The Obstetricians' Obstetrician*. With Lady Turnbull's permission, we use the photograph of that occasion on the facing page.

Alec developed a secondary malignancy and become ill in 1989. In July of the following year, a great scientific meeting was held in Oxford at which all his friends gathered. He died in August 1990.

This book is a memorial to Alec Turnbull. It is hoped that it will go through many editions. Alec's influence is still with us in obstetrics; in all he touched, he left his mark for the betterment of women in childbirth. We shall all be remembering and paying respect to a great British obstetrician for we all owe Alec a debt.

Geoffrey Chamberlain
Swansea
2001

Philip Steer
London
2001

Preface

The origins of this textbook are described on page ix in the appreciation of Alec Turnbull. It started when the two original editors, Professor Alec Turnbull and Professor Geoffrey Chamberlain, were in Chandiga in the Punjab. They were discussing the need for a full comprehensive account of British obstetrics for postgraduate education. They planned out the contents, returned to England and so the first edition was born in 1989. Unfortunately, Alec Turnbull developed a secondary malignancy in the same year, and so when another edition was required in 1995, the remaining editor oversaw the production and changed the title to honour Sir Alec Turnbull. Now, in the next millennium, that second edition has been updated and so we turn to a third edition.

The senior editor, Professor Geoffrey Chamberlain, has retired from clinical obstetrics and so thought he should have another editor with him who was deep in the shifting world of obstetrics. Professor Philip Steer was invited to join; he is a professor at the Chelsea and Westminster Hospital, which is now part of an Imperial College School of Medicine and is active in many research areas in obstetrics and neo-natology, having recently completed three years as President of the British Association of Perinatal Medicine.

Another innovation was to form an Editorial Board to whom manuscripts were circulated and whose comments were used to add final polish to the work. The Board was Professor Gérard Bréart of INSERM in Paris, Professor Allan Chang of Hong Kong, Mr. Mark Johnson, Senior Lecturer in Obstetrics and Obstetrics Medicine at the Chelsea and Westminster Hospital and Professor James Neilson, Professor of Obstetrics in Liverpool. This innovation has improved the work considerably and the two senior editors are greatly indebted to the members of the Editorial Board for their (usually) quick turn around of material and their comments.

The need for a third edition was based on the large demand from obstetricians throughout the English speaking world for an update on material published previously in 1989 and 1994 for the subject has moved on rapidly in obstetrics. This edition reflects that for there is new material in all chapters while some chapters have been replaced by others considered by the editors to be more important in the understanding in the new obstetrics. Whilst the majority of the chapter authors come from teaching hospitals in the British Isles we also include work from France, South Africa, Australia and Hong Kong.

We have again structured the book chronologically. First is basic science, which now includes maternal genetics and immunology. Antenatal care contains chapters pertaining to care of the normal followed by the abnormal. A section on labour follows, again divided into normal and abnormal. After this, the puerperium is considered. Finally, there is a brief but comprehensive account of the statistics of childbirth and its medico-legal problems. The last chapter helps the reader who wants to perform and publish research on the subject.

We have enjoyed producing this volume but it would not have been possible without the help of many people. Our secretaries have worked hard and we particularly would like to thank Mrs Caron McColl who dealt with many drafts of the chapters. We are very happy with the co-operation of the publishers Churchill Livingstone. The constant support of Tim Kimber and Miranda Bromage has lead us and our authors along a straight and narrow path and we are proud of the production, which has resulted. We have consulted widely and are grateful for the advice, which has been given. As always, we are happy to receive letters, faxes or e-mails about this new edition and we will try to answer any questions you may pose.

Geoffrey Chamberlain
Swansea
2001

Philip Steer
London
2001

Contributors

Nazar N. Amso, PhD, FRCOG
Department of Obstetrics & Gynaecology
University of Wales College of Medicine, Cardiff, UK

Rekha Bajoria, PhD, MD, MRCOG
University of Manchester & St Mary's Hospital
Manchester, UK

Phillip Bennett, BSc, PhD, MD, MRCOG
Professor of Obstetrics & Gynaecology
Institute of Reproductive and Development Biology
Imperial College School of Medicine, London, UK

Eve M. Blair, PhD
Research Officer to the Western Australian Cerebral Palsy
Register
Senior Research Officer
TVW Telethon Institute for Child Health Research, Perth,
Australia

John Bonnar, MA, MD, FRCPI, FRCOG
Emeritus Professor of Obstetrics and Gynaecology
Trinity College, University of Dublin
Trinity Centre for Health Sciences
St James's Hospital, Dublin, Ireland

Gérard Bréart, MD
Professor
Research Unit Director,
Epidemiological Research Unit on Women and Children's
Health, Paris, France

Fiona Broughton-Pipkin, MA
Professor of Perinatal Physiology
Department of Gynaecology
Queen's Medical Centre, Nottingham, UK

Helen Budge, MA, BM, BCh, MRCP, MRCPCH
Lecturer in Child Health
Academic Division of Child Health
University Hospital
Queen's Medical Centre, Nottingham, UK

Allan Chang, PhD, MBBS, FRCOG, FRACOG
Professor
Department of Obstetrics and Gynaecology
The Chinese University of Hong Kong, Hong Kong

Jean Chapple, MB, ChB MCommH FFPHM DRCOG DCH MFFP
Consultant in Perinatal Epidemiology
and Honorary Senior Lecturer
Imperial College School of Medicine, London, UK

Roger V. Clements, FRCS, FRCOG
Founding Governor Expert Witness Institute
Editor Clinical Risk
Consultant Obstetrician and Gynaecologist, London, UK

Katy Clifford, MA, MD, MRCOG
Consultant Obstetrician and Gynaecologist
St Mary's Hospital, London, UK

Anna Cockell, MD, MRCOG
Consultant in Genetics and Fetal Medicine
Fetal Medicine Unit, Institute of Child Health and
University College Hospital London
London, UK

Rachel Collis, MBBS FRCA
Consultant Obstetric Anaesthetist
University Hospital of Wales, Cardiff, UK

Phillip Cox, PhD, MBBS, FRCPath
Consultant Perinatal Pathologist
Birmingham Women's Hospital
Birmingham, UK

Patricia Crowley, FRCPI, FRCOG
Senior Lecturer
Department of Obstetrics & Gynaecology
Coombe Women's Hospital, Dublin, Ireland

John Davison, BSc, MD, MSc, FRCOG
Consultant Obstetrician & Professor of Obstetric Medicine
University Department of Obstetrics & Gynaecology
Royal Victoria Infirmary, Newcastle-upon-Tyne, UK

Michael de Swiet, MD, FRCP, FRCOG
Consultant Physician
Professor of Obstetric Medicine
Imperial College School of Medicine
Queen Charlotte's Hospital, London, UK

Noel Dilly, GM, MB, BS, FRCOphth
Chairman
Department of Anatomy and Development Biology
St George's Hospital Medical School, London, UK

James Drife, BSc, MD, FRCS (Ed), FRCOG
Department of Obstetrics and Gynaecology
Leeds General Infirmary, Leeds, UK

William Dunlop, PhD, MBChB, FRCOG, FRCS (Ed)
Department of Obstetrics and Gynaecology
Royal Victoria Infirmary, Newcastle-upon-Tyne, UK

Nicholas Fisk, PhD, FRCOG, FRANZCOG, DDU
Professor of Obstetrics and Gynaecology
Institute of Reproductive and Developmental Biology
Division of Paediatrics, Obstetrics and Gynaecology
Imperial College School of Medicine, Queen Charlotte's &
Chelsea Hospital
Hammersmith Hospital Campus, London, UK

Gillian Forrest, MB, BS, FRCPsych, FRCPCH
Consultant Child Psychiatrist
Park Hospital for Children, Oxford, UK

Harold Fox, MD, FRCPath, FRCOG
Emeritus Professor of Reproductive Pathology
Department of Pathological Sciences
University of Manchester, Manchester, UK

Ian Greer, MD, FRCP (Glas), FRCP(Edin), FRCP(Lond), FRCOG, MFFP
Regius Professor and Head of Department
Department of Obstetrics and Gynaecology
University of Glasgow, Glasgow, UK

François Goffinet, PhD, MD
Obstetrician
Epidemiological Research Unit on Women and Children's
Health, Paris, France

Marion Harvey Hall, MD, FRCOG
Consultant Obstetrician & Gynaecologist
Clinical Professor in the University of Aberdeen
Aberdeen Maternity Hospital, Aberdeen, UK

Michael Harmer, MD, FRCA
Professor of Anaesthesia and Honorary Consultant
Anaesthetist
University of Wales College of Medicine, Cardiff, UK

Anne Harper, MD, FRCOG
Senior Lecturer
School of Medicine, Obstetrics and Gynaecology
Queen's University, Belfast, UK

Philip Hay, MBBS, FRCP
Department of Genitourinary Medicine
St George's Hospital, London, UK

G. Justus Hofmeyr, MBBCh, MRCOG
Professor and Head
Department of Obstetrics and Gynaecology
Effective Care Research Unit
University of the Witwatersrand, Johannesburg, South
Africa

Peter Howie, MD, FRSE, FRCP, FRCOG
Professor of Obstetrics and Gynaecology
Ninewells Hospital and Medical School, Dundee, UK

Frank E. Hytten, MD, PhD, FRCOG
Previously Head of Division of Perinatal Medicine
Clinical Research Centre, Harrow, Middx

Mark Johnson, PhD, MRCP, MRCOG
Senior Lecturer/Honorary Consultant
Imperial College School of Medicine
Chelsea & Westminster Hospital, London, UK

The Late R Kumar
Section of Perinatal Psychiatry
Institute of Psychiatry, Denmark Hill, London, UK

Ashley King, MA, MD, MRCP, MRCPath
King's College Fellow in Medical Sciences
Research Group in Human Pathology
University of Cambridge, Cambridge, UK

Tze Kin Lau, MBChB, MD, MRCOG
Associate Professor
Department of Obstetrics and Gynaecology
The Chinese University of Hong Kong, Hong Kong

Elizabeth A. Letsky, MB BS, FRCPath, FRCOG, FRCPCH
Consultant Perinatal Haematologist/Hon Senior Lecturer,
ICSM
Queen Charlotte's & Chelsea Hospital, London, UK

Yung Wai Loke, MA, MD, FRCOG (Hon)
Professor of Reproductive Immunology
Department of Pathology, University of Cambridge
Research Group in Human Reproductive Immunobiology
Cambridge, UK

William Martin, DM, MRCOG
Consultant in Fetal Medicine, Department of Fetal Medicine
Birmingham Women's Hospital, Birmingham, UK

James Purdie Neilson, BSc, MB ChB, MD, FRCOG
Professor of Obstetrics and Gynaecology
University of Liverpool
Honorary Consultant Obstetrician and Gynaecology
University Department of Obstetrics and Gynaecology
Liverpool Women's Hospital, Liverpool, UK

Catherine Nelson-Piercy, MA (Cantab), FRCP
Consultant Obstetric Physician
Department of Obstetrics,
Guys & St Thomas' Hospital, London, UK

Ann Oakley, MA, PhD
Professor of Sociology and Social Policy
Director of Social Science Research Unit
Institute of Education, University of London, London, UK

Lorien O'Dowd, MBBS, BSc, MRCPsych
Specialist Registrar in Psychiatry
Bethlem and Maudsley Hospitals, London, UK

Sandy Oliver, PhD, BA (Hons),
Honorary Visiting Fellow
UK Cochrane Centre
Senior Research Officer
Social Science Research Unit
Institute of Education, University of London, London, UK

Philip Owen, MB, BCh, MD, MRCOG
Consultant Obstetrician and Gynaecologist
North Glasgow NHS University Trust, Glasgow, UK

Lesley Ann Page, MSc BA RM RN RNT RMT
Head, Department of Midwifery
C&W Health Centre of British Columbia
Professor, Department of Family Practice
University of British Columbia
Vancouver, Canada

Pran Pandya, MBBS, MD, MRCOG
Consultant in Obstetrics and Fetal Medicine
Fetal Medicine Unit
Obstetric Hospital
University College London Hospitals, London, UK

Martin Pera, PhD, BA
Associate Professor
Institute of Reproduction and Development, Victoria,
Australia

Leslie Regan, MD, FRCOG
Professor of Obstetrics and Gynaecology
Department of Reproductive Science and Medicine
ICSM at St Mary's Hospital, London, UK

Charles H. Rodeck, BSc, MBBS, DSc (Med), FRCOG, FRCPath, fMedSci
Professor and Head of Department of Obstetrics and
Gynaecology
University College London Hospitals, London, UK

Michael Rogers, MD
Department of Obstetrics/Gynaecology
Prince of Wales Hospital, Shatin, Hong Kong

Henry Sathananthan, PhD, BSc
Honorary Associate Professor
Institute of Reproduction and Development, Victoria,
Australia

Michael Sharland, MB BSc, MD, FRCPCH, MRCP, DTM&H
Consultant in Paediatric Infectious Disease
Paediatric Infectious Disease Unit
St George's Hospital, London, UK

Robert Shaw, MD, FRCS(Ed), FRCOG, MFFP
Head of Department of Obstetrics & Gynaecology
Welsh School of Medicine, Cardiff
President
Royal College of Obstetricians and Gynaecologists

Richard Smith, MRCOG
Clinical Research Fellow
Institute of Reproductive and Development Biology
Imperial College School of Medicine
Queen Charlotte's & Chelsea Hospital
Hammersmith Hospital Campus, London, UK

Fiona Stanley, AC, MSc, MD, Hon. DSc, FFPHM, FAFPHM, FRACP, FRACOG, FASSA
Director
TWV Telethon Institute for Child Health Research
Professor of Paediatrics
University of Western Australia, Perth, Australia

Philip J. Steer, BSc, MD, FRCOG
Academic Head of Maternal Fetal Medicine
Imperial College School of Medicine
Clinical Director of Perinatal Services
Chelsea and Westminster Hospital, London, UK

Terence Stephenson, BSc, BM, BCh, DM, FRCP, FRCPCH
Professor of Child Health
Head of Academic Division of Child Health
Academic Division of Child Health
University Hospital, Queen's Medical Centre
Nottingham, UK

William Thompson, BSc, MD, FRCOG
Emeritus Professor of Obstetrics and Gynaecology
Queen's University, Belfast, UK

Alan Trounson, PhD
Professor and Deputy Director
Institute of Reproduction and Development, Victoria,
Australia

Austin H. N. Ugwumadu, MB, MRCOG
Consultant Obstetrician & Gynaecologist
Honorary Senior Lecturer
Department of Obstetrics & Gynaecology
St George's Hospital, London, UK

Stephen A. Walkinshaw, BSc (Hons), MD, MRCOG
Consultant in Maternal-Fetal Medicine,
Fetal Centre,
Women's Hospital Liverpool, Liverpool, UK

Martin Whittle, MD, FRCOG, FRCP (Glas.)
Head of Division of Reproductive and Child Health
University of Birmingham, Birmingham, UK

Catherine Williamson, MRCP
Wellcome Advanced Fellow
MRC Clinical Sciences Centre
Imperial College School of Medicine
Hammersmith Hospital, London, UK

Section 1
BASIC SCIENCE IN OBSTETRICS

1

The continuum of obstetrics

Geoffrey Chamberlain

Obstetrics is the art and science of caring for women and their unborn progeny during pregnancy, labour and the immediate puerperium. In previous times there was much craft but not much science, but now the balance is being redressed with an increasing amount of well-understood science although a lot of craft is still required to deal with the mechanical problems. The one has not given way to the other, rather, science has augmented the practical side of childbirth.

THE PAST

Early times

Long before physicians took an interest in obstetrical matters, midwives or guid women were supervising labour. With no formal training but a variable heritage of experience, such women have been working since biblical times (Genesis 25.17 and Genesis 38.28) and were well known in the Egyptian and Greek civilisations. Training was usually obtained by learning from a more experienced guid woman—the apprentice system—but there was no checking of standards. Other than some ill-defined teaching by Egyptian female priests, the first formal training for midwives was laid down by Hippocrates in the fifth century BC, followed by intermittent efforts in Italy and Greece in the second and third century AD (for example, Soranus of Rome). The Dark Ages (from AD500–1300) are so called not because nothing happened then, but because there is little recorded historical evidence of those days. Monasteries flourished and kings and nobles lived good lives while the ordinary people went about their daily tasks with little change, and no records, for a thousand years. Childbirth was part of this and few trained midwives were recorded. Doctors were not involved. There was nothing they could do to help women in any adverse circumstances at childbirth and so they did not consider that medical care for maternity mattered. In Europe, one or two centres trained midwives; in Italy, Trotula in the eleventh century was a shining example in teaching and maintaining midwifery standards.

In the UK, William Chamberlen, an immigrant Huguenot, started a midwifery school in Southampton in 1590. A uniform compilation of midwifery training, however, was not undertaken until the Midwives Acts were passed in 1908.

Doctors came into obstetrics comparatively late. At first they were resisted by midwives who saw them as competing for fees, but gradually a team approach evolved so that both professionals worked together. One feature that may have catalysed the rise of the accoucheur was the abundant extra-marital activity of the courts of France and England during the later seventeenth century. In both countries, monarchs and their courts led a merry life of multiple coitus which, in the days before effective contraception, led to many pregnancies. In both countries, in consequence, obstetricians were used because of the confidentiality and secrecy required to handle the results of royal dalliance. From such insalubrious beginnings rose to fame several of the great obstetricians of the seventeenth and eighteenth centuries. These men invented and refined instruments to assist delayed labours—the obstetric forceps. Their wider use brought doctors into obstetrics for now they could do something which was sometimes helpful.

The first aid service for delivery

Forceps came into use with Peter Chamberlen, son of William Chamberlen, although possibly as a re-invention of a much earlier instrument used for extracting dead babies. A century of manipulative skills followed with increasingly complex instruments being evolved to help deal with problems. Women did not have access to effective anaesthesia at this time and so a vaginal delivery had to be successful, even at the expense of the baby's life. Nearly all manipulations were very intrusive, requiring long apprenticeship and much training for practice. Obstetricians were great mechanics, inventing ingenious instruments to extract babies from awkward corners. Some appliances were modifications of existing tools and the destructive instruments of the previous generation. Most well-known obstetricians had their own instrument maker (usually the blacksmith) around the corner to make their own version of the various instruments. They would promote the use of these in their own practice. If they were influential and had apprentices, the latter would be taught the skills of using their master's eponymous instruments, thus perpetuating the innumerable ramifications of the obstetrical armamentarium which flourished into the nineteenth and early twentieth centuries.

Safer caesarean section came in the mid 1800s after inhalation anaesthesia was first used in 1851 by James Young Simpson. The increase in the use of the abdominal route of delivery for prolonged labour, so bypassing a more difficult vaginal delivery, sounded the knell of mechanistic obstetrics. The attitude of vaginal delivery at all costs persisted for a few decades since obstetricians were still concerned about intraperitoneal infection. Puerperal sepsis (childbed fever) killed women after vaginal delivery, and peritoneal infection after abdominal operative delivery was a death sentence until chemotherapy and antibiotics were introduced from the 1930s. Maternal mortality was sharply reduced as a result and only then could obstetricians start to consider a caesarean section as a comparatively safe alternative to a vaginal delivery.

The beginnings of science

All science depends upon measurement. Among the first steps in obstetrics was the measurement of various aspects of the pelvis by Levret in 1753. Like many enthusiasts, he overelaborated the complexities of pelvic axes and planes. Smellie, in the following years, first proposed a measurement which

has been continued into current obstetrics, the diagonal conjugate (anteroposterior diameter) of the pelvis. All sorts of measuring instruments were used and external pelvimetry became fashionable, but was mostly dismissed after the analysis of Michaelis in 1851. *In vivo* measurements followed the invention of X-rays by Roentgen. The first radiographic pelvimetries were performed by Albert in 1897, giving way in modern practice to spiral computed tomography, ultrasound, or magnetic resonance imaging (MRI) on the rare occasions when pelvimetry is necessary.

A surge in biophysical fetal estimations in obstetrics started with fetal heart auscultation in the early nineteenth century but really came to prominence with the work of the Glaswegian obstetrician, Ian Donald, in the 1950s. He, more than any other single person, introduced biophysics into obstetrics with the use of ultrasound measurement of the fetus. His work will forever stand as a landmark. Following his introduction of ultrasound into many aspects of pregnancy care, systems of measuring fetal growth from serial readings were followed by dynamic measurements of blood flow (mainly as velocity) in the fetal and placental vessels.

Biochemistry in medicine owes much to another obstetrician, Robert Barnes of St George's Hospital, London. He was an obstetric physician from 1875 to 1907. During this time he set up the first hospital-based biochemical laboratory in the world for the measurement of levels of body constituents such as sodium, potassium, proteins and urea in human blood. Another great advance came after the Second World War when miniaturisation of biochemical processes, automation and the use of radioactive labels allowed steroid biochemistry to forge ahead. While the value of the steroid markers as a measure of fetal well-being in late pregnancy has mostly been overshadowed by ultrasound, the assessment of pregnancy-associated placental proteins is helping in the management of first-trimester problems. Again, measurement is leading research.

The enumeration and analysis of chromosomes and their genes has blossomed in the last few years. Amniocentesis to retrieve fetal fibroblasts for assessment of numbers of chromosomes to exclude trisomy 21 has been overtaken by sophisticated gene probes and assessment of one nucleus from an eight-cell embryo by gene amplification using DNA polymerase. With this comes new ethical problems for parents and professionals.

Epidemiology, the measurement of large numbers of people, has been a major part of modern obstetrics. The counting of heads started with epidemics of infectious diseases in the Victorian period and progressed to quantify birth rates and death rates. From 1830 these measurements were under the control of the Registrar General's Office in England and equivalent bodies in other parts of the United Kingdom. The Office of Population Censuses and Surveys, now the Office for National Statistics (ONS), performs this task for England and Wales. Obstetrics epidemiology in this country has led the rest of the world. Measures of fetal and antenatal outcome are collected, providing a rapid medical audit of populations of women, procedures and professional groups. Comparisons can be made from one centre to another or even from one country to another, provided the data compare like with like. The ready acceptance of randomised controlled trials and meta-analysis of results by obstetricians has allowed even more sophisticated analyses with more valid results; multi-centre studies are mostly run through the National Perinatal Epidemiology Unit in Oxford, leading to much more efficient data gathering.

Clinical care

Statistical methods have not always been used in the evaluation of systems of management; antenatal care, for example, evolved piecemeal. Starting in Edinburgh at the turn of the century, current practice owes much to Dame Doreen Campbell in the mid 1920s. It was she who, in London, laid down the pattern of antenatal visits followed today in most of the Western world.

The place of delivery has shifted from the home to the institution. This is partly the result of the trend of hospitalisation of much Western medicine, with primary care becoming a service dealing mostly with ambulatory care or diagnosis only. Further, most obstetricians, general practitioners or midwives concerned with the unexpected serious complications that might arise suddenly in labour, wish to have rapid access to the full facilities required if labour deviates from the normal. Institutional delivery in the UK has increased from 20% in the 1920s to 98% at present. A move by some to return to home births is occurring, for women often feel they have more control over events when they are not in hospital. Provided those women electing to deliver in their homes have been selected and screened for absence of high risk factors, have good antenatal care and are properly supported by midwives during labour, they and their babies are probably at no greater risk than if they deliver in an institution. It is the unbooked mothers who incur high rates of mortality and morbidity.

In the hospital too the midwife is the principal professional for the birth of normal deliveries in the UK. Three-quarters of women are cared for in labour and delivered by midwives. Among the other quarter, midwives still care for the women and help the obstetrician. Following a period when the role of midwives diminished in the UK, they now are reasserting their place as independent practitioners working alongside obstetricians. The emphasis on midwife care has been catalysed in the UK by the initiative *Changing Childbirth* (1993), steered through the Department of Health by Baroness Cumberledge.

CONTEMPORARY OBSTETRICS

The years of the Second World War (1939–1945) provide a convenient division between the end of a long period of conservative maternity care and the beginning of contemporary obstetrics. The older practice was dominated by fear of maternal death: rightly so—the maternal mortality rate in England and Wales had remained between 4 and 5 per 1000 births for a century until 1937. The introduction of sulphonamides and newer antibiotics, widespread blood transfusion and other advances led to a dramatic reduction in maternal mortality rates (see Ch. 48). As a result, obstetricians returning to practice after the end of the war in 1945 realised that with the maternal mortality rate dropping they could now concentrate more on the fetus, improving perinatal morbidity and mortality. This change in philosophy and the wider availability of more sensitive measuring methods led to a renaissance of scientific obstetrics.

ADVANCES IN PERINATAL CARE

Perinatal medicine

One of the earliest obstetricians to practise what developed into perinatal medicine was Professor Dugald Baird in Aberdeen. He classified the clinical causes of perinatal death and demonstrated the importance of good maternal health as well as expert perinatal care in achieving a low perinatal mortality rate. By describing the circumstances of perinatal death, he drew attention to those obstetric conditions for which better management was needed to improve fetal outcome. The conditions initially stressed were labour disorders such as a prolonged first stage, manipulative vaginal delivery, preterm labour and prolonged pregnancy. Disorders of pregnancy carrying special risks for the fetus included severe pre-eclampsia, antepartum haemorrhage, rhesus disease and maternal medical disorders such as diabetes. He naturally recognised fetal abnormality as a major cause of fetal death but, like others at that time, considered that much of this was unavoidable.

Biochemical assessment of fetus and placenta

For many years it was considered that poor placental function was the probable explanation for complications such as intrauterine fetal death in pregnancy, intrauterine death of the fetus during labour or unexpected birth asphyxia. However it was not possible to make any measurements of placental function or fetal well-being until the mid 1950s, when reliable methods were developed by Arnold Klopper and Jim Brown in Edinburgh for measurement of pregnanediol and oestrogens in maternal urine. At first, urinary pregnanediol was used to assess placental function, but this was soon superseded by urinary oestriol which gave an indication not only of placental function but also of fetal well-being (a feto-placental function test). Scientists made great efforts to provide quicker and simpler methods of measuring oestriol in urine and blood, while clinicians hastened to apply these methods widely in practice. Other hormones, such as human placental lactogen, were measured in the quest for the best biochemical method for assessing the condition of the fetus and placenta. After about 20 years, the popularity of this biochemical approach waned because of the increasing realisation that the assessment provided was incomplete, for it measured the metabolism of the placenta but not its exchange capacity. The two bear a loose relationship but a variable one: with urinary oestriol, for example, the daily background coefficient of variation is almost 40%.

Nevertheless, attempts to assess the fetus by biochemical means showed obstetricians how important it was to have reliable knowledge of the condition of the intrauterine fetus. Better biophysical methods were becoming available and finally, in 1984, St. George's Hospital in London took the plunge and formally reported that discontinuing oestriol assay in the third trimester in clinical practice had no effect on perinatal outcome.

Many biochemical measurements are still of value, including serum alpha-fetoprotein assay in maternal blood and amniotic fluid. High levels in early second-trimester pregnancy indicate increased risks of fetal open neural tube defect and of later fetal compromise. Unduly low levels of serum alpha-fetoprotein and raised serum oestriol and human chorionic gonadotrophin in late first-trimester pregnancy were developed as the triple test to screen for and indicate increased risks of Down's syndrome in the fetus.

Biophysical assessment of fetus and placenta

Biophysical methods of making direct observation of the intrauterine conditions have proved more valuable than biochemical ones, which tend to be indirect. Diagnostic ultrasound, pioneered by Ian Donald in Glasgow, has made possible accurate measurements of the parameters of normal and abnormal fetal growth with advancing pregnancy. Pathological growth restriction of the fetus is detectable by measurements made at serial scans. The first scanners provided only a static picture but now most function in real time and can assess fetal function in a dynamic fashion. Frank Manning and Larry Platt in the USA utilised real-time ultrasound to derive a fetal biophysical profile, which gives a dynamic assessment of the fetus. While the full profile is not widely used in the UK, the essential elements are. Doppler ultrasound techniques now enable the characteristics of blood flow or velocity in specific vessels of the fetal and placental circulation to be assessed with considerable accuracy and prognostic ability.

Another important biophysical measurement, first developed in Germany by Fred Hammacher, is fetal cardiotocography. Fetal heart rate is recorded continuously and the tracing is related to a recording of uterine contractions, originally measured by the changes in intrauterine pressure. Although this method was first developed for use in labour, the application of sophisticated ultrasound techniques has enabled it also to be used throughout the second half of pregnancy. It has become a technique of major importance for assessment of the fetus.

Even more recent is the introduction of cordocentesis, by which samples of blood are taken from the umbilical artery or vein using a needle passed, under ultrasound control, through the maternal abdomen into the uterus and then into the cord. This was first developed in France by Daffos in the early 1980s and has since been used extensively in the UK, USA, Europe and Scandinavia in the intrauterine assessment of the potentially jeopardised fetus.

While it is now possible to assess the condition of the fetus with some precision in most cases, it must be remembered that in a minority of cases even the most careful and skilful assessment may be misleading, and that repeated assessment is especially important when there is any uncertainty.

Antenatal diagnosis

Intrauterine diagnosis of the sex of the fetus was first reported by Fritz Fuchs in Copenhagen in the mid 1950s when the performed amniocentesis and centrifuged the amniotic fluid so enabling cells of fetal origin in the fluid to be cultured and the fetal karyotype determined. Progress was initially slow but improvements in fetal fibroblast cell culture meant that by the mid 1960s the method was reliable enough for the clinical use of amniocentesis. National studies on the safety of amniocentesis in the USA, Canada and the UK indicated that the risks were low enough to be clinically acceptable. Since then, amniocentesis has become the standard technique for prenatal diagnosis. It was initially used mainly for the diagnosis of chromosomally determined abnormalities such as trisomy 21 (Down's syndrome), but the development of screening to direct its application has been patchy and so the incidence of Down's syndrome at birth has only been reduced slowly over the past 20 years or so. Chorionic villus sampling at 11–12 weeks gives swift results because of direct chromosomal analysis of the much larger number of cells obtained than by amniocentesis. Research is now achieving the isolation of fetal cells from the mother's circulation in 70% of cases and the karyotyping of these cells may warn of chromosomal abnormalities as early as 8 weeks' gestation. While such investigations are diagnostic, screening with ultrasound (nuchal translucency) is showing markers of chromosomal fetal abnormalities and other conditions such as cardiac malformation which can identify a subset of the population for diagnostic invasive tests.

Advances have been made in the application of DNA technology to clinical diagnosis so that disorders associated with gene abnormalities and deletions are now increasingly detectable. Fetal cells, obtained at amniocentesis or chorionic villus sampling, provide small samples of fetal tissue. From these samples results can be obtained rapidly and a reliable diagnosis can be made of fetal disorders such as sickle cell disease, thalassaemia major, Duchenne's muscular dystrophy, cystic fibrosis or Huntington's chorea. Ova fertilised by in vitro methods can provide a cell from an eight-cell embryo to allow post-fertilisation gene diagnosis and so warn against replacement of that embryo in the mother.

By contrast, the first demonstration that serum and amniotic fluid alpha-fetoprotein levels were elevated in women carrying a baby with an open neural tube defect (NTD) led to the rapid application of maternal serum alpha-fetoprotein screening. This, coupled with ultrasound confirmation of the diagnosis, made possible screening programmes which have been associated with a considerable reduction in the incidence of NTD. Although this reduction had started spontaneously before the tests were introduced, the availability of NTD screening procedures has contributed to the reduced incidence of these disorders. Since ultrasound examination can warn of NTD by itself, many units have given up alpha-fetoprotein screening and depend entirely on routine fetal anomaly scanning at 20 weeks to detect NTD and other fetal abnormalities. However, the association between elevated alpha-fetoprotein at 16 weeks and later pregnancy complications, such as fetal growth retardation and preterm labour, and between very low alpha-fetoprotein at 16 weeks and Down's syndrome, represents an additional reason for considering alpha-fetoprotein screening at 16–18 weeks' gestation. In many parts of the world ultrasound services are not expert enough to take their part in the accurate estimate of gestational age needed to interpret any AFP results.

CONTROL OF FERTILITY

Scientific advances are making it increasingly possible for women to bear the number of children they wish, rather than being at the mercy of their natural fertility. In the mid 1950s, the first combined oral contraceptive preparations became available and were improved rapidly. Major side effects were found to be dose-related and so equally effective lower-dose preparations were introduced. Improved intra-uterine devices also became available but medico-legal problems are now causing the manufacturers to reduce production. Hormone-impregnated intrauterine devices are now used as a source of continuous release, while deep intramuscular and subcutaneous depots of progesterone provide good contraception.

The technique of laparoscopic sterilisation was pioneered in France by Raoul Palmer and popularised in the UK by Patrick Steptoc. This quickly replaced laparotomy for sterilisation. Therapeutic abortion for a series of indications was legalised in England, Wales and Scotland in 1967.

The UK birth rate reached its peak in 1964 and then fell steadily until 1977 as a result of many factors, helped by the increased availability of contraception, sterilisation and pregnancy termination. Since 1980 the general fertility rate (see Ch. 46) has been maintained at around this level with small fluctuations. There has been a slight shift to the older mother, particularly among first pregnancies.

PERINATAL MORTALITY AND MORBIDITY

Perinatal mortality has continued to fall steadily in the UK. Surveys performed in 1958 and 1970 clarified many aspects of causation and pointed to the directions in which further improvements could be achieved; in those surveys the perinatal mortality rates were 38.7 and 24.8 per thousand total births respectively. Better methods of fertility control helped women to avoid pregnancy at extremes of age and parity or if there was an unduly high risk of perinatal death. The perinatal mortality rate combines the stillbirth and first week neonatal death rates and is therefore expressed as the rate per 1000 live and stillbirths. In 1998 the rate in England and Wales was 8.0 per 1000 total births (see Ch. 47).

NEONATAL INTENSIVE CARE

Among the many specialties with which obstetricians collaborate, in none do they work closer than with neonatology.

Peter Dunn in Bristol carried out much pioneering work on the care of the preterm baby, and with his colleagues founded the British Association of Perinatal Medicine. The clinical use of new knowledge of neonatal cardiorespiratory and metabolic functions, combined with impressive technology, has made possible an increasing rate of high-quality survival of extremely immature babies. Advances in neonatal surgery have corrected many congenital fetal disorders previously thought to be lethal.

OBSTETRIC ANAESTHESIA

Anaesthesia and analgesia are essential to good obstetric practice (Ch. 28). Although the number of women having general anaesthesia for vaginal operative delivery has been reduced in recent years, there has been an increase in the use of regional methods, especially epidural anaesthesia. Currently about 20% of women in the UK use this form of analgesia; in some maternity units the figure is as high as 60–70%. In the early 1960s the technique of paracervical block was popular but proved less effective for the mother and sometimes dangerous to the fetus; it has largely been abandoned in the UK. Apart from providing anaesthesia for operative delivery, anaesthetists are now much involved with intensive care in obstetrics since conditions such as severe pre-eclampsia or eclampsia and excessive bleeding (with or without coagulation defects) require intensive care and anaesthetists are very skilled in this field.

CONTROL OF LABOUR

The use of a continuous intravenous oxytocin infusion was first reported in 1947 by Geoffrey Theobald in the UK, and in the same year by Louis Helman in the USA. Vincent du Vingeaud in 1955 received the Nobel Prize for his work on oxytocin, however oxytocin was not widely used at first because of the relative unreliability of the extracts available. With the synthesis of pure oxytocin (Syntocinon) in 1955 (see Ch. 35), various investigators recognised that intravenous administration could be used more efficiently than previously for the induction of labour and for augmentation of uterine contractions in a slowly progressing labour of spontaneous onset. Alec Turnbull published in 1967 and 1968 studies from Aberdeen which triggered the use of oxytocin titration for induction and augmentation of labour. The philosophy of active management of labour, in which almost 50% of multiparae have their labour augmented by intravenous oxytocin to promote rapid progress, was pioneered at the National Maternity Hospital in Dublin by Kieran O'Driscoll. Oxytocin works best when the membranes are ruptured. Amniotomy and intravenous oxytocin administration reigned supreme as initiators or stimulators of uterine contractions for over 10 years until the mid 1970s when, after work by Sultan Karim at Queen Charlotte's Hospital, vaginal administration of prostaglandins achieved initiation of labour without amniotomy; this was more gradual and apparently physiological than labour provoked using amniotomy and oxytocin. Prostaglandin E_2 proved to have fewer side effects than prostaglandin $F_{2\alpha}$. Given intravenously, prostaglandins have no advantages over oxytocin, but when administered extra-amniotically, or intravaginally in appropriate doses, they are as effective and more acceptable to women for the induction of labour than the more invasive amniotomy and intravenous oxytocin administration. Augmentation of labour still remains essentially the province of Syntocinon, although the experimental use of prostaglandins such as misoprostol has begun.

WOMEN'S WISHES

Throughout the 1960s, advances in obstetric care involved the introduction of many technological innovations. Many women were concerned by what they regarded as unnecessary interference in what was a physiological process, and by the potentially serious complications of some of the technology. They felt that women were no longer in control of their own labour. The caesarean section rate rose steadily and although perinatal mortality was reduced slightly, the two rates were not necessarily related to each other.

In the UK, obstetricians and women's organisations continued on a collision course until the mid 1970s when there was a major confrontation. Women's organisations vilified obstetric technology on the television, on radio and in the newspapers, while obstetricians defended their record of improving results although many innovations had not been subjected to trials to assess their efficacy. Subsequently there was a significant reduction in the use of interventions that could not be clearly justified. Obstetricians recognised that they had failed to convince women of the value of many useful advances in technique.

Women are now increasingly involved in the decision-making processes of pregnancy management and any research studies to improve the outcome. Obstetricians need to convince women of the necessity of using the high-technology methods when there is a high risk for the mother or her infant. In many units there has been a considerable reduction in the use of interventions previously thought to be essential, including episiotomy, epidural anaesthesia, induction of labour and electronic fetal heart rate monitoring in labour. Women have encouraged their husband or partner to be present during labour and at the birth of the baby. Analgesic drug use in labour has been reduced, with some multiparous women requiring no analgesia at all. Ambulation in labour has been encouraged, as has delivery with the mother in any position she cares to adopt.

All these changes in practice seem to have lightened the atmosphere in UK maternity hospitals, many of which are now more orientated towards fulfilling the expectations of pregnant women and their families, even when this involves accepting requests for less usual forms of management such as recent requests for caesarean section to prevent damage to the pelvic floor from vaginal birth (see Ch. 37). Childbirth is a major life event and must be treated as such. It is important that the woman is centre stage and that all the attendants, their equipment and their science are supportive.

While most pregnancies end with the mother and baby fit and well, the baby may be born dead or may die in the neonatal period. It used to be customary to protect the mother from as much of the experience as possible by not letting her see the dead baby, keeping her away from other women and discharging her from hospital as soon as possible. Although this was well meant, it is now recognised that such management caused untold misery to bereaved mothers. Grief is usually an intense process but, once completed, normal life can start again. The mother and father should be properly counselled and given an opportunity to talk about their feelings of loss in the weeks or months after the baby's death.

THE FUTURE

Women in the developed world are having fewer babies and obstetricians will continue to add the finer tuning of safety, comfort and control to the natural process. With fewer perinatal and maternal deaths, even more individual attention will be paid to those women at higher risk. Perhaps fetal and maternal monitoring will be applied more rationally. Individual methods will be more carefully assessed so that we reject the less useful tests but apply more widely those investigations that can be shown to be powerful in their capacity to predict problems with reasonable precision. If obstetricians concentrate on detecting and protecting this smaller group of higher-risk pregnancies, the majority of healthy women will be cared for by other members of the obstetric team. In the British Commonwealth, these will be the midwives, whose natural place in caring for the normal will be better fulfilled as they find their rightful place in obstetrics.

In providing better support for the woman who is having a baby, a new wave of education and understanding is starting in the developed world, especially through the internet, home to the websites of many consumer and patient support groups. This will spread knowledge so that women are more aware and in a better position to discuss what is happening with their doctor, midwife or traditional birth attendant. The Victorian barriers between the professional and the woman will continue to break down and a wider and better understanding will take their place. In non-drug analgesic techniques, we will refine and use what can be more widely applied.

The most important problems facing obstetricians in the Western world are the prevention of preterm delivery and of intrauterine growth restriction. These two overlapping but distinct conditions need much more research into their causes before correct preventive measures can be applied; this will be much more effective than the current emphasis on treating the established conditions (see Ch. 45). The place of subclinical infection in preterm birth needs to be addressed, as does the level of oxidative stress in pre-eclampsia.

In the future, obstetrics will probably use many more non-invasive techniques of a biophysical nature. Functions of fetal heart and brain and of uterine muscle will be more precisely measured, so possibly a more correct understanding of fetal and maternal physiology in pregnancy will follow. The indirect assessment of the body state from blood gas and acid–base levels will have to continue until better measures are perfected. Probably these too will be derived non-invasively by magnetic resonance imaging rather than by blood samples taken from the body.

In the developing world, many of the obstetrical problems converge with political ones. The provision of health care for such large numbers so widely spread is a major hurdle. Those who come from countries that went through the Industrial Revolution two centuries ago must remember that suggestions for the improvement in health care took their place among other social priorities in building a country's economy. Politicians perceive different goals from those given priority by the health professionals. If they are good politicians, they seek the good of the whole of society, of which health is but a part and obstetrics a subpart of that good. Nonetheless, health care professionals know that maternal and child health preventive measures will in the long run yield greater returns per unit of money spent than virtually anything else. Some politicians grasp this principle, but forget that they must also provide some improvements in care for the present generation of women and their babies. They must build for the future but not turn their backs on the present.

KEY POINTS

- Obstetrics has come a long way from basic first aid midwifery. It now occupies a position embracing the practical skills of the past, an increasing scientific component and much application of the humanity of one human looking after another.
- These three features must be in all obstetric carers although in individuals one may predominate over the others.
- The woman having the baby is always centre stage. Her medical and midwifery attendants are *corps de ballet*.
- The basis of all obstetrical science is an accurate measurement.
- The basis of comparisons is often the randomised controlled trial. Some of these are capable of providing meta-analysis to add to the strength of their predictive power.
- The fetal origins of adult disease are probably the most exciting and potentially useful area of research at present.
- The major problem facing obstetricians in the developed world is very early preterm delivery leading to neonatal immaturity.
- The major problems facing the developing world are at three levels:
  1. the status of women and their entitlement to care
  2. the practical problems of those with no or semi-skilled attendants
  3. improvement of literacy, nutrition and background health.

2

Anatomy of the female pelvis

Noel Dilly

INTRODUCTION

This chapter contains a clinically oriented introduction to functional anatomy of the female pelvic and genital organs, starting with the bony walls.

THE PELVIC CAVITY

The pelvic cavity is that part of the abdominal cavity surrounded by the bony pelvis. It is bounded inferiorly by the urogenital diaphragm separating the pelvis from the perineum. The pelvis contains the organs of reproduction, the bladder and the terminal portion of the gut.

The urogenital diaphragm and perineum are penetrated by the urethra, the vagina and the anal canal. The urethra and vagina are surrounded by a series of structures, which together constitute the vulva (Fig. 2.1).

The bony pelvis surrounds a cavity shaped like a pudding basin lying on its side, such that the anterior superior iliac spine and the pubic symphysis are in the same vertical plane. The brim of the cavity is made from the promontory and alae

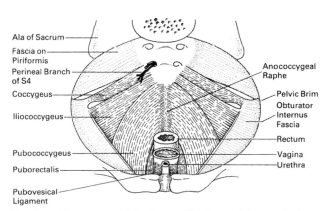

Fig. 2.1 The urogenital diaphragm. The floor of the pelvis slopes steeply forwards and plays an important role in continence and childbirth.

of the sacrum, the arcuate line of the ilium, the pectineal line of the pubis; the pubic crest lies at about 30° to this plane. The upper border of the symphysis pubis, the spine of the ischium, a useful landmark for local anaesthesia of the pudendal nerve,

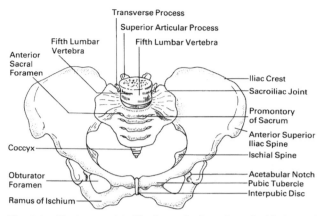

Fig. 2.2 The bony pelvis. The bones both enclose the birth canal and provide support for the body on the legs. There are notable sexual differences between the male and female bony pelvis.

and the tip of the coccyx define a plane that can just be reached by the tip of a finger placed in the vagina (Fig. 2.2).

The major obstetric feature in the bony pelvis is that it is not distensible; only minor degrees of movement are possible at the pubic and sacroiliac joints.

THE PELVIC JOINTS

The sacroiliac joint is a synovial joint between the articular surfaces of the ilium and the sacrum. The facets have interlocking facies and, at least posterosuperiorly, the two bones are united by fibrous tissue typical of a fibrous joint, especially in later life. Indeed, in old age bony fusion may take place. The joint has considerable support from its associated ligaments.

The symphysis pubis is a secondary cartilaginous joint. The adjoining surfaces of the pubic bones are covered with hyaline cartilage, between which there is a disc of fibrocartilage joining the two bones. The joint is further strengthened by ligaments superiorly, and inferiorly by direct fibres, but anteriorly and obliquely by interdigitating fibres that interlace with fibres from the rectus abdominis and external oblique muscles.

There is an increase in movements of these joints, especially during the third trimester of pregnancy. The net result is to increase the sagittal diameter of the outlet and true conjugate. Studies of these movements suggest that, as far as pelvic capacity is concerned, squatting during uterine contractions and lying recumbent between them may be a helpful routine during the second stage of labour; this could widen the outlet. The dimensions of the birth canal are critical during childbirth. The diameters of the pelvis vary in different regions of the canal (Table 2.1). The pelvic cavity is widest transversely at the inlet and anteroposteriorly at the outlet. Most attempts to classify the shape of the pelvis fail because there appears to be a continuous series of pelves, extending from the classical gynaecoid, the anteroposteriorly flattened and platypelloid.

The pelvic aspect of the bony pelvis is covered mostly by muscles—superiorly by the psoas and iliacus muscles, below

Table 2.1 Changes in the diameters of the pelvis

Level of pelvis	Approximate diameter of bony pelvis (cm)		
	Anteroposterior	Oblique	Transverse
Brim	11	12	13
Midcavity	12	12	12
Outlet	13	12	11

the pelvic brim by the obturator internus muscle and posteriorly by pyriformis and coccygeus muscles arising from the anterior surface of the sacrum. The fascia covering these muscles is a tough membrane attached to the periosteum at the edges.

The pelvic floor is a V-shaped gutter of muscles which is higher posteriorly than anteriorly. The base of the V is formed by the midline raphe of these muscles. The raphe and muscles are penetrated by the urethra, vagina and rectum. The direction of the muscle fibres forming the anterior part of this diaphragm of muscles is backwards and medially, such that they form a series of slings encircling the posterior aspects of the penetrating structures and thus have a potential sphincter-like action (Fig. 2.3). There is a hole anteriorly between the muscles arising from the posterior aspect of the pubis. This gap is closed by the pubovesical ligaments, between which passes the deep dorsal vein of the clitoris. The muscles arise peripherally from a continuous line starting at the spine of the ischium, which proceeds as the white line over the fascia covering the medial aspect of obturator internus, and from the body of the pubis.

The function of this gutter during labour is to deflect anteriorly the first part of the baby which comes into contact with it and later to rotate it so that the shortest diameter lies transversely at the outlet of the bony pelvis (Fig. 2.4). The muscles of the pelvic diaphragm are supplied in the main by the perineal branch of S4, and anteriorly by branches from the inferior rectal and perineal nerves. The function of these muscles is to respond to changes in intra-abdominal pressure, assisting in maintaining faecal and urinary continence. In micturition and defecation the relevant portion of the muscle is

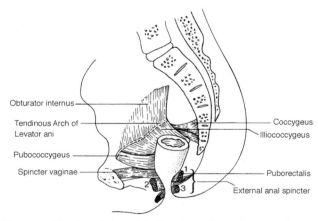

Fig. 2.3 Muscles of the pelvic floor. The slings of muscle that surround and separate the major body outlets have an important role as sphincters.

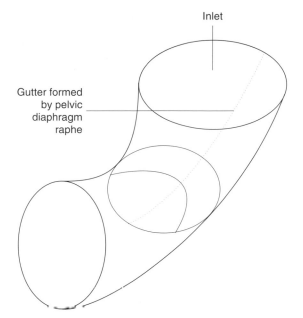

Fig. 2.4 The curve of the human birth canal.

relaxed, but the remainder maintains its tone to prevent prolapse of the pelvic organs.

The fascia of the pelvic floor is little more than loose areolar tissue. Separating the pelvic floor from the pelvic peritoneum are the pelvic viscera. The space around these organs provides room for distension of the bladder and rectum.

BLOOD VESSELS OF THE PELVIS

The pelvic contents and walls are supplied by branches of the internal iliac artery and are drained to the internal iliac veins. The vessels lie within the parietal pelvic fascia and only those branches that leave the pelvis pierce this membranous structure. The internal iliac artery divides into a large anterior branch and a smaller posterior branch, the anterior branch supplying the pelvic viscera (Fig. 2.5).

The venous drainage is via the internal iliac veins to the inferior vena cava, but there are anastomoses through the superior rectal and inferior mesenteric veins to the portal system. There is also a drainage passage of the internal vertebral plexus via the lateral sacral veins to the internal iliac veins, the flow in which can be reversed by raised intra-abdominal pressure. This is a potential route of spread of pelvic inflammatory and malignant disease.

THE NERVES OF THE PELVIS

Besides nerves of passage such as the obturator nerve, the nerves whose function lies with the pelvis are branches of the sacral plexus and the pelvic autonomic system. The sacral plexus is a broad structure formed by the fusion of nerves from L4 to S4 and lies lateral to the anterior sacral foramina. It lies upon the piriformis muscle and is covered anteriorly by the parietal pelvic fascia.

The pudendal nerve that is sensory to the pudenda arises from S2, S3 and S4; it then passes backwards between the piriformis and coccygeus around the sacrospinous ligament and enters the ischiorectal fossa. The perineal branch of S4 passes between the coccygeus and iliococcygeus to be distributed to the external anal sphincter and the perianal skin.

The pelvic autonomic plexus lies on the side wall of the pelvis lateral to the rectum.

Sympathetic fibres

The sympathetic fibres are derived from the hypogastric plexus and a contribution from the upper sacral ganglia of the sympathetic trunk. The plexus is ganglionated. About half of the fibres in the hypogastric plexus are preganglionic and synapse in these ganglia; the rest are post-ganglionic and do not synapse.

Parasympathetic fibres

The parasympathetic nerves travel with some branches of this plexus and arise by several rootlets from the anterior surfaces of S2, S3 and sometimes S4. They do not synapse here but in the walls of the viscera.

The autonomic system is organised so that the sympathetic fibres are vasoconstrictor and the parasympathetic fibres are motor to the smooth muscle of the bladder and gut, and secretomotor to the gut glands. The sympathetic fibres are motor to the bladder and anal canal sphincters, and to the smooth muscle of the seminal vesicles in the male. The course of pain and sensory fibres is complex and not fully understood. Most pain fibres travel with the sympathetic system, especially those from the gut and the gonads. However, pain fibres from the bladder and rectum, as well as those conveying the sensation of distension, probably travel in the nervi erigentes. Pain fibres from the cervix also follow this course, but those from the body of the uterus travel mainly in the hypogastric nerves, especially to thoracic dorsal roots 11 and 12.

THE LYMPHATIC DRAINAGE OF THE PELVIS

The lymphatics in the pelvis originate as tiny lymphocapillaries that form complex nets of interconnecting vessels. They

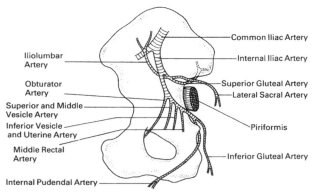

Fig. 2.5 The blood supply to the pelvic viscera is derived in the main from the internal iliac artery.

are without valves and their walls consist solely of endothelial plates. These networks join to form lymphatic vessels with smooth muscle in their walls and have valves. Eventually lymph vessels lead to lymph nodes. The lymphatics of the perineum, together with those of the lower limb, go to a collection of lymph nodes below the inguinal ligament. Some of the deeper lymphatics of the buttock follow the superior and inferior gluteal arteries and penetrate into the pelvic cavity (Fig. 2.6). In general these lymphatics are found between the membranous layer of superficial fascia and the deep fascia. The nodes are classified into three major groups—superficial inguinal, deep inguinal and pelvic lymph nodes.

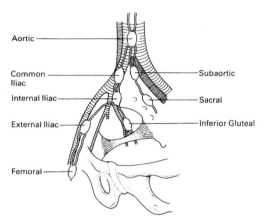

Aortic

Common Iliac

Internal Iliac

External Iliac

Femoral

Subaortic

Sacral

Inferior Gluteal

Fig. 2.6 The lymphatic drainage of the pelvis and associated structures.

Superficial lymph drainage

The superficial inguinal nodes radiate outwards from the saphenous opening, in the form of the letter T. The stem of the T is made by the group associated with the terminal part of the great saphenous vein, while the arms of the T follow the inguinal ligament. The vulva drains initially to the medial horizontal group. In most cases the vulval lymphatics do not cross the crural fold of the labia, but reach the contralateral nodes by traversing the mons pubis.

From the posterior part of the vulva and the perineum the lymphatics drain into the thigh and the lower lymph nodes, together with those from the lower limb. The deep inguinal nodes lie in relation to the junction between the femoral vein and the great saphenous vein after it has passed through the deep fascia at the saphenous opening. It is no longer believed that all efferent drainage from the inguinal region passes through this group.

Internal iliac lymph system

The pelvic lymph nodes are usually related to the major blood vessels and are named with them. The internal iliac vessels drain the pelvic contents. Unfortunately there are several common variations amongst the veins, and the distribution of the lymphatics may vary with the veins. Variations include how the vessels join with each other and the territories they drain. There is frequently variation between the two sides of

the pelvis. Usually nodes are named external iliac when related to the external iliac artery. All nodes inferior to the external iliac vein and anterior to the internal iliac artery are named interiliac. Lymph nodes behind the anterior division of the internal iliac artery are called the internal iliac group. As there are three main arteries entering the pelvis—one paired, the common iliac arteries, and two single, the median sacral and the superior haemorrhoidal arteries—there are three possible routes for lymphatic drainage.

The external iliac nodes

This system is much confused, as several surgical and anatomical texts describe the same structures, giving them differing names. Basically there is a system of chains of nodes and vessels surrounding the external iliac artery and vein with a few related nodes associated with them. Although these lymph chains are interconnected it is usual to describe them as anterior–superior, intermediate and posteromedial. The associated glands are those within the inguinal canal, those associated with the inferior epigastric artery and those associated with the first part of the obturator artery. They are named after their associated vessels. It is the posteromedial group that is the important lymphatic relay for the genital tract and the cervix.

The internal iliac nodes, like the arterial supply, are in two main divisions: those from the pelvic viscera and those from the buttock and leg. As the viscera within the pelvis are separated from the pelvic wall, the peripheral lymph nodes are associated with the walls of the organs rather than with the pelvic wall. Both the internal and external iliac system of lymphatics drain to the common iliac nodes. They are most easily visualised as a continuation of the three chains of nodes surrounding the external iliac vessels. These chains continue to the bifurcation of the aorta, where they anastomose freely with each other and with those from the other side. The symmetry of the two sides is disturbed by the left common iliac vein. Besides this system there are a few nodes associated with the median sacral artery, and with the superior haemorrhoidal artery. The median sacral vessels join the common iliac lymphatics at the bifurcation of the aorta.

It is important to realise that this classification in terms of adjacent vessels gives very little clue to the drainage of these nodes; structures like the urethra and vagina straddle the territories of several vessels. Even structures such as the bladder and uterus, which are supplied by the visceral division of the internal iliac artery, drain to nodes associated with other vessels.

It is a reasonable generalisation that the lymphatic drainage of the pelvic viscera follows the vessels that supply them. The posteromedial group of the external iliac lymph nodes is functionally more related to the visceral branches of the internal iliac artery than to the external iliac artery territory.

THE VULVA

The vulva consists of the vaginal orifice, the urethral orifice and those structures associated with them which make up the floor of the anterior part of the pelvic outlet. It extends upwards to include the mons pubis (Fig. 2.7). It is supported by the largely transverse fibres of the inferior fascia of the urinogenital diaphragm, a part of the perineal membrane. This fascia has three holes: one just behind the pubic bone, one for the urethra and one for the vagina. It is strengthened posteriorly by the perineal body, an aponeurosis for the fibres of the perineal, levator ani and external and internal anal sphincter muscles.

Above this membrane lies the deep perineal pouch and beneath it the superficial pouch that contains the terminal portions of the vagina and urethra as well as their associated structures, the clitoris, the bulb of the vestibule, the vestibular glands, the superficial perineal muscles and their nerves and vessels.

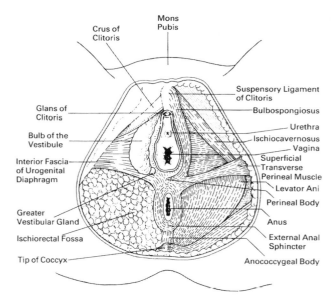

Fig. 2.8   The perineum. A view from below of the pelvic outlet showing its boundaries and triangles.

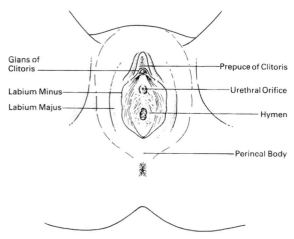

Fig. 2.7   The female external genitalia. This represents the classical portrait of the female external genitalia, but in life the labia majora are normally in contact with each other, except during intercourse and labour.

The perineum

The perineum is the pelvic outlet below the pelvic diaphragm. It is usually divided by a line joining the anterior end of the ischial tuberosities into an anterior urogenital area and a posterior anal triangle. The anal triangle contains the anal canal and the surrounding ischiorectal fossae. It is bound posterolaterally by the sacrotuberous ligaments. The fossa itself is filled with fat. Its lateral wall is the fascia over obturator internus and the edge of the sacrotuberous ligaments; medially the fossae are separated by the perineal body, the anal canal and the anococcygeal body (Fig. 2.8).

The pudendal nerve and vessels leave the pelvis through the greater sciatic foramen then often hook around the ischial spine. They re-enter the perineum through the lesser sciatic foramen into the pudendal canal, where they run forwards to supply the perineum.

The urogenital triangle

The perineal membrane is a narrow shelf of fibrous tissue attached along the pubic rami. Anteriorly the crurae of the clitoris are attached to it. Each crus is covered by the ischio-

cavernosus muscle. Medial to each crus is the erectile tissue of the bulb of the vestibule and separating the bulbs on either side are the openings of the urethra and vagina. The bulbs fuse anteriorly in front of the urethral orifice and extend to the glans of the clitoris. The bulbospongiosus muscle lies superficial to the bulb, extending from the perineal body where it also covers the vestibular glands forwards around the vagina and urethra to the clitoris (Figs 2.8, 2.9).

The perineal body is the fibrous tissue aponeurosis of the fibres of the bulbospongiosus, the transverse perinei, the sphincter vaginae and the external anal sphincter. It is somewhat mobile but provides support for the levator ani above.

The nerve supply of the urogenital triangle is derived from the ilioinguinal nerve, the perineal branch of the posterior cutaneous nerve of the thigh and the pudendal nerve. The ilioinguinal nerve supplies the anterior part of the labia majora, the posterior part being supplied by the posterior

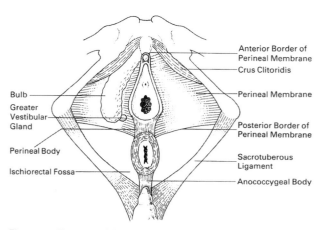

Fig. 2.9   The superficial layers of the urogenital triangle. The bulbospongiosus and ischiocavernosus muscles have been removed to reveal the structure of the clitoris and the glands associated with it.

13

cutaneous nerve of the thigh laterally. Its remaining area, together with the labia minora, is supplied medially by branches of the pudendal nerve. The clitoris is supplied by one of the terminal branches of the pudendal nerve, the dorsal nerve of the clitoris.

The mons pubis

The mons pubis is an area over the pubic bone which develops at puberty as a secondary sexual characteristic. The pubic hair is usually distributed upon its surface in a characteristic triangular fashion but a significant proportion of normal woman have male-type distribution with the hair extending up the midline of the lower abdomen. The probable functions of the mons include acting as a buffer between the male and female pubic bones during intercourse and as a source of arousal responses when stimulated. It is also said to provide tissue for the increase in size of the labia minora as they expand during coitus.

The labia majora

The labia majora are a pair of fatty folds which are continuous anteriorly with the mons. Posteriorly they peter out but small continuations come together between the vagina and the anus. In the adult their outer surfaces are covered with pubic hair and their medial surfaces are usually in apposition, closing off a potential aperture called the pudendal cleft. This apposed surface contains many large sebaceous and sweat glands.

The labia majora consist of skin-covered loose fibrofatty tissue similar to that of the mons, but containing some muscle, as well as the termination of the round ligament of the uterus.

The labia minora

The labia minora are a pair of fleshy folds containing erectile tissue, usually contained within the folds of the labia majora and separated from them by a deep cleft. They surround the vestibule of the vagina. Posteriorly in the virgin the labia minora join each other with a delicate fold of skin called the fourchette just deep to the labia majora. Anteriorly they divide into a pair of folds that split to enclose the clitoris. The outer surface is hairy and contains many sweat and sebaceous glands but the inner hairless surface is covered by a poorly keratinized stratified squamous epithelium with sweat and sebaceous glands. The labia minora contain extensive vascular spaces surrounded by delicate connective tissue and a little smooth muscle. Their probable functions are to increase the depth of the vaginal canal during intercourse and afterwards probably to help in maintaining the vaginal continence to the ejaculate. They are a potent source of stimuli resulting in sexual arousal.

The vestibule

The vestibule is the space between the labia minora, bounded anteriorly by the clitoris and posteriorly by the fold of skin joining the labia minora, the fourchette. Opening into the vestibule are the vagina, the urethra and the ducts of the great and lesser vestibular glands. The bulborectal glands with their alkaline mucus secretion also drain into the vestibule posteriorly. The vaginal orifice may contain a hymen or hymenal remnants. Its lining is similar to the vaginal epithelium and is stratified squamous non-keratinized epithelium. Its glands are one of the major natural sources of lubrication during coitus.

The clitoris

The clitoris is a small but variable-sized organ made mainly of erectile tissue situated at the anterior end of the vestibule. It is suspended from the lower border of the pubic arch by a small triangular ligament. It is made from two corpora cavernosa, the cavernous blood spaces of which are separated from each other by fibromuscular trabeculae. Each corpus cavernosum arises from a crus near the ischiopubic ramus and this crus is palpable. The free extremity of the clitoris is made up of a rounded mass of erectile tissue—the glans—which, when not aroused, is normally covered by the anterior folds of the labia minora to form a prepuce. This prepuce contains vast numbers of sebaceous and sweat glands. However, the glans of the clitoris has neither sweat nor sebaceous glands.

The clitoris is an important source of stimuli and is responsible for sexual arousal and reflex lubrication; it contains a considerable number of mechanoreceptors.

Vestibular bulb

The vestibular bulb consists of two masses of erectile tissue, one on either side of the vaginal orifice. They are covered by the bulbospongiosus muscle and lie deep in the labia majora. They are joined by a commissure in front of the vagina, which is in contact with the lower surface of the urinogenital diaphragm.

Musculature of the vulva

Superficially these muscles are the transverse perinei, the bulbospongiosus and the ischiocavernosus muscles, and deeper, the parts of the urinogenital diaphragm surrounded by the superficial and deep layers of fascia. The deeper muscles are the deep transverse perinei and the sphincter urethrae. The superficial muscles are slender and delicate; the transverse perinei run horizontally from the inferior ramus of the ischium to the perineal body superficial to the posterior part of the inferior fascia of the urinogenital diaphragm. On each side, the bulbospongiosus comes from the perineal body and passes forwards encircling the external end of the vagina, superficial to the bulb and the greater vestibular glands. It ends in the dorsal aspect of the connective tissue capsule of the corpus cavernosus of the clitoris.

The deep transverse perinei also meet at the perineal body. The sphincter urethrae fibres encircle not only the anterior and lateral parts of the urethra but also the corresponding parts of the vagina.

Nerve supply

Nerves come from the anterior divisions of the anterior rami of the second, third and fourth sacral spinal nerves. The principal named nerve is the pudendal nerve but the labia and the adjacent skin of the perineum also have a sensory supply from the perineal branch of the posterior cutaneous nerve of the thigh.

The pudendal nerve is a mixed nerve. Its inferior rectal branch provides the sensory supply to perianal skin and the lower part of the anal canal, and the vital motor supply to the external anal sphincter.

The pudendal nerve itself divides into two branches in the anterior part of the pudendal canal, the dorsal nerve of the clitoris and the perineal nerve. The dorsal nerve of the clitoris runs above the inferior fascia of the urinogenital diaphragm alongside the ischiopubic ramus. It then passes out between the anterior border of the urogenital diaphragm and the pubis to reach the clitoris and glans (Fig. 2.10).

The perineal nerve gives motor branches to the striated muscles of the vulva, some of the anterior fibres of the external anal sphincter and the levator ani. Its sensory terminations are a pair of posterior labial nerves.

The vulva contains large numbers of special nerve endings and a corresponding rich supply of sensory nerves. Many of these specialised endings are mechanoreceptors, but they are absent from the region of the vestibule surrounding the vagina where there is a dense arborisation of free nerve endings.

Most of the sensory fibres are conveyed by the pudendal nerve, but those in the mons and the anterior parts of the labia majora go to the lumbar plexus via the ilioinguinal and genitofemoral nerves. Some fibres from the posterior parts of the labia majora are conveyed with the perineal branch of the posterior femoral cutaneous nerve to the sacral plexus.

There is also a dense autonomic nerve supply—the postganglionic sympathetic fibres arising from the hypogastric plexus, and the pelvis plexus; these are distributed to their endings via the pudendal nerve. The parasympathetic fibres come from S2, S3 and S4, as the nervae erigentes to join with the pelvic plexus; they are distributed with either the pelvic blood vessels or the pudendal nerves.

Blood supply

The arteries spring mainly from the internal iliac artery with a significant contribution from the femoral artery. The internal pudendal artery arises from the internal iliac artery and runs in the pudendal canal to the labia majora where it forms a very rich anastomosis with the deep external pudendal branches from the femoral artery. There are also communications between the vessels on either side.

The pudendal artery gives off the inferior rectal artery, which supplies the anal skin and musculature around the anal canal but provides blood for only a small area — the posterior aspect of the lower end of the vagina. Although the pudendal artery is near the ischiopubic ramus, it gives off branches that penetrate the inferior fascia of the urinogenital diaphragm to supply the labia, the erectile tissue of the bulb, the lower end of the vagina and associated muscles. Its final branches are the deep and dorsal arteries of the clitoris. It is the deep branch that is the main supply to the corpus cavernosus. The branches of the femoral artery, the superficial and deep external pudendal vessels, pass medially to reach the anterior portion of the labia majora.

The venous drainage of this area is basically a vast intercommunicating plexus that drains to the internal pudendal veins and hence to the internal iliac veins, with a small part of the anterior region of the labia majora draining to the greater saphenous vein.

Lymphatic drainage

The initial drainage from the vulva, the lower part of the urethra, the vagina and anal canal is mostly to the medial group of superficial inguinal lymph nodes. From here they drain into the deep inguinal lymph nodes in the femoral canal. The glans clitoridis drains directly into these nodes. There is considerable overlap in the drainage, which is bilateral. This overlap is of crucial importance during radical surgery for malignant disease.

THE VAGINA

The vagina is a distensible fibromuscular tube extending from the vestibule to the cervix of the uterus. It runs backwards and upwards with the anterior and posterior walls in close contact. The lining epithelium is thrown into transverse folds or rugae. It is probably the slack in these folds that accommodates the considerable distension of the vagina during intercourse and, later, parturition so that the vagina does not tear.

The vagina is related anteriorly to the base of the bladder and the urethra. It is separated from the bladder base by loose connective tissue, but the urethra is firmly bound to the adventitia of the anterior surface of the lower two-thirds of the vagina. Where the vagina is related to the bladder base it

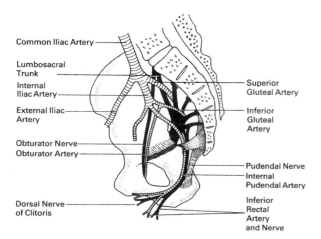

Fig. 2.10 Pelvic nerves and blood supply of the pudenda. The major nerve is the pudendal, but it is supplemented by the posterior cutaneous nerve of the thigh, the ilioinguinal and genitofemoral nerves.

Common Iliac Artery
Lumbosacral Trunk
Internal Iliac Artery
External Iliac Artery
Obturator Nerve
Obturator Artery
Dorsal Nerve of Clitoris
Superior Gluteal Artery
Inferior Gluteal Artery
Pudendal Nerve
Internal Pudendal Artery
Inferior Rectal Artery and Nerve

is separated from it in part by the two ureters, as their terminal portions pass in front of the anterior fornix.

Posteriorly the vagina is related to the rectum and the recotouterine pouch of Douglas. The lowermost part of the vagina is separated from the anal canal by the mass of dense connective tissue, the perineal body (Fig. 2.11).

Laterally the upper vagina is related to the pelvic fascia and the lower part is embraced by the anteromedial fibres of pubococcygeus and the urinogenital diaphragm. Near its outermost extremity the bulb of the vestibule, the greater vestibular glands and the bulbospongiosus muscles are its lateral relations.

The epithelium lining the vagina lies upon a dense fibrous lamina propria. The epithelium is stratified, squamous and non-keratinized and does not contain mucous glands; it should never be referred to as vaginal mucosa.

The submucosa consists of loosely arranged connective tissue with many elastic fibres and numerous large venous spaces together with occasional lymphoid patches. The muscularis is relatively thin, with both longitudinal and circular smooth muscle, and is continuous above with the uterine muscle. The outer layer of the vagina, the adventitia, is a fibrous tissue coat that binds the vagina to the surrounding structures.

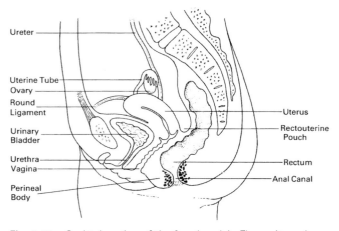

Fig. 2.11 Sagittal section of the female pelvis. The peritoneal covering of the pelvic organs is organised much as if a cover had been draped over them. Note the close relationship between the posterior fornix of the vagina and the rectouterine pouch.

Blood supply

The vagina has a rich and variable blood supply. The major vessels are the uterine arteries and the vaginal branches of the internal iliac arteries. From the anastomosis of these vessels azygos arteries extend on the anterior and posterior surfaces of the vagina. Other contributions, especially to the lower end of the vagina, are from the artery to the bulb, the pudendal arteries and the middle and inferior rectal vessels. Because the vagina is distensible these vessels have a very tortuous course in its contracted state. The venous drainage, in common with the other pelvic viscera, starts as a series of plexuses associated with the vesicle, rectal and uterine

plexuses and drains eventually by vaginal veins to the internal iliac veins.

Lymphatic drainage

Drainage for the upper two-thirds is different from that for the lower third and for the anterior wall differs from the posterior wall. From the upper two-thirds the drainage is to the internal and external iliac lymph nodes. The difference between the anterior and posterior walls is that, while drainage from the anterior wall is direct to the internal iliac nodes, that from the posterior wall relays first in a node lying in the connective tissue between the vagina and rectum. From the lower third of the vagina, lymph drains to the superficial inguinal nodes on both sides.

Nerve supply

The major nerve supply to the vagina is autonomic, arising from the pelvic plexuses, but the lower end has a sensory supply from the pudendal nerve.

The sympathetic fibres come from the lower lumbar sympathetic ganglia via the hypogastric plexus. The parasympathetic outflow is through the second, third and fourth sacral nerves. The fibres are distributed mainly in company with the arterial supply. The parasympathetic ganglia are found between the bladder and vagina and in association with the lateral walls of the vagina. Most nerve endings are undecorated, but Pacinian corpuscles are found within the vaginal adventitia.

THE UTERUS

The uterus is usually described in terms of cervix, body and fundus. In the nulliparous woman it is pear shaped and measures about $7.5 \times 5 \times 2.5$ cm. There is a cavity which communicates with the peritoneal cavity via the fallopian tubes and with the cavity of the vagina via the cervical canal. The fundus is that part of the uterus which lies above the openings of the tubes, while the tapering body lies below the fundus. It is somewhat flattened anteroposteriorly and is continuous with the cervix below. The cervix protrudes into the vault of the vagina. The gap between the cervix and the vaginal wall is called the fornix of the vagina; it is deepest posteriorly.

The uterus is described as having four layers. First, there is an outer peritoneal or serous coat, below which is a subserous connective tissue layer that is most dense where the various ligaments attach to the cervix. Third is the myometrium, the muscle layer of the uterus; it is the thickest layer, made up of interlacing bundles of smooth muscle fibres separated by connective tissue sheets containing blood vessels. This layer is about 15 mm thick in the nulliparous uterus of the adult. The fourth, innermost, layer is the endometrium, surrounding the cavity of the uterus; the endometrium undergoes considerable changes during the menstrual cycle.

The cervix has a central canal that extends from the internal os, where it becomes continuous with the cavity of the uterus, to the external os, where it becomes continuous with the cavity of the vagina. It forms a narrow bottleneck between these two organs.

The cervix is divided from the corpus by a fibromuscular junction, the internal os, which acts as a sphincter; its competence is important, especially during the second trimester of pregnancy.

The cervix projects into the vagina, surrounded by a gutter-like fornix. The vaginal cervix has a short anterior lip and a longer posterior lip. It is penetrated by the endocervical canal, which joins the uterine cavity to the vagina. The canal is fusiform in shapes is flattened from front to back, measures 7 mm across at its widest part and is about 3 cm long.

Anteriorly the supravaginal part is separated from the bladder by the connective tissue layer, the parametrium. The uterine arteries run in this tissue while the ureter runs downwards and forwards within the parametrium about 2 mm from the cervix.

Posteriorly the supravaginal cervix is covered with the peritoneum lining the rectouterine pouch of Douglas. The cervix is supported posteriorly by the uterosacral ligaments, which extend from this part of the cervix to the second, third and fourth sacral vertebrae. The cardinal ligaments support the cervix laterally and are the major support of the cervix and uterus.

The cervix shares its blood supply with that of the body of the uterus. The venous drainage is lateral into a plexus on either side of the cervix and from there into veins that follow the arteries.

The nerve supply to the cervix is autonomic, with the densest innervation being at the level of the internal os and most of these fibres supplying the smooth muscle in this region. The fibres appear to follow the arterially derived vessels. In contrast with the body of the uterus, many of these nerve fibres are cholinesterase positive. There are both adrenergic and cholinergic fibres within the cervix: their distribution is very similar, but overall there are fewer cholinergic fibres. Most of these fibres disappear after the menopause. Sensory fibres travel with both divisions of the autonomic nervous system.

The cervix has a rich lymphatic drainage with a three-layered arrangement of beds of vessels: a subepithelial bed, a stromal bed and a serosal bed which gives rise to a series of larger vessels that drain along the base of the broad ligament. The most anterior are closely related to the uterine artery and eventually reach the external iliac nodes. Slightly posteriorly the vessels also follow the uterine artery to its origin, where they join the internal iliac nodes. The most posterior group leaves the cervix posterolaterally and passes along the uterosacral fold to reach the nodes situated over the sacrum.

The bulk of the cervix consists mainly of fibrous tissue containing varying proportions of smooth muscle—usually about 10%, but it can vary between 2 and 40%.

Blood supply

This is through the uterine arteries supported superiorly by the terminal branches of the ovarian arteries. The uterine artery arises from the internal iliac artery, passing medially across the pelvic floor and lying in the base of the broad ligament. As the artery reaches the uterus near the supravaginal part of the cervix, it passes above the ureter and turns upwards to pass close to the lateral side of the body of the uterus as far as the entrance of the fallopian tube into the uterus. Here it anastomoses with the ovarian artery. Throughout its course it gives off many branches that penetrate the wall of the uterus (Fig. 2.12).

The venous drainage of the uterus consists of a plexus of veins that starts in the broad ligament, spreading out across the pelvic floor to communicate with the rectal and vesicle plexuses and draining into the internal iliac veins.

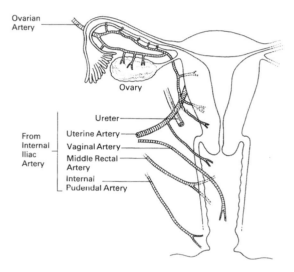

Fig. 2.12 Blood supply of the genitalia. The uterus has an anastomotic supply from both the ovarian and uterine arteries, both vessels running in the broad ligament.

Lymphatic drainage

In general this follows the arteries.

Nerve supply

This system is poorly understood. The main sensory fibres from the cervix run in the nervi erigentes from the sacral segments 2 and 3, while those from the body of the uterus travel with the hypogastric plexus to the lower thoracic segments. Some sensory fibres from the fundus travel in the ovarian and renal plexuses to reach their dorsal nerve roots of T11 and T12.

Peritoneal relations

The uterus is draped in a fold of peritoneum which extends forwards to cover the bladder and backwards to the rectum. It spreads laterally as the broad ligament, and the peritoneum then spreads to cover the pelvic wall. It is as if these organs had been pushed up into the pelvic cavity from below, carrying the peritoneum to various degrees into the cavity of the pelvis.

Anteriorly the peritoneum extends downwards as far as

the attachment of the base of the bladder at the level of the internal os, where the uterine attachment of the peritoneum is loose and may be easily separated. Posteriorly the uterus is completely covered by peritoneum continuous with that over the posterior fornix of the vagina, forming the anterior wall of the pouch of Douglas.

Fascia and ligaments of the uterus

These ligaments contain a remarkably high proportion of smooth muscle besides the usual collection of collagen. The cardinal and uterosacral ligaments assist the fibrous tissue in fixing the anterior aspect of the uterus to the bladder base and in maintaining the stability of the bladder. This connective tissue extends inferiorly to bind the urethra to the anterior wall of the vagina. It is probable that the broad and round ligaments have little function in uterine stability.

The uterosacral ligaments, arising from the supravaginal part of the cervix, pass backwards, embracing the rectum, to be attached to the front of the lower part of the sacrum. Posteriorly the vaginal and anal canals are separated but bound together by the fibromuscular mass of the perineal body. The lateral ligaments, the main ligaments of uterine stability, extend laterally from the cervix to the side wall of the pelvis (Fig. 2.13). The round and broad ligaments are associated with the body of the uterus. The round ligament arises from the junction between the body of the uterus and the uterine tube passes via the broad ligament where it raises a ridge on the anterior surface. It eventually runs along the inguinal canal to the labium majus of the vulva. It is mostly made up of smooth muscle. It probably functions as an anchor for the uterus in the anteverted position during recumbent sleep and against the pressure of a full bladder.

The broad ligament is not a ligament but a fold of peritoneum extending between the side of the body of the uterus and the lateral wall of the pelvis. Superiorly, there is a free border, while inferiorly it merges with the pelvic floor. It contains the ovarian artery and uterine tube, the round and ovarian ligaments superiorly, and the uterine artery medially. There are extensive lymphatics associated with the arteries. The ovary is attached to the posterior surface of the broad ligament by the mesovarium, a fold of peritoneum from the posterior side of the ligament (Fig. 2.14).

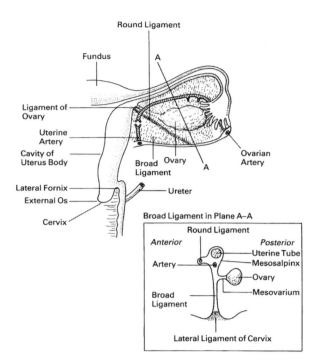

Fig. 2.14 Ovary and broad ligament from the back showing the relations of structures within the broad ligament. There are multiple small branches from the ovarian artery to the fallopian tube.

THE UTERINE TUBES

The uterine (fallopian) tubes are between 10 and 14 cm long, lying for the middle three-quarters in the upper border of the broad ligament. The lateral extremity is free of the broad ligament and is in close association with the surface of the ovary. The end is open and expanded with a bunch of finger-like processes, the fimbriae. There can be more than one ostium to a fallopian tube. Often one of the fimbriae—the ovarian fimbria—is longer than the others and is attached by its tip to the ovary.

The uterine tube is usually considered to have four regions: the fimbriated infundibulum outside the broad ligament, a dilated ampulla, followed by a narrow isthmus with a lumen 1–2 mm in diameter within the broad ligament, and finally an intramural part of the tube which lies within the muscular wall of the uterus. Thus the cavity of the uterus is continuous with the peritoneal cavity. However, the circular muscle at the uterine end of the fallopian tube is thickened and is regarded by some as a sphincter controlling the flow of fluids from the uterus into the tube. The tube is capable of producing secretions; the nature of these secretions is poorly known, but the amounts vary during the ovarian cycle, being greatest in the post-ovulation phase. The nutritional and oxygen needs of the developing embryo come from these fluids in the first few days of life.

The tube consists of smooth muscle surrounding a mucous membrane, which is ciliated and thrown into many complex longitudinal folds. The isthmus differs in that here the lumen is narrow, the folds disappear and there are fewer cilia.

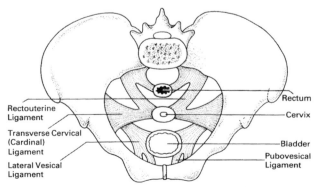

Fig. 2.13 Pelvic ligaments. The transverse or cardinal ligament is probably the major supporting structure of the cervix.

The tube has a rich blood supply via many small branches from the ovarian artery and its inner end from the uterine artery. The veins of the tube drain to the pampiniform plexus, while the lymphatics follow the course of the ovarian arteries in reverse.

THE OVARIES

The ovaries lie free within the cavity of the pelvis; they are without a covering of peritoneum except along the equatorial attachment of the mesovarium. The ovary is attached to the uterus at its upper angle by the ligament of the ovary. This mass of fibrous tissue and smooth muscle lies between the two layers of the broad ligament.

The ovary lies obliquely, with its upper pole medial and its lower pole lateral. It touches the side wall of the pelvis between the internal and external iliac vessels and lies upon the obturator nerve. The peritoneum, against which the ovary lies, is supplied by the obturator nerve. The ovary receives its blood from the ovarian arteries—direct branches of the abdominal aorta—while the ovarian veins form a plexus in the mesovarium that eventually drains into a pair of veins which run with the ovarian artery. Those from the left unite to form a single vein that drains into the left renal vein. Those on the right fuse and join the inferior vena cava.

The ovarian lymph drainage follows the course of the ovarian artery.

Structure

The ovary consists of a cuboidal epithelium surrounding a fibrous stroma. Initially each ovary contains about 3 million potential ova which have migrated along the dorsal mesentery during development.

In the newborn baby the ovaries are very large compared with the uterus. They increase in weight some 20 times before maturity, but the relative growth of the uterus is such that by puberty the ovaries are relatively much smaller than the uterus. There is practically no recognisable germinal tissue in the fully involuted ovary after the menopause.

THE BLADDER

In life, the base of the bladder lies flat; this flat area is greater than the area of the trigone but is of prime importance in maintaining urinary continence. There are said to be three sphincters controlling micturition: an internal urinary sphincter, urethral one and an external urinary sphincter. The internal sphincter is complex. It probably does not exist as a discrete entity but is composed of a series of muscular folds of the bladder. It is really the tone of the detrusor loop from the outer longitudinal layer of bladder muscle that forces the urethra backwards and it is the tone of the base plate that forces the trigone forwards into the concavity formed by the circular fibres of the fundus. Thus the trigone comes to lie in front of the urethral orifice, so that as long as the base plate remains flat the bladder neck remains closed.

In order to convert the base plate into a funnel-like tube during voiding, considerable force is required. The human is probably alone amongst animals in being able to hold urine for a considerable time after bladder filling has reached the point where the bladder would empty reflexly. This can even be achieved during sleep. At birth this bladder control is not possible because the base plate is rounded and does not fit into the concavity formed by the detrusor. In stress incontinence it is probably a sagging of the anterior vaginal wall that causes a descent of the bladder, distorting it in the base and so reducing its ability to resist increases in intra-abdominal pressure.

The bladder wall is made of smooth muscle fibres which run in spirals. The apparently randomly arranged muscle fibres produce a series of trabeculated ridges which at cystoscopy show through the bladder lining. The muscle as a whole is called the detrusor. The lining of the bladder is thick and lax and is a transitional epithelium which is urine-proof because of the specialised junctions between the inner edges of the adjacent cells. There is said to be a ring of fibres around the internal urethral orifice. The lining has neither glands nor muscularis mucosa.

The blood supply to the bladder is from the superior and inferior vesicular arteries, assisted by a few branches from the pubic branch of the inferior epigastric artery.

The veins of the bladder become a plexus at the base of the bladder. The vesicle plexus communicates with veins in the broad ligament and drains to the internal iliac veins.

The lymph drainage follows the course of the arteries.

Nerve supply is autonomic from the pelvic plexus, the parasympathetic segments are S2, S3 and S4 and the fibres reach the plexus via the nervi erigentes. The sympathetic nerves are inhibitory to the detrusor muscle and motor to the internal sphincter.

THE URETHRA

This tube extends from the bladder to the vestibule, a distance in the normal non-pregnant adult female of about 5 cm. It penetrates the urinogenital diaphragm. The vagina is closely related to it posteriorly and the urethra is closely bound to the vagina in its lower two-thirds; the upper part is loose and held only by loose connective tissue. The urethra is a very distensible organ which has muscular, submucous and mucous layers; the smooth muscle is made up of an outer circular and inner longitudinal layer. In its lower part there is a ring of striated muscle fibres, the sphincter urethrae. The submucosa is remarkable in that it contains numerous venous channels surrounded by loose elastic connective tissue. The mucous membrane itself is thrown into a series of longitudinal folds with an especially prominent one posteriorly.

The epithelium is stratified and columnar in the middle third of the urethra, merging with bladder epithelium upwards and with the stratified squamous non-keratinized epithelium of the vestibule inferiorly. There are numerous small and a pair of large periurethral glands that drain via short ducts into its lumen.

The blood supply of the main part of the urethra is from branches of the vaginal vessels and the upper part is supplied by terminations of the vesicle arteries. The venous plexuses have a corresponding drainage, either to the vesicle veins or to the venous plexuses of the vulva.

The urethral sphincter has inner longitudinal and outer circular smooth muscle layers around the urethra and some striated paraurethral muscle. It is normally closed except during micturition, when the inner longitudinal muscle contracts, shortening the urethra and therefore increasing the bore of its lumen.

The external urinary sphincter is located between the layers of the urinogenital diaphragm. It is made up of striated muscle innervated by the pudendal nerve. It can stop the voluntary urinary stream.

The lymph drainage is either to inguinal nodes or to the internal and external iliac nodes. The nerve supply is autonomic from the pelvic and hypogastric plexuses.

THE RECTUM

The rectum, despite its name, is anything but straight. It curves to follow the anterior curve of the sacrum and deviates towards the left in its middle part, whereas the upper and lower thirds lie in the midline. The rectum begins at the level of the third segment of the sacrum and extends as far as the perineal body, where it becomes the anal canal. The rectum has no mesentery but its upper third has pelvic peritoneum on its anterior and lateral surfaces, the middle third only on its anterior surface and the lowest third has no contact with the peritoneum.

Unlike the large intestine, the external layer of longitudinal muscle is complete over the surface of the rectum. Internally the junctions between the curves of the rectum are marked by horizontal folds, the valves of Houston. These folds contain circular muscle of the gut.

Anorectal lymphatic drainage

The rectosigmoid and upper rectum drain via the mesentery to the inferior mesenteric group of nodes. The middle and lower part of the rectum drains both to the mesenteric group and to the internal iliac nodes. The anal canal below the levator ani muscle drains across the thigh to the inguinal and gluteal nodes.

The rectum has an autonomic nerve supply which is sympathetic directly from the pelvic plexus and parasympathetic via S2 and S3 and the nervi erigentes.

CONCLUSIONS

The anatomy of the female urogenital tract is highly dynamic and undergoes huge changes at all stages of the reproductive cycle, from the vast increase in size of the labia minora during copulation to the recovery of the prepregnant uterine size after parturition. The tract is under the control of multiple influences—psychogenic, emotional, sensory, autonomic and hormonal—but seems capable of fulfilling its role in reproduction in the absence of many of them. Its design faults, if they may be considered as such, are the shape of the bony pelvic canal at different levels, demanding, in the human, rotation of the fetal head as it descends and the great vulnerability to the effects of infection of the narrow lumen of the fallopian tubes.

ACKNOWLEDGEMENTS

I have borrowed heavily from the standard anatomical textbooks and from the advice of my colleagues. The standard diagrams are in such a highly evolved state that it would be a research project in itself to trace them to their origins. I have done little except tinker with their details. To these unknown original artists and ancestors I offer my sincere thanks.

KEY POINTS

- The bony pelvis has to combine weight bearing of the upper body through each hip joint with the functions of child bearing.
- The bony pelvis is not distensible, and has only minor degrees of movement at its joints.
- The muscles of the pelvic diaphragm make up a gutter, penetrated in three places by the rectum, vagina and urethra.
- Uterine function is to retain the pregnancy for 38 weeks and then expel it in 12 hours.
- The two major reproductive deficiencies of the femal pelvis are its long shape and the narrowness of the fallopian tubes.

3

Fertilisation, early development and implantation

Alan O. Trounson, Martin F. Pera, A. Henry Sathananthan

INTRODUCTION

Fertilisation marks a decisive event in the reproductive process—a continuum starting with the formation of primordial germ cells that are multipotential (Shamblott et al 1998), germ cell migration, differentiation into male and female gamete precursor (Buehr 1997, Swain & Lovell-Badge 1999) cells, their unique maternal and paternal imprinting (Surani et al 1986) and further differentiation and growth (gametogenesis) into mature gametes. Gametes have the full potential to unite at fertilisation, activating the oocyte and controlling the initial preimplantation development phase that can occur independently of the maternal reproductive system (Trounson et al 1982). In this early phase of embryo development the new embryonic genome becomes progressively activated, demethylated and then remethylated, following which the first differentiated lineage appears (trophectoderm). Segregation of the trophectoderm lineage occurs by positional influence in the actively dividing spherical ball of cells (morula), to create either inside cells or outside cells with specific polar characteristics (Johnson & Ziomek 1981). At this stage, the nascent blastocyst (Fig. 3.1) requires the maternal reproductive tract for further normal development, implanting in the uterine endometrium on day 8 after fertilisation. As a consequence, normal human embryo development *in vitro* (outside the body) is limited to the first 6 days after fertilisation. Maintenance of embryos in culture after this time results in abnormalities of development, chaotic differentiation and failure to establish an integrated body plan. It is possible that maternally derived factors are required for regulation of these processes *in vivo*.

PREPARATION OF THE OOCYTE FOR FERTILISATION

Oocyte maturation

The growing oocyte needs to reach a critical size (by definition the full size of the normally ovulated oocyte) before it can respond to gonadotrophin-mediated activators by resumption of meiosis and the final phase of oocyte maturation. Normally, human ovarian follicles are 18–24 mm in diameter when they are exposed to the endogenous LH surge that induces ovulation. However, it is apparent that follicles as small as 8 mm that are leading the cohort in growth *in vivo* contain oocytes that can be induced to mature in response to the administration of endogenous gonadotrophin (human chorionic gonadotrophin—hCG). These oocytes fertilise and develop normally to blastocysts in culture *in vitro*, and to term when replaced in a human female host (Trounson et al 2001). The acquisition of developmental competence by the oocyte, which occurs early in the follicular phase, means that recovery of oocytes suitable for both *in vitro* fertilisation (IVF)

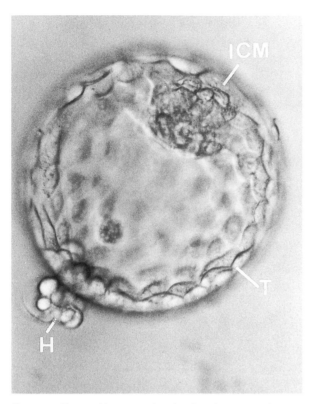

Fig. 3.1 Human blastocyst that developed to term when transferred singly to the patient's uterus. T = Trophectoderm; ICM = inner cell mass; H = hatching from the zona.

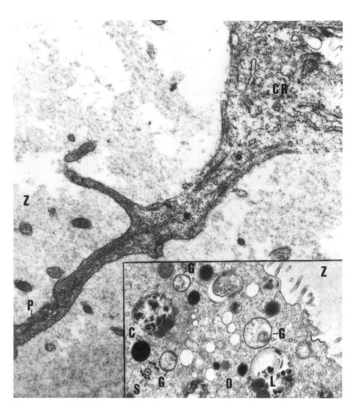

Fig. 3.2 Follicle (corona) cell process extending through the zona pellucida of an immature oocyte (TEM, × 20 000). Inset: Such processes end up within the oocyte in circular gap junctions, where physiological exchanges could occur between the two cells (TEM, × 11 760). This egg was injected with sperm. C = cortical granule; CR = corona cell; G = gap junction; L = lysosome; O = ooplasm; S = sperm tail; Z = zona.

and *in vitro* maturation (IVM) (Chian et al 1999) can be accomplished during most of the follicular phase.

Oocyte maturation is a complex process that involves signals from the follicle support cells and is initiated by a removal of inhibition by the granulosa cells in response to the preovulatory surge of LH. The inhibitory influences on resumption of meiosis of the granulosa cells in the immediate vicinity of the oocyte (cumulus and corona radiata cells) cease when their cytoplasmic processes are withdrawn from the zona pellucida and from direct connection with the oocyte (Fig. 3.2). It is believed that the follicle cells maintain high intracytoplasmic cAMP within the oocyte through sustained secondary messenger input via the intracytoplasmic connections. Their withdrawal is coincident with the initiation of protein synthesis and phosphorylation/dephosphorylation cascades in the oocyte that lead to dephosphorylation and activation of p34^{cdc2} kinase activity and phosphorylation of cyclin B. These molecules exist as an inactive heterodimer under the influence of several genes, including weeI, that functions to maintain the tyrosine 15 residue in a phosphorylated state. The active form is known as M-phase promoting factor (MPF) and inactive form as pre-MPF. The active dephosphorylated p34^{cdc2} and phosphorylated cyclin β heterodimer can be first detected at the time of germinal vesicle breakdown (GVBD). Activation and deactivation of MPF is associated with nuclear remodelling, the active form being associated with metaphase of the cell cycle. Consequently, MPF activation is probably the factor responsible for GVBD

(Trounson et al 2001). MPF activity rises at metaphase I of meiosis and is inactivated to allow anaphase I and telophase I to occur, culminating in metaphase II and expulsion of the first polar body with reactivation of MPF this is stabilized by mos, a product of the c-mos proto-oncogene. This is recognised as the completion of oocyte maturation and human oocytes are usually ovulated at or just before the completion of the meiotic process. A number of other important genes are activated in human oocytes at the beginning of and during oocyte maturation, including those associated with mitogen activated protein (MAP) kinase (Trounson et al 2001).

Human oocytes can be matured successfully *in vitro* but under the present conditions, there is a lack of synchrony in the initiation of GVBD and completion of maturation that may be due to variation in the transcriptional competence of oocytes, maintenance of inhibition by follicle support cells or the lack of appropriate culture conditions *in vitro*. However, if the oocytes receive the LH activation stimulus *in vivo*, they mature rapidly and in synchrony when removed 30–36 hours later (Trounson et al 2001, Chian et al 1999). This suggests that LH priming in the intact follicle *in vivo* is necessary to establish the initial developmental competence of the human oocyte.

Oocytes are recovered for IVF by follicular aspiration from the ovary some time before ovulation. In some of these oocytes, the second polar body is not visible and waiting for 4–5 h before insemination significantly increases the likelihood of fertilisation. For intracytoplasmic sperm injection (ICSI) (Van Steirteghem et al 1993) oocytes are injected with sperm only if they have a second polar body visible. Those oocytes that still have a germinal vesicle visible need to be matured *in vitro* for around 24 h (Trounson et al 2001) and those with no germinal vesicle or second polar body should be cultured for 3–8 h until the polar body is extruded. Insemination or injection of immature oocytes can lead to an increase in fertilisation abnormalities and developmental defects.

FERTILISATION

Sperm capacitation and the acrosome reaction

Ejaculated sperm are modified in the female reproductive tract to enable them to bind to, and fertilise, ovulated oocytes. This process is called capacitation and involves cAMP-dependent phosphorylation, the presence of the extracellular cations calcium and sodium, and an increase in intracellular pH (which occurs by activation of the exchange of Na$^+$ and H$^+$, which in turn promotes the efflux of H$^+$ and influx of Ca^{2+}). Capacitation is a reversible process, and can be recognised by changes to the ultrastructure and antigenicity of sperm head membranes (Trounson & Bongso 1996). Human sperm capacitate spontaneously when washed free of seminal plasma and incubated in simple chemically defined media, and the only protein required is albumin. Capacitated sperm are able to locate the ovulated oocyte–cumulus mass in the ampulla of the fallopian tube and, even though there may be very few sperm in the vicinity of the oocyte at any one time, fertilisation is very efficient. Sperm release hyaluronidase to aid penetration of the cumulus–oophorus matrix and the fertilising sperm acrosome reacts with the surface of the zona pellucida (the extracellular matrix that surrounds the oocyte cell) (Fig. 3.3). The zona is composed of at least three major glycoproteins: ZP1, ZP2 and ZP3. The ZP3 and ZP2 molecules are filaments that are structurally cross-linked with ZP1 to form a network. ZP3 binds to capacitated sperm aggregating receptors on the sperm head, inducing G protein signalling that activates protein phosphorylation, increases intracellular calcium ions (Ca^{2+}) through voltage-sensitive Ca^{2+} channels, and increases intracellular pH. Three signal transduction pathways that lead to protein phosphorylation and the acrosome reaction have been identified: the adenylate cyclase–cAMP–protein kinase A pathway; the phospholipase C–diacylglycerol–protein kinase C pathway; and the guanylate cyclase–cGMP–protein kinase G pathway (Trounson & Bongso 1996). The molecular identity of the sperm zona receptor remains unknown but there are several candidates, including β-galactosyltransferase, sperm protein 56 and zona receptor kinase.

Importantly, sperm–oocyte binding is species specific and gametes are unable to recognize any other species. The glycoprotein ZP3 is the sperm receptor and its specificity is determined by O-linked sugar residues that are responsible for sperm zona binding (Wassarman 1999). The acrosome reac-

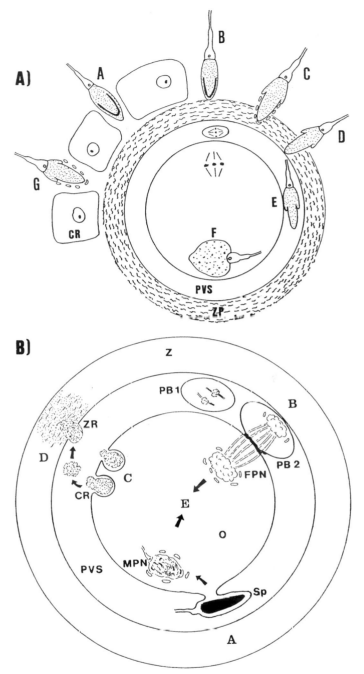

Fig. 3.3 (A) Sperm changes during fertilisation.
A: Acrosome-intact sperm between corona radiate (CR) cells; B: acrosome-intact sperm bound to the zona (ZP); C: acrosome-reacting sperm activated by ZP3; D: acrosome-reacted sperm penetrating the zona; E: acrosome-reacted sperm in the perivitelline space (PVS) fusing with the oocyte plasma membrane; F: incorporated sperm with expanded head and decondensing chromatin; G: acrosome-reacted non-fertilising sperm in corona cells.
(B) Major events that occur at fertilisation.
A: Sperm–oocyte fusion (SP) and incorporation; B: completion of meiosis by expulsion of the second polar body (PB2); C: excytosis of the cortical granules (CR); D: zona reaction to prevent polyspermy (ZR); E: migration of the male (MPN) and female (FPN) pronuclei to the centre of the oocyte. Z = zona pellucida; O = ooplasm; PB1 = first polar body; PVS = perivitelline space. (Reproduced from Sathananthan et al 1996, with permission.)

tion is a vesiculation process triggered by ZP3 that results in the fusion of the oocyte plasma membrane with the outer acrosomal membrane over the acrosomal cap and equatorial segment of the sperm head (Fig. 3.3). The acrosome is a specialised organelle of the sperm, similar to the lysosome of an ordinary cell. When the acrosome reaction occurs, hydrolytic enzymes are released, and those bound to the inner acrosomal membrane are exposed to enable the rapidly moving sperm cell to penetrate the zona. This is achieved by a combination of physically grinding a hole, proteolytic digestion to open the pathway, and secondary binding to the ZP2 molecule at the equatorial segment during zona penetration to assist the direction of sperm passage. The enzymes hyaluronidase and pro-acrosin/acrosin have been identified as acrosomal enzymes that are likely to be involved in sperm digestion of the zona and entry into the oocyte, although acrosin gene-deficient mice are still able to fertilise oocytes. Sperm require hyperactive motility for penetration of the zona. The physical activity of sperm is important in the drilling and penetration of the zona. Without capacitation, the acrosome reaction, and hyperactive motility, passage through the zona cannot occur (Yanagimachi 1994).

Process of fertilisation *in vivo* and *in vitro*

During the mid-cycle fertile period, sperm appear in the fallopian tubes within minutes of their deposition in the vagina. Thereafter, further sperm make their way from the vagina and progress through the fallopian tubes over the next 36–72 h. Under normal circumstances there are sufficient capacitated sperm to ensure that at least some encounter oocytes in the tubal ampulla and initiate fertilisation. However, idiopathic infertility occurs frequently (15–30% of infertile couples) and this can be efficiently treated by gamete intrafallopian transfer (GIFT), in which oocytes and sperm are transferred together to the tubal ampulla. This suggests that sperm transport is diminished in these couples, and that insufficient sperm numbers arrive and/or stay in the tube to produce fertilisation. Idiopathic infertility is now usually treated by IVF because the success rates are equivalent to those of GIFT, and laparoscopy is avoided. Sperm transport during the early follicular phase, luteal phase and menses is dramatically reduced because of structural, biochemical and volumetric changes in cervical mucus.

Sperm reaching the ampulla–isthmus junction of the fallopian tube may be drawn to the oocyte by some chemotactic mechanism, although it is rare to find many supernumerary sperm in the zonae of oocytes *in vivo*. The acrosome-reacted sperm that penetrate the zona pellucida lose their motility after entry into the perivitelline space (Fig. 3.3). The surface of the oocyte has numerous microvilli that protrude from the oocyte surface and, in a process akin to phagocytosis, the finger-like microvilli fuse with the equatorial segment of the sperm head and initiate the fusion process. Sperm are engulfed by the oocyte tangentially and the whole sperm head, midpiece and tail are drawn into the cytoplasm (Sathananthan et al 1985). It is likely that gamete fusion is an integrin-mediated process involving $\alpha6\beta1$ integrin on the oocyte plasma membrane and the ADAM (Fertilin 1 and 2)

protein on sperm. Fertilin β has a disintegrin domain which contains a RGD like cell binding domain that interacts with integrin receptors. The α chain of fertilin contains a fusion domain but this is non-functional in primates, including the human.

More recent evidence in the mouse implicates CD9, a widely expressed tetraspannin that organises multimolecular complexes at the cell surface, in fusion via interaction with $\alpha6\beta1$ integrin. CD9 gene knockout mice are infertile and sperm enter the perivitelline space but do not fuse with the oocyte. Sperm–oocyte fusion is generally species specific, except for human sperm–hamster oocyte fusion, and this specificity is likely to be regulated by mediator molecules or specific carbohydrate side chains.

The oocyte responds rapidly to sperm fusion by depolarising the sperm membrane and initiating a wave of exocytosis which liberates the contents of the cortical granules that have migrated to the plasma membrane during oocyte maturation (Fig. 3.3). These contain trypsin-like enzymes that alter the structural arrangements within the zona, blocking the progression of any sperm in the zona and changing the receptor activity of ZP3. In the human, the block to polyspermy is primarily due to the zona reaction induced by gamete fusion and secondarily due to changes in the plasma membrane. The sperm induces activation of the oocyte either as a result of gamete fusion or by release of a protein that induces release of intracellular calcium stores in the oocyte. The activation of the oocyte can be visualised as oscillating waves of calcium ions released as a result of sperm receptor interaction and increase in IP3 or the direct influence of a protein (oscillagen or a truncated form of c-kit). Oocyte activation induces the extrusion of the second polar body and completion of the second reduction division and deactivation of MPF by degrading cyclin B. In the presence of deactivated MPF, nuclei are remodeled with chromatin decondensation and the formation of pronuclear membranes around the decondensing male and female chromatin. The two pronuclear and polar bodies are visible 3–6 h after insemination. They migrate to the centre of the oocyte by 8–10 h after insemination and remain until dissolution of the pronuclear membranes at syngamy 20–28 h after insemination. DNA replication occurs in the pronuclear stage of the embryonic zygote.

The mitotic cell cycle is initiated by the reactivation of MPF involving the series of protein dephosphorylation and phosphorylation events established as a regular sequence during oocyte maturation. Rising MPF levels remodel the pronuclei by initiating chromatin condensation and dissolution of the pronuclear membrane.

Maternal and paternal chromosomes are mixed for the first time at syngamy and the replicated chromosomes align on the first embryonic metaphase plate attached by microtubules in a barrel-shaped spindle. The spindle microtubules are nucleated by the centrosomes that are composed of two centrioles aligned perpendicular to one another, surrounded by dense material (pericentriolar substance). In the human the sperm contains a single functional centriole in the neck region and this is contributed to the centrosome that remains in close association with the male pronucleus. The sperm centriole has a major role in cell cleavage and is located at one pole of the first mitotic spindle at syngamy. This paternally inherited centriole is inherited by all daughter cells and has a primary role in embryonic cleavage and development (Sathananthan et al 1996).

The first cleavage division occurs 3–6 h after disappearance of the pronuclear membranes, with the cleavage furrow separating the replicated telophase chromosomes equally into each daughter cell beginning 20–28 h after insemination (Trounson & Bongso 1996). This effectively ends the fertilisation process and initiates embryogenesis. Cleavage is accompanied by inactivation of MPF through cyclin degradation induced by calmodulin-dependent protein kinase II, by intracellular calcium waves and the reformation of a nucleus with decondensed interphase chromatin.

Fertilisation *in vitro* may be achieved in the human by washing ejaculated sperm free of seminal plasma using centrifugation and resuspension in simple chemically defined media (this process is known as 'swim-up' procedure) or buoyant density-gradient centrifugation and resuspension of the motile sperm fraction in culture medium. Washed motile sperm are added to oocytes usually at 2×10^5 motile sperm per ml. Lower concentrations of sperm are needed in smaller volumes of medium containing oocytes as droplets (50–200 µl) under oil or in capillary tubes. It is now common to inseminate oocytes for only 1–2 h, then to wash and culture the oocytes with adhering sperm and corona cells for 12–18 h in fresh culture medium without additional sperm. With normospermic patients these insemination methods are efficient and result in 50–75% fertilized pronuclear oocytes. The microdroplet or capillary tube insemination systems were recommended for patients with reduced semen quality (reduced motility and sperm concentration in semen or increased abnormal morphological forms of sperm) (Trounson & Bongso 1996). However, these potential inhibitors of fertilisation are now often dealt with by ICSI (Van Steirteghem et al 1993), as are problems such as immobilising or agglutinating antibodies and generalised functional problems such as acrosome reaction defects (Baker et al 2000).

The major differences between IVF and fertilisation *in vivo* are the presence of numerous sperm in the vicinity of the zona. In the absence of cumulus cells, sperm will attempt to enter the zona at all angles instead of the usual oblique or tangential entry mode. High sperm numbers in the insemination medium can increase polyspermic fertilisation. IVF removes the selectivity of the human reproductive tract for the fertilising spermatozoon but has no apparent effect on embryo developmental competence.

It has now been well established (Van Steirteghem et al 1998) that the selection of a single sperm for microinjection into the oocyte (ICSI) enables high rates of fertilisation for patients with only a few abnormal or immature sperm cells. There is a marked decrease in fertilisation with completely immotile sperm (some of which may have damaged DNA) or those that are unable to activate oocyte and decondense their chromatin. Sperm recovered from the epididymis or testis can be used for ICSI to successfully fertilise oocytes without any apparent problems for embryo development and the health of the babies that result. There are, however, problems associated with the use of sperm precursor cells such as round spermatids and secondary spermatocytes in the human. In the case of the former, the proportion of embryos that develops to term is low and inconsistent. In the case of the latter, the secondary spermatocyte is diploid, which presents an additional challenge for the oocyte to form a normal haploid male pronucleus. In contrast, in mice both precursor cells have been used successfully to produce live offspring (Yanagimachi 1998). Sperm DNA is still being methylated during maturation in the testis and epididymis and there may be important species differences that prevent immature human spermatids and spermatocytes from contributing normally to fertilisation and development.

Abnormalities of fertilisation

There is a wide range of abnormalities observed in fertilisation *in vitro* (Trounson & Bongso 1996) that include polyspermy, digyny, fragmentation and various forms of suppression (e.g. polar body extrusion, male and/or female pronuclei formation). Pronuclei do not necessarily appear synchronously, and examination of the oocyte at any one point in time can result in errors of diagnosis when single or multiple pronuclei are seen (Trounson & Bongso 1996). Oocytes with a single pronucleus can develop to blastocysts and to term, particularly if two polar bodies are present. Oocytes with two male pronuclei form tripolar spindles that usually (~60%) result in immediate cleavage to three cells rather than two cells, and lead to chaotic chromosome numbers in the cells of the embryonic blastomeres. Less frequently (~25%) they will cleave to two cells with a triploid chromosome complement in all blastomeres. Occasionally they revert to diploid status with expulsion of a set of chromosomes. Fertilised digynic oocytes usually cleave to two cells and develop as triploids. Triploids are usually lost during early embryo development or are aborted.

Embryos that contain a multiple set of paternal genes (triploids or androgenones) are more likely to develop abnormally. As a probable consequence of an abnormal complement of imprinted genes, these embryos have excessive trophoblast development and reduced or absent fetal development. These embryonic defects may predispose patients to the development of trophoblastic disease (hydatiform moles and choriocarcinoma). Tripronuclear oocytes are always discarded in clinical IVF practice when identified at the zygote stage. At later cleavage divisions (e.g. 8-cell) triploidy can be identified by embryo biopsy and fluorescent *in situ* hybridisation (FISH) or fluorescent polymerase chain reaction (FPCR). Triploid embryos are capable of development to blastocysts with apparently normal morphology.

Human oocytes can be parthenogenetically activated but their cleavage is usually disorganised, probably because of the absence of the paternal centriole. Haploidy has been observed in a human blastocyst but this was originally derived from a normal dipronuclear oocyte (Magli et al 2000). In this case, a haploid chromosome complement may have been lost during early development but the cells retained the paternal centriole.

EMBRYONIC DEVELOPMENT

Preimplantation embryos

Human embryos divide and develop in culture media into two cells at 20–30 h after insemination, four cells by 44–48 h, eight cells by 72 h (third day), compacted morulae by the fourth day and cavitating-expanding blastocysts on the fifth day, with expanded and hatching (escaping from the zona) blastocysts on the sixth day (Trounson & Bongso 1996). Embryos that lag in development or that fragment (Alikani et al 1999) during cleavage have reduced viability. Other defects, including multiple nuclei in blastomeres, vacuoles in the cytoplasm, unequal cleavage of blastomeres and rapid cleavage are also associated with chromosomal abnormalities and loss of continued development and implantation.

The human embryonic genome is activated between the four-cell and eight-cell stage (Braude et al 1988) and progressively new transcripts and proteins appear as the embryo advances in development. At the eight-cell stage the blastomeres compact with one another as cell surface changes produce adhesion molecules that bond the cell mass together, creating outside cells that become polar, and inside cells that are apolar. These outside cells of the 16- to 32-cell morula become the trophectoderm cells and the inside cells become the inner cell mass cells (Fig. 3.1) of the nascent blastocyst (Johnson & Ziomek 1981). Polarity of some gene products may be observed in the oocyte, zygote and cleavage-stage embryo but it is not certain if these characteristics are critical for development because the mammalian embryo can be manipulated to rearrange intracellular components and cell position without apparently affecting development. When compacting blastomeres flatten on one another, microvilli become polarised to the outside and the plane of division dictates the fate of the daughter cells (Fig. 3.4). The cleavages

are either radial or tangential, giving rise to polar outside trophectoderm or the apolar inner cell mass, mediated by E cadherin redistribution. Cadherin is activated by some form of post-translational modification at the eight-cell stage. Tight junctions are formed between outside cells and characteristic trophectoderm is evident around the 64-cell stage. Tight junction proteins, adherent junction proteins and desmosomal proteins are present at sites of contact between trophectoderm cells. The blastocoelic cavity is formed by activation of sodium ion pumping. The cytokine FGF-4 induces differentiation of embryonic cells into trophectoderm, and transcription of this gene is first observed at the morula stage. The cognate receptor FGFr-2 also appears at this time, and at the blastocyst stage FGF-4, produced by the inner cell mass, drives trophoblast proliferation through the FGFr-2 receptor (Tanaka et al 1998).

Trophectoderm differentiates under the influence of the transcription factor mash2. Mural trophectoderm cells not in contact with the inner cell mass become polytene through endoreduplication. The polar trophectoderm in contact with the inner cell mass forms the chorion. The expanding blastocyst swells with increasing expansion of the blastocoelic cavity, eventually rupturing the thinning zona pellucida, and the embryo squeezes out of the ruptured zonae in culture on day 6–7 after insemination. If left in culture *in vitro*, the continuously expanding blastocyst will float in isotonic culture medium for 1 or 2 days before seeking attachment to the culture vessel or a monolayer of coculture feeder cells (Bongso et al 2000). Human blastocysts need to be returned to the maternal uterine environment by day 6 after insemination for continued normal development (Jones et al 1998).

Chromosomal aneuploidy in human preimplantation embryos

Large-scale cytogenetic analyses show that normal men have a frequency of about 9% chromosomal abnormalities in their sperm. Cytogenetic studies show that human oocytes have around 20% anomalies in chromosome number and structure and, as a result, 30% or more of two-to-four-cell embryos are chromosomally abnormal (Trounson & Bongso 1996). More recent studies using FISH for 5–9 different chromosomes that usually include X, Y, 13, 16, 18, 21 and 22 show a much higher rate of aneuploidy from biopsied blastomeres or polar bodies. Most embryos biopsied at the eight-cell stage for FISH have 50% or more numerical chromosomal abnormalities and, in women of increasing age over 37 years, these increase to 75% or more. While it is possible that the FISH technique overestimates aneuploidy because of signal failure, there is a high concordance between the aneuploidy error biopsied from one cell of an eight-cell embryo and the aneuploidy present in inner cell mass cells of the blastocyst (Magli et al 2000). Mixaploidy is also apparent in up to 25% of embryos and is usually represented in lineages of the inner cell mass (Magli et al 2000). The estimated error rate due to technical and mixaploid factors is considered to be less than 10%. It is not apparent that aneuploid cells present in a euploid embryo are preferentially partitioned to the trophectoderm. However, it

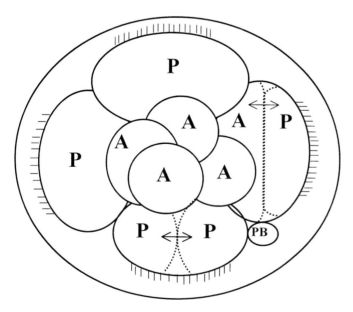

Fig. 3.4 Inside-apolar cells (A) and outer-polar cells (P) formed during compaction at eight-cell stage with cleavage division giving rise to polar or apolar (↔) daughter cells depending on the plane of cleavage. PB = polar body.

is likely that these are less fit cells that are lost during development.

The high rate of aneuploidy in human oocytes that increases with maternal age (>37 years) is thought to be due to mechanisms of anaphase lagging or non-disjunction of whole bivalents during meiosis, but it has also been suggested that precocious division of chromosomal univalents at anaphase I results in single chromatids at metaphase II, and that this is a major cause of trisomy and monosomy (Trounson & Bongso 1996). It is possible that maternal ageing affects transcription or translation of key anaphase proteins that could also destabilise the spindle microtubule assembly and bivalent and univalent chromatin separation mechanisms.

Inner cell mass cells and embryonic stem cells

If the inner cell mass of human blastocysts is immunosurgically isolated from the trophectoderm on days 6–7, they can be cultured on selected batches of fetal fibroblasts under conditions that prevent their differentiation into endoderm, trophectoderm or extra-embryonic endoderm. Maintenance of the culture conditions and continuous passage of the disaggregated colonies can result in the establishment of pluripotent embryonic stem (ES) cells that are immortal. These cells represent the completely undifferentiated precursor for all human cell lineages and somatic cell types and are an immensely valuable resource for research and potential human benefit. Human ES cells are different from inner cell mass cells and their exact counterpart in the embryo, if it exists, has not been identified. ES cells can be indefinitely expanded without differentiation (Thomson et al 1998). Under conditions that induce differentiation, they are able to produce mature somatic cells representing three major germ layers (ectoderm, mesoderm and endoderm) and, under specific conditions can form a pure somatic cell type (Reubinoff et al 2000), for example mature neurons (Fig. 3.5).

ES cells provide an opportunity to further explore human development that has been inaccessible for research in the past. Discovery of the intrinsic and extrinsic factors that govern cell multiplication and differentiation and those factors that maintain them as stem cells or direct them into lineage decisions towards a finite phenotype will be extremely valuable for many aspects of human medicine. The cells will be used for new drug discoveries and for toxicology, and eventually they may be used for tissue engineering and transplantation.

Axis formation and the elaboration of the embryonic body plan

Differentiation of the inner cell mass is accompanied by spatial rearrangement of cells forming the embryonic–abembryonic axis through asymmetric placement of inner cell mass cells and a bilateral asymmetry known as the animal vegetal axis (Fig. 3.6). At the egg cylinder stage there is a proximal and distal axis and later the anterior–posterior, dorsal–ventral and left–right axes are defined. The embryonic body plan cannot be formed by human ES cells *in vitro*,

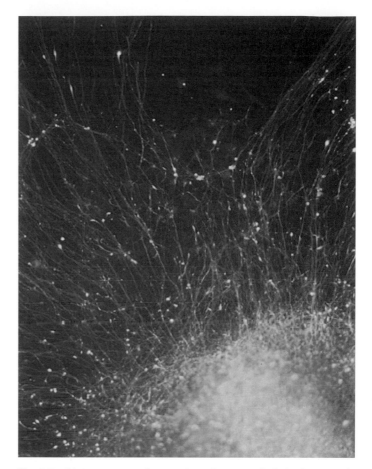

Fig. 3.5 Mature neurons from embryonic stem cell-derived neuronal progenitors. Neural precursor cells were isolated from human embryonic stem cell cultures, and grown under conditions which support the growth of neural stem cells. The resulting neurospheres were then allowed to attach to a culture dish under conditions which support neuronal differentiation. Maturing neurons emanating from attached neurospheres are stained with an antibody against the 160 kDa neurofilament protein.

nor when xenotransplanted to the kidney capsule, and there is no evidence of formation of organised embryoid bodies as seen in cultured mouse ES cells (Reubinoff et al 2000). It is possible that maternal factors are required to direct axis formation and elaboration of the human embryo's distinctive body structure.

Polarity within embryonic cells is a feature of early embryo development (Antczak & Van Blerkom 1997) and it is thought that polar distribution of cytoplasmic determinants are important for axis orientation. The inner cell mass is more ovoid than round in structure and the axis of orientation can be related to the position of the polar body. In the intact implanting embryo, cells that arise near the polar body contribute to the distal egg cylinder, while those on the opposite side end up in a more proximal location. These tissues will ultimately induce the anterior region of the embryo.

In the mouse, the inner cell mass grows and undergoes a process of cavitation to form the cap-like structure of epiblast known as the egg cylinder. Cavitation may occur by selective

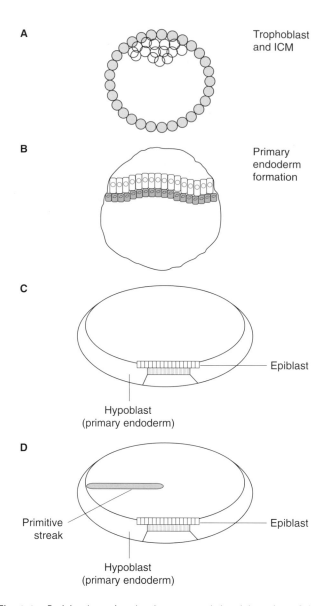

A — Trophoblast and ICM

B — Primary endoderm formation

C — Epiblast / Hypoblast (primary endoderm)

D — Primitive streak / Epiblast / Hypoblast (primary endoderm)

Fig. 3.6 Peri-implantation development and the elaboration of the body plan. Evidence of asymmetry in the mammalian conceptus from the earliest stages of development (two-cell stage) suggests that maternal factors may act in patterning the body plan well before the blastocyst stage. During the formation of the blastocyst, the first differentiation event sets aside the trophoblast lineage from the pluripotent cells of the inner cell mass (a). Next, the primitive endoderm or hypoblast forms below the epiblast (b). The epiblast in the human embryo is in the form of a flat disc. Primitive endoderm will play a crucial role in embryonic axis determination, through cell–cell interactions with the overlying epiblast (c). The primitive streak forms at the posterior end of the embryo, and mesodermal cells ingress through it to form the germ layers in the process of gastrulation (d).

cell death or by extrusion of fluid by the nascent epithelium of the epiblast. In the human the epiblast is not in the form of a cup but instead is a flat sheet of cells (Fig. 3.6).

It is apparent that the extraembryonic tissues are very important for patterning the body. The anterior visceral endoderm patterns the anterior epiblast and determines its fate. This portion of the extraembryonic endoderm originates from the distal tip of the egg cylinder and migrates proximally and anteriorly during subsequent development. The anterior visceral endoderm is essential for the formation of the head.

The process of gastrulation begins at the future posterior end of the embryo; this is where the primitive streak forms in the human at about 14 days after fertilisation (Fig. 3.6). The primitive streak defines the posterior end of the embryo. Cells of the primitive streak move in between epiblast and the visceral endoderm to form the mesoderm. Definitive endoderm cells appear between mesoderm and visceral endoderm at the tip of the primitive streak. The mesoderm of the streak is patterned along its length such that the proximal mesoderm will be predominantly extraembryonic, the middle portion will form lateral plate and paraxial mesoderm, and the distal portion will form axial mesoderm.

The anterior aspect of the primitive streak contains the node that organises the body plan. The node contains precursors of the prechordal mesoderm, the notochord and the embryonic endoderm. In the mouse the node can induce a new axis if moved by micromanipulation, but this lacks anterior structures. The precursor of the node is termed the early gastrula organiser (EGO) and is present in the posterior epiblast outside the primitive streak. The EGO can induce some neural tissue. The combined activity of the anterior visceral endoderm and the EGO are required to induce the full neuraxis.

IMPLANTATION

Blastocyst attachment to the endometrium

The developing embryo passes through the isthmus and enters the uterus 68–80 h after ovulation. The embryo will remain free floating in the uterine cavity for a further 3–4 days. The polar trophoblast cells adjacent to the inner cell mass are involved in the primary adhesion to endometrial cells. Carbohydrate–selectin interactions are involved in adhesion of human embryos to endometrial cells. P-selectin is found on human embryos and the major selectin ligand α (2–3) sialylLe-x is expressed by the luminal epithelial cells (Kimber & Spanswick 2000). The H-type-1 antigen, which is a fucosylated sugar (Fucα1–2Galβ1–3GlcNAcβ1-), is thought to be an initial attachment ligand in mice and is expressed on the human luminal ethelilium (Kimber & Spanswick 2000). The Le-y carbohydrate antigen (Fucα1–2Galβ1–4[Fucα1–3]GlcNAcβ1-) may also be involved in blastocyst attachment. The group of lectins known as galectins are major non-integrin laminin binding proteins and are present on trophectoderm of mouse blastocysts but not inner cell mass. However, mice lacking galectin-1 or galectin-3, or both, are fertile.

Heparin sulphate proteoglycan (HSPG) has been considered a likely molecule involved in blastocyst adhesion and perlecan (a basement membrane form of HSPG) is present on mouse blastocysts after hatching from the zona. Human epithelial cells express heparin/HSPG-interacting protein

(HIP), non-covalently associated with the external membrane, which could bind trophoblast HSPG Perlecan-HIP could be involved in human blastocyst attachment (Fig. 3.7). Other molecules that have been proposed to be involved in attachment include heparin-binding EGF-like growth factor (HB-EGF) and CD-44. HB-EGF may interact with ErbB4 EGF-receptor and HSPG, promoting trophectoderm adhesion and has a role in promoting trophoblast outgrowth; CD-44 isoforms may form bridging ligands with abundant sialylated and sulphated carbohydrates on the apical surface of human luminal epithelium (Kimber & Spanswick 2000).

Once the polar trophectoderm is firmly tethered to the luminal epithelium other cell adhesion molecules are thought to promote further interactions. These include integrins, their ligands and the trophinin–tasin–bystin complex. This complex has been shown to be a unique intrinsic membrane protein that binds trophoblast cells to an endometrial adenocarcinoma cell line. Trophinin and tasin are expressed by human endometrium on day 16/17 at their apical surface. A number of α and β integrin subunits are expressed by embryos and trophoblast (see Kimber & Spanswick 2000). Integrin αvβ3 interacts with fibronectin, vitronectin, tenascin, osteopontin, thrombospondin and a cryptic domain of laminin. All these ligands are found in the trophoblast adhesion and invasion pathway. In the human there is a changing pattern of integrin units expressed by different populations of cytotrophoblast during differentiation, and invasion suggestive of a specific sequence of interactions with different extracellular matrix molecules occurs during implantation. For example, α6 integrin is restricted to

cytotrophoblast stem cells and is downregulated during invasion but α5β1 and α1β1 integrins are upregulated during invasion. It is apparent that implantation involves a regulated balancing of adhesion and invasion-inducing mechanisms of cytotrophoblast. This is driven by integrin cell surface expression controlling interactions between laminin/collagen and their adhesion receptors and fibronectin–integrin binding that promotes migration or invasion (Fig. 3.7).

Trophoblast proliferation and differentiation

Blastomeres positioned on the outside of the compacting morula become the trophoblast and the transcription factor Oct4 (expressed by undifferentiated early cleavage embryos, inner cell mass cells and ES cells) is extinguished in trophectoderm. In Oct4-deficient embryos all cells develop to trophoblast, independent of blastomere position (Nichols et al 1998). There are usually more than 100 trophoblast cells in the blastocyst and extraordinary proliferation of these cells occurs after implantation. The signals for trophoblast multiplication arise from the inner cell mass and embryonic ectoderm and act only locally. The proliferating polar trophoblast is therefore most active, and later the extraembryonic ectoderm (trophoblast) of the chorion also proliferates rapidly. The factor responsible is the fibroblast growth factor FGF4, which is under the influence of the transcription factor genes *Cdx2* and *Eomes*, expressed in trophoblast stem cells.

Trophoblast cells differentiate into either syncytiotrophoblast or extravillous cytotrophoblast (equivalent to tro-

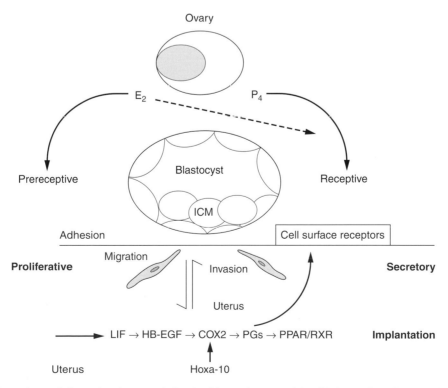

Fig. 3.7 Human implantation and the molecular cascade involved in uterine receptivity. (Redrawn from Paria et al 2000, with permission.)

phoblast giant cells in mice) cells and require downregulation of *Cdx2* and *Eomes* and upregulation of specific regulatory transcription factors (Nichols et al 1988). The extravillous cytotrophoblast cells are polyploid, inherently invasive and interact with the maternal circulatory system. They extensively invade the uterine arteries, replacing the muscular artery walls to produce low-resistance blood flow to the implantation site. Extravillous cytotrophoblast cells express the genes *Mash2*, *1d2* and *E-factor* and it is likely they are downregulated as the cytotrophoblast cells differentiate into invasive cell types (Cross 2000). The gene *Stra13* (Id gene) is upregulated during differentiation of cytotrophoblast cells.

Synctiotrophoblast, which constitutes the bulk of the labyrinthine layer of the placenta, develops from villous cytotrophoblast stem cells and fuses into syncytial-like cells or differentiates down the extravillous (invasive) pathway. The ability of cytotrophoblast cells to fuse into a syncytium is stimulated by epidermal growth factor (EGF). However, EGF receptor-deficient mice do not have an apparent defect in the synctiotrophoblast labyrinth, suggesting that EGF is not essential for synctiotrophoblast differentiation.

A number of mutations in mice in genes including *D1x3*, *Esx1*, *Fgfr2*, *JunB*, *Rxr-a*, *Hgf*, *c-Met*, *Vcam1* and *Wnt2* alter morphogenesis in the labyrinthine layer. Some genes function in chorioallantoic fusion and subsequent labyrinth growth and morphogenesis (*Vcam1* and *Fgfr2*), development of spongiotrophoblast and labyrinth (*Wnt2* and *Hgf*) and vascularisation in the labyrinth (*Esx1*, *JunB*, *Arnt* and *Vhl*) (Cross 2000).

Rapid trophoblast proliferation in the few days after implantation is accompanied by erosion of maternal stromal tissue. Both syncytiotrophoblast and cytotrophoblast cells are invasive. The villous syncytium is a polarised epithelium that transports nutrients to the embryo and fetal blood supply and removes fetal waste products. The main features of the placenta are present by day 21 after ovulation.

Uterine receptivity and molecular signalling in implantation

Implantation requires stromal decidualisation and human embryos embed in the antimesometrial stroma with the inner cell mass directed antimesometrially. Progesterone is essential for human implantation, but oestrogen may not be (Trounson 1992). Uterine receptivity is defined as the 'window' when blastocysts are able to implant. A non-receptive uterus does not respond to the presence of a blastocyst, as illustrated by delayed implantation in ovariectomised rodents (Paria et al 2000) or diapausing blastocysts in the uterus of some marsupials. This state can be maintained by continuous progesterone influence. In the human, the receptivity of the uterus can be induced with progesterone following preparation with oestrogen (Lutjen et al 1984), an effect which appears to be largely independent of maternal age. The breadth of the receptivity window is not known but it is wider than first envisaged because human blastocysts can implant at 5–10 days (or more) after initiation of exogenous progesterone treatment in women who lack ovarian function.

Targeted deletion of genes has shown that expression of leukaemia inhibitory factor (*LIF*), *Hoxa-10* and *COX-2* are essential for implantation in the mouse. Progesterone, and possibly oestrogen, direct *LIF* expression for preparation of a receptive uterus that is responsive to the presence of a blastocyst. The blastocyst attachment reaction depends on HB–EGF interaction with heparin sulphate proteoglycans and/or *ErbBs* in a paracrine/juxtacrine manner, and the correct expression of *COX-2* at the site of blastocyst-uterine apposition. The homeobox gene *Hoxa-10* is critical for stromal induction of *COX-2*; hence *COX-2* appears to be a convergent downstream signalling pathway for implantation (Paria et al 2000). Prostaglandins are also essential for implantation and these lipid mediators are generated by cyclo-oxygenase. Prostaglandins produced by nuclear cyclo-oxygenase can activate peroxisome proliferator-activated receptors (PPARs) of the nuclear hormone receptor superfamily; these are necessary for vascular changes in the maternal endometrium observed at implantation. PPARs heterodimerise with retinoid X receptors (RXRs) for transcriptional regulation and synergistic activation of target genes that require both ligands. PPAR8, RXRα and RXRβ are all expressed in the mouse uterus at the site of implantation (Paria et al 2000).

Implantation and embryo quality

It has been considered that defects in uterine receptivity control human fertility. However, maternal age has a relatively minor effect on conception involving oocytes or embryos from younger women. In addition, pregnancy rates increase with increasing numbers of embryos transferred if embryos are randomly selected from a large cohort of embryos produced by IVF. Furthermore, cytogenetic evidence would indicate 40% or more of human embryos are aneuploid and that most of these have a very reduced developmental competence. Implantation rates of 20–30% are now not uncommon in human IVF without identification of the aneuploid embryos. After genetic screening some clinics claim up to 50% implantation rates. With several embryos transferred, pregnancy rates are claimed to be 60% or higher. Under these circumstances, it is difficult to demonstrate a major effect of impaired uterine receptivity on conception and pregnancy. It is likely that embryo quality, including chromosomal and genetic normality, regularity of the cell cycle and cleavage interval, absence of significant fragmentation, nuclear multiplication, cytoplasmic vacuoles and nucleated cell number, determines the probability of conception, implantation and development to term.

Unlike those of many other species, early cleavage stage human embryos (two-cells or more) will survive and develop in the uterus. Even fertilized one-cell zygotes survive exposure to the uterine environment. As a result, human embryos from one cell to blastocysts can be grown in culture *in vitro* or be transferred to the uterus for further development. Growing embryos to the more advanced stages enables selection of chromosomally and genetically normal embryos and evaluation of their morphology and rate of development. Selection of euploid blastocysts that are expanding on day 5 after insemination will increase implantation rates substantially.

Further increases in viability and implantation rates may be achieved by selecting those with normal gene expression patterns, particularly for genes expressed in trophoblast for cell adhesion, migration/invasion and proliferation.

KEY POINTS

- Fertilisation is the union of mature male and female gametes, activating an oocyte and initiating the preimplantation phase.
- Normally, sperm appear in the lateral end of the fallopian tubes within minutes of deposition in the vagina.
- Oocytes respond to sperm fusion with rapid depolarisation of the surface membranes, thus blocking polyspermy. Multiple sets of paternal genes lead to abnormal development.
- After 68–80 hours' passage down the oviduct, the embryo is free in the uterine cavity for 72–96 hours before implantation.
- The blastocyst adheres to the endometrium and trophoblast cells lead the implantation process under the influence of progesterone and prostaglandins.

REFERENCES

Alikani M, Cohen J, Tomkins G, Garrisi J, Mack C, Scott RT 1999 Human embryo fragmentation in vitro and its implications for pregnancy and implantation. Fertil Steril 71:836–842

Antczak M, Van Blerkom J 1997 Oocyte influences on early development: the regulatory proteins leptin and STAT3 are polarized in mouse and human oocytes and differentially distributed within the cells of the preimplantation stage embryo. Mol Hum Reprod 3:1067–1086

Baker G, Liu DY, Bourne H 2000 Assessment of the male and preparation of sperm for ARTs. In: Trounson AO, Gardner DK (eds) Handbook of In Vitro Fertilization, 2nd edn. CRC Press, Boca Raton, pp 99–126

Bongso A, Sakkas D, Gardner DK 2000 Coculture of embryos with somatic helper cells. In: Trounson AO, Gardner DK (eds) 'Handbook of In Vitro Fertilization,' 2nd edn. CRC Press, Boca Raton, pp 181–203

Braude PR, Bolton VN, Moore S 1988 Human gene expression first occurs between 4- and 8-cell stages of preimplantation development. Nature (Lond) 332:459–461

Buehr M 1997 The primordial germ cells of mammals: some current perspectives. Exp Cell Res 232:194–207

Chian RC, Gülekli B, Buckett WM, Tan SL 1999 Priming with human chorionic gonadotropin before retrieval of immature oocytes in women with infertility due to the polycystic ovary syndrome. N Engl J Med 341:1624–1626

Cross JC 2000 Genetic insights into trophoblast differentiation and placental morphogenesis. Cell Dev Biol 11:105–113

Johnson M, Ziomek C 1981 The foundation of two distinct cell lineages within the mouse morula. Cell 24:71–80

Jones GM, Trounson AO, Lolatgis N, Wood C 1998 Factors affecting the success of human blastocyst development and pregnancy following IVF and embryo transfer. Fertil Steril 70:1022–1029

Kimber SJ, Spanswick C 2000 Blastocyst implantation: the adhesion cascade. Cell Dev Biol 11:77–92

Lutjen P, Trounson A, Leeton J, Findlay J, Wood C, Renou P 1984 The establishment and maintenance of pregnancy using in vitro fertilization and embryo donation in a patient with primary ovarian failure. Nature (Lond) 307:174–175

Magli MC, Jones GM, Gras L, Gianaroli L, Korman I, Trounson AO 2000 Chromosome mosaicism in aneuploid embryos that develop to morphologically normal blastocysts in vitro. Hum Reprod 15: 1781–1786

Nichols J, Zevnik B, Anastassiadis K et al 1998 Formation of pluripotential stem cells in the mammalian embryo depends on the POU transcription factor Oct4. Cell 95:379–391

Paria BC, Lim H, Das SK, Reese J, Dey SK 2000 Molecular signaling in uterine receptivity for implantation. Cell Dev Biol 11:67–76

Reubinoff BE, Pera MF, Fong CY, Trounson A, Bongso A 2000 Embryonic stem cell lines from human blastocysts: somatic differentiation in vitro. Nature Biotech 18:399–404

Sathananthan AH, Ng SC, Jackson P, Dharmawardena V, Trounson A 1996 Sperm penetration, incorporation, fertilization and microfertilization in assisted reproduction. In: Sathananthan AH (ed) Visual Atlas of Human Sperm Structure and Function for Assisted Reproductive Technology. Singapore, National University of Singapore, pp 193–277

Sathananthan AH, Ratnam SS, Ng SC, Tarin JJ, Gianaroli L, Trounson A 1996 The sperm centriole: Its inheritance, replication and perpetuation in early human embryos. Hum Reprod 11:345–356

Sathananthan AH, Trounson AO, Wood C (eds) 1985 Ultrastructural Atlas of Human Fertilization and Embryonic Development. Praeger, Philadelphia

Shamblott MJ, Axelman J, Wang S et al 1998 Derivation of pluripotent stem cells from cultured human primordial germ cells. Proc Natl Acad Sci 95:13726–13731

Surani MAH, Barton SC, Norris ML 1986 Nuclear transplantation in the mouse: heritable differences between parental genomes after activation of the embryonic genome. Cell 45:127–136

Swain A, Lovell-Badge R 1999 Mammalian sex determination: a molecular drama. Genes Dev 13:755–767

Tanaka S, Kunath T, Hadjantonakis AK, Nagy A, Rossant J 1998 Promotion of trophoblast stem cell proliferation by FGF4. Science 282:2072–2075

Thomson JA, Itskovitz-Eldor J, Shapiro SS et al 1998 Embryonic stem cell lines derived from human blastocysts. Science 282:1145–1147

Trounson A 1992 The development of the technique of oocyte donation and hormonal replacement therapy: is oestrogen really necessary for the establishment of and maintenance of pregnancy? Reprod Fertil Dev 4:671–679

Trounson A, Bongso A 1996 Fertilization and development in humans. Curr Top Dev Biol 32:59–101

Trounson AO, Mohr LR, Wood C, Leeton J 1982 Effect of delayed insemination on in vitro fertilization, culture and transfer of human embryos. J Reprod Fertil 64:285–294

Trounson A, Anderiesz C, Jones G 2001 Maturation of human oocytes in vitro and their developmental competence. Reproduction 121: 51–75

Van Steirteghem AC, Nagy Z, Joris H et al 1993 High fertilization and implantation rates after intracytoplasmic sperm injection. Hum Reprod 8:1061–1066

Van Steirteghem A, Nagy P, Joris H et al 1998 Results of intracytoplasmic sperm injection with ejaculated, fresh and frozen-thawed epididymal and testicular spermatozoa. Hum Reprod 13, suppl 1:134–142

Wassarman PM 1999 Mammalian fertilization: molecular aspects of gamete adhesion, exocytosis, and fusion. Cell 96:175–183

Yanagimachi R 1994 Mammalian fertilization. In: Knobil E, Neil JD, Markert CL, Greenwald GS, Pfaff DN (eds) The Physiology of Reproduction, 2nd edn. Raven Press, NY, pp 189–317

Yanagimachi R 1998 Intracytoplasmic sperm injection experiments using the mouse as a model. Hum Reprod 13, suppl 1:87–98

4

The placenta, membranes and umbilical cord

Harold Fox

THE PLACENTA

The placenta as expelled from the uterus is generally regarded as a complete organ. This, the fetal placenta, is not, however, the total structure; there is also a vitally important maternal component—the placental bed and the uteroplacental vessels.

Development of the fetal placenta

The fertilised ovum enters the uterine cavity as a morula that rapidly converts into a blastocyst and detaches from its surrounding zona pellucida. The outer cell layer of the blastocyst proliferates to form the primary trophoblastic cell mass from which cells infiltrate between those of the endometrial epithelium. The latter degenerates and the trophoblast thus comes into contact with the endometrial stroma. This process of implantation is complete by the 10th or 11th postovulatory day. In the seven-day conceptus, the trophoblast forms a peripheral circumferential plaque which rapidly differentiates into two layers, an inner layer of large, mononuclear cytotrophoblastic cells with well-defined, limiting membranes, and an outer layer of multinucleated syncytiotrophoblast, which is a true syncytium. That the syncytiotrophoblast is derived from the cytotrophoblast, not only at this early stage but throughout gestation, is now well established. Even when trophoblast is growing rapidly, DNA synthesis and mitotic activity occur only in the nuclei of the cytotrophoblastic cells, the syncytiotrophoblast being a postmitotic, terminally differentiated tissue. The syncytiotrophoblast appears to be formed by a breaking down of the limiting membrane of the cytotrophoblastic cells.

Between the 10th and 13th postovulatory days, a series of intercommunicating clefts, or lacunae, appear in the rapidly enlarging trophoblastic cell mass (Fig. 4.1). These are probably formed as a result of engulfment within the trophoblast of endometrial capillaries. These lacunae soon become confluent to form the precursor of the intervillous space and it has been widely thought that, as maternal vessels are progressively eroded, this becomes filled with maternal blood. It has, however, been suggested in recent years that at this stage only maternal plasma perfuses the intervillous space, a true maternal blood flow into the intervillous space not becoming established until the 12th week of gestation (Hustin 1995, Jauniaux et al 1995), a view not without its critics (Moll 1995). The lacunae are incompletely separated from each

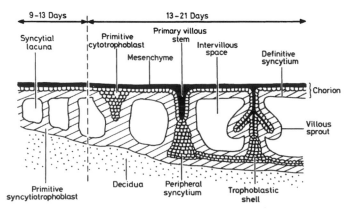

Fig. 4.1 Diagrammatic representation of the development of the placenta during the first 21 days of gestation. Reproduced with permission from Fox (1997a).

33

other by trabecular columns of syncytiotrophoblast which, between the 14th and 21st postovulatory days, tend to become radially orientated and come to possess a central cellular core that is produced by proliferation of the cytotrophoblastic cells at the chorionic base. These trabeculae are not true villi but serve as the framework, or scaffolding, from which the villous tree will later develop. The placenta at this time is a labyrinthine rather than a villous organ and the trabeculae act as primary villous stems (Boyd & Hamilton 1970). The cytotrophoblast continues to grow into the decidua, where it becomes attached. At the same time, a mesenchymal core appears within the villous stems. This core is formed by extension of the extra-embryonic mesenchyme. Later, the villous stems become vascularised, with the vessels developing *in situ* from mesenchyme within the core. The villous stems eventually differentiate into the body stalk and the inner chorionic mesenchyme.

The distal part of the villous stems is now formed almost entirely by cytotrophoblastic cells, which form columns anchored to the decidua of the basal plate. The cells in these cytotrophoblastic cell columns proliferate and spread laterally to form a continuous cytotrophoblastic shell that splits the syncytiotrophoblast into two layers, the definitive syncytium on the fetal aspect of the shell and the peripheral syncytium on the maternal side. The definitive syncytium persists as the lining of the intervillous space, but the peripheral syncytium eventually degenerates and is replaced by fibrinoid material (Nitabuch's layer). The establishment of the cytotrophoblastic shell is a mechanism to allow for rapid circumferential growth of the developing placenta, and this leads to an expansion of the intervillous space, into which sprouts extend from the primary villous stems. These offshoots consist initially only of syncytiotrophoblast, but as they enlarge they pass through the stages previously seen during the development of the primary villous stems: intrusion of cytotrophoblast, formation of a mesenchymal core, and eventual vascularisation. These sprouts are the primary stem villi and, as they are true villous structures, the placenta is by the 21st postovulatory day a vascularised villous organ. The primary stem villi later grow and divide to form secondary and tertiary stem villi, and these latter eventually break up into the terminal villous tree.

Between the 21st postovulatory day and the end of the fourth month of gestation, there is not only continuing growth but also considerable remodelling of the placenta. The villi orientated towards the uterine cavity degenerate and form the chorion laeve, while the thin rim of decidua covering this area gradually disappears to allow the chorion laeve to come into contact with the parietal decidua of the opposite wall of the uterus. The villi on the side of the chorion orientated towards the decidual plate proliferate and progressively arborise to form the chorion frondosum, which develops into the definitive fetal placenta. During this period there is some regression of the cytotrophoblastic elements in the chorionic plate and in the trophoblastic shell, while the cytotrophoblastic cell columns largely degenerate and are replaced by fibrinoid material (Rohr's layer); clumps of cells persist, however, as 'cytotrophoblastic cell islands'.

The placental septa appear during the third month of gestation: they protrude into the intervillous space from the basal plate and divide the maternal surface of the placenta into 15–20 lobes. These septa are simply folds of the basal plate, formed partly as a result of regional variability in placental growth and partly by the pulling up of the basal plate by the anchoring columns, which have a poor growth rate (Boyd & Hamilton 1970). The basal plate is formed principally by the remnants of the trophoblastic shell embedded in fibrinoid material, and it therefore follows that the septa are similarly constituted, although some decidual cells may also be carried up into the folds. The septa are simply an incidental byproduct of the architectural remodelling of the placenta, and have no physiological or morphological role to play.

By the end of the fourth month of gestation, the fetal placenta has achieved its definitive form and undergoes no further anatomical modification. Growth continues, however, until term and is the result principally of the continuing branching of the villous tree and formation of fresh villi.

Development of the maternal placenta

During the early weeks of gestation, cytotrophoblastic cells stream out from the tips of the anchoring villi, penetrate the trophoblastic shell, and extensively colonise the decidua and adjacent myometrium of the placental bed. These cells are known as the 'interstitial extravillous cytotrophoblast;' in addition, trophoblastic cells stream into the lumens of the intradecidual portions of the spiral arteries of the placental bed, where they form intraluminal plugs and constitute the 'intravascular extravillous cytotrophoblast'. These endovascular trophoblastic cells destroy and replace the endothelium of the maternal vessels and then invade the media, with resulting destruction of the medial elastic and muscular tissue (Brosens et al 1967); the arterial wall becomes replaced by fibrinoid material that appears to be derived partly from fibrin in the maternal blood and partly from proteins secreted by the invading trophoblastic cells. This process is complete by the end of the first trimester, at which time these 'physiological' changes within the spiral arteries of the placental bed extend to the myometriodecidual junction. There then appears to be a pause in this process, but between the 14th and 16th week of gestation there is a resurgence of endovascular trophoblastic migration, with a second wave of cells moving down into the intramyometrial segments of the spiral arteries, extending as far as the origin of these vessels from the radial arteries. Within the intramyometrial portion of the spiral arteries, the same process that occurs in their intradecidual portion is repeated, i.e. replacement of the endothelium, invasion and destruction of the medial musculo-elastic tissue, and fibrinoid change in the vessel wall. The end-result of this trophoblastic invasion of, and attack on, the vessels is that the thick-walled muscular spiral arteries are converted into flaccid, sac-like uteroplacental vessels (Fig. 4.2) that can passively dilate in order to accommodate the greatly augmented blood flow through this vascular system that is required as pregnancy progresses.

Although the function of the intravascular population of extravillous trophoblastic cells appears clear, that of the interstitial extravillous trophoblastic cells is obscure. The number of these cells has been seriously underestimated in

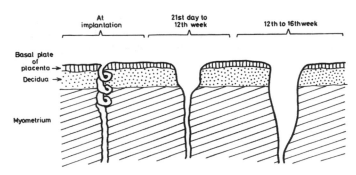

Fig. 4.2 Diagrammatic representation of the conversion of the spiral arteries in the placental bed into uteroplacental vessels. Reproduced with permission from Fox (1997a).

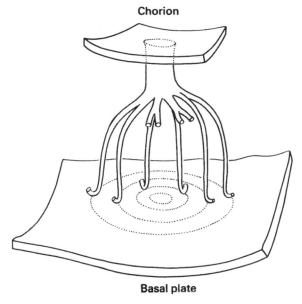

Fig. 4.3 Diagrammatic representation of a fetal lobule. The stem villi are arranged in a circular fashion around a central hollow core. Reproduced with permission from Fox (1997a).

the past, for it is now known that they are a major component of the placental bed. The interstitial trophoblastic cells tend to aggregate around the spiral arteries, and it has been suggested that they prime these vessels to allow them to react to their eventual invasion by endovascular trophoblast (Pijnenborg et al 1983); if this is indeed the function of these cells, then their mode of action on the vessels is unknown.

Although more recent studies suggest that trophoblastic invasion of the placental bed vessels may not be as temporally rigidly restricted as was originally thought (Pijnenborg 1994), it is nevertheless clear that the extravillous population of trophoblastic cells plays a key role in placentation. Through these cells the placenta establishes its own low-pressure high-conductance vascular system, simultaneously ensuring an adequate maternal blood flow to itself and an ample supply of oxygen and nutrients to the fetus. It is far from clear why only arteries, and not veins, in the placental bed are invaded by trophoblasts. Furthermore, the factor(s) controlling the well-timed waves of intravascular trophoblast movement and the limitation of interstitial trophoblastic invasion to the inner third of the myometrium are poorly understood.

Anatomy of the fetal placenta

The fetal placenta is made up of a number of subunits that are now generally known as lobules. The injection studies of Wilkin (1965) have shown that the primary stem villi break up just below the chorionic plate into a number of secondary stem villi which, after running parallel to the chorionic plate for a short distance, divide into a series of tertiary stem villi. The lobules are derived from these tertiary stem villi, which sweep down through the intervillous space to anchor onto the basal plate; during their course through the intervillous space they give off multiple branches that ramify into the terminal villous network. As the tertiary stem villi pass down towards the basal plate, they are arranged in a circular fashion around the periphery of an empty cylindrical space; the lobule thus forms a hollow globule (Fig. 4.3) with the bulk of the terminal villi mainly in the outer shell of this globular structure and the centre of the lobule relatively empty and free of villi. The lobules are separated from each other by interlobular areas that are in continuity with the subchorial space.

There has been considerable confusion as to the meaning of the term cotyledon when applied to the human placenta. This name should not be used to describe the lobes seen on the maternal surface; these are merely the areas lying between the septa and lack any other morphological significance. The term cotyledon should be restricted to the functional unit of the placental villous tree, which is best defined as that part of the villous tree that is derived from a single, primary stem villus (Ramsey & Donner 1980). A primary stem villus can, however, give rise to a varying number of secondary stem villi and thus to a differing number of lobules, because there is no fixed relationship between cotyledons and lobules. Thus, centrally placed cotyledons may contain as many as five lobules, while those situated laterally may have only one or two lobules. The situation has, however, been made unduly complicated by the fact that some morphologists have applied the term cotyledon to the maternal surface lobes, and others have also used this name to describe the lobule. The human placenta is not really a cotyledonary structure, and there is a strong case for abandoning the term cotyledon when referring to the human placenta.

KEY POINTS

- Development of the placenta is complete by the end of the fourth gestational month but growth continues until term.
- The placenta establishes its own blood supply as the extravillous cytotrophoblast converts the spiral arteries into uteroplacental vessels.
- Maternal blood flow into the intervillous space may not be established until the 12th week of gestation.
- The functional subunit of the placenta is the lobule. The lobes seen on the maternal surface of the placenta are not cotyledons but simply indicate where the septa formed.

The maternal uteroplacental circulatory system

Maternal blood enters the intervillous space via arterial inlets in the basal plate and is then driven by the head of maternal pressure towards the chorionic plate as a funnel-shaped stream (Fig. 4.4). The driving head of maternal pressure is gradually dissipated, a process aided by the baffling effect of the villi, and lateral dispersion of the blood occurs (Ramsey & Donner 1980). This forces the blood already present in the intervillous space out through basally sited wide venous outlets, into the endometrial venous network. India ink injection studies originally suggested that the maternal blood entered the intervillous space as a jet or spurt, but cineangiography has shown that these terms give an undue impression of both speed and intermittency. The maternal blood enters the space 'much as water from an actively flowing brook penetrates a reed-filled marsh' (Ramsey & Donner 1980).

The physiological basis for this circulatory system is a series of pressure differentials. The pressure in the maternal arterioles is higher than the mean intervillous space pressure which, in turn, exceeds that in the maternal veins during a myometrial diastole. This entire system is, however, a low-pressure one, for whereas in most organs there is a progressive decrease in the diameter of the arteries as they approach their target tissues, the reverse is true for the placenta. The uteroplacental vessels assume an increasing diameter as they approach their entry into the intervillous space. There is, therefore, a considerable drop in pressure from the proximal to the distal portion of these vessels, and the full arterial pressure is not transmitted to the intervillous space. The placenta itself offers little flow resistance to maternal blood and has a high vascular conductance; there is thus very little fall in pressure across the intervillous space, and the main factor governing the rate of maternal blood flow in a normal pregnancy is the vascular resistance within the radial arteries. Despite the fact that the pressure difference between the arterial and venous sides of the intervillous space is small, it is apparently sufficient to drive arterial blood towards the chorionic plate, to stop short-cutting of the stream into adjacent venous outlets, and to prevent mixing of neighbouring arterial inflows.

Cineangiography has shown that the individual uteroplacental arteries act independently of each other. They are not all patent and do not discharge blood simultaneously into the intervillous space. Furthermore, during myometrial contractions, the afferent blood flow through the intervillous space may be markedly reduced or can even cease. This is probably caused by compression and occlusion of the veins draining the intervillous space, but ultrasound studies have shown that during a myometrial contraction the intervillous space distends (Blecker et al 1975), so the fetus is not severely deprived of an oxygen supply during myometrial systole.

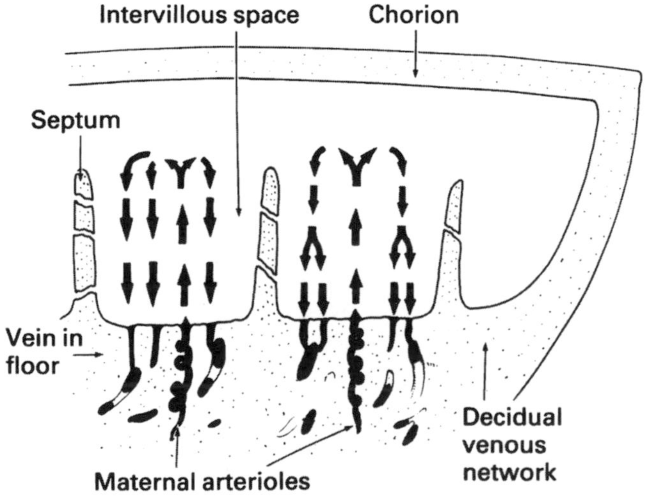

Relationship of maternal circulatory system to fetal lobule

The haemodynamic system originally proposed by Ramsey & Donner (1980) postulated that the maternal blood flow into the intervillous space was through randomly situated arterial inlets, but it has since become clear that this is not the case and that a definite relationship exists between the maternal vessels and the fetal lobules. This is not coincidental, because it is probable that the lobules tend to develop preferentially around the flow from eroded maternal vessels. The exact nature of this relationship is still not fully determined, and two contrasting schemes have been proposed. Some have thought that arterial inlets into the intervillous space are so situated that the inflow from each uteroplacental vessel is into the central, villus-free space of a fetal lobule (Wigglesworth 1967) and that the maternal blood then flows laterally through the lobule into the interlobular area from which it is drained by basal venous outlets (Fig. 4.5). Others consider that the maternal vessels open, not into the central space of a lobule, but into the interlobular spaces (Gruenwald 1973) and that the maternal blood then encircles the lobules in streams to form a shell around them, entering and leaving the lobule while doing this and before draining through the basal outlets (Fig. 4.6).

Fig. 4.4 Diagrammatic representation of the circulation of maternal blood through the placenta. Reproduced with permission from Fox (1997a).

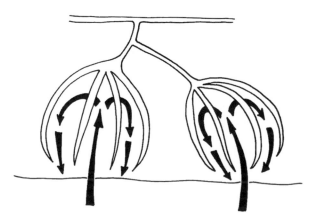

Fig. 4.5 Diagrammatic representation of the relationship between the maternal blood flow (black arrows) and the fetal lobule as envisaged by Wigglesworth. Reproduced with permission from Fox (1997a).

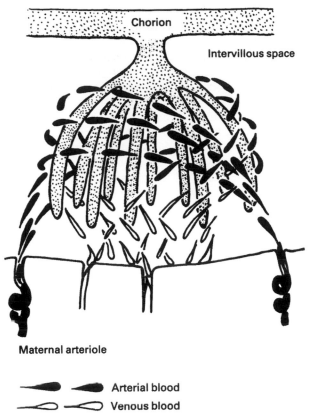

Fig. 4.6 Diagrammatic representation of the relationship between the maternal blood flow (black) and the fetal lobule (stippled) as envisaged by Gruenwald. Reproduced with permission from Fox (1997a).

Whichever of these two concepts is correct, it is clear that maternal–fetal exchange takes place principally in those villi that form the shell of the lobule, and that it is only here that a true functional intervillous space, which is probably only of capillary calibre, exists; elsewhere, in the subchorial lake, the interlobular spaces and the central intralobular spaces, villi are either sparse or absent, and these areas are, in functional terms physiological dead spaces.

KEY POINTS

- Maternal blood flow through the placenta depends upon a series of pressure differentials.
- In vascular terms the placenta is a low-resistance high-conductance organ.
- The functional intervillous space is probably only of capillary calibre and much of the intervillous space is physiological dead space.

Basic villous structure

The histological appearances of the placental villi vary with the gestational age and with the stage of development and maturation of the villous tree. Nevertheless, there is a basic

villous structure which is independent of these variables (Fox 1986). The outer surface of the villi is covered by a trophoblastic mantle which consists of two layers, an outer layer of syncytiotrophoblast and an inner layer of cytotrophoblastic (Langhans') cells (Fig. 4.7). The latter cells are cuboid, polyhedral or ovoid and have well-marked cell borders. These cells are prominent and form a complete layer in early pregnancy and are still present in the terminal villi of the mature placenta though they are less conspicuous than in the immature placenta. It should be noted that although the cytotrophoblastic cells are dispersed in the mature placenta and no longer form a complete layer their absolute number is not decreased and, indeed, continues to increase throughout pregnancy. The cytotrophoblastic cells are, as already remarked, the stem cells of the syncytiotrophoblast and although largely quiescent in late pregnancy retain their

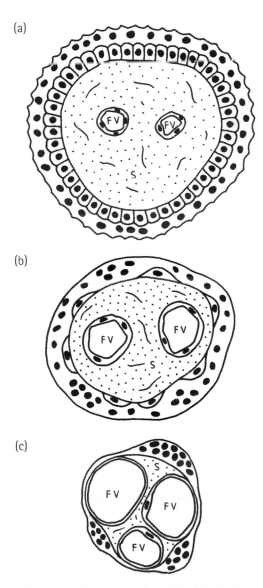

Fig. 4.7 Diagrammatic representation of the histological appearances of the predominant villus type seen in the placenta. (a) During the first trimester, (b) during the second trimester, (c) during the third trimester. FV, fetal vessels; S, villous stroma. Reproduced with permission from Fox (1986).

capacity to multiply and thus represent an inactive germinative layer which can undergo a resurgence of proliferative activity if the need occurs to replace damaged or destroyed syncytiotrophoblast.

No cell boundaries are visible between the nuclei of the syncytiotrophoblast, which, in early pregnancy, forms a layer of uniform thickness around the periphery of the villus. Microinjection studies have shown that substances flow freely throughout this layer and the syncytiotrophoblast forms a continuous uninterrupted cytoplasmic layer that extends over the entire surface of the villous tree and completely lines the intervillous space. It is of note that the syncytiotrophoblast is in direct contact with maternal blood and thus functions as an endothelium: the structure of the syncytiotrophoblast is quite unlike that of an endothelial cell but studies with monoclonal antibodies have shown that, despite their morphological dissimilarity, syncytiotrophoblast and endothelial cells share otherwise specific antigens and an ability to synthesise nitric oxide.

In villi from term placentas the syncytial nuclei are irregularly dispersed and often appear aggregated to form multinucleated protrusions from the villous surface, these being known as syncytial knots (Fig. 4.8). Syncytial knots should be differentiated from syncytial sprouts which are present from the early stages of pregnancy and mainly represent the initial stages in the development of lateral villi. Some apparent syncytial knots are artefacts resulting from tangential cutting of the villous surface trophoblast; however in true syncytial knots the nuclei are small and densely staining and electron microscopy shows that they have a degenerate, senescent appearance. These appearances are in sharp contrast to those of the dispersed syncytial nuclei in a villus bearing a knot which have a normal appearance. When considering the pathogenesis of true syncytial knots it must be borne in mind that the syncytiotrophoblast is derived from the cytotrophoblast and that mitotic activity within the villous cytotrophoblast is marked in early pregnancy but continues, though to a progressively diminishing degree, into the third trimester. It follows, therefore, that the syncytial nuclei in any given villus are produced at varying stages of pregnancy and are, in respect to age, a heterogeneous population. The ultrastructural findings suggest that the oldest nuclei in the syncytium are eventually aggregated together to form knots, which may therefore be considered to represent a sequestration of unwanted aged nuclei.

In some areas of many villi of the mature placenta the syncytiotrophoblast is focally thinned and anuclear; such areas overlie a dilated fetal capillary and may, on light microscopy, appear to fuse with the vessel wall to form what is now known as a vasculo-syncytial membrane (Fig. 4.9). These membranous areas of the syncytiotrophoblast differ markedly from the non-thinned areas of the syncytium in their content of enzymes, in their ultrastructure and in their surface characteristics; it is almost certain that they are specialised zones of the trophoblast for the facilitation of gas transfer across the placenta.

The villous trophoblast is separated from the underlying stroma by the trophoblastic basement membrane which has a fibrillary structure and measures between 20 and 50 nm in thickness: the main components of the membrane are collagen IV, laminin and heparan sulphate.

The villous stroma contains undifferentiated mesenchymal cells, mature mesenchymal (reticulum) cells, fibroblasts, myofibroblasts, pre-collagen and collagen fibres, the relative proportions of which vary with the gestational age and the stage of development of the villous tree.

Also present in the villous stroma are Hofbauer cells (Castellucci & Zaccheo 1989); these cells may be round, ovoid or reniform, measure about 25 μm in diameter and have an eccentrically placed nucleus and vacuolated cytoplasm (Fig. 4.10). Hofbauer cells not only have the typical morphological, histochemical and functional characteristics of macrophages, but share with such cells the defining feature of possessing a surface IgG receptor and expressing class II MHC molecules. They are present in the villi at a very early

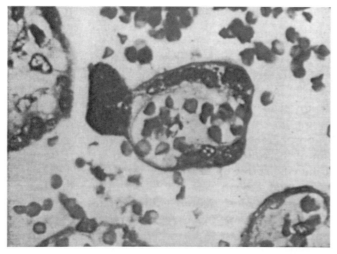

Fig. 4.8　A terminal villus bearing a syncytial knot which appears as a multinucleated protrusion from the free surface of the trophoblast. Reproduced with permission from Fox (1997a).

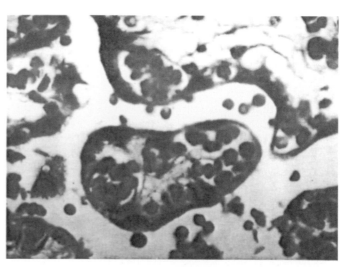

Fig. 4.9　A terminal villus with a vasculo-syncytial membrane (on the right). Reproduced with permission from Fox (1997a).

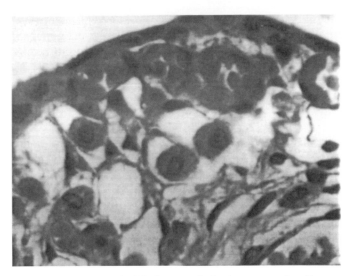

Fig. 4.10 Several typical Hofbauer cells in the stroma of a villus. Reproduced with permission from Fox (1997a).

stage of development and persist throughout pregnancy, though the presence of these cells tends to become masked as the villous stroma becomes denser as gestation progresses, their presence only becoming overt if the meshes of the stroma are widened by oedema fluid. The presence of these cells in the villi before they are vascularised suggests that Hofbauer cells differentiate from mesenchymal cells in early pregnancy; at a later stage of gestation, however, this original population of Hofbauer cells may be supplemented by cells derived from fetal bone marrow-derived monocytes. These cells are probably a heterogeneous population, and the fact that they can show mitotic activity suggests that a subset of these populations is an independent self-replicating population. Hofbauer cells are capable of both immune and non-immune phagocytosis, can trap maternal antibodies crossing over into the placental tissues, and are probably an important source of cytokines within the placenta. Other suggested functions, such as maintenance of placental water balance, involvement in transport mechanisms, a possible endocrine function and a role in the control of vasculogenesis, remain speculative.

The exact time at which villous fetal vessels first appear is variable but by the end of the second month well-formed vessels lined by large immature endothelial cells are present. The vessels within the terminal villi of the mature placenta are of capillary size though many appear sinusoidally dilated. The endothelial cells are attached to each other by tight junctions and are supported by a delicate basal lamina which contains fibronectin, laminin and type IV collagen.

Temporal variation in villous structure: growth and maturation of the villous tree

Placental villi are usually described in terms of their changing appearance as pregnancy progresses, comparing, for instance, typical first-trimester villi with those in third-trimester placentas. It has always been recognised that this temporal variability in villous appearances was a reflection of the continuous development and branching of the villous tree but it is only relatively recently that the relationship between the growth of the villous tree and the villous appearances has been formally codified (Fig. 4.11), largely as a result of work by Kaufmann and his colleagues (Kaufmann 1982, Castellucci et al 1990, Kosanke et al 1993). Thus five types of villi can be identified:

1. **Mesenchymal villi.** These represent a transient stage in placental development: they can differentiate into either mature or immature intermediate villi. They comprise the first generation of newly formed villi and are derived from trophoblastic sprouts by mesenchymal invasion and vascularisation. They are found mainly in the early stages of pregnancy but a few may still be found at term in the centres of the lobules. They have complete trophoblastic mantles with many cytotrophoblastic cells and regularly dispersed nuclei in the syncytiotrophoblast. Their loose, immature-type stroma is abundant and contains a few Hofbauer cells together with poorly developed fetal capillaries.

2. **Immature intermediate villi.** These are peripheral extensions of the stem villi. They are the predominant form seen in immature placentas and often persist in small groups in the centres of the lobules in mature placentas where they represent a persistent growth zone. These villi have a well-preserved trophoblastic mantle in which cytotrophoblastic cells are numerous; the syncytial nuclei are evenly dispersed and there are no syncytial knots or vasculo-syncytial membranes. They have an abundant loose stroma that contains many Hofbauer cells; capillaries, arterioles and venules are present.

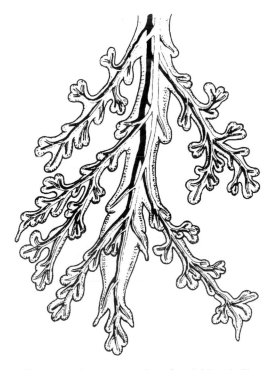

Fig. 4.11 Diagrammatic representation of a peripheral villous tree. The large central stem villus runs down to terminate in a bulbous immature intermediate villus. The lateral branches from the stem villus are the mature intermediate villi from which the terminal villi protrude. After Kaufmann (1982) with permission.

3. Stem villi. These comprise the primary stems which connect the villous tree to the chorionic plate, up to four generations of short thick branches and further generations of dichotomous branches. Their principal role is to serve as a scaffolding for the peripheral villous tree. Up to one-third of the total volume of the villous tissue of the mature placenta is made up of this villous type, the proportion of such villi being highest in the central subchorial portion of the villous tree. Histologically, the stem villi have a compact stroma and contain either arteries and veins or arterioles and venules while superficially located capillaries may also be present.

4. Mature intermediate villi. These are the peripheral ramifications of the villous stems from which the vast majority of terminal villi directly arise. They are large (60–150 μm in diameter) and contain capillaries admixed with small arterioles and venules, the vessels being set in a very loose stroma which occupies more than half of the villous volume. The syncytiotrophoblast has a uniform structure, no knots or vasculo-syncytial membranes being present. Up to a quarter of the villi in a mature placenta are of this type.

5. Terminal villi. These are the final ramifications of the villous tree and are grape-like outgrowths from mature intermediate villi. They contain capillaries, many of which are sinusoidally dilated to occupy most of the cross-sectional diameter of the villus (Fig. 4.12). The syncytiotrophoblast is thin, the syncytial nuclei are irregularly dispersed, syncytial knots may be present and vasculo-syncytial membranes are commonly seen. These terminal villi begin to appear at about the 27th week of gestation and account for 30–40% of the villous volume, 50% of the villous surface area and 60% of villi seen in cross section at term. It has been suggested that these villi are not outgrowths in the true sense of the word but are formed as a result of disproportionate longitudinal growth of the capillaries within an intermediate villus as compared to that of the villus as a whole. The subsequent looping of the capillaries causes them to obtrude from the villous surface and, with their covering of trophoblast, form the terminal villi. The terminal villi are optimally differentiated for materno-fetal transfer and there can be no doubt that they are the site at which most transport across the placenta occurs.

The pattern of development of the villous tree envisaged by Kaufmann and his colleagues is as follows:

1. During the early weeks of pregnancy all the villi are of the mesenchymal type.
2. Between the seventh and eighth weeks mesenchymal villi begin to transform into immature intermediate villi and these subsequently transform into stem villi.
3. Development of additional immature intermediate villi from mesenchymal villi gradually ceases at the end of the second trimester but these immature intermediate villi continue to mature into stem villi and only a few persist to term as growth zones in the centres of the lobules.
4. At the beginning of the third trimester, mesenchymal villi switch from transforming into immature intermediate villi and start transforming into mature intermediate villi. These latter serve as a framework for the terminal villi which begin to appear shortly afterwards and predominate at term. The terminal villi do not result from trophoblastic proliferation but develop when longitudinal capillary growth outstrips longitudinal villous growth, thus causing bulging and protrusions into the intervillous space.

KEY POINTS

- The villous cytotrophoblast is the stem cell of the villous syncytiotrophoblast, the latter being a true syncytium.
- Vasculo-syncytial membranes are areas of trophoblast thinning which facilitate gas transport.
- The histological appearances of the placenta vary as pregnancy progresses. This is a reflection of the continuing growth and maturation of the placental villous tree.
- The terminal villi, optimally adapted for materno-fetal transfer, begin to appear at the 28th week of gestation and predominate in the term placenta.

Growth, maturation and ageing of the placenta

The progressive elaboration of the villous tree results in a predominance of terminal villi in the mature placenta. Such villi have been conventionally classed as 'third-trimester villi' and a comparison of their structure with the predominant type of villi in the first trimester, immature intermediate villi, has led many to suggest that the changes in villous structure represent an ageing process.

The maturation of the villous tree results in a predominant villous form that is optimally adapted for materno-fetal transfer diffusion mechanisms. The morphological changes result in a very considerable increase in trophoblastic surface area and a significant reduction in the harmonic mean of the diffusion distance between maternal and fetal blood with a resulting increase in the conductance of oxygen diffusion. It

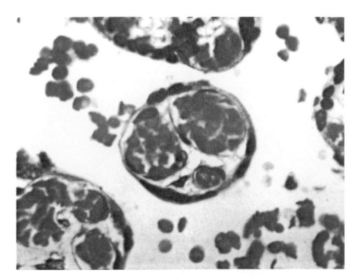

Fig. 4.12 A terminal villus with sinusoidally dilated fetal vessels. Reproduced with permission from Fox (1997a).

should be stressed that it is not mere pedantry to distinguish between maturation, which results in increased functional efficiency, and ageing which results in decreased functional efficiency. There are, in fact, no light or electron microscopic features in the villi that can be considered indicative of an ageing process (Fox 1997b).

It has, however, been maintained that placental growth and DNA synthesis cease at about the 36th week of gestation but, in reality, total placental DNA levels continue to rise in a linear fashion until and beyond the 40th week of pregnancy. This finding is in accord with histological evidence of fresh villous growth in the term placenta, with flow cytometric demonstration of continuing DNA synthesis and with morphometric studies that have demonstrated a continuing expansion of the villous surface area and progressive branching of the villous tree up to and beyond term. Placental growth certainly slows during the last few weeks of gestation, but this decline in growth rate is neither invariable nor irreversible, because the placenta can continue to increase in size if faced with an unfavourable maternal environment (e.g. pregnancy at high altitude, severe maternal anaemia), while the potential for a recrudescence of growth is shown by the proliferative response to ischaemic syncytial damage. Those arguing that a decreased placental growth rate during late pregnancy is evidence of senescence often appear to be comparing the placenta to an organ such as the gut, in which continuing viability is dependent on a constantly replicating stem cell layer producing short-lived postmitotic cells. A more apt comparison would be with an organ such as the liver, which is formed principally of long-lived postmitotic cells and which, once an optimal size has been attained to meet the metabolic demands placed on it, shows little evidence of cell proliferation while retaining a latent capacity for growth activity. There seems no good reason why the placenta, once it has reached a size sufficient to meet its transfer function adequately should continue to grow; the term placenta, with its considerable functional reserve capacity, has more than met this aim.

Functional adequacy of the placenta

The most important role of the placenta is to transfer oxygen and nutrients from the maternal circulation to the fetal blood. Many have thought that the placenta frequently fails to meet the demands placed upon it and that the resulting condition of placental insufficiency is responsible for many instances of fetal hypoxia, growth retardation or death. In reality the placenta rarely becomes insufficient for it has a very considerable functional reserve capacity (Fox 1997a). Histopathological studies and experimental studies clearly indicate that the placenta can withstand a very considerable reduction in the population of functioning villi without any evidence of a decline in physiological capacity. Very few pathological lesions of the placenta are sufficiently extensive to dissipate this functional reserve and it is difficult to accept that intrinsic placental damage is an important factor in the aetiology of inadequate materno-fetal transfer. It has, in fact, become increasingly clear that the common factor in most cases of presumed placental insufficiency is a reduced mater-

nal uteroplacental blood flow which is, in turn, due to inadequate conversion of the spiral arteries into uteroplacental vessels by extravillous trophoblast during the early stages of pregnancy (Khong et al 1986, Fox 1997c, 1998).

THE FETAL MEMBRANES—AMNION AND CHORION

The conversion of the early morula to a blastocyst is facilitated by the formation of a central fluid-filled cavity. This separates the primary trophoblastic cell mass, which develops into the placenta and extraplacental chorion, from those cells that give rise to the embryo, yolk sac and amnion. These latter cells form the inner cell mass which, during the 8th and 9th days after ovulation, arranges itself into a bilaminar disc with the inner layer, i.e. that facing the blastocyst cavity forming the primitive embryonic endoderm while the outer forms the primitive embryonic ectoderm. The amniotic cavity, appears as a slit-like space between the embryonic ectoderm and the adjacent cytotrophoblast and this enlarges to form a small cavity by the 12th postovulatory day. At the same time endodermal cells migrate out from the deepest layer of the embryonic disc to line the blastocyst cavity and thus form the primary yolk sac.

Extraembryonic mesenchyme, possibly derived from trophoblast, subsequently appears (Fig. 4.13) to separate the yolk sac from the blastocyst wall and most of the roof of the amniotic cavity from the trophoblast of the chorion. The extraembryonic mesenchyme forms a loose reticulum in which small cystic spaces appear which gradually enlarge and fuse to form the extraembryonic coelom which splits the extraembryonic mesenchyme into two layers. The progressive enlargement of the extraembryonic coelom (Fig. 4.14) separates the amnion from the inner aspect of the chorion except at the caudal end of the embryo where an attachment of extraembryonic mesenchyme persists to form the body stalk from which the umbilical cord develops. Subsequently the amniotic cavity enlarges at the expense of the extraem

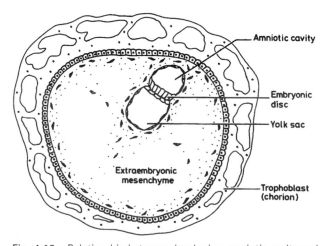

Fig. 4.13 Relationship between developing amniotic cavity and extraembryonic mesenchyme. Reproduced with permission from Fox (1986).

41

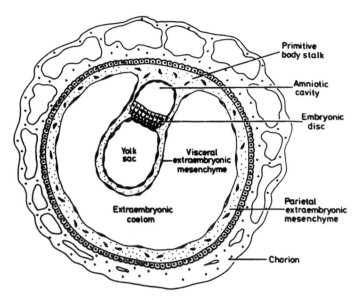

Fig. 4.14 Relationship between developing amniotic cavity, extra-embryonic mesenchyme, extraembryonic coelom and primitive body stalk. Reproduced with permission from Fox (1986).

bryonic coelom and the developing embryo bulges into this enlarged amniotic cavity. The yolk sac becomes partially incorporated into the embryo where it gives rise to the gut, the part outside the embryo becoming incorporated into the lower end of the body stalk. Further expansion of the amniotic cavity (Fig. 4.15) leads to almost total obliteration of the extraembryonic coelom with fusion of the extraembryonic mesenchyme covering the amnion with that lining the chorion, the single fused amniochorion now being fully formed.

On histological examination the amniochorion consists of five layers, these being (from fetal to maternal side):

1. amniotic epithelium
2. amniotic connective tissue
3. spongy layer
4. chorionic connective tissue
5. trophoblast.

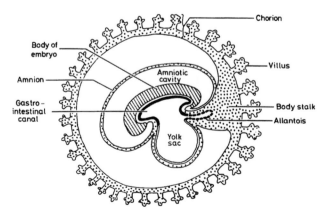

Fig. 4.15 Relationship between the expanding amniotic cavity and the developing embryo. Reproduced with permission from Fox (1986).

The amniotic epithelial cells form a mechanically stable layer; they do not, however, serve only a mechanical function for they play an important role in water transport and appear to have a significant secretory capacity.

THE UMBILICAL CORD

The umbilical cord, often regarded simply as a mechanical conduit between the fetus and the placenta, also plays a role in the movement of water and other substances between the fetal circulation and the amniotic fluid. The basic structure of the cord is, however, simple; it consists of two arteries and a vein embedded in Wharton's jelly which is covered by amniotic epithelium. Wharton's jelly consists of an abundant ground substance, rich in mucopolysaccharides, in which are embedded collagen fibres, mast cells and sparse flat stellate cells arranged concentrically around the vessels. Clearly, Wharton's jelly has as its salient function a mechanical cushioning effect which protects the umbilical vessels from trauma; nevertheless it is metabolically very active tissue and probably serves more than just a mechanistic role.

The average length of the cord is between 54 and 61 cm. It is thought that the minimum length of the cord that allows a normal cephalic delivery is 32 cm and that 100 cm is the maximum length which does not predispose to complications such as knotting, torsion or prolapse. Male babies tend to have longer cords than do females and this may be related to greater intrauterine movement of male fetuses for there is clear clinical and experimental evidence that fetal movement has a stimulatory effect on the longitudinal growth of the cord.

With the notable exception of velamentous insertion, the site of insertion of the cord is of no clinical significance.

CONCLUSIONS

The placenta establishes its own blood supply and its development is complete by the end of the fourth month of gestation; thereafter, growth is by a process of continuing branching of the villous tree and formation of fresh villi. Many of the ills that can beset a pregnancy have their roots during the early stages of gestation when there may be inadequate conversion of spiral arteries to uteroplacental blood vessels with a consequent limitation of maternal blood supply to the fetoplacental unit. The placenta is a highly adapted organ for feto-maternal transfer purposes: it does not age as pregnancy progresses, it has a very considerable functional reserve capacity and rarely, if ever, does it become functionally inadequate, most cases of presumed placental insufficiency being, in reality, examples of inadequate maternal blood flow to the placenta.

Acknowledgements
Figures 4.2, 4.7, 4.13, 4.14 and 4.15 were drawn by Dr Carolyn J.P. Jones. I am indebted to Dr P. Wilkin for supplying me with Figure 4.1.

KEY POINTS

- The placenta establishes its own blood supply via the extravillous trophoblastic cells which convert the spiral arteries of the placental bed into uteroplacental vessels.
- Throughout pregnancy there is a progressive elaboration and functional maturation of the villous tree.
- The placenta does not undergo an ageing process as pregnancy progresses.
- The placenta has a considerable functional reserve capacity and rarely, if ever, becomes inadequate because of any intrinsic disease or lesion. Most cases of presumed placental insufficiency are the result of inadequate placentation during early pregnancy with a subsequent restriction of maternal blood flow to the placenta.

REFERENCES

Blecker OP, Kloosterman GJ, Mieras DJ, Oosting J, Salle HJA 1975 Intervillous space during uterine contractions in human subjects: an ultrasonic study. Am J Obstet Gynecol 123:697–699

Boyd JD, Hamilton WJ 1970 The human placenta. Heffer, Cambridge

Brosens I, Robertson WB, Dixon HG 1967 The physiological response of the vessels of the placental bed in normal pregnancy. J Pathol Bacteriol 93:569–579

Castellucci M, Zaccheo D 1989 The Hofbauer cells of the human placenta: morphological and immunological aspects. Prog Clin Biol Res 269:443–451

Castellucci M, Scheper M, Scheffen I, Celona A, Kaufmann P 1990 The development of the human placental villous tree. Anat Embryol 181:117–128

Fox H 1986 Development of the placenta and membranes. In: Dewhurst J, De Swiet M, Chamberlain G (eds) Basic sciences in obstetrics and gynaecology. Churchill Livingstone, Edinburgh, pp 33–41

Fox H 1997a Pathology of the placenta, 2nd edn. WB Saunders, Philadelphia

Fox H 1997b Aging of the placenta. Arch Dis Child 77:F165–F170

Fox H 1997c Placentation in intrauterine growth retardation. Fetal Maternal Reviews 9:61–71

Fox H 1998 Abnormal placentation. Curr Opin Obstet Gynecol 8:212–216

Gruenwald P 1973 Lobular structure of hemochorial primate placentas, and its relation to maternal vessels. Am J Anat 136:133–152

Hustin J 1995 Vascular physiology and pathophysiology of early pregnancy. In: Bourne TH, Jauniaux E, Jurkovic D (eds) Transvaginal colour doppler. Springer, Berlin, p 47

Jauniaux E, Jurkovic D, Campbell S 1995 Current topic: in vivo investigation of the placental circulation by Doppler echography. Placenta 16:323–331

Kaufmann P 1982 Development and differentiation of the human placental villous tree. Bibliotheca Anatomica 22:29–39

Khong TY, de Wolf F, Robertson WB, Brosens I 1986 Inadequate maternal vascular response to placentation in pregnancies complicated by pre-eclampsia and by small-for-gestational-age infants. Br J Obstet Gynaecol 93:1049–1059

Kosanke G, Castellucci M, Kaufmann P, Mironov VA 1993 Branching patterns of human placental villous trees: perspectives of topological analysis. Placenta 14:591–604

Moll W 1995 Invited commentary: absence of intervillous blood flow in the first trimester of human pregnancy. Placenta 16:333–334

Pijnenborg R 1994 Trophoblast invasion. Reprod Med Rev 3:53–73

Pijnenborg R, Bland JM, Robertson WB, Brosens I 1983 Uteroplacental arterial changes related to interstitial trophoblast migration in early human pregnancy. Placenta 4:397–414

Ramsey EM, Donner MW 1980 Placental vasculature and circulation. WB Saunders, Philadelphia

Wigglesworth JS 1967 Vascular organization of the human placenta. Nature 216:1120–1121

Wilkin P 1965 Pathologie du placenta. Masson, Paris

5

Structural development of the embryo and fetus

Phillip Cox

The contribution of the author of the equivalent chapter in the second edition, on which this chapter draws extensively, is gratefully acknowledged.

INTRODUCTION

In Chapter 3 events from fertilisation to implantation are considered. Briefly, following fertilisation, the zygote undergoes a series of cell divisions to form a ball of cells, the morula. Within the morula a fluid-filled blastocyst cavity develops. At one pole of the blastocyst cavity lies a collection of cells, the inner cell mass, from which the embryo develops. At this stage, between the sixth and eighth day after fertilisation, human implantation takes place (Fig. 5.1).

Shortly after implantation the cells facing the blastocyst cavity become cuboidal and form a single layer of primary embryonic endoderm. The cells of the remainder of the inner cell mass then become columnar and separate from the overlying trophoblast, forming the amniotic cavity. The columnar cells are the precursors of the embryonic ectoderm and also give rise to the embryonic mesoderm (Fig. 5.2). Thus, by 9–13 days after fertilisation the inner cell mass has formed a bilaminar embryonic disc. The remainder of the conceptus goes on to form the placenta and fetal membranes.

The lining of the blastocyst cavity undergoes squamous differentiation to become extraembryonic endoderm, in conti-

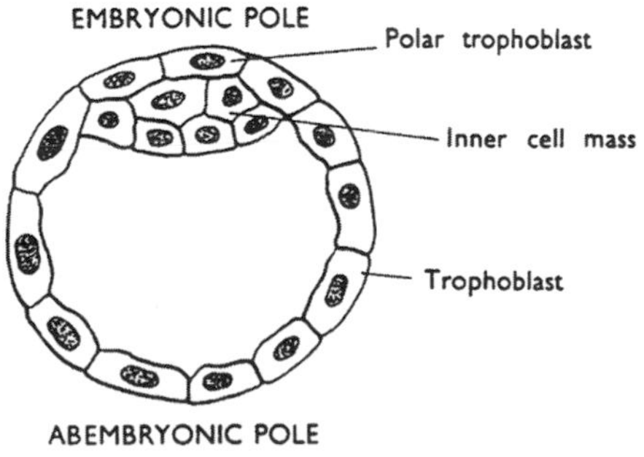

EMBRYONIC POLE

- Polar trophoblast
- Inner cell mass
- Trophoblast

ABEMBRYONIC POLE

Fig. 5.1   The human blastocyst. (From Beck et al 1985, with permission.)

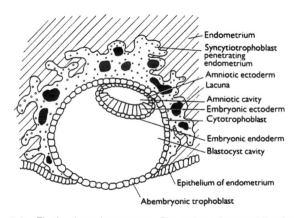

- Endometrium
- Syncytiotrophoblast penetrating endometrium
- Amniotic ectoderm
- Lacuna
- Amniotic cavity
- Embryonic ectoderm
- Cytotrophoblast
- Embryonic endoderm
- Blastocyst cavity
- Epithelium of endometrium
- Abembryonic trophoblast

Fig. 5.2   The implanted conceptus. The embryo forms a bilaminar disc, above which the amniotic cavity lies. (From Beck et al 1985, with permission.)

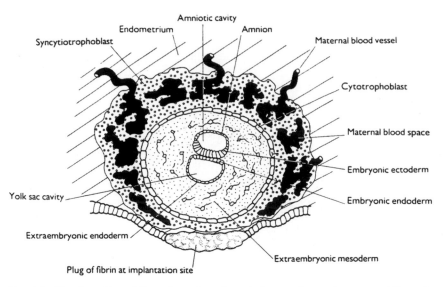

Fig. 5.3 The formation of the extraembryonic endoderm and mesoderm around the yolk sac. (From Beck et al 1985, with permission.)

nuity with the cuboidal embryonic endoderm. The cavity is now the yolk sac. The extraembryonic endoderm is separated from trophoblast by loose extraembryonic mesoderm, within which develops the extraembryonic coelom (Fig. 5.3). The embryo, yolk sac and amniotic cavity are then suspended in this fluid-filled cavity, attached only by the connecting stalk (Fig. 5.4).

Craniocaudal orientation of the embryo is marked by a columnar area of endoderm in the future cranial end of the embryo, the prochordal plate, which, together with the overlying ectoderm, forms the buccopharyngeal membrane.

FORMATION OF THE TRILAMINAR EMBRYO

Fourteen days after fertilisation, proliferation and migration of ectodermal cells backwards and medially leads to formation of the primitive streak at the posterior part of the embryonic midline (Fig. 5.5). Cells within the streak spread laterally

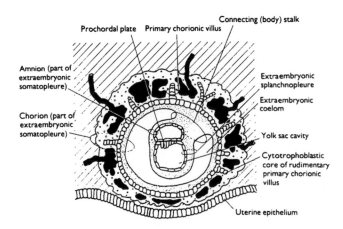

Fig. 5.4 Day 15: chorionic vesicle after the formation of the extraembryonic coelom. (From Beck et al 1985, with permission.)

and forwards between ectoderm and endoderm as intraembryonic mesoderm, becoming continuous with the extraembryonic mesoderm at the lateral border of the embryonic disc. The mesodermal cells become continuous across the midline in front of the prochordal plate, although in the plate itself ectoderm and endoderm remain in contact, forming the buccopharyngeal membrane. Similarly, behind the primitive streak, the endoderm and ectoderm remain adherent forming the cloacal membrane (Fig. 5.5). At 16 days the primitive knot forms at the anterior end of the primitive streak, from which arises the notochordal process running backwards from the posterior edge of the prochordal plate (Fig. 5.6). At 17–18 days ectoderm overlying and anterior to the notochordal process forms a thickened neural plate, from which the neural tube arises (Fig. 5.7). The paraxial mesoderm, on either side of the notochord, becomes segmented to form 44 somites. Anteriorly this area of thickened mesoderm remains unsegmented. Laterally, the mesoderm forms lateral plate mesoderm and between lies the intermediate mesoderm, from which the nephrogenic cord arises (Fig. 5.8). The allantois, a diverticulum of the yolk sac, grows into the connecting stalk immediately behind the cloacal membrane.

The genetic basis of regional specification in mammalian development is being elucidated gradually. For example, a series of closely linked developmental control genes, the *Hox* genes, are expressed in the primitive streak and somite stages of development. These code for transcription factors that regulate the expression of further sets of genes and are fundamentally important in basic pattern formation. A large literature has been established (Gehring 1987, Hunt et al 1991) discussion of which is beyond the scope of this chapter.

THE INTRAEMBRYONIC COELOM AND FORMATION OF THE BODY FOLDS

Cavitation of the lateral plate and anterior mesoderm at 19–20 days of development results in formation of the

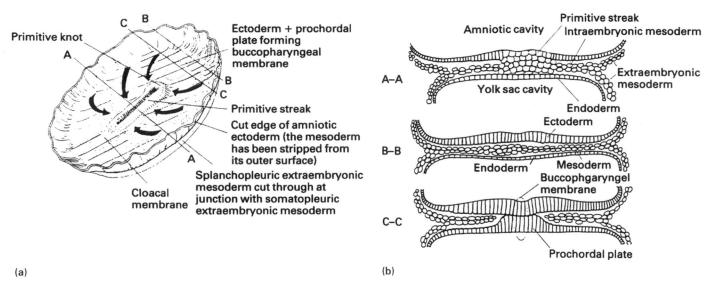

Primitive knot

Ectoderm + prochordal plate forming buccopharyngeal membrane

Primitive streak

Cut edge of amniotic ectoderm (the mesoderm has been stripped from its outer surface)

Splanchopleuric extraembryonic mesoderm cut through at junction with somatopleuric extraembryonic mesoderm

Cloacal membrane

Primitive streak
Amniotic cavity
Intraembryonic mesoderm

Extraembryonic mesoderm

Yolk sac cavity

Endoderm

Ectoderm

Endoderm
Mesoderm
Buccophgaryngel membrane

Prochordal plate

(a)

(b)

Fig. 5.5 (a) Diagram of the embryonic disc revealed by cutting away the overlying amnion. Intraembryonic ectoderm is represented as being transparent, showing the stippled intraembryonic mesoderm beneath. Note the absence of mesoderm from the region of the buccopharyngeal and cloacal membranes. Arrows indicate the direction of migration of cells towards the primitive streak. (b) Transverse sections through the embryo shown in Fig. 5.5(a) at A-A, B-B and C-C. (From Beck et al 1985, with permission.)

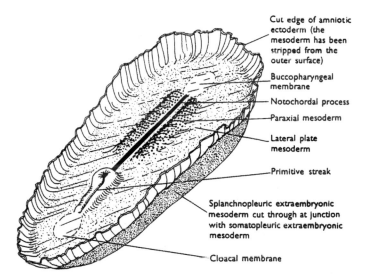

Cut edge of amniotic ectoderm (the mesoderm has been stripped from the outer surface)

Buccopharyngeal membrane

Notochordal process

Paraxial mesoderm

Lateral plate mesoderm

Primitive streak

Splanchnopleuric extraembryonic mesoderm cut through at junction with somatopleuric extraembryonic mesoderm

Cloacal membrane

Fig. 5.6 A more advanced stage of development than that shown in Fig. 5.5(a). The notochord is elongated and the paraxial mesoderm is heaped up on either side of it as the somites begin to form. (From Beck et al 1985, with permission.)

intraembryonic coelom (Fig. 5.9), which communicates with the extraembryonic coelom on either side (Fig. 5.8) in the region of the future midgut.

Bulging of the embryonic disc into the amniotic cavity, during the fourth week after fertilisation, results in cranio-caudal and lateral folding of the embryo (Figs 5.8, 5.10). As a consequence, a primitive endodermally lined foregut is formed within the head fold and a hindgut with an allantoic diverticulum is present in the tail fold. Between them the midgut is continuous inferiorly with the yolk sac. The lateral

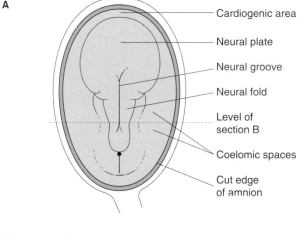

A

Cardiogenic area

Neural plate

Neural groove

Neural fold

Level of section B

Coelomic spaces

Cut edge of amnion

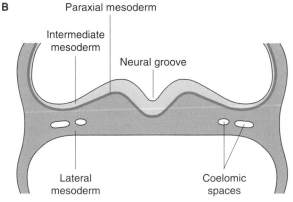

B

Paraxial mesoderm

Intermediate mesoderm

Neural groove

Lateral mesoderm

Coelomic spaces

Fig. 5.7 Embryo of 18 days, illustrating development of the neural plate. (A) Dorsal view, exposed by removal of the amnion; (B) transverse section through the embryonic disc at the levels shown. (After Moore, The Developing Human. Clinically Oriented Embryology. 3rd edn. WB Saunders, Philadelphia.)

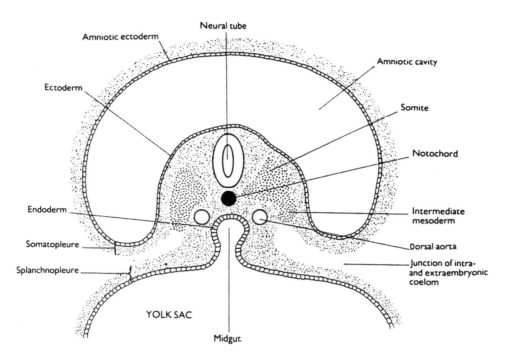

Fig. 5.8 The embryonic disc is beginning to bulge into the amniotic cavity, forming lateral folds. The intraembryonic mesoderm has split to form the intraembryonic coelom, which is continuous at the edges of the disc with the extraembryonic coelom (see Fig. 5.9, A-A). (From Beck et al 1985, with permission.)

folds close to divide the midgut from the remainder of the yolk sac, producing an elongated vitellointestinal duct (Fig. 5.11), which atrophies as pregnancy proceeds.

Within the head fold the caudal wall of the pericardial cavity forms an important landmark, the septum transver-

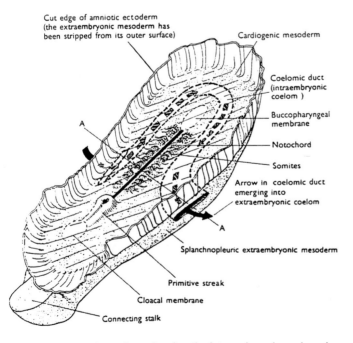

Fig. 5.9 19–20-day embryo showing the intraembryonic coelom. A section through A-A is shown in Fig. 5.8. (From Beck et al 1985, with permission.)

sum (Fig. 5.10), a broad ventral mesentery for the caudal foregut, marking the anterior limit of the midgut.

Through formation of the tail fold the connecting (or body) stalk comes to lie on the ventral surface of the embryo. This will form the umbilical cord and will incorporate the tip of the allantois and the remnant of the vitellointestinal duct (Fig. 5.10).

Defective folding and body wall closure results in maldevelopment of the umbilical cord and severe abdominal wall defects, the so-called 'body stalk' anomaly or 'limb-body wall' complex (Fig. 5.12). Defective formation of the septum transversum is probably responsible for the pentalogy of Cantrell, a complex upper abdominal and lower thoracic defect. If the vitellointestinal duct fails to regress completely a Meckel's diverticulum (Fig. 5.13), Meckel's band or umbilicoileal fistula is the result.

DEVELOPMENT OF THE MAJOR ORGAN SYSTEMS

This is a brief overview of some of the most important events in organ development and their relationship to some of the more common congenital malformations. For a more detailed discussion of human development the reader is referred to specialist texts (Beck et al 1985); the important clinical sequelae are discussed in Chapter 43.

The mesodermal somites

Segmentation of the paraxial mesoderm (see above) leads to the progressive formation of approximately 44 pairs of

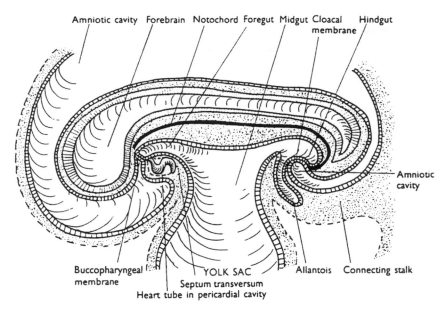

Amniotic cavity　Forebrain　Notochord　Foregut　Midgut　Cloacal membrane　Hindgut

Amniotic cavity

Buccopharyngeal membrane　YOLK SAC　Allantois　Connecting stalk

Septum transversum

Heart tube in pericardial cavity

Fig. 5.10　Sagittal section through the embryo during the fourth week, showing the formation of the head and tail folds. (From Beck et al 1985, with permission.)

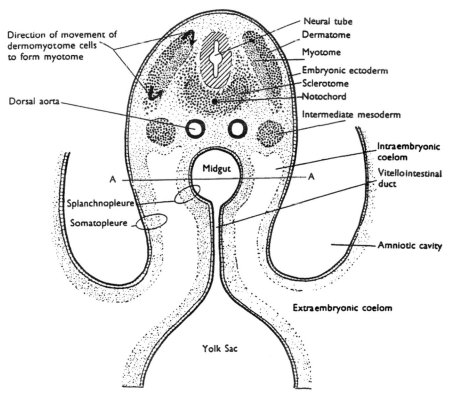

Direction of movement of dermomyotome cells to form myotome

Neural tube
Dermatome
Myotome
Embryonic ectoderm
Sclerotome
Notochord
Intermediate mesoderm

Dorsal aorta

Intraembryonic coelom
Vitellointestinal duct

Midgut

A　　　　A

Splanchnopleure
Somatopleure

Amniotic cavity

Extraembryonic coelom

Yolk Sac

Fig. 5.11　Transverse section through the embryo after the formation of the lateral folds in the region of the midgut. (From Beck et al 1985, with permission.)

somites (Fig. 5.9). These form the basic segmental structure of the body and somite-derived tissue will spread medially to form vertebrae, dorsally to form the extensor musculature of the back and ventrally into the body wall to form ribs, intercostal muscles and abdominal muscles. The dermis of the skin is also of somite origin; without it the skin would remain a thin and semi-transparent somatopleure and eventually would lose its viability. The somites form in a craniocaudal sequence, the occipital somites appear at about 21 days and caudal somites remain visible until 40–45 days.

The ventromedial part of each somite forms the sclerotome (Sensenig 1949); its cells surround the neural tube (Fig.

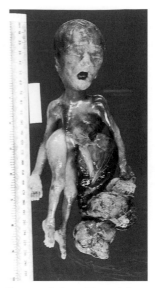

Fig. 5.12 Body stalk anomaly in a 17-week fetus, the result of defective folding of the early embryo. Note that the covering of the abdominal contents is continuous with the placental membranes.

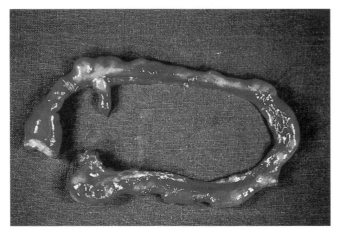

Fig. 5.13 Meckel's diverticulum of the small intestine, a remnant of the vitellointestinal duct.

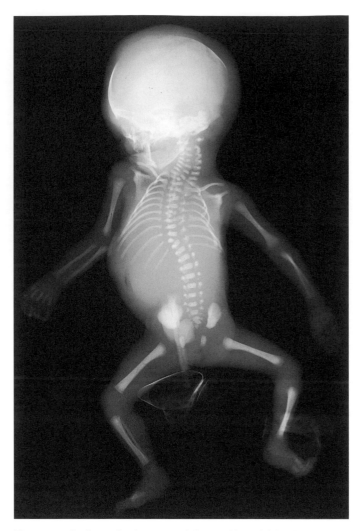

Fig. 5.14 Radiograph of a 25-week fetus with multiple abnormal vertebrae.

5.11) and the notochord. Sclerotomal differentiation appears to be dependent upon inductive signals from the notochord. The vertebral bodies develop from fusion of the caudal portion of one sclerotome with the cranial portion of the next. Chondrification of the sclerotome begins at around 7 weeks in the cervical region and is followed by ossification between T5 and S2 in the eighth week, between C5 and T4 and L5 and S2 after 12 weeks, in C2 and C4 and S3 by about 16 weeks, at C1 and S4 after 20 weeks and at S5 at about 28 weeks. At birth the vertebrae have three ossification centres—one in the centrum and one on each side of the neural arch. Abnormal sclerotomal development results in hemi- and block vertebra as may be seen in the VATER and MURCS associations (Fig. 5.14). Agenesis of the sacrum, as seen in some of the infants of diabetic mothers, may result from failure of induction of caudal sclerotomes by the notochord, perhaps due to premature regression of the notochord as seen in some mouse mutants (Greene et al 1998) (Fig. 5.15).

Somitic tissue remaining after segregation of the sclerotome (Fig. 5.11) differentiates into an inner myotome and an outer dermatome. The spindle-shaped myoblasts of the myotome form the skeletal musculature of the body wall and spine. The myotomes of certain somites adopt an atypical location giving rise, for example, to tongue, diaphragmatic and pelvic floor musculature. In the whole of the trunk (including the pectoral and pelvic girdles), as myoblasts migrate they are followed by their segmental nerves so that it becomes a simple matter to deduce the origin of any trunk muscle.

By 12 weeks the dermis is established from the dermatomes, which also carry their segmental nerve supply with them. By 10 weeks the nail anlagen appear, as do lanugo hairs. By 20 weeks the vernix caseosa is present and at around 28 weeks of gestation the scalp and eyebrow hairs develop. If dermatomyotomal migration is defective, the body wall remains thin and fragile and may break down. This is thought to be the cause of some major abdominal wall defects, such as cloacal and bladder exstrophy.

As in birds, the limb musculature of mammals probably develops from the somites. Limb buds appear at the somite stage of development (Fig. 5.16) and at about 5 weeks the prominences of the future knee and elbow region can be recognized, projecting both laterally and backwards. Hand and foot plates appear as flattened expansions and between 36 and 38 days the digital rays become apparent. The limb bones differentiate from the mesenchyme of the limb bud. The limb buds grow in such a way that they appear to rotate in different directions (Fig. 5.17) so that the preaxial border of the hand is located laterally and that of the foot medially. Much is now known about the molecular biology of patterning of limb development and the detail is beyond the scope of this chapter (for review see Ferretti & Tickle 1997). However, specification of proximal to distal segments and pre- to postaxial position is under the control of gradients of signalling molecules produced within closely defined regions of the limb bud. In experimental models, interruption of the proximo-distal gradients leads to terminal transverse defects of limbs, whereas interference with the pre-axial to postaxial gradients leads to polydactyly or oligodactly. Separation of digits is, to a large extent, the result of apoptosis of cells between the digital rays, and thus syndactyly (fusion of digits) is regarded as a failure of this process of programmed cell death.

The nervous system

As mentioned above, at 17–18 days of development the neural plate differentiates within the surface ectoderm under the inductive influence of the underlying mesoderm. At this stage a pattern of gene expression appears, specifying the fate of the different regions of the neural plate. Concurrently, neural folds arise at the edges of the neural plate with a longitudinal neural groove between (Figs 5.7, 5.18a). The neural folds meet in the midline, initiating neural tube closure in the cervical region at day 21 (Fig. 5.18b). Closure proceeds cranially and caudally, until by day 25 only the anterior and posterior neuropores remain open. Final closure

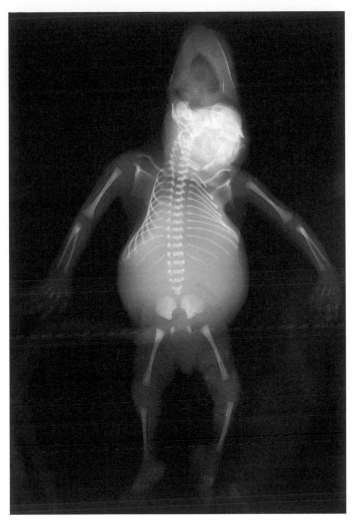

Fig. 5.15 Radiograph showing sacral agenesis in a 22-week fetus of a diabetic mother.

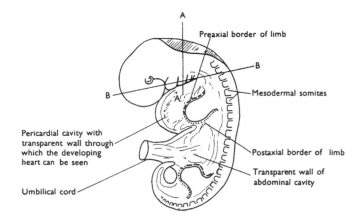

Fig. 5.16 An embryo in the somite stage of development (about 33 days) before invasion of the body wall by cells from the somites. The limb buds have just begun to develop. (From Beck et al 1985, with permission.)

Preaxial border of limb

Mesodermal somites

Pericardial cavity with transparent wall through which the developing heart can be seen

Postaxial border of limb

Transparent wall of abdominal cavity

Umbilical cord

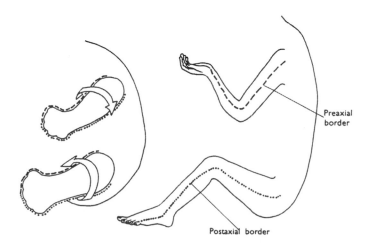

Fig. 5.17 Stages in the development of the limbs to show their changes in position. (From Beck et al 1985, with permission.)

Preaxial border

Postaxial border

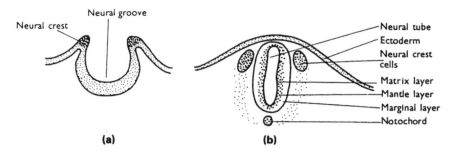

Fig. 5.18 (a) The neural groove and neural crest. (b) The three layers of the neural tube can be distinguished. (From Beck et al 1985, with permission.)

is complete by day 30. As the neural tube closes a population of neural crest cells delaminate from the tips of the neural folds. These cells form the peripheral nervous system, cutaneous melanocytes and facial connective tissues and are also involved in cardiac development. The unspecialised ectoderm closes over the neural tube, such that it lies beneath the surface.

By the time of neuropore closure (by 25 days) differential growth in the cranial neural tube results in three well defined subdivisions of the brain—the forebrain (prosencephalon), midbrain (mesencephalon) and hindbrain (rhombencephalon; Fig. 5.19)—and the cervical and midbrain flexures.

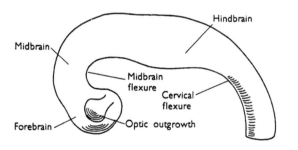

Fig. 5.19 The cranial end of the neural tube at 28 days, showing the primitive forebrain, midbrain and hindbrain. (From Beck et al 1985, with permission.)

Thinning of the roof of the hindbrain at 35 days results in the pontine flexure over the fourth ventricle (Fig. 5.20). Further segmentation divides the prosencephalon into the two telencephalic vesicles, which will give rise to the cerebral hemispheres and basal ganglia, and the diencephalon, from which the thalamus and hypothalamus arise (Fig. 5.21). In the hindbrain the metencephalon and myelencephalon become defined. The former is the origin of the pons and cerebellum, while the latter develops into the medulla. The telencephalic vesicles increase rapidly in size and soon hide the diencephalon completely. The lamina terminalis joining the developing hemispheres is a region in which commissural fibres develop, and the corpus callosum begins to develop here (Figs 5.22, 5.23). Projection fibres develop and fill up the space between the telencephalon and diencephalon until eventually these two parts of the forebrain fuse so that the projection fibres and the developing corpus striatum lie immediately lateral to the thalamus (Fig. 5.24). The cerebellum begins to develop at 6 weeks from dorsolateral swellings of the metencephalon, these fuse in the midline over the fourth ventricle by 12 weeks and its main lobes are large and clearly delineated by the fourth month.

Following neural tube closure, there is very rapid proliferation of the cells lining the neural tube and differentiation into neural and glial lineages. The immature cells form the periventricular germinal matrix, from where neurons migrate to their final positions. In the spinal cord and brainstem the distances involved are not large; however, in the cerebrum, precursors of cortical neurons have considerable

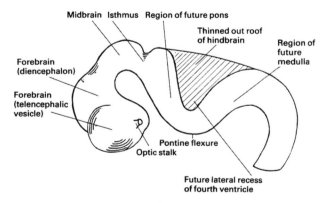

Fig. 5.20 The brain at 37 days. The pontine flexure is further developed and the telencephalic vesicles are forming. (From Beck et al 1985, with permission.)

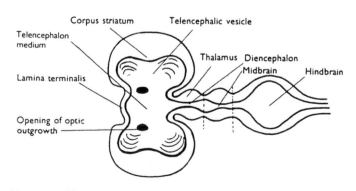

Fig. 5.21 Diagrammatic horizontal section through the developing brain. (From Beck et al 1985, with permission.)

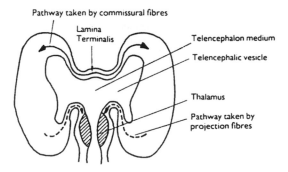

Fig. 5.22 Diagrammatic horizontal section through the developing forebrain to show how the commissural fibres use the lamina terminalis as a pathway while the projection fibres bend sharply round into the diencephalon. (From Beck et al 1985, with permission.)

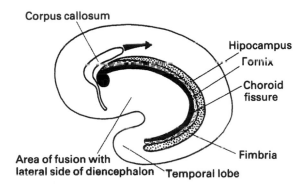

Fig. 5.23 Diagram of the medial side of the telencephalic vesicle detached from the mesencephalon. Growth of the caudal part of the telencephalic vesicle has formed the temporal lobe. The corpus callosum grows caudally. (From Beck et al 1985, with permission.)

distances to travel. Neuronal migration occurs in waves, the neurons being directed to their final positions by radially arranged glial cells with one foot process attached to the ventricular lining and the other to the pial surface of the brain.

In addition to cell proliferation and migration, programmed cell death plays an important role in the development of the nervous system, probably by removing unwanted populations of cells. The choroid plexuses are formed from the vascular mesenchyme covering the developing brain, which becomes invaginated in the medial walls of the developing cerebral hemispheres (see Fig. 5.24). The events described above happen early in gestation. At 7 weeks there is already a large corpus striatum and thalamus, and at 8 weeks the meninges have formed and the cerebral cortex is differentiating. By 12–16 weeks the brain begins to resemble that of the adult and the corpus callosum together with the other commissures are formed. From 16 weeks to full term the cerebral gyri and sulci appear, the insula sinks below the surface and considerable myelination takes place, though this is not complete until well after birth. By about 16 weeks the neuronal cell complement of the brain is almost complete, and subsequent rapid growth involves multiplication of glia and increasing myelinsation.

Abnormalities of neural development

Defective neural tube closure. Defects of neural tube closure are the most common congenital malformations of the central nervous system. Failure of closure of the cranial neuropore results in anencephaly (Fig. 5.25), while myclomeningocele occurs when the caudal neuropore remains open (Fig. 5.26). Total failure of neural tube closure leads to the much rarer craniorachischisis (Fig. 5.27). Genetic influences are clearly important in controlling closure, as demonstrated by the occurrence of neural tube defects in a number of mouse mutants and human genetic disorders. However, neural tube closure is also sensitive to mutagens such as valproate. More recently it has been shown that mechanical influences may also affect closure of the caudal neuropore. In curly tail mice, failure of closure results from excessive curvature of the body; when this is corrected

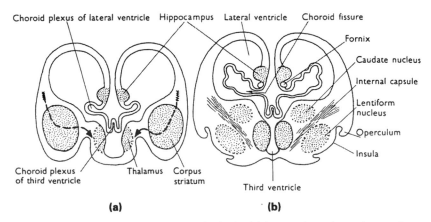

Fig. 5.24 Frontal section through the forebrain. (a) Arrows show the pathway taken by projection fibres through the corpus striatum and into the diencephalon. (b) Fusion has taken place between the lateral sides of the diencephalon and the medial side of the telencephalon lateral to the thalamus. The corpus striatum is divided into lentiform and caudate nuclei. The choroid fissure is developing in relation to the hippocampus and fornix. (From Beck et al 1985, with permission.)

53

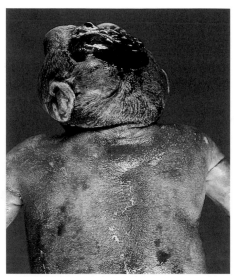

Fig. 5.25 Anencephaly in an 18-week fetus—the cranial vault is absent and the cerebrum is absent. Residual vascular tissue covers the skull base.

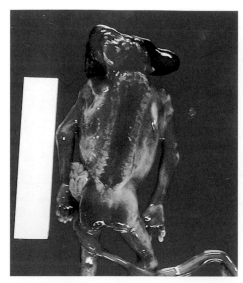

Fig. 5.27 Craniorachischisis—major failure of neural tube closure.

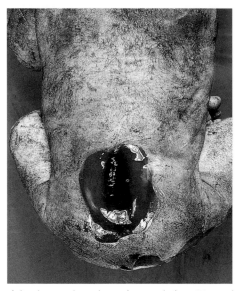

Fig. 5.26 A lumbosacral myelomeningocoele in a 20-week fetus.

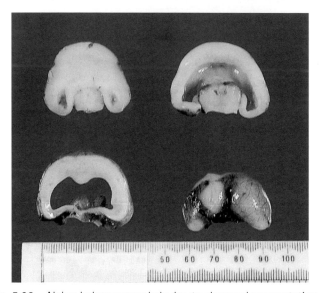

Fig. 5.28 Alobar holoprosencephaly due to abnormal segmentation of the forebrain vesicle. The abnormal forebrain has a single holosphere and common ventricular cavity.

artificially closure proceeds normally (Brook et al 1991). Closed neural tube defects such as meningocoeles and encephalocoeles probably result from defective development of the skeletal elements rather than the neural tube.

Abnormalities of major brain structures. Failure of segmentation of the telencephalon into left and right cerebral hemispheres results in holoprosencephaly (HPE). In its most severe form there is a single forebrain mass (alobar HPE) (Fig. 5.28), while in lesser forms the telencephalon is partially or completely separated into left and right halves (semilobar and lobar HPE). HPE may result from a failure of early forebrain patterning and is associated with a number of distinct genetic loci (Muenke & Beachy 2000). In HPE abnormal development of the craniofacial skeleton is common, severe forms being associated with cyclopia (a single midline eye) and an

absent nose or single nostril, while in milder variants there may be hypotelorism (close-set eyes) or a single central incisor.

The corpus callosum is formed by commissural fibres linking the cerebral hemispheres across the lamina terminalis. Development starts in the frontal region and proceeds posteriorly (Fig. 5.23). Isolated complete or partial absence of the corpus callosum (ACC) is relatively common and may occur in 'normal' individuals; however, ACC also occurs in association with other abnormalities of the central nervous system.

Total cerebellar agenesis is a rare malformation, which may be due to defective early patterning of the hindbrain. In contrast, hypoplasia or aplasia of the cerebellar vermis is relatively common and is associated with cystic dilatation of the fourth ventricle (Dandy-Walker malformation) (Fig. 5.29). The abnormality is probably due to incomplete fusion of the

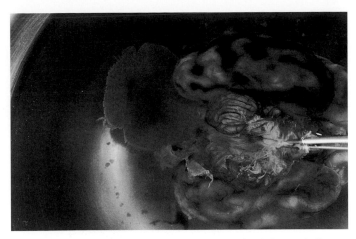

Fig. 5.29 Dandy-Walker malformation—agenesis of the cerebellar vermis and a cystic fourth ventricle.

cerebellar anlage in the dorsal midline. Dandy-Walker malformation is frequently associated with other abnormalities of the central nervous system.

Neuronal migration defects. Abnormal neuronal migration can result in lissencephaly or glioneuronal heterotopia. In type 1 lissencephaly (Miller–Dieker) the cerebral cortex is broad and poorly demarcated from the underlying white matter, and lacks the normal six-layered structure. In many cases a microdeletion on chromosome 17 is present. In type 2 lissencephaly migration appears excessive, extending into the overlying meninges in a disordered fashion. The abnormality may be present throughout the central nervous system and may be associated with hydrocephalus and retinal dysplasia. Focal areas of arrested neuronal migration result in laminar or nodular heterotopia, which may be the source of epileptic seizures.

Deficient proliferation/excessive cell death. Microencephaly, with otherwise normal development of the brain, may be due to deficient proliferation of precursors or more likely, excessive cell death. This may either be of genetic origin or due to external influences, such as toxins or congenital infection.

The face, mouth, palate and branchial region

At about the 20-somite stage (Fig. 5.16) the stomatodaeum, or primitive mouth, has been delineated. The mesenchyme covering the forebrain is seen to form its cranial boundary, the mandibular arches are lateral and the pericardial cavity is placed inferiorly. These topographical relations can be seen in sagittal section in Figure 5.10. With the breakdown of the buccopharyngeal membrane the ectodermally derived stomatodaeum becomes continuous with the endodermally lined foregut. The transition occurs at the level of Rathke's pouch but leaves no visible sign after the disappearance of the buccopharyngeal membrane.

Figure 5.30 illustrates the subsequent development of the face (Slarkin 1979). The mandibular arches fuse below the stomatodeal opening and a dorsal wing from each mandibular arch gives rise to the maxillary process on that side.

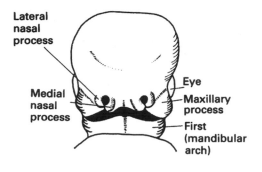

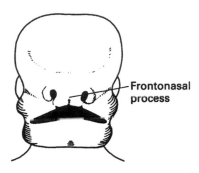

Fig. 5.30 The developing face. (From Beck et al 1985, with permission.)

Bilateral thickenings in the ectoderm, the olfactory placodes, sink beneath the surface each to lie in the floor of a nasal sac. The external opening of the sac forms the external nares with mesodermal thickenings—the medial and lateral nasal processes—on each side of it. The two medial nasal processes fuse to form the frontonasal process, and the maxillary processes, growing medially, fuse with the lateral edges of the frontonasal process.

The nasal sac establishes continuity with the stomatodaeum posteriorly to form the primitive posterior nares and the mesoderm of the maxillary processes becomes continuous with that of the frontonasal process to form the upper lip and primitive palate (Fig. 5.31). Most of the palate is formed behind from the palatal processes that grow medially from the inner surface of the maxillary processes (Fig. 5.31). From their initial position on either side of the tongue the palatal

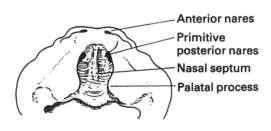

Fig. 5.31 Horizontal section through the head of an embryo to show the the developing palate. The palatal processes grow medially and will eventually meet the nasal septum in the midline (From Beck et al 1985, with permission.)

processes rise to fuse with each other and with the edge of the nasal septum in the midline (Fig. 5.32).

Underdevelopment of the frontonasal process is responsible for midline cleft lip and premaxillary agenesis, seen in trisomy 13 and severe forms of holoprosencephaly (Fig. 5.33), while defective fusion between a maxillary process and the frontonasal process is responsible for the more common unilateral cleft lip (Fig. 5.34). Similarly, midline clefts of the posterior palate are due to failure of the palatal processes to fuse. Such fusion defects may be the result of undergrowth of the components that contribute to the palate and lip, abnormalities of the epithelium (e.g. of adhesion molecule expression) or mechanical effects.

The branchial (or pharyngeal) arches are a series of mesenchymal thickenings on the lateral surface of the embryonic face. In contrast to the rest of the embryo, the mesenchyme of the future face is largely derived from cranial neural crest rather than mesoderm. The two most cranial arches are

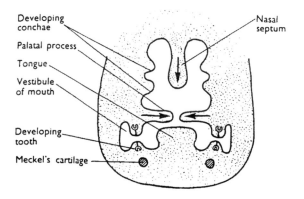

Fig. 5.32   Coronal section through the head to show the formation of the palate and nasal septum. The diagram is simplified – in a real embryo the tongue at first lies between the palatal processes so that its dorsum is in contact with the free border of the nasal septum. (From Beck et al 1985, with permission.)

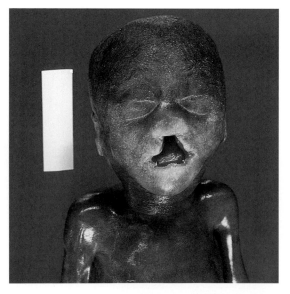

Fig. 5.33   Agenesis of the premaxilla giving a midline facial cleft in a fetus with trisomy 13.

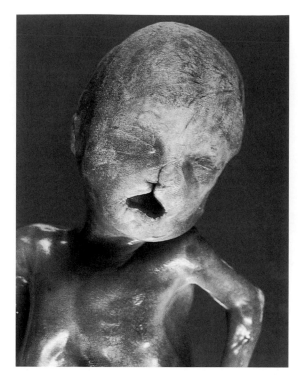

Fig. 5.34   Unilateral cleft lip and palate due to failed fusion between the frontonasal process and the right maxillary process.

clearly marked but, behind these, the arches become progressively smaller and completely overgrown by the second arch so that the smooth surface of the neck is established (Fig. 5.35). The external groove between the first and second arches forms the external auditory meatus.

Each branchial arch contains an aortic arch artery, a cranial nerve, muscle and skeletal tissue (Fig. 5.36). Altogether there are six branchial arches, although the fifth is rudimentary: the first gives rise to the muscles of mastication (Vth cranial nerve) and the malleus and incus in the middle ear; the second to the muscles of facial expression (VII), the stapes and styloid process; the third to the stylopharyngeus muscle (IX) and hyoid bone; and the fourth and sixth to the pharyngeal and laryngeal muscles (X) and cartilages. Skeletal

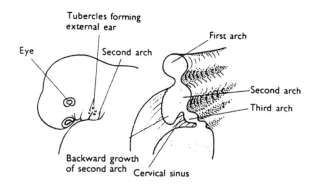

Fig. 5.35   Diagram to show how backward growth of the second arch forms the cervical sinus. Its obliteration will form the smooth line of the neck. (From Beck et al 1985, with permission.)

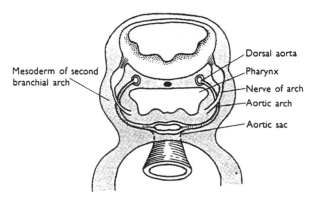

Fig. 5.36 A section through the pharynx at the level of the second branchial arch (A–A in Fig. 5.16), seen from the front. Each arch contains a nerve and an artery. (From Beck et al 1985, with permission.)

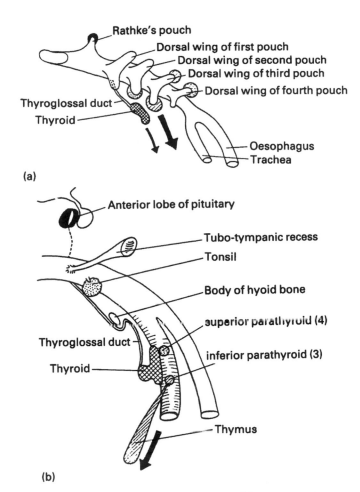

Fig. 5.38 Side view of the pharynx to show: (a) the origin of the endodermal proliferations giving rise to the pharyngeal pouch derivatives. Also shown is Rathke's pouch and the thyroid outgrowth. (b) The fate of the structures depicted in (a). (From Beck et al 1985, with permission.)

elements of branchial arch origin are depicted in Fig. 5.37; the arch arteries are discussed below in connection with the cardiovascular system.

Between the branchial arches lie the endodermally lined branchial pouches, which, at first, are continuous with the cavity of the pharynx. Pouch 1 becomes the eustachian tube and middle ear. The endodermal lining of the remaining pouches differentiates into various important structures situated chiefly in the neck (these are illustrated in Fig. 5.38, which also illustrates the development of the pituitary and thyroid glands). The thyroid anlage originates in the root of the tongue and descends in the neck, becoming attached to the ventral part of pouch 4. Here it gains cells from the ultimobranchial body, which will form the calcitonin-secreting C cells of the parathyroid gland.

The cardiovascular system

The vascular system, including the heart, is formed initially from endothelial tubes which develop in mesenchyme within

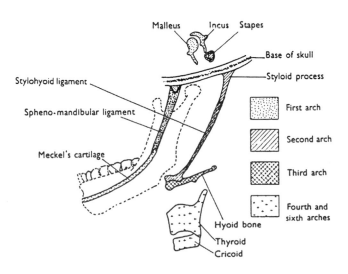

Fig. 5.37 The derivatives of the skeletal elements of the branchial arches. (From Beck et al 1985, with permission.)

both the embryo and the extraembryonic tissues. The scattered endothelial tubes link up to form a primitive circulatory system. Paired heart tubes form in the mesenchyme rostral to the prochordal plate and fuse to produce a single tube, which invaginates the anterior portion of the intraembryonic coelem to form the pericardial cavity (Fig. 5.39). Formation of the head fold brings the heart to lie caudal to the head within the pericardium, ventral to the foregut and delineated posteriorly by the septum transversum (Fig. 5.40). The first peristalsis-like heartbeats begin on day 21. The heart tube is divided into four primitive chambers, of which the most caudal (the sinus venosus) is still embedded in the septum. The cranially situated bulbus cordis leads into a short wide segment, the truncus arteriosus, which, further forward, runs into an aortic sac. Paired branchial arch arteries develop in a cranial–caudal sequence, connecting the ventral and dorsal aortas (O'Rahilly 1971). The vessels of the first and second arches are destined to regress, the third arch vessels form the common and internal carotid arteries, those of the fourth arch contribute to the right subclavian artery and aortic isth-

57

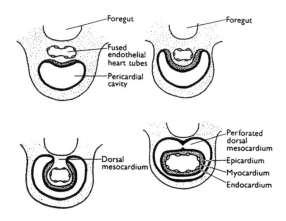

Fig. 5.39 The heart develops from a pair of endothelial tubes which fuse and invaginate the pericardial cavity. The dorsal mesocardium, which is thus formed, becomes perforated so that the heart tube runs freely through the pericardial cavity. (From Beck et al 1985, with permission.)

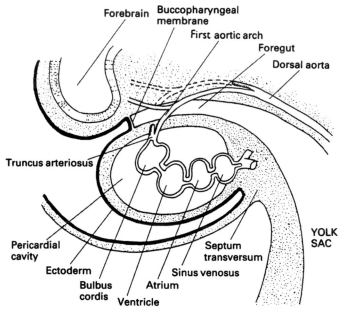

Fig. 5.40 The heart tube consists of four chambers. The first aortic arch arteries only have developed at this stage. (From Beck et al 1985, with permission.)

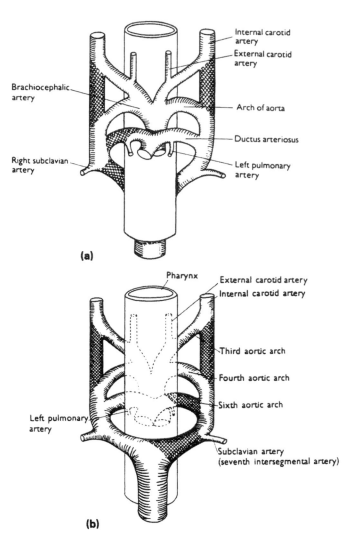

Fig. 5.41 The relation of the aortic arch arteries to the pharynx viewed from in front (a) and from behind (b). The cross-hatched vessels will later disappear. (From Beck et al 1985, with permission.)

mus, while the sixth arch arteries contribute to the pulmonary trunk and ductus arteriosus (L) (Fig. 5.41).

From its inception the heart tube grows faster than the pericardium. As it is fixed both cranially and caudally it becomes kinked in both the anteroposterior and the transverse planes (Fig. 5.42a). At about 25–26 days the bulbus cordis and ventricle lie ventral to the atrium and sinus venosus. Endocardial cushions have begun to form in the atrioventricular canal. A further lateral twist of the tube brings the bulbus cordis to lie to the right of the ventricle so that the two form a common chamber in which a depression corre-

sponding to the interventricular septum can already be seen (Fig. 5.42b).

At this stage the sinus venosus has become asymmetrical due to shunting of the venous return from the head and neck to the right by development of the brachiocephalic vein. As a result of the relative decrease in size of the left horn, it is now the right horn of the sinus venosus that opens into the posterior wall of the common atrial cavity, rather to the right side, by a slit which is guarded by two venous valves (Fig. 5.43).

At about 32 days the growth of the septum primum from the dorsum of the atrial wall begins the formation of the interatrial septum (Fig. 5.43). The septum primum grows towards the endocardial cushions, which have fused to partition the atrioventricular canal. As fusion with the cushions is completed, the septum primum becomes perforated, producing the foramen secundum. A second, thicker, membrane then grows out from the dorsal wall of the right side of the atrial chamber, adjacent to the septum primum. This septum secundum is incomplete, having an opening, the foramen ovale, for which the septum primum forms a flap valve. The

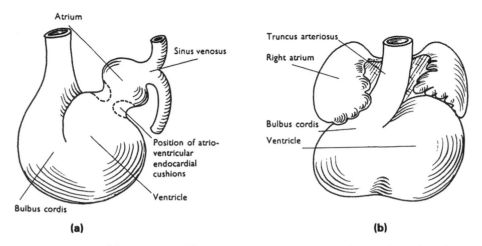

Fig. 5.42 Lateral (a) and anterior (b) views of the developing heart after the formation of the acute bends in the heart tube. (a) is at a slightly earlier stage of development than (b). (From Beck et al 1985, with permission.)

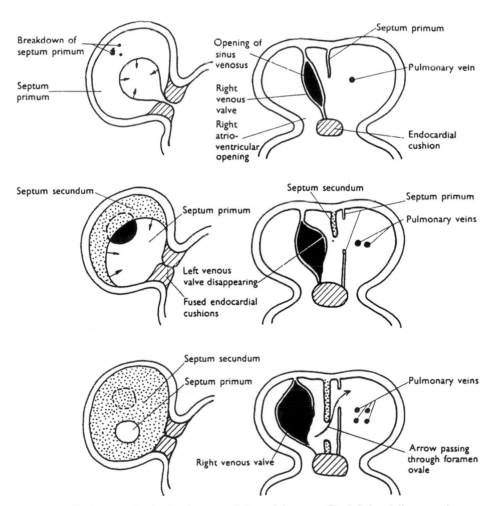

Fig. 5.43 Three stages in the development of the atrial septum. The left-hand diagrams show the right side of the developing septum and the right-hand diagrams show a coronal section in the plane of the atria. The septum secundum is stippled. (From Beck et al 1985, with permission.)

fully functional foramen ovale is present towards the end of the organogenetic period, though the septum secundum is quite well developed by about 46 days. Two other changes take place in the atria; on the left the origins of the pulmonary vein become incorporated into the atrial wall to form its smooth-walled part and on the right the sinus venosus is incorporated into the right atrium. The right horn of the sinus venosus forms the smooth posterior portion of the right atrium and into it opens the coronary sinus, which is the original left horn of the sinus venosus.

Septation of the bulboventricular cavity is illustrated in Fig. 5.44. At about 42 days of development a spiral aorticopulmonary septum, formed by fusion of bulbar ridges, divides the common outflow tract (truncus arteriosus). A muscular interventricular septum arises near the apex of the ventricle and its concave upper border fuses with the lower ends of the bulbar ridges and a contribution from the atrioventricular cushion, which form the membranous part of the interventricular septum. Thus blood from the left ventricle empties exclusively into the aorta and from the right into the pulmonary trunk. Septation of the ventricles is complete at about 46 days of development.

With such a complex series of folding, rotation and fusion events required for normal cardiac development, it is hardly surprising that congenital heart defects are relatively common. Probably the most frequently encountered abnormality is the perimembranous ventricular septal defect due to failure of fusion of the various elements of the membranous and muscular ventricular septum. Defects in the muscular septum are probably the result of excessive cell death. In contrast, the atrioventricular septal defect, characteristic of Down's syndrome (trisomy 21) is due to underdevelopment of the endocardial cushions in the atrioventricular canal (Fig. 5.45).

Abnormalities of the cardiac outflow are also relatively frequent. In transposition of the great arteries, the aorta arises from the right ventricle and the pulmonary trunk from the left. This appears to be the result of misalignment of the aorticopulmonary septum, which is straight rather than spiral. Misalignment also occurs in the tetralogy of Fallot, where the aorta overrides the septum and the pulmonary trunk is

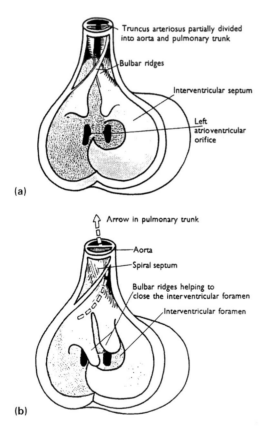

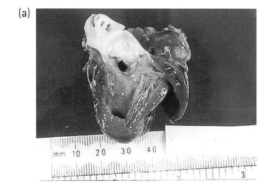

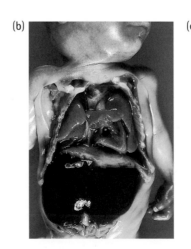

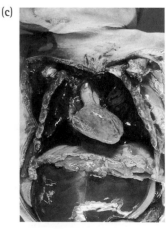

Fig. 5.44 (a) The heart viewed open from the front to show the spiral bulbar ridges. (b) Fusion of the right and left bulbar ridges has formed a separate aorta and pulmonary trunk. The interventricular foramen is partly closed and will later completely close by further development of the bulbar ridges and by proliferation of the tissues of the atrioventricular cushions. After closure of the interventricular septum the right atrioventricular orifice will open exclusively into the right ventricle and the left orifice into the left ventricle. (From Beck et al 1985, with permission.)

Fig. 5.45 Congenital heart defects. (a) Perimembranous ventricular septal defect. (b) Atrioventricular septal defect in trisomy 21. (c) In transposition of the great arteries the aorta arises from the right ventricle and the pulmonary trunk from the left.

narrow. Tetralogy of Fallot and interruption of the aortic arch are frequently found in individuals with small deletions at chromosome 22q11. Absence of the thymus and parathyroid glands and palatal clefts are other features of this 22q11 microdeletion syndrome, and it has been suggested that the malformations are due to an effect on cranial neural crest-derived tissues which contribute to the craniofacial mesenchyme and the mesenchyme of the cardiac outflow tract (Creazzo et al 1998).

The coelom, lungs and diaphragm

The coelem develops within the lateral and most rostral mesenchyme of the early embryo to form a horseshoe-shaped cavity (Fig. 5.9). Formation of the body folds brings the anterior part of the cavity, which is crossed by the heart tube, to lie ventrally (Fig. 5.10). This will be the pericardial sac. The lateral arms of the horseshoe lie to either side of the fore- and midgut (Fig. 5.11).

Development of the lower respiratory tract begins with formation of a groove in the floor of the pharynx. This groove enlarges to become a laryngotracheal diverticulum, from which arise left and right lung buds, which are lined by foregut endoderm with a covering of splanchnic mesenchyme. These buds grow out into the arms of the coelomic cavity, the pleuropericardial canals (Fig. 5.46). Folds of mesenchyme—the pleuropericardial folds—containing the cardinal veins and enlarged by the developing lung buds, partition the cranial part of the coelem into pericardial and pleural parts. Similar pleuroperitoneal folds, caudal to the lung buds separate the pleura from the peritoneum. By a process of dichotomous branching of the lung buds the bronchial tree, and later the bronchioles, alveolar ducts and alveoli, develop to form the mature lung structure (Fig. 5.47). Localised dis-

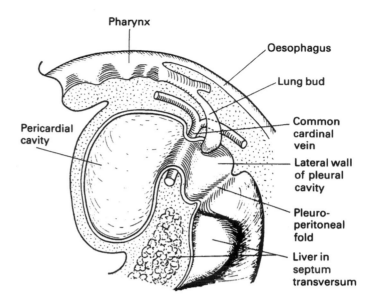

Fig. 5.46 Parasagittal section through the region of the septum transversum to show the right lateral wall of the pericardial cavity and the right coelomic duct (pleural cavity). (From Beck et al 1985, with permission.)

ruption of this progressive, regular branching, which appears to be regulated by interactions between the epithelial and mesenchymal components of the developing lung (McGowan 1992), results in the various forms of congenital cystic adenomatoid malformation (Fig. 5.48). Lung growth is dependent upon adequacy of lung fluid, fetal respiratory movements and space. Thus severe oligohydramnios, particularly in the mid-trimester, may result in hypoplasia of the

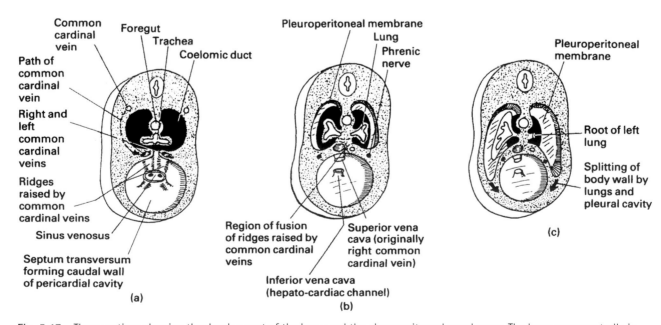

Fig. 5.47 Three sections showing the development of the lungs and the pleuroperitoneal membranes. The lungs grow ventrally in the direction of the arrows in (c). (From Beck et al 1985, with permission.)

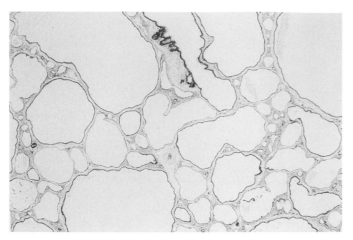

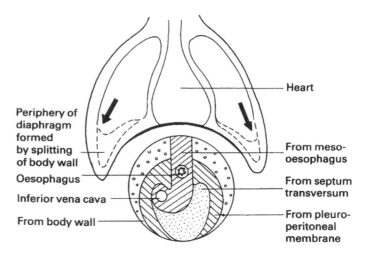

Fig. 5.48 Histological appearance of a congenital cystic adenomatoid malformation of lung—irregular cystic airspaces due to abnormal branching of the developing lung.

Fig. 5.50 Coronal section (above) showing how the lungs split the body wall to form the peripheral portion of the diaphragm. The arrows show the direction of lung growth in this plane. The lower diagram shows the embryonic constituents of the adult diaphragm viewed from above. (From Beck et al 1985, with permission.)

lungs. Similarly, a baby with severe neuromuscular disease, a space-occupying lesion in the chest (e.g. abdominal contents via a diaphragmatic hernia or pleural effusions) or a malformed thorax may suffer from pulmonary hypoplasia (Fig. 5.49).

Development of the diaphragm requires components from a variety of sources (Fig. 5.50). The main fibrous central tendon is derived from the septum transversum. The pleuroperitoneal folds, which initially separate the pleural cavity from the peritoneum, form only a minor part of the final diaphragm at the lateral edge of the central tendon. The muscular diaphragm is derived from the body wall, while the dorsal mesentery of the oesophagus contributes the crura. Failure of the pleuroperitoneal membranes to fuse with the septum transversum is responsible for the typical posterolateral diaphragmatic defect, which allows herniation of abdominal contents into the thoracic cavity (Fig. 5.51).

The urogenital system

When the tail fold is formed the cloacal membrane, marking the caudal limit of the hindgut, comes to lie on the ventral aspect of the embryo (Fig. 5.52). The proximal end of the allantois now opens into the cloaca just anterior to the cloacal membrane and takes part in the formation of the apex of the adult bladder. The mesenchyme between the allantois and the hindgut grows caudally to fuse with the cloacal membrane, partitioning the cloaca into a ventral urogenital

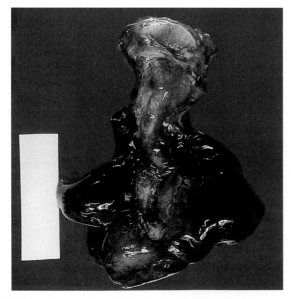

Fig. 5.49 Pulmonary hypoplasia due to oligohydramnios.

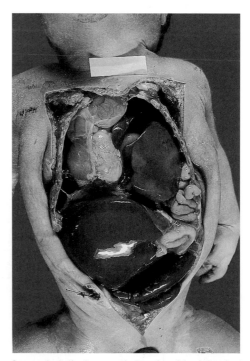

Fig. 5.51 Congenital diaphragmatic hernia with abdominal contents in the left side of the thorax.

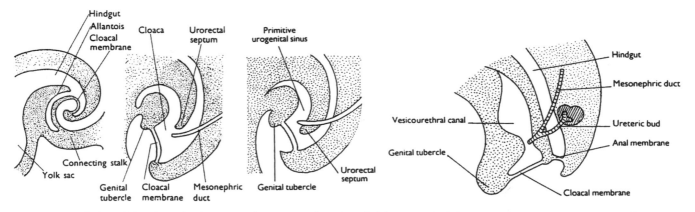

Fig. 5.52 The splitting of the cloaca by the urorectal septum to form the primitive urogenital sinus; also shown is the ureteric bud. (From Beck et al 1985, with permission.)

sinus which will form the bladder and urethra, and a dorsal rectum and anal canal. At about 8 weeks the membrane closing the anal canal ruptures. Thus the hindgut is in communication with the amniotic cavity.

The kidneys develop from the nephrogenic cord, a derivative of the intermediate mesoderm extending caudally from the cervical region of the embryo in the dorsal wall of the coelomic cavity. First to develop is a primitive pronephros, which quickly regresses. This is followed by development, late in the fourth week, of the mesonephros, which may function for a few weeks (Fig. 5.53). While the mesonephric kidney involutes the mesonephric duct persists in males to form the epididymis and ductus deferens. In addition, at around 5 weeks, a ureteric bud arises from the caudal portion of each mesonephric duct. This ureteric bud grows into the caudal portion of the nephrogenic cord, the metanephric blastema, and branches to form the pelvicalyceal system and collecting ducts of the definitive kidney. At the end of each branch the ureteric bud induces the mesenchyme of the blastema to

undergo epithelial transformation, initially forming a metanephric vesicle, which gives rise to the Bowman's capsule, proximal and distal convoluted tubules and loop of Henle of the nephron. Continuity is established between the collecting duct and tubule, while invagination of Bowman's capsule by capillaries forms the glomerulus (Fig. 5.54). New glomeruli continue to be formed up to around 36 weeks of pregnancy, after which time the metanephric blastema has disappeared. The molecular embryology of the interaction between the ureteric bud is some way towards being understood, and some of the important genes, such as WT-1 (the Wilms' tumour gene), are known. Failure of the inductive process may result in absence of one or both kidneys (renal agenesis) or renal dysplasia (Fig. 5.55).

At between 5 and 6 weeks a second longitudinal duct (Fig. 5.53) develops lateral to the mesonephric duct. This is the paramesonephric (Müllerian) duct, which will form much of the reproductive system in the female.

The primitive urogenital sinus becomes subdivided by the

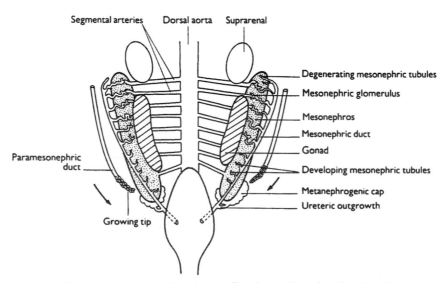

Fig. 5.53 The mesonephros and its relations. The glomeruli are functional at this stage but will disappear later. (From Beck et al 1985, with permission.)

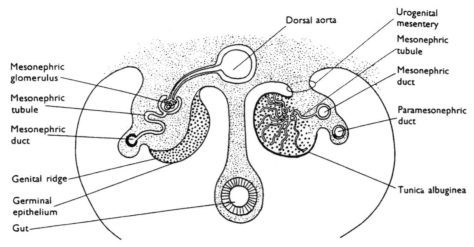

Fig. 5.54 The interior of the adult right atrium seen from in front. Reproduced with permission from Beck et al (1985).

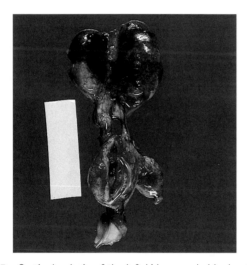

Fig. 5.55 Cystic dysplasia of the left kidney, probably due to abnormal induction between the ureteric bud and metanephric blastema. The right kidney showed solid dysplasia.

entrance of the mesonephric ducts at about 28 days into an upper portion (the vesicourethral canal), from which the bladder and part of the urethra develop, and a lower definitive urogenital sinus. The lower part has a short, narrow cylindrical pelvic portion lying above a laterally compressed phallic portion (Fig. 5.56). The phallic portion extends forwards onto the ventral surface of a midline mesodermal swelling covered by ectoderm (called the genital tubercle), which develops at about 5 weeks. At first this is similar in males and females (Fig. 5.57). Further growth in the region between the genital tubercle and the umbilicus leads to the development of the infraumbilical abdominal wall which will become invaded by tissues of dermatomyotome origin. The bladder is derived mainly from the vesicourethral canal with the lower ends of the mesonephric ducts contributing to the

trigone, while the allantois, which largely regresses, makes a small contribution to its apex. In the female the entire urethra is derived from the vesicourethral canal. In the male the urethra distal to the ejaculatory ducts originates from the pelvic and phallic portions of the definitive urogenital sinus, while the glandular urethra is of ectodermal origin. Congenital posterior urethral valves, a malformation confined to males, may represent a malalignment of the parts of the urethra derived from the vesicourethral canal and the urogenital sinus.

Gonadal elements develop from two sources. The stromal tissues are derived from the mesodermal gonadal ridges that form medial to the nephrogenic ridges on the dorsal body wall (Fig. 5.53); the germ cells migrate to the gonadal primordia from their origin in the yolk sac wall. Differentiation of the testes and the male genital tract from the indeterminate primordia is under the influence of genes on the Y chromosome. Absence of these influences results in activation of the default pathway leading to female gonadal and genital development (Sinclair et al 1990).

In the male, the epididymis and ductus deferens are derived from the mesonephric (Wolffian) duct (Figs 5.53, 5.58). In females the paramesonephric (Müllerian) ducts persist and their caudal portions fuse to form the fallopian tubes, uterus and upper vagina (Fig. 5.59).

Internal sexual phenotype can be recognised by as early as 11 weeks gestation, and male and female gonads can be distinguished histologically by 7–8 weeks. However, the external sexual organs may be difficult to differentiate before 12–14 weeks.

The digestive system

Following formation of the body folds, the developing gut pulls away from the dorsal body wall to form its dorsal mesentery. The ventral mesentery develops due to separation from the septum transversum (Fig. 5.60). The endoderm-derived epithelium of the gut is enclosed in splanchnic meso-

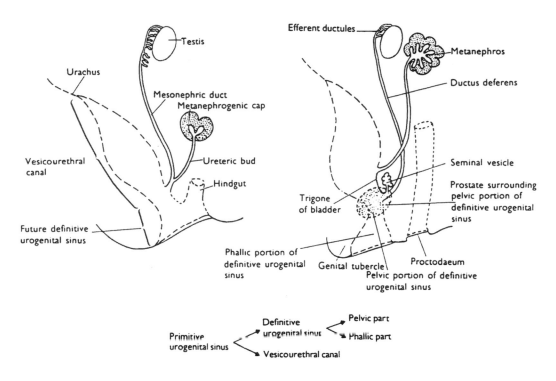

Fig. 5.56 The development of the bladder and internal genitalia. The endodermal derivatives are dotted. The flow chart shows how the primitive urogenital sinus becomes divided. (From Beck et al 1985, with permission.)

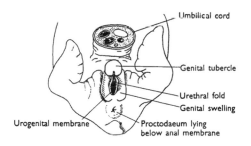

Fig. 5.57 The external genitalia at the end of the second month. There is little development of the infraumbilical abdominal wall at this stage; the genital tubercle reaches up as far as the umbilicus. (From Beck et al 1985, with permission.)

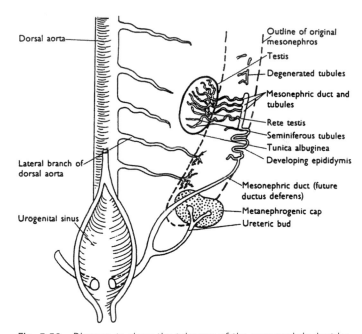

Fig. 5.58 Diagram to show the takeover of the mesonephric duct by the testis and the development of the metanephros. (From Beck et al 1985, with permission.)

derm, which provides the connective tissue, vasculature and muscle coats. The neuronal plexuses are formed by cranial–caudal invasion of the developing intestine by neural crest cells, predominantly from the vagal region (Grand et al 1976). Failure of this process of colonisation is thought to be the cause of aganglionosis of the distal intestine (Hirschsprung's disease).

Rapid growth of the liver results in physiological herniation of the developing gut into the extraembryonic coelem in the root of the body stalk (Fig. 5.61). With growth of the body cavity, the midgut returns to the abdomen at 8–9 weeks' gestation. The process of herniation and return is associated with three rotations of 90°, so that the gut comes to lie in its final position by around 11 weeks. Fusion of the mesentery of the ascending and descending colon with the

dorsal body wall results in fixation of these segments (Fig. 5.62).

Focal atresia of the intestine is relatively common. Oesophageal atresia is most frequently related to abnormal formation of the laryngotracheal groove and is frequently

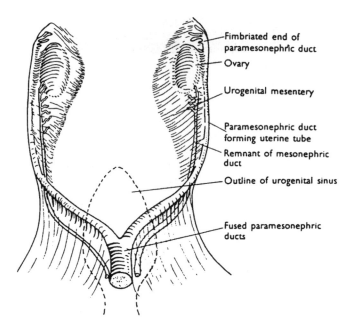

Fig. 5.59 Development of the urogenital mesentery into the broad ligament of the uterus. The mesonephros, together with its ducts and tubules, has almost completely disappeared. (From Beck et al 1985, with permission.)

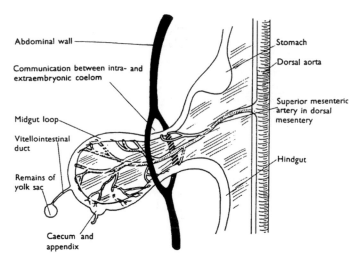

Fig. 5.61 Side view of the midgut loop herniated out into the extraembryonic coelom. (From Beck et al 1985, with permission.)

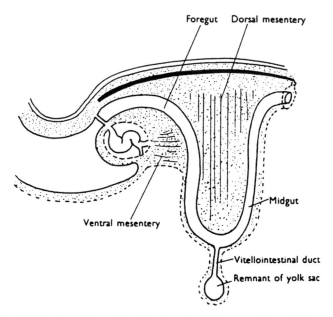

Fig. 5.60 Formation of the dorsal and ventral mesenteries of the gut. (From Beck et al 1985, with permission.)

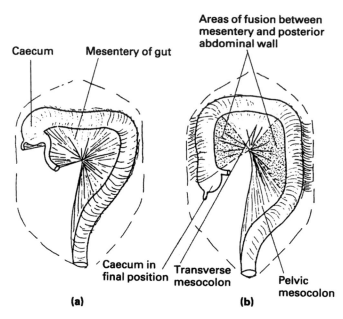

Fig. 5.62 (a) The colon and its mesentery immediately after the return of the midgut loop. (b) The final stage of rotation of the gut. The caecum has attained its final position and the ascending and descending colon have become retroperitoneal. (From Beck et al 1985, with permission.)

associated with a tracheo-oesophageal fistula distal to the atretic segment (Fig. 5.63). Atresia of the duodenum and of the anorectal canal is due to defective canalisation of the primitive gut at points of transient occlusion (Fig. 5.64). These malformations may be associated with genetic abnormalities, such as trisomy 21 (Down's syndrome). More severe forms of anorectal atresia are often associated with

other abnormalities of cloacal and Müllerian development such as rectovesical and rectovaginal fistulas, cloacal or vesical exstrophy and with abnormalities of the sacral spine. In contrast, atresia of the midgut is generally regarded as a vascular disruption, due to interruption of the mesenteric blood supply, and is thus non-genetic (Fig. 5.65).

The liver, biliary tree, gall bladder and pancreas develop from outgrowths at the junction of the fore- and midgut into the dorsal and ventral mesenteries (Severn 1971). The

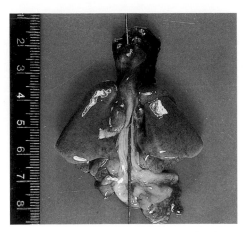

Fig. 5.63   Tracheo-oesophageal fistula with atresia of the oesophagus.

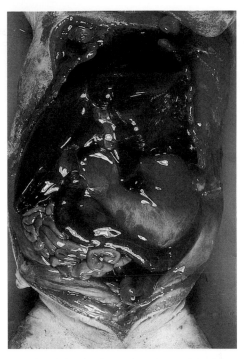

Fig. 5.64   Atresia of the duodenum in a fetus with trisomy 21, leading to gross dilatation of the stomach.

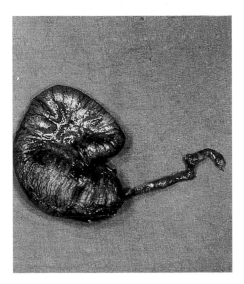

Fig. 5.65   Ileal atresia due to vascular disruption.

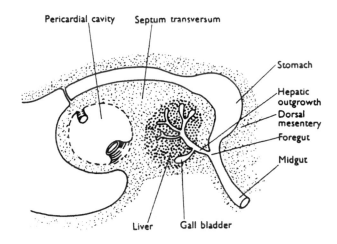

Fig. 5.66   The hepatic outgrowth grows into the ventral mesentery from the end of the foregut. Liver cells invade the septum transversum. (From Beck et al 1985, with permission.)

pancreas has dorsal and ventral primordia, which rotate and fuse at around 8 weeks' gestation (McLean 1979). The liver grows rapidly in the ventral mesentery and invades the septum transversum (Fig. 5.66). The liver primordium becomes colonised by haemopoietic stem cells that originate in the wall of the yolk sac. The liver is the major source of haemopoiesis for the embryonic and fetal periods until the bone marrow takes over this function in the third trimester.

Malformations of the liver, biliary tree and pancreas are uncommon. Abnormal development of the intrahepatic biliary tree, the so-called 'ductal plate' malformation (Fig. 5.67), is associated with a number of genetic disorders, including Meckel syndrome and autosomal recessive polycystic kidney disease. Extrahepatic biliary atresia is probably a disruption rather than a malformation and there is some evidence to indicate a viral aetiology.

RELATIONSHIP OF THE TIMING OF GENETIC AND TERATOGENIC INFLUENCES TO DEVELOPMENTAL ABNORMALITIES

The precise temporal sequence of developmental events means that the timing of any insult will critically influence the pattern of congenital malformation which results. Organogenesis is effectively complete by 11 weeks' gestation, so all major structural defects are the result of events before this. The only exceptions are abnormalities produced by disruption or deformation of otherwise normally formed tissues. Examples of disruption include ileal atresia, amputations due

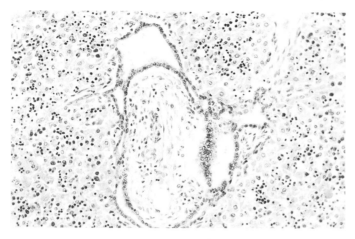

Fig. 5.67 Histological appearance of ductal plate malformation of the liver—dilated and irregular bile ducts in a portal tract.

to amniotic bands and haemorrhagic and ischaemic disruptions of the brain; deformation is most commonly due to oligohydramnios, which leads to the typical 'Potter's' facial appearance (Fig. 5.68) and limb deformity, together with pulmonary hypoplasia.

Once structural development is complete (at 11 weeks), the fetus enters a period of very rapid growth. From a weight of 10 g and crown–rump length of 50 mm at 11 weeks the fetus grows to 1000 g and 250 mm by 28 weeks. Thus adverse influences on the fetus in the fetal period, such as teratogens or viral infection, lead to impaired growth rather than congenital malformation.

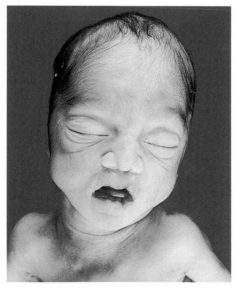

Fig. 5.68 The facial appearance of a fetus subjected to prolonged oligohydramnios ('Potter facies'). Note the low-set ears, epicanthic folds, receding mandible and flattened nose. The infant also had talipes and hypoplastic lungs.

CONCLUSIONS

An understanding of human embryology is essential for the investigation of the fetus with congenital anomalies. As the morphogenesis of the major organ systems is well advanced by the end of the first month after fertilisation, interventions to prevent the development of abnormalities (e.g. neural tube defects) must be given periconceptually. The embryo is most vulnerable to teratogenic influences between conception and the end of the third month of pregnancy.

KEY POINTS

- Early human embryology proceeds through two-layered and three-layered embryonic disc stages, followed by three-dimensional folding to produce a solid embryo with body cavities.
- Most major malformations are the result of events occurring between the fourth and eighth weeks of development.
- Neural tube closure is normally complete by day 30 of development.
- Cardiac morphogenesis is complete by developmental day 46. Cardiac morphogenesis involves folding, rotation, differential growth and fusion events.
- Events after 10 weeks of development tend to affect fetal growth rather than structure. Exceptions to this are disruptions (e.g. amniotic bands) and deformations (e.g. oligohydramnios).

REFERENCES

Beck F, Moffat DB, Davies DP 1985 Human embryology, 2nd edn. Blackwell, Oxford

Brook FA, Shum AS, Van Straaten HW, Copp AJ 1991 Curvature of the caudal region is responsible for failure of neural tube closure in the curly tail (ct) mouse embryo. Development 113:671–678

Creazzo TL, Godt RE, Leatherbury L, Conway SJ, Kirby ML 1998 Role of cardiac neural crest cells in cardiovascular development. Annu Rev Physiol 60:267–286

Ferretti P, Tickle C 1997 The limbs. In: Thorogood P (ed.) Embryos genes and birth defects. Wiley, Chichester

Gehring W 1987 Homeoboxes in the study of development. Science 236:1245–1252

Grand RJ, Watkins JB, Troti FM 1976 Progress in gastroenterology. Development of the human gastrointestinal tract. A review. Gastroenterology 70:790

Greene ND, Gerrelli D, Van Straaten HW, Copp AJ 1998 Abnormalities of floor plate, notochord and somite differentiation in the loop-tail (Lp) mouse: a model of severe neural tube defects. Mech Dev 73:59–72

Hunt P, Whiting J, Muchamore I, Marshall H, Krumlauf R 1991 Homeobox genes and models for patterning the hindbrain and branchial arches. Development (suppl I): 187–197

McGowan SE 1992 Extracellular matrix and the regulation of lung development and repair. FASEB J 6:2895–2904

McLean JM 1979 Embryology of the pancreas. In: Howart HT, Sarles H (eds) The exocrine pancreas. Saunders, London, p 3

Muenke M, Beachy PA 2000 Genetics of ventral forebrain development and holoprosencephaly. Curr Opin Genet Dev 10(3):262–269

O'Rahilly R 1971 The timing and sequence of events in human cardiogenesis. Acta Anatomica 79:70

Sensenig EC 1949 The early development of the human vertebral column. Contributions to Embryology, Carnegie Institute 33:23

Severn CB 1971 A morphological study of the development of the human liver. I. Development of the hepatic diverticulum. Am J Anat 131:133

Sinclair AH, Berta P, Palmer MS et al 1990 A gene from the human sex-determining region encodes a protein with homology to a conserved DNA-binding motif. Nature 346:240–244

Slarkin HC 1979 Developmental craniofacial biology. Lea & Febiger, Philadelphia

6

Maternal physiology in pregnancy

Fiona Broughton Pipkin

The contribution of the author of the equivalent chapter in the second edition, on which this chapter draws extensively, is gratefully acknowledged.

Pregnancy is the biggest physiological upheaval of a woman's life. The luteal phase of every ovulatory menstrual cycle is a preparation for pregnancy and, should conception occur, nothing will ever be quite the same again. The physiological changes of pregnancy are strongly proactive, not reactive. It appears in many respects as if a first pregnancy that proceeds beyond the first trimester is a trial run; whether or not it results in a live baby, adaptations have been made to the mother's physiology which never revert to the never-pregnant state. First pregnancies are associated with a lower mean birthweight, increased rate of complications and raised perinatal mortality. This chapter attempts to give an overview of adaptations to specific systems and also more general concepts, in order to provide a basis for the rational application of antenatal care.

MATERNAL CHARACTERISTICS THAT AFFECT ADAPTATION

Gravidity is an important determinant of the mother's response; the maternal reaction may also be affected by her age, obstetric history, overt or covert illness (acute or chronic), and the present or earlier environment. One or more previous normal pregnancies probably imply that adaptation to the current pregnancy will be normal and complete. Changes in uterine vessels and possibly in the maternal immune response are permanent and help to ensure satisfactory adaptation.

A first pregnancy need not go to term to have a beneficial effect on the outcome of subsequent pregnancies: spontaneous miscarriage of the first pregnancy ensures that mean birthweight in a subsequent pregnancy is similar to that of a parous woman. Therapeutic termination has a similar effect. A previous spontaneous miscarriage also protects against pregnancy-induced hypertension, but not so completely as one that is therapeutically terminated or reaches viability (Strickland et al 1986). This presumably reflects the impact of the underlying pathology which led to the spontaneous miscarriage. Further miscarriages do not confer additional protection. Curiously, however, increasing gravidity increases the risk of spontaneous miscarriage.

Maternal age influences adaptation to pregnancy. Women can conceive in any decade from the first to the sixth; it may not be calendar age so much as the number of years following menarche or how long it will be before the the menopause that is important. The probability of conceiving an aneuploid fetus is possibly determined by the interval between conception and the menopause. Spontaneous miscarriage and an empty gestation sac are both more frequent at the extremes of reproductive age.

Before the menarche, increase in pelvic size is slower than increase in height. After the menarche, growth in height continues for only 2 years whereas pelvic diameter continues to enlarge for 5–12 years. By the time women reach 18, the age of the menarche and pelvic capacity are not well related, but those who have an early menarche are shorter and have a smaller pelvis than those who start to menstruate when they are older. This difference is not of great clinical significance in most societies. If, however, a girl conceives when she is in her early teens she is not only small but her pelvis is even less capacious than would be expected from her height, so that if she survives the pregnancy the chances of her sustaining a vesicovaginal fistula are high. Nature may be partly on her side, however, for among a group of Nigerian girls who were pregnant at 13–16 years, more than half grew 2–16 cm in height during the pregnancy; this reduced the proportion who had mechanical problems in labour. The rest of her body is less likely to adapt satisfactorily to the pregnancy. In every society, pregnancy-induced hypertension is more common in young mothers and in those over 35 years old. It is not a situation in which youngest is best: 18–25 years of age is probably the period for optimal physiological adaptation.

The older woman has other problems. Her development is complete but the physiological changes of ageing or concurrent disease may prevent the development of a totally healthy pregnancy, although only a minority exhibit frank pathology. She may have developed habits with cumulative effects; for example, the higher risk of restricted fetal growth in women of 35 or more who smoke may be a consequence of the effects of tobacco on the cardiovascular system. With increasing age the possibility of fetal chromosome anomalies and of dizygotic twins rises. After the age of 35 blood vessels become less flexible, and with increasing age both systolic and diastolic blood pressures rise. In the childbearing age group this is rarely of clinical significance but it is worth remembering that at any age a primigravida with a normal pregnancy has a higher blood pressure than a multigravida.

Many diseases are covert in the childbearing ages; abnormalities of carbohydrate metabolism, bacteriuria, chronic renal disease, hypertension, undiagnosed thrombophilic tendency and many other disorders may be undetected before conception, yet affect the mother's reaction to pregnancy. Treatment of disease may also modify reactions. Significant numbers of women are on long-term treatment with steroids, non-steroidal analgesics, drugs affecting the adrenergic system or other drugs which can affect their mechanisms of adaptation. Treatment of involuntary infertility with gonadotrophins or other drugs may have an effect, but little is known about this apart from an increased rate of miscarriage. Many of these women, however, are poor reproducers who can be recognised by their history of recurrent miscarriage or other obstetric problems as being less likely to respond physiologically to the stimulus of pregnancy.

Social class and reproductive performance are related: the lower the social class the worse the pregnancy outcome. Since adaptation and outcome are also related, it is likely that social class does affect how well the mother adapts, but there is little direct evidence for this. Physiological investigations and reference ranges of normality do not often define the social class of the population on which they are based. Young age at first conception, high parity which depletes stores, smoking, inappropriate diet, not knowing what care and advice is available—all are associated with lower social class and may affect adaptation. Even the effect of smoking is related to social class. While reduced birthweight is found in smokers of all social classes, increased perinatal mortality is present only in smokers of classes III, IV and V. Raised blood pressure at conception affects adaptation, and at age 36 (an age relevant to childbearing), hypertension is more common in lower than upper social classes. Studies of the non-pregnant may be relevant to the mechanism of the effects of social class on maternal adaptation. Iron stores are frequently low

in women of lower social class, and cell-mediated immune responses are less effective in iron deficiency. Other less well defined deficiencies may also affect adaptation. Fibrinogen levels in the blood are raised in lower social class men and women. Raised fibrinogen increases viscosity, which in pregnancy is associated with poor outcome. Although many data such as these suggest that there is a social class effect on maternal adaptation to pregnancy, accurate and specific information is incomplete.

Heavy work may also affect adaptation. Certainly in pregnancy the respiratory system does not respond to increasing workloads as well as in the non-pregnant, although training increases physical work capacity and uterine blood flow during exercise in both pregnant sheep and women. Africans who work hard adopt methods that are economical in energy use. Such satisfactory dynamic adaptation may reflect good physiological adjustment to pregnancy, but only indirectly.

The effects of social class and of ethnic origin are not always clearly differentiated. In part this results from difficulty of allocating women in one ethnic group to another ethnic group's social classification. If an Asian husband was a qualified accountant before moving to the UK where he runs a shop, what is his real social class? Religion may also be associated with differences in traditions and practices. In diet there are variations that could affect birthweight and other measures of adaptation; for example, intakes of vitamin D, total folate, vitamin B_6, zinc and magnesium were much lower in pregnant women studied in Birmingham who originated from the Indian subcontinent than those consumed by pregnant European women. Intermarriage between close relatives reduces mean birthweight. Hindus have lighter babies than Europeans, even when the weights are adjusted for maternal size and the other variables relevant to birthweight. This is not caused by calorie deficiency as both groups have equal intake from different diets. Essential nutrients can be in short supply or the balance of constituents may be relevant. High fibre content reduces blood oestrogen, which is associated with delay in sexual maturation. Migration unavoidably alters environmental factors which are relevant to maternal health, and frequently leads to gradual alterations in diet and social behaviour. Whatever the mechanism, migration appears also to affect maternal adaptation. For example, mean birthweight falls in Jewish women who move from North Africa to Israel; the longer they live in Israel, the more it falls (Yudkin et al 1983).

Ethnic variations also influence some basic physiological differences. Black Nigerians have a smaller non-pregnant blood volume than Europeans, so that, while an increase of 1270 ml during pregnancy is a 55% increase, it is considerably less than occurs in Europeans. Black African peoples appear not to have a renal dopamine response to sodium as it is not required in warm and humid climates but the relevance of this and other differences to pregnancy has not been fully explored. Some features of other communities have, however, been examined in detail. While Indian Asians have lipid changes in pregnancy which are almost identical with those of whites, Asians require a higher level of insulin in the blood to maintain the same blood sugar. Asians have a lower blood pressure but a similar pattern of change during pregnancy to Europeans. Vegetarian Asians have low serum vitamin B_{12} levels without suffering ill effects possibly because of effective enterohepatic circulation of the vitamin. This wide range of ethnic similarities and differences is relevant to the construction of reference ranges and to the recognition that normality is not the same for each ethnic group or even for ethnic subgroups.

The number of fetuses in the uterus determines the extent of many adaptive changes. While electrolyte concentrations, osmolality and other indices of the *milieu intérieur* are the same in single and multiple pregnancy, the increase in blood volume is 30% greater with twins and 50% greater with quadruplets. Plasma volume increases proportionately more with twins than singletons, so haemodilution is greater. Total body water increase is greater with twins, even in the first trimester, so that weight gain is increased by more than that of the additional conceptus. Cardiac output, glomerular filtration rate, uterine blood flow and tidal volume increases are greater than in singletons. Women carrying twins have more potential stresses on almost all of their systems than mothers of singletons.

METABOLISM

Extra energy is required during pregnancy to fuel the growth of the conceptus and for the increased work that the mother must do because she is pregnant. The total requirement has been calculated to be 80 000 kcal, of which 36 000 is for maintenance metabolism. This estimate may be too high. Studies in the Gambia and in Scotland suggest that the additional energy required for a successful pregnancy is 13 000–20 000 kcal. The difference between the calculated and observed requirements arises because the calculation assumes a steady increase in resting metabolic rate which does not occur. Among the well nourished, or those whose diet has been supplemented, there is little change in the first 10 weeks of pregnancy, a gradual rise from then until 36 weeks of 50–100 kcal/day, and an increase of 200–300 kcal/day in the final 4 weeks. By late pregnancy, individual resting metabolic rates studied longitudinally from before conception have increased from approximately 450 to 3400 kJ/day. Total and active energy expenditure during pregnancy varies enormously between individuals, even in apparently homogeneous groups, ranging from small falls to not inconsiderable rises. Resting metabolic rate and total energy expenditure in North Americans were on average 15–26% higher during pregnancy than postpartum, after adjustment for fat-free mass, fat mass, and energy balance. In rural Africans with a low food intake, resting metabolism falls in the first 2 weeks' and may not return to prepregnancy levels until 25–30 weeks' gestation. In these women, the total energy cost of pregnancy may be as little as 1000 kcal, although this is associated with low birthweight.

Weight gain in pregnancy is usually in the range of 10–12 kg. It comprises increases in maternal body water, fat and other tissues. At term, 40% of the weight gained is in the fetus, amniotic fluid, placenta and uterus (Fig. 6.1). The rate of weight gain is fairly steady throughout pregnancy and in the last trimester the mean is about 0.4 kg/week. The total gained during pregnancy is slightly greater in younger women, and possibly in primigravidae than in multigravidae, but the difference is not large enough to affect the clinical significance of weekly weight gain. Overall weight gain has a positive association with birthweight. There may be a fall in weight during the first trimester because of nausea and vomiting, but this is usually made up quickly from about 15 weeks. While the physiology of early morning sickness is uncertain, it is associated with a satisfactory outcome for the pregnancy. One reason for this is that restriction of calorie intake in early pregnancy leads to increased growth of the placenta, perhaps in compensation. Restoration of calorie intake in the second and third trimesters (as happened in a large cohort of women in the Dutch famine of the 1940s) leads to an overall increase in birthweight, presumably because the larger placenta is more efficient. Those who report vomiting to their doctor are less likely to miscarry or have a preterm or stillborn child. Other common reasons for failure to gain weight in physiological amounts are dieting, vomiting due to oesophageal reflux, or diarrhoea. Excessive weight gain is sometimes a consequence of reducing or stopping smoking.

Fat deposition accounts for about 3.5 kg of weight gain. Fat accumulates in the abdominal wall, upper back, hips and thighs. Fat deposition is most rapid between 20 and 30 weeks and is possibly less in those who have generalised oedema. In well-nourished women, maternal body fat near term does not contribute significantly to the baby's birthweight. The other tissues that contribute to weight gain are shown in Figure 6.1.

Pregnancy is hyperlipidaemic and glucosuric. These physiological changes in lipid and carbohydrate metabolism are accompanied by related alterations in amino acids. Together they increase the availability of glucose for the fetus (its preferred source of energy) while the mother utilises lipids. These metabolic modifications start soon after conception and increase to become most marked in the second half of pregnancy, coinciding with increasing fetal requirements for growth. The uterus and placenta also require carbohydrate, fat and amino acids for their metabolic activity as well as for their growth in size.

Carbohydrates and insulin resistance

By 6–12 weeks' gestation, fasting plasma glucose concentrations have fallen by 0.11 mmol/l, and by the end of the first trimester the increase in blood glucose following a carbohydrate load is less than in the non-pregnant state (Fig. 6.2; Lind et al 1973). This increased sensitivity stimulates glycogen synthesis and storage, deposition of fat and transport of amino acids into cells. It also produces a fall in glycosylated haemoglobin which, because glycosylation takes some weeks, does not occur until early in the middle trimester but then is maintained until term: the reduction is from 7.4% of haemoglobin in early pregnancy to 6.6% at term. There does not appear to be any alteration in the absorption of glucose from the gut or in the half-life of insulin, and the insulin response is well maintained (Fig. 6.3).

After mid-pregnancy, resistance to the action of insulin

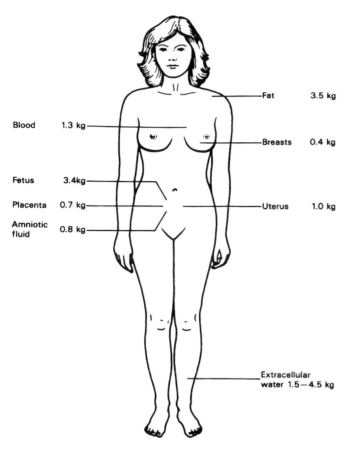

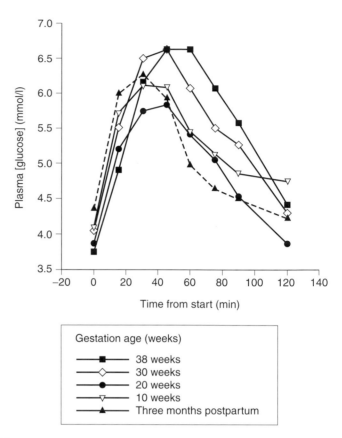

Fig. 6.1 The tissues that form the major part of weight gain in pregnancy (after Hytten 1980). There is considerable variation: the range in normal pregnancy is from 0 to 23 kg. Mean weight gain in primigravidae is 12.5 kg.

Fig. 6.2 Mean plasma glucose concentrations in 19 women before and after the ingestion of 50 g glucose after an overnight fast. Note the differences in response from early pregnancy, with a decreased peak during the first half of pregnancy and increased peak thereafter. Note also the increase in the area under the curve as pregnancy progresses. (Data from Lind et al 1973.)

develops progressively and plasma glucose concentrations rise. A carbohydrate load at this time results in a higher rise in plasma insulin than earlier, to three to four times the prepregnant level (Fig. 6.4). The plasma glucose concentration also rises to higher levels than before 20 weeks and the rise lasts for longer: the peak of a glucose tolerance test is then at 60 rather 30 minutes and the return to fasting levels is delayed (Fig. 6.2).

Since glucose readily crosses the placenta by facilitated diffusion, and the fetus utilises glucose as its primary energy substrate, this rise in maternal concentration is presumably beneficial to the fetus. During the third trimester of a normal pregnancy, there is a significant decrease of umbilical venous glucose concentration and a significant increase of the maternal–fetal glucose concentration difference. A significant correlation between fetal and maternal glucose concentrations is also apparent. Despite the high and prolonged rises in postprandial plasma glucose, the fasting level in late pregnancy remains below the non-pregnant even though the basal endogenous glucose production rises by 30% during pregnancy. Fasting plasma insulin levels reach their maximum at around 32 weeks but the decrease in sensitivity to its action persists until delivery. This reduces maternal utilisation of glucose and induces glycogenolysis and gluconeogen-

esis as well as the utilisation of lipids as energy sources. One consequence of these changes is the potential for the rapid development of ketosis by the pregnant woman, especially during the hard work of labour. Pre-eclampsia is associated with even more pronounced insulin resistance, which persists until at least the third month postpartum (Kaaja et al 1999). Whether the insulin resistance may indeed antedate the pregnancy, and predispose to the development of pre-eclampsia, has yet to be determined.

Insulin resistance can be caused by decreased insulin sensitivity, decreased insulin responsiveness, or both. Factors acting at the pre-receptor level could reduce free insulin concentration, at receptor level there could be decreases in affinity or receptor density, while at the post-receptor level there might be changes in how the hormone–receptor complex functions or in the final response. The insulin secretory capacity appears to be unaltered, as is its half-life; there might be reduced gastrointestinal potentiation of insulin secretion in late pregnancy. Adipocytes seem to be highly reflective of changes in insulin action *in vivo* and have therefore been used to study insulin receptors. The density of high-affinity insulin receptors is decreased by about two-thirds in normal term pregnancy, but their kinase activity is unaltered. They do, however, show a threefold decrease in insulin sensitivity

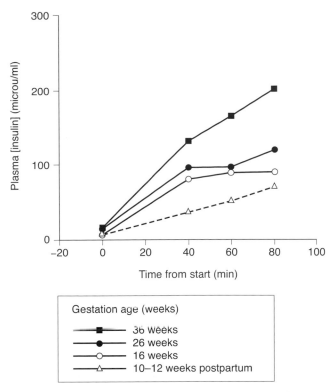

Fig. 6.3 Maternal plasma glucose concentrations were held at approximately 11 mmol/l for up to 80 min in 10 women at different stages of gestation and 3 months postpartum. Their basal plasma glucose concentrations were: 4.8 mmol/l postpartum and 4.1, 4.3 and 4.5 mmol/l at 16, 26 and 36 weeks' gestation. The stimulus evoked a progressively greater insulin response, showing that the insulin secretory capacity itself is well maintained during pregnancy. (Data from Lind et al 1973.)

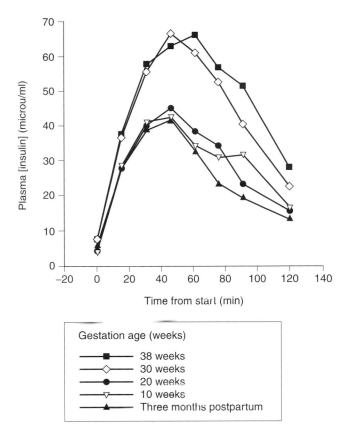

Fig. 6.4 Mean plasma insulin concentrations in 19 women before and after the ingestion of 50 g glucose after an overnight fast. There is a progressive rise in insulin response during gestation, and the area under the curve increases. (Data from Lind et al 1973.)

for glucose transport. Glucose transport into adipocytes and skeletal muscle is the function of two related glucose transport proteins: GLUT1 and GLUT4. GLUT4 is insulin responsive, so reduced expression, increased degradation or defects in activity might contribute to the insulin resistance of pregnancy, as has been identified outside pregnancy. GLUT4 protein concentrations in the adipose tissue of pregnant women have indeed been reported to be significantly lower than those in non-pregnant women.

The resistance to the action of insulin is presumably largely endocrine driven. Plasma cortisol rises in pregnancy since oestrogen increases cortisol binding globulin synthesis, which in turn stimulates adrenal cortisol synthesis. A positive correlation has been demonstrated between the increase of plasma cortisol concentrations during normal pregnancy and the concomitant decrease in glucose tolerance. However, there is no correlation between the rise in cortisol and the changes in insulin and glucagon response to glucose in pregnancy. In non-pregnant women, unlike men, plasma aldosterone correlates directly with visceral adipose tissue mass and inversely with insulin sensitivity. These associations are independent of plasma renin activity. Both plasma renin and aldosterone rise markedly in pregnancy, and a dissociation between plasma aldosterone and renin is well documented at

this time (see below). The mechanism for an effect of aldosterone on insulin responsiveness is unclear, and this may simply be an epiphenomenon. Neither glucagon nor the catecholamines, which can influence insulin resistance outside pregnancy, rise significantly in pregnancy. Leptin has been implicated in altered insulin sensitivity outside pregnancy, but appears not to play a role during gestation. Growth hormone concentrations are also unaltered or even decreased, but human placental lactogen (hPL) is present in high concentration. It is likely that this contributes to the reduced maternal peripheral insulin sensitivity. It has been shown to stimulate insulin release and inhibit glucose uptake. However, hPL did not enhance lipolysis in adipocytes from pregnant women. The increased levels of oestrogen and progesterone may also be involved, since progesterone increases the level of serum insulin without altering the concentration of glucose.

Ethnicity or diet, or both, may be relevant. Vegetarian Hindu Indians have lower serum hPL and higher serum glucose than Europeans. Well-nourished African women have the same increase in insulin sensitivity as Europeans early in pregnancy but do not develop insulin resistance in the second half of pregnancy. While there may be inherent metabolic differences between races, diet is also relevant. The increase in plasma glucose following a glucose load is reduced by regular consumption of the vegetable karela (bitter gourd) which is eaten by many Indians. If the carbohydrate intake is restricted to pulses, the postprandial rise in blood sugar is less than that which follows the ingestion of bread, pasta or similar foods. Obesity in any ethnic group is relevant; fasting insulin is raised, insulin response is greater and glucose disposal is slower in the overweight.

Amino acids

Amino acids are required by both mother and fetus for growth and for energy. The amino acid levels rise following a meal but not so much as in the non-pregnant and for a shorter time. The plasma concentration of most amino acids falls during pregnancy. This starts in the second half of the menstrual cycle and continues into the pregnancy and until the third trimester. The decrease is greater than that produced by physiological haemodilution. It is most marked in the gluconeogenic amino acids such as alanine. In part this may result from transport across the placenta; also, increased insulin response during pregnancy may accelerate the uptake of amino acids by the mother for gluconeogenesis. There is also loss from the kidneys (see The renal system, p. 83).

Pregnancy is an anabolic state so urea synthesis is reduced, possibly because of decreased hepatic extraction of circulating amino acids. The protein breakdown that occurs with fasting is reduced. The concentrations of proteins in the maternal serum fall markedly: by 20 weeks the total protein concentration has fallen from 7.0 g to 6.0 g per 100 ml. Most of this is from the fall in serum albumin.

Lipids

The increase in circulating lipids is one of the most striking metabolic changes of pregnancy. In a normal pregnancy there is an approximate threefold increase in triglycerides and fatty acids and a 50% increase in LDL cholesterol. HDL cholesterol is also increased. The increase in triglycerides and VLDL cholesterol is positively correlated with the mother's body mass index—weight (kg) divided by height^2 (m) (Knopp et al 1982). It is related to gravidity but not to maternal age. Plasma concentrations tend to underestimate the magnitude of the total increase because of the increase in plasma volume during pregnancy. As with glucose and amino acids, there is loss from the maternal circulation into and across the placenta so the changes in intermediate metabolism are more complex than simple alterations in plasma levels. There are different patterns of increase; some lipid levels rise to three or four times the prepregnant level, some hardly at all; some peak by mid-pregnancy and some not until 36 weeks. After delivery the plasma levels return to normal, but this may take 6 months for some lipids and is affected by whether or not the mother breast-feeds and by the use of oral contraceptives.

Fat is deposited early in pregnancy but from mid-pregnancy it is used as a source of energy, mainly by the mother so that glucose is available for the growing fetus. The absorption of fat from the intestine is not directly altered during pregnancy but the reduction in intestinal motility may allow more time for the absorption of fat. The enterohepatic circulation is reduced with increased excretion of cholesterol in the bile. These changes are controlled by the balance of maternal hormones.

Leptin is a hormone of molecular weight ~16 000 kDa. It is a long-chain helical cytokine with structural similarities with the interleukins. In the non-pregnant state, the *ob* gene, which codes for leptin, is only expressed in white adipose tissue, where its expression is stimulated by insulin and glucocorticoids. The leptin receptor is present in the hypothalamus, where it appears to react with neuropeptide Y, and in peripheral tissues. Leptin acts as a sensor alerting the brain to the extent of body fat stores (Tritos & Mantzoros 1997). In pregnancy, the cytotrophoblast can express both leptin and leptin receptor from early gestation; such expression appears to be regulated by a placenta-specific upstream enhancer. 17β-oestradiol stimulates placental leptin synthesis *in vitro*. It has been speculated that placental leptin may have angiogenic and immunomodulatory activities, which affect the placenta in an autocrine or paracrine manner. Placental leptin expression continues to rise in late pregnancy. Maternal plasma leptin concentrations rise some threefold during pregnancy, and are correlated with body mass index and mid-arm circumference. They fall early in the puerperium, but remain considerably raised during lactation. It is assumed that the increased plasma concentrations may have a role in regulating maternal energy balance.

The increased insulin sensitivity of early pregnancy increases the activity of lipoprotein lipase (LPL) so fat is deposited. As insulin secretion increases and resistance develops, however, fat mobilisation is activated through increased tissue lipase and maintained by oestriol, oestradiol, progesterone and hPL, but not by human chorionic gonadotrophin (hCG). Although general lipoprotein lipase activity decreases after mid-pregnancy the LPL concentrations in the uterus and in the placenta increase, as they do in the mammary tissue. Part of the increase in VLDL during pregnancy may be a consequence of the reduction in hepatic lipase and LPL so that clearance of VLDL is reduced although the hypertriglyceridaemia is principally caused by increased entry of triglyceride-rich lipoprotein into the circulation (Knopp et al 1982).

Total plasma cholesterol falls by 5% early in pregnancy, reaching its lowest point at 6–8 weeks. There is considerable individual variation in this, as in all lipid changes in pregnancy. Following the initial fall there is a progressive rise to term (Fig. 6.5). Total cholesterol increases by 24–206%; in VLDL it is raised by 36% and in LDL by 50–90%. HDL cholesterol is raised by 10–23% at term, having risen to 30% in mid-gestation and then fallen. Triglyceride concentrations are raised by 90–570% at term (Darmady & Postle 1982, Knopp et al 1982). The increase in triglyceride is mainly in VLDL and LDL; HDL triglyceride rises by a third at the end of the second trimester, the rise then stops and the accompanying rise in HDL cholesterol is reversed although HDL protein is not reduced. The fall in HDL is in HDL 2 and not in HDL 3 since it is HDL 3 which accepts free cholesterol from cells. This cholesterol is esterified and transferred into the core of the particle which increases its content of lipids so that it is transformed into HDL 2. The level of HDL 2 indicates the flux of cholesterol through HDL 3. This requires the enzyme LCAT and apoprotein A I; apoprotein A II modulates the reaction.

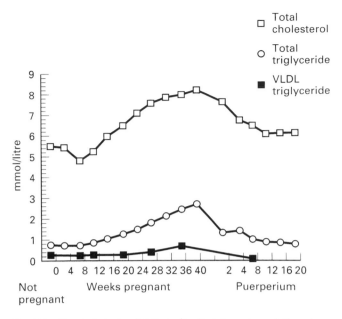

Fig. 6.5 Total cholesterol falls in the first 8 weeks and then rises progressively to term. Triglycerides do not show the initial fall but rise progressively to term. (After Darmady & Postle 1982, Knopp et al 1982.)

Apoprotein A I levels rise during pregnancy; those of apo II do not. LCAT activity increases during pregnancy; that of apo II does not. The increase in LCAT activity is only by 20–25%; this occurs in the last trimester of pregnancy coinciding with the maximal increase of triglyceride and VLDL levels and the decline in HDL. The esterification of cholesterol continuously decreases from the 14th until the 28th week, accompanying the rise in cholesterol and LDL. These changes may be the result of an increased turnover of cholesterol and VLDL with reduction in removal of cholesterol from lipoprotein, giving an increased supply of cholesterol to most tissues. The fall in HDL 2 from 28 weeks coincides with a steep rise in VLDL (Fahraeus et al 1985). Plasma fasting triglycerides peak at 36 weeks, at this point being 2–4 times the non-pregnancy level. The VLDL content of triglyceride cholesterol also peaks at 36 weeks. Steroid production by the placenta in late pregnancy may be 500 mg or more in 24 hours, which is equivalent to 50% of the daily synthesis of steroids in the non-pregnant so that demand for cholesterol may then exceed supply and account for the fall in late pregnancy. An additional factor in this fall may be the increasing LPL activity in the uterus and in the mammary tissues at that time.

The hyperlipidaemia of normal pregnancy is not atherogenic, even though lipid levels move well into the zone which would cause anxiety in the non-pregnant, because the pattern of increase is not that of atherogenesis. Although lipoprotein A increases until 22 weeks it then falls steadily until it reaches non-pregnant levels at term. Apoprotein A I rises but A II does not change, apoprotein B does rise but proportionately less than apoprotein A I or HDL 3, LDL is rich in triglyceride but poor in apoprotein: these are different from atherogenic alterations in lipids. Pregnancy may, however, unmask pathological hyperlipidaemia. The lipid changes of pregnancy may be exaggerated in women with pre-existing hypercholesterolaemia, even when they are on an appropriate diet. Diet during pregnancy does not affect the increase in lipid but there are ethnic variables. Lipid concentrations are lower in black North Americans (and other non-White ethnic groups) than in White North Americans.

Birthweight, placental weight and maternal weight gain are directly related to VLDL and triglyceride levels at the end of pregnancy and inversely to apoprotein A I and A II. Birthweight is negatively correlated with the levels of triglycerides in the umbilical vein. Cord blood lipids are one-half or one-quarter of maternal levels. The umbilical venous levels of cholesterol, triglycerides, HDL cholesterol and apoprotein A I are all higher than those in the umbilical artery.

After delivery, plasma free fatty acids fall to non-pregnant levels within 3 days but LDL and apoprotein B are still raised at 20 weeks. Total triglycerides begin to fall within 2 weeks and continue to do so. There is great variation in the time taken for triglycerides to return to non-pregnant levels, part of this depending on whether or not the mother is lactating. In those who are lactating the fall takes about 6 weeks, whereas it takes around 18 weeks in those who never established lactation (Darmady & Postle 1982). Prolactin is relevant to this since it increases mammary LPL activity so that, along with intrinsic synthesis of fatty acids, the mother can secrete 250–400 calories per day into the milk as lipids. HDL cholesterol too is significantly higher in lactating mothers. Total cholesterol is raised after delivery in all mothers; unlike the rise during pregnancy it can be reduced by dieting. The fractional rate of removal of cholesterol from lipoproteins by CETP and LCAT rises and is still above prepregnant values at 8 weeks. The slow fall in LDL may be a consequence of low oestradiol levels in the puerperium, VLDL being converted to LDL. As with the increase in pregnancy, the variation in return to prepregnant levels is not only between individuals but also between individual lipids.

Lipid peroxidation and free radicals

Lipids undergo peroxidation in all tissues as part of normal cellular function. Lipid peroxides are significant because their uncontrolled production can result in oxidative stress, with considerable damage to the integrity of the cell membrane. The site of the process is the cell membrane, where polyunsaturated fats are peroxidised. This occurs during the synthesis of prostacyclin, thromboxane and other metabolites. In physiological amounts these stimulate cyclo-oxygenase, but in excess they inhibit both this enzyme and prostacyclin synthase so that prostacyclin synthesis is reduced. Thromboxane synthase, however, is not affected by the excess of lipid peroxides. The damage to cell membranes occurs both locally and at a distance because plasma lipoprotein may also undergo peroxidation and be transported to vulnerable tissues within the brief half-life (a few minutes) of the peroxides. Such damaging effects of free radical activity are countered by vitamin E which is a free radical scavenger and by such antioxidants as superoxide dismutase, glucose 6-phosphate-dehydrogenase, glutathione peroxidase, ceruloplasmin and glutathione transferase. Plasma proteins and uric acid also buffer free radicals.

During normal pregnancy, increases in plasma lipid peroxides appear by the second trimester in step with the general rise in lipids and may taper off later in gestation. As the peroxide levels rise so do those of vitamin E and some other antioxidants: this rise is proportionately greater than that of peroxides so physiological activities are protected (Wang et al 1991). However, levels of β-carotene and retinol fall during pregnancy. Vitamin A, the carotenoids and provitamin A carotenoids are effective antioxidants, especially in conditions of low Pao_2, such as are found in the placenta. Lipid peroxidation is active in the placenta also, increasing with gestation; there too antioxidant defences are required to protect both mother and fetus from free radical activity since the placenta contains high concentrations of unsaturated fats.

THE CARDIOVASCULAR SYSTEM

Many of the cardiovascular adaptations to normal pregnancy are initiated in the luteal phase of every ovulatory cycle and are then maintained and amplified should conception occur. They are thus proactive and not reactive. For example, prospective studies of ovulatory cycles show significant falls in mean arterial pressure and total peripheral resistance in the mid-luteal phase, with increased heart rate, cardiac output, renal plasma flow and glomerular filtration rate (Davison & Noble 1981, Chapman et al 1997). The renin–angiotensin system (RAS) is also activated. These changes are all amplified should conception occur.

The total peripheral resistance falls significantly by at least 6 weeks' gestational age (Robson et al 1989, Duvekot et al 1993, Chapman et al 1998) and reaches a nadir 40% below non-pregnant values by mid-gestation. This very early effect may be caused by an increase in circulating vasodilators such as prostacyclin or kallikrein, the urinary excretion of which is markedly raised by the end of the first trimester. A recent prospective study during the menstrual cycle and first trimester (Fig. 6.6) suggests, however, that most of the rise of prostacyclin above non-pregnant concentrations is achieved during the second, rather than the first, half of the first trimester. Similarly, neither oestrogens nor progesterone rise above luteal phase levels until later in the first trimester. A withdrawal of sympathetic tone seems unlikely, given the marked effect of ganglion blockade on the blood pressure later in pregnancy.

Table 6.1 summarises some of the major cardiovascular changes seen during normal pregnancy. If the first cardiovascular response to pregnancy is the fall in vascular resistance, such a decrease in afterload would be perceived as a relative circulatory underfilling, associated with a fall in arterial blood pressure and increase in heart rate and stroke volume. The heart rate rises first, being significantly raised by 5 weeks' amenorrhoea (Duvekot et al 1993). The cardiac output would therefore be expected to rise, which it does (Fig. 6.7). There is also a small increase in myocardial contractility in pregnancy. Most of the pregnancy-associated rise in cardiac output occurs during the first trimester (Duvekot et al 1993, Chapman et al 1998). Cardiac output rises by about

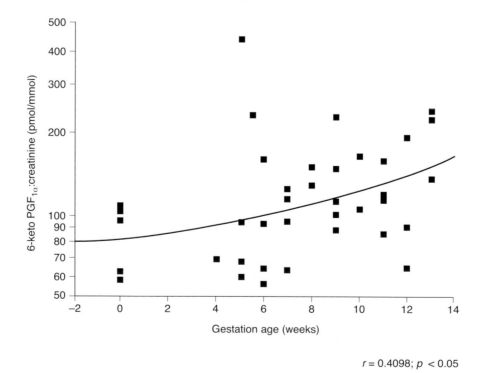

$r = 0.4098$; $p < 0.05$

Fig. 6.6 The urinary prostaglandin 6-keto $F_{1\alpha}$: creatinine ratio was determined prospectively during the follicular phase of the menstrual cycle and at least five times during the first trimester of pregnancy in six primigravid women. The ratio rose significantly over this time. (From Al Kadi 2001.)

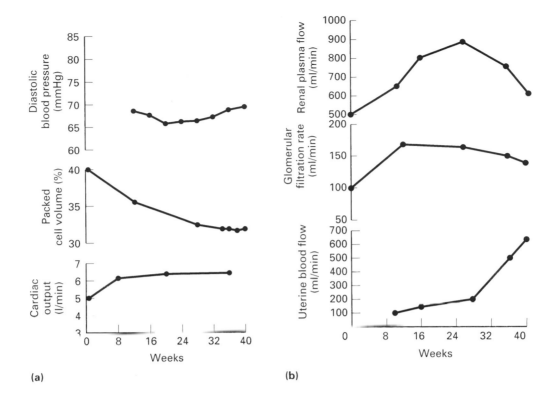

Fig. 6.7 (a) *Cardiac output* is related to body size so there is wide variation at the beginning of pregnancy but in the average woman it is 5 l/min. During pregnancy cardiac output increases by 1.5–3 l/min, most of this occurring in the first trimester. Changes in cardiac output are independent of changes in blood volume (Rovinsky & Jaffin 1965).
Packed cell volume: with haemodilution the packed cell volume decreases progressively in normal pregnancy until around 34 weeks, and then rises slightly. If the woman takes oral iron during the pregnancy the packed cell volume is 0.5–3% higher.
Diastolic blood pressure falls early in pregnancy, the lowest levels being at 16–20 weeks, then rising to term. The values shown here are for multigravid women with singleton pregnancies: in primigravid mothers mean diastolic pressure is 1–3 mmHg higher at all gestational ages (Christianson 1976). Systolic pressure shows a similar pattern but the later increase is less.
(b) *Uterine blood flow* is 12–15 ml/100 g conceptus throughout pregnancy. As the myometrium and its contents enlarge, total flow increases. Intervillous flow near term is 65–120 ml/100 g placenta/min.
Glomerular filtration rate and renal plasma flow: both increase during pregnancy but while the glomerular filtration rate remains raised for the whole of the pregnancy, renal plasma flow falls in the third trimester.

Table 6.1 Percentage change in some cardiovascular variables during pregnancy. Data are derived from studies in which pre-conception values were determined. The mean values shown are those at the end of each trimester, and are thus not necessarily the maxima. Note that most changes are near maximal by the end of the first trimester. (Data from Robson et al 1989, 1991.)

	First trimester	Second trimester	Third trimester
Heart rate (bpm)	+11	+13	+16
Stroke volume (ml)	+31	+29	+27
Cardiac output (l/min)	+45	+47	+48
Systolic BP (mmHg)	−1	+1	+6
Diastolic BP (mmHg)	−6	−3	+7
MPAP (mmHg)	+5	+5	+5
Total peripheral resistance (resistance units)	−27	−27	−29

BP, systemic blood pressure; MPAP, mean pulmonary artery pressure.

50% from a baseline of ~5 l/min, and reaches a plateau during the third trimester. Established labour may increase it by a further 2 l/min, partly because of the blood expressed from the uterus during each contraction. The very early fall in plasma osmolality presumably indicates water retention, in an attempt to rectify the sensed hypovolaemia. The early activation of the renin–angiotensin system (RAS), which is one of the first hormone systems to recognise pregnancy, is presumably also a response to this stimulus, as well as to the direct natriuretic effect of progesterone. The normal pregnant woman is protected from the potential pressor effects of the raised circulating angiotensin II concentrations by a specific fall in pressor sensitivity to the hormone, which is established by 10 weeks' gestation.

The plasma volume has increased significantly by 6 weeks' gestation (Chapman et al 1998), and by the late third trimester has increased from its baseline 2600 ml by about 50% in a first pregnancy and 60% in a second or subsequent pregnancy. It is greater in multiple than in single pregnancies, and in women who exercise regularly. Pregnancy outcome correlates with the degree of plasma volume expansion. The bigger the expansion, the bigger, on average, the birthweight of the baby. Conversely, the expansion is relatively less when pregnancy is complicated by pre-eclampsia or (normotensive) intrauterine fetal growth restriction or in women who habitually abort. Measurements made in pre-eclampsia must be viewed with some caution; the Evans Blue dye is usually used to measure plasma volume in pregnancy, to avoid using radioisotopes, and the vasculature in pre-eclampsia is more leaky than in normal pregnancy. The matter of whether this reduced plasma volume is primary or secondary has recently been advanced by the demonstration by van Beek et al (1998) that primiparous women who had developed pre-eclampsia during their pregnancy still had relatively contracted plasma volumes by comparison with parous women who had remained normotensive. The total extracellular fluid volume rises by about 16% by term; the percentage rise in plasma volume is thus disproportionate to the whole. The plasma volume: interstitial volume ratio therefore rises in normal pregnancy but the relative contraction of plasma volume in pre-eclampsia, in the presence of a maintained total extracellular fluid volume, reverses this rise, and the ratio is then lower than in non-pregnant women. Factors that may drive this increase in plasma volume are discussed below (see Renal function).

The heart rate (HR) variability falls in normal pregnancy (Blake et al 2000) because of an increase of 10–15 beats/min in the resting baseline rate (variability falls with increasing rate in both the pregnant and non-pregnant). The baroreflex sensitivity, the linkage between changing arterial pressure and HR, has not been intensively studied in pregnancy, and there are conflicts between earlier data and later ones using more sophisticated measurement techniques. Recent studies using cross-spectral analysis and non-invasive blood pressure monitoring have reported a decrease in baroreflex sensitivity from the second trimester of normal pregnancy, and in the third trimester, by comparison with non-pregnant women or the same subjects postpartum. The changing cardiovascular response to head-up tilt as pregnancy progresses also suggests a fall in baroreflex sensitivity.

The heart is rotated forwards and pushed upwards as the diaphragm rises, so that the apex beat appears in the fourth, rather than the fifth, intercostal space. Its volume increases by about 12% which seems to result from the rise in venous filling, rather than from hypertrophy. Systolic ejection murmurs are common from mid-pregnancy, even in healthy primigravidae. The positional changes of the heart are associated with changes in the electrocardiogram, with a leftward deviation in the electrical axis, low-voltage QRS complexes, and a flattened or even inverted T wave in lead III such as is seen in ischaemic heart disease.

The measurement of the systemic arterial blood pressure in pregnancy is fraught with problems. Mercury sphygmomanometry is an imprecise and frequently inaccurate way of measuring a notoriously variable parameter. In pregnancy, it overestimates both systolic and diastolic pressure, by about 7 and 12 mmHg respectively. A perception that Korotkoff Phase V (disappearance) may be less reliable in pregnancy has been increasingly questioned over the last decade, and a number of carefully controlled studies have now led to the recommendation that Phase V be routinely used in pregnancy (de Swiet & Shennan 1996). Oscillometric monitors remove variability due to observer error, but the suitability of any particular type for use in pregnancy must be validated. Ambulatory blood pressure monitoring has a place in the management of the women believed to be at risk of developing pregnancy-associated hypertension but requires considerable investment in equipment and training. It should be remembered that ambulatory blood pressure monitoring gives lower readings than those obtained by conventional methods. Whichever method of measuring blood pressure is used, it is important that a standardised technique be used, with an appropriately-sized cuff at the level of the left atrium. Reference levels for normality should be appropriate both to the technique used to measure the blood pressure, and to the circumstances in which the blood pressure is measured.

However measured, there is a small fall in systolic, and a greater fall in diastolic blood pressure during the first half of pregnancy (Fig. 6.7), resulting in an increased pulse pressure. In normotensive pregnancy, there is a pronounced circadian rhythm of both systolic and diastolic pressure, with the nadir at around 4 am (Ayala et al 1997). Interestingly, women who go on to develop pregnancy-related hypertension show significantly greater changes in amplitude of this circadian rhythm, even in the first trimester (Ayala et al 1997). It is important that the blood pressure be recorded at the first antenatal clinic visit to give a baseline against which any subsequent change can be assessed. The blood pressure rises steadily during the second half of gestation, in both normal and future hypertensive women. Even in normotensive women, there is some overshoot of non-pregnant values by late gestation. In late gestation, the blood pressure falls by an average of 10% in some two-thirds of women, and by 30–50% in about one woman in 12 (the supine hypotensive syndrome) when the woman lies supine; this is presumed to be caused by compression of the inferior vena cava, and perhaps the aorta, by the pregnant uterus. There is a protective mechanism in the collateral venous return to the heart via the paravertebral and azygos vessels, and to some venous return from the uterus via the ovarian veins.

Changes in venous pressure occur in the lower circulation because of the mechanical pressure of the uterus on the iliac veins and the inferior vena cava and the hydrodynamic effects of venous return from the uterus. In late gestation, the pressure of the fetal head also contributes. The venous pressure in the legs rises from around 9 cm H_2O in early pregnancy to some 24 cm H_2O by term. The combination of increased distensibility (see below) and pressure predisposes the pregnant woman to the development of varicose veins in her legs, vulva, rectum and pelvis. Owing to the anatomy of the vascular system, the effect is greater in the left leg than in the right, probably accounting for the fact that 80% of venous thromboses in pregnancy occur in the left leg. The pulmonary circulation is able to absorb high rates of flow without an increase in pressure; it is, therefore, not surprising that pressure in the right ventricle, and the pulmonary arteries and capillaries, does not change during pregnancy. Pulmonary resistance, like systemic resistance, falls in early pregnancy, and does not change thereafter.

There is progressive venodilatation throughout a normal pregnancy. There are increases in both venous distensibility and capacitance to accommodate the increased flow on the venous side. The forearm blood flow rises by up to 30% in normal pregnancy (Anumba et al 1999). In non-pregnant women, venous capacitance is greater in the leg than in the forearm, but in pregnancy this difference is lost, presumably because of the haemodynamic effect of the gravid uterus. The local generation of nitric oxide may be involved; there is increased nitric oxide activity in the veins of the dorsum of the hand in pregnancy. Blood flow itself is a major regulator of endothelial nitric oxide synthesis, and it has been shown that nitric oxide responses to flow are enhanced in small arteries from fat biopsies in healthy pregnant women by comparison with those from non-pregnant subjects. The forearm vascular response to nitric oxide synthase inhibition is also enhanced in normal pregnancy by comparison with non-pregnant women, again suggesting a role for nitric oxide in the vasodilatation of pregnancy (Anumba et al 1999).

THE RESPIRATORY SYSTEM

The investigation of the respiratory system by currently available methods is not entirely satisfactory, and some of the published data are contradictory. It appears that the vital capacity is only a little increased in pregnancy, but tidal volume rises by ~40% from ~500 to ~700 ml. Inspiratory capacity increases by about 300 ml. There is therefore a fall in expiratory reserve and in the residual volume, which falls by ~20%. The shape of the chest changes during pregnancy as the lower ribs flare out and the subcostal angle widens dramatically. The diaphragm rises, and breathing in pregnancy is probably more diaphragmatic in nature. Neither FEV_1 nor peak expiratory flow rate is affected by pregnancy, even in women with asthma. This is probably because progesterone relaxes smooth muscle and there are increased concentrations of PGE_1 and prostacyclin, which are bronchodilators, offsetting the effects of the reduction in total lung capacity and the potentially bronchoconstrictor effects of increased $PGF_{2\alpha}$.

There is an increase in oxygen consumption of between 30 and 40 ml/min by late pregnancy, from a baseline level of around 220 ml/min. This is partitioned between the mother (extra cardiac, renal and respiratory work and uterine and breast development) and the feto-placental unit, the latter, of course, making up a progressively greater proportion as pregnancy progresses. Both the cardiac and renal increments stabilise early in gestation, as their maximal adaptation to pregnancy occurs then. The overall increment is only about 15% at term, and since the increase in oxygen-carrying capacity of the blood (see Haematology) is some 18%, there is actually a fall in arterio-venous oxygen difference. Pulmonary blood flow, of course, rises in parallel with cardiac output; this will of itself enhance gas transfer. In early pregnancy, the minute ventilation rises by about 30%, with a slower rise to a maximum of 40–50% above non-pregnant values by term. This is achieved by the rise in tidal volume, rather than respiratory rate. The rise is largely driven by progesterone which appears to sensitise the medulla oblongata to carbon dioxide, but the reduced plasma osmolality and increased circulating levels of angiotensin II and vasopressin have also been suggested as being implicated.

Another contribution to the lowered Pco_2 may be the stimulatory effect of progesterone on carbonic anhydrase, which facilitates carbon dioxide transfer. These hormones increase from very early pregnancy and relative overbreathing also begins early, washing out carbon dioxide from the lungs. The Pco_2 is at its lowest in early gestation, another example of the generally proactive nature of adaptations to pregnancy. Indeed, similar changes are seen in every menstrual cycle. By term, when the carbon dioxide load has risen because of the fetal contribution, the Pco_2 has risen to about 30 mmHg (4 kPa), by comparison with 35–40 mmHg (4.7–5.3 kPa) in the non-pregnant woman. The rise in sensitivity to CO_2 is very marked: a 1 mmHg rise results in a rise in ventilation of about 1.5 l/min in the non-pregnant woman, but some 6 l/min during pregnancy.

Anaesthesia is affected by these physiological changes. If the normally hyperventilating pregnant woman hypoventilates under general anaesthesia, she requires less inhalational agents than are required by a woman who is not pregnant. The cardiovascular and respiratory changes of pregnancy do not have deleterious effects during air travel.

The fall in maternal Pco_2 allows more efficient placental transfer of carbon dioxide from the fetus, which has a Pco_2 of around 55 mmHg (7.3 kPa). It is also, however, one of the pregnancy adaptations with cost to the mother, since she may experience dyspnoea, giddiness and nausea (Garcia-Rio et al 1996). Indeed, it appears that women who have a relatively high Pco_2 outside pregnancy may be particularly susceptible to dyspnoea when pregnant, and especially when taking exercise (Garcia-Rio et al 1996). It has been suggested that regular moderate physical exercise (to a heart rate of around 145–150 beats/min) during mid to late pregnancy reduces both ventilatory demand and respiratory perception of effort in late gestation. Associated with the fall in Pco_2 is a fall in plasma bicarbonate concentration (to around

18–22 mmol/l by comparison with 24–28 mmol/l) which contributes to the fall in plasma osmolality and plasma sodium concentration in the face of a requirement to conserve sodium (see Renal function). The fall in plasma bicarbonate also has some repercussions on peripheral venous pH, which rises slightly, from ~7.35 to ~7.38.

The increased alveolar ventilation results in a much smaller rise in P_{O_2} than the fall in P_{CO_2}, from around 96.7 to 101.8 mmHg (12.9–13.6 kPa). This increase is offset by the rightward shift of the maternal oxyhaemoglobin dissociation curve caused by an increase in 2,3-diphosphoglycerate (2,3-DPG) in the erythrocytes. This facilitates oxygen unloading to the fetus, which has both a much lower P_{O_2} (25–30 mmHg; 3.3–4.0 kPa) and a marked leftward shift of the oxyhaemoglobin dissociation curve because of the lower sensitivity of fetal haemoglobin to 2,3-DPG.

COMPOSITION OF THE THE BLOOD

Pro rata, the plasma volume increases considerably more than the red cell mass; this leads to a fall in the various measures which include the plasma volume, such as the packed cell volume (Fig. 6.7), the haemoglobin concentration and the red cell count. Since the cardiac output rises much more than the oxygen consumption, the arterio-venous oxygen difference is actually lower in pregnancy until about the last month, and in a normal pregnancy the oxygen-carrying capacity of the blood is entirely adequate. Indeed, a fall in packed cell volume from around 36% in early pregnancy to 32% in the third trimester is a sign of normal plasma volume expansion, while a static packed cell volume, or one that increases, is often a sinister sign. The circulating red cell mass increases by 20–30% during pregnancy, the size of the increase depending on whether or not oral iron is taken. It rises by about 240 ml in women with singleton pregnancies who do not take iron supplements (~17%) and by 400 ml in those who do (~29%) (Pritchard et al 1960). In women expecting twins the increase is about 680 ml and in triplets 900 ml. A recent meta-analysis, using the Cochrane database, found that among fertile women, only 20% have iron reserves of >500 mg, which is the required minimum during pregnancy, 40% have iron stores of 100–500 mg, and 40% have virtually no iron stores (Milman et al 1999). The median dietary iron intake is also below that recommended. The conclusion was that, in spite of concerns about unnecessary iron supplementation, there is a valid case for the routine measurement of serum ferritin at the first antenatal clinic visit, and supplementation where indicated. A recent careful study has confirmed that, for purposes of screening in pregnancy, serum ferritin is the best single indicator of iron storage. Serum iron falls, the absorption of iron from the gut rises and iron-binding capacity rises in a normal pregnancy, since there is increased synthesis of transferrin. Cellular iron uptake is facilitated by transferrin receptor (TfR)-mediated endocytosis, and, unless there is hyperplastic erythropoiesis, the serum TfR level is a sensitive parameter of early tissue iron deficiency. Interestingly, in early pregnancy, approximately 11% of women had serum TfR levels below the reference range, but serum TfR increased significantly from early to late pregnancy, even in women with persisting iron stores.

The rise in red cell mass results from an increase in both the number and size of the red cells, which have a normal 120-day lifespan. It is accompanied by an increase in the reticulocyte count to 2% or more. Among pregnant women not taking iron, red cell volume shows an increase from 82–85 to 87–88 fl, whereas in those taking such supplementation, with or without folic acid, it rises to 88–90 fl. These are mean changes, but by the third trimester some individuals may have red cells of 100 fl or more yet no abnormality in their bone marrow. A possible advantage of these large red cells would be better transport of oxygen and carbon dioxide. A disadvantage would be reduced deformability of the cells in the capillary circulation although the raised fibrinogen concentration in pregnancy may counteract this tendency. Erythrocyte deformability decreases significantly by the end of the first trimester, falling to about half of the non-pregnant value by 16 weeks and then returning to non-pregnant deformability by term. Deformability decreases still further in pre-eclampsia.

At the end of the first trimester, the red cell hydration is lower than in the non-pregnant woman, even though plasma osmolality is itself 10 mosmol/kg lower. However, red cell hydration increases thereafter, and by term is higher than in the non-pregnant. This suggests that the increased size of the red cells is unlikely, at least in early pregnancy, to be caused by the fall in plasma oncotic pressure leading to increased red cell uptake of water. It could be a result of release of relatively immature cells from the marrow, which tend to be large. The marrow is hyperplastic with an increase in immature erythroid precursors. The concentration of fetal haemoglobin (HbF) increases by 1–2% during pregnancy, because of an increase in the number of red cells containing HbF (which are also large). Iron is incorporated more quickly into red cells during pregnancy than in the non-pregnant woman.

The physiological mechanisms that produce the increase in circulating haemoglobin are not yet clear. Plasma erythropoietin rises by about 25% during pregnancy in iron-replete women, and by about 55% in women not taking iron supplementation, but the reticulocyte count increases and the iron stores decrease before this rise occurs. Human placental lactogen and other hormones which increase early in pregnancy probably have erythropoietic actions.

The 10 or more periods of menstruation which are suppressed contribute 250 mg of iron saved toward the cost of conception, but this does not balance the 300–500 mg required for the increase in maternal haemoglobin or the 500 mg required for fetus and placenta. This deficit could be compounded by a reduction in iron absorption and by the loss of folic acid and other nutrients in the urine. The renal clearance of folic acid doubles, and plasma folate falls to about half non-pregnant values by term, although red cell folate concentrations fall less markedly. Maternal stores of these are, however, usually adequate for normal adaptation to pregnancy. Some of these are quickly replenished after delivery, but it may take months for iron stores to return to normal. Frequent pregnancies can prevent this replenishment, especially if diet is inadequate; this may produce anaemia in multigravidae.

If the mother has a haemoglobinopathy, her haematological responses to pregnancy may be modified. Those with beta-thalassaemia trait have a smaller increase in their red cell mass because of the disorder of haemoglobin synthesis. This is not improved by iron supplementation unless there are other signs of iron deficiency.

Even relatively mild maternal anaemia (below 9 g/dl) is associated with increased placental:birthweight ratios and decreased birthweight. Severe anaemia in pregnancy is an important contributor to maternal and perinatal morbidity and mortality. In sub-Saharan Africa severe anaemia in pregnancy is very common, the main causes being iron and folate deficiency associated with several factors, of which malaria is one of the most important and also potentially one of the most susceptible to treatment. A trial in Kenya showed that intermittent treatment with the antimalarial sulfadoxine–pyrimethamine, given a couple of times during pregnancy when women attended for antenatal care, reduced severe anaemia in primigravidae by nearly 40% and halved the incidence of low birthweight. It has been suggested that, since malaria in pregnancy in endemic areas is usually asymptomatic and often associated with a negative peripheral blood film, the condition needs to be treated or prevented as a matter of routine in all women at risk of infection.

The white cells do not show a uniform pattern of change during pregnancy. The total white cell count rises in pregnancy. Neutrophil numbers rise synchronously with the oestrogen peak of an ovulatory menstrual cycle and, if conception occurs, continue to rise to peak at about 33 weeks, after which their count stabilises. They reach a mean value of about $6.8 \times 10^9/1$, but there is a wide range and they may increase to $20 \times 10^9/1$ in normal pregnancy. The neutrophil number peaks during labour and in the early puerperium. Neutrophil metabolic activity increases, as does phagocytic function. The number of eosinophils, basophils, and monocytes in each millilitre of blood does not change significantly during pregnancy, but with the increase in circulating volume the total numbers of these cells are increased. Lymphocyte counts do not change but their function is suppressed. This renders the pregnant woman more susceptible to viral infections, malaria and leprosy.

Platelet count and platelet volume remain within the normal non-pregnant range in the majority of pregnancies even though platelet survival is reduced. In 8–10% of normal pregnancies, however, the platelet count falls below $150 \times 10^9/1$ without ill effects on the fetus or neonate (Burrows & Kelton 1990). This probably is a consequence of physiological increased fibrinolysis within the uteroplacental circulation to maintain blood flow. Platelet reactivity is increased in the second and third trimesters and does not return to normal until 12 weeks after delivery. Platelet α_2-adrenergic receptor number and affinity do not change in normal pregnancy.

Coagulation

Even normal pregnancy may be regarded as being a state of continuing low-grade coagulopathy. The topic is extensively reviewed in Chapter 20. Several of the potent procoagulatory factors rise from at least the end of the first trimester, some very markedly; for example, factors VII, VIII and X all rise,

and absolute plasma fibrinogen doubles, while antithrombin III, an inhibitor of coagulation, falls. The erythrocyte sedimentation rate rises early in pregnancy owing to the increase in fibrinogen and other physiological changes: 100 mm in an hour is not uncommon in normal pregnancy. Concentrations of the high-molecular-weight fibrin–fibrinogen complex rise. It seems likely that protein C, which inactivates factors V and VIII, is unchanged in pregnancy, but concentrations of protein S, one of its co-factors, fall during the first two trimesters. Plasma fibrinolytic activity is decreased during pregnancy and labour but returns to non-pregnant values within an hour of delivery of the placenta, suggesting strongly that the control of fibrinolysis during pregnancy is significantly affected by placentally derived mediators.

Table 6.2 summarises sequential changes in various coagulation and fibrinolytic variables throughout normal pregnancy.

Table 6.2 Percentage changes in some coagulation (upper) and fibrinolytic variables and fibronectin levels are expressed from postpartum data in the same women. The mean values shown are those at the end of each trimester, and are thus not necessarily the maxima. Note the very large rises in PAI-2 (placental type PAI) and TAT III complexes in the first trimester. (Data from Halligan et al 1994.)

	First trimester	Second trimester	Third trimester
PAI-1 (mg/ml)	−10	+68	+183
PAI-2 (mg/ml)	+732	+1804	+6554
t-PA (mg/ml)	−24	−19	+63
Protein C (% activity)	−12	+10	+9
AT III (% activity)	−21	−14	−10
TAT III	+362	+638	+785
Fibronectin (mg/l)	+3	−12	+53

PAI-1 and PAI-2, plasminogen activator inhibitors 1 and 2; t-PA, tissue plasminogen activator antigen; AT III, antithrombin III; TAT III, thrombin–antithrombin III complex.

THE RENAL SYSTEM

The kidneys increase in size in pregnancy since both vascular volume and interstitial space increase. By the third trimester, renal parenchymal volume has risen by about 70% and the kidneys are 1–2 cm longer and their weight 20% greater than in the non-pregnant state. There is marked dilatation of the calyces, renal pelvis and ureters in a majority of women, and there may be kinking of the ureters. These changes are more marked on the right side, and in parous than nulliparous women. They should not extend below the pelvic brim where it is crossed by the iliac artery. The dilatation probably results from a combination of hormonal factors and, in later gestation, from the effects of the enlarging uterus. The ureteric changes are not accompanied by a decrease in ureteric tone as was originally imagined. Indeed, there is increased tone in the upper ureter and hypertrophy of the smooth muscle, but the rate of urine flow does decrease. Bladder tone does, however, decrease, and its capacity increases. Ureteric reflux is uncommon in normal pregnancy since there is proliferation of Waldeyer's sheath around the ureter at its entry to the bladder. Vesico-ureteric reflux does, nevertheless, occur in up to 3% of women in late pregnancy because of ureteral displacement by the enlarging uterus. The relaxation of the bladder supports can result in stress incontinence, which is also associated with a lack of urethral elongation.

A majority of the changes taking place in renal haemodynamics are, yet again, foreshadowed during the menstrual cycle and, in pregnancy, largely completed by the end of the first trimester. The effective renal plasma flow (ERPF) is increased by at least 6 weeks' gestation (Fig. 6.7; Chapman et al 1998); it rises thereafter to some 80% by mid-pregnancy, then falls to ~65% above non-pregnant values (Fig. 6.7). This increase is thus proportionally greater than the increase in cardiac output, presumably reflecting specific vasodilatation. The urinary excretion of the major renal metabolite of prostacyclin, prostaglandin 6-keto $F_{1\alpha}$, rises fourfold during the first trimester, and the higher rise in renal plasma flow (RPF) may well be a result of this. The glomerular filtration rate (GFR) also increases dramatically (Fig. 6.7). In an elegant longitudinal study over non-conception and conception cycles in 9 women, Davison & Noble (1981) showed there to be an increase in GFR, measured by endogenous creatinine clearance, of some 20% during the luteal phase of the menstrual cycle; this was maintained when conception occurred. The rise in GFR was of the order of 25% by 4 weeks after the last menstrual period (LMP) and 45% by the ninth week, only rising thereafter by 5–10% (Davison & Noble 1981). Unlike the rise in ERPF, the GFR only falls slightly to term. This means that the filtration fraction falls during the first trimester, is largely maintained at this level during the second, and rises towards non-pregnant values in the third trimester. It might be speculated that these major increments exhaust the renal reserve, but serial studies during and after pregnancy have shown the renal response to amino acid infusion to be proportionally similar in pregnant and non-pregnant women.

These changes in haemodynamics have profound effects on the concentration of certain plasma metabolites and electrolytes, which must be remembered when considering clinical laboratory data in pregnancy. Thus, plasma creatinine concentration falls significantly by the fourth week post LMP (Davison & Noble 1981) and continues to fall to mid-pregnancy. Creatinine clearance (but not GFR as measured by infusion techniques) begins to fall during the last couple of months of pregnancy, resulting in a rise in plasma (creatinine) and implying altered renal handling of creatinine. The normal laboratory ranges established for non-pregnant subjects are thus inappropriate. For example, mean plasma creatinine falls from around 73 mmol/l to a nadir of 47 mmol/l while plasma urea falls from a mean of ~4.3 mmol/l to a nadir of 3.1 mmol/l.

The GFR is a function of the single nephron glomerular filtration rate and the number of glomeruli; since the latter does not change, the former must. Pregnancy hyperfiltration appears to result largely from the increments in RPF with a minor contribution from decreases in capillary oncotic pressure. There may also be a rise in glomerular membrane poros-

ity during pregnancy. The late fall in RPF in the face of a largely maintained GFR strongly suggests a mechanism acting at the efferent arterioles. Two renal hormones have effects which might contribute to this: angiotensin II (A II) and atrial natriuretic peptide hormone (ANP). A II is known to be a major factor regulating efferent arteriolar resistance. It has been known for many years that A II exerts differential effects on the renal and systemic circulations in late pregnancy. In late pregnancy, the infusion of A II results in a rise in filtration fraction, by comparison with similar infusions at 26–35 weeks, which result in a fall. Similarly, the infusion of ANP during the third trimester of pregnancy results in a fall in RPF without a concomitant fall in GFR, and hence a rise in filtration fraction. There is considerable discussion about whether ANP concentrations do rise in pregnancy and, if so, when they peak. The assay methodology of Irons et al (1996) was very carefully validated for use in pregnancy, and suggested that ANP did indeed show an increase in late gestation.

Total body water rises by about 20% during pregnancy (~8.5 l); curiously, the magnitude of this rise may not be dependent on parity. This is not the result of a change in the way in which the kidney handles water, but of a major alteration in the way in which the body's volume sensor functions. There is a very sharp fall in plasma osmolality between weeks 4 and 6 post conception. The osmotic thresholds for thirst and arginine vasopressin (AVP) release decrease in parallel, although that for thirst remains 2–5 mosmol/kg higher than that for AVP release. The decreased threshold for drinking stimulates increased water intake and dilution of body fluids. AVP release is not suppressed at the usual level of body tonicity, and so AVP continues to circulate and the extra water intake is retained. Thus plasma osmolality falls until it is below the osmotic thirst threshold, and a new steady state with little change in water turnover is established. The volume-sensing AVP release mechanisms evidently adjust as pregnancy progresses so that each new volume status is sensed as normal, with the appropriate response to acute change. The placenta synthesises a cystine aminopeptidase (vasopressinase), the rise in plasma concentration of which results in a fourfold increase in the metabolic clearance of AVP. Failure to appreciate the very high plasma levels of vasopressinase in pregnancy resulted in some of the earlier confusion in the literature. The mechanisms responsible for the altered osmoregulation in pregnancy have not been formalised, but human chorionic gonadotropin can lower the osmotic thresholds for both thirst and AVP secretion outside pregnancy.

In pregnancy, the kidneys are more sensitive to maternal posture in relation to water excretion than in non-pregnancy. A seated pregnant woman has a greater diuretic response to water intake in early pregnancy, but a lesser response when she stands. Water drunk by a pregnant woman who is mobile during the day tends to accumulate in the legs only to be excreted when she lies down, partly accounting for the high incidence of nocturia during pregnancy. Indeed, it has been observed that a majority of normal pregnant women show dependent oedema in late pregnancy. In normal pregnancy, this is associated with increased birthweight and reduced perinatal mortality. The increase in body water deduced from the amount calculated to be present in the fetus, amniotic fluid, placenta and maternal tissues is 2.5–3 litres short of the actual increase. The deficit is caused partly by oedema fluid and partly by increased hydration of the connective tissue ground substance. This leads to laxity and swelling of connective tissue and consequent changes in joints which occur mainly in the last trimester and are not related to maternal age. It is, however, more marked in those having second than first babies. These joint changes, together with the postural changes consequent on the alteration in the centre of gravity, produce much of the backache and other aches which are so common in pregnancy. The symphysis pubis may become very lax and extremely painful (especially during walking) but this has physiological benefit because as it occurs the capacity of the pelvis increases. Generalised tissue swelling produces corneal swelling and intraocular pressure changes, gingival oedema and the common and persistent symptoms (nasal stuffiness) arising in the cranial sinuses resulting from their increased vascularity. It may also produce tracheal oedema, which can lead to problems with anaesthesia if intubation is required. The carpal tunnel syndrome often develops.

The pregnant woman accumulates some 950 mmol sodium during the course of pregnancy. This is done in the face of high circulating concentrations of progesterone which, because of its very strong structural similarity with aldosterone, competes with it at the distal tubule. There are also marked increases in GFR and a relatively alkaline urine. If left unchecked, this would result in sodium loss, rather than retention. This is partly compensated for by a marked activation of the renin–angiotensin system (RAS). This activation results in increased synthesis and release of aldosterone from the first trimester, yet another phenomenon foreshadowed in the luteal phase of the menstrual cycle. Interestingly, however, by at least the second trimester there appears to be no correlation between components of the RAS and aldosterone, and both plasma and urinary aldosterone increase substantially more than plasma renin activity. Perhaps the receptor sensitivity to angiotensin II is maintained in the adrenal, unlike vascular sensitivity (see above), or the adrenal could be sensitised by the rise in ACTH in pregnancy. There is quite marked dissociation between components of the RAS and aldosterone in response to acute stimuli; for example, the effect of sodium loading in pregnancy is considerably more marked on aldosterone than on plasma renin activity. However, both the RAS and aldosterone do respond appropriately to both sodium loading and sodium depletion during pregnancy. Simultaneous with the rise in aldosterone and the weaker mineralocorticoid, deoxycorticosterone, is a rise in the potentially natriuretic prostacyclin and a small rise in atrial natriuretic peptide (ANP). Since right atrial area does not rise until the third trimester, and there is the appearance of 'underfill' even in the presence of a much expanded blood volume, the small increase in ANP until late pregnancy is not surprising. It is assumed that glomerulotubular balance must change in pregnancy to allow the sodium retention which actually occurs. There is a fall of some 4–5 mmol/l in plasma sodium by term, but plasma chloride does not change.

Even more curious is that some 350 mmol potassium are retained during pregnancy in the face of the much increased GFR, substantially raised aldosterone concentrations and a relatively alkaline urine. The regulation of potassium excretion in pregnancy has not been studied to the same extent as that of sodium. It appears that renal tubular potassium reabsorption adjusts appropriately to the increased filtered potassium load.

Serum uric acid concentration falls by about a quarter in early pregnancy, with an increase in its fractional excretion secondary to a decrease in net tubular reabsorption. The kidney excretes a progressively smaller proportion of the filtered uric acid, so a rise in serum uric acid concentration during the second half of pregnancy is normal, although it is enhanced in women developing pre-eclampsia. Angiotensin II inhibits urate excretion outside pregnancy, but this effect is also blunted as early as the first trimester of pregnancy. A similar pattern is seen in relation to urea, which is also partly reabsorbed in the nephron.

Glucose passes freely across the glomerulus and may be excreted at levels 10 times higher than those seen normally outside pregnancy. In normal non-pregnant women, the maximum reabsorptive capacity of the proximal tubule is ~1.6–1.9 mmol/min, and the quantity of filtered glucose does not exceed the capacity of the tubule to reabsorb it. In pregnancy, however, the reabsorption of glucose is less complete and glycosuria is common. If the urine of pregnant women is tested sufficiently often glycosuria will be detected in 50%. Teleologically, this seems strange in view of the fetus' use of glucose as its primary energy substrate and the demands which this makes on maternal glucose homeostasis. The excretion of lactose and fructose is also increased in pregnancy, through a similar mechanism.

It is also counter-intuitive that the excretion of most amino acids should increase in pregnancy, since these are used by the fetus as the building blocks from which it synthesises protein. The pattern of excretion is not constant: some, such as glycine and histidine, show an early increase in excretion which is maintained to term; others, such as tyrosine and phenylalanine, show an early increase which subsequently declines; yet others, such as methionine and isoleucine, show only small changes. The excretion of arginine falls; this might be related to the proposed rise in nitric oxide synthesis in pregnancy. Again, the mechanism is inadequate tubular reabsorption in the face of a 50% rise in GFR. Excretion of the water-soluble vitamins is also increased.

Urinary calcium excretion is 2–3-fold higher in normal pregnancy than in the non-pregnant state, even though there is a need to conserve calcium for both maternal and fetal development and maternal serum total calcium rises. Tubular reabsorption is enhanced in pregnancy, as is intestinal reabsorption of calcium, presumably under the influence of the increased concentrations of 1,25-dihydroxyvitamin D (Seely et al 1997).

As mentioned above, the arterial pH rises from early in normal pregnancy, by about 0.04, while plasma bicarbonate concentrations fall by ~4 mmol. However, renal bicarbonate reabsorption and hydrogen ion excretion appear to be unaltered during pregnancy. It appears that pregnant women can acidify their urine as normal, but in pregnancy the urine is usually mildly alkaline.

Protein excretion rises throughout pregnancy owing to the increased GFR, changes in glomerular permselectivity and alterations in tubular function. Total protein excretion, and that of albumin, are significantly increased by 20 weeks of pregnancy, and continue to rise to at least 36 weeks. This later rise is accelerated in women developing pre-eclampsia. Thus, in late pregnancy, an upper limit of normal of 300 mg total protein excretion/24 h collection is accepted. The use of dipstick methodology to quantitate proteinuria in pregnancy has been shown to give highly variable data.

The changes in renal function influence the mother's day-to-day living. Micturition increases in frequency from early in gestation, with nocturia developing as pregnancy progresses. As well as the postural effects (see above), fetal movements and insomnia contribute to nocturia.

Table 6.3 summarises sequential changes in some aspects of renal function throughout normal pregnancy.

Table 6.3 Percentage change in some measurements of renal function during pregnancy. Changes are expressed from postpartum data in the same women. The mean values shown are those at the end of each trimester and are thus not necessarily maxima. (Data from Dunlop & Davison 1977, Dunlop 1981.)

	First trimester	Second trimester	Third trimester
ERPF (ml/min)	+75	+86	+61
GFR (ml/min)	+51	+55	+53
Filtration fraction (%)	−13	−13	−3
Reabsorption UA (ml/min)	+13	+26	+46
Plasma (uric acid) (µmol/l)	−23	−19	−8

ERPF, effective renal plasma flow; GFR, glomerular filtration rate; UA, uric acid.

THE GASTROINTESTINAL SYSTEM

Salivary secretion is usually within the normal non-pregnant range but is occasionally excessive although it is more of a nuisance to the mother than a threat to her fluid balance. Gastric secretion is reduced as is the motility of the stomach. The latter used to be considered to cause delayed emptying, particularly in labour with the risk of regurgitation during the induction of anaesthesia. It is now widely recognised that intrapartum changes in gastric emptying are entirely the result of analgesic drug administration. Nevertheless, the whole intestinal tract has decreased motility: this may be the explanation for increased absorption of water and salt and other substances. Gut transit time returns to non-pregnant levels in the third trimester. The increase in water absorption produces a tendency to constipation, although oral iron may also contribute. Another symptom, so common that many mothers do not complain of it, is heartburn (reflux), producing regurgitation of acid mouthfuls with retrosternal or epigastric pain. This is a consequence of increased intragastric pressure without concomitant increase in tone of the oesophageal cardiac sphincter. It is greater in heavier patients. There may also be reflux of bile into the stomach

because of pyloric incompetence; this responds to treatment with aluminium hydroxide rather than magnesium sulphate. The underlying mechanism may be increased progesterone or decreased concentrations of the hormonal peptide motilin.

The histological appearance of the liver does not change during pregnancy. In some respects hepatic function increases during pregnancy, in that plasma globulin and fibrinogen concentrations increase despite the diluting effect of the increase in plasma volume. Albumin concentration falls by 22%, from ~3.5 to 2.5 g/100 ml, but the synthetic rate rises between 12 and 28 weeks so that the total albumin mass increases by 19%, reaching a plateau at 28 weeks. It is normal for serum alkaline phosphatase concentrations to rise to values which may be double those outside pregnancy, but most of this is an isoenzyme of placental origin and the γ-glutamyl transpeptidase concentration does not increase. Again, a knowledge of what is normal in pregnancy, by comparison with the non-pregnant state, is needed for the correct interpretation of laboratory results. Transaminase values are largely unaltered in normal pregnancy although some studies have suggested that the upper limit of normal should be reduced by 2.5%. Total globulin increases, so the hormone-binding globulins rise. The excretion of both bromsulphthalein and bilirubin is impaired in late pregnancy, so the clearance of compounds metabolised via microsomal oxidation may be impaired. While hepatic blood flow does not change, the velocity patterns in the hepatic vein flatten. This may result in part from the mild cholestasis which is physiological in pregnancy. Hepatic malfunction may be falsely suggested by reddening of the palms or by the appearance of spider naevi.

Although the gall bladder increases in size and empties more slowly during pregnancy, there is no change in the constitution of the bile. There is stasis of bile in dilated biliary canaliculi but no cellular necrosis or alteration in the secretion of bile. Cholestasis may be associated with generalised pruritus which responds to treatment with cholestyramine, very rarely does it produce jaundice; it is, however, associated with raised postprandial serum glucose. The cholestasis is probably a hormonal effect since it also occurs in users of oral contraceptives and postmenopausal hormone replacement.

Taste often alters early in pregnancy and the change can occur even before a period has been missed. There may be the sensation of a metallic taste, similar to that experienced in liver disease, a loss of taste for something usually enjoyed, or a craving for a food or other substance not normally eaten, such as wall plaster. Such cravings (pica) may be an expression of nutritional lack but many have no such potentially therapeutic effect. Some are potentially hazardous. Eating mothballs is not uncommon; this may produce a fetal haemolytic anaemia. Many cravings are concealed by the mother and may be discovered only after delivery.

Pharmacokinetics
The increase of total body water, the fall in plasma albumin concentration, the slowing of gastric emptying and the rise in GFR in pregnancy all contribute to marked changes in the disposition and handling of drugs. The distribution volume of water-soluble drugs increases. Albumin is the major protein

binding acidic drugs such as salicylates and warfarin, and the fall in plasma albumin concentration is compounded by the rise in free fatty acid concentration in late pregnancy. Binding can vary widely between individuals, and when the therapeutic concentration has to be maintained within narrow limits as, for example, with phenytoin administration, saliva monitoring may be more useful than measuring plasma concentration. Progesterone is an enzyme inducer, but there are inconsistent changes in metabolic liver enzyme activity between individuals. Drugs with a high hepatic extraction ratio have unchanged elimination rates during pregnancy as hepatic blood flow does not change. When the hepatic extraction ratio is below ~0.7, however, extraction rates may be increased, unaltered or decreased depending on the individual characteristics of each drug. It appears likely that the placenta also has an important role in metabolising drugs in pregnancy. This topic is covered in considerable detail by Loebstein et al (1997).

VASCULAR REACTIVITY

A reduced pressor response to angiotensin II in normal pregnancy was first noted nearly 40 years ago and has since been repeatedly confirmed. It seems to be initiated in the luteal phase and is well established by 10 weeks' gestation (Gant et al 1973). The density of angiotensin II receptors on platelets also falls markedly from early pregnancy. A number of comparative studies have shown this effect to be specific for angiotensin II, and not to occur with noradrenaline (norepinephrine). The reduced sensitivity to angiotensin II presumably protects against the potentially pressor levels of angiotensin II found in normal pregnancy; plasma noradrenaline is not increased in normal pregnancy. Vasopressin is believed to contribute to the maintenance of blood pressure mainly under conditions of severe hypotension. The pressor response to vasopressin has not been studied in human pregnancy but is unchanged in pregnant rats; again, vasopressin concentrations do not change in pregnancy.

Women with pre-eclampsia show an increase in pressor sensitivity to both angiotensin II and noradrenaline, an increase which antedates the onset of the clinically identified disease. There is a generalised increase in total peripheral resistance in preeclampsia, which will itself enhance the effect of any vasoconstrictor; there is also some evidence for increased intracellular free calcium concentrations, which again have a non-specific amplificatory effect.

There are differences in the responsiveness of the myometrial and omental resistance vessels to vasodilators, both in pregnant and non-pregnant women; pregnancy per se does not alter this. Omental arteries show a consistently greater endothelium-dependent relaxation to bradykinin (BK) than the myometrial arteries. On the other hand, pregnancy does differentially affect BK-mediated vasodilatation in small subcutaneous fat arteries pre-constricted with noradrenaline, being associated with a greater response. This illustrates the difficulty of selecting suitable control vessels for any studies of function. The endothelially mediated vasodilator response to BK of myometrial vessels pre-constricted with vasopressin is not effected through the cyclo-oxygenase pathway, but may be partly dependent on nitric oxide. Nitric oxide appears to play a significant role in modulation of myogenic tone and flow-mediated responses in the resistance vasculature of the uterine circulation in normal pregnancy. Endothelially mediated vasodilatation is impaired in pre-eclampsia.

Pregnancy per se also seems not to alter the response of intramyometrial arteries to a variety of vasoconstrictors (A II, noradrenaline, vasopressin and the TxA2-mimic 1991). A II is a highly potent vasoconstrictor in human pregnant myometrial arteries, but tachyphylaxis rapidly develops. The response to noradrenaline in these vessels is enhanced by concomitant nitric oxide synthase inhibition. Endothelin is also a potent contractile agent in myometrial resistance arteries at term.

THE ENDOCRINE SYSTEM

The autonomy of the mother's endocrine system is very much challenged by pregnancy. This challenge is necessary to provide an optimal environment for the development of the fetus, the next generation. The placenta is a powerhouse of hormone production from the earliest days of gestation. The placenta is considered in more detail in Chapter 4. Suffice it to say here that human chorionic ganadotrophin appears to be the signal for pregnancy; human embryos in culture can synthesise measurable quantities from around 7 days after conception. The placental trophoblast can synthesise hormones that are usually synthesised in other tissues, such as adrenocorticotrophic hormone (ACTH), progesterone, parathyroid hormone-related protein and renin in forms that are either identical or almost identical to those synthesised elsewhere, hormone receptors, and releasing hormones and their receptors. Since these are immensely potent agents and their synthesis appears to be largely regulated only by the availability of precursors, it is not surprising that the mother's physiology is taken over. The placenta synthesises large amounts of steroids, some of which, such as oestriol, are unique, but it appears that the maternal capacity for steroid synthesis is in any case underused before conception. The raised oestrogen concentration of pregnancy enhances hepatic synthesis of the binding globulins for such hormones as thyroxine, corticosteroids and the sex steroids. This in turn is associated with a rise in the total plasma content of the hormones, although the free fraction does not necessarily rise. The increased plasma content might act both as a store of hormone and protect the fetus from the potentially harmful effects of high transplacental concentrations.

The hypothalamus and pituitary gland
The hypothalamus is a coordinator of endocrine and neural control, regulating the maintenance of the internal environment. It receives input from the periphery, has extensive connections with the limbic system, has thermo- and osmoreceptors, and appears to be central to the regulation of food intake and energy homeostasis. Output from the hypothalamus controls the pituitary gland, and most hypothalamic hormones are stimulatory rather than inhibitory.

It is curious that human pregnancy seems not to depend heavily on the pituitary gland, since ovulation induction is successful in women with hypopituitarism, and hypophysectomy during the third month is compatible with the continuation of pregnancy. Perhaps the very high degree of similarity between placental and pituitary hormone synthesis is an explanation. For example, human placental lactogen (placental production), and growth hormone and prolactin share a high degree of structural homology. The pituitary increases in weight by 30% in first pregnancies and by 50% in subsequent conceptions. Even this normal increase can produce headache. It also increases the gland's sensitivity to haemorrhage, a feature accentuated by the lack of a direct arterial supply to the anterior pituitary. Since blood is delivered via the portal system, in which the pressure is lower than the systemic arterial pressure, the effects of any hypotension will be greater in the anterior pituitary circulation; hypotension may be aggravated by thrombotic tendencies or necrotic swelling. This can lead to postpartum hypopituitarism (Sheehan's syndrome).

The increase in weight of the pituitary results from differential changes in number of several cell types. The number of lactotrophs is increased while the number of growth hormone and gonadotrophin-secreting cells is reduced, their secretion possibly being suppressed by high levels of cortisol or human placental lactogen. Plasma prolactin begins to rise within a few days of conception and by term may be 10–20 times as high as in the non-pregnant woman. The secretion of other anterior pituitary hormones may be unchanged or reduced. Thyroid-stimulating hormone secretion is not different from that in the non-pregnant woman (except that it is possibly lower in the first trimester) and it responds normally to thyrotropin-releasing hormone from the hypothalamus. There is, however, a blunted response of follicle-stimulating hormone to gonadotrophin-releasing hormone (GnRH). This shows a progressive decrease, finally leading to no response 3 weeks after ovulation. The luteinising hormone response also disappears, but not until some weeks after the loss of GnRH response. This blunting of GnRH response may be caused by human chorionic gonadotrophin, which starts to rise before oestrogen levels rise, and before progesterone or prolactin rises significantly. The pituitary content of luteinising and follicle-stimulating hormones also falls.

ACTH concentrations rise during pregnancy, even though the raised cortisol concentrations would be expected to decrease them. Dexamethasone also does not suppress ACTH secretion as effectively as it does in non-pregnant women. Although this might be due to an altered hypothalamic sensitivity, it seems more likely that the placental synthesis of ACTH results in a breakdown of normal control mechanisms. The placental production of ACTH, and of a corticotrophin-releasing hormone (CRH) effectively identical to hypothalamic CRH, is not suppressible by exogenous steroids. Although maternal systemic CRH concentrations rise during pregnancy to very high concentrations, most is bound rather than free (active). The proportion of free CRH, however, rises rapidly towards term, suggesting a role in the initiation of parturition. Plasma vasopressin does not change in pregnancy, but it has also been suggested to contribute to stress-induced increases in pituitary ACTH release during pregnancy. ACTH does not cross the placenta.

The adrenal gland

The maternal adrenal glands do not enlarge during pregnancy but there is an increase in width of the zona fasciculata, with histological changes there suggesting increased secretion. Progesterone has an antiglucocorticoid effect. Both the plasma total and the unbound cortisol and other corticosteroid concentrations rise in pregnancy, from about the end of the first trimester (Wintour et al 1978); urinary cortisol excretion is doubled. The half-life of cortisol in the plasma is prolonged and its metabolic clearance rate is reduced. This might account for the increased response of cortisol and 17-hydroxycorticosterone (17-OHCS) to ACTH while urinary 17-OHCS and ketosteroid are unchanged. There is no change in glucocorticoid receptor numbers in the cells during pregnancy but the high levels of progesterone may compete for binding sites. Other corticosteroids show similar patterns during normal pregnancy (Wintour et al 1978). Excess glucocorticoid exposure in utero appears to inhibit fetal growth in both animals and humans. The increased circulating maternal cortisol concentrations might therefore be predicted to be deleterious to the fetus, since one would expect steroids to cross the placenta readily; however, the normal placenta synthesises a pregnancy-specific 11β-hydroxysteroid dehydrogenase, which converts cortisol and corticosterone to cortisone and 11-dehydrocortisone. Fetal circulating cortisol concentrations are thus much lower than maternal until close to term.

The marked rise in secretion of the mineralocorticoid aldosterone in pregnancy has already been mentioned. Synthesis of the weaker mineralocorticoid 11-deoxycorticosterone is also increased by the eighth week of pregnancy, and actually increases proportionally more than any other cortical steroid (Wintour et al 1978). Since this increased synthesis is not suppressible by any of the normal manoeuvres (changes in salt balance, administration of dexamethasone), it seems likely again that there is an ectopic source, presumably the placenta.

Plasma catecholamine concentrations are a measure of adrenergic activity at any given time, with plasma noradrenaline reflecting predominantly sympathetic nerve activity and adrenaline (epinephrine) that of the adrenal medulla. The measurement of plasma catecholamines has inherent difficulties, but there is now a broad consensus that plasma catecholamine concentrations fall from the first to the third trimesters. There is some blunting of the rise in noradrenaline seen on standing and isometric exercise in pregnancy, but the adrenaline response is unaltered.

The thyroid gland

The raised GFR of pregnancy results in a doubling of the renal clearance of iodide, with a fall in plasma inorganic iodide. There is a threefold rise in the thyroid's clearance of iodine, however, allowing the absolute iodine uptake to remain within the non-pregnant range. The compensatory follicular hyperplasia may result in a frank goitre when there is a degree of dietary iodine deficiency. The thyroid remains normally responsive to stimulation by thyroid-stimulating hormone (TSH) and suppression by triiodothyronine (T_3). It appears that there is a small fall in TSH in the first trimester, followed by a rise thereafter. hCG and TSH share a common α subunit, so hCG can also stimulate the TSH receptors. A placental form of the hypothalamic thyrotrophin-releasing hormone (TRH) has been identified, but no placental TSH, so the placental TRH would have to act through the mother's pituitary. There is a doubling in thyroid-binding globulin levels during pregnancy, but other thyroid-binding proteins do not increase. Overall, free plasma T_3 and thyroxine (T_4) remain at the same levels as outside pregnancy (although total levels are raised), and the majority of pregnant women are euthyroid. Free T_4 may fall in late gestation, but again, results vary with the methodology used. Calcitonin (CT) is another thyroid hormone, synthesised by the parafollicular cells in response to a rise in extracellular free calcium concentration (see below).

The parathyroid glands

Extracellular free calcium acts directly on the parathyroid cell to regulate the secretion of parathyroid hormone (PTH). One of the main functions of PTH is to regulate the renal synthesis of 1,25-dihydroxyvitamin D, the major active metabolite of vitamin D, which enhances calcium reabsorption from the kidney and gut and its mobilisation from bone. By term, there is a transplacental flux of about 6.5 mmol/day calcium and 4.6 mmol/day of inorganic phosphate, requiring considerable modification in maternal mineral homeostasis. There is an early, marked rise in urinary calcium excretion, due to the raised GFR, so that intestinal absorption has to increase from basal values of around 20–25% to a maximum of 50% by 24 weeks, after which it stabilises. There is a fall in intact PTH during pregnancy, but a doubling of 1,25-dihydroxyvitamin D and a rise in CT and PTH-related protein. The increase in serum 1,25-dihydroxyvitamin D values is probably a key factor in providing for the increased calcium requirements in pregnancy. PTHrP rises in the first trimester, stimulating 1,25 dihydroxyvitamin D synthesis, even though iPTH is falling at that time.

Renal hormones

The activation of the renin–angiotensin system has already been considered both in relation to the cardiovascular system and the renal system. In brief, plasma active renin and angiotensin II concentrations have risen significantly by the end of the first trimester, and largely plateau thereafter, while plasma angiotensinogen II (A II) continues to increase to term. This is thought to be both a response of renin secretion to the natriuretic effects of progesterone, and of angiotensinogen synthesis under the action of oestrogens.

Erythropoietin (EPO) synthesis occurs mainly in the peritubular capillary lining cells of the kidneys. It stimulates proliferation and differentiation of erythroid progenitor cells and regulates the number of erythrocytes in peripheral blood. Its concentration is reciprocally related to that of haemoglobin. Synthesis of EPO appears to be stimulated by hCG. Its concentration rises from the first trimester, peaking at around week 24 and falling somewhat thereafter.

The pancreas

The size of the islets of Langerhans and the number of β cells increase during pregnancy, as does the number of receptor sites for insulin. The functions of the pancreas in pregnancy have been considered in relation to the gastrointestinal system and insulin resistance elsewhere in this chapter.

Other endocrine effects

The mood swings and altered psyche of pregnancy are usually attributed to the enormous endocrine changes. Progesterone is associated with tiredness and dyspnoea; the overbreathing may also result in giddiness and feelings of nausea. Many pregnant women are, however, almost euphoric, a state which is thought to be attributable to the raised corticosteroids of pregnancy. This has been particularly studied postpartum. Raised maternal cortisol concentrations have been found to be associated with baby blues, while lower levels characterised women who exhibited mild hypomania (the highs).

THE SKIN

The most obvious change in the skin is pigmentation in some areas. The development of a linea nigra and darkening of the nipple and areola are almost universal, although the depth of pigmentation varies in different people and different ethnic groups. Facial chloasma is almost as common. All are caused by increased secretion of pituitary melanocyte-stimulating hormone. A suntan acquired during pregnancy lasts longer than at any other time. Spider naevi are also common and some reddening of the palms is found in most mothers. Both are oestrogen effects. The striae that develop on the abdomen, breasts and elsewhere are a response to increased circulating corticosteroids. There is generalised vasodilatation to assist in losing the extra heat produced by maternal, placental and fetal metabolism.

Fingernails grow more quickly during pregnancy. Hair does not but the rate at which hair is shed is reduced. The excess hair is lost in the puerperium, to the consternation of many mothers who worry that they may be going bald. Subcutaneous fat increases but the generalised increase in skinfold thickness results from oedema and increased vascularity. Intensely itchy papules sometimes appear during normal pregnancy—pregnancy prurigo—and disappear spontaneously either before or after delivery; there does not appear to be underlying pathology.

EXERCISE

Exercise is good for the mother. Both her pulse rate and oxygen consumption are raised in proportion to the severity of the exercise: provided the pulse rate does not rise above 150–160 per minute there is little risk. There is little effect on the blood pressure or temperature, nor is there an increase in uterine contractions with activities involving only the upper part of the body although there may be with whole-body exercise. Myometrial, placental and umbilical flow may be affected, but there is no agreement about the extent of this. A transient reduction in flow occurring during exercise may produce a compensatory increase in placental size and weight, and in birthweight. Even if there is a reduction in flow, it does not harm the healthy fetus whose heart rate and its variability rise with exercise. Another positive effect of exercise is to raise plasma beta-endorphin: this is maintained in labour and reduces the maternal perception of pain. Physical training is associated with lower plasma insulin concentrations and increased sensitivity to insulin in skeletal muscle and adipose tissue of those with non-insulin-dependent diabetes mellitus. It has therefore been suggested that such exercise as swimming, which uses a high number of muscle groups, may be of particular benefit in pregnancy, in view of the insulin resistance which develops. Impact sports or those that lead to exhaustion, however, are probably best avoided. Reduced joint stability and changes in the centre of gravity (and therefore stability) make skiing or horse riding even more risky than usual.

AFTER PREGNANCY

The physiology of the puerperium is covered more fully in Chapter 39. The rate of return to non-pregnant values is not uniform and, as noted earlier, may never be complete. Carbohydrate metabolism is close to prepregnant levels within 24 hours of delivery but it may take months for iron stores to recover. Cardiac output is back to normal within 2 weeks and venous distensibility within 3–12 weeks, but stroke volume does not revert to normal until 24 weeks after delivery. Cervical ectropion (erosion) may persist for a year while circulating volume reverts within days. These data are not academic since a cervical ectropion found at the 6-week postnatal visit is not abnormal and a haemoglobin estimation 2 days after delivery is an accurate reflection of the maternal situation. Joint changes may take 3–5 months to return to normal. The rate of involution is dependent on whether or not the mother is breast-feeding.

Some changes are peculiar to the puerperium rather than a loss of adaptation. In one-third of women who have had normotensive pregnancies, diastolic blood pressure rises to 90 mmHg or more 48 hours after delivery. Oestrogen synthesis falls, remaining low during breast-feeding, and may produce vaginal atrophy. The white cell count rises to 20×10^9 or more. Thyroid function is frequently altered, possibly in as many as one-fifth of mothers. This may be asymptomatic or produce overt hyperthyroidism or hypothyroidism, but often only lassitude. Function almost always returns to normal spontaneously, but this may take 6 months.

Although the puerperium is defined as the 6 weeks following delivery, it takes considerably longer than this for all the physical and psychological changes of pregnancy to return as close to their previous state as they will do. Repeated childbearing at short intervals may prevent this ever happening. The variability of the return towards non-pregnant values must be taken into account in any research which attempts to use the mother as her own control after pregnancy. This is particularly relevant in, for example, studies of the genetics of pre-eclampsia, in which a return to 'normal'

values of blood pressure, renal, hepatic and haemostatic function is a prerequisite for accurate phenotyping. Three months should be the minimum, and 6 months may be preferable.

CONCLUSION

This chapter has attempted to give an overview of an enormous, and rapidly expanding, topic. It has been impossible to do more than sketch in an outline, with a little detail reflecting the author's particular interests. The reader who desires more detail is referred to *Clinical Physiology in Obstetrics* (Chamberlain & Broughton-Piplen 1998). It is becoming increasingly apparent that high-quality care of the pregnant woman will have an impact on the health of the baby into full adulthood. Such quality care requires a good understanding of basic principles; the author hopes that this chapter is at least a step towards such understanding.

KEY POINTS

- Most changes in the mother's physiology are proactive, not reactive, and many are initiated during the luteal phase of the conception cycle.
- Pregnancy is almost entirely hormonally driven. The trophoblast is a largely autonomous hormone factory, synthesising not only steroids but also prostanoids, polypeptides, enzymes and cytokines. These are essential to a successful outcome.
- Cardiac output rises while systemic blood pressure and total peripheral resistance fall. Alveolar ventilation and red cell mass increase. There is a marked rise in kidney function.
- Normal pregnancy is associated with marked hyperlipidaemia which is not atherogenic; lipid peroxides also rise. Considerable insulin resistance develops.
- Pre-eclampsia appears in many respects to be a response to failed or inadequate adaptation to pregnancy, originating very early in gestation.

REFERENCES

Al Kadi H 2001 Ms PhD, University of Nottingham

Anumba D, Robson S, Boys R, Ford G 1999 Nitric oxide activity in the peripheral vasculature during normotensive and preeclamptic pregnancy. Am J Physiol 277:H848–H854

Ayala DE, Hermida Ramon C, Mojon Artemio, Fernandez JR, Iglesias M 1997 Circadian blood pressure variability in healthy and complicated pregnancies. Hypertension 30:601–610

Blake M, Martin A, Manktelow B et al 2000 Changes in baroreceptor sensitivity for heart rate during normotensive pregnancy and the puerperium. Clin Sci 98:259–268

Burrows R, Kelton J 1990 Thrombocytopenia at delivery: a prospective survey of 6715 deliveries. Am J Obstet Gynecol 162:731–734

Chamberlain G, Broughton-Piplen F (Ed) 1998 Clinical Physiology in Obstetrics. Blackwells Oxford.

Chapman A, Zamudio S, Woodmansee W et al 1997 Systemic and renal hemodynamic changes in the luteal phase of the menstrual cycle mimic early pregnancy. Am J Physiol 273:F777–F782

Chapman A, Abraham W, Zamudio S et al 1998 Temporal relationships between hormonal and hemodynamic changes in early human pregnancy. Kidney Int 54:2056–2063

Christianson RE 1976 Studies on blood pressure during pregnancy. I Influence of parity and age. Am J Obstet Gynecol 125:509–513

Darmady J, Postle A 1982 Lipid metabolism in pregnancy. Br J Obstet Gynaecol 89:211–215

Davison J, Noble M 1981 Serial changes in 24 hour creatinine clearance during normal menstrual cycles and the first trimester of pregnancy. Br J Obstet Gynaecol 88:10–17

de Swiet M, Shennan A 1996 Blood pressure measurement in pregnancy. Br J Obstet Gynaecol 103:862–863

Dunlop W 1981 Serial changes in renal haemodynamics during normal human pregnancy. Br J Obstet Gynaecol 88:1–9

Dunlop W, Davison J 1977 The effect of normal pregnancy upon the renal handling of uric acid. Br J Obstet Gynaecol 84:13–21

Duvekot J, Cheriex E, Pieters F, Menheere P, Peeters L 1993 Early pregnancy changes in hemodynamics and volume homeostasis are consecutive adjustments triggered by a primary fall in systemic vascular tone. Am J Obstet Gynecol 169:1382–1392

Fahraeus L, Larsson-Cohn U, Wallentin L 1985 Plasma lipoproteins including high density lipoprotein subfractions during normal pregnancy. Obstet Gynecol 66:468–472

Gant N, Daley G, Chand S, Whalley P, Macdonald P 1973 A study of angiotensin II pressor response throughout primigravid pregnancy. J Clin Invest 52:2682–2689

Garcia-Rio F, Pino J, Gomez L, Alvarez-Sala R, Villasante C, Villamor J 1996 Regulation of breathing and perception of dyspnea in healthy pregnant women. Chest 110:446–453

Halligan A, Bonnar J, Sheppard B, Darling M, Walshe J 1994 Haemostatic, fibrinolytic and endothelial variables in normal pregnancies and pre-eclampsia. Br J Obstet Gynaecol 101:488–492

Hytten FE 1980 Weight gain in pregnancy. In: Hytten FE, Chamberlain GVP (eds) Clinical physiology in obstetrics. Blackwell, Oxford, pp 193–233

Irons D, Baylis P, Davison J 1996 The metabolic clearance of atrial natriuretic peptide during human pregnancy. Am J Obstet Gynecol 175:449–454

Kaaja R, Laivuouri H, Laakso M, Tikkanen M, Ylikorkala O 1999 Evidence of a state of increased insulin resistance in preeclampsia. Metabolism 48:892–896

Knopp R, Berglin R, Wahl P, Walden C, Chapman M, Irvine S 1982 Population-based lipoprotein lipid reference values for pregnant women compared to nonpregnant women classified by sex hormone usage. Am J Obstet Gynecol 143:626–637

Lind T, Billewicz W, Brown G 1973 A serial study of changes occurring in the oral glucose tolerance test during pregnancy. J Obstet Gynaecol Br Commonwealth 80:1033–1039

Loebstein R, Lalkin A, Koren G 1997 Pharmacokinetic changes during pregnancy and their clinical relevance. Clin Pharmacokinet 33:328–343

Milman N, Bergholt T, Byg K, Eriksen L, Graudal N 1999 Iron status and iron balance during pregnancy. A critical reappraisal of iron supplementation. Acta Obstet Gynecol Scand 78:749–757

Pritchard J, Wiggins K, Dickey J 1960 Blood volume changes in pregnancy and the puerperium. I. Does sequestration of red blood cells accompany parturition? Am J Obstet Gynecol 80:956–963

Robson S, Hunter S, Boys R, Dunlop W 1989 Serial study of factors influencing changes in cardiac output during human pregnancy. Am J Physiol 256:H1060–H1065

Robson S, Hunter S, Boys R, Dunlop W 1991 Serial changes in pulmonary haemodynamics during human pregnancy: a non-invasive study using Doppler echocardiography. Clin Sci 80:113–117

Rovinsky JJ, Jaffin H 1965 Cardiovascular hemodynamics in pregnancy. I. Blood and plasma volumes in multiple pregnancy. Am J Obstet Gynecol 93:1–13

Seely E, Brown E, DeMaggio D, Weldon D, Graves S 1997 A prospective study of calciotropic hormones in pregnancy and post partum: reciprocal changes in serum intact parathyroid hormone and 1,25-dihydroxyvitamin D. Am J Obstet Gynecol 176: 214–217

Strickland D, Guzick D, Cox K, Gant N, Rosenfield C 1986 The relationship between abortion in the first pregnancy and development of pregnancy-induced hypertension in the subsequent pregnancy. Am J Obstet Gynecol 154:146–148

Tritos N, Mantzoros C 1997 Leptin: its role in obesity and beyond. Diabetologiz 40: 1371–1379

van Beek E, Ekhart T, Schiffers P, van Eyck J, Peeters L, de Leeuw P 1998 Persistent abnormalities in plasma volume and renal hemodynamics in patients with a history of preeclampsia. Am J Obstet Gynecol 179:690–696

Wang Y, Walsh S, Guo J, Zhang J 1991 The imbalance between thromboxane and prostacyclin in preeclampsia is associated with an imbalance between lipid peroxides and vitamin E in maternal blood. Am J Obstet Gynecol 165:1695–1700

Wintour E, Coghlan J, Oddie C, Scoggins B, Walters W 1978 A sequential study of adrenocorticosteroid level in human pregnancy. Clin Exp Pharmacol Physiol 5:399–403

Yudkin PL, Harlap S, Baras M 1983 High birthweight in an ethnic group of low socioeconomic status. Br J Obstet Gynaecol 90:291–296

7

Immunology in pregnancy

Y.W. Loke, Ashley King

The contribution of the author of the equivalent chapter in the second edition, on which this chapter draws extensively, is gratefully acknowledged.

INTRODUCTION

The term immunity (Latin *immunis* = exempt) was coined from the observation that individuals who had recovered from certain infections were thereafter protected from the disease. From this originated the science of immunology which was, therefore, mainly concerned with elucidating how the body defended itself against infections. The factors involved in this defence were later found to reside in the serum as well as certain cells of the protected individual, thereby defining respectively the *humoral* and *cellular* basis of immunity. Furthermore, it became clear that there are two levels of immunity: innate (or natural) and adaptive (or acquired). Innate immunity calls upon the basic anatomical and physiological features inherent in an organism which are protective, such as epithelial barriers, phagocytic cells and the inflammatory reaction. Adaptive immunity, in contrast, is a process mounted by an infected host especially to eliminate the invasive foreign microorganisms or substances. The crucial difference between the two is that acquired immunity is specific and has memory whereas innate immunity is relatively non-specific and carries no memory of a previous encounter with a foreign organism. These two types of immunity do not occur independently but are complementary to each other so that each augments the activity of the other.

More detailed studies of the generation of the adaptive immune response revealed that, for a foreign substance to be recognised by the host, it has to be degraded into small peptides which are then re-expressed on the cell surface complexed with other molecules. These latter are encoded by genes of the major histocompatibility complex (MHC) and are known in humans as human leucocyte antigens (HLA).

There are two major classes of these antigens—class I and class II. There are multiple forms (alleles) of these antigens (polymorphism) so that every individual's HLA is different. For this reason, an organ graft from a donor will be rejected by a recipient if the two are not compatible for these antigens. This observation led to the science of transplantation immunology. There are excellent recent textbooks of the immune system which can be consulted (Janeway et al 1999, Goldsby et al 2000, Parham 2000).

What is the relevance of all this to obstetricians? There are many aspects of immunology that have a direct bearing on the specialty. For example, successful pregnancy itself is an immunological paradox because of the antigenic incompatibility between the embryo and its mother. Some pathological conditions associated with pregnancy appear to have an underlying immunological aetiology. The transfer of immunity from mother to fetus is a crucial event in the protection of the latter against infection. A proper understanding of these processes requires some knowledge of the underlying immunological mechanisms involved. The present chapter will focus on those areas of basic immunology that are pertinent to reproduction.

INNATE IMMUNE SYSTEM

Physical barriers such as the skin and mucous membrane can prevent the entry of pathogens, providing a first line of defence.

Physiological barriers such as the acid secretions in the stomach and soluble proteins like lysozyme in tears are usually successful deterrents of microbial colonisation. Very few organisms can survive the acid condition of the stomach. Lysozyme is a hydrolytic enzyme that is able to cleave the peptidoglycan layer of the cell walls of bacteria and thus lyse them.

There are other soluble factors which may play a role in innate defence, an important one being complement. The complement system consists of a group of proteins in serum that can be activated sequentially in a cascade fashion in which the product of one step becomes the enzyme catalyst for the next step. There are nine components of complement (C1–C9). In innate immunity, complement can be activated by contact with the surface of pathogens to set off the cascade, a process known as the alternative pathway of activation. The cleaved-off fragments after activation (e.g. C3a) are powerful mediators of the acute inflammatory response resulting in vasodilatation, accumulation of extracellular fluid and infiltration of phagocytic cells, all of which are important for defence.

There are two main types of cells involved in innate defence: phagocytic cells and natural killer cells.

The phagocytic cells comprise blood neutrophils and monocytes and tissue macrophages. These cells can ingest whole microorganisms and digest them. The initial event is attachment to the microbe via receptors expressed on the surface of the phagocytes followed by invagination of both the receptor and microbe into the cell. A variety of receptors are involved. One is the mannose receptor (MR), which can recognise certain carbohydrates present on the surface of microorganisms. Other receptors are those for the Fc portion of immunoglobulins (FcR) and for the C3b fragment of complement (CR3). These are components of the humoral arm of the acquired immune response and act as opsonins (= to make more palatable) which enhance attachment of the microbe to the phagocyte and, hence, subsequent ingestion. This is a good example of how the adaptive immune response can cooperate with the innate immune response.

The importance of phagocytes in innate defence can be seen in patients with the congenital condition known as leucocyte adhesion deficiency (LAD) in which neutrophils fail to accumulate in areas of infection because a mutation of the β2 subunit of the integrin adhesion molecule on the surface of these cells prevents their migration. These patients suffer from recurrent infections and may die at an early age.

Once ingested, the microbe is bound in a vesicle (phagosome) which fuses with the lysosomal contents of the cell (phagolysosome) and is digested. Digestion occurs via two mechanisms, one of which is oxygen independent while the other is oxygen dependent. The first of these depends on enzymes within the cell. The second mechanism occurs by the generation of hydrogen peroxide in a process known as metabolic burst. Individuals with chronic granulomatous disease, a congenital condition, fail to initiate the metabolic burst after phagocytosis because of an enzyme defect and are highly susceptible to infections. Similarly, in the autosomal recessive Chediak–Higashi syndrome, patients fail to form phagolysosomes after phagocytosis and they also succumb readily to infections.

The other cell type playing a role in innate defence are the natural killer (NK) cells. As the name implies, these cells are capable of spontaneous cytolytic activity against target cells without having to be activated. The original observation was that NK cells killed targets that were deficient in HLA class I molecules, such as tumour cells and virus-infected cells, where cell surface class I expression is frequently downregulated. This led to the theory known as the missing self hypothesis, which postulated that NK cells eliminated cells not expressing self HLA class I molecules and that their role, therefore, is to police the body and destroy any aberrant cells by sensing the presence of normal levels of self HLA class I molecules. However, this missing self hypothesis subsequently required some modification when it became clear that individual NK cell clones could discriminate between different HLA class I alleles and not merely recognise the presence or absence of class I molecules. There is, thus, a greater degree of functional complexity than originally envisaged. The potential significance of this will be discussed later when considering the fetal–maternal relationship. Besides spontaneous cytotoxicity, NK cells also kill targets that have been coated with antibody by binding to the Fc portion via an Fc receptor designated as CD16 (cf. opsonisation in phagocytosis). This mechanism is called antibody-dependent cell-mediated cytoxicity (ADCC) and is a further example of how acquired immunity cooperates with innate immunity. Apart from their cytotoxicity, NK cells can also affect target cells by the production of soluble proteins called cytokines.

ACQUIRED IMMUNE SYSTEM

Generation of the acquired immune response requires two main types of cells: lymphocytes and antigen-presenting cells (APC). There are two major populations of lymphocytes: B lymphocytes (B cells) and T lymphocytes (T cells). Both types of lymphocytes originate from haematopoietic cells in the bone marrow. While B cells continue to mature in the bone marrow, T cells migrate to the thymus where they undergo a process of selection and further differentiation. The bone marrow and thymus are designated as *primary lymphoid tissues* from where lymphocytes emerge to colonise specialised structures such as the spleen, lymph nodes, tonsils and Peyer's patches. These latter are collectively known as *secondary lymphoid tissues* and it is here that mature lymphocytes become stimulated to respond to foreign pathogens or substances.

The T cell is central to the generation of acquired immune responses. T cells express a T cell receptor (TCR) that is capable of recognising a foreign molecule or antigen. There are two subpopulations of T cells with differing functions: T helper (Th) cells and T cytotoxic (Tc) cells which can be distinguished by their expression of membrane glycoproteins designated CD4 for Th cells and CD8 for Tc cells. When a foreign antigen is introduced it is taken up by specialised cells called 'antigen-presenting cells' processed into small peptides and subsequently displayed on the surface of these cells in association with HLA class II molecules (see later). This complex of class II molecule and foreign peptide is recognised by the TCR of Th cells which become activated to produce a variety of cytokines. There are two subtypes of Th cells designated Th1 and Th2. The cytokine and hormonal environment in which the Th cells differentiate determines which subset develops. These are distinguished by the cytokines each subset secretes. Th1 cells (IL-2 and IFN-γ) bias the immune response towards activation of macrophages and CD8 Tc cells, while those from Th2 cells (IL-4, IL-5 and IL-10) encourage B cell differentiation and generalised antibody production. The type of immune response to a pathogen is thus determined by triggering either the cell-mediated (Th1) or the humoral (Th2) arms of the immune response.

THE MAJOR HISTOCOMPATIBILITY COMPLEX (MHC)

The MHC is a large complex of genes with multiple loci on chromosome 6. It encodes two major classes of membrane proteins known as human leucocyte antigens (HLA). These are designated as class I and class II. The HLA class I molecules are glycoproteins found on the surface of nearly all nucleated cells in association with a smaller molecular weight protein called β_2-microglobulin (β_2m). At present, six class I loci with demonstrable protein products have been identified. Three (HLA-A, B, C) are grouped as classical and three (HLA-E, F, G) as non-classical loci. The classical loci are highly polymorphic, that is there are large numbers of different alleles at each locus so that each individual expresses a unique combination of these HLA molecules on the cell surface. Disparity for these molecules between donor and recipient is the cause of graft rejection. In contrast, the non-classical HLA-E, F, G exhibit virtually no polymorphism so that these HLA class I proteins are almost identical in all individuals. There are three class II loci (DR, DP, DQ) and these are also all highly polymorphic. Class II molecules are not as ubiquitous as class I and are expressed only by certain cells such as B lymphocytes and antigen-presenting cells.

These MHC molecules are crucial for the generation of the adaptive immune response. Both HLA class I and class II molecules have a cleft that binds the antigenic peptides which may be derived from exogenous antigens (binding to class II molecules) or endogenous antigens (binding to class I molecules). A foreign exogenous antigen, such as a bacterium, when first introduced is endocytosed or phagocytosed by host MHC class II-expressing antigen-presenting cells. After processing, the smaller peptide fragments are bound to the cleft within the class II molecule and transported to the cell surface where they are recognised by CD4 Th cells. Similarly, a foreign endogenous antigen, such as viral proteins produced within the infected cells, is also degraded into peptides but is bound to the cleft of MHC class I molecules and will be recognised by CD8 Tc cells. It can be seen, therefore, that T lymphocytes always recognise a foreign antigen in association with either self MHC class I or class II molecules, a phenomenon known as MHC restriction. The reason why T cells respond in this seemingly complicated way is that it ensures that the response is not inappropriately directed at self components, thereby leading to autoimmunity.

The need to bind a wide spectrum of foreign peptides for protection against all kinds of pathogens is thought to be the evolutionary drive that has led to the high degree of poly-morphism of the MHC loci. This has created two major problems. One is the contemporary problem of graft rejection because, in an outbred human population, no two individuals will have the same MHC, except for identical twins. The second problem is in reproduction because the fetus has inherited half its genes from the father and is, therefore, analogous to a transplant in the uterus. So how does the fetus evade rejection by the mother? This question was first raised by Medawar (1953) but the answer has remained elusive.

KEY POINTS: THE IMMUNE RESPONSE

- Important cells in innate immunity are phagocytes and NK cells.
- Phagocytes ingest microorganisms by a variety of receptors and digest them.
- NK cells are cytolytic to target cells and can produce cytokines.
- Acquired immunity requires two populations of cells: T cells and B cells.
- T cells are involved in cell-mediated immunity while B cells produce antibodies.
- T cells are central to the generation of acquired immunity by expressing receptors capable of recognising foreign antigens.
- The MHC is a large complex of genes with multiple loci on chromosome 6 which encodes class I and class II HLA.
- MHC molecules are crucial for the generation of the acquired immune response by binding to antigens and presenting them for recognition by T cells.

DEVELOPMENT OF THE PLACENTA

Viviparity is a major advance in the evolution of vertebrate reproductive strategy because it allows the fetus to develop inside the maternal uterus protected from the dangers inherent in the external environment (Loke & King 1996). This form of reproduction is made possible by the formation of a specialised organ, the placenta, where maternal nutrients are delivered to the fetus and gaseous exchange takes place. Placentation is initiated when the blastocyst makes contact with the epithelial lining of the uterine mucosa, leading to a series of events known as implantation (Loke & King 1999). This involves fetally derived placental trophoblast cells invading the maternal uterine decidua. Thus, the fetus itself does not come into direct contact with the mother. It is the fetal placenta which does so. Furthermore, it is the population of trophoblast cells of the placenta which forms the ultimate interface between fetal and maternal tissues. This anatomical fact should be borne in mind when considering the fetal–maternal immunological relationship (Loke & King 1995). Indeed, the placenta is a very efficient barrier against the transmission of cells between the fetal and maternal circulations. Any cells that do cross usually do so at parturition; this explains why maternal sensitisation, for example against the RhD antigen, normally occurs after the first pregnancy.

The first element to differentiate in the blastocyst is the

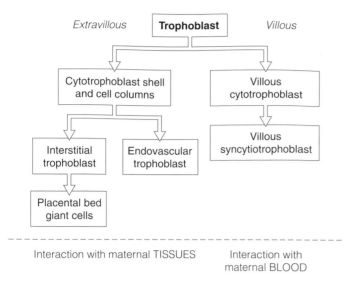

Fig. 7.1 Trophoblast differentiating along the villous and extravillous pathways. Villous trophoblast comes into contact with maternal blood in the intervillous space while extravillous trophoblast invades maternal uterine tissues.

trophectoderm. From this layer, trophoblast cells differentiate along two main pathways: villous and extravillous (Fig. 7.1). Villous trophoblast ultimately covers all the chorionic villi of the definitive placenta and is concerned mainly with the transport of oxygen and nutrients from mother to child; it is also the source of hormones such as hCG. This villous trophoblast consists of an inner layer of mononuclear cytotrophoblast cells, which sits on a basement membrane, and an outer multinucleated layer of syncytiotrophoblast. It is this latter which lines the entire intervillous space and comes into contact with maternal blood in a manner similar to endothelial cells. At the tips of some villi, cytotrophoblast cells break through the syncytium and fix the villi to the underlying uterine decidua to begin the extravillous pathway of differentiation. Initially these cytotrophoblast cells remain as a solid core known as cytotrophoblast cell columns. These spread laterally and fuse with neighbouring columns to form the cytotrophoblast shell which encircles the entire embryonic sac. Invading trophoblast cells arise from this shell and stream into the uterine mucosa as isolated interstitial trophoblast. These trophoblast cells can be seen to move towards and eventually surround the decidual spiral arteries which begin to show endothelial swelling with destruction of the muscular media and replacement with fibrinoid material. These changes are not seen in decidual vessels away from the implantation site (Kam et al 1999). By eight weeks of pregnancy, interstitial trophoblast has extensively colonised the full thickness of the uterine mucosa to reach the decidual–myometrial border. As the trophoblast cells move deeper into the decidua, they become multinucleated. These cells are known as placental bed giant cells and can be regarded as the terminally differentiated end-point of the extravillous pathway (as syncytiotrophoblast is for the villous pathway).

Besides interstitial trophoblast, the cytotrophoblast shell also is the source of endovascular trophoblast. Where the

shell comes to lie over the openings of the uterine spiral arteries, trophoblast cells form a plug, seemingly occluding the lumen. From these plugs, trophoblast moves in a retrograde manner down the inside of the spiral arteries 'like wax dripping down a candle', so that these vessels become lined partly by residual endothelial cells and partly by trophoblast. Interestingly, the walls of decidual veins are not similarly invaded by trophoblast. However, these veins do contain isolated syncytial cells (syncytial knots) which have become detached from the chorionic villi into the intervillous space. These knots are deported into the maternal circulation and become trapped in the blood vessels of the lungs where they are eventually lysed. A similar route is taken by choriocarcinoma, which explains why pulmonary deposits are the most frequent sites of metastases.

It can be seen that the function of the extravillous trophoblast populations (cytotrophoblast cell columns, interstitial trophoblast, endovascular trophoblast and placental bed giant cells) is to convert the maternal spiral arteries from muscular high-resistance vessels to dilated structures capable of high conductance (Fig. 7.2). This change is crucial to the normal growth and development of the feto-placental unit, and inadequate vascular transformation by trophoblast is the underlying defect in pre-eclampsia and some cases of intrauterine growth restriction (IUGR) and unexplained stillbirth.

TROPHOBLAST EXPRESSION OF MHC ANTIGENS

Since the genes responsible for recognition of non-self in graft rejection are from the highly polymorphic MHC, it is pertinent to look at the expression of these genes in trophoblast. The two layers of villous trophoblast (cytotrophoblast and syncytiotrophoblast) do not express either HLA class I or class II molecules. In contrast, all the extravillous trophoblast populations express HLA class I but not class II antigens (Table 7.1). Thus, there are essentially two fetomaternal interfaces which differ immunologically. While the maternal systemic immune system is likely to encounter a villous trophoblast population that is immunologically neutral, the maternal local uterine immune system can potentially be stimulated by the HLA class I antigens expressed by extravillous trophoblast (Loke & King 1995).

Table 7.1 Expression of HLA molecules by trophoblast: villous trophoblast is HLA class I and class II negative while extravillous trophoblast is HLA class II negative but expresses class I HLA-C, E and G; this has immunological implications because villous trophoblast interacts with the maternal systemic immune response while extravillous trophoblast interacts with the maternal local uterine immune response

Villous trophoblast	Extravillous trophoblast
HLA class I negative	HLA class I positive (HLA-C, E, G)
HLA class II negative	HLA class II negative
Interacts with maternal systemic immune response	Interacts with maternal local uterine immune response

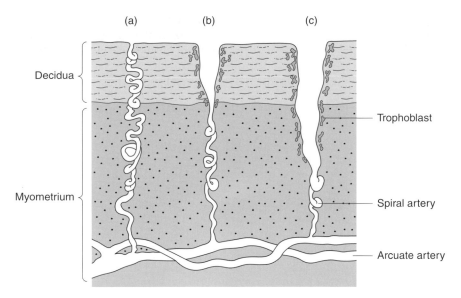

(a)　　　(b)　　　(c)

Decidua

Myometrium

Trophoblast

Spiral artery

Arcuate artery

Fig. 7.2 Diagram showing uterine spiral arteries which supply the placenta. (a) Arteries in the non pregnant state are tightly coiled. (b) During the first trimester, invading extravillous trophoblast cells replace the muscle and elastic tissue of the wall of the decidual segment of the artery, resulting in dilatation. (c) By the latter half of pregnancy, both the decidual and deeper myometrial segments of the artery are transformed in this way. This results in an increased flow of blood delivered at low pressure. Inadequate vascular transformation might lead to clinical conditions such as intrauterine growth restriction, stillbirth and pre-eclampsia.

The immunological implications have created much interest in elucidating the nature and function of the extravillous trophoblast HLA class I molecule. It is now generally accepted that extravillous trophoblast expresses a total of three class I molecules: one classical (HLA-C) (King et al 2000a) and two non-classical (HLA-E) (King et al 2000b) and (HLA-G) (Loke et al 1997). This is a rather unusual combination compared to other nucleated cells and, indeed, the functions of these trophoblast class I antigens are not known. Of the three, HLA-G has, so far, received most attention because of its unusual characteristics (Loke et al 1999). Its expression appears to be restricted to extravillous trophoblast and it is not found on other fetal or adult cells, which suggests a trophoblast-specific function. The only other non-trophoblast cell which has been observed to express HLA-G is a subpopulation of medullary epithelial cell in the thymus (Mallet et al 1999). This could provide a mechanism for the induction of central tolerance to HLA-G. HLA-G can bind peptides in the same way as classical class I molecules (Diehl et al 1996) but shows negligible polymorphism, particularly in the residues that make up the peptide-binding cleft (Hiby et al 1999). Therefore, there does not appear to be the same degree of evolutionary pressure for increasing the diversity of peptides presented by HLA-G as there is for HLA-A and HLA-B which present a diverse array of peptides to T cells. In contrast to HLA-G, HLA-E expression is not restricted to extravillous trophoblast but has a more ubiquitous pattern of tissue distribution although it shares with HLA-G the characteristic of limited polymorphism. HLA-E is a sentinel molecule which provides information on the level of expression of all other HLA class I molecules. This is achieved by HLA-E using the leader sequence peptide from other HLA class I molecules to bind in its cleft (Braud et al 1999). The classical class I HLA-C is also atypical when compared with the other classical molecules in having low surface expression and being less polymorphic than HLA-A and HLA-B. However, paternally-derived HLA-C alleles have been detected in extravillous trophoblast so these molecules would be expected to be recognised by the maternal immune system (King et al 2000a). HLA-C is therefore of particular interest as it is the only HLA class I molecule which is polymorphic and expressed by trophoblast, and the paternal HLA-C can differ with different pregnancies. The implications of this are slowly being unravelled by recent research (see below).

KEY POINTS: IMMUNOLOGY OF TROPHOBLAST

- Trophoblast differentiates along two main pathways: villous and extravillous.
- Villous trophoblast covers the chorionic villi and contacts maternal blood in the intervillous space while extravillous trophoblast invades into decidua.
- Villous trophoblast does not express HLA class I or class II molecules.
- Extravillous trophoblast does not express HLA class II molecules but expresses three HLA class I molecules: HLA-C, E, G.
- HLA-G protein expression is restricted to extravillous trophoblast.
- HLA-C is polymorphic but HLA-E and G are not.

MATERNAL SYSTEMIC IMMUNE RESPONSE DURING PREGNANCY

Sera from multiparous women are a major source of anti-HLA antibodies used for crossmatching in tissue-typing laboratories, and T cells from pregnant women frequently show sensitised responses to paternal lymphocytes (Sargent 1993). From these observations it can be concluded that, during pregnancy, the mother is not immunosuppressed and she can mount both a humoral and a cell-mediated immune response against paternal HLA antigens. However, the immunogenic source of maternal sensitisation is unlikely to be placental trophoblast because villous trophoblast which is in direct contact with maternal blood does not express HLA class I or class II molecules, while extravillous trophoblast in contact with uterine tissue expresses mainly non-classical HLA class I. A more likely stimulus probably comes from fetal cells that have crossed into the maternal circulation from fetomaternal bleeds, which generally occur during delivery in the same way as maternal sensitisation against the rhesus antigen on fetal red cells. This conclusion is supported by the finding that maternal HLA antibodies occur late in first pregnancies and are more easily detectable in multiparous women (Regan et al 1991). The most pertinent observation of all is that the presence of maternal sensitisation has no discernible effects on the outcome of pregnancy (Sargent et al 1987). This is presumably because the placenta presents no targets for maternal antibodies or cells to act on since villous trophoblast expresses no HLA antigens at all while the extravillous trophoblast HLA molecules are sufficiently monomorphic so as not to be recognised. Thus, the placenta can be considered as an efficient immunological barrier in the face of an intact maternal immune response.

However, observations from animal models of pregnancy have suggested that, while maternal immune responses may be intact, this response is quantitatively and qualitatively altered (Vacchio & Jiang 1999). Experiments with transgenic mice have shown a downregulation of T cell receptors in maternal blood specific for paternal allospecificity (Tafuri et al 1995). Also, during pregnancy, maternal immune responses appear to be deviated from a Th1 to a Th2 type (i.e. from a cell-mediated to a humoral response), and it has been suggested that this Th2 response is beneficial in some way to pregnancy, perhaps by the production of appropriate cytokines (Wegmann et al 1993). This was shown in mice experimentally infected with the intracellular protozoan Leishmania (normally a Th1 response). Pregnancy was found to impair resistance of mice to infections by Leishmania (Krishnan et al 1996a) and, in the reciprocal situation, a successful response against Leishmania led to increased implantation failure and fetal resorption (Krishnan et al 1996b). In human pregnancy there is only indirect evidence in support of immunodeviation. For example, among the autoimmune diseases, rheumatoid arthritis, which is due to a Th1 response, usually shows remission during pregnancy whereas systemic lupus erythematosus (SLE), which involves a Th2 response, is worse during pregnancy (Buyon 1998). It has also been reported that T cells cloned from women with recurrent miscarriages produce low levels of Th2 cytokines such as IL-4 and IL-10 (Piccinni et al 1998). There is still much confusion in this area because it remains unclear what antigens are responsible for triggering this Th2 response during pregnancy. The idea that a pregnant woman may be required to mount an appropriate immune response against her conceptus to ensure success of her pregnancy has led to the regimen of treating women with recurrent miscarriages by injecting them with their husbands' lymphocytes, the rationale being to induce these women to generate this putative, potentially beneficial immune response (Mowbray et al 1985). However, recent data from a multicentre randomised trial have shown that this kind of immunotherapy does not show any beneficial effects, and it was recommended that it should no longer be offered to patients (Ober et al 1999).

MATERNAL LOCAL IMMUNE RESPONSE IN THE UTERUS

At the implantation site, the pregnant uterine mucosa (decidua) is infiltrated by large numbers of lymphoid cells with an unusual morphology and phenotype. They have been referred to as large granular lymphocytes (LGL) because of the prominent granules in their cytoplasm. These LGL are CD56^{bright} CD16$^-$, suggesting that they are natural killer (NK) cells but distinct from peripheral blood NK cells which are CD56^{dim} CD16$^+$ (King et al 1998, King 2000). Macrophages are also abundant at the implantation site whereas T and B cells are sparse. Thus, it is cells of the innate immune system (NK cells and macrophages) that predominate and not cells of the adaptive immune system (T and B cells). The total number of NK cells in the uterine mucosa varies throughout the menstrual cycle (Fig. 7.3). There are very few during the proliferative phase. They increase significantly in number throughout the secretory phase and remain in large numbers in the decidua during the early stages of gestation. They are particularly abundant in decidua basalis (where the placenta implants) compared with decidua parietalis (away from the implantation site) and come into close contact with the invading extravillous trophoblast cells. This temporal and spatial association between decidual NK cells and placental trophoblast had led to the proposal that their interaction is pivotal in the control of implantation (King & Loke 1991).

The mechanisms of this NK cell–trophoblast interaction are not known but the recent identification of NK cell receptors and their ligands has suggested possible ways by which this can occur (Lanier 1998). Three structurally distinct families of receptors have been defined. The first to be described belongs to the immunoglobulin superfamily and is known as KIR (killer cell immunoglobulin-like receptor). Through variation of their cytoplasmic domains, interaction with ligands will trigger either an inhibitory or activating response by the NK cell. The second receptor identified (CD94/NKG2) belongs to the C type lectin superfamily. These are heterodimers consisting of an invariant CD94 which associates with different members of the NKG2 family resulting in contrasting functions. For example, CD94/NKG2A induces an inhibitory signal preventing cytolysis by the NK cell while CD94/NKG2C is activating. Again, as in KIR, this dichotomy in function arises

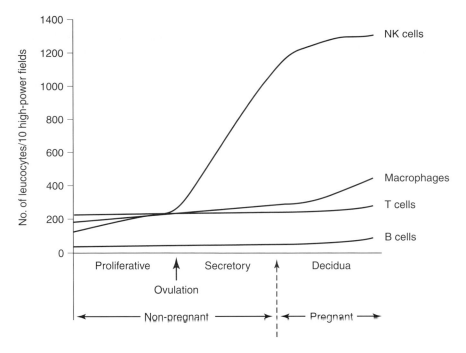

Fig. 7.3 Numbers of leucocytes present in the uterine mucosa during the non-pregnant menstrual cycle and in the early decidua. The data were obtained by immunohistological staining for natural killer (NK) cells, T cells, B cells and macrophages and subsequent direct counting of these cells in tissue sections. (From Loke & King 1997.)

from variation in the cytoplasmic domains of the NKG2 molecules (Fig. 7.4). The most recently described receptor is ILT (immunoglobulin-like transcripts) which is also a member of the immunoglobulin superfamily and is expressed by many leucocytes (B cells and monocytes) besides NK cells. As with the other receptors, there are inhibitory and activating forms of ILT.

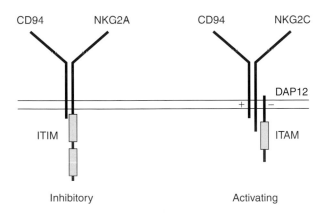

Fig. 7.4 Structures of the CD94/NKG2 family of lectin-like receptors. CD94 associates with members of the NKG2 family to form heterodimers. CD94/NKG2A is inhibitory due to the presence of immunoreceptor tyrosine-based inhibitory motifs (ITIM) in the cytoplasmic domain. CD94/NKG2C is activatory and has a charged residue in the transmembrane region through which it associates with a signalling molecule, DAP-12, which contains an immunoreceptor tyrosine-based activation motif (ITAM). (From King et al 2000a.)

All these NK receptors can recognise HLA class I molecules. The class I locus that seems to be most influential to KIR function is HLA-C although there is preliminary evidence that one member may recognise HLA-G. The ligand for CD94/NKG2 is now established to be HLA-E. So far, two members of the ILT family (ILT2 and ILT4) are reported to bind to a wide range of HLA class I molecules including HLA-G. Since HLA-C, HLA-E and HLA-G are precisely the three class I molecules expressed by extravillous trophoblast, a potential mechanism is therefore in place for decidual NK cells to interact with trophoblast (King et al 2000c). The outcome of this interaction is still unclear, but it is thought that NK cell derived cytokines will affect how deeply extravillous trophoblast cells transform the spiral arteries (Loke & King 2000).

The overall conclusion is that the immunological mechanisms involved in implantation are not the same as those encountered in organ transplantation. Implantation appears to be influenced by an evolutionary older innate allorecognition system rather than by the contemporary adaptive T cell immune system (Loke & King 1997).

TRANSFER OF MATERNAL ANTIBODIES TO THE FETUS

Antibodies from the mother can cross the placenta into the fetal circulation (Loke 1978). This is a very important means of defence against infection for the fetus in utero and during the first few months after birth as illustrated by the increased susceptibility to infection in neonates born to mothers with hypogammaglobulinaemia. These maternal antibodies are gradually catabolised over the first few months of life to be replaced by the infant's own actively acquired antibodies which are developed as a result of coming into contact with antigens in the environment. Of the five classes of immunoglobulins, only IgG can cross the placenta. This is because the mechanism of transfer is a receptor-mediated process. The layer of syncytiotrophoblast through which the antibody has to cross expresses a receptor specific for the Fc region of IgG (FcγR) and not for any of the other immunoglobulin classes. Interestingly, this FcγR is not the same as that expressed by other cells such as phagocytes, NK cells or mast cells. Instead, the syncytiotrophoblast receptor is structurally very similar to an HLA class I molecule and is known as FcRn (Simister & Story 1997).

The first step in the transfer is a non-specific fluid phase endocytosis by syncytiotrophoblast which has numerous microvilli on the surface, thus presenting a large absorptive area. This is followed by specific binding of IgG to FcRn in the acidified environment of the endocytic vesicles. This complex protects the IgG molecule from intracellular degradation. When it reaches the fetal side, the IgG is released under the neutral pH conditions and makes its way into the fetal vessels which lie in close proximity to the overlying layer of syncytiotrophoblast (Simister 1998).

Since the mechanism of transfer is via the Fc portion of the immunoglobulin molecule, the question arises as to how the placenta can distinguish between beneficial IgG (that combats infection) and potentially harmful IgG (that is directed at fetal antigens) since the antigen recognition sites reside in the Fab portion of the molecule. There is some evidence that the placenta can discriminate between the two, at least to some extent, but not always. It seems to do so by expressing relevant fetal antigens, probably in the cells of the chorionic villous mesenchyme through which the antibodies have to pass before reaching the fetal vessels, and mopping up all those potentially harmful antibodies directed at fetal antigens. Thus arose the concept of the placenta acting as an immunological sponge (Swinburne 1970).

This selection cannot occur if the placental cells do not express the relevant antigens. Such a situation is seen with the blood group antibodies, of which the most important are those directed against RhD. When a RhD-negative mother is sensitised by red blood cells from a RhD-positive fetus, she will produce anti-RhD antibodies which are IgG and will therefore cross the placenta into the fetal circulation. These maternal antibodies destroy fetal red cells, giving rise to haemolytic disease of the newborn. Fortunately, the 'natural' ABO blood group antibodies are IgM and, therefore, cannot cross the placenta so that maternal–fetal incompatibility for these blood group antigens does not normally lead to haemolytic disease. The alloantigenic system on fetal platelets can also stimulate an incompatible mother to make IgG antibodies which, when transferred across the placenta, can lead to thrombocytopenia in the fetus or newborn.

Besides alloantibodies, another group of potentially harmful maternal antibodies are IgG autoantibodies directed at her own cellular components. Again, this is probably due to the fact that there are no equivalent antigens in the placenta to mop up these antibodies because many of these antigens are organ-specific. One example is the autoantibody directed at the receptor on thyroid cells for TSH which is the cause of hyperthyroidism (Graves disease). When transmitted to the fetus, it will cause a similar syndrome of neonatal thyrotoxicosis (Mckenzie 1964). This is usually transient and resolves when all the maternal antibodies are catabolised. Another example is the autoantibody to the choline esterase receptor which, when transmitted from the mother, gives rise to myasthenia gravis in the infant. There are other autoimmune diseases, such as systemic lupus erythematosus (SLE), which are associated with a broad array of autoantibodies directed at a variety of tissue components, especially blood cells. These autoantibodies lead to haematological symptoms in the fetus or newborn baby, such as haemolytic anaemia and thrombocytopenia (Chaplin et al 1973). Destruction of fetal blood components, therefore, may be caused by either an alloimmune or an autoimmune mechanism. An interesting IgG autoantibody present in approximately 25% of SLE patients is the anti-RO antibody. It causes complete heart block in the fetus which, unlike other conditions caused by maternal antibodies, does not resolve. Furthermore, the mother herself shows no evidence of cardiac disease so this antibody appears to react only to antigens in the fetal bundle of His and not to adult cardiac cells.

From the preceding discussion it is clear that, although the major role of maternal antibodies is to protect the developing fetus from infections, their transfer can sometimes lead to unwanted and damaging consequences. This occurs because the mechanism of transmission of these antibodies across the placenta is via the Fc region so that the selection is according to antibody class rather than specificity.

KEY POINTS: MATERNAL IMMUNE RESPONSE

- Maternal sera contain anti-HLA antibodies and sensitised T cells against paternal antigens. Their presence has no discernible effects on the outcome of pregnancy.
- Immune response during pregnancy is said to be deviated from a Th1 to a Th2 response.
- The decidua is infiltrated by a unique population of NK cells which are phenotypically and functionally different from NK cells in blood.
- Decidual NK cells express three families of receptors capable of recognising HLA-C, E and G expressed by extravillous trophoblast.
- It is proposed that interaction between decidual NK cell receptors and trophoblast HLA class I molecules could provide a mechanism for controlling trophoblast invasion.

IMMUNOLOGICAL ASPECTS OF RECURRENT MISCARRIAGE

Recurrent miscarriage is usually defined as the consecutive loss of three or more pregnancies before 20 weeks' gestation (Regan 1992). It is estimated that the problem affects up to 0.5% of all couples. A variety of causes have been proposed including chromosomal abnormalities of the fetus, uterine anomalies in the mothers, endocrine disorders, infections and environmental pollutants. The antigenic disparity between the mother and her fetus means that the possibility of an immunological cause has always attracted much attention. Both alloimmune and autoimmune reactions have been suggested.

According to the hypothesis that an appropriate Th2 maternal immune response towards her genetically dissimilar conceptus is required for successful pregnancy, failure to mount such a response would be expected to lead to pregnancy failure. Women who suffer from recurrent miscarriages are thought to be poor responders. Thus, the regimen of immunotherapy described earlier is designed to boost this putative response although the overall consensus now is that this form of treatment is not effective. One reason offered for maternal hyporesponsiveness is that the fetal HLA phenotype is insufficiently different from that of the mother to generate a response. This, in turn, has led to a search to determine whether couples who suffer from recurrent miscarriage share more HLA antigens than couples with successful pregnancies. The published data are highly conflicting and do not permit any definite conclusion (Bellingard et al 1995, Jin et al 1995, Sbracia et al 1996, Brennan 1997, Ober et al 1998).

A common autoimmune disorder found in women of reproductive age is SLE. Recurrent miscarriage is a well-recognised complication of the disease. The sera from these women contain a variety of autoantibodies but the ones that seem to have the greatest association with fetal loss are the two antiphospholipid antibodies, lupus anticoagulant and anticardiolipin. Some women with these antibodies do not exhibit overt clinical signs of SLE although they may develop symptoms later; the term antiphospholipid syndrome has been adopted to define this group (Rai & Regan 1997). The mechanism of action of these antibodies is thought to be dysregulation of the coagulation pathway leading to thrombosis of the uteroplacental vessels. This results in poor placental perfusion and even infarction of the placenta and eventual fetal death. Owing to this thrombogenic action, current treatment is to administer either low-dose aspirin or a combination of low-dose aspirin with the anticoagulant heparin. The latter appears to be more effective, improving the subsequent live birth rate of these patients to 70% compared to 40% with aspirin alone, although there is some risk of growth restriction among the infants born (Backos et al 1999). The antigenic targets for antiphospholipid antibodies have still not been clearly defined. Some studies have shown that these antibodies are not directed at phospholipids at all but are against phospholipid-binding plasma proteins which act as carriers (Roubey 1994). Others have found evidence that these antibodies can bind to phospholipids on the surface of trophoblast cells (Yamamoto et al 1996), suggesting that an alternative mode of action could be by direct disruption of implantation.

Supportive evidence that recurrent miscarriage could have an immunological aetiology is provided by analysis of the lymphoid cell population in the endometrium from these patients in a non-pregnant cycle. Changes in the numbers of endometrial lymphocytes have been observed compared with women with successful pregnancies (Quenby et al 1999). In particular, there is a decrease in the usual population of $CD56^{bright}$ $CD16^-$ NK cells with a concomitant increase in $CD56^{dim}$ $CD16^+$ NK cells (Lachapelle et al 1996). The conclusion is that recurrent aborters do have a distinct cellular profile in their endometrium which antedates implantation, indicating an altered immune environment within the uterus.

IMMUNOLOGICAL ASPECTS OF PRE-ECLAMPSIA

Pre-eclampsia is a systemic disease characterised by widespread endothelial activation resulting in diverse symptoms including proteinuria, hypertension and peripheral oedema. It occurs primarily in first pregnancies and is found in all ethnic groups worldwide. Furthermore, it is a disease associated with the presence of placental tissue only, and in situations in which there is increased placental mass (twins, hydatidiform mole) there is an increased incidence of pre-eclampsia (Perloff 1998).

The pathogenesis of the disease can be considered in three stages:

1. Detailed histological studies of the placental bed have revealed that there is defective transformation by trophoblast of the spiral arteries feeding the intervillous space. This results in partial retention of the muscular wall so that the vessels do not have the high conductance necessary for increased blood flow required for the developing fetoplacental unit.
2. The decreased blood flow to the growing placenta results in disordered formation of the complex villous tree which continues to form throughout most of pregnancy. The reduced branching then results in defective transport of nutrients and oxygen. The fetus will not grow and develop normally and growth will be restricted. Fetal death in utero may result from hypoxia.
3. The ischaemic placenta triggers maternal systemic endothelial activation by an unknown mechanism. Candidate factors have included villous syncytial membranes and cytokines.

Many of the epidemiological, genetic and clinical features of pre-eclampsia suggest that there is an 'immunological' basis to this disease (Lie et al 1998). It occurs principally in first pregnancies unless there is a change of partner when the risk in subsequent pregnancies is similar to that of the first. This suggests that previous exposure to placental (or fetal cells) bearing paternal antigens is protective. A long period of exposure to sperm from the reproductive partner may also be protective (Robillard et al 1994) which may explain the increased incidence of pre-eclampsia seen with pregnancies resulting from sperm donation (Smith et al 1997, Dekker et al 1998). That paternal factors are important is also seen in the lack of concordance of the disease in monozygotic twins, indicating that maternal genetic predisposition alone cannot explain the pathogenesis of the disease. Fathers who change partners also carry an increased risk of pre-eclampsia developing in their partners in the next pregnancy. More recently, it has emerged that the greatest risk for pre-eclampsia (>30%) is seen in women who have received donated oocytes (Abdalla et al 1998, Soderstrom-Antilla et al 1998). In these pregnancies the implanting blastocyst is totally allogeneic to the mother and shares no 'self' antigens, in contrast to the normal semi-allogeneic embryo.

The immunological mechanisms involved have not been established. Since the primary defect in pre-eclampsia is failure of transformation of spiral arteries by extravillous trophoblast, it is possible that interaction of HLA class I molecules expressed by extravillous trophoblast with uterine NK cells could lead to different degrees of invasion in different pregnancies. In particular, trophoblast paternally-derived HLA-C will vary in different pregnancies. Furthermore, the NK receptors for HLA-C, the KIR, are inherited as a KIR NK genotype which will also differ in different women. Some combinations of fetal HLA-C and maternal KIR might result in inadequate trophoblast invasion.

IMMUNITY TO SPERM AND INFERTILITY

It has long been demonstrated in experiments both on animals and in human patients suffering from infertility that the presence of antisperm antibodies is correlated with impaired reproductive success (Bronson 1999). However, published data remain highly conflicting so the significance of this correlation is still unclear. There are several reasons for this confusion. Firstly, antisperm antibodies are relatively ubiquitous and not all of them are relevant to infertility. Only those that are directed at sperm surface antigens would be expected to play a role in infertility and not those that recognise internal antigens. Secondly, antisperm antibodies belong to different immunoglobulin classes (e.g. IgG, IgM, IgA) which can influence sperm activity in different ways. Finally, there appears to be a dichotomy in the concentration of antisperm antibodies in serum and in the reproductive tract. It is the concentration in the latter that influences reproduction.

Antisperm antibodies can be found in the male or female. It is generally believed that sperm antigens are sequestered by the blood–testis barrier and thereby normally prevented from recognition by the host's immune system. This tolerance can be broken if there is disruption of the barrier such as prevention of egress of sperm from the testis. Thus, approximately half the men who have undergone vasectomy have detectable sperm antibodies in their sera. Although women regularly come into contact with spermatozoa during coitus, they do not normally make antisperm antibodies. Yet the female reproductive tract is not an immunologically privileged site since it can mount an immune response to infective organisms. The absence of a response to sperm is thought to result from immunosuppressive substances in semen. Why some women and not others are stimulated to make antisperm antibodies is not known.

There are two possible mechanisms by which antisperm antibodies can lead to infertility. One is that these antibodies directed at gamete receptors or ligands block interaction and penetration of the egg by sperm. The other is reduction of sperm motility, thereby interfering with their ability to penetrate cervical mucus and subsequent transport into the uterus. Impairment of sperm transport may be amenable to treatment. Intrauterine insemination, by placing large numbers of sperm directly into the uterine cavity has been tried, the rationale being to increase the likelihood that sperm will enter the fallopian tube to come into contact with an egg. An alternative method of treatment is IVF, which would be expected also to circumvent any defect in sperm mobility due to antisperm antibody.

CHIMERISM

It is now established that lymphocytes from the mother or the fetus can cross the placenta during pregnancy in both directions (Aractingi et al 2000). This is presumably the major source of maternal sensitisation for the production of anti-HLA antibodies against paternal MHC antigens. Surprisingly, some of these cells can survive for a remarkably long time, with a report of fetal cells found in the mother 27 years later (Bianchi et al 1996). Since these are immunocompetent cells, the question arises as to what might be the consequence of this reciprocal chimerism. The induction of a graft-versus-host reaction (GVHR) in the fetus, such as runting, is well recognised in animal studies. In humans, the occurrence of severe immunodeficiency in neonates may be an example of this. What happens in the mother is less well documented. There is now a suspicion that some maternal autoimmune diseases might, in fact, be caused by surviving fetal cells attacking her antigenically incompatible tissue as in a reverse GVHR. One such example could be the disease scleroderma whose clinical manifestations are similar to those seen in GVHR. Indeed, the presence of large numbers of fetal cells has been demonstrated in skin lesions of these patients (Artlett et al 1999). The possibility that some autoimmune diseases are really alloimmune diseases is intriguing. It would seem that the close immunological relationship between the fetus and its mother during pregnancy can lead to long-term subtle and far-reaching effects in both fetus and mother which may not be immediately obvious.

CONCLUSION

Ever since the recognition that transplant rejection is immunological, the paradox of the survival of the allogeneic mammalian conceptus has intrigued biologists from a wide variety of disciplines. In spite of a great deal of research, the solution remains tantalisingly elusive. It is now realised that this is because human reproduction is not governed by the laws of contemporary transplantation immunology. Instead, it seems to involve an evolutionary older immune system which is probably unique to the placenta and the uterus so that the trophoblast–decidua interaction is not directly comparable to the graft–host interaction. The cellular and molecular mechanisms are now slowly being unravelled. This is, perhaps, the most exciting area of research in reproductive immunology. Once there is an understanding of how successful pregnancy is maintained, then an explanation might be found for those pregnancy diseases where this immunological equilibrium is disrupted, such as infertility, miscarriage, intrauterine growth restriction and pre-eclampsia.

Outstanding questions

- What are the functions of trophoblast HLA-C, E and G molecules?
- How do decidual NK cells interact with trophoblast HLA class I molecules and what is the outcome of this interaction?
- Can pathological conditions of pregnancy be correlated with defects in trophoblast–NK cell interaction?

KEY POINTS: IMMUNOPATHOLOGY

- Transfer of maternal alloantibodies or autoantibodies may cause disease in the fetus.
- Maternal autoimmune disorders may be associated with recurrent miscarriage.
- Many features of pre-eclampsia suggest that it may have an immunological aetiology.
- Antisperm antibodies could lead to infertility.
- Establishment of chimerism could have long-term immunological consequences.

REFERENCES

Abdalla HI, Billett A, Kan AKS, Baig S, Wren M, Korea L, Studd JWW 1998 Obstetric outcome in 232 ovum donation pregnancies. Br J Obstet Gynaecol 105:332–337

Aractingi S, Uzan S, Dausset J, Carosella ED 2000 Microchimerism in human diseases. Immunol Today 21:116–118

Artlett CM, Smith JB, Jimenez SA 1999 New perspectives in the etiology of systemic sclerosis. Mol Med Today 5:74–78

Backos M, Rai R, Baxter N, Chilcott IT, Cohen H, Regan L 1999 Pregnancy complications in women with recurrent miscarriage associated with antiphospholipid antibodies treated with low dose aspirin and heparin. Br J Obstet Gynaecol 106:102–107

Bellingard V, Hedon B, Eliaou JF, Seignalet J, Clot J, Viala JL 1995 Immunogenetic study of couples with recurrent spontaneous abortions. Eur J Obstet Gynecol Reprod Biol 60:53–60

Bianchi DW, Zickwolf GK, Weil GJ, Sylvester S, DeMaria MA 1996 Male fetal progenitor cells persist in maternal blood for as long as 27 years postpartum. Proc Natl Acad Sci U S A 93:705–708

Braud VM, Allan DS, McMichael AJ 1999 Functions of non-classical MHC and non-MHC-encoded class I molecules. Curr Opin Immunol 11:100–108

Brennan P 1997 HLA sharing and history of miscarriage among women with rheumatoid arthritis. Am J Hum Genet 60:738–740

Bronson RA 1999 Antisperm antibodies: a critical evaluation and clinical guidelines. J Reprod Immunol 45:159–183

Buyon JP 1998 The effects of pregnancy on auto-immune diseases. J Leukoc Biol 63: 281–287

Chaplin H, Cohen R, Bloomberg G, Kaplan HJ, Moore JA, Dorner I 1973 Pregnancy and idiopathic haemolytic anaemia: a prospective study during 6 months gestation and 3 months post-partum. Br J Haematol 24:219–229

Dekker GA, Robillard PY, Hulsey TC 1998 Immune maladaptation in the etiology of preeclampsia: a review of corroborative epidemiologic studies. Obstet Gynecol Surv 53:377–382

Diehl M, Munz C, Keilholz W, Stevanovic S, Loke YW, Holmes N, Rammensee H-G 1996 Non-classical HLA-G molecules are classical peptide presenters. Curr Biol 6:305–314

Goldsby RA, Kindt TJ, Osborne BA 2000 Immunology, 4th edn. WH Freeman, New York

Hiby SE, King A, Sharkey A, Loke YW 1999 Molecular studies of trophoblast HLA-G: polymorphism, isoforms, imprinting and expression in pre-implantation embryo. Tissue Antigens 53:1–13

Janeway CA, Travers P, Walport M, Capra JD 1999 Immunobiology. The immune system in health and disease, 4th edn. Churchill Livingstone, London

Jin K, Ho HN, Speed TP, Gill TJ 1995 Reproductive failure and the major histocompatibility complex. Am J Hum Genet 56:1456–1467

Kam EPY, Gardner L, Loke YW, King A 1999 The role of trophoblast in the physiological change in decidual spiral arteries. Hum Reprod 14:2131–2138

King A 2000 Uterine leukocytes and decidualization. Hum Reprod Update 6:28–36

King A, Loke YW 1991 On the nature and function of human uterine granular lymphocytes. Immunol Today 12:432–435

King A, Burrows T, Verma S, Hiby SE, Loke YW 1998 Human uterine lymphocytes. Humn Reprod Update 4:480–485

King A, Burrows TD, Hiby SE et al 2000a Surface expression of HLA-C antigen by human extravillous trophoblast. Placenta 21:376–387

King A, Allan DSJ, Joseph S et al 2000b HLA-E is expressed on trophoblast and interacts with CD94/NKG2 receptors on decidual NK cells. Eur J Immunol 30: 1623–1631

King A, Hiby SE, Gardner L et al 2000c Recognition of trophoblast HLA class I molecules by decidual NK cell receptors. Trophoblast Res 14:S81–S85

Krishnan L, Guilbert LJ, Russell AS, Wegmann TG, Mosmann TR, Belosevic M 1996a Pregnancy impairs resistance of C57BL/6 mice to Leishmania major infection and causes decreased antigen-specific IFN-γ responses and increased production of T helper 2 cytokines. J Immunol 156:644–652

Krishnan L, Guilbert LJ, Wegmann TG, Belosevic M, Mosmann TR 1996b T helper 1 response against Leishmania major in pregnant C57BL/6 mice increases implantation failure and fetal resorptions. J Immunol 156:653–662

Lachapelle M-H, Miron P, Hemmings R, Roy DC 1996 Endometrial T, B and NK cells in patients with recurrent spontaneous abortion. J Immunol 156:4027–4034

Lanier LL 1998 NK cell receptors. Ann Rev Immunol 16:359–393

Lie RT, Rasmussen S, Brunborg H, Gjessing HK, Lie-Nielsen E, Irgens IM 1998 Fetal and maternal contributions to risk of pre-eclampsia: population based study. BMJ 316: 1343–1347

Loke YW 1978 Immunology and immunopathology of the human foetal–maternal interaction. Elsevier/North Holland, Amsterdam

Loke YW, King A 1995 Human implantation: cell biology and immunology. Cambridge University Press, Cambridge

Loke YW, King A 1996 Immunology of human implantation: an evolutionary perspective. Hum Reprod 11:283–286

Loke YW, King A 1997 Immunology of human placental implantation: clinical implications of our current understanding. Mol Med Today 3:153–159

Loke YW, King A 1999 Implantation. In: Rodeck CH, Whittle MJ (eds) Fetal medicine: basic science and clinical practice. Churchill Livingstone, London, pp 87–92

Loke YW, King A 2000 Decidual NK cell interaction with trophoblast: cytolysis or cytokine production? Biochem Soc Trans 28:196–198

Loke YW, King A, Burrows T et al 1997 Evaluation of trophoblast HLA-G antigen with a specific monoclonal antibody. Tissue Antigens 50:135–146

Loke YW, Hiby SE, King A 1999 Human leucocyte antigen-G and reproduction. J Reprod Immunol 43:235–242

Mckenzie JM 1964 Neonatal Graves' disease. J Clin Endocrinol 24:660–668

Mallet V, Blaschitz A, Crisa L et al 1999 HLA-G in the human thymus: a subpopulation of medullary epithelial but not CD83+ dendritic cells express HLA-G as membrane-bound and soluble protein. Int Immunol 11:889–898

Medawar PB 1953 Some immunological and endocrinological problems raised by the evolution of viviparity in vertebrates. In: Society for Experimental Biology. Academic Press, New York, pp 320–328

Mowbray JF, Gibbings C, Liddell H, Reginald PW, Underwood JL, Beard RW 1985 Controlled trial of treatment of recurrent miscarriage with paternal cells. Lancet i: 941–943

Ober C, Hyslop T, Elias S, Weitkamp LR, Hauck WW 1998 Human leukocyte antigen matching and fetal loss: results of a 10 year prospective study. Hum Reprod 13:33–38

Ober C, Karrison T, Odem RR et al 1999 Mononuclear-cell immunisation in prevention of recurrent miscarriages: a randomised trial. Lancet 354:365–369

Parham P 2000 The immune system. Garland Publishing/Elsevier Science, London

Perloff JD 1998 Hypertension and pregnancy-related hypertension. Cardiol Clin 16:79–101

Piccinni MP, Beloni L, Livi C, Maggi E, Scarselli G, Romagnani S 1998 Defective production of both leukaemia, inhibitory factor and type 2 T helper cytokines by decidual T cells in unexplained recurrent abortion. Nat Med 4:1020–1024

Quenby S, Bates M, Doig T, Brewster J, Lewis-Jones DI, Johnson PM, Vince G 1999 Pre-implantation endometrial leukocytes in women with recurrent miscarriage. Hum Reprod 14:2386–2391

Rai R, Regan L 1997 Antiphospholipid antibodies, infertility and recurrent miscarriage. Curr Opin Obstet Gynecol 9:279–282

Regan L 1992 Recurrent early pregnancy failure. Curr Opin Obstet Gynecol 4:220–228

Regan L, Braude PR, Hill DP 1991 A prospective study of the incidence, time of appearance and significance of anti-paternal lymphocytotoxic antibodies in human pregnancy. Hum Reprod 6:294–298

Robillard P, Hulsey TC, Alexander GR, Keenan A, de Caunes F, Papiernik E 1994 Paternity patterns and risk of pre-eclampsia in the last pregnancy in multiparae. J Reprod Immunol 24:1–12

Roubey RAS 1994 Autoantibodies to phospholipid-binding plasma proteins: a new view of lupus anticoagulants and other 'antiphospholipid' autoantibodies. Blood 84:2854–2867

Sargent IL 1993 Maternal and fetal immune responses during pregnancy. Exp Clin Immunogenet 10:85–102

Sargent IL, Arenas J, Redman CWG 1987 Maternal cell-mediated sensitisation to paternal HLA may occur, but is not a regular event in normal human pregnancy. J Reprod Immunol 10:111–120

Sbracia M, Mastrone M, Scarpellini F, Grasso JA 1996 Influence of histocompatibility antigens in recurrent spontaneous abortion couples and on their reproductive performances. Am J Reprod Immunol 35:85–92

Simister NE 1998 Human placental Fc receptors and the trapping of immune complexes. Vaccine 16:1451–1455

Simister NE, Story CM 1997 Human placental Fc receptors and the transmission of antibodies from mother to fetus. J Reprod Immunol 37:1–23

Smith GN, Walker M, Tessier JL, Millar KG 1997 Increased incidence of preeclampsia in women conceiving by intrauterine insemination with donor versus partner sperm for treatment of primary infertility. Am J Obstet Gynecol 177:455–458

Soderstrom-Antilla V, Tiitinen A, Foudila T, Hovatta O 1998 Obstetric and perinatal outcome from oocyte donation: comparison with in vitro fertilization pregnancies. Hum Reprod 13:483–490

Swinburne LM 1970 Leucocyte antigens and placental sponge. Lancet 2:592–594

Tafuri A, Alferink J, Möller P, Hämmerling GJ, Arnold B 1995 T cell awareness of paternal alloantigens during pregnancy. Science 270:630–633

Vacchio MS, Jiang S-P 1999 The fetus and the maternal immune system: pregnancy as a model to study peripheral T-cell tolerance. Crit Rev Immunol 19:461–480

Wegmann TG, Lin H, Guilbert I, Mosmann TR 1993 Bidirectional cytokine interactions in the maternal–fetal relationship: is successful pregnancy a T_H2 phenomenon? Immunol Today 14:353–356

Yamamoto T, Takahashi Y, Geshi Y, Sasamori Y, Mori H 1996 Antiphospholipid antibodies in preeclampsia and their binding ability for placental villous lipid fractions. J Obstet Gynaecol Res 22:275–283

Section 2
NORMAL ANTENATAL CARE

8

Prepregnancy and antenatal care

Marion H. Hall

The practice of health care should at the beginning of the third millennium include only elements that are of established benefit and which represent good value for money to those commissioning health care on behalf of the tax payer. Does prepregnancy or antenatal care fit this description? To answer this question we need to know whether health gain, including women's perception of their own health, will result. We also need to know whether intervention should be offered to all prepregnant or pregnant women or only to high-risk groups, whether all eligible women can be reached and whether any additional costs required for the intervention will be offset by savings in the prevention or treatment of ill health. A net increase in cost may not be worth incurring if the money could be more effectively used elsewhere.

PREPREGNANCY CARE

Reaching the target population

Starting with prepregnancy care, no one could disagree that it would be ideal if every couple approached pregnancy in optimal health, but the real question is whether it is appropriate or effective to offer unsolicited or solicited prepreg-

nancy advice, and to whom the advice should be offered. One difficulty is in identifying the target population, which could theoretically include all women of reproductive age, and all postpubertal men of any age, who have not been sterilised. However, although men may be involved in consultations before pregnancy, the few health-related actions that they may be asked to make are usually designed to improve fertility, rather than pregnancy outcome. On the rare occasions when men are taking drugs such as finasteride, which may, if excreted in semen, be harmful to pregnant women, protective use of condoms would preclude conception. Even if only women are to be targeted it has been calculated (Boon & Hull 1995) that to reach one woman who is actually going to become pregnant a general practitioner would have to interrogate, test or advise, during general medical consultations, 78 women. This is unlikely to be feasible. More promising approaches might be to target consultations concerning infertility, pregnancy termination, miscarriage or contraception (these consultations are calculated to reach one prepregnant woman per 28 consultations (Boon & Hull 1995), but even then the woman who is going to become pregnant may not believe that she is, or may become, pregnant sooner than she expects. If there is a long delay, healthy behaviour may not be sustained. Alternatively, health promotion could be (as it often is) aimed at the general public, or at secondary school children. Environmental measures (such as fertification of food or water with minerals, vitamins and micronutrients) may also be considered.

Even when the health advice proposed is based on high-quality randomised controlled trials (RCTs), difficulty in reaching the target population may prevent useful intervention. Perhaps the best-documented example is the policy (Expert Advisory Group 1992) for universal pre/periconceptual folic acid to prevent primary occurrence of central nervous system (CNS) malformation. This recommendation arose from a rather small RCT in Hungary (Czeizel & Dudas 1992) which showed a significantly lower rate of CNS malformation in the offspring of women randomised to receive a small dose of preconceptional folic acid than in controls. There is some dispute as to whether the effect is of true primary prevention by correcting a vitamin deficiency, by promoting miscarriage of damaged fetuses, or by an effect on fertility (Hock & Czeizel 1997, Wald & Hackshaw 1997). The Hungarian study was considered in the context of previous trials and quasi-experimental studies showing a beneficial effect of a larger dose of folic acid in reducing the recurrence rate of CNS malformation. The target group for the intervention in those studies (women with prior CNS malformation) was easy to identify and compliance with therapy a relatively small problem. In contrast, however, initiatives for prevention of primary occurrence have been rather unsuccessful: numerous audits (Sutcliffe et al 1994, De Jong-Van den Berg 1995, Metson et al 1995, Sharpe & Young 1995, Wild et al

1997, Huttly et al 1999) have shown that a minority of women know of the advice, and a smaller minority managed to take the folic acid preconception (taking it later is rarely of value because the neural tube closes at 21–26 days after conception). One factor in this disappointingly low uptake of advice is that about a third of pregnancies are unplanned. Also, the tablets are not prescribed, and the cost of over-the-counter purchase, while not very great, may have deterred some potential users. It is likely that the women who actually took prophylactic preconceptual folic acid were at lower risk of having a baby with CNS malformation than those who did not for social, nutritional and other reasons. Compliers tend to have more favourable health characteristics and behaviours than non-compliers. It is no surprise then, that there is no evidence that UK advocacy of preconceptual folic acid has contributed to the fall in CNS malformation rates (Kadir et al 1999) (Fig. 8.1). Fortification of bread, flour or other appropriate staple foods with folic acid is feasible in order to ensure universal coverage of the population including prepregnant women, but it is not agreed what the minimum requirements are. Even among pregnant women, not everyone would benefit from the folic acid supplements. It may be that folic acid is required only by the 5% of the population with impaired methionine synthase function, which results in hyperhomocysteinaemia (vd Put et al 1995). There is an issue of potential harm to a very small number of non-pregnant individuals with undiagnosed B_{12} deficiency anaemia, who might sustain subacute combined degeneration of the spinal cord. Food fortification is policy in the USA (McCarthy 1996) but not, at the time of writing, in the UK.

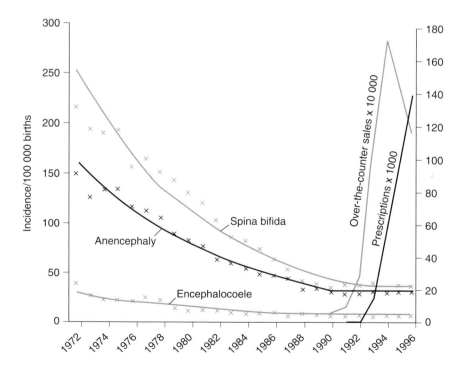

Fig. 8.1 True incidence (×) and modelled incidence (——) of spina bifida, anencephaly and encephalocoele per 100 000 births in England and Wales 1972–1996, and number of prescriptions dispensed and preparations sold over the counter containing 400–500 µgs of folic acid 1992–1996. (From *BMJ* 1999; 319: 92–93, with permission.)

Women with medical disorders

The difficulties encountered in population coverage should in theory be less when dealing with women with medical disorders, who would be expected to be in regular contact with a doctor, and prepregnancy intervention therefore more feasible. Medical problems are discussed in more detail in other Chapters but some groups who could benefit from advice or intervention are:

- Women with very severe disorders for whom pregnancy would be very dangerous—e.g. Eisenmenger's syndrome.
- Women with phenylketonuria, who need to know how important it is to adhere to their phenylalanine-restricted diet especially in the early weeks of pregnancy.
- Women with diabetes. In view of the evidence (Steel et al 1990, Kitzmiller et al 1991) that good diabetic control before conception may reduce the likelihood of dysmorphogenesis, and that hormonal contraception may make good control more difficult to achieve, diabetics are usually asked to use non-hormonal contraception until their HbAIC levels are satisfactory. This is discussed in Ch. 18, but it should be noted that the evidence of benefit is based on comparison between women who attended for preconception care and those who did not. The latter group had several other recorded unfavourable characteristics (such as smoking more) and no doubt others not recorded. It has always been claimed that an RCT would be unethical, but in view of persisting reports of suboptimal glycaemic control in early pregnancy (Casele & Laifer 1998) even in women with prior pregnancy complications, there may be scope for research including trials (informed by qualitative studies) of interventions focusing on the group not now complying with recommendations. Without proof of efficacy, intensive efforts to reach and influence this difficult group are not likely to be successful.
- Women being prescribed essential but potentially fetotoxic medicines need to discuss whether to continue their therapy and how to optimise therapy to minimise harm to the fetus. Women with epilepsy, for example, should have their therapy reviewed to make as sure as possible that they do not experience convulsions; monotherapy will reduce the risk of dysmorphogenesis, as will use of dietary supplementation with high doses (5 mg daily) folic acid preconception. Women on warfarin because of artificial heart valves should be warned of the risk of dysmorphogenesis, and should consider transferring to heparin at least during the first trimester.

Previous obstetric history

Because many complications such as ectopic pregnancy, preterm labour, growth restriction, pre-eclampsia, complications of the third stage of labour and rhesus isoimmunisation have a tendency to recur, they may be a topic for discussion at a prepregnancy consultation. Explanation and discussion about previous pregnancy events and complications should logically occur in the puerperium of the previous pregnancy but are often omitted. Advice should usually be given by an obstetrician with previous case records available. Such discussion could result in a decision not to embark on another pregnancy, though there are very few circumstances in which the obstetrician would need to advise that (placenta accreta could be such a case). Only where there is a need for very early intervention, such as an early scan to confirm intrauterine gestation, would there be an advantage in consultation before conception. Most other discussions could occur in early pregnancy and plans made for appropriate intervention, such as cervical cerclage for some women with prior preterm labour, extra antenatal visits for those with previous pre-eclampsia, hospital booking for confinement for those with a previous caesarean section, or plans for serial scans, amniocentesis and/or intrauterine transfusion in rhesus isoimmunisation.

Genetic problems

Where genetic counselling and investigation has established a recurrence or risk of serious or lethal malformation, a prepregnancy consultation may be useful to make final decisions about whether to conceive at all, whether to consider preimplantation diagnosis or donor insemination, to discuss the timing and accuracy of prenatal diagnosis, the current prognosis and any available intervention for a fetus or a newborn suffering from the relevant condition. Some of these discussions could also occur in early pregnancy, but some couples will feel more secure if a plan has been made in advance.

Normal women

When women without any risk factors seek prepregnancy advice, the main issue (apart from prophylactic folic acid, discussed above) is to check that she is immune to rubella. If immunisation is required, contraception should be used for 3 months thereafter, as it is a live vaccine, although the evidence suggests that rubella vaccine is not teratogenic, and there is no need to advise termination of pregnancy if the vaccine is given inadvertently in the first trimester. There is good evidence of a small benefit from antismoking advice from a doctor at any consultation but there are no RCTs of prepregnancy advice on cessation of smoking. However, it seems sensible to give this advice because there is evidence from observational studies that fertility is reduced and the ectopic pregnancy rate increased in smokers. Evidence of an increased risk of fetal malformation with periconceptual smoking is weak. Women (and their partners) with a firm intention to quit smoking may find it easier to do so when not yet involved in the excitement of pregnancy but there is really no evidence of this. It goes without saying that abuse of alcohol or illegal drugs should be strongly discouraged, but the scenario of alcoholics or illegal drug users seeking prepregnancy consultation is unrealistic.

Although eloquent descriptions of the many possible functions of prepregnancy clinics have been published, the problem about research to establish the usefulness of such clinics is the heterogeneous character of the clientele—a mixture of the worried well, who may not conceive but will have a good prognosis even without any advice, and the women with major problems who would have a poor prognosis even with good advice.

In summary, then, general practitioners and midwives should make sure that preconceptual intake of folic acid is discussed, rubella immunity tested with immunisation as required and advice on giving up smoking given in women undergoing miscarriage, termination, infertility investigation, using prescribed contraception, or indeed in women seeking a consultation for any reason. It may, however, be that population-based measures such as food fortification, infant immunisation or tobacco taxation and regulation of tobacco advertising to reduce smoking will be more effective than prepregnancy clinics as such. Obstetricians can usefully counsel women who are at actual or perceived increased risk of occurrence or recurrence of pregnancy or medical complications. While this can and should be done postpartum, it can also be undertaken at a prepregnancy clinic. If the conditions under review are medical, a joint clinic with a physician is essential and most large maternity units now offer this service, staffed by a maternal and fetal medicine subspecialist.

ANTENATAL CARE

Once a woman is pregnant it is no longer satisfactory to consider separately each medical problem and its resolution. The effectiveness of individual components of care can and should be properly evaluated, usually by RCT, but women must be offered an organised programme of care, mainly so that they know what to expect but also to facilitate rational deployment of health care resources. This does not mean that all women need the same care, nor that caregivers should continue with outmoded and pointless routines. A welcome feature of the last decade of the twentieth century was that at last some RCTs of different ways of organising care were undertaken, which may facilitate much-needed change.

Antenatal care is such a venerable part of the midwifery–obstetric armamentarium that it is sometimes seen as sacrilege to challenge or question anything. But, although it is neither practical nor desirable to go back to the drawing board completely, it is worth considering all the components of antenatal care in the context of the criteria that are now required to be met by the National Screening Committee for all *new* screening programmes. Of these, perhaps the key principles are that there should be a detectable risk factor, disease marker, latent period or early symptomatic stage; that the distribution of test or factor values in the target population should be known and a suitable cut-off level defined and agreed; that effective treatment for patients identified through early detection should be shown to lead to better outcomes than late treatment; and that there should be RCT evidence of more good than harm (both physical and psychological) from the screening programme. Although antenatal care consists mainly of a multifaceted screening programme, very few components of current antenatal care would meet any or all of these criteria. For example, there is virtually no trial evidence to guide the obstetrician's recommendation or practice following one caesarean section. Although there is observational evidence of high rates of vaginal delivery in the next pregnancy, irrespective of the indication for the first section, there is wide and unjustified variation in what is actually recommended.

In some clinical scenarios it is difficult to ascertain the effect of a risk factor because it is modified by treatment. If women identified as being at high risk are treated effectively, this may then diminish the apparent value of the risk factor (the treatment paradox). If, on the other hand, the treatment is actually harmful, the risk factor will appear to have an even better predictive value than it really does. This is why RCTs (where the criteria for treatment, nature of the intervention and the outcomes are strictly defined) are so informative, and this should be the gold standard.

Another key feature of recent research on antenatal care is the importance attached to ascertaining women's views, which are as important as clinical effectiveness as an outcome measure for RCTs. Until the 1970s it was taken for granted that women would feel reassured and informed by antenatal care, and it is only fairly recently that serious efforts have been made to research this. Research can be done in many different ways: by consulting health professionals who often have the confidence of women, such as midwives; by consulting lay organisations of women (most of whom have been pregnant), such as the National Childbirth Trust or the Maternity Alliance; or by advertising for responses, as was done by the Health Committee of the House of Commons. The trouble with all of these is that they may give too much weight to groups with strongly held views, who are not necessarily representative. That problem was avoided by the expert group advising on *Changing Childbirth* who commissioned a MORI poll of women who had recently been pregnant. Unfortunately, however, this poll was never published, so there was no opportunity for external scrutiny of the questions and the answers. It is well known that public opinion polls can elicit apparently contradictory results by asking leading or highly selective questions. Ascertainment of women's views will be most robust if surveys or questionnaires are formulated by social scientists, who are well acquainted with the concerns and the preferred terminology of the women concerned (often explored by prior qualitative research), and if the questionnaire instruments are carefully piloted and checked for validity and reliability. Any questionnaire to be used during or after pregnancy should have a range of normal values for pregnancy. A good response rate makes the results more generalisable.

There is a particular problem in obtaining women's views of antenatal care, which is that if surveys are done at (say) 36 weeks' gestation, women delivering earlier are omitted, as may be key events occurring in late pregnancy. On the other hand, if women are asked after delivery about their antenatal care, their view may be coloured by the events of delivery and the puerperium. It would be only natural if a woman whose baby had died, for example, was inclined to look for faults and omissions in her antenatal care. Nevertheless, it is most commonly after their delivery that women are surveyed about antenatal care (though women with perinatal losses are usually omitted).

It is logical to consider first the identification of risk and problems in early pregnancy (the 'booking' visit) then secondly the subsequent routine care for women without serious problems and finally the way in which care can best be organised.

The booking visit

Information should be recorded on a document to be held by the woman, as this empowers her to take more responsibility for her own care with less risk of loss of the record. The essential components to be explored and recorded are:

- Calculation of gestational age
- Maternal physical characteristics
- Maternal medical history
- Maternal obstetric history
- The woman's own wishes for care and confinement
- Social problems
- Routine and selective investigations.

From these, a logical plan can be negotiated as to what care should be provided routinely, by whom it should be given and where it should take place.

Gestational age

Most women currently use over-the-counter pregnancy testing, which is highly accurate, to confirm that they are pregnant. The determination of the expected date of delivery is usually quite straightforward, by adding 280 days to the first day of the last menstrual period; however, this is not accurate in women with infrequent menstruation or who have recently stopped oral contraception, or who have conceived while taking it. It has become customary to offer an early pregnancy scan to confirm gestational age by measuring size (which has little biological variation in the early weeks of pregnancy). The arguments for this practice are:

- Women and their partners like to see the fetus and to know when to expect delivery – though some women prefer to believe their menstrual date, even when this is inexact.
- Women with previous ectopic pregnancy or miscarriage can be reassured that the pregnancy is intrauterine and ongoing, and unanticipated missed miscarriage can be diagnosed early.
- The performance of serum screening tests for chromosomal anomaly is enhanced by scan dating.
- The optimal time for later fetal anomaly scanning can be chosen.
- In the very unlikely event of a serious complication arising in the second or early third trimester, decisions about when to deliver the mother for fetal reasons may be better informed.
- Because of the fact that when menstrual information is unreliable, the gestational age by scan is usually less than the menstrual estimate, false-positive inductions for postmaturity can be minimised.
- Increasingly, markers for fetal malformation (such as nuchal translucency), or occasionally an actual diagnosis, can be identified, facilitating early management decisions.
- Multiple pregnancy and its chorionicity can be determined early.

All of this adds up to a rather small health gain from routine (as opposed to selective) first-trimester scanning. However, this lack of cost effectiveness is unlikely to influence the many units that have it in place. It is always more difficult to withdraw an established service than to think carefully about whether to introduce it, and midwives and obstetricians increasingly depend on scan results at the expense of clinical examination. Many of the above objectives could be met by routine scanning at 20 weeks, when most structural malformations can be identified, with first-trimester scanning restricted to specific indications.

Maternal characteristics

Mean age at first delivery fell from 1950 until the mid 1970s but has been rising since then. There is no obvious logical cut-off for what constitutes increased age as a risk factor for complications, but 35 years is often used. Because obstetricians intervene much more commonly in older women (and this may improve outcome) it is difficult to quantify the real risk, but there is probably no need for any special antenatal care for older women who are otherwise well. However, although neither pre-eclampsia nor eclampsia is more common in older primigravidas, older women are over-represented among maternal deaths from hypertension, and surveillance should be careful if complications do occur. Eclampsia is more common in very young women; youth is probably not a real risk factor, but a marker for under-utilisation of antenatal care. Short stature is a risk factor for a need for intervention at delivery, not during the antenatal period. Specialist review may be reasonable at around 37–38 weeks, but in first deliveries a trial of labour would usually be advised. For parous women, the prognosis is largely dependent upon the events of previous deliveries. Women with a very low BMI, whether due to gastrointestinal disease or eating disorder, are at risk of having a small baby; dietetic and other specialist advice may be useful but is not of proven value (Kramer 1998). Women who are overweight are at risk of developing pregnancy-induced hypertension and may be offered more than the minimum number of blood pressure checks in late pregnancy (see later in this chapter). A suitably large cuff should be used.

A proportion of smokers will have given up of their own volition, either before conception or as soon as they realise that they are pregnant. Those who are still smoking at booking are the hard core: RCTs with cotinine validation have shown, however, that an active programme of professional advice and support can marginally increase the proportion of those who do manage to stop, but with evidence of only a small increase in birthweight. There is no evidence on the efficacy of advice on alcohol consumption, but midwives and doctors should alert women to the need to restrict consumption, and particularly to avoid binge drinking. Women using illegal drugs are usually offered methadone substitution/reduction/withdrawal via special clinics with social work and psychiatric input.

General medical examination is not now usually routinely performed, except in women with a medical history or current symptoms, but the blood pressure, spine and conjunctiva should be checked.

Maternal medical history

Significant medical disorders are discussed in chapters 16–23, and care by an obstetrician and physician team usually offered. However, the need for continued contact with their own midwife and general practitioner must also be met.

Maternal obstetric history

Women with single previous obstetric problems can usually be given a well informed prognosis for the recurrence risk (typically two to three times the population risk) but may need sympathetic discussion of its practical significance. Even when there is no real risk of recurrence, detailed consideration of problems and interventions in previous pregnancies may help women to work through what happened last time. Those with multiple problems can be given only an approximate estimate of what is likely to happen.

Where there has been previous uterine surgery (usually caesarean section) the woman should be seen by a specialist to discuss the prognosis for delivery based on:

- the expected risk of recurrence of the indications for the first section
- the very small risk of uterine rupture in labour and
- the woman's own hopes and desires.

A similar but more complex discussion is needed for women who have had more than one caesarean—and also some vaginal deliveries.

Some causes of perinatal death have much higher risks of recurrence than others, but the woman's natural anxiety will often mean that extra surveillance and support is indicated even if there is little likelihood of recurrence.

The woman's own views

It is customary to invite women to make a record of their wishes for the management of the pregnancy and delivery. Most such *birth plans* concentrate on the delivery rather than the antenatal period, but some women, for example, wish to have scans only when absolutely essential, and others have a strong desire to avoid antenatal hospital admission. The problem about deciding on the *birth plan* in early or even late pregnancy is that the sensitivity and specificity of the risk factors is low. It can be argued therefore that women may experience considerable disappointment if things do not go according to their plan. On the other hand, given the difficulty that women have often felt in asserting themselves in the face of professional advice, especially in active labour, it is probably a good thing for them to think through their ideal scenario well in advance, with full knowledge that it is impossible to forecast accurately what will happen. Although some women will formulate their plan without reference to professionals, it is certainly incumbent on any professional asked for advice (usually the midwife) to make sure that women are adequately informed of the evidence base for routine intervention where it exists.

Social problems

Many social problems can contribute to adverse outcomes such as preterm delivery and growth restriction. However, there are very few relevant interventions of proven value. For example, if a woman is homeless, unsupported by her partner or employed doing heavy work or night work, extra health care may not be what she needs, although a sensitive community midwife will try to be as supportive as possible and make appropriate social work referrals. There is some trial evidence from the USA of both short and long-term benefit from home visits, but this was in a setting where many of the women would not be eligible for standard antenatal care, so it may not be applicable to the UK, where home visits are offered routinely, and are not considered as a special intervention. Domestic violence is increasingly recognised as a problem that may present or become worse in pregnancy, but which may be missed unless sensitive enquiries are made when the woman is alone (i.e. not in the presence of the putative abuser). If required, information about refuges and social work help should be supplied.

Routine and selective investigations

All tests and investigations should be discussed with the pregnant woman, and should be performed only with her consent. The investigations that are usually undertaken at booking but which may need to be repeated are shown in Table 8.1. Not all are cost effective.

The full blood count is routinely checked at booking as a baseline, because iron-deficiency anaemia may occur later in pregnancy due to fetal demands. The blood group is ascertained at booking, mainly to identify the Rhesus-negative woman, who should be offered anti-D at 28 and 34 weeks to prevent isoimmunisation (Crowther & Keirse 1998). The information will also facilitate emergency crossmatching of blood, should that be required around delivery. The presence of antibodies needs to be further investigated in respect of the risk to the fetus of haemolytic disease (discussed elsewhere) and in respect of likely difficulties in crossmatching if that is required.

Testing for syphilis, which is extremely rare, is nevertheless held to be cost effective (Welch 1998) because of the treatability of the condition, which, when untreated, has very serious implications for the fetus as well as the mother and father.

Table 8.1 Routine and selective investigations

Investigation	Timing
Routine:	
Full blood count	Booking, 28 weeks
Blood group	Booking
Antibodies	Booking and as advised by laboratory
Test for syphilis	Booking
Rubella (if immunity not established by two previous tests)	Booking
HBs Ag	Booking
Selective:	
Hb electrophoresis	Booking
MSSU	Booking
HIV/Hepatitis C	Booking
Screening for fetal anomaly	As per local protocol

Rubella immunity should be the norm for women entering pregnancy because of adolescent immunisation (now being superseded by infant immunisation of both sexes) but it is important to detect the few women who are not immune so that they can be offered immunisation after delivery. The only reason for doing the test at booking is that the information may be useful if possible clinical infection occurs.

The National Screening Committee has recommended that all women should be offered screening for hepatitis B so that the newborn babies of infected mothers can be immunised to reduce their risk of becoming carriers. This is 90–95% effective. Again, if this test has been missed at booking, it can effectively be performed even in late pregnancy. The benefits of screening for hepatitis C are less certain and it is currently offered only to high-risk groups such as intravenous drug users.

Testing urine for glucose is justified mainly to diagnose the very few women who develop type 1 diabetes during pregnancy, while the presence of proteinuria may be a presenting sign of pre-eclampsia (though it is usually antedated by hypertension).

Routine blood screening for gestational diabetes has been widely advocated but is not justified by current evidence. An important large multicentre study (Hyperglycaemia Adverse Pregnancy Outcome) is currently under way and should eventually allow more rational policy determination, as short-, medium- and long-term effects will be studied. One advantage of blood screening is that regular urine testing for glucose is not then necessary.

Selective investigations may sometimes be appropriately offered routinely. Haemoglobin electrophoresis should be offered to those whose ethnic background makes haemoglobinopathy likely, and in populations where women of African, Afro-Caribbean, Asian or Mediterranean background form a significant minority routine screening may be more sensible. It has recently been reported that, at haemoglobinopathy prevalences of greater than 2.5%, community screening is self financing, as is antenatal screening with follow-up counselling (Cronin et al 2000).

Screening for asymptomatic bacteriuria (with treatment of those found positive) is clearly effective in reducing the rate of subsequent pyelonephritis (though probably not of preterm labour) but whether it is cost effective depends upon how common pyelonephritis is—in many populations screening is offered only to women with a previous history of urinary infection (see Chapter 23).

Selective screening of pregnant women for HIV has proved very unsatisfactory; although there are well recognised high-risk groups, many cases are missed. The case for universal screening has recently been very much strengthened by the accumulating RCT evidence of benefit, in terms of reduced vertical transmission, of interventions such as antenatal zidovudine, operative delivery, abstention from breast-feeding, etc. Benefit for maternal health is less certain, but universal screening is now government recommended policy. Screening for fetal anomaly is discussed elsewhere, but should be coordinated with the other investigations offered.

Routine return antenatal visits

The two main purposes of *routine* return antenatal visits for low-risk women are:

- to detect asymptomatic conditions (mainly malpresentation, growth restriction and pre-eclampsia)
- health education and maternal reassurance.

How frequent should routine *visits be?*
Detection of asymptomatic conditions   Detection of malpresentation justifies one visit at around 37 weeks' gestation, so that women with breech presentation can be referred for external cephalic version, which reduces the term prevalence of breech presentation and hence of caesarean section (Hofmeyr 1989).

Screening for growth disorders by fundal height measurement or scan has not been shown to improve outcome but is considered here because growth restricted babies are overrepresented among perinatal deaths. In low-risk women it may justify two antenatal visits, one in the third trimester. However, fundal height can also be measured at visits which are primarily for other reasons. This also applies to screening for macrosomy (though there is no agreed definition and no recognised helpful intervention).

The main determinant of routine visit frequency and timing is therefore pre-eclampsia, which fulfils most, if not all, of the criteria for screening. It has an agreed definition. It is fairly common (up to 5% in nulliparous and 1–2% in parous women) and, in a proportion of cases, serious (still a major cause of maternal and perinatal mortality). There is usually a prodromal phase before eclampsia—though this phase was not present in as many as 38% of cases in the 1992 National Audit of Eclampsia) (Douglas et al 1994), and women can be seriously ill and die without having eclampsia (e.g. from cerebral haemorrhage). In cases of pre-eclampsia, hypertension usually antedates proteinuria, and can be regarded as prodromal, but many women with hypertension do not go on to develop pre-eclampsia; pregnancy-induced hypertension alone is not associated with increased maternal or perinatal mortality. Are there useful interventions that can be made if the condition is diagnosed promptly? The condition cannot be cured except by delivery, but close monitoring allows optimal timing of intervention, and the manifestations (such as hypertension) can be treated. There is trial evidence that expectant management is preferable to aggressive management in many women with onset between 28 and 34 weeks but up to 30% may require very prompt delivery.

Reliable biochemical or biophysical prediction of pre-eclampsia is not yet available. The problems with clinical screening (blood pressure measurement and urine analysis for protein) are:

- The clinical presentation can be at any gestation in the second and third trimesters but becomes more common as gestational age increases, so that the vast majority of women present towards the end of the third trimester.
- When the condition presents early it is often more severe, particularly for the fetus, because the complications of preterm birth may be added to those of pre-eclampsia.

- Whatever the frequency and timing of visits, clinical screening has more chance of early detection of slowly progressing cases than fulminating cases. In slowly progressing cases, treatment may be less urgent.
- The possibility of detriment to the false positives (the women who have pregnancy-induced hypertension but no proteinuria) must be considered.

The UK 1929 model of antenatal care, with an average of 13–14 visits for all women irrespective of parity, inevitably results in a very low incidence (at any one visit) of new diagnosis of hypertension, and an even smaller incidence of early identification of pre-eclampsia, especially in parous women. It is still widely practised in the UK, however, and great store has rightly been set by historical data showing a reduction in maternal mortality over the last 70 years. Antenatal care has probably made an important contribution to the decline, though improvements in surveillance, therapy and the ability to deliver women preterm may have been equally important. Other countries (such as France) with many fewer visits (Mascarhenas et al 1992) have also achieved good results. Studies with historical controls (Hall et al 1985, Berglund & Lindmark 1998) have shown no clinical detriment from a reduction in routine visits (using the proportion of cases of pre-eclampsia presenting for the first time in labour as an indicator), but it is only recently that trial evidence has become available. There are now six published RCTs comparing reduced visit schedules for low-risk women with current practice (traditional care) (Binstock & Wolde-Tsadik 1994, McDuffie et al 1996, Munjanja et al 1996, Sikorski et al 1996, Walker & Koniak-Griffin 1996, BACS 2000), including around 22 400 women in the UK, USA and Zimbabwe. Most women were eligible, and between 48% and 100% were recruited (one trial, the largest (Munjanja et al 1996), randomised clinics, not individual women). In all of the studies the *control* (conventional care) women experienced fewer visits than initially planned but the experimental group (reduced frequency of visits) still had between two and three visits fewer than the control group.

It is difficult to devise an appropriate clinical outcome measure for any detrimental or beneficial effect of visit frequency upon pre-eclampsia, as it is not biologically plausible that fewer visits would influence the incidence of the condition, though late detection might make management more difficult.

Several different outcome measures were used to assess the effect upon pre-eclampsia of reduced visit numbers.

- Incidence of hypertension (Binstock & Wolde-Tsadik 1994, Walker & Koniak-Griffin 1996) or pre-eclampsia (McDuffie et al 1996, BACS 2000).
- Referrals for pre-eclampsia (Munjanja et al 1996).
- Rates of delivery within 24 hours, induction or caesarean section because of pre-eclampsia (Sikorski et al 1996).
- Maternal and perinatal mortality, birthweight (all collected in the knowledge that trials would not be expected to show any significant difference).

None of the studies showed any adverse medical effects of reduced visit schedules on any clinical outcome, whether relating to pre-eclampsia or not. In some, women receiving fewer visits felt deprived of attention (see Ch. 8). The results of a large WHO trial are awaited.

The argument that trial results are invalid because they did not have the power to exclude a rise in maternal mortality cannot be sustained because this would be the case for virtually every obstetric trial that has ever been performed (currently the rate of maternal mortality attributable to pre-eclampsia in the UK is around nine per million). To a lesser extent the same applies to perinatal mortality (currently the rate of perinatal mortality attributable to hypertension in Scotland is 0.6 per 1000 births). The problem of prompt recognition of fulminating pre-eclampsia should be addressed by making sure that women are aware of the possible symptoms (Douglas & Redman 1994), that they know how to contact a midwife or doctor in the event of experiencing such symptoms and that prompt and appropriate action is taken by all concerned.

Health education and maternal reassurance Educational initiatives should be scientifically evaluated according to whether women actually attend, whether their knowledge improves, whether they feel informed, and whether healthier behaviour (and ultimately better health) results.

Health education should cover changes in normal pregnancy, recognition of abnormality, preparation for delivery (including visits to hospital), preparation for parenthood and infant feeding. It is likely to be more necessary and useful in first pregnancies than in subsequent ones. Although some women and their partners enjoy classes, others do not and must be offered information and discussion during antenatal care. However, although there may be a very few women who really need very frequent educational input, the need for this is rarely an appropriate determinant of the frequency of routine visits. It is nevertheless essential to know women's views about this.

Not all trials are informative about women's views of the health education and reassurance provided. For example, the largest trial (Munjanja et al 1996) randomised clinics, not women, and women's views were not researched; the smallest (Walker & Koniak-Griffin 1996) is so lacking in methodological details that it is not useful. In the four useful trials (Binstock & Wolde-Tsadik 1994, McDuffie et al 1996, Sikorski et al 1996, BACS 2000) questionnaires were administered at varying times and intervals, and response rates varied from 51 to 95%. Nevertheless, women's views on visit numbers are remarkably consistent (Table 8.2). Although the majority thought the number of visits they had had was just right, there was a significant tendency for the intervention arms (with fewer visits) to include a larger proportion (typically around 30%) who would have liked more visits. Conversely more of the control women (10–16%) would have liked fewer.

Women's satisfaction with care was generally high but in one trial (Sikorski et al 1996), although the intervention women were more likely to choose the same schedule next time than the controls, this study showed that in five out of 25 psychosocial measurements women following the reduced schedule were significantly more worried. However, the actual differences in the mean scores for the two groups were

Table 8.2 Percentage distribution of women's views about visit numbers in randomised controlled trials of reduced visits (intervention) with traditional care (control)

Trial	Too few		Just right		Too many	
	Control	Intervention	Control	Intervention	Control	Intervention
Binstock & Wolde-Tsadik (1994)	6	27	84	71	10	2
Sikorski et al (1996)	16	33	68	65	16	3
McDuffie et al (1996)	1	7	83	89	16	2
BACS (2000)	17	28	73	67	10	5
Jewell et al (2000)	17	28	74	69	10	5

small, and a 3-year follow-up study (Clement et al 1999) found no evidence of persisting problems. A similar analysis was made in more detail, with much higher response rates, in another study (BACS 2000) and no significant evidence of psychosocial problems was found. Further reassurance on this topic is available from two recent trials of devolved care (Tucker et al 1996, Turnbull et al 1996) in which, although visit numbers were not a specified outcome, the experimental groups had significantly fewer visits than the controls, but were happy with, or preferred, that style of care.

It does not seem to be possible (Clement et al 1999) easily to identify groups of women who would be more likely to prefer reduced visits, and offering women additional visits on request was not successful (BACS 2000) as women felt unable to request additional visits once told they were not required on medical grounds.

In summary, there is now good evidence that a modest reduction in routine visits is associated with good clinical outcome, and is acceptable to women. Savings may result but a full economic analysis including women's costs has not been done. Table 8.3 shows the minimum number of routine return visits recommended for a low-risk parous woman (one who is not hypertensive at booking, has not had pre-eclampsia in a previous pregnancy and has a singleton pregnancy). Nulliparous, and parous women who have had previous pre-eclampsia, should be offered additional visits at 36 and 41 weeks. Other factors that might influence decisions about additional visits are multiple pregnancy, extremes of maternal age, obesity and/or high weight gain, family history of hypertension. Once hypertension or proteinuria has occurred the care must be individualised.

Organisation of care

Once the content of antenatal care has been agreed (including the recommended frequency and timing of visits) the issues arise of who should provide the care and whether it can be delivered in a community setting (GP surgery, health centre or the woman's home) or requires hospital attendance. Appropriate considerations include:

- clinical outcomes
- woman's views
- cost and cost effectiveness
- likely volume of work
- training, experience and the philosophy of staff.

Many different arrangements for care provision currently exist and some recent initiatives towards woman-centred

Table 8.3 Minimum schedule of routine antenatal attendances for low-risk parous women (not including scan and blood tests)

Gestation	Content
First trimester	Provide written and verbal information on recommended dietary changes, folic acid, smoking, pregnancy symptoms, bleeding in early pregnancy, fetal anomaly screening, maternity benefits and local options for antenatal care and delivery. Identify 'low risk' status after basic history. Establish gestational age. Baseline weight and blood pressure
20 weeks	Check blood pressure, urine, fundal height. Discuss fetal anomaly screening results. Provide written and verbal information on symptoms of pre-eclampsia and awareness of fetal movements
26 weeks	Check blood pressure, urine, fundal height
30 weeks	Check blood pressure, urine, fundal height
34 weeks	Check blood pressure, urine, fundal height, presentation. Discuss plans and wishes for labour, birth and infant feeding
38 weeks	Check blood pressure, urine, fundal height, presentation
41 weeks	Check blood pressure, urine, fundal height, presentation. Discuss the circumstances in which induction is recommended

Women in their first pregnancy should have additional blood pressure and urine checks at 36 and 40 weeks

care, performed mainly by midwives, were based largely on observational, survey or anecdotal evidence. Relevant RCT trial evidence is now available encompassing most of these dimensions and recommendations can therefore be stronger.

The three relevant trials are one that compared midwife/GP antenatal care for low-risk women in nine settings in Scotland with traditional shared care (in which women routinely saw a specialist) (Tucker et al 1996), one comparing integrated midwifery care for low-risk women throughout pregnancy, delivery and the puerperium, in one Scottish city hospital, with traditional shared care where women routinely saw specialists (Turnbull et al 1996) and a Swedish trial in which a routine booking visit to the doctor was replaced by a planning conference (Berglund & Lindmark 1999). It is important to note that none of these trials is informative about the safety of home confinement because all the women were delivered in specialist hospitals. Furthermore, no conclusion is possible as to whether midwife care is better or worse than GP care: this was not the subject of randomisation. In one trial (Tucker et al 1996) the mix of midwifery and GP care was left to individual practices, and in both arms of the trial it was more or less shared equally. In the other Scottish trial (Turnbull et al 1996) GPs made only a small contribution to care (12–14% of visits), with no difference between the two arms of the trial.

Both Scottish trials had excellent participation rates (>80%) and the Swedish trial had cluster randomisation, so the question of participation did not arise. Non-participants did not differ from participants in any major way and few (<5%) had missing records, though unfortunately shared care cards were missing for between 18 and 40% in one trial (Turnbull et al 1996). In all trials there were clear differences between the experimental and control arms in terms of care provided so an intervention did take place and the primary care staff adhered more closely to the recommended care plan in terms of visit numbers. Low-risk women were correctly identified by primary care staff but overall 33–51% of the new care pattern women had to be referred for a specialist opinion when problems arose and 17–33% had their care transferred permanently (but the higher figure includes intrapartum transfers). Continuity of care was better and defaulting less frequent in the primary care sector in one trial (Tucker et al 1996) in which it was reported. In all trials it was anticipated that clinical outcomes would be as good in the new care arm as in the shared care arm and this proved to be the case.

The woman's view of care received was studied only in the Scottish trials. It was ascertained objectively by social scientists not involved in patient care and showed satisfaction with both arms in each trial, but there were more favourable responses for the new style of care, especially in the group receiving midwifery care (Turnbull et al 1996).

Economic evaluation showed a clear advantage for the new care group in one trial (Ryan et al 1997), both for NHS and women's and Society's costs, but Turnbull et al (1996) found no NHS cost difference between midwife-managed care and specialist-led shared antenatal care (though postpartum care provided by midwives was significantly more expensive). At current pay levels, it seems self-evident that it will cost less for most routine antenatal care for low-risk women to be provided by midwives, and the trial evidence is that it will be cost effective.

In sparsely populated rural areas the volume of work for individual members of staff will always be small, but in urban practices it is logical that expertise can more easily be maintained by midwives practising only midwifery than by GPs with much wider responsibility, although GPs will still be providing general medical services as appropriate. Simple arithmetic (Keirse 1989) demonstrates that it is impossible for specialists who undertake all routine care of normal women to maintain expertise in the management of complications, but the trials show that even amongst low-risk women a considerable proportion do need to see a specialist as and when problems arise. Arrangements must be in place

Table 8.4 Referral protocols for problems arising in pregnancy

Problem	Plan
Hyperemesis with ketosis	Admit
Glycosuria +	Random plasma glucose
Fasting plasma glucose >5.5 mmol/l or glucose <2 hours after food >7.0 mmol/l	Book glucose tolerance test
Haematuria	MSSU, treat, refer if persists
Proteinuria (trace or +) without hypertension	MSSU, HVS
Proteinuria (++)	Admit
Diastolic blood pressure (90 mmHg)	Domiciliary check next day
Sustained diastolic (90 mmHg)	Refer to specialist
Hb <100 g/l	Treat, refer if no response
Minor haemorrhage <20 weeks	Rest
Minor haemorrhage 20 or more	Refer to specialist
Major haemorrhage	Admit
Deep venous thrombosis	Admit
Polyhydramnios	Refer to specialist
Reduced fetal movements	Check fetal heart. Refer urgently
Intrauterine death	Admit
Abnormal presentation after 36 weeks	Refer to specialist
Preterm rupture of membranes	Admit
Term rupture of membranes	Admit within 24 hours
Prolonged pregnancy (T + 7)	Refer to specialist
Weight gain 28–34 weeks >0.8 kg/week	Weekly BP from 34 weeks
Weight gain 16–28 weeks <0.4 kg/week	
Fundal height 3 cm less than mean	Refer to specialist at 30 weeks for a growth scan if any
Smoking	two of these features are present
Height <1.52 metres	
Weight <50 kg at 20 weeks	

for easy access to specialist advice for primary-care staff in rural areas, and in the future telemedicine may have a part to play. Women should be able to see an obstetrician if they wish.

Apart from considerations of clinical efficacy and cost, the training, experience, and philosophy of staff is relevant to the provision of the best possible care for women. Some tasks within routine antenatal care could be delegated to a lower level of skill than that of a trained midwife, but to arrange care in this way would conflict not only with continuity but also with the woman's confidence in a professional who knows her as a person, is oriented towards pregnancy and parturition as normal, and yet can recognise problems and deal with them.

CONCLUSIONS

Prepregnancy advice is within the province of GPs or health visitors, except in women with medical or previous obstetric problems who should, if necessary, see an obstetrician or other specialist. If this has not been done before pregnancy, referral should occur in early pregnancy. Protocols as to what constitutes a problem should be agreed between all staff concerned, and trials show that primary care staff can safely use these, and can also refer appropriately if problems arise. An example of a referral protocol is shown in Table 8.4. This is very similar to the referral protocol used by Tucker et al (1996) and is currently in use in Grampian, Scotland, having been agreed by midwives, GPs and obstetricians. Such referrals need not necessarily result in a permanent transfer of care to specialist staff, and it is important to make sure that when problems are resolved women can return to the care of the midwife or GP.

As primary care (especially midwifery care) is preferred by normal women, and seems to be cheaper, it should be the normal model of care. There is no RCT evidence as to whether care at the woman's home is more effective or more acceptable. It seems likely that it is more expensive in terms of midwives' time, but is normally offered for one visit, often the booking visit and later as appropriate (for women who have difficulty in attending elsewhere, have defaulted from visits, or have been advised to rest at home).

GPs will usually arrange confirmation of pregnancy, review the medical history, make a physical examination as necessary and refer to specialists as appropriate, provide general medical services and may wish to participate in routine care including referrals because of problems arising in pregnancy.

Obstetricians should see women with complicated previous obstetric histories to discuss recurrence risks and prognosis, to arrange additional care and to discuss mode and place of delivery. Women with medical problems, special problems (such as substance misuse) or other risk factors such as short stature or advanced age, should also be reviewed in early pregnancy and those with problems arising during pregnancy seen as appropriate. Obstetricians should be responsible for counselling women recalled because of serum or scan screening results, and for the organisation of screening programmes. It is the responsibility of the obstetrician, usually in collaboration with the primary care team and neonatologist.

KEY POINTS

- Prepregnancy care can be effective only if it is possible to reach the target population; this presents major problems, especially for women without medical disorders.
- Antenatal care is a multifaceted screening programme, each component of which should meet the criteria for new screening programmes.
- Randomised controlled trials must include women's views of care as an outcome.
- There is no evidence that a modest reduction in the frequency of routine antenatal visits adversely affects clinical outcomes of pre-eclampsia.
- For low-risk women, *routine* antenatal care provided entirely in the community (by midwives and GPs) has good clinical outcomes, is usually preferred by women and may be cheaper. However 50% of low-risk women need antepartum specialist referral at some time.

REFERENCES

BACS 2000

Berglund A, Lindmark GC 1998 Health service effects of a reduced routine programme for antenatal care. An area-based study. Eur J Obstet Gynecol Reprod Biol 77:193–199

Berglund A, Lindmark G 1999 Midwife managed care – impact on use of health services. An area based randomised controlled trial. In: Berglund A (ed) Consequences of programme changes in antenatal care. Uppsala University Press, Uppsala

Binstock MA, Wolde-Tsadik F 1994 Alternative prenatal care. J Reprod Med 39:1–6

Boon C, Hull S 1995 Preconceptional supplementation is impracticable. BMJ 311:256–257

Casele HL, Laifer SA 1998 Factors influencing preconception control of glycemia in diabetic women. Arch Intern Med 158:1321–1324

Clement S, Candy J, Sikorski J, Wilson J, Smitten N 1999 Does reducing the frequency of routine antenatal visits have long term effects? Follow up of participants in a randomised controlled trial. Br J Obstet Gynaecol 106:367–370

Crowther CA, Keirse MJNC 1998 Anti-D administration in pregnancy (Cochrane Review). In: Cochrane Library, Issue 4. Oxford: Update Software, 2000.

Cronin EK, Normand C, Henthorn JS, Graham V, Davies SC 2000 Organisation and cost-effectiveness of antenatal haemoglobinopathy screening and follow up in a community-based programme. B J Obstet Gynaecol 107:486–491

Czeizel AE, Dudas I 1992 Prevention of the first occurrence of neural-tube defects by periconceptional vitamin supplementation. N Engl J Med 327:1832–1835

De Jong-Van den Berg LTW, Cornel MC, Tystra T, Buitendijk SE 1995 Folate prophylaxis in pregnancy. Lancet 346:1227–1228

Douglas KS, Redman CWG 1994 Eclampsia in the United Kingdom. BMJ 309:1395–1400

Expert Advisory Group 1992 Folic acid and the prevention of neural tube defects. Department of Health, Scottish Office Home and Health Department, Welsh Office, Department of Health and Social Services, Northern Ireland

Hall MH, McIntyre SM, Porter M 1985 Antenatal care assessed. Aberdeen University Press, Aberdeen

Hock EB, Czeizel AE 1997 Can terathanasia explain the protective effect of folic acid supplementation on birth defects? Lancet 350:513–515

Hofmeyr J 1989 Breech presentation and abnormal lie in late pregnancy. In: Chalmers I, Enkin M, Keirse MJNC (eds) Effective Care in Pregnancy and Childbirth. Oxford University Press, Oxford, pp 653–666

Huttly WJ, Wald NJ, Walters JC 1999 Folic acid supplementation before pregnancy remains inadequate. BMJ 319:1499

Jewell D, Sharp D, SandersJ, Peters TJ 2000 A randomised controlled trial of flexibility in routine antenatal care. Br J Obst Gynae 107:1241–1247

Kadir RA, Sabin C, Whitlow B, Brockbank E, Economides D 1999 Neural tube defects and periconceptual folic acid in England and Wales: retrospective study. BMJ 319:92–93

Keirse MJNC 1989 Interaction between primary and secondary care during pregnancy and childbirth. In: Chalmers Enkin M, Keirse MJNC (eds) Effective Care in Pregnancy and Childbirth. Oxford University Press, Oxford, pp 197–201

Kitzmiller JL, Gavin LA, Gin GD et al 1991 Preconception care of diabetes. Glycemic control prevents congenital anomalies. J Am Med Assoc 265:731–736

Kramer MS 1998 Nutritional advice in pregnancy (Cochrane Review). In: Cochrane Library, Issue 4. Oxford: Update Software, 2000.

Lumley J, Oliver S, Waters E 1998 Smoking cessation programs implemented during pregnancy (Cochrane Review). In: Cochrane Library, Issue 4. Oxford: Update Software, 2000.

Mascarhenas L, Eliot BW, MacKenzie IZ 1992 A comparison of perinatal outcome, antenatal and intrapartum care between England and Wales and France. Br J Obstet Gynaecol 99:955–958

McCarthy M 1996 USA plans to add folic acid to food products. Lancet 347:682

McDuffie R, Beck A, Bischoff K et al 1996 Effect of frequency of prenatal care visits on perinatal outcome among low risk women: A randomised controlled trial. J Am Med Assoc 275:847–851

Metson D, Kassianos GS, Kremer MG, Broomfield C, Tobin M, Cruise J 1995 Supplementation with folic acid. BMJ 310:942

Munjanja SP, Kindmark G, Nystrom L 1996 Randomised controlled trial of a reduced visits programme of antenatal care in Harare, Zimbabwe. Lancet 348:364–369

Ryan M, Ratcliffe J, Tucker J 1997 Using willingness to pay to value alternative models of antenatal care. Soc Sci Med 44:371–380

Sharpe G, Young G 1995 Most pregnant women do not take folic acid. BMJ 311:256

Sikorski J, Wilson J, Cleiment S, Das S, Smeeton N 1996 A randomised controlled trial comparing two schedules of antenatal visits: the antenatal care project. BMJ 312:546–553

Steel JM, Johnstone FD, Hepburn DA, Smith AF 1990 Can prepregnancy care of diabetic women reduce the risk of abnormal babies? BMJ 301:1070–1074

Sutcliffe M, Wild J, Perry A, Schorah CJ 1994 Prevention of neural tube defects. Lancet 344:1578

Tucker JS, Hall MH, Howie PW et al 1996 Should obstetricians see women with normal pregnancies? A multicentre randomised controlled trial of routine antenatal care by General Practitioners and midwives compared with shared care led by obstetricians. BMJ 312:554–559

Turnbull D, Holmes A, Shields N et al 1996 Randomised controlled trial of efficacy of midwife managed care. Lancet 38:213–218

vd Put NMJ, Steegers-Theunissen PM, Frosst P et al 1995 Multated methyltetra hydrofolate reductase as a risk factor for spina bifida. Lancet 346:1070–1071

Wald NJ, Bewer C 1995 Folic acid and the prevention of neural tube defects. BMJ 310:1019–1020

Wald N, Hackshaw A 1997 Folic acid and prevention of neural tube defects. Lancet 350:665

Walker DS, Koniak-Griffin D 1996 Evaluation of reduced frequency prenatal visit schedule for low risk women at a free-standing birthing center. Midwifery 12:120–128

Welch J 1998 Antenatal screening for syphilis. BMJ 317:1605–1606

Wild J, Sutcliffe M, Schorah CJ, Levene MI 1997 Prevention of neural tube defects. Lancet 350:30–31

Young D, Lees A, Twaddle S 1997 The costs to the NHS of maternity care: midwife-managed vs shared. Br J Midwifery 5:465–472

9

Sporadic and recurrent miscarriage

Lesley Regan, Katy Clifford

The contribution of the author of the equivalent chapter in the second edition, on which this chapter draws extensively, is gratefully acknowledged.

INTRODUCTION

Sporadic miscarriage is the most common complication of pregnancy: approximately 25% of women lose a pregnancy at some time in their reproductive lives. This may be at any stage of development but the term miscarriage is used for all losses occurring up to 24 weeks' gestation.

Recurrent miscarriage is defined as the loss of three or more consecutive early pregnancies irrespective of the gestation. It is a heterogeneous condition with no single pathological condition underlying all cases and it follows that no single therapy will be applicable to every case. The optimal management of couples presenting with recurrent pregnancy failure has been difficult to determine. Although the aetiology of recurrent miscarriage can be broadly categorised into genetic, infective, structural, endocrine, immune and idiopathic causes, there is disagreement amongst clinicians as to the numerical contribution of each of these factors. The paucity of randomised controlled trials for the treatment of recurrent miscarriage has led to the use of empirical treatments—a situation that is no longer acceptable in current evidence-based medical practice. This chapter will review the epidemiology and aetiology of miscarriage and discuss the appropriate investigations and management options that can be supported by peer-reviewed studies.

PREVALENCE OF SPORADIC AND RECURRENT MISCARRIAGE

A distinction should be made between an overt miscarriage that is recognised by the patient and the subclinical loss of a pregnancy before the ensuing menses. It is consistently reported that 12–15% of all clinically recognised pregnancies fail spontaneously (Warburton & Fraser 1964, Regan et al 1989, Hemminski & Forsass 1999). However, the rate of subclinical loss may be much higher than this. In a study of 221 women attempting conception using sensitive urinary hCG assays the overall pregnancy loss rate after implantation was 31% (Wilcox et al 1988). However, in 22% of women the pregnancy ended before it was detected clinically. The fate of a fertilised ovum has been estimated by Kline et al (1989) and is summarised in Figure 9.1. It can be seen that for every 1000 conceptions only 500 live births result (excluding elective terminations of pregnancy), the majority being lost before the pregnancy is clinically recognised.

The majority of sporadic miscarriages occur in the first trimester and are termed early pregnancy losses; only 2–5% of pregnancies miscarry after fetal heart activity has been detected on ultrasound (Cashner et al 1987, Mackenzie et al 1988). Late miscarriage (the loss of a fetus that has reached an ultrasound size compatible with at least 13 weeks' gesta-

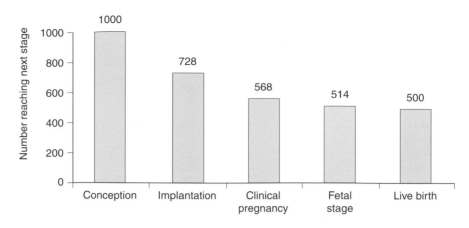

Fig. 9.1 The fate of 1000 fertilised ova (after Kline et al 1989).

tion) is a rare event. In contrast to sporadic pregnancy loss, late or mid-trimester miscarriage is a more common finding amongst recurrent miscarriers, with 22–37% of such women having experienced at least one late loss in the past (Clifford et al 1994, Drakeley et al 1998).

Assuming that 15% of pregnancies fail spontaneously, the likelihood of three consecutive losses can be predicted to be 0.3% from chance alone. The observed rate of recurrent miscarriage is higher, approximately 1%, and together with the observation that the risk of miscarriage increases with each successive pregnancy loss it is reasonable to conclude that a systematic abnormality underlies some cases of recurrent miscarriage.

Several studies have attempted to quantify a woman's risk of pregnancy loss after each successive miscarriage (Table 9.1). Past obstetric history is the most important indicator for future pregnancy outcome, the risk of miscarriage increasing with each successive loss. The risk of miscarriage also increases with maternal age. There is a sharp increase in the rate of miscarriage as women reach their late thirties. Women aged 40 years have a 30% chance of miscarrying a clinically recognised pregnancy (Alberman 1988). This is in part caused by the direct effect of maternal age on the frequency of autosomal trisomies but there is also an increase in euploid losses (Stein et al 1980).

AETIOLOGY AND INVESTIGATION OF MISCARRIAGE

Genetic factors

At least 50% of sporadic losses are the result of a fetal chromosomal abnormality (Boue et al 1975, Simpson & Bombard 1987). This may be an underestimate of the true incidence of fetal aneuploidy as there are difficulties in culturing aborted tissue. There is an age-related rise in the rate of fetal aneuploidy, reaching 80% in women over 40 years of age who miscarry. The most commonly found chromosomal abnormality is an autosomal trisomy, which accounts for over 50% of cytogenetically abnormal miscarriages. Apart from chromosome 1, trisomies for every chromosome have been reported, the most frequently found being a trisomy of chromosome 16. Although karyotyping of the products of conception is rarely indicated after a sporadic miscarriage, it is imperative to send tissue for chromosome analysis from women with recurrent miscarriage since they are not protected from random episodes of pregnancy loss. The finding of an abnormal fetal karyotype provides a definitive cause for the miscarriage and for those women involved in treatment trials the cytogenetic results direct the advice offered to them for future management.

Table 9.1 The risk of miscarriage after successive pregnancy losses

	Number of pregnancies observed	Risk of miscarriage according to number of previous losses				
		0	1	2	3	≥4
Naylor & Warburton 1979	14 000	11%	23%	29%	33%	—
Regan 1988	226	5%	12%	29%	36%	—
Parazzini et al 1988	66	—	—	20%	40%	54%
Knudsen et al 1991	300 500	11%	16%	25%	45%	54%
Quenby & Farquharson 1993	125	—	—	11%	13%	41%

Although fetal chromosomal abnormalities are the most common cause of sporadic miscarriage it is not clear whether this is the case in recurrent miscarriage. Studies of the conceptuses from recurrent miscarriers have reported large variations in the proportion of losses that are chromosomally abnormal, with published figures of between 18% and 57% (Strobino et al 1986, Stern et al 1996, Daniely et al 1998). It has been suggested that the lower figures for fetal aneuploidy from earlier studies may have resulted from a high prevalence of contamination with maternal tissue giving misleading results (Bell et al 1999). There is a tendency for successive abortuses to be karyotypically normal or karyotypically abnormal (Boue et al 1973) and some couples are at risk of recurrent aneuploidy. However, the risk of a further pregnancy loss appears to be greater when the index pregnancy has a normal karyotype (Simpson 1980), suggesting that some recurrent miscarriage sufferers have an underlying systematic cause for their pregnancy losses.

Couples in which one or other partner carries a chromosome anomaly are at risk of repeated miscarriages with the loss of pregnancies with an abnormal karyotype. The most common type of parental chromosome rearrangement is a balanced translocation. This is usually either a balanced reciprocal translocation where the overall number of chromosomes is unchanged, or a Robertsonian translocation where there are only 45 chromosomes but the genetic information is intact. The conceptuses of such parents carry a high risk of an unbalanced translocation and the pregnancies are usually lost in the first trimester. The prevalence of parental chromosome abnormalities is consistently reported to be 3–5% in couples with recurrent miscarriage (Stray-Pedersen & Stray-Pedersen 1984, De Braekeleer & Dao 1990, Clifford et al 1994) in contrast to a prevalence of between 0.7% and 0.8% in unselected newborn infants.

Although parental peripheral blood karyotyping is expensive, the profound effect of a parental chromosome rearrangement on the prognosis for future pregnancy outcome justifies this test in any protocol for investigation of recurrent miscarriage. Affected couples should receive specialist genetic counselling and be advised of the need for prenatal diagnosis in subsequent ongoing pregnancies. Preimplantation genetic diagnosis may offer an alternative treatment option for these individuals in specialist assisted conception units.

Infective causes

Many severe maternal infections have been reported to cause sporadic miscarriage. The mechanisms are unclear but have been postulated to be due to maternal pyrexia or bacteraemia. However, a recent prospective study found that women experiencing a first-trimester miscarriage were no more likely to have a clinical infection than those having a successful pregnancy (Simpson et al 1996). The role played by infective organisms, in particular genital tract infection, in the aetiology of recurrent miscarriage is unclear. The majority of organisms implicated do not persist for long enough to produce repeated miscarriages, or alternatively are found in high prevalence in the normal population. Isolation of

Ureaplasma urealyticum from the genital tract has been reported to be associated with recurrent early pregnancy loss (Stray-Pedersen & Stray-Pedersen 1984) but other studies have shown this organism to be highly prevalent in the general population (Carey et al 1991) and, further, eradication of the organism has no effect on the outcome of pregnancy (Harger et al 1983).

Bacterial vaginosis (BV), a polymicrobial anaerobic infection, has been implicated in the aetiology of preterm labour and late miscarriage (Hay et al 1994, Lhahi-Camp et al 1996); however antibiotic treatment for BV carriers during pregnancy only benefits those women with a history of previous preterm loss (McDonald et al 1997). This suggests that BV does not cause miscarriage unless it is accompanied by another insult, as yet undetermined. In a recent study of patients undergoing IVF, BV was implicated in the aetiology of first-trimester loss (Ralph et al 1999). This appeared to be accounted for by an increase in the rate of preclinical pregnancy loss, as distinct from clinical miscarriages, raising the possibility that infection with BV adversely affected early embryonic development. To date there are no reports on the value of treating BV in such women.

Structural causes

Müllerian duct defects

Anatomical abnormalities of the uterus, such as congenital Müllerian duct anomalies, have long been quoted as a cause of recurrent miscarriage, both in early pregnancy and in the mid-trimester. The numerical contribution of these uterine structural abnormalities in the aetiology of recurrent miscarriage has been difficult to ascertain. The prevalence of structural abnormalities in women with normal reproductive histories identified at the time of laparoscopic sterilisation is approximately 3% (Simon et al 1991). The prevalence in recurrent miscarriers varies according to the method of investigation employed but has been quoted as ranging from 3% to 27% (Stray-Pedersen & Stray-Pedersen 1984, Stephenson 1996, Li 1998). The most sensitive method of investigation has yet to be agreed: hysterosalpingography has been superseded by hysteroscopy (Raziel et al 1994) but whether this is superior to ultrasonography remains to be established. The use of 3D ultrasound is encouraging (Jurkovic et al 1995) and appears to be a useful non-invasive tool for the investigation of uterine morphology, although it is not yet widely available.

If Müllerian duct defects cause early pregnancy loss, the embryo must be presumed to implant in an avascular area of endometrial cavity leading to arrested development and early pregnancy failure. To account for recurrent episodes of early pregnancy loss this process must occur in sequential pregnancies, which seems unlikely.

The lack of any randomised trials of surgical intervention for congenital uterine abnormalities has led to further controversy since there is no clear evidence that prospective pregnancy outcome is improved. Further, open surgical correction carries the risk of pelvic and intrauterine adhesion formation, and subsequent infertility rates may be as high as 30% (Bennett 1987). Hysteroscopic resection of intrauterine septa is likely to be a more promising therapeutic option but to date randomised studies are lacking.

Cervical incompetence

Cervical incompetence is a condition in which painless dilatation of the cervix leads to miscarriage in the absence of uterine contractions or haemorrhage. The role played by cervical incompetence in the aetiology of second-trimester loss remains contentious. Traditionally, cervical cerclage has been considered on the basis of a history of mid-trimester painless cervical dilatation or rupture of the membranes, as the diagnosis in the non-pregnant state is unreliable. However, the only large randomised controlled trial failed to give clear evidence that cerclage improved live birth rates (MRC/RCOG Working Party on Cervical Cerclage 1993). This multicentre trial is difficult to interpret as women were only included in the study if the clinician was uncertain whether to perform cerclage. Women with a clear history of cervical incompetence were excluded (as they received cerclage in any case) and many women with a dubious history were randomised. It is probable that many women in the trial would not be considered for a cervical suture in normal practice today.

The use of transvaginal sonography in pregnancy to look for progressive shortening of the cervix and funnelling of the upper cervix prior to overt cervical dilatation may improve diagnostic accuracy and allow a more selective use of cerclage (Fox et al 1996). Transabdominal cervical cerclage has been advocated as a treatment for recurrent mid-trimester loss, with the objective of closing the internal os at the junction with the isthmus of the uterus (Gibb & Salaria 1995). Randomised controlled trials of this treatment are awaited.

While the role of cervical incompetence in the aetiology of mid-trimester loss remains controversial, there is general agreement that cervical incompetence is not a cause of recurrent early pregnancy loss.

Social and environmental factors

Although some chemical and toxic agents have been associated with miscarriage (Katz & Kuller 1994), a history of exposure to such agents is rarely encountered in a clinical setting. Heavy alcohol consumption has been associated with an increased risk of miscarriage in some studies (Sokol et al 1980) but not in others (Parazzini et al 1994). Smoking has been reported to be a risk factor for miscarriage (Parazzini et al 1991, Chatenoud et al 1998) and the risk appears to increase with the number of cigarettes smoked. However, the contribution that these habits make to the overall problem of recurrent miscarriage is small.

Alloimmune factors

The hypothesis that some women fail to mount a protective immune response to pregnancy, resulting in rejection of the genetically dissimilar fetus, has been proposed but lacks concrete evidence to support it. It was originally proposed that there is a maternal immune response to the conceptus that must be blocked in order for the pregnancy to progress nor-

mally, and that in the absence of this 'blocking' response pregnancy loss occurs. The concept that it is necessary to develop detectable antipaternal cytotoxic antibodies (APCA) in order for a pregnancy to be successful has since been disproved (Regan & Braude 1987, Regan 1988). However, the belief that a protective response could be provoked by deliberate immunisation with exogenous antigen (usually paternal leucocytes) led to the development of immunotherapy as a treatment for recurrent miscarriage. To date there has only been one randomised controlled trial documenting a significant benefit from immunotherapy (Mowbray et al 1985) and meta-analyses of immunotherapy trials have produced conflicting results (The Recurrent Miscarriage Immunotherapy Trialists Group 1994, Jeng et al 1995). A recent well-designed randomised double-blind trial of 171 women with unexplained recurrent miscarriage who received immunisation with either paternal white cells or saline showed no benefit from treatment (Ober et al 1999). An intention-to-treat analysis showed the success rate (pregnancy progressing beyond 28 weeks) to be 36% in the treatment group and 48% in the control group ($p=0.1$). Analysis of women who conceived gave a success rate of 46% in the treatment group compared to 65% in the control group ($p=0.03$) with significantly more losses in the treatment group. The potential risks of immunotherapy, including blood-borne virus transmission, anaphylaxis, hepatitis and its sequelae, and transfusion reactions, led to the conclusion that immunotherapy should not be recommended for the treatment of recurrent miscarriage (Royal College of Obstetricians and Gynaecologists 1998, Ober et al 1999).

The use of intravenous immunoglobulin (IVIG) infusions as an alternative to immunotherapy for unexplained recurrent miscarriage has also been explored. Once again, a clear underlying hypothesis of the mechanism of action is lacking, and so far randomised controlled trials and a meta-analysis have failed to show any significant benefit (Christiansen 1998, Daya et al 1998, Stephenson et al 1998).

Endocrine dysfunction

Generalised endocrine disease

Diabetes mellitus has historically been considered to be an important cause of recurrent miscarriage. Whilst poorly controlled diabetics do have an increased rate of early miscarriage (Miodovnik et al 1990), there is good evidence that well-controlled diabetes is not associated with an increased risk of early pregnancy loss (Mills et al 1988). It follows that subclinical carbohydrate intolerance is not a risk factor for recurrent early miscarriage.

Thyroid dysfunction has previously been cited as a cause of recurrent miscarriage (Winikoff & Malinek 1975, Stray-Pedersen & Stray-Pedersen 1984) but direct evidence is lacking and thyroid function tests are rarely abnormal in these women. There does appear to be an association between antithyroid antibodies and recurrent pregnancy loss (Kutteh et al 1999) although this may well reflect a generalised autoimmune abnormality rather than a specific endocrine dysfunction. Further, the presence of antithyroid antibodies in women with recurrent miscarriage appears to have no effect on pregnancy outcome compared to women who are antithyroid antibody negative (Rushworth et al 1999).

Luteal phase defect

Luteal phase defect (LPD) remains a controversial and poorly defined endocrine disorder that has been associated with both infertility and early pregnancy loss. There has been much debate about the definition, diagnosis, clinical relevance and value of treatment of LPD. It was originally suggested that inadequate progesterone secretion (in either amount or duration) from the corpus luteum in the luteal phase led to retarded maturation of the endometrium that was incapable of supporting an implanting embryo (Jones 1976). Noyes and co-workers (1950) proposed that the diagnosis of LPD be made if endometrial development lagged two or more days behind the chronologic date of the cycle originally calculated from basal body temperature charts and the date of the next menstrual period. Since then, histological dating of the endometrium has been considered by many to be the gold standard for the diagnosis of LPD. However, subsequent studies have identified flaws in this methodology. Peters and co-workers in 1992 reported that the prevalence of LPD in infertile women and women with recurrent miscarriage varied according to the method of timing of the cycle and was low when ultrasound evidence of the precise day of ovulation was used. There was no significant difference in the prevalence of out-of-phase biopsies between these women and fertile controls, indicating that LPD was not an important cause of infertility or recurrent early pregnancy failure.

The clinical relevance of LPD has also been widely questioned. In a study of preconceptual cycles, urinary metabolites of oestrogen and progesterone were assayed and no difference in patterns was seen between cycles leading to a successful pregnancy and cycles ending in early pregnancy failure (Baird et al 1991). In another interesting study of 54 endometrial biopsies inadvertently taken in the cycle of conception, there was no difference in the prevalence of out-of-phase biopsies in cycles that ended in miscarriage and cycles that led to ongoing pregnancies (Wentz et al 1986). This study provides convincing evidence that histological endometrial retardation has no predictive value for the outcome of pregnancy.

Finally, the treatment of LPD is also contentious since good-quality randomised controlled trials are scarce. Supplementation of the luteal phase with progestogens has been the most common treatment modality tried, but other drugs have been explored including clomiphene citrate and gonadotrophins, usually human chorionic gonadotrophin (hCG). No randomised controlled trials have demonstrated a benefit of progestational agents in terms of successful pregnancy rates, and the authors of meta-analyses of this therapy have published differing conclusions (Daya 1989, Goldstein et al 1989). Similarly, the use of hCG in LPD has not been proven in randomised trials.

From the above we can conclude that LPD is a controversial condition that is at best poorly defined and difficult to diagnose accurately. Many clinicians now question the relevance of LPD to fertility and the establishment of successful pregnancy. In summary, progestational agents should not be recommended for the treatment of either recurrent or threatened miscarriage (Royal College of Gynaecologists Study Group 1997).

Hypersecretion of luteinising hormone

Evidence accumulating from the mid 1980s suggests that hypersecretion of luteinising hormone (LH) has an adverse effect on fertility and pregnancy outcome. Women with recurrent miscarriage and infertility have a high prevalence of ultrasound-diagnosed polycystic ovaries (PCO), in most studies in the region of 50% (Jacobs et al 1987, Balen et al 1993a, Clifford et al 1994, Liddell et al 1997), compared to a background rate of PCO of between 14% and 23% in a 'normal' population of women of reproductive age (Polson et al 1988, Farquhar et al 1994, Koivunen et al 1999).

It appeared to be the presence of LH hypersecretion that was responsible for the poor reproductive outcome in these women rather than a polycystic ovarian morphology per se. Women with high LH levels have been reported to have reduced rates of fertilisation, lower conception rates and higher miscarriage rates when undergoing IVF and ovulation induction (Stanger & Yovich 1985, Howles et al 1987, Homburg et al 1988, Punnonen et al 1988, Hamilton-Fairley et al 1991). The adverse effect of LH hypersecretion has also been documented in spontaneous cycles. A large prospective study of 193 women planning a pregnancy reported that a single raised mid-follicular phase serum LH level was associated with a lower conception rate than in women with normal LH concentrations (Regan et al 1990). Moreover, those women who did conceive with raised LH levels experienced a significantly higher miscarriage rate than those conceiving with normal LH levels (65% versus 12%; $p < 0.005$).

It has been suggested that the effect of LH on reproductive outcome could be mediated via an adverse effect on the oocyte (Stanger & Yovich 1985, Homburg & Jacobs 1989, Jacobs 1991), or on the endometrium, principally via abnormal androgen secretion (Tulppala et al 1993a, Okon et al 1998), or both.

Following the hypothesis that high LH levels are detrimental to the establishment of early pregnancy, many workers have examined the reproductive outcome after suppression of elevated LH concentrations with analogues to LHRH. Several studies of women undergoing assisted conception have documented improved pregnancy and live birth rates after LH suppression (Abdalla et al 1990, Balen et al 1993, Homburg et al 1993). However, this appears not to be the case for fertile women with recurrent miscarriage who hypersecrete LH. A recent randomised controlled trial reported that there was no apparent benefit from LH suppression in these women, and an important finding was a live birth rate of 76% amongst the control groups (Clifford et al 1996; Fig. 9.2).

In summary, although LH hypersecretion is associated with recurrent miscarriage it appears not to be the direct cause of reproductive failure, as there is no benefit from reducing LH levels. It is possible that factors other than LH (such as abnormal androgen or insulin secretion) influence the pregnancy outcome in these women. Meanwhile the search for a specific endocrinopathy that dictates pregnancy

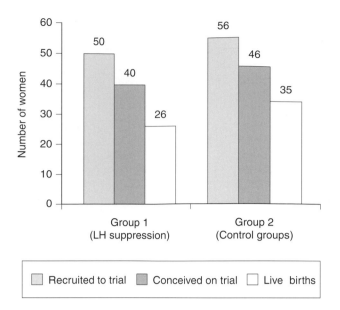

Fig. 9.2 LH suppression in women with recurrent miscarriage and high LH—conception and live birth rate over six cycles (after Clifford et al 1996).

Table 9.2 Clinical features of the primary antiphospholipid antibody syndrome

Obstetrics and gynaecology
Recurrent miscarriage
Infertility
Pre-eclampsia
Placental abruption
Intrauterine growth restriction
Chorea gravidarum

Dermatological
Livedo reticularis
Cutaneous necrosis

Vascular
Venous thrombosis
Arterial thrombosis
Mitral valve disease
Thrombotic endocarditis

Neurological
Transient ischaemic attacks
Cerebrovascular disease
Migraine
Epilepsy
Multiple sclerosis

outcome in women with PCO continues. However, the beneficial effect of supportive care observed in the above study raises the question of whether any pharmacological intervention is needed for these women (Clifford et al 1996).

Autoimmune factors

It is now well established that circulating antiphospholipid antibodies (aPL), the most important of which are the lupus anticoagulant (LA) and anticardiolipin antibodies (ACA), are associated with recurrent pregnancy failure at all stages of pregnancy. Although the adverse effects of aPL on the out come of pregnancy were first noted in women with systemic lupus erythematosus (Gatenby 1989), the primary antiphospholipid syndrome (PAPS) is now established as an important cause of recurrent miscarriage (Hughes 1983, Harris et al 1986, Asherson et al 1989). The features of the syndrome are raised circulating aPL in association with recurrent fetal loss, arterial or venous thrombosis, and other features detailed in Table 9.2. The pathophysiology of aPL is uncertain. The adverse effects of aPL may be mediated via thrombosis and fibrin deposition in many vessels including the uteroplacental circulation. This may be caused by inhibition of endothelial prostacyclin production, enhanced thromboxane release from platelets, reduced antithrombin III production or a decrease in the activation of protein C (Triplett 1992). There is also evidence of a direct effect of aPL on trophoblast function leading to impaired implantation (Lyden et al 1992, Rote et al 1998). Fetal demise can occur at all stages of the pregnancy and there is an association with pre-eclampsia, intrauterine growth restriction (IUGR) and placental abruption.

The prevalence of PAPS in women with recurrent miscarriage is 15% compared to 2% in women with normal obstetric histories (Pattison et al 1991, Rai et al 1995a). Untreated women with PAPS have a poor prognosis: a recent prospective study documented a fetal loss rate of 90% (Rai et al 1995b). The majority of these losses were noted to be in the first trimester after the establishment of fetal heart activity. A variety of treatments have been advocated for women with PAPS, including corticosteroids, low-dose aspirin, heparin and immunoglobulins. Most studies have been uncontrolled and are therefore open to criticism. However, a randomised controlled trial of corticosteroids in pregnancy in women with PAPS has shown that there is no benefit from steroid treatment (Laskin et al 1997) and further there is significant maternal and fetal morbidity associated with their use (Cowchock et al 1992, Silver et al 1993).

The mainstay of treatment for pregnant women with PAPS is low-dose aspirin in combination with subcutaneous heparin. Two studies, one randomised (Rai et al 1997) and one non-randomised (Kutteh 1996), both reported that the live birth rate amongst women with PAPS is improved to 40% when they are treated with low-dose aspirin but that this is further and significantly increased to 70% when treated with aspirin in combination with heparin (Fig. 9.3). The beneficial effects of aspirin and heparin have been confirmed in a larger cohort study (Backos et al 1999a). The use of prolonged heparin in pregnancy has given rise to concerns about the development of osteopenia. In a longitudinal study of women with aPL who were treated with heparin throughout pregnancy, the results using the powerful diagnostic imaging technique of dual photon X-ray absorptiometry were reassuring (Backos et al 1999b). Although a reduction in bone mineral density (BMD) of up to 3.7% was noted

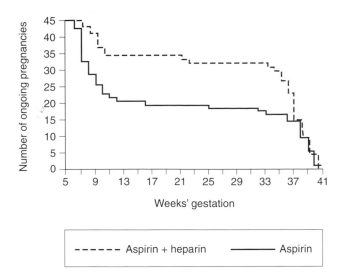

Fig. 9.3 Survival plot of pregnancies treated with aspirin and aspirin plus heparin (after Rai et al 1997).

Table 9.3 Studies of women with no identifiable cause for their miscarriages

Authors	Number of women with unexplained losses
Stray-Pedersen & Stray-Pedersen 1984	85/195 (44%)
Parazzini et al 1988 (≥2 losses included)	95/158 (60%)
Gilchrist et al 1991 (≥2 losses included)	93/171 (54%)
Tulppala et al 1993	35/63 (51%)
Quenby & Farquharson 1993 (≥2 losses included)	162/203 (80%)
Clifford et al 1994	237/500 (47%)
Stephenson 1996	84/197 (43%)

amongst the heparin-treated women, this is similar to the decrease in BMD observed in untreated pregnancies.

Inherited thrombophilia

Thrombophilic defects have recently been identified as potential causes of both early and late miscarriage and adverse pregnancy outcome. Retrospective surveys of women with inherited thrombophilia have reported an increased fetal loss rate in the past obstetric history (Preston et al 1996, Sanson et al 1996, Kupferminc et al 1999). There are as yet no prospective studies documenting an adverse pregnancy outcome in such women, and a causal role for thrombophilic defects remains unconfirmed. Activated protein C resistance (APCR) is the most common inherited thrombophilia, with a prevalence in the general population of 3–5% (Bertina et al 1994). In up to 90% of cases it is due to a single point mutation in the factor V gene resulting in a mutated factor V, known as factor V Leiden. Factor V Leiden is resistant to inactivation by activated protein C, a natural inhibitor of coagulation, and therefore a state of increased thrombin generation occurs. Women with recurrent mid-trimester losses have been shown to have a prevalence of APCR of 20% (Rai et al 1996), raising the possibility that intravascular coagulation may underlie some cases of second-trimester miscarriage.

Hyperhomocysteinaemia is a condition in which elevated blood homocysteine concentrations are associated with occlusive arterial and venous disease. It results either from an autosomal recessive inborn error of metabolism or from an acquired disorder (usually secondary to folate deficiency). Hyperhomocysteinaemia has been reported to be a risk factor for recurrent miscarriage, including early pregnancy loss, with a reported prevalence of 12–21% in two small studies (Wouters et al 1993, Quere et al 1998). Further work in this area is needed, especially as this condition is potentially amenable to treatment with folic acid and vitamin B_{12}.

Unexplained recurrent miscarriage

The number of women with recurrent miscarriage who have negative results after thorough investigation has been documented in several series (Table 9.3). Despite different investigative protocols the proportion of women with unexplained losses in most studies lies between 43% and 60%. One recent series reported that in 80% of women there was no identifiable cause after investigation, although it should be noted that this study included women with only two previous miscarriages (Quenby & Farquharson 1994).

The prognosis in unexplained recurrent miscarriage has been reported by several authors (Table 9.4) and several factors appear to influence the outcome in the next pregnancy. The number of previous losses has been shown to affect outcome (Gilchrist et al 1991, Quenby & Farquharson 1994, Clifford et al 1997) with a steady increase in the risk of subsequent miscarriage for each previous loss. In the largest recent study of unexplained recurrent pregnancy loss, the miscarriage rate in the next pregnancy rose from 29% after three losses to 52% after six or more losses (Clifford et al 1997). The effect of past reproductive performance on future pregnancy outcome mirrors that seen in large observational series of unselected women entering pregnancy. It follows that studies that include women who have had only two previous miscarriages will report a better prognosis in the next pregnancy than studies that use the more rigorous definition of three consecutive losses. Maternal age also influences the prognosis for the future. A pronounced effect is seen after the mid thirties: more than 50% of women over 40 years lose the next pregnancy irrespective of the number of previous losses (Clifford et al 1997). Most studies report that the presence of a previous live birth in the history does not appear to have a significant effect on outcome, with a similar prognosis after both primary and secondary recurrent miscarriage (Gilchrist et al 1991, Clifford et al 1997).

The most striking observation is that supportive therapy or *'tender loving care'* (TLC) in the setting of a dedicated early pregnancy clinic confers a highly significant beneficial effect on pregnancy outcome in women with unexplained recurrent miscarriage (Stray-Pedersen & Stray-Pedersen 1984, Liddell et al 1991, Clifford et al 1997). In these studies, women who received supportive therapy in the first trimester had a 72–86% chance of a successful pregnancy without any

Table 9.4 Pregnancy outcome in unexplained recurrent miscarriage and the effect of supportive care

Authors	Overall live birth rate	Effect of supportive care		
Tupper & Wiel 1962	21/38 (55%)	TLC	16/19	(84%)
		No TLC	5/19	(26%)
Stray-Pedersen & Stray-Pedersen 1984	40/61 (66%)	TLC	32/37	(86%)
		No TLC	8/24	(33%)
Parazzini et al 1988 (≥2 losses included)	47/66 (71%)	–		
Gilchrist et al 1991 (≥2 losses included)	62/69 (90%)	–		
Liddell et al 1991	41/53 (77%)	TLC	38/44	(86%)
		No TLC	3/9	(33%)
Tulppala et al 1993	21/35 (60%)	–		
Clifford et al 1997	133/201 (66%)	TLC	115/160	(72%)
		No TLC	18/41	(44%)

TLC, tender loving care.

pharmacological treatment (Table 9.4). Although these studies were not randomised, the consistency of the data suggests that this is a genuine phenomenon although the mechanism of action is not clear. An adverse effect of stress on uterine blood flow has been postulated (Liddell et al 1991) but to date evidence is lacking.

The observation that TLC alone improves the outcome in the next pregnancy explains why a large placebo response is observed in new therapeutic trials for recurrent miscarriage. Women with unexplained recurrent miscarriage entering such trials must be expected to do well irrespective of the treatment intervention as they receive increased vigilance and care as a trial participant.

MANAGEMENT

Sporadic miscarriage

Bleeding in early pregnancy is the commonest complication of pregnancy, occurring in up to 25% of pregnancies. When a woman presents with bleeding in early pregnancy the clinician must attempt to assess the pregnancy and give a prognosis. Where examination reveals an open cervix with the obvious passage of products of conception, the diagnosis of an inevitable or incomplete miscarriage is uncomplicated. Ultrasound examination is usually the first investigation to be performed, and transvaginal ultrasound (TVS) is at present the best available tool to assess early pregnancy. An intrauterine gestation sac can be visualised on TVS as early as 4.5 weeks amenorrhoea and fetal cardiac activity can be reliably detected from 6 weeks (or when the crown–rump length is at least 5 mm). The finding of a viable intrauterine pregnancy carries an excellent prognosis, with a subsequent miscarriage rate of 2% when detected between 9 and 11 weeks amenorrhoea (Mackenzie et al 1988). TVS can also identify other features of early pregnancy that can be correlated with subsequent outcome, such as the presence of an intrauterine haematoma, fetal bradycardia and a discrepancy between the gestational sac diameter and the crown–rump size. The more abnormal features present, the higher the likelihood of subsequent early pregnancy failure (Falco et al 1996).

Maternal serum β-hCG assays can be useful in the investigation and assessment of early pregnancy, although more particularly in the detection of ectopic gestations. A discriminatory level of around 1000 iu/l is used to determine those pregnancies in which an intrauterine gestation sac should be visualised by TVS.

Other biochemical tests, including progesterone and pregnancy-associated plasma protein A (PAPP-A), have been advocated in the assessment of early pregnancy but at present they cannot be considered as part of routine management.

Recurrent miscarriage

Women with recurrent miscarriage should ideally be seen in a specialist miscarriage clinic where there are established protocols for investigation and management. Structured history sheets have been recommended (Li 1998) and details of previous pregnancy losses can be documented by the patient prior to the consultation to avoid distress at the first appointment (Clifford et al 1994). At the first appointment the couple should be seen together and sufficient time should be allowed for a detailed discussion. Information booklets that explain the proposed investigations, a brief summary of the causes of recurrent miscarriage and future prognosis should be available. Support personnel such as dedicated secretarial staff, specialist nurses and counsellors are important. Current evidence-based investigations for recurrent miscarriage are shown in Table 9.5.

In future pregnancies, direct access to an early pregnancy clinic is invaluable. Women with recurrent miscarriage have been shown to benefit from serial first-trimester ultrasound scans for fetal growth in the setting of a dedicated early pregnancy clinic. If the next pregnancy fails, obtaining fetal tissue for karyotypic analysis is imperative. Not only does it provide an explanation for the miscarriage if the karyotype is abnormal but the results are also important for guidance for future pregnancies.

CONCLUSION

Sporadic miscarriage is the commonest complication of pregnancy and is associated with a good prognosis for future

Table 9.5 Recommended investigations after recurrent miscarriage

Evidence-based investigations	Research-based investigations
Karyotype both partners	Thrombophilia screen
Karyotype products of conception	Assess ovarian morphology Mid-follicular LH
Establish uterine morphology (ultrasound/hysteroscopy)	Screen for bacterial vaginosis
Antiphospholipid antibodies (lupus anticoagulant and anticardiolipin antibodies)	

pregnancies. Recurrent miscarriage is less frequently encountered and is best managed in a specialist clinic. Such clinics have the opportunity to develop protocols for the investigation and management of the condition, audit the outcome of subsequent pregnancies, provide a comprehensive multidisciplinary approach to the management of recurrent miscarriage and conduct research investigations into potential new treatments. Recent studies have identified that antiphospholipid antibodies and other thrombophilic defects are emerging as important causes of repeated pregnancy failure.

After thorough investigation approximately 50% of women with a history of recurrent miscarriage will have negative results. The future pregnancy outcome for these women is good and supportive therapy alone is the treatment of choice in the next pregnancy. To avoid the pitfalls of the past, empirical treatment of women with recurrent miscarriage should be avoided and new therapies should only ever be tested in the setting of a randomised trial.

KEY POINTS

- A quarter of women have a miscarriage in their reproductive life.
- Recurrent miscarriage is the loss of three or more pregnancies before 24 weeks. There is no simple cause but half are associated with fetal chromosomal abnormalities.
- Well-controlled endocrine diseases such as diabetes or thyroid dysfunction are not associated with raised miscarriage rates, and alloimmune factors do not seem to be significant.
- High levels of antiphospholipid antibodies are associated with spontaneous miscarriages, as are thrombophilic defects.
- Women with true recurrent miscarriages should be investigated at specialist miscarriage clinics.

REFERENCES

Abdalla HI, Ahuja KK, Leonard T et al 1990 Comparative trial of luteinizing hormone-releasing hormone analog/human menopausal gonadotropin and clomiphene citrate/human menopausal gonadotropin in an assisted conception program. Fertil Steril 53:473–478

Alberman E 1988 The epidemiology of repeated abortion. In: Beard RW, Sharp F (eds) Early pregnancy loss: mechanisms and treatment. Royal College of Gynaecologists, London, pp 9–17

Asherson RA, Khamasta MA, Ordi-Ross J et al 1989 The 'primary' antiphospholipid syndrome: major clinical and serological features. Medicine 68:366–374

Backos M, Rai R, Baxter N et al 1999a Pregnancy complications in women with recurrent miscarriage associated with antiphospholipid antibodies treated with low dose aspirin and heparin. Br J Obstet Gynaecol 106:102–107

Backos M, Rai R, Thomas E et al 1999b Bone density changes in pregnant women treated with heparin: a prospective, longitudinal study. Hum Reprod 14:2876–2880

Baird DD, Weinberg CR, Wilcox AJ et al 1991 Hormonal profiles of natural conception cycles ending in early, unrecognized pregnancy loss. J Clin Endocrinol Metab 72:793–800

Balen AH, Tan SL, Jacobs HS 1993a Hypersecretion of luteinising hormone: a significant cause of infertility and miscarriage. Br J Obstet Gynaecol 100:1082–1089

Balen AH, Tan SL, MacDougall J et al 1993b Miscarriage rates following in-vitro fertilisation are increased in women with polycystic ovaries and reduced by pituitary desensitisation with buserelin. Hum Reprod 8:959–964

Bell KA, Van Deerlin PG, Haddad BR, Feinberg RF 1999 Cytogenetic diagnosis of 'normal 46 XX' karyotypes in spontaneous abortions frequently may be misleading. Fertil Steril 71:334–341

Bennett MJ 1987 Congenital abnormalities of the fundus. In: Bennett MJ, Edmonds DK (eds) Spontaneous and recurrent abortion. Blackwell Scientific, Oxford, pp 109–129

Bertina RM, Koeleman BP, Koster T et al 1994 Mutation in blood coagulation factor V associated with resistance to activated protein C. Nature 369:64–67

Boue J, Boue A, Lazar P, Gueguen S 1973 Outcome of pregnancies following a spontaneous abortion with chromosomal anomalies. Am J Obstet Gynecol 116:806–812

Boue J, Boue A, Lazar P 1975 Retrospective and prospective epidemiological studies of 1500 karyotyped spontaneous human abortions. Teratology 12:11–26

Carey JC, Blackwelder WC, Nugent RP et al 1991 Antepartum cultures for Ureaplasma urealyticum are not useful in predicting pregnancy outcome. Am J Obstet Gynecol 164:728–733

Cashner KA, Christopher CR, Dysert GA 1987 Spontaneous fetal loss after demonstration of a live fetus in the first trimester. Obstet Gynecol 70:827–830

Chatenoud L, Parazzini F, di Cintio E et al 1998 Paternal and maternal smoking habits before conception and during the first trimester: relation to spontaneous abortion. Ann Epidemiol 8:520 526

Christiansen OB 1998 Intravenous immunoglobulin in the prevention of recurrent spontaneous abortion: the European experience. Am J Reprod Immunol 39:77–81

Clifford K, Rai R, Watson H, Regan L 1994 An informative protocol for the investigation of recurrent miscarriage: preliminary experience of 500 consecutive cases. Hum Reprod 9:1328–1332

Clifford K, Rai R, Watson H et al 1996 Does suppressing luteinising hormone secretion reduce the miscarriage rate? Results of a randomised controlled trial. BMJ 312:1508–1511

Clifford K, Rai R, Regan L 1997 Future pregnancy outcome in unexplained recurrent miscarriage. Hum Reprod 12:387–389

Cowchock FS, Reece EA, Balaban D et al 1992 Repeated fetal losses associated with antiphospholipid antibodies: a collaborative randomized trial comparing prednisolone with low-dose heparin treatment. Am J Obstet Gynecol 166:1318–1323

Daniely M, Aviram-Goldring A, Barkai G, Goldman B 1998 Detection of chromosomal aberration in fetuses arising from recurrent spontaneous abortion by comparative genomic hybridization. Hum Reprod 13:805–809

Daya S 1989 Efficacy of progesterone support for pregnancy in women with recurrent miscarriage. A meta-analysis of controlled trials. Br J Obstet Gynaecol 96:275–280

Daya S, Gunby J, Clark DA 1998 Intravenous immunoglobulin therapy for recurrent spontaneous abortion: a meta-analysis. Am J Reprod Immunol 39:69–76

De Braekeleer M, Dao TN 1990 Cytogenetic studies in couples experiencing repeated pregnancy losses. Hum Reprod 5:519–528

Drakeley AJ, Quenby S, Farquharson RG 1998 Mid-trimester loss—appraisal of a screening protocol. Hum Reprod 13:1975–1980

Falco P, Milanao V, Pilu G et al 1996 Sonography of pregnancies with first trimester bleeding and a viable embryo: a study of prognostic indicators by logistic regression analysis. Ultrasound Obstet Gynecol 7:165–169

Farquhar CM, Birdsall M, Manning P et al 1994 The prevalence of polycystic ovaries on ultrasound scanning in a population of randomly selected women. Aust NZ J Obstet Gynaecol 34(1):67–72

Fox R, James M, Tuohy J, Wardle P 1996 Transvaginal ultrasound in the management of women with suspected cervical incompetence. Br J Obstet Gynaecol 103:921–924

Gatenby PA 1989 Systemic lupus erythematosus and pregnancy. Aust NZ J Med 19:261–278

Gibb D, Salaria DA 1995 Transabdominal cervicoisthmic cerclage in the management of recurrent second trimester miscarriage and preterm delivery. Br J Obstet Gynaecol 102:802–806

Gilchrist DM, Livingston JE, Hurlburt JA, Wilson RD 1991 Recurrent spontaneous pregnancy loss—investigation and reproductive follow-up. J Reprod Med 36:184–188

Goldstein P, Berrier J, Rosen S et al 1989 A meta-analysis of randomised control trials of progestational agents in pregnancy. Br J Obstet Gynaecol 96:265–274

Hamilton-Fairley D, Kiddy D, Watson H et al 1991 Low-dose gonadotrophin therapy for induction of ovulation in 100 women with polycystic ovary syndrome. Hum Reprod 6:1095–1099

Harger JH, Archer DF, Marchese SG et al 1983 Etiology of recurrent pregnancy losses and outcome of subsequent pregnancies. Obstet Gynaecol 62:574–581

Harris EN, Chan JK, Asherson RA et al 1986 Thrombosis, recurrent fetal loss, and thrombocytopenia. Arch Intern Med 146:2153–2156

Hay PE, Lamont RF, Taylor-Robinson D et al 1994 Abnormal bacterial colonisation of the genital tract and subsequent preterm delivery and late miscarriage. BMJ 308: 295–298

Hemminki E, Forssas E 1999 Epidemiology of miscarriage and its relation to other reproductive events in Finland. Am J Obstet Gynecol 181:396–401

Homburg R, Jacobs HS 1989 Etiology of miscarriage in polycystic ovary syndrome. Fertil Steril 51:196–197

Homburg R, Armar NA, Eshel A et al 1988 Influence of serum luteinising hormone concentrations on ovulation, conception and early pregnancy loss in polycystic ovary syndrome. BMJ 297:1024–1026

Homburg R, Levy T, Berkovitz D et al 1993 Gonadotrophin-releasing hormone agonist reduces the miscarriage rate for pregnancies achieved in women with polycystic ovarian syndrome. Fertil Steril 59:527–531

Howles CM, Macnamee MC, Edwards RG 1987 Follicular development and early luteal function of conception and non-conceptional cycles after human in-vitro fertilization: endocrine correlates. Hum Reprod 2:17–21

Hughes GVR 1983 Thrombosis, abortion, cerebral disease and the lupus anticoagulant. BMJ 287:1088–1089

Jacobs HS 1991 The LH hypothesis. In: Shaw RW (ed) Polycystic ovaries: a disorder or a symptom. Parthenon Publishing, Carnforth, Lancs, pp 91–98

Jacobs HS, Porter R, Eshel A, Craft I 1987 Profertility uses of luteinising hormone releasing hormone agonist analogues. In: Vickery BH, Nestor JJ (eds) LHRH and its analogs. MTP Press, Lancaster, pp 303–322

Jeng GT, Scott JR, Burmeister LF 1995 A comparison of meta-analytic results using literature vs individual patient data. Paternal cell immunization for recurrent miscarriage. JAMA 274:830–836

Jones GS 1976 The luteal phase defect. Fertil Steril 27:351–356

Jurkovic D, Geipel A, Gruboeck K et al 1995 Three dimensional ultrasound for the assessment of uterine anatomy and detection of congenital anomalies: a comparison with hysterosalpingography and two-dimensional sonography. Ultrasound Obstet Gynecol 5:233–237

Katz VL, Kuller JA 1994 Recurrent miscarriage. Am J Perinatol 11:386–397

Kline J, Stein Z, Susser M 1989 Conception to birth. Oxford University Press, New York, pp 43–68

Knudsen UB, Hansen V, Juul S, Secher NJ 1991 Prognosis of a new pregnancy following previous spontaneous abortions. Eur J Obstet Gynaecol Reprod Biol 39:31–36

Koivunen R, Laatikainen T, Tomas C et al 1999 The prevalence of polycystic ovaries in healthy women. Acta Obstet Gynecol Scand 78:137–141

Kupferminc MJ, Elder A, Steinman N et al 1999 Increased frequency of genetic thrombophilia in women with complications of pregnancy. N Engl J Med 340:9–13

Kutteh WH 1996 Antiphospholipid antibody-associated recurrent pregnancy loss: treatment with heparin and low-dose aspirin is superior to low-dose aspirin alone. Am J Obstet Gynecol 174:1584–1589

Kutteh WH, Yetman DL, Carr AC et al 1999 Increased prevalence of antithyroid antibodies identified in women with recurrent pregnancy loss but not in women undergoing assisted reproduction. Fertil Steril 71:843–848

Laskin C, Bombardier C, Hannah M et al 1997 Prednisone and aspirin in women with autoantibodies and unexplained fetal loss. N Engl J Med 337:148–153

Lhahi-Camp JM, Rai R, Ison C et al 1996 Association of bacterial vaginosis with a history of second trimester miscarriage. Hum Reprod 11:1575–1578

Li TC 1998 Recurrent miscarriage: principles of management. Hum Reprod 13:478–482

Liddell HS, Pattison NS, Zanderigo A 1991 Recurrent miscarriage—outcome after supportive care in early pregnancy. Aust NZJ Obstet Gynaecol 31:320–322

Liddell HS, Sowden K, Farquhar CM 1997 Recurrent miscarriage: screening for polycystic ovaries and subsequent pregnancy outcome. Aust NZJ Obstet Gynaecol 37:402–406

Lyden TW, Vogt E, Ng AK et al 1992 Monoclonal antiphospholipid antibody reactivity against human placental trophoblast. J Reprod Immunol 22:1–14

McDonald HM, O'Loughlin JA, Vigneswaran R et al 1997 Impact of metronidazole therapy on preterm birth in women with bacterial vaginosis (Gardnerella vaginalis): a randomised, placebo controlled trial. Br J Obstet Gynaecol 104:1391–1397

Mackenzie WE, Holmes DS, Newton JR 1988 Spontaneous abortion rate in ultrasonographically viable pregnancies. Obstet Gynecol 71:81–83

Mills JL, Simpson JL, Driscoll SG et al 1988 Incidence of spontaneous abortion among normal women and insulin-dependent diabetic women whose pregnancies were identified within 21 days of conception. N Engl J Med 319:1617–1623

Miodovnik M, Mimouni F, Siddiqi TA et al 1990 Spontaneous abortions in repeat diabetic pregnancies: a relationship with glycaemic control. Obstet Gynaecol 75:75–78

Mowbray JF, Gibbings C, Liddell H et al 1985 Controlled trial of treatment of recurrent spontaneous abortion by immunisation with paternal cells. Lancet i:941–943

MRC/RCOG Working party on Cervical Cerclage 1993 Final report of the Medical Research Council/Royal College of Obstetricians and Gynaecologists Multicentre Randomised Trial of Cervical Cerclage. Br J Obstet Gynaecol 100:516–523

Naylor AF, Warburton D 1979 Sequential analysis of spontaneous abortion. II. Collaborative study data show that gravidity determines a very substantial rise in risk. Fertil Steril 31:282–286

Noyes RW, Hertig AT, Rock J 1950 Dating the endometrial biopsy. Fertil Steril 1:3–25

Ober C, Karrison T, Odem RR et al 1999 Mononuclear-cell immunisation in prevention of recurrent miscarriages: a randomised trial. Lancet 354:365–369

Okon MA, Laird SM, Tuckerman EM et al 1998 Serum androgen levels in women who have recurrent miscarriages and their correlation with markers of endometrial function. Fertil Steril 69:682–690

Parazzini F, Acaia B, Ricciardiello O et al 1988 Short-term

reproductive prognosis when no cause can be found for recurrent miscarriage. Br J Obstet Gynaecol 95:654–658

Parazzini F, Bocciolone L, Fedele L et al 1991 Risk factors for spontaneous abortion. Int J Epidemiol 20:157–161

Parazzini F, Tozzi L, Chatenoud L et al 1994 Alcohol and risk of spontaneous abortion. Hum Reprod 9:1950–1953

Pattison NS, Chamley LW, McKay EJ et al 1991 Antiphospholipid antibodies in pregnancy: prevalence and clinical association. Br J Obstet Gynaecol 100:909–913

Peters AJ, Lloyd RP, Coulam CB 1992 Prevalence of out-of phase endometrial biopsy specimens. Am J Obstet Gynecol 166:1738–1745

Polson DW, Wadsworth J, Adams J, Franks S 1988 Polycystic ovaries—a common finding in normal women. Lancet ii:870–872

Preston FE, Rosendaal FR, Walker ID et al 1996 Increased fetal loss in women with heritable thrombophilia. Lancet 348:913–916

Punnonen R, Ashorn R, Vilja P et al 1988 Spontaneous luteinising hormone surge and cleavage of in-vitro fertilised embryos. Fertil Steril 49:479–482

Quenby SM, Farquharson RG 1993 Predicting recurring miscarriage: what is important? Obstet Gynecol 82:132–138

Quenby S, Farquharson RG 1994 Human chorionic gonadotrophin supplementation in recurring pregnancy loss: a controlled trial. Fertil Steril 62:708–710

Quere I, Bellet H, Hoffet M et al 1998 A woman with five consecutive fetal deaths: case report and retrospective analysis of hyperhomocysteinaemia prevalence in 100 consecutive women with recurrent miscarriages. Fertil Steril 69:152–154

Rai RS, Regan L, Clifford K et al 1995a Antiphospholipid antibodies and beta 2 glycoprotein I in 500 women with recurrent miscarriage: Results of a comprehensive screening approach. Hum Reprod 10:2001–2005

Rai R, Clifford K, Cohen H et al 1995b High prospective fetal loss rate in untreated pregnancies of women with recurrent miscarriage and antiphospholipid antibodies. Hum Reprod 10:3301–3304

Rai R, Regan L, Hadley E et al 1996 Second trimester miscarriage is associated with resistance to activated protein C. Br J Haematol 92:489–490

Rai R, Cohen H, Dave M, Regan L 1997 Randomised controlled trial of aspirin and aspirin plus heparin in pregnant women with recurrent miscarriage associated with phospholipid antibodies (or antiphospholipid antibodies). BMJ 314:253–257

Ralph SG, Rutherford AJ, Wilson JD 1999 Influence of bacterial vaginosis on conception and miscarriage in the first trimester: cohort study. BMJ 319:220–223

Raziel A, Arieli S, Bukovsky I, Caspi E, Golan A 1994 Investigation of the uterine cavity in recurrent aborters. Fertil Steril 62:1080–1082

The Recurrent Miscarriage Immunotherapy Trialists Group 1994 Worldwide collaborative observational study and meta-analysis on allogenic leukocyte immunotherapy for recurrent spontaneous abortion. Am J Reprod Immunol 32:55–72

Regan L 1988 A prospective study of spontaneous abortion. In: Beard RW, Sharp F (eds) Early pregnancy loss: mechanisms and treatment. Royal College of Gynaecologists, London, pp 23–42

Regan L, Braude PR 1987 Is antipaternal cytotoxic antibody a valid marker in the management of recurrent abortion? Lancet ii:1280

Regan L, Braude PB, Trembath PR 1989 Influence of past reproductive performance on risk of spontaneous abortion. BMJ 299:541–545

Regan L, Owen EJ, Jacobs HS 1990 Hypersecretion of luteinising hormone, infertility and miscarriage. Lancet ii:1141–1144

Rote NS, Vogt E, DeVere G et al 1998 The role of placental trophoblast in the pathophysiology of the antiphospholipid antibody syndrome. Am J Reprod Immunol 39:125–136

Royal College of Gynaecologists Study Group 1997 Recommendations arising from the 33rd Study Group. In: Grudzinskas JG, O'Brien PMS (eds) Problems in early pregnancy: advances in diagnosis and management. RCOG Press, Dorchester, pp 327–331

Royal College of Obstetricians and Gynaecologists 1998 The management of recurrent miscarriage. RCOG Clinical Guidelines, RCOG Press, Dorchester

Rushworth FH, Backos M, Rai R et al 1999 Prospective pregnancy outcome in untreated recurrent miscarriers with thyroid autoantibodies. European Society for Human Reproduction & Embryology, Tours, France, 1999. Hum Reprod, 14, Abstract book 1, Abstr P 169, p 225

Sanson B, Friederich PW, Simioni P et al 1996 The risk of abortion and stillbirth in antithrombin-, protein C- and protein S-deficient women. Thromb Haemost 75:387–388

Silver RK, MacGregor SN, Sholl JS et al 1993 Comparative trial of prednisolone plus aspirin vs. aspirin alone in the treatment of anticardiolipin antibody-positive obstetric patients. Am J Obstet Gynecol 169:1411–1417

Simon C, Martinez L, Pardo F et al 1991 Mullerian defects in women with normal reproductive outcome. Fertil Steril 56:1192–1193

Simpson JL 1980 Genes, chromosomes and reproductive failure. Fertil Steril 33:107–116

Simpson JL, Bombard AT 1987 Chromosomal abnormalities in spontaneous abortions: Frequency, pathology and genetic counselling. In: Bennett MJ, Edmonds DK (eds) Spontaneous and recurrent abortion. Blackwell Scientific, Oxford, pp 51–76

Simpson JL, Gray RH, Queenan JT et al 1996 Further evidence that infection is an infrequent cause of first trimester spontaneous abortion. Hum Reprod 11:2058–2060

Sokol RJ, Miller SI, Reed G 1980 Alcohol abuse during pregnancy: an epidemiologic study. Clin Exp Res 4:135–145

Stanger JD, Yovich JL 1985 Reduced in-vitro fertilization of human oocytes from patients with raised basal luteinizing hormone levels during the follicular phase. Br J Obstet Gynaecol 92:385–393

Stein Z, Kline J, Susser E et al 1980 Maternal age and spontaneous abortion. In: Porter IH, Hook EB (eds) Human embryonic and fetal death. Academic Press, New York, pp 107–127

Stephenson MD 1996 Frequency of factors associated with habitual abortion in 197 couples. Fertil Steril 66:24–29

Stephenson MD, Dreher K, Houlihan E et al 1998 Prevention of unexplained recurrent spontaneous abortion using intravenous immunoglobulin: a prospective, randomized, doubleblinded, placebo-controlled trial. Am J Reprod Immunol 39:82–88

Stern JJ, Dorfmann AD, Gutierrez-Najar AJ et al 1996 Frequency of abnormal karyotypes among abortuses from women with and without a history of recurrent spontaneous abortion. Fertil Steril 65:250–253

Stray-Pedersen B, Stray-Pedersen S 1984 Etiologic factors and subsequent reproductive performance in 195 couples with a prior history of habitual abortion. Am J Obstet Gynecol 148:140–146

Strobino BR, Fox HE, Kline Z et al 1986 Characteristics of women with recurrent spontaneous abortions and women with favourable reproductive histories. Am J Publ Health 76:986–991

Triplett DA 1992 Obstetrical implications of antiphospholipid antibodies. In: Stirrat GM, Scott JR (eds) The immune system in disease. Baillieres Clin Obstet Gynaecol 6(3): 507–518

Tulppala M, Stenman UH, Cacciatore B, Ylikorkala O 1993a Polycystic ovaries and levels of gonadotrophins and androgens in recurrent miscarriage: prospective study in 50 women. Br J Obstet Gynaecol 100:348–352

Tulppala M, Palosuo T, Ramsay T et al 1993b A prospective study of 63 couples with a history of recurrent spontaneous abortion: contributing factors and outcome of subsequent pregnancies. Hum Reprod 8:764–770

Tupper C, Weil RJ 1962 The problem of spontaneous abortion: The treatment of habitual abortion by psychotherapy. Am J Obstet Gynecol 83:421–424

Warburton D, Fraser FC 1964 Spontaneous abortion risks in man: data from reproductive histories collected in a medical genetics unit. Hum Genet 16:1–25

Wentz AC, Herbert CM, Maxson WS et al 1986 Cycle of conception endometrial biopsy. Fertil Steril 46:196–199

Wilcox AJ, Weinberg CR, O'Connor JF et al 1988 Incidence of early pregnancy loss. N Engl J Med 319:447–453

Winikoff D, Malinek M 1975 The predictive value of thyroid 'test profile' in habitual abortion. Br J Obstet Gynaecol 82:760–766

Wouters MG, Boers GH, Blom HJ et al 1993 Hyperhomocysteinaemia: a risk factor in women with unexplained recurrent early pregnancy loss. Fertil Steril 60:820–825

10

Fetal assessment in the third trimester: fetal growth and biophysical methods

Philip Owen

The contribution of the author of the equivalent chapter in the second edition, on which this chapter draws extensively, is gratefully acknowledged.

INTRODUCTION

Late pregnancy fetal assessment is aimed at identifying the fetus at increased risk of antepartum hypoxia and acidosis. Many of these pregnancies will be identified because of coexisting maternal illness such as preeclampsia or on the basis of clinical events such as antepartum haemorrhage. In Scotland in 1994–1998, stillbirths continued to occur at a rate of 6 per 1000 total births with no indication of a decline over the previous 20 years despite advances in our understanding of various aspects of fetal response to acute and chronic hypoxia (Fig. 10.1). Against this background it is important to recognise the need for more clinically useful measures of pregnancy risk stratification and to institute a schedule of fetal monitoring appropriate to the perceived degree of risk and gestational age. Screening for the growth-restricted fetus is generally poorly performed and inaccurate; properly performed it can become the cornerstone of late pregnancy fetal assessment. Once a clinically important deviation from normal fetal growth is identified, serial monitoring of the bio-physical response of the fetus to its intrauterine environment aims to guide the obstetrician towards the appropriate timing and mode of delivery.

BIRTHWEIGHT ACHIEVEMENT

The determinants of birthweight

The determinants of birthweight are multifactorial, reflecting the balance reached between the natural growth potential of the fetus and its environment, the latter being controlled by placental and maternal factors. A large number of well-recognised maternal, fetal, medical, environmental, infective and toxicological factors are associated with the birth of a small for gestational age (SGA) baby, many of which are inter-related. Studies of twins and siblings have identified the extent of these influences and describe the approximate proportionate influences on birthweight variation (e.g. maternal height and weight, proportion of body fat), maternal genotype (24%), fetal genotype (18%), maternal environmental

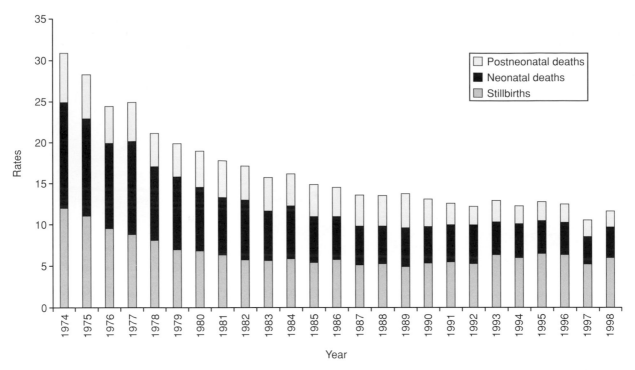

Fig. 10.1 Stillbirth, neonatal and postneonatal mortality rates for Scotland 1974–1998. The definition of stillbirth was changed from after 28 weeks to after 24 weeks in October 1992. (From Scottish Stillbirth and Infant Death Report 1998, ISD Publications, Edinburgh.)

influences (20%) and maternal disease (10%) (Beattie & Whittle 1993). It is notable that, contrary to much lay belief, paternal height has little relevance (<5%).

Birthweight, perinatal and long-term outcome

The term **small for gestational age (SGA)** fetus or baby is a descriptive one, identifying a predetermined proportion of pregnancies classified as such depending upon whether the 10th, 5th or 3rd percentile is taken as a cut-off point. This concept has been widely adopted in the obstetric and paediatric literature but is only an arbitrary distinction of normality and abnormality based upon birthweight and gestational age, where birthweight is the sole indicator of growth achievement and nutritional status. It is widely accepted that the SGA fetus or infant is at increased risk of serious morbidity and mortality but care must be taken in interpreting some of the older literature when corrections for gestational age have not been made.

Antenatal identification of the small baby remains a worthwhile task only if the small baby is at particular risk. In a large study of over 44 000 births, Patterson et al (1986) described an increasing incidence of poor perinatal outcome with falling birthweight centiles. Nevertheless, most cases of adverse outcome had birthweights above the 10th centile, such that birthweight centile can only be considered a weak predictor of adverse perinatal outcome in the individual case. A higher incidence of antenatal mortality amongst SGA fetuses not identified as such prior to delivery is described and reflects an improved outcome (attributed to closer fetal surveillance

and more frequent elective preterm delivery) amongst those identified (Wennergren et al 1988). Disappointingly, despite increasing the antenatal identification of the SGA fetus, randomised trials of screening with third-trimester ultrasound fetal biometry have failed to demonstrate any significant benefits in terms of perinatal outcome (Larsen et al 1992). This may result partly from the generally good outcome in SGA fetuses as a whole, which means that studies would need to be very large to be able to show any benefit of prebirth identification. Amongst SGA (birthweight <5th percentile) term newborn the incidence of early neonatal problems such as hypoglycaemia and need for admission to the special care nursery is less than 10%. (Jones & Roberton 1986).

Information relating birthweight for gestational age to neurodevelopmental outcome is available but needs to be interpreted with caution, as studies do not always adjust for confounding factors such as socioeconomic status. Small for gestational age infants perform less well on a wide range of psychometric tests, have an excess of abnormalities of behaviour and temperament, and show more abnormalities on neurological examination compared to non-SGA matched controls (Neligan et al 1976). Socioeconomic or family factors are recognised to exert an important influence on outcome but were not controlled for. When socioeconomic status is also matched, there were no differences in intellectual outcome between the cases and controls at 11 years of age (Hawdon et al 1990). In a further investigation of children identified as neurodevelopmentally delayed, there was a significantly lower adjusted birthweight compared to unaffected controls. However, only 20% of the disabled group had birthweights below the 10th centile and the association of maternal prenatal complications with disability was stronger than simply being SGA (Taylor & Howie 1989).

One of the difficulties in attempting to make comparisons between studies addressing neurodevelopmental outcome is establishing uniform criteria that determine neurodevelopmental normality and abnormality. One approach is to consider children with cerebral palsy (CP), a diagnosis which can be made with reasonable certainty on the basis that the disability is chronic, characterised by aberrant control of movement or posture, appears early in life and is not the result of progressive disease. Ellenberg & Nelson (1979) compared the gestational ages and birthweights of children with CP and children free of CP among a prospectively studied cohort of 54 000 singleton births. They described an increase in the risk of CP with shorter gestational age and lower birthweight. When birthweight was adjusted for gestational age, very few infants fell below the 10th centile for gestational age although, as a group, infants with CP also born prematurely had lower centile birthweight distributions than those born at term.

If one accepts that different types of growth restriction (reflected by different anthropometric features at birth) are a consequence of insults to the fetus at differing times in gestation (Villar & Belizan 1982, Fay & Ellwood 1993), then an insult in the first half of pregnancy seems more likely to result in a child with CP than a later insult. This may be because of the susceptibility of the developing brain in early pregnancy or because a combination or sequence of events is necessary which must begin in early pregnancy and be exacerbated by a persistently adverse intrauterine environment. However, from these considerations it would appear that being SGA, by itself, is a poor predictor of adverse short- or long-term outcome.

Alternative measures of fetal growth achievement

An alternative measure of fetal growth achievement is to employ anthropometric measurement of the newborn in an effort to identify infants experiencing intrauterine malnourishment (Miller & Jekel 1989). The Ponderal Index (PI) is a ratio of weight to body length and is one of several methods of evaluating neonatal nutritional status independent of birthweight (for example, subscapular skinfold thickness has also been used). These birthweight independent measures may help to identify babies that are growth restricted but not SGA.

A simpler measure, which does not require additional neonatal measurements to be made, is to compare the actual birthweight with that which would have been expected by analysing the physiological variables influencing birthweight. Wilcox et al (1993) were able to quantify the influences of a range of maternal and fetal variables upon term birthweight. This permits the calculation of the individualised birthweight ratio (IBR) which is a ratio of the actual birthweight achieved to the expected birthweight. Reclassification of growth-restricted pregnancies according to an IBR lower than the 10th centile identifies a higher proportion of infants with anthropometric features of intrauterine growth restriction (IUGR) than does birthweight less than the 10th centile. Furthermore, a number of SGA infants are reclassified as not being growth restricted on the basis that their IBR is above the 10th centile and there are no anthropometric features of IUGR. Although this approach is pragmatically useful, there are concerns that correcting for example for a body mass index of less than 19 may not be appropriate, and the issue of whether one should correct for presumably pathological variables such as smoking remains unresolved.

Nutritional status at birth and perinatal outcome

Infants with anthropometric features of intrauterine growth restriction (IUGR) such as low PI or low skinfold thickness are more likely to have experienced intrapartum fetal distress, neonatal morbidity and mortality (Patterson & Pouliot 1987). Amongst infants of low birthweight, those with a low PI have a higher mortality rate compared to those with a normal PI (Hoffman & Bakketeig 1984). Non-SGA infants with low PI delivering at term experience significantly higher rates of intrapartum fetal distress and caesarean section than SGA infants with normal PI whereas infants of low birthweight and low PI experience the highest rates of fetal distress (Fay et al 1991). When birthweight is adjusted to account for physiological variables amongst term deliveries (IBR), those infants with a low IBR but normal birthweight by traditional criteria have a higher incidence of abnormal fetal heart rate patterns in labour, increased incidence of operative delivery for fetal distress and higher rates of neonatal resuscitation, compared to infants with normal IBR values (Sanderson et al 1994).

The implication from these studies is that it is intrauterine malnourishment as reflected by abnormal neonatal morphometric features, rather than simply birthweight per se, that identifies the fetus at risk of intrauterine hypoxia. When considering intrauterine growth and its measurement it is important to recognise that unadjusted birthweight is not an appropriate sole arbiter of fetal growth achievement and that alternative and more relevant methods of quantifying and describing fetal growth achievement exist.

ESTIMATING FETAL SIZE AND GROWTH

Making and understanding the distinction between fetal size and growth is fundamental to the interpretation of different methods of quantification. Size signifies the magnitude of a fetus at a given point in gestation and allows the obstetrician to gain a very general impression of fetal growth up to that point in time. Fetal growth implies that an attempt has been made to quantify and describe the magnitude of an increment in fetal dimensions over a specified interval in gestation. The distinction is important since methods of quantifying size are inappropriate for describing growth, and vice versa.

Measurements of several fetal parameters have been described for the estimation of fetal weight; formulae incorporating measures of the fetal head and abdominal circumference are most predictive (Chien et al 2000). There will inevitably be an inherent error (usually $\pm 15\%$) in ultrasonic estimation of fetal weight which will vary according to the size of the fetus, gestational age and quality of measurements. These limitations need not deter the clinician from employing estimated fetal weight in clinical practice but it is essential that decision making takes account of the range of error that is inherent in this practice. Calculating ratios of the dimensions of fetal body parts such as the head to abdominal circumference ratio or fetal PI does not provide any additional clinically useful information.

Fetal size is usually categorised according to an intrauterine weight centile but alternatively, and preferably, it can be expressed as a standard deviation score (Z score). Either approach allows fetal measurements to be expressed in relation to a given set of standards and permits the comparison of measurements independently of gestational age (Kurmanavicius et al 1999a,b). Regardless of how fetal size is expressed, standards constructed from cross-sectional data are appropriate for estimating fetal size (Figs 10.2, 10.3). The methodology applied to the construction of size (cross-sectional) standards is important since failure to adhere to the recommended criteria can easily result in misleading standards. The criteria for designing a study aiming to establish size standards have been described and include the following key recommendations (Altman & Chitty (1994):

1. Cases should be representative of the obstetric population to which the standards will eventually be applied and should be selected solely for the purpose of constructing the reference data (including clinically indicated measurements is not appropriate).

2. Each case should be included once only in order to avoid over-representation of individual cases.

3. There should be an even spread of the number of cases across the gestational age window(s) of interest.

4. Exclusion criteria should be limited to fetuses with serious congenital anomalies. Removing cases because they are large or small at the time of measurement or following delivery will adversely affect the degree to which the standards truly reflect the population studied.

5. The sample size at each gestational age will influence the precision with which the centile estimates can be made and should be estimated in advance. The method of statistical analysis should be both appropriate to the data and appropriately described.

Few published reference ranges for ultrasound fetal biometry fulfil these criteria and, together with the poor performance of fetal size estimation in the prediction of important measures of perinatal outcomes, this limits the clinical value of estimating fetal size in the third trimester.

An advance upon the traditional practice of describing

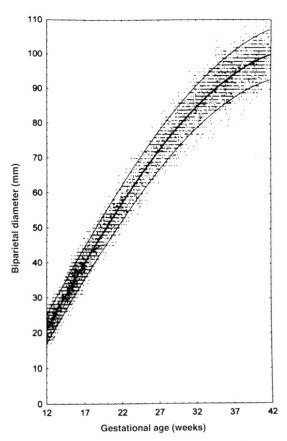

Fig. 10.2 Biparietal diameter versus gestational age (Kurmanavicius et al 1999a). The lines indicate the mean ± and standard deviations from the mean.

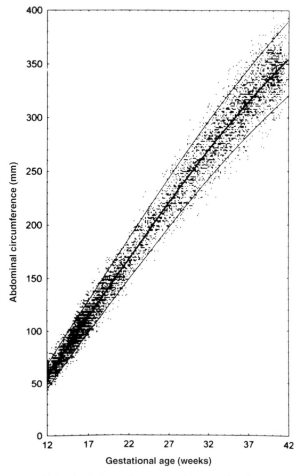

Fig. 10.3 Abdominal circumference versus gestational age (Kurmanavicius et al 1999b). The lines represent the mean ± standard deviations from the mean.

fetal size with reference to a population standard is the development of individualised growth curves (Gardosi et al 1992), a method whereby fetal size can be quantified with respect to the degree of under- or over-achievement of an appropriately estimated, physiologically *ideal* birthweight. The *term optimal weight (TOW)* is predicted from a computer program that makes adjustments for a number of physiological variables including fetal gender, parity, maternal weight, height, ethnic group and smoking. By applying a proportional weight equation across the range of gestation and anchoring it to the TOW at 280 days, a gestation-related optimal weight (GROW) curve can be derived (Fig. 10.4). The growth

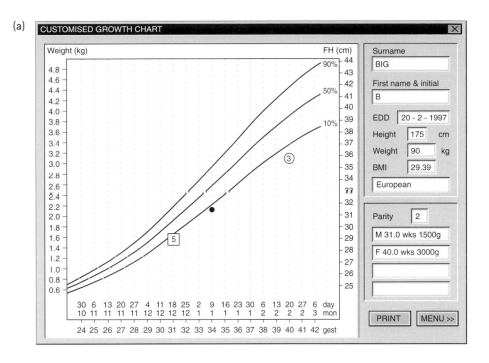

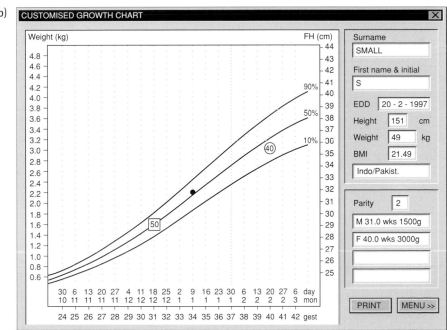

Fig. 10.4 Customised growth charts. (**a**) Mrs Big, showing the weight centiles of two previous babies (5th and 3rd) and a fetal weight estimation in the current pregnancy at 34 weeks (2.1 kg, 7th centile, black circle). (**b**) Mrs Small's chart with the same data plotted but showing different centiles (50th and 40th for previous pregnancies, 53rd centile for the current pregnancy, black circle) as the norm for fetal growth has been adjusted according to the different pregnancy characteristics. (From www.gest.net/charts.htm.)

achievement of the individual fetus at a particular gestation can subsequently be judged against a range of weight centiles generated specifically for that fetus, such that if it is believed to be small (<10th customised weight centile) it is more likely to demonstrate clinical features of true intrauterine growth restriction and adverse perinatal outcome than if it was judged against the routinely available unadjusted population birthweight standards (de Jong et al 1997).

The correlation between correctly determined symphysis–fundal height (SFH) measurements and fetal weight means that customised fetal weight standards can be applied to entire antenatal populations resulting in more appropriate use of antenatal monitoring resources (Gardosi & Francis 1999). These observational studies are interesting and represent an important advance in our understanding of the importance of birthweight achievement but there are as yet no published randomised trials upon which to recommend or discourage the introduction of these methods into clinical practice.

Normal fetal growth

Growth is a dynamic process describing changes in dimensions over time. Clinical methods such as palpation, maternal weight gain and the measurement of SFH are prone to considerable variability, measurement errors and weakness of association such that they cannot be considered sufficiently precise for the purpose of serial measurement. Ultrasound lends itself to serial measurements on the grounds that it is more reproducible, widely available and acceptable to the mother. Standards for fetal growth are most appropriately constructed from longitudinal data which permit a more valid examination of the growth patterns of individual fetuses as well as fetus-to-fetus variations. In order to diagnose a significant and possibly pathological deviation of growth, carefully derived and appropriately constructed reference ranges

for fetal growth applicable to a given population are necessary.

The construction of reference ranges suitable for describing fetal growth rather than size requires serial measurements obtained from longitudinal studies. A small number of studies have attempted to establish normal growth data using prospectively collected data from unselected pregnancies. The appropriate method for the construction of reference standards for longitudinal data and the subsequent categorisation of an individual fetus' growth as normal or abnormal is controversial and several published methods have been found to be flawed (Royston & Altman 1995).

A relatively simple approach is to estimate fetal growth velocity at different gestational ages based upon standards derived from the analysis of serially measured low-risk pregnancies. Fetal weight velocity increases from the late second trimester to a maximum mean velocity of 26.9 g/day over the 32–36 weeks' gestation interval with a subsequent progressive decline to 24.1 g/day over the 36–40 weeks' gestation interval (Fig. 10.5, Table 10.1) (Owen et al 1996). Once the gestational age means and standard deviations are established, it is then possible to quantify and describe fetal growth velocity as a standard deviation (Z) score, provided the gestational age at the last measurement and the time interval between the measurements are known. For example, if a fetus has an estimated weight of 1300 g at 28 weeks' gestation and an estimated weight of 1900 g 28 days later, then the mean growth velocity is 21.4 g/day. The mean and standard deviation at 32 weeks are 24.9 and 3.3 respectively, therefore the velocity Z score is

$$\frac{21.4 - 24.9}{3.3} = -1.1$$

A Z score of zero is the mean and scores of 1.3 and −1.3 approximate to the 90th and 10th percentiles respectively.

Expressed in this manner, fetal growth velocity has been

Table 10.1 Mean daily increment (with SD) of fetal measurements and estimated fetal weight (FWt); BPD, Biparietal diameter; FAA, fetal abdominal area; FL, femur length (from Owen et al 1996)

Weeks	BPD (mm/day)		FAA (cm²/day)		FL (mm/day)		FWt (g/day)	
	Mean	SD	Mean	SD	Mean	SD	Mean	SD
26	0.464	0.086	0.461	0.110	0.36	0.05	16.9	2.5
27	0.469	0.093	0.468	0.090	0.35	0.06	18.3	3.1
28	0.466	0.082	0.483	0.090	0.34	0.06	19.9	3.0
29	0.433	0.068	0.492	0.120	0.33	0.05	20.7	2.9
30	0.411	0.085	0.530	0.125	0.32	0.06	22.2	3.6
31	0.398	0.063	0.545	0.140	0.30	0.05	23.6	4.1
32	0.357	0.065	0.584	0.100	0.30	0.06	24.9	3.3
33	0.336	0.065	0.623	0.160	0.30	0.05	26.4	4.6
34	0.312	0.064	0.615	0.150	0.28	0.05	26.3	4.3
35	0.278	0.056	0.617	0.150	0.27	0.04	26.9	4.7
36	0.264	0.060	0.600	0.140	0.25	0.05	26.9	4.7
37	0.231	0.055	0.583	0.170	0.24	0.05	25.6	5.9
38	0.209	0.050	0.580	0.150	0.21	0.05	25.6	5.3
39	0.180	0.056	0.540	0.200	0.21	0.05	24.4	6.6
40	0.162	0.069	0.540	0.160	0.20	0.04	24.1	5.3

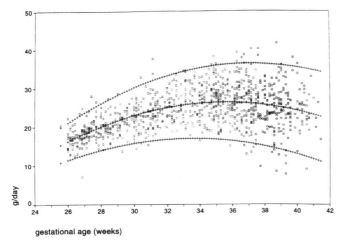

Fig. 10.5 Fetal growth velocity with mean ± 2SD superimposed (Owen et al 1996).

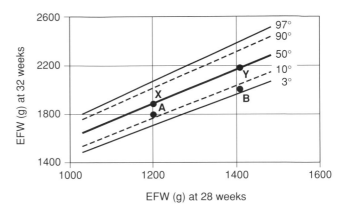

Fig. 10.6 An example of conditional centiles demonstrating the influence of size at 28 weeks' gestation upon the expected size at 32 weeks and the categorisation of the same growth increment for two fetuses (see text) (Owen & Ogston 1998).

applied to the prediction of intrapartum fetal distress and true intrauterine growth restriction with encouraging results (Owen et al 1997, Owen & Khan 1998). Although the calculation of growth velocity is relatively simple it is important to recognise some practical limitations of the technique. The variation in measurements (particularly if more than one sonographer is involved) and the influence of the between-measurement time interval (Mongelli et al 1998) will inevitably influence the precision and reproducibility of growth estimation.

In addition to these potential drawbacks, growth velocity does not take into account the fact that the change in fetal dimensions over a period of time is not independent of the size of the fetus at the earlier gestational age, for example the magnitude of the normal growth increment from 28 weeks to 34 weeks will be smaller for a fetus weighing 1200 g at 28 weeks than for another fetus weighing 1400 g at 28 weeks. By employing appropriate statistical techniques (Royston & Altman 1995), it is possible to construct reference ranges of conditional centiles which are designed to reflect and adjust for the influence of fetal size upon subsequent growth (Owen & Ogston 1998) (conditional centiles being so named because the centile position of the second measurement is *conditional* upon the initial fetal size). An example of conditional centiles is presented in Figure 10.6. Fetus A weighs 1200 g at 28 weeks at its 50th conditional weight centile four weeks later is 1900 g (point X) (Owen & Ogston 1998). Fetus B is heavier at 28 weeks at 1400 g and its 50th conditional weight centile four weeks later is 2150 g (Y). If both fetuses increase in weight by 600 g over the 28–32 week period, then they will both have achieved the same growth velocity but fetus A will be above the 10th conditional centile at 32 weeks (point A) whereas fetus B will be below its 10th conditional centile (point B). Describing the growth increment of an individual fetus in this manner is attractive because it individualises the quantification of the increment to take account of maternal and fetal physiological variables affecting fetal growth, albeit indirectly via fetal size itself.

At the present time, growth velocity and conditional cen-

tile ranking are interesting techniques for quantifying fetal growth; however, further studies demonstrating a useful clinical advantage of these techniques compared with single fetal size estimates and other biophysical methods are required before they can be justifiably adopted into clinical practice

KEY POINTS: FETAL GROWTH

- Small for gestational age (SGA) is a descriptive term and does not imply pathology.
- Intrauterine growth restriction (IUGR) implies a meaningful failure to fulfil growth potential.
- Growth-restricted infants may or may not be small for gestational age.
- Traditional size charts are not appropriate for interpreting serial fetal measurements.
- Alternative standards such as growth velocity, conditional centiles or individualised growth assessment are required to quantify fetal growth achievement.

FETAL MOVEMENT COUNTING

It is established clinical practice to enquire of mothers whether or not they are feeling regular and frequent fetal movements, since continuing fetal activity is a reassuring, albeit crude, indicator of fetal well-being. Conversely, amongst pregnancies resulting in antepartum stillbirth apparently due to impaired placental function, fetal death is preceded by a reduction in movements for several days and then a cessation of movements up to two days prior to demise (Sadovski & Yaffe 1973).

In an attempt to quantify maternally perceived fetal activity and relate it to perinatal performance, Pearson & Weaver (1976) developed the Cardiff Kick Chart whereby mothers recorded the time taken each day to feel 10 movements. Fetal activity declines towards term but the threshold of 10 movements consistently identifies less than 3% of pregnancies. Failure to perceive 10 movements during a 12-hour period

(9am to 9pm) should prompt attendance for further biophysical assessment. The results confirmed that antepartum fetal demise was preceded by the cessation of fetal activity, giving rise to the hope that this would become a cheap and widely applicable method for the prevention of antepartum stillbirth.

The value of routine formal fetal movement counting has been addressed in two randomised trials. The initial trial demonstrated a significant reduction in fetal loss in the counting group (Neldam 1983) but this was not found in the much larger multicentre trial (Grant et al 1989). Although it is not an effective method for screening fetal well-being in the general obstetric population, the value of fetal movement counting remains to be assessed in pregnancies previously identified as being at increased risk of late antepartum stillbirth.

CARDIOTOCOGRAPHY

Obstetricians have long looked for antenatal tests that would identify the fetus at risk of intrauterine hypoxia and death. Ideally such a test should not only be reliable, but performed easily and repeatedly. The result should be available immediately and the cost should be minimal. While many biochemical tests, such as estimations of oestriol and placental lactogens, have been carried out in the past, these are poor predictors of fetal outcome and are no longer widely used.

Currently, the most commonly used antenatal test of fetal well-being is cardiotocography. The sophisticated equipment needed for fetal heart rate recording and the significance of the various changes that occur in heart rate are the results of many years of observations and research.

The introduction of continuous fetal heart rate recording in the 1960s and 1970s changed the pattern of monitoring in labour. Subsequent developments included the first antenatal cardiotocograph equipment (using the phonocardiograph) and enabled descriptions of the fetal heart rate characteristics associated with fetal compromise in the antepartum period to be made (Hammacher 1966). Kubli et al (1969) noted the association of late decelerations, baseline tachycardia and loss of variability with fetal compromise. The contraction stress test (CST) began to be evaluated in the USA for monitoring the fetus antenatally while the non-stress test (cardiotocography; CTG) was being used in Europe.

Methodology

Antenatal cardiotocography employs external (indirect) methods of monitoring the fetal heart rate. The signals obtained are often small, sometimes discontinuous and constantly shifting, and therefore the qualities of tracing are often not as good as those obtained by direct methods, such as the fetal scalp electrode used during labour. Three techniques have been evaluated to obtain fetal heart recordings antenatally, namely phonocardiography, fetal electrocardiography and ultrasound Doppler cardiography.

Phonocardiography

In phonocardiography the signal is obtained by pressing a microphone on the maternal abdomen; the natural fetal heart sounds are amplified and converted into electrical signals. In theory this should allow the fetal heart signal to be identified clearly, however, in practice, sound generated by the placenta, umbilical vessels and maternal intra-abdominal vessels is also picked up by the abdominal microphone and may mask the fetal heart sounds. Although satisfactory recordings of the fetal heart rate may be obtained using this method, the recording is affected by many factors; it is found to be difficult to use in practice and has a high incidence of poor-quality tracings.

Fetal electrocardiography

By placing electrodes on the maternal abdominal wall it is possible to record the fetal ECG. However, the maternal ECG is also recorded; elimination of this maternal ECG complex requires electronic filtration of the signals and amplification of the fetal component before a clear fetal heart rate recording can be obtained. With an abdominal fetal ECG, the fetal R waves of the fetal ECG complex are used as trigger signals but the potential of this part of the ECG signal varies throughout pregnancy.

From the 18th week of gestation until the 27th, the R-wave potential is high. Following this, there is a decline to a minimum potential at 30 weeks' gestation. Between 27 and 34 weeks' gestation it is not possible to obtain continuous fetal heart rate tracings in 70% of cases (Steer 1986). Thereafter the fetal R-wave potential increases until delivery. This variation is thought to be due to the effect of vernix caseosa altering the electrical resistance of the fetal skin. Several studies have reported the successful use of abdominal ECG to record the fetal heart, particularly when used in the last four weeks of pregnancy.

Ultrasound fetal cardiotocography

Ultrasound fetal cardiotocography is the most commonly used method for recording the fetal heart rate antenatally. It utilises the physical principle of the Doppler effect in which sound waves hitting a moving object are reflected back at an altered frequency. Using this principle, the movements of the ventricular wall cause a definite ultrasound frequency shift; these physical movements can be used to generate well-defined trigger pulses.

Initially, the ultrasound transducers used consisted of a single transmitter and a single piezoelectric crystal receiver. This combination of narrow beam transducers had the disadvantage that the ultrasound beam required precise positioning to produce a good signal. Broad-beam array transducers, consisting of several pairs of transmitters and receiver crystals that detect the movement of a large area of the fetal heart wall and produced smaller, slower frequency shifts compared with those produced by the fetal heart valves themselves are a reliable method of recording the fetal heart provided autocorrelation detection and averaging are used. However, because of this averaging, ultrasound fetal cardiotocography with a broad-beam transducer cannot be used to make a true assessment of beat-to-beat variability of the fetal heart. Short-term variability (variation over 10–15 beats) can be assessed adequately. Therefore, assessment of baseline variability is possible in clinical practice providing the recordings are of good quality. Its ease of use and relatively non-invasive nature have resulted in this method becoming the most useful in clinical practice, with good recordings being obtained relatively easily, independent of gestational age. Although it is widely regarded as non-invasive, it should be remembered that the fetus is being exposed to up to 10 mW/cm^2 of sound energy. At present, it is not known whether such irradiation is harmful.

Physiology of fetal heart rate recordings

The parasympathetic and sympathetic components of the autonomic nervous system control fetal cardiac behaviour. The regulation of fetal heart rate is also influenced by vasomotor centres, chemoreceptors baroreceptors and cardiac autoregulation. Pathological events such as fetal hypoxia modify these influences and fetal cardiac responses.

Baseline fetal heart rate
Fetal heart rate falls with increasing gestational age and also becomes more variable. The decrease in fetal heart rate is due to the development of vagal tone, the mean baseline fetal heart rate being a reflection of the balance of sympathetic and parasympathetic autonomic influences. The mean normal baseline fetal heart rate in late pregnancy is about 135 beats per minute (bpm), with a normal range between 110 and 150 bpm. It should be noted that the normal range of baseline rate described by FIGO (Federation Internationale Gynecologie et Obstetrique) is 110–150, 10 bpm lower than the traditional UK range of 120–160 bpm. The correct normal range is probably a mixture of the two. Fetal hiccuping is a common occurrence in late pregnancy and is often described by the mother as a repetitive, jerky movement. Hiccuping is associated with a temporary rise in the baseline fetal heart rate of up to 5 bpm (Woerden et al 1989). Persistent or prolonged episodes of fetal movement may result in a pseudo-tachycardia ('the jogging fetus') and can be differentiated from a pathological tachycardia by the maternal recording of numerous fetal movements and the return to a normal baseline rate when the fetus is at rest.

A baseline tachycardia of over 150 bpm is associated with maternal fever or chorio-amnionitis; in the latter there may also be loss of variability. In the presence of chronic fetal hypoxia the fetal heart rate is within the normal range (Kubli & Ruttgers 1972), in contrast to the situation in acute or subacute fetal hypoxia where there is a baseline tachycardia which may result from an increase in the levels of circulating fetal catecholamines. The maternal administration of beta-mimetic drugs such as ritodrine leads to a mild fetal tachycardia.

Fetal tachyarrhythmias are uncommon but are a potentially reversible cause of hydrops fetalis. Supraventricular tachycardia is commoner than atrial fibrillation although both may be intermittent, making prolonged examination necessary if a rhythm disturbance is suspected (Owen & Cameron 1997). Fetal heart rates between 100 and 120 bpm are regarded as fetal bradycardia. If the variability is normal, it is usually a reflection of increased vagal tone. If observed spasmodically it may suggest cord compression. Persistent

marked bradycardia (<60 bpm) may be associated with congenital heart defects or reflect complete heart block secondary to transplacentally acquired autoantibodies. Baseline bradycardia is rarely associated with antepartum hypoxia (Young et al 1979) unless placental abruption is present.

Fetal heart rate variability
Under normal physiological conditions the interval between successive heart beats (beat-to-beat variation) is different. This has been referred to as short-term variability; it increases with advancing gestational age. In current practice, because of the widespread use of ultrasound, beat-to-beat averaging is widely used, and in this context short-term variation is taken as the variation between epochs of 3–5 seconds, rather than being true beat-to-beat variation (Wheeler et al 1979). The value of normal short-term variation depends on the epoch length chosen for measurement. Visual inspection of the cardiotocograph shows oscillations occurring approximately 2–6 times per minute. Their amplitude is usually 5–15 bpm, and they are best referred to as 'baseline variation'.

In addition to gestational age, heart rate variability is influenced by fetal sleep states, accelerations and decelerations. Under normal physiological conditions the fetal heart rate variability is the product of opposing sympathetic and parasympathetic influence on the heart. The fetus is known to undergo quiet–active cycles of 60–70 minutes, the quiet phase (sleep state 1F; quiet sleep state) typically lasting from 20 to 30 minutes and characterised by the absence of fetal movements and low fetal heart rate variability. It is important not to misinterpret this appearance as pathological; once the active fetal sleep state returns, accelerations and increased fetal heart rate variability become evident. The development of differentiated quiet–active sleep cycles reflects maturing fetal brain activity and usually occurs between 28 and 32 weeks' gestation (Wheeler et al 1979). Thus the CTG often appears relatively featureless before 28 weeks. Active sleep is associated with fetal limb and rapid eyeball movements, similar to adult dreaming sleep. The low PO_2 in the fetus means that the fetal brain remains relatively quiescent (uses less oxygen); animal studies and intrapartum human studies show that the fetus is hardly ever awake in the adult sense.

Several investigators have shown a relationship between reduced variability and chronic fetal hypoxia; both mild and severe fetal hypoxia acidosis may result in loss of variability (Flynn et al 1979). However, it should be noted that fetal hypoxia without significant acidosis actually causes an increase in fetal heart rate variability, and this is sometimes a source of confusion for the inexperienced. Drugs that cause depression of the central nervous system, such as benzodiazepines and opiates, are also associated with reduced fetal heart rate variability.

Sinusoidal fetal heart rate pattern
The sinusoidal pattern is typically associated with an anaemic fetus as a result of rhesus sensitisation or fetal exsanguination and is accordingly very rare. Sinusoidal fetal heart rate pattern resembles a sine wave of fixed periodicity of

2–5 cycles/min, usually with profound loss of short-term variability (Young et al 1980). Original publications describing this unusual pattern invariably reported a very high rate of perinatal loss (Rochard et al 1976). In a prospective study, Murphy et al (1991) distinguished pseudo-sinusoidal patterns from sinusoidal ones on the basis of episodes of baseline oscillations of constant amplitude alternating with episodes of normal baseline reactivity. Such episodes are often associated with fetal sucking identified by ultrasound; in contrast to the true sinusoidal pattern they are not symmetrical and are not accompanied by a loss of baseline variability. Also, true sinusoidal patterns usually have an amplitude greater than 25 bpm.

Fetal heart rate accelerations

Accelerations are increases in rate of more than 15 bpm for more than 15 seconds and are usually associated with fetal movement but sometimes with external stimuli or uterine contractions. They are rarely present in the hypoxic fetus (Wood et al 1979). The presence of accelerations suggests intact fetal sympathetic activity and is therefore a major component in the evaluation of antenatal cardiotocography or non-stress tests. The magnitude of the acceleration is directly related to the nature of the associated fetal movement (Table 10.2). Both accelerations and fetal movement are associated with the active sleep state. Accelerations are not directly caused by fetal movements, for example they still occur in fetuses paralysed pharmacologically to enable cordocentesis.

Table 10.2 Influence of fetal movements upon baseline fetal heart rate (from van Woerden and van Geijn. In: Nijhuis JG (ed) Fetal behaviour. Oxford Medical 1992)

Fetal movement	Increase in FHR (beats/min; mean ± SD)
Regular mouthing	9 ± 2
Head movements	15 ± 4
Arm movements	16 ± 3
Trunk movements	18 ± 6
Sucking	16 ± 4
Compilations of movements	22 ± 8

Fetal heart rate decelerations

Decelerations of a transient nature are a frequent occurrence. The non-recurring early or mildly variable type, often in association with uterine activity or following fetal movement, are usually associated with normal fetal outcome (Kidd et al 1985a). Late and recurrent decelerations are of hypoxic origin and should be more than 15 bpm and lasting 10 seconds or more (Kidd et al 1985a). Decelerations in the presence of loss of baseline variability are more likely to be associated with fetal hypoxia. Occasional late decelerations without any other abnormal fetal heart rate characteristics, such as loss of variability, are not an indication for intervention (Kidd et al 1985b). Marked decelerations may also result from the maternal supine hypotensive syndrome due to underperfusion of the uteroplacental circulation and can be quickly corrected by adjusting maternal position. Many researchers have reported the association of repeated late decelerations

and fetal death, particularly in high-risk cases; late decelerations, particularly in association with loss of heart rate variability, are a sign of a poor prognosis (Visser et al 1980).

Based on the physiology and pathophysiology of fetal heart rate recording, the following criteria could be used in the diagnosis of fetal hypoxia in the antepartum period. A normal trace is one with a baseline of 120–150 bpm with a variability of 5–25 bpm, with at least two accelerations of an amplitude of more than 15 bpm over a 15–20-minute interval. There should be no decelerations, except for an occasional sporadic mild variety. An abnormal fetal heart rate pattern is any pattern that does not conform to this definition. In general terms, abnormalities in relation to baseline rate, variability, accelerations and decelerations have different implications, but the more of these four that are abnormal, the worse the prognosis.

Performing non-stress cardiotocography and its interpretation

The woman should be comfortable either in a left lateral position or semi-recumbent to avoid supine hypotension. The maternal blood pressure and pulse rate should be recorded prior to performing the test. An external ultrasound transducer for the recording of fetal heart rate and tocodynamometer for recording of uterine activity are attached to the maternal abdomen. The ultrasound transducer is placed to obtain the best fetal heart signal. The tocodynamometer is usually placed towards the fundus of the uterus.

The recording is carried out over a period of 20–60 minutes depending on the pattern observed. External stimulus by palpation or gentle movement of the fetus can be performed if the non-stress test remains non-reactive (absence of fetal heart rate accelerations) after 20 minutes although usually this is insufficient to change the fetal sleep state. Vibroacoustic stimulators ('buzzers') are sometimes used to provoke accelerations. However, they increase fetal oxygen consumption and may be dangerous if the fetus is in a seriously hypoxic environment.

For clinical purposes the antenatal fetal heart rate patterns can be divided into:

1. normal
2. showing transient abnormality
3. suspicious
4. abnormal, requiring intervention.

The tracing is regarded as normal when the baseline is within normal range, has normal variability and when accelerations and fetal activity are present and there are no significant decelerations with contractions (Fig. 10.7). Shallow spiked occasional decelerations are not an ominous sign, and are especially common in the preterm fetus. A transient reduction in variability and lack of accelerations may be related to a quiet fetal sleep state, or medications given via the mother (Fig. 10.8). A fall in maternal blood pressure may also be the cause. Tests of fetal stimulation can be considered in these situations.

Suspicious tests are associated with reduced fetal activity and reactivity (accelerations with fetal movement). There

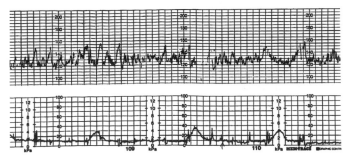

Fig. 10.7 Normal non-stress test showing fetal movement and uterine activity, normal fetal heart rate with normal long-term variability and accelerations.

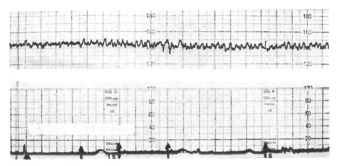

Fig. 10.8 Antenatal non-stressed fetal heart rate recording showing reduced long-term variability with no accelerations. Arrows are event markers during fetal movements. Tracing is an effect of sedative drugs.

may be reduced variability and accelerations may be absent. Sporadically occurring non-repeating late decelerations may occur despite the presence of fetal activity and reactivity (Fig. 10.9). Mild repeated decelerations in the presence of accelerations are suspicious and require the test to be repeated. Fetal heart rate tracings showing a marked reduction in variability and an absence of accelerations with isolated or recurrent decelerations should be regarded as abnormal (Figs 10.10, 10.11).

The need for a uniform method of interpretation of ante-

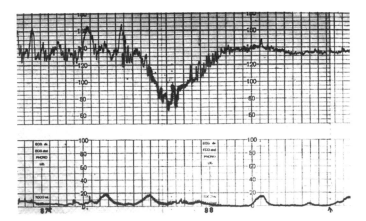

Fig. 10.9 Isolated marked late deceleration of fetal heart rate which had previously followed a normal reactive pattern. Tracing is of suspicious but doubtful significance and should be repeated.

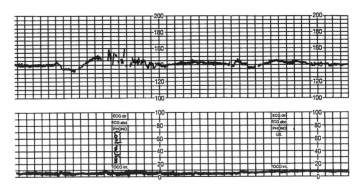

Fig. 10.10 Fetal heart rate with low-amplitude decelerations, complete loss of variability and no fetal reactivity. No fetal movements are marked. Tracing suggestive of severely abnormal state.

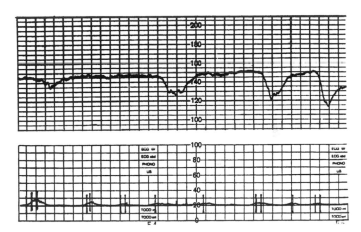

Fig. 10.11 Antenatal heart rate tracing showing loss of variability with recurrent decelerations following fetal movements. Tracing suggests fetal hypoxic state.

natal cardiotocography is obvious since it will make the test more comparable and the task of teaching staff in training easier. Guidelines for the standardisation of methodology, application, terminology and interpretation are available (Rooth et al 1987). Alternatively, a number of scoring systems have been proposed, each including different criteria and with varying degrees of sophistication, in an effort to establish uniformity of interpretation.

A relatively simple method is described by Pearson & Weaver (1978) and is based on a 6-point score which includes the three variables of baseline fetal heart rate (FHR), FHR in response to fetal movements and FHR in response to Braxton Hicks contractions; baseline variability is not a component of the scoring system (Table 10.3). There is a significant relationship between the six point score on the day before delivery and both condition at birth and birthweight centile. Furthermore, objective analysis demonstrates a progressive change in each of the three scoring components as fetal condition deteriorates; there is an initial loss of response to contractions followed by the absence of FHR accelerations, the cessation of movements and finally changes in the baseline FHR itself.

Table 10.3 The scoring system for antenatal cardiotocography (Pearson & Weaver 1978)

	Score		
	0	1	2
Baseline FHR (beats/minute)	Less than 100 *or* more than 150	100–120 or 160–180	120–160
Movements	None	Present	Present
FHR change	–	No change	Acceleration
Contractions ± FHR change	Deceleration	No change	Acceleration

The assessment of cardiotocographs using scoring systems improves the inter- and intra-observer reliability compared to subjective assessment (Trimbos & Keirse 1978). However, comparing a number of scoring systems against a subjective assessment of the cardiotocographs as either reactive or non-reactive demonstrates subjective categorisation to be superior to formal scoring when attempting to predict a range of measures of poor outcome (Flynn et al 1982).

Simplified scoring systems are a useful method for instructing less experienced staff in the recognition and relative importance of various features of the antenatal cardiotocograph, but once experienced at interpretation the trained eye will be able to differentiate abnormal patterns occurring as a consequence of physiological variation from those demonstrating features consistent with persistent hypoxia.

Computer analysis of fetal heart rate recordings

Computer analysis provides an objective and reproducible numerical evaluation of the fetal heart rate recording in an effort to overcome some of the limitations of subjective interpretation. Attempts at computerised analysis were initially hampered by high signal loss resulting in failure times averaging 40% (Dawes et al 1981). However, by employing the technique of autocorrelation with interactive advice to the operator, signal loss is dramatically reduced with resulting improvement in record keeping and saving of time. There is a close correlation between computer assessment and visual assessment of cardiotocographs; there may be episodes of computer misclassification of tracings as false-positive, but reassuringly no false-negatives (Cheng et al 1992). When compared to visual interpretation, computerised analysis by the Oxford Sonicaid System 8000 resulted in a shorter testing time and a reduction in the use of second-line testing with the biophysical profile (Bracero et al 1999).

The advantages of a computerised analysis lie in its objectivity and greater reproducibility which lends itself to the analysis of serial changes in baseline FHR, short-term variability and quantification of number of accelerations and decelerations. The final interpretation of these changes and the decision when and how to deliver the fetus remains a clinical decision made by the obstetrician.

Antenatal stress tests incorporating the cardiotocograph

Oxytocin challenge tests. The contraction stress test (CST) or oxytocin challenge test is performed in the same manner as the non-stress test with the addition of an infusion of oxytocin if spontaneous uterine activity is not recorded after 20 minutes of testing. The infusion aims to provoke three uterine contractions within 10 minutes. A considerable literature has accumulated concerning the CST in the management of high-risk pregnancies, demonstrating an incidence of false-positive tests of between 5% and 10% with a similar range of hyperstimulation. The correlation of a positive test with subsequent intrapartum events is poor and the test is invasive and time consuming. It has been recommended as a second-line test following equivocal non-stress cardiotocography (Keegan & Paul 1980) but has largely been replaced by alternative methods of biophysical assessment.

Nipple stimulation during human lactation institutes a neurohypophyseal reflex resulting in the release of oxytocin. Stimulation of the nipples in late pregnancy produces a uterine contraction and this forms the basis of the nipple CST which is potentially cheaper, less invasive and less time-consuming than the oxytocin CST. The technique has been evaluated and found to have a hyperstimulation rate around 4%, a failure rate of 4–15% and poor correlation with intrapartum events and neonatal outcome (Huddleston et al 1984). This method of stress testing has not gained widespread popularity.

Vibroacoustic stimulation involves the application of an artificial larynx over the uterus; an auditory stimulus is created in order to provoke fetal heart rate accelerations when the tracing is initially non-reactive (Reid & Miller 1977). The test is considered negative if a fetal heart rate acceleration of 15 bpm or more is evoked. The test cannot be reliably applied to the very immature fetus since there is no consistent response before 30–31 weeks' gestation. A positive vibroacoustic test has been found to be highly sensitive in predicting a subsequent abnormal oxytocin CST and possessing similar positive predictive value for the development of intrapartum fetal distress as the oxytocin CST (Schiff et al 1992). The fetal recoil test relies upon generating a fetal startle response following sound stimulation. A test is considered negative and reassuring when a palpable fetal response occurs. In a series of 100 consecutive NST, a reassuring recoil test had a 98% positive predictive value for a subsequent reactive NST (Strong et al 1992).

Other developments include the introduction of a digital system for distant heart rate recording and subsequent rapid transmission by telephone to the hospital which overcomes any difficulties experienced by the patient in having to attend the clinic (Gough et al 1986). The complete recording of fetal heart rate carried out by the mother at home is transmitted to hospital in less than 30 seconds and stored on computer for later analysis. The introduction of such a system can result in a reduction in hospital admissions and improved patient satisfaction (Moore & Sill 1990).

Clinical application of antenatal cardiotocography

In an attempt to prevent antepartum stillbirths and positively identify those fetuses with insufficient reserve to withstand the hypoxic stress of labour, obstetricians have looked for a reliable test to identify those pregnancies at risk. Antepartum fetal heart rate monitoring has become widely accepted over the last few years, but the stillbirth rate remains high. In an unselected population the risk of antenatal fetal death is one in 1000 within one week of a normal cardiotocograph (Schifrin et al 1979).

The incidence of normal and pathological cardiotocographs varies according to the nature of the population being considered. Amongst high-risk pregnancies non-reactive cardiotocographs are usually regarded as being significantly associated with adverse intrapartum factors and neonatal outcome (Lenstrup & Hasse 1985). However, several randomised trials of antenatal cardiotocography have not confirmed this association (Brown et al 1982, Lumley et al 1983, Kidd et al 1985b) although not all these trials were reporting on frequent and repeated fetal heart testing. Their results were mainly related to one or two isolated cardiotocographs prior to delivery or death of the fetus.

The concept of fetal assessment with antenatal fetal heart testing demands frequent testing, particularly in the compromised fetus, since the fetal heart rate changes occur in a progressive fashion with an increasing duration of low fetal activity periods. However, in situations of acute hypoxia, fetal death may occur shortly after a normal reactive tracing is obtained. In terms of predicting adverse intrapartum neonatal events the false-negative rate varies from 2% to 20%. A normal tracing is therefore not reassuring in all cases but a pathological tracing relates closely to poor fetal outcome. When an abnormal tracing is obtained in the very premature fetus, the consequences of intervening may be disastrous if the fetus is not acidotic (false-positive CTG) and additional methods of assessment should be employed such as umbilical artery Doppler velocimetry or a biophysical profile.

As the natural course of chronic fetal hypoxia is slow, antenatal fetal heart rate monitoring is likely to be less informative than ultrasound growth velocity or umbilical artery velocimetry. However, in high-risk cases with suspected growth restriction or maternal disease such as hypertension, daily or even twice daily testing is probably appropriate. The multinational Growth Restriction Intervention Trial (GRIT) project is currently assessing whether ultrasound growth velocity, umbilical artery blood velocity assessment, or CTG pattern is the best indicator of the need for delivery. The mode of delivery will be influenced by the severity of the abnormality of the fetal heart pattern together with other clinical features such as gestational age, previous obstetric history and presentation.

KEY POINTS: CARDIOTOCOGRAPHY (CTG)

- The CTG remains the cornerstone of antenatal fetal assessment.
- Interpretation of the CTG must take account of risk factors for fetal hypoxia, gestational age and fetal physiology.
- Formal scoring of the CTG improves reliability of interpretation but does not improve its clinical usefulness over subjective assessment.
- Frequency of testing is dictated by the nature of the clinical indication for fetal assessment.

DOPPLER ULTRASOUND

Introduction

Investigation of the fetal cardiovascular and haemodynamic system has become a clinical reality with the advent of advanced ultrasound technology enabling evaluation of patterns of blood flow velocity within the uterine, placental and fetal arterial and venous circulations. Since the first report of the application of the Doppler principle to the human fetal circulation (Fitzgerald & Drumm 1977), a large experience with this technique has been reported with respect to the prediction of the fetus at risk of developing growth restriction, antepartum and intrapartum asphyxia, perinatal mortality and neonatal morbidity. Many of the earlier studies employed relatively simple equipment in order to obtain and process signals from the umbilical circulation, whereas study of most of the fetal vessels requires sophisticated equipment and a degree of operator skill and expertise.

Principles

Sound waves returning from a moving object (e.g. a column of erythrocytes) have an altered frequency with respect to the incident beam and this difference or frequency shift is dependent upon the direction and velocity of the moving object. This phenomenon was first described by Johann Christian Doppler (1803–1853), an Austrian physicist after whom the Doppler effect is named. The shifted frequencies obtained are not only directly proportional to the velocity of the moving blood cells but also proportional to the cosine of the angle of insonation (the angle between the ultrasound beam and the column of blood).

In order to calculate the amount of blood flowing in a vessel, accurate estimation of the angle of insonation and the diameter of the vessel must be possible. Significant errors in estimating these parameters together with errors in estimating fetal weight mean that the measurement of actual blood flow is unlikely to be useful in clinical practice at least with current methodological limitations. Alternatively, semiquantitative assessment of the flow velocity waveform (FVW) can be made and this has been widely adopted. The waveform obtained is the result of several different factors including fetal cardiac contraction force, density of blood, vessel wall elasticity and peripheral or downstream resistance. The fetal and umbilical circulations are typified by low-resistance flow patterns demonstrating continuous forward flow where the velocity in diastole is inversely related to peripheral resistance (Fig. 10.12).

Although both systolic and diastolic frequencies are dependent upon the angle of insonation, ratios comparing the pulsatile or systolic element of the waveform to the continuous or diastolic element are independent of the angle, making this a useful index of changes in peripheral resistance. Alternatives to the S/D or A/B ratios include the pulsatility index and the resistance index (or Pourcelot index) (Fig. 10.13). As the end-diastolic velocities decrease, all the indices rise and the changes in the values obtained correlate closely between the different indices (Thompson et al 1986). Theoretically, the pulsatility index is preferred since it can still quantify the FVW in the absence of diastolic flow, although in practice A/B ratios are commonly used whilst waveforms with absent or reverse end-diastolic flow (AREDF) are classified separately.

A variety of Doppler ultrasound methods exist, with three types being employed in clinical practice: continuous wave (CW), pulsed wave (PW) and colour flow mapping (CFM). Continuous wave Doppler emits and receives an ultrasound beam continuously, has a low acoustic energy output and is

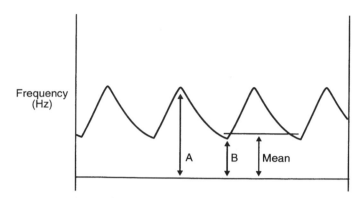

Fig. 10.13 Characteristics of the umbilical artery flow velocity waveform. A, Peak systolic frequency, B, end-diastolic frequency. Pulsatility index = (A–B)/Mean; Resistance Index = (A–B)/A. (From Mires et al 1990.)

relatively inexpensive. Obtaining a FVW with CW Doppler is a blind technique, however, and it cannot discriminate between signals from different locations which may result in mixed waveforms. Despite this, CW equipment has been

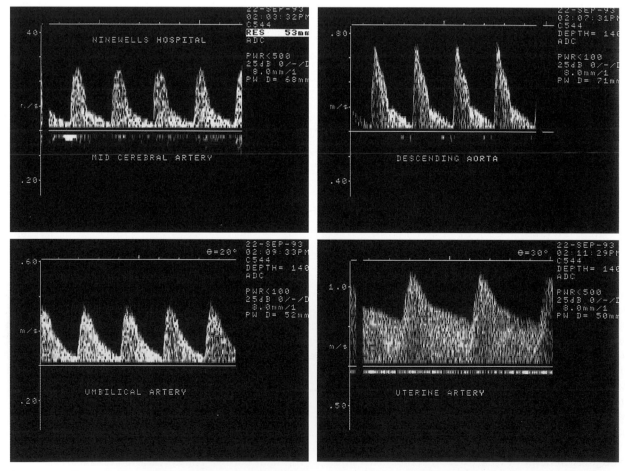

Fig. 10.12 Flow velocity waveforms obtained from the umbilical, fetal aortic and middle cerebral arteries and maternal uterine artery at 19 weeks' gestation. (Courtesy of Dr A.D. Christie, Dundee.)

widely employed in the study of the umbilical circulation where it produces results similar to those obtained by PW equipment.

Pulsed wave Doppler differs in that pulses of ultrasound energy are emitted. By varying the time interval of the pulses it becomes possible to determine the distance of the signal origin from the transducer by range-gating. Combining PW Doppler with real-time ultrasound provides a duplex system, with the obvious advantage that the vessel to be examined is positively identified before it is sampled.

Colour flow mapping is a further refinement of the duplex system whereby two-dimensional velocity flow images are superimposed on the real-time image. Special signal processing techniques permit colour coding of the direction of the flow with different degrees of shading according to the magnitude of the Doppler shift. Although the equipment necessary for CFM is relatively expensive, it permits more precision in vessel location and identification including the fetal arterial and venous circulations.

Umbilical artery flow velocity waveforms

The umbilical arteries were the first fetal vessels to be studied with Doppler ultrasound, the signals being readily obtained with CW Doppler. Subsequently, FVW from these vessels have been widely investigated in the hope that they would provide an appropriate test of fetal well-being in the complicated pregnancy and also as a screening test for the development of problems in the low-risk population. The ease with which signals can be obtained is reflected by good reproducibility in the measurement of the waveforms (Schulman et al 1989). FVW should be obtained with the mother lying at rest in a semi-recumbent position during periods of fetal apnoea and quiescence since the impedance indices are modified by fetal breathing and elevated fetal heart rates (Mires et al 1987).

Relationship of the flow velocity waveform to placental pathology

The umbilical artery FVW is characterised by continuous forward flow typical of a low-resistance circuit; as gestation increases there is a gradual fall in the resistance indices due to enlargement of the placenta with a corresponding expansion of its vascular tree (Fig. 10.14). A reduction in end-diastolic velocity suggests increased resistance to blood flow originating in the placenta and this pattern is seen in pregnancies complicated by growth restriction and fetal compromise (Trudinger et al 1985).

Vascular abnormalities are known to be present in the placenta of the growth-restricted fetus, and histological examination of placentas from pregnancies with abnormal FVW has revealed obliteration of tertiary stem villus arteries and deficient functional differentiation (Giles et al 1985). It is possible to demonstrate a correlation between the percentage of obliterated placental vessels and the resistance to umbilical artery flow, providing an anatomical basis for the observed FVW changes seen in many complicated pregnancies (Fok et al 1990). An alternative explanation, supported by scanning electronic microscope studies of the placentas of fetuses

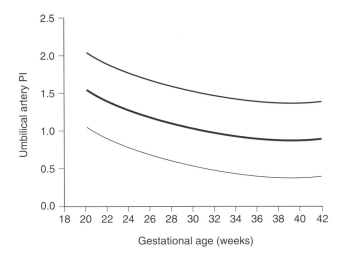

Fig. 10.14 Umbilical artery pulsatility index versus gestational age (5th, 50th and 95th centiles) (Arduini & Rizzo 1990).

demonstrating severe umbilical artery FVW abnormalities, is of abnormal trophoblast proliferation and abnormal development of the terminal villi (Krebs et al 1996).

Placental pathologies such as these would be expected to give rise to an abnormal fetal acid–base status through hypoxia. A relationship between very high impedance ratios and umbilical venous hypoxia and acidosis has been demonstrated by obtaining fetal blood at cordocentesis and at prelabour caesarean section (Tyrrell et al 1989, Weiner 1990).

Clinical application of umbilical artery Doppler
Prediction of the pregnancy compromised by hypoxia and acidosis. Examination of the umbilical artery FVW has been evaluated in the prediction of the small for gestational age fetus; although there is an association between abnormal impedance indices and birthweight, the true association probably lies between impedance and compromise due to asphyxia, with birthweight being an intervening variable (Haddad et al 1988). Fetal biometry with standard real-time ultrasound is superior to Doppler in the identification of the small fetus (Chambers et al 1989).

It is well recognised that pregnancies with abnormal FVW are at increased risk of several aspects of perinatal morbidity, including increased rates of preterm delivery, abnormal FHR in labour, operative delivery and admission to and duration of stay in neonatal units. In a blind prospective study of apparently growth-restricted fetuses an abnormal FVW reliably identified the distressed fetus, with the appearance of abnormal FVW preceding FHR abnormalities by at least nine days (Reuwer et al 1987). A similar relationship between abnormal FVW and antepartum late FHR decelerations is described: FVW abnormalities appeared before the decelerations in 27 of 29 growth-restricted fetuses with a median duration of the interval being 17 days but with a wide range of 0–60 days (Bekedam et al 1990).

Umbilical artery FVW analysis appears to be a more sensitive predictor of fetal compromise than antepartum cardiotocography when compromise is taken to be a 5-minute Apgar score of less than 5 or birthweight less than the 10th centile for gestation (Trudinger et al 1986). When compared with the antepartum CTG in the surveillance of suspected SGA pregnancies, FVW analysis results in fewer hospital admissions, inductions of labour and emergency caesarean sections for fetal distress, although there are no significant differences in gestational age at delivery or Apgar scores (Almstrom et al 1992). Similar reductions in the rates of fetal distress in labour and emergency caesarean section were found in a randomised controlled trial of FVW analysis, with the conclusion that the availability of Doppler results in more appropriate obstetrical decision making (Trudinger et al 1987). The routine, rather than selective, use of Doppler in high-risk pregnancies does not result in an iatrogenic increase in preterm delivery and does in fact reduce the frequency of depressed Apgar scores at birth and of serious neonatal morbidity (Tyrrell et al 1990).

Whereas an abnormal FVW appears to identify the SGA fetus at risk of perinatal hypoxia, for Doppler to be an appropriate test of fetal well-being, the finding of a normal FVW should be reassuring by identifying the constitutionally small fetus that is not affected by placental pathology. Burke et al (1990) examined 179 ultrasonically diagnosed SGA pregnancies and found that of the 119 physically normal fetuses with normal flow, there was only one unfavourable outcome. Certainly, the presence of a normal Doppler study places the SGA fetus in a much lower risk category than those with an abnormal FVW. A normal Doppler result can be taken to be a reassuring sign when monitoring the SGA fetus but it must be considered along with the other individual features of the pregnancy in order to optimise the outcome since a normal Doppler result does not exclude subsequent intrapartum fetal distress in all cases.

Extreme abnormalities of the flow velocity waveform. Extreme elevation of resistance to flow results in a FVW with no end-diastolic component or even reversal of flow in the umbilical artery (Fig. 10.15). The frequency of absence of end-diastolic flow is low, between 3% and 7% in high-risk groups. Although there is only a small number of these pregnancies, they have a high incidence of hypoxia and acidosis. In a series of 59 fetuses with absence of end-diastolic flow in the umbilical artery FVW referred for assessment of severe growth restriction, cordocentesis revealed 25 to be hypoxic, 5 acidotic and 22 both acidotic and hypoxic; only 7 fetuses had normal acid–base status (Nicolaides et al 1988).

Not surprisingly, fetuses with absence of end-diastolic flow have a poorer outcome than those with elevated ratios alone. Growth restriction and chronic hypoxia are almost invariably present, resulting in high rates of perinatal mortality. Battaglia et al (1993) found a 60% perinatal mortality rate among 26 growth-restricted fetuses with absence of end-diastolic flow or reversed flow, highlighting the ominous nature of this class of FVW. This is further reflected in delivery being almost exclusively by caesarean section for fetal distress and a significantly higher rate of abnormal neurological signs in the neonatal period compared with a group matched for gestational age with normal FVW (Weiss et al 1992).

The management of such cases must be individualised to

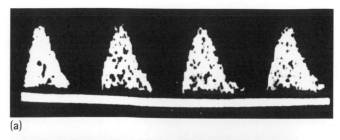

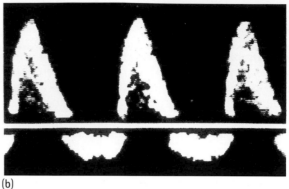

Fig. 10.15 Examples of absent end-diastolic flow (a) and reversed end-diastolic flow (b) in the umbilical artery.

take into account other obstetric features, particularly gestation and the confidence with which congenital and karyotypic abnormalities can be excluded. Absence of end-diastolic flow is not only seen in pregnancies complicated by maternal hypertension and abnormal placental function, but also in some pregnancies with lethal malformations and chromosomal disorders (Wenstrom et al 1991). Careful consideration should be given to detailed anatomical screening and obtaining a fetal karyotype before considering operative delivery in cases of absence of end-diastolic flow where maternal disease is not evident.

It is possible for end-diastolic velocities to reappear with subsequent apparent improvement in perinatal outcome, implying a possible future therapeutic avenue to reduce the hypothesised reversible spasm in the vessels of the placental villi. Such a temporary reappearance of end-diastolic velocities is described after the maternal administration of corticosteroids for the purpose of accelerating fetal lung maturity (Wallace & Baker 1999). There is currently no evidence to suggest that this observation reflects a therapeutic advantage to the fetus (beyond promoting surfactant production) but it is important to recognise this phenomenon when evaluating pregnancies receiving this treatment.

Doppler studies of fetal vessels

Fetal aorta

Flow velocity waveforms from the descending aorta in late pregnancy were first described 20 years ago by Eik-Nes et al (1982). In normal pregnancy the blood flow velocity profile remains above zero throughout the cardiac cycle with the presence of a notch in the waveform which coincides with closure of the aortic valve. There appears to be a small increase in end-diastolic velocities with advancing gestation, although this has not been found in all studies (Fig. 10.16).

There is an association between apparent fetal growth restriction and an abnormal aortic FVW. The absence of end-diastolic velocities precedes abnormalities of the FHR in pregnancies complicated by hypertension, suggesting that aortic FVW analysis might have a role in fetal assessment (Jouppila & Kirkinen 1984). Amongst small fetuses, absence or reversal of diastolic flow is predictive of birthweight more than two standard deviations below the gestation mean and is a sensitive indicator of the need for operative delivery due to fetal distress. However, the aortic FVW may not be a better predictor of growth restriction or neonatal outcome than the umbilical artery FVW alone (Gudmundsson & Marsal 1991).

A close association between aortic mean velocity and abnormal acid–base status in utero exists in the growth-restricted fetus, implying that hypoxia results in peripheral vasoconstriction (Soothill et al 1986). Such a peripheral vasoconstriction, with associated reduction in visceral perfusion, has been used to explain the increased rate of necrotising enterocolitis (NEC) reported in growth-restricted fetuses with absence of aortic end-diastolic flow (AEDF) when compared to those with persisting diastolic flow (Hackett et al 1987). However, more recent papers have failed to confirm the association of AEDF with NEC. Absence of aortic end-diastolic flow is associated with a significantly greater risk of fetal haemorrhage (pulmonary, gastrointestinal or intraventricular) and perinatal death, with only 15% of pregnancies experiencing an uncomplicated neonatal course. It is not surprising therefore that abnormal aortic FVW are associated with neurodevelopmental impairment in childhood (Marsal & Levy 1992).

Fetal carotid and intracranial arteries

The advent of colour flow mapping has enabled the study of FVW in the vessels of the head and neck of the human fetus. The FVW of the carotid and cerebral arteries always displays forward flow in normal pregnancy with a small reduction in the impedance indices as gestation advances so that the brain is supplied by a low-resistance vascular bed with increased perfusion towards term (Wladimiroff et al 1986) (Fig. 10.17). Caution must be exercised during cranial Doppler examination not to apply too much pressure over the fetal skull since raising the intracranial pressure in this way can alter the FVW (Vyas et al 1990a).

Studies of asphyxiated primate and lamb fetuses have demonstrated a redistribution of cardiac output, favouring the cardiac and cerebral circulations at the expense of the abdominal viscera and carcass (Behrman et al 1970). This 'brain-sparing' effect is believed to exist in genuine intrauterine growth restriction where the infant's head size appears to be disproportionately large in relation to its wasted trunk.

A similar brain-sparing effect can be demonstrated in the human fetus whereby a reduction in the impedance indices of the carotid and cranial vessels is seen in growth restriction frequently associated with elevated impedance in the thoracic aorta and umbilical artery. By obtaining blood at cordocentesis in SGA fetuses, Vyas et al (1990b) examined the relationship between middle cerebral artery (MCA) FVW and acid–base status, demonstrating a positive relationship between the degree of hypoxia and reduction in FVW impedance. An abnormal MCA waveform identifies the SGA fetus at increased risk of an abnormal outcome but the MCA may not be suitable for serial monitoring since it reaches maximum dilatation with mild hypoxia only. Although cerebral FVW changes frequently precede FHR changes the interval may be as long as two weeks (Arduini et al 1992). The vasodilatory response of the cerebral circulation to hypoxia is not only a predictor of short-term morbidity but also points to an increased risk of neonatal neurological abnormalities (Rizzo et al 1989).

Doppler examination of the fetal venous circulation

Examination of the fetal arterial circulation has become commonplace whereas attention has only more recently turned

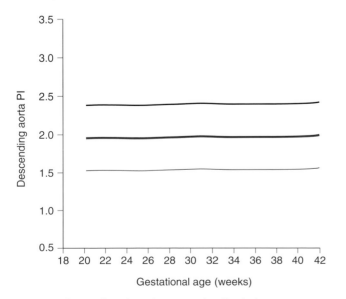

Fig. 10.16 Descending thoracic aorta pulsatility index versus gestational age (5th, 50th and 95th centiles) (Arduini & Rizzo 1990).

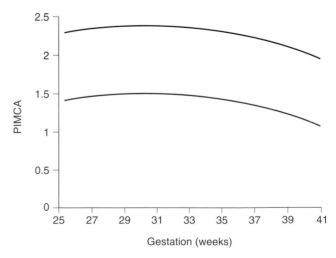

Fig. 10.17 Normal limits of pulsatility index (± 2SD) in the middle cerebral arteries versus gestational age (Wijngaard et al 1989).

towards the fetal venous system. The advent of colour Doppler equipment allows the vessel of interest to be positively identified, permitting reproducible signals to be obtained from the venous as well as the arterial circulation. The vessels of most clinical interest are the umbilical vein and the ductus venosus, the latter being the continuation of the former through the liver before joining the inferior vena cava under the diaphragm.

Continuous, non-pulsatile forward flow is the norm in the umbilical vein although subtle pulsations synchronous with cardiac contractions are described in the minority of normal pregnancies towards term; these may represent transmitted pulsations from the umbilical arteries. The ductus venosus is much narrower than the umbilical vein and the waveform changes abruptly to a much higher velocity, pulsatile pattern. The waveform in the ductus venosus can be described in relation to the phases of right-sided cardiac activity (Fig. 10.18). Quantifying venous blood flow is subject to large errors, and variations in the sampling site of the ductus venosus can result in large variations in waveform patterns. For these reasons, waveform analysis is restricted to qualitative description or the use of ratios of velocities. It is essential that standardisation of sampling sites and absence of fetal breathing is established, and the technique of venous Doppler analysis is more demanding than the acquisition and analysis of arterial waveforms.

Abnormalities of the fetal venous waveforms are seen very late in the sequence of biophysical changes related to chronic hypoxia. Marked umbilical venous pulsations are frequently an ominous sign associated with a number of fetal pathologies including severe growth restriction, fetal hydrops and congenital cardiac anomalies. The aetiology for this pulsatile flow is incompletely understood but possibly represents retrograde transmission of pressure waves across the ductus venosus causing a rhythmic decrease in umbilical venous flow (Gudmundsson 1999). Pulsatile umbilical venous flow identifies a group at much higher risk of death compared to fetuses with similar pathologies but without pulsatile flow.

Abnormalities of the ductus venosus waveform are also a late manifestation of progressive chronic hypoxia and are invariably associated with fetal growth restriction. The interval from demonstrating redistribution of arterial flow to abnormalities of the FHR tracing is variable and might be prolonged, limiting its clinical application. Abnormalities of the ductus venosus waveform have been proposed as an intermediate sign of impending fetal compromise which would represent an important advance in our ability to time delivery with more precision. Absence or even reversal of flow in the ductus venosus during atrial contraction indicates impaired cardiac function in association with fetal acidosis (Fig. 10.19) and appears to identify the fetus at risk of developing abnormal FHR recordings or impending death (Hecher et al 1995, Rizzo et al 1996). Unfortunately this is unlikely to be a consistent finding across all gestational ages and in all fetal conditions limiting its clinical value to a specific group of well-defined pregnancies (Hofstaetter et al 1996).

To date, examination of the fetal venous system has provided insights into the progressive nature of chronic fetal hypoxia. Observational studies suggest a role for examination of the ductus venosus waveform in the timing of delivery of fetuses recognised as compromised who demonstrate redistribution of arterial blood flow. Further evaluation of this new application of Doppler is necessary to determine its role amongst the existing methods of biophysical assessment.

KEY POINTS: DOPPLER

- Analysis of arterial waveforms is used to describe the degree of resistance to blood flow.
- A normal umbilical artery waveform in a SGA pregnancy identifies a subgroup at low risk of fetal death.
- Extreme abnormalities of the umbilical waveform identify a fetus at high risk of hypoxia, acidosis and severe growth restriction.
- Examination of the fetal arterial and venous circulations has not yet been demonstrated to improve clinical management or perinatal outcome.

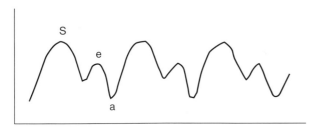

(a)

(b)

Fig. 10.18 Example of normal ductus venosus Doppler waveform (a) with diagrammatic representation of the principal features (b). 'S' represents ventricular systole, 'e' represents early diastole and 'a' represents late diastole. (Adapted from Hecher K 1995.)

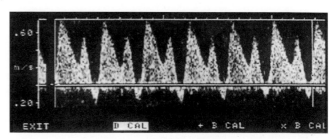

Fig. 10.19 Example of abnormal ductus venosus Doppler waveform demonstrating reversal of flow during late diastole. (From Harrington et al 1995.)

AMNIOTIC FLUID VOLUME MEASUREMENT

Amniotic fluid volume measurement is widely employed as an indicator of fetal well-being during the third trimester. Clinical evaluation is imprecise at other than the extremes of liquor volume and assessment relies upon ultrasound measurement. Amniotic fluid is not static but is in a dynamic state, its composition and volume changing as gestational age advances. The amniotic fluid volume broadly reflects chronic changes in intrauterine oxygenation. Reduced liquor volume in chronic hypoxia is believed to be the result of a redistribution of fetal organ perfusion towards the brain and away from the abdominal viscera including the fetal kidneys. Doppler studies of the renal arteries of apparently growth-restricted fetuses with reduced liquor demonstrate increased resistance to renal blood flow, lending support to the hypothesis that reduced renal perfusion may result in reduced fetal urine production and subsequent oligohydramnios (Arduini & Rizzo 1991).

The precise determination of amniotic fluid volume requires direct access to the amniotic cavity and the subsequent introduction of a marker solution of known volume and concentration. These techniques are not appropriate for clinical practice and so ultrasound is employed to estimate qualitatively and semi-quantitatively liquor volume. Subjective qualitative assessment relies upon operator experience to identify abnormal degrees of fetal crowding and echo-free spaces. By its very nature, such an assessment does not lend itself to objective evaluation as a test of fetal well-being and semi-quantitative descriptions are preferred.

The maximum vertical pocket (MVP) is the on-screen distance of the largest pocket of amniotic fluid, measured at right angles to the contour of the uterine wall. An MVP of less than 2 cm or greater than 8 cm represents oligohydramnios or polyhydramnios respectively (Williams 1993). The two-diameter pocket is an elaboration of the MVP, describing the product of multiplying the vertical and transverse diameters of the single largest pool. The amniotic fluid index (AFI) is a semi-quantitative measure summating the MVP from each arbitrary quadrant of the uterine volume and bears a closer relationship to actual amniotic volume than does the MVP (Phelan et al 1987).

A variety of reference ranges for the AFI have been described, but most suffer from deficiencies in study design including the use of measurements from clinically indicated scans and post-delivery birthweight exclusions. Measurements collected from a longitudinal study of 101 low-risk pregnancies have been presented for the purpose of interpreting a single measurement and demonstrate the change in AFI with advancing gestational age (Nwosu et al 1993) (Fig. 10.20). The interpretation of changes in the AFI of an individual fetus is more complex and their clinical significance not yet established but appropriate standards are described (Owen & Ogston 1996).

The association of both oligohydramnios and polyhydramnios with fetal anomalies is well recognised and can often be anticipated as consequences of impaired or absent production or circulation of amniotic fluid. As an antenatal test of fetal well-being in the absence of recognised fetal

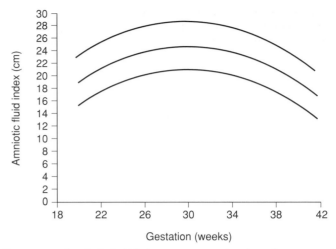

Fig. 10.20 Amniotic fluid index versus gestational age (mean ± 2SD). (From Nwosu et al 1993.)

anomalies, oligohydramnios is associated with an increased risk of preterm delivery, antenatal and intrapartum fetal distress and delivery by caesarean section amongst high-risk pregnancies. Unfortunately, this association is weak both for the AFI and the two-diameter pocket, such that amniotic fluid measurement alone is unable usefully to predict any of a range of indicators of hypoxia-related adverse perinatal outcomes (Magann et al 1999). Despite these limitations, the estimation of amniotic fluid volume is widely performed in antenatal fetal surveillance but is generally considered as one component of the assessment which will include one or more other measures such as fetal biometry, umbilical artery Doppler, cardiotocography or its incorporation into the biophysical profile.

THE FETAL BIOPHYSICAL PROFILE

The biophysical profile (BPP) is a method of determining fetal well-being by employing real-time ultrasound and cardiotocography. Originally described by Manning et al (1980), the BPP has been widely adopted and evaluated as a clinical tool in the prediction of antenatal fetal demise and perinatal morbidity and mortality.

The clinical basis for employing the BPP arises from the observation that combining several fetal parameters improves the predictive value of an abnormal test above that obtained by employing a single variable. The original BPP assigned an arbitrary score of 0 or 2 according to the presence or absence of each of five variables (Table 10.4). A total score of 8 or 10 is considered normal, a score of 6 considered equivocal and an indication for repeat assessment, and a score of 4 or less deemed abnormal and an indication for delivery according to the clinical circumstances.

Physiology

The physiological basis for using the BPP lies in the fact that coordinated fetal activities such as breathing and movement

Table 10.4 Variables included in the biophysical profile

	Score
Non-stress test	
Reactive; at least 2 FHR accelerations >15 bpm in a 20-minute period	2
Non-reactive; 1 FHR acceleration or nil	0
Fetal breathing movements	
FBM present; at least one episode of prolonged breathing (>60 s) within 30-minute period	2
FBM absent; absence of above	0
Gross fetal body movements	
FM present; at least three discrete episodes of fetal movement within a 30-minute period	2
FM absent; <3 or absence of movements	0
Fetal tone	
Normal; extremities and neck held in flexion. At least one episode of completed limb extension and flexion	2
Abnormal; extremities in extension. Fetal movement not followed by return to flexion	0
Amniotic fluid volume	
Normal; largest pocket of fluid >1 cm in vertical diameter	2
Decreased; absence of above. Crowding of fetal parts	0
Total score	0–10

Reproduced with permission from Manning et al (1980).

require an intact and, therefore by implication, non-hypoxic central nervous system. Whilst hypoxia and acidosis are certainly responsible for producing abnormal fetal behaviour, other factors may be responsible and awareness of these influences is essential before inappropriate conclusions regarding fetal welfare are made.

The presence of different fetal behavioural states is well recognised and the influence of this physiological variation should be appreciated when performing the BPP. The time taken to achieve a satisfactory BPP depends strongly on whether the fetus is in state 1F (quiet sleep) or states 2F and 4F (active states); biophysical recording should be extended to at least 40 minutes before the BPP is considered suspicious (Pillai & James 1990).

Fetal breathing movements may be absent for up to 120 minutes in the healthy term fetus (Patrick et al 1980) and are influenced by gestation such that the time spent breathing increases from 12% at the start of the third trimester to 50%

by the end. Fetal breathing is inhibited by maternal cigarette smoking and stimulated by maternal hyperglycaemia, necessitating the standardisation of patient preparation before testing.

Clinical application

Clinical testing of the BPP began with a prospective study of 216 high-risk patients in which the test results were withheld and not allowed to influence clinical decision making (Manning et al 1980). The last result of each test variable before delivery was related to markers of fetal hypoxia and perinatal mortality (PNMR), with the result that the PNMR was zero when all variables were normal (score 10) and 600/1000 when all the variables were abnormal (score 0). Subsequently, Baskett et al (1984) applied the BPP in the management of 2400 high-risk pregnancies and calculated the perinatal morbidity and mortality according to the most recent BPP score (Table 10.5).

False-negative outcomes (i.e. perinatal death within a week of a normal test) are recognised to occur but are very uncommon, with a normal BPP being reassuring of fetal health. In a series of 19 221 referred high-risk pregnancies, there were only 14 deaths unrelated to major fetal anomalies, giving a false-negative rate of 0.72/1000 (Manning et al 1987a). However, the positive predictive value of an abnormal test for perinatal death has a high false-positive rate (i.e. abnormal score with normal outcome), resulting in the potential for unnecessary intervention and its associated maternal and neonatal morbidity.

There does appear to be a progressive evolution of changes in the BPP as intrauterine hypoxia and acidosis worsens. By examining the relationship between the results of BPP performed immediately before prelabour caesarean section and subsequent umbilical artery acid–base values, the appearance of a non-reactive CTG and the absence of fetal breathing movements have been demonstrated to be the first manifestations of hypoxia and acidosis (Vintzileos et al 1991). Such a progression of changes, whereby fetal movements and tone are the last of the variables to be affected, has also been confirmed in growth-restricted fetuses undergoing cordocentesis (Ribbert et al 1990).

The original BPP did not take the composition of the score into account and this has formed the basis of several criticisms of Manning's original test. The arbitrary scoring system whereby each parameter is accorded the same importance

Table 10.5 Distribution of biophysical profiles and their relationship to perinatal morbidity and mortality in a high-risk population

BPP score	n	Fetal distress (%)[a]	Apgar <7 at 5 min (%)	Birthweight <3rd centile	Perinatal death (%)
Normal (8–10)	1938 (97.1)	123 (7)	24 (1.2)	103 (5.3)	5 (0.3)
Equivocal (6)	34 (1.7)	7 (23.3)	1 (2.9)	10 (29.4)	2 (5.9)
Abnormal (0–4)	24 (1.2)	12 (66.7)	8 (33.3)	10 (41.7)	7 (29.2)

Reproduced with permission from Baskett et al (1984).
[a]Calculated for the 1811 fetuses who underwent labour.

means that an apparently abnormal score of 4 can be achieved by a number of combinations. If it is achieved by a reactive CTG and normal liquor volume then the fetus is not showing evidence of acute or chronic hypoxia, rather the low score is more likely to be the result of normal periodicity of fetal activity and intervention is not warranted.

Modifications to Manning's original biophysical profile
There is inevitably an interdependence of the test variables and, whilst most possible combinations can be seen, score composition is important when considering the test's predictive accuracy (Manning et al 1990). This has resulted in several modifications of the original BPP in order to rationalise the use of human and equipment resources without impairing test performance.

Fetal assessment based solely on real-time ultrasonographic examination has been proposed and Manning et al (1987b) have previously found that the CTG was unnecessary when all the ultrasound parameters were normal, thus reducing the use of the CTG to only 2.7% of 7851 tests. Although this may be attractive with respect to saving time and patient convenience, the CTG is a long-established tool that is widely accepted and thought to be understood by obstetricians and is generally more available than the BPP.

By limiting the number of variables included in a test, the potential for error is reduced, time is saved and interpretation is simplified. Disregarding the presence or absence of fetal movements does not adversely influence the test performance (Devoe et al 1992). Walkinshaw et al (1992) found that a BPP comprising the CTG, amniotic fluid volume and fetal breathing movements performed as well as the full BPP in predicting acidosis at delivery in SGA infants. In fact, reducing the BPP further to include the CTG and ultrasound evaluation of amniotic fluid volume alone, with no additional biophysical assessment unless the CTG is unreactive, may be appropriate for routine clinical practice (Eden et al 1988). This is based on the fact that a reactive CTG largely excludes the possibility of fetal acidosis at the time of testing and the absence of FHR decelerations with an adequate liquor volume is reassuring with regard to the exclusion of chronic hypoxia and the likelihood of a cord accident.

An extension of this is the creation of a two-tier approach to fetal biophysical assessment whereby the indication for assessment and periodic ultrasound growth are employed to influence the necessity, nature and frequency of fetal testing. By employing such an approach, a reduction in the workload of CTG testing by more than 60% and BPP by more than 75% could be achieved when managing high-risk pregnancies (Mills et al 1990).

The biophysical profile in relation to Doppler ultrasound
In most obstetric units in which biophysical profile scoring is being employed, it is unlikely to be utilised in isolation from Doppler studies of the uteroplacental circulation since the facilities for Doppler examination are usually present with modern ultrasound equipment. The relationship between umbilical artery Doppler indices and the BPP in high-risk pregnancies has been described such that if the umbilical artery FVW is normal then there are no cases with persis-

tently abnormal BPP scores and a persistently abnormal BPP is always associated with absent end-diastolic flow (Tyrrell et al 1990, James et al 1992). The umbilical artery FVW is superior to either the BPP or FHR variation analysis in predicting fetal distress in labour and acidosis at birth in SGA infants (Nordstrom et al 1989, Soothill et al 1993).

KEY POINTS: FETAL BIOPHYSICAL PROFILE (BPP)

- Non-hypoxic variables such as gestational age, maternal medication and diabetes mellitus can influence the BPP result.
- Risk of fetal death within I week of a normal BPP is approximately 1 per 1000.
- The full BPP is time consuming; a modified assessment with AFV measurement and CTG is a useful alternative.

FETAL ASSESSMENT IN DIABETIC PREGNANCIES

The perinatal mortality rate of pregnancies complicated by diabetes mellitus is now only marginally elevated above that of the non-diabetic population provided that optimal care is provided to a compliant population. Unexpected fetal death is now uncommon amongst well-controlled, non-macrosomic pregnancies but remains a problem amongst pregnancies complicated by macrosomia, polyhydramnios and growth restriction secondary to maternal vascular complications. As a consequence, biophysical fetal assessment has become commonplace in diabetic pregnancy although there is no evidence from randomised trials to support routine third-trimester testing.

Assessment of fetal growth with serial biometry and assessment of amniotic fluid volume is commonplace and can be expected to improve the detection of fetuses with growth restriction and the presence of polyhydramnios. It is debatable whether plotting routine serial ultrasound on cross-sectional charts of fetal biometry provides any clinically useful improvement in the prediction of macrosomia beyond symphysis–fundal height measurements (Johnstone et al 1996) but this remains common clinical practice. There are currently no published reports of the appropriate assessment of longitudinal measurements in diabetic pregnancies.

The cardiotocograph remains the cornerstone of antenatal testing in diabetic pregnancy. The baseline FHR is slightly higher and the number of FHR accelerations lower in diabetic pregnancies compared to non-diabetic controls (Devoe et al 1994). More frequent absent episodes of high-frequency variation mean that diabetic pregnancies more frequently fail to meet the criteria for normality in computerised CTG analysis (Tincello et al 1998). It has been proposed that the CTG be routinely performed twice weekly in uncomplicated diabetic pregnancy because of the observation of stillbirths occurring within four to seven days of a reactive test (Landon & Gabbe 1996).

A number of observational studies have described the performance of the biophysical profile (BPP) in monitoring the fetus in diabetes mellitus. Fetal activity is modified even in the presence of well-controlled diabetes, demonstrating more frequent episodes of fetal breathing and less time spent in body movements compared to gestational age matched non-diabetic controls (Devoe et al 1994). The interpretation of amniotic fluid volume will be complicated by the tendency to higher volumes in diabetic pregnancies. Despite these complicating factors, the incidence of an abnormal test (score of seven or less) is only 3% (Dicker et al 1988, Devoe et al 1994) and a normal test is very reassuring with a very high negative predictive value. In common with its performance in other high-risk pregnancies, an abnormal BPP score is not a good predictor of adverse outcome but this may be because abnormal tests have resulted in prompt delivery (Dicker et al 1988). Currently there is no evidence to demonstrate that the BPP is superior to the CTG alone although the BPP may be considered a useful second-line test in the presence of a non-reactive CTG.

Umbilical artery Doppler FVW analysis has been evaluated in diabetic pregnancies by a number of published studies demonstrating that the impedance ratios of diabetic pregnancies appear to be independent of maternal glycosylated haemoglobin concentration or mean glucose levels (Johnstone et al 1992). In the presence of fetal growth restriction due to maternal hypertension, nephropathy or vasculopathy, abnormal waveforms are associated with adverse perinatal outcome as they are in other non-diabetic high-risk pregnancies, but the demonstration of a normal FVW does not exclude the possibility of fetal compromise and unexpected fetal death (Tyrrell 1988, Johnstone et al 1992). The explanation appears to lie in the fact that antenatal fetal compromise in diabetic pregnancy is multifactorial, where a metabolic component may play a greater role in causing eventual fetal demise than borderline impairment of placental perfusion (Salvesen et al 1992).

At present, there are no randomised or comparative trials upon which to recommend one programme of antenatal fetal assessment over another. Diabetic pregnancies are relatively uncommon and, with good glycaemic control, the rate of antepartum stillbirth of non-malformed fetuses is low so that definitive studies are unlikely to be performed. In the absence of data to support the practice of routine third-trimester testing it can be argued that fetal testing should be restricted to women whose diabetes has been inadequately controlled, where there is evidence of diabetic vasculopathy, or where fetal growth restriction, macrosomia, polyhydramnios or maternal hypertension is present.

CONCLUSIONS

Despite considerable technological advances and the widespread availability of antenatal care, antepartum stillbirths of apparently normally formed fetuses continue to be both tragic and frustrating occurrences. A significant proportion of stillbirths occur in women with no apparent obstetric risk factors and, as such, are unlikely to benefit from the routine introduction of biophysical fetal assessment. Screening for the

small-for-gestational age infant by clinical or ultrasound methods does not materially improve perinatal outcome on a population basis although the introduction of individualised growth assessment shows considerable promise in being able to identify a sub-population who may benefit from closer biophysical assessment. In the past, fetal growth assessment has been based upon the use of inappropriate standards and without recognition of the limitations of the accuracy and reproducibility of fetal biometry. Appropriate standards now exist for the purpose of describing fetal growth and demonstrate potential in being able to identify those pregnancies at greatest risk of adverse outcome.

Antepartum fetal heart rate monitoring remains the most widely accepted diagnostic test for the assessment of the fetus at risk of hypoxia. For monitoring an apparently normal pregnancy, the non-stress test has been found to be inappropriate and is difficult to justify. In designated high-risk pregnancies, the test is used serially and identifies fetuses at risk of hypoxia having normal outcome in 90% of cases, whilst a pathological test, particularly one where there is loss of variability with decelerations, is associated with fetal compromise in nearly all cases. However, the test needs to be performed frequently in order to identify the changing fetal heart rate pattern associated with hypoxia, and interpretation is subject to error.

Doppler ultrasound has enabled the obstetric sonographer to gain considerable insight into the understanding of the vascular changes underlying intrauterine hypoxia and growth restriction. Although it is not appropriate to apply umbilical Doppler as a screening tool to an entire antenatal population (Goffinet et al 1997), it is useful in clinical practice in differentiating constitutionally small fetuses from those at increased risk from impaired placental function, enabling the obstetrician to take a more rational approach to patient management. Randomised trials of umbilical Doppler in high-risk pregnancies have demonstrated a reduction in perinatal mortality when the results are made available to the clinicians (Neilson 1993). Doppler examination of fetal arteries and veins is indicated in only a small percentage of complicated pregnancies but serial evaluation demonstrates trends suggestive of evolving fetal acidosis and often enables the obstetrician to determine the appropriate timing of delivery with more confidence.

The biophysical profile has undergone many suggested modifications since its original description but remains time-consuming and labour-intensive. A major advantage of performing detailed ultrasound as part of fetal assessment is the detection of previously undiagnosed fetal anomalies which will influence pregnancy management. Although a normal test is very reassuring, determining abnormality with certainty may require prolonged scanning since fetal activity is prone to physiological fluctuations. Allowing for the fact that the number of women involved in randomised trials of the BPP is relatively small, the available results do not support its use as a test of fetal well-being in high-risk pregnancies (Neilson & Alfirevic 1993). Where facilities exist, Doppler ultrasound is preferable to the BPP as a second-line test of fetal well-being since it is performed more easily and abnormalities of the FVW precede an abnormal BPP. It would appear reasonable to reserve comprehensive BPP scoring for those fetuses with an abnormal umbilical artery Doppler examination or a CTG which remains non-reactive after prolonged recording.

KEY POINTS

- Birthweight is only one measure of fetal growth achievement; adjusting birthweight to account for physiological variables identifies more accurately those infants at risk of adverse perinatal outcomes.
- Fetal growth is a dynamic process that needs to be quantified with reference to appropriately constructed standards. Charts of fetal size are appropriate for quantifying fetal size but not growth.
- It is not appropriate to subject all pregnancies to biophysical testing. Current methods of testing are designed for, and should be applied to, pregnancies complicated by maternal illness (hypertension, diabetes mellitus) or fetal growth restriction. The performance of biophysical assessment for other indications is less well described.
- All biophysical tests have a high negative predictive value (absence of adverse outcome in the presence of a normal test).
- With the exception of the most abnormal results, biophysical tests have a poor positive predictive value (presence of an adverse outcome in the presence of an abnormal test).
- Randomised controlled trials have demonstrated a reduction in the perinatal mortality rate of high-risk pregnancies managed with umbilical artery Doppler analysis.
- Randomised controlled trials of the CTG and BPP do not demonstrate improvement in perinatal mortality but the studies are small or do not apply to current practice.
- There is no one programme of fetal assessment that can be recommended for all high-risk pregnancies. The nature and frequency of testing will be dictated by perceived clinical risk of fetal hypoxia and antepartum death together with local availability of testing resources.

REFERENCES

Almstrom H, Axellsson O, Cnattingius S et al 1992 Comparison of umbilical-artery velocimetry and cardiotocography for surveillance of small-for-gestational age fetuses. Lancet 340:936

Altman DG, Chitty LS 1994 Charts of fetal size. 1. Methodology. Br J Obstet Gynaecol 101:29–34

Arduini D, Rizzo G 1990 Normal values of Pulsatility Index from fetal vessels: a cross-sectional study of 1556 healthy fetuses. J Perinat Med 18:165–172

Arduini D, Rizzo G 1991 Fetal renal artery velocity waveforms and amniotic fluid volume in growth retarded and post-term fetuses. Obstet Gynecol 77:370–374

Arduini D, Rizzo G, Romanini C 1992 Changes of pulsatility index from fetal vessels preceding the onset of late decelerations in growth-retarded fetuses. Obstet Gynecol 79:605

Baskett TF, Gray JH, Prewett SJ, Young LM, Allen AC 1984 Antepartum fetal assessment using a fetal biophysical profile score. Am J Obstet Gynecol 148:630

Battaglia C, Artini PG, Galli PAD, Ambrogio G, Droghini F, Genazzani R 1993 Absent or reversed end-diastolic flow in umbilical artery and severe intrauterine growth retardation. An ominous association. Acta Obstet Gynecol Scand 72:167

Beattie RB, Whittle MJ 1993 The aetiology of intrauterine growth retardation. Curr Obstet Gynaecol 3:184–189

Behrman RE, Lees MH, Peterson EN, de Lannoy CW, Seeds AE 1970 Distribution of the circulation in the normal and asphyxiated fetal primate. Am J Obstet Gynecol 108:956

Bekedam DJ, Visser GHA, van der Zee AGJ, Snijders RJM, Poelmann-Weesjes 1990 Abnormal velocity waveforms of the umbilical artery in growth retarded fetuses: relationship to antepartum late heart rate decelerations and outcome. Early Hum Dev 24:79

Bracero LA, Morgan S, Byrne DW 1999 Comparison of visual and computerized interpretation of non stress test results in a randomized controlled trial. Am J Obstet Gynecol 181:1254–1258

Brown VA, Sawers RS, Parsons FJ, Duncan SLB, Cooke ID 1982 The value of antenatal cardiotocography in the management of high risk pregnancy: a randomised control trial. Br J Obstet Gynaecol 98:716

Burke G, Stuart B, Crowley P, Scanaill SN, Drumm J 1990 Is intrauterine growth retardation with normal umbilical artery blood flow a benign condition? BMJ 300:1044

Chambers SE, Hoskins PR, Haddad NG, Johnstone FD, McDicken WN, Muir BB 1989 A comparison of fetal abdominal circumference measurements and doppler ultrasound in the prediction of small for dates babies and fetal compromise. Br J Obstet Gynaecol 96:803

Cheng LC, Gibb DMF, Ajayi RA, Soothill PW 1992 A comparison between computerised (mean range) and clinical visual cardiotocographic assessment. Br J Obstet Gynaecol 99:817

Chien PFW, Owen P, Khan K 2000 Validity of ultrasound estimation of fetal weight. Obstet Gynecol 95:856–860

Dawes GS, Visser GHA, Goodman JDS, Vevene DH 1981 Numerical analysis of the human fetal heart rate; the quality of ultrasound records. Am J Obstet Gynecol 141:43

de Jong CLD, Gardosi J, Dekker GA, Colenbrander GJ, van Geijn HP 1997 Application of a customised birthweight standard in the assessment of perinatal outcome in a high risk population. Br J Obstet Gynaecol 104:531–535

Devoe LD, Alaaeldin AY, Gardner P, Dear C, Murray C 1992 Refining the biophysical profile with a risk-related evaluation of test performance. Am J Obstet Gynecol 167:346

Devoe LD, Youssef AA, Castillo RA, Croom CS 1994 Fetal biophysical activities in third-trimester pregnancies complicated by diabetes mellitus. Am J Obstet Gynecol 171:298–305

Dicker D, Feldberg D, Yeshaya A, Peleg D, Karp M, Goldman JA (1988) Fetal surveillance in insulin-dependent diabetic pregnancy: Predictive value of the biophysical profile. Am J Obstet Gynecol 159:800–804

Eden PD, Seifert LS, Kodack LD, Trofatter KF, Killam AP, Gall SA 1988 A modified biophysical profile for antenatal fetal surveillance. Obstet Gynecol 71:365

Eik-Nes SH, Marsal K, Brubakk AO, Kristofferson K, Ulmstein M 1982 Ultrasonic measurement of human fetal blood flow. J Biomed Eng 4:28–36

Ellenberg JH, Nelson KB 1979 Birth weight and gestational age in children with cerebral palsy or seizure disorders. Am J Dis Child 133:1044–1048

Fay RA, Ellwood DA 1993 Categories of intrauterine growth retardation. Fet Mat Med Rev 5:203–212

Fay RA, Dey PL, Saadie CM et al 1991 Ponderal Index: a better definition of the at risk group with intrauterine growth problems than birth-weight for gestational age in term infants. Aust NZJ Obstet Gynaecol 31:17–19

Fitzgerald DE, Drumm JE 1977 Non-invasive measurement of human fetal circulation using ultrasound: a new method. BMJ 2:1450

Flynn AM, Kelly J, O'Connor M 1979 Unstressed antepartum cardiotocography in the management of the fetus suspected of growth retardation. Br J Obstet Gynaecol 86:106

Flynn AM, Kelly J, Matthews K, O'Connor M, Viegas O 1982 Predictive value of, and observer variability in several ways of reporting antepartum cardiotocography. Br J Obstet Gynaecol 89:434

Fok RY, Pavlova Z, Benirschke K, Paul RH, Platt LD 1990 The correlation of arterial lesions with umbilical artery Doppler velocimetry in the placentas of small-for-dates pregnancies. Obstet Gynecol 75:578

Gardosi J, Francis A 1999 Controlled trial of fundal height measurement plotted on customised antenatal growth charts. Br J Obstet Gynaecol 106:309–317

Gardosi J, Chang A, Kalyan B, Sahota D, Symonds EM 1992 Customised antenatal growth charts. Lancet 339:283–287

Giles WB, Trudinger BJ, Baird PJ 1985 Fetal umbilical artery flow velocity waveforms and placental resistance: pathological correlation. Br J Obstet Gynaecol 92:31

Goffinet F, Paris-Llado J, Nisand I, Breart G 1997 Umbilical artery Doppler velocimetry in unselected and low-risk pregnancies: a review of randomised controlled trials. Br J Obstet Gynaecol 104:425–430

Gough NAG, Dawson AAJ, Tomins TJ 1986 Antepartum fetal heart rate recording and subsequent fast transmission by a distributed microprocessor based dedicated system. Int J Biomed Comput 18:61

Grant AM, Elbourne DR, Valentin L, Alexander S 1989 Routine formal fetal movement counting and risk of antepartum late death in normally formed singletons. Lancet ii:345

Gudmundsson S 1999 Importance of venous flow assessment for clinical decisionmaking. Eur J Obstet Gynecol Reprod Biol 84:173–178

Gudmundsson S, Marsal K 1991 Blood velocity waveforms in the fetal aorta and umbilical artery as predictors of fetal outcome: a comparison. Am J Perinatol 8:1

Hackett GA, Campbell S, Gamsu H, Cohen-Overbeek T, Pearce JF 1987 Doppler studies in the growth retarded fetus and prediction of neonatal necrotizing enterocolitis, haemorrhage and neonatal morbidity. BMJ 294:13

Haddad NG, Johnstone FD, Hoskins PR, Chambers SE, Muir BB, McDicken WN 1988 Umbilical artery Doppler waveform in pregnancies with uncomplicated intrauterine growth retardation. Gynaecol Obstet Invest 26:206

Hammacher K 1966 Fruherkennung intrauteriner Gefahrenzustana durch Elektophonokardiographie und Tokographie. In: Elert R, Huter K (eds) Die Parophylaxe fruhkindlicher Hirnschaden. Thieme, Stuttgart

Harrington K, Hecher K, Campbell S 1995 The fetal haemodynamic response to hypoxia. In: Harrington K, Campbell S (eds) Doppler ultrasonography in obstetrics. Edward Arnold, London

Hawdon JM, Hey E, Kolvin I, Fundudis T 1990 Born too small—is outcome still affected? Dev Med Child Neurol 32:943–953

Hecher K 1995 The fetal venous circulation. In: Harrington K, Campbell S (eds) Doppler ultrasonography in obstetrics. Edward Arnold, London

Hecher K, Snijders R, Campbell S, Nicolaides K 1995 Fetal venous, intracardiac and arterial blood flow measurements in intrauterine growth retardation: relationship with fetal blood gases. Am J Obstet Gynecol 173:10–15

Hoffman HJ, Bakketeig LS 1984 Heterogeneity of intrauterine growth retardation and recurrence risks. Semin Perinatol 8:15–24

Hofstaetter C, Gudmundsson S, Dubiel M, Dudenhausen JW, Marsal K 1996 Ductus venosus velocimetry in high risk pregnancies. Eur J Obstet Gynecol Reprod Biol 70:135–140

Huddleston JF, Sutcliffe G, Robinson D 1984 Contraction stress test by intermittent nipple stimulation. Obstet Gynecol 63:669

James DK, Parker MJ, Smoleniec JS 1992 Comprehensive fetal assessment with three ultrasonographic characteristics. Am J Obstet Gynecol 166:1486

Johnstone FD, Steel JM, Haddad NG, Hoskins PR, Greer IA, Chambers S 1992 Doppler umbilical artery flow velocity waveforms in diabetic pregnancy. Br J Obstet Gynaecol 99:135

Johnstone FD, Prescott RJ, Steel JM, Mao JH, Chambers S, Muir N 1996 Clinical and ultrasound prediction of macrosomia in diabetic pregnancy. Br J Obstet Gynaecol 103:747–754

Jones RAK, Roberton NRC 1986 Small for dates babies; are they really a problem? Arch Dis Child 61:877–880

Jouppila P, Kirkinen P 1984 Increased vascular resistance in the descending aorta of the human fetus in hypoxia. Br J Obstet Gynaecol 91:853

Keegan KA, Paul RH 1980 Antepartum fetal heart rate testing, IV. The non-stress test as a primary approach. Am J Obstet Gynecol 136:75

Kidd LC, Patel NB, Smith R 1985a Non-stress antenatal cardiotocography—a prospective blind study. Br J Obstet Gynaecol 92:1152

Kidd LC, Patel NB, Smith R 1985b Non-stress antenatal cardiotocography—a prospective randomised clinical trial. Br J Obstet Gynaecol 92:1156

Krebs C, Macara LM, Leiser R, Bowman AWF, Greer IA, Kingdom JCP 1996 Intrauterine growth restriction with absent end-diastolic velocity in the umbilical artery is associated with maldevelopment of the terminal villous tree. Am J Obstet Gynecol 175:1534–1542

Kubli F, Ruttgers H 1972 Semi-quantitative evaluation of antepartum fetal heart rate. Int J Gynaecol Obstet 10:182

Kubli FW, Hon EH, Khazin AF, Takemura H 1969 Observations on heart rate and pH in the human fetus during labour. Am J Obstet Gynecol 104:1190

Kurmanavicius J, Wright EM, Royston P, Wisser J, Huch R, Huch A, Zimmerman R 1999a Fetal ultrasound biometry: 1. Head reference values. Br J Obstet Gynaecol 106:126–135

Kurmanavicius J, Wright EM, Royston P, Zimmerman R, Huch R, Huch A, Wisser J 1999b Fetal ultrasound biometry: 1. Abdomen and femur length reference values. Br J Obstet Gynaecol 106:136–143

Landon MB, Gabbe G (1996) Fetal surveillance and timing of delivery in pregnancy complicated by diabetes mellitus. Obstet Gynecol Clin North Am 23(1):109–123

Larsen T, Larsen JF, Petersen S, Greisen G 1992 Detection of small-for-gestational age fetuses by ultrasound screening in a high-risk population; a randomised controlled study. Br J Obstet Gynaecol 99:469–474

Lenstrup C, Hasse N 1985 Predictive value of antepartum fetal heart rate non-stress test in high risk pregnancy. Acta Obstet Gynecol Scand 64:133

Lumley J, Lester A, Anderson I, Renou P, Wood C 1983 A randomised trial of weekly cardiotocography in high risk obstetric patients. Br J Obstet Gynaecol 90:1018

Magann EF, Chauhan SP, Kinsella MJ, McNamara MF, Whitworth NS, Morrison JC 1999 Antenatal testing among 1001 patients at high risk: The role of ultrasonographic estimate of amniotic fluid volume. Am J Obstet Gynecol 180:1330–1336

Manning FA, Platt LD, Sipos L 1980 Antepartum fetal evaluation: development of a fetal biophysical profile. Am J Obstet Gynecol 136:787

Manning FA, Morrison I, Harman CR, Lange IR, Menticoglou S 1987a Fetal assessment based on fetal biophysical profile scoring: experience in 19 221 referred high-risk pregnancies II. Am J Obstet Gynecol 157:880

Manning FA, Morrison I, Lange IR, Harman CR, Chamberlain P 1987b Fetal biophysical profile scoring: selective use of the nonstress test. Am J Obstet Gynecol 156:709

Manning FA, Morrison I, Harman CR, Menticoglou SM 1990 The abnormal fetal biophysical profile score V. Predictive accuracy according to score composition. Am J Obstet Gynecol 162:918

Marsal K, Levy D 1992 Intra-uterine blood flow and postnatal neurologic development in growth retarded fetuses. Biol Neonate 62:258

Miller HC, Jekel JF 1989 Malnutrition and growth retardation in newborn infants. Pediatrics 83(3):443

Mills MS, James DK, Slade S 1990 Two-tier approach to biophysical assessment of the fetus. Am J Obstet Gynecol 163:12

Mires GJ, Dempster J, Patel NB, Crawford JW 1987 The effect of fetal heart rate on umbilical artery flow velocity waveforms. Br J Obstet Gynaecol 94:665

Mires GJ, Patel N, Dempster J 1990 Review: the value of fetal umbilical artery flow velocity waveforms in the prediction of adverse fetal outcomes in high risk pregnancies. J Obstet Gynaecol 10:261

Mongelli M, Ek S, Tambyrajia R 1998 Screening for fetal growth restriction: a mathematical model of the effect of time interval and ultrasound error. Obstet Gynecol 92:908–912

Moore KH, Sill R 1990 Domiciliary fetal monitoring in a district maternity hospital. Aust NZJ Obstet Gynaecol 30:36

Murphy KW, Russell V, Collins A, Johnson P 1991 The prevalence, aetiology, and clinical significance of pseudo-sinusoidal fetal heart rate patterns in labour. Br J Obstet Gynaecol 98:1093

Neilson JP 1993 Doppler ultrasound (all trials). In: Enkin MW, Keirse MJNC, Renfrew MJ, Neilson JP (eds) Pregnancy and childbirth module. Cochrane Database of Systematic Reviews. Review No. 07337 February, Oxford

Neilson JP, Alfirevic Z 1993 Biophysical profile for antepartum fetal assessment. In: Enkin MW, Keirse MJNC, Renfrew MJ, Neilson JP (eds) Pregnancy and childbirth module. Cochrane Database of Systematic Reviews: Review No. 07432. April, Oxford

Neldam S 1983 Fetal movements as an indicator of fetal well-being. Dan Med Bull 30:274

Neligan GA, Kolvin I, Scott D, Garside RF 1976 Born too soon or born too small. A follow up study to seven years of age. SIMP, Heinemann Medical, London

Nicolaides KH, Bilardo CM, Soothill PW, Campbell S 1988 Absence of end diastolic frequencies in umbilical artery: a sign of fetal hypoxia and acidosis. BMJ 297:1026

Nordstrom UL, Patel NB, Taylor DJ 1989 Umbilical artery waveform analysis and biophysical profile. A comparison of two methods to identify compromised fetuses. Eur J Obstet Gynecol Reprod Biol 30:241

Nwosu EC, Welch CR, Manasse PR, Walkinshaw S 1993 Longitudinal assessment of amniotic fluid index. Br J Obstet Gynaecol 100:816–819

Owen P, Cameron A 1997 Fetal tachyarrhythmias. Br J Hosp Med 58:142–144

Owen P, Khan K 1998 Fetal growth velocity in the prediction of intrauterine growth retardation in a low risk population. Br J Obstet Gynaecol 105:536–540

Owen P, Ogston S 1996 Standards for the quantification of serial changes in the amniotic fluid index. Ultrasound Obstet Gynecol 8:403–407

Owen P, Ogston S 1998 Conditional centiles for the quantification of fetal growth. Ultrasound Obstet Gynecol 11:110–117

Owen P, Donnet L, Ogston S, Christie AD, Patel N, Howie PW 1996 Standards for ultrasound fetal growth velocity. Br J Obstet Gynaecol 103:60–69

Owen P, Harrold A, Farrell T 1997 Fetal size and growth velocity in the prediction of intrapartum caesarean section for fetal distress. Br J Obstet Gynaecol 104:445–449

Patrick J, Campbell K, Carmichael L 1980 Patterns of human fetal breathing during the last ten weeks of pregnancy. Obstet Gynecol 65:24

Patterson RM, Pouliot MR 1987 Neonatal morphometrics and perinatal outcome: Who is growth retarded? Am J Obstet Gynecol 157:691–693

Patterson RM, Prihoda TJ, Gibbs CE, Wood RC 1986 Analysis of birth weight percentile as a predictor of perinatal outcome. Obstet Gynecol 68:459–463

Pearson JF, Weaver JB 1976 Fetal activity and fetal wellbeing; an evaluation. BMJ 1:1305

Pearson JF, Weaver JB 1978 A six point scoring system for antenatal cardiotocographs. Br J Obstet Gynaecol 85:321

Phelan JP, Smith CV, Broussard P 1987 Amniotic fluid volume assessment using the four-quadrant technique in the pregnancy between 36 and 42 weeks' gestation. J Reprod Med 32:540–545

Pillai M, James D 1990 The importance of the behavioural state in biophysical assessment of the term human fetus. Br J Obstet Gynaecol 97:1130

Reid J, Miller F 1977 Fetal heart rate acceleration in response to acoustic stimulation as a measure of fetal wellbeing. Am J Obstet Gynecol 129:512

Reuwer PJHM, Sijmons EA, Rietman GW, van Tiel MWM, Bruinse HW 1987 Intrauterine growth retardation: prediction of perinatal distress by Doppler ultrasound. Lancet i:415

Ribbert LSM, Snijders RJM, Nicolaides KH, Visser GHA 1990 Relationship of fetal biophysical profile and blood gas values at cordocentesis in severely growth-retarded fetuses. Am J Obstet Gynecol 163:569

Rizzo G, Arduini D, Luciano R et al 1989 Prenatal cerebral Doppler ultrasonography and neonatal neurologic outcome. J Ultrasound Med 8:237

Rizzo G, Capponi A, Talone PE, Arduini D, Romanini C 1996 Doppler indices from inferior vena cava and ductus venosus in predicting pH and oxygen tension in umbilical blood at cordocentesis in growth-retarded fetuses. Ultrasound Obstet Gynecol 7:401–410

Rochard F, Chiforene B, Gone-Poponpil F, Legrand H, Blottiere J, Sureau C 1976 Non stress fetal heart rate monitoring in the antepartum period. Am J Obstet Gynecol 126:699

Rooth G, Huch A, Huch R 1987 Guidelines for the use of fetal monitoring. Int J Gynaecol Obstet 25:159–167

Royston P, Altman DG 1995 Design and analysis of longitudinal studies of fetal size. Ultrasound Obstet Gynecol 6:307–312

Sadovski E, Yaffe H 1973 Daily fetal movement recording and fetal prognosis. Obstet Gynecol 41:845

Salvesen DR, Higueras MT, Brudenell JM et al 1992 Doppler velocimetry and fetal: heart rate studies in nephropathic diabetics. Am J Obstet Gynecol 167:1297–1303

Sanderson DA, Wilcox MA, Johnson IR 1994 The individualised birthweight ratio; a new method of identifying intrauterine growth retardation. Br J Obstet Gynaecol 101:310–314

Schiff E, Lipitz S, Sivan E, Barkai G, Mashiach S 1992 Acoustic stimulation as a diagnostic test; comparison with the oxytocin challenge test. J Perinat Med 20:275

Schifrin B, Foy G, Amato J, Kates R, McKenna J 1979 Routine FHR monitoring in the antepartum period. Obstet Gynecol 54:21

Schulman H, Winter D, Farmakides G et al 1989 Pregnancy surveillance with Doppler velocimetry of uterine and umbilical arteries. Am J Obstet Gynecol 160:192

Soothill PW, Nicolaides KH, Bilardo CM, Campbell S 1986 Relation of fetal hypoxia in growth retardation to mean blood velocity in the fetal aorta. Lancet i:1118

Soothill PW, Ajayi RA, Campbell S, Nicolaides KH 1993 Prediction of morbidity in small and normally grown fetuses by fetal heart rate variability, biophysical profile score and umbilical artery Doppler studies. Br J Obstet Gynaecol 100:742

Steer PJ 1986 Evaluation of cardiotocographs. BMJ 292:827

Strong TH, Jordan DL, Marden DW 1992 The fetal recoil test. Am J Obstet Gynecol 567:1382

Taylor DJ, Howie PW 1989 Fetal growth achievement and neurodevelopmental disability. Br J Obstet Gynaecol 96:789–794

Thompson RS, Trudinger BJ, Cook CM 1986 A comparison of Doppler ultrasound waveform indices in the umbilical artery 1. Indices derived from the maximum velocity waveform. Ultrasound Med Biol 12:835

Tincello DG, el-Sapagh KM, Walkinshaw SA 1998 Computerised analysis of fetal heart rate recordings in patients with diabetes mellitus: the Dawes-Redman criteria may not be valid indicators of fetal well-being. J Perinat Med 26(2):102–106

Trimbos JM, Keirse MJNC 1978 Observer variability in the assessment of antepartum cardiotocograms. Br J Obstet Gynaecol 85:900

Trudinger BJ, Giles WB, Cook CM, Bombardieri J, Collins L 1985 Fetal umbilical artery flow velocity waveforms and placental resistance: clinical significance. Br J Obstet Gynaecol 92:23

Trudinger BJ, Cook CM, Jones L, Giles WB 1986 A comparison of fetal heart rate monitoring and umbilical artery waveforms in the recognition of fetal compromise. Br J Obstet Gynaecol 93:171

Trudinger BJ, Cook CM, Giles WB, Connelly A, Thompson RS 1987 Umbilical artery flow velocity waveforms in high-risk pregnancy. A randomised, controlled trial. Lancet 1:188

Tyrrell SN 1988 Doppler studies in diabetic pregnancy. BMJ 296:428

Tyrrell SN, Obaid AH, Lilford RJ 1989 Umbilical artery Doppler velocimetry as a predictor of fetal hypoxia and acidosis at birth. Obstet Gynaecology 74:332

Tyrrell SN, Lilford RJ, Macdonald HN, Nelson EJ, Porter J, Gupta JK 1990 Randomized comparison of routine versus highly selective use of Doppler ultrasound and biophysical scoring to investigate high-risk pregnancies. Br J Obstet Gynaecol 97:909

Villar J, Belizan JM 1982 The timing factor in the pathophysiology of the intrauterine growth retardation syndrome. Obstet Gynecol Surv 37:499–507

Vintzileos AM, Fleming AD, Scorza WE et al 1991 Relationship between fetal biophysical activities and umbilical cord blood gas values. Am J Obstet Gynecol 165:707

Visser GHA, Redman CWG, Huisjess J, Turnbull AC 1980 Non-stress antepartum heart rate monitoring; implications of decelerations after spontaneous contraction. Am J Obstet Gynecol 138:429

Vyas S, Campbell S, Bower S, Nicolaides KH 1990a Maternal abdominal pressure alters fetal cerebral blood flow. Br J Obstet Gynaecol 97:740

Vyas S, Nicolaides KH, Bower S, Campbell S 1990b Middle cerebral artery flow velocity waveforms in fetal hypoxaemia. Br J Obstet Gynaecol 97:797

Walkinshaw S, Cameron H, MacPhail S, Robson S 1992 The prediction of fetal compromise and acidosis by biophysical profile scoring in the small for gestational age fetus. J Perinat Med 20:227

Wallace EM, Baker LS 1999 Effect of antenatal betamethasone administration on placental vascular resistance. Lancet 353:1404–1407

Weiner CP 1990 The relationship between the umbilical artery systolic/diastolic ratio and umbilical blood gas measurements in specimens obtained by cordocentesis. Am J Obstet Gynecol 162:1198

Weiss E, Ulrich S, Berle P 1992 Condition at birth of infants with previously absent or reverse umbilical artery end-diastolic flow velocities. Arch Gynaecol Obstet 252:37

Wennergren M, Wennergren G, Vilbergsson G 1988 Obstetric characteristics and neonatal performance in a four year small for gestational age population. Obstet Gynecol 72:615–620

Wenstrom KD, Weiner CP, Williamson RA 1991 Diverse maternal and fetal pathology associated with absent diastolic flow in the umbilical artery of the high-risk fetus. Obstet Gynecol 77:374

Wheeler T, Cooke E, Murrills A 1979 Computer analysis of fetal heart rate variation during normal pregnancy. Br J Obstet Gynaecol 86:186

Wijngaard van den JA, Groenenberg IA, Wladimiroff JW, Hop WC 1989 Cerebral Doppler ultrasound of the human fetus. Br J Obstet Gynaecol 96:845–849

Wilcox MA, Johnson IR, Maynard PV, Smith SJ, Chilvers CED 1993 The individualised birthweight ratio; a more logical outcome measure of pregnancy than birthweight alone. Br J Obstet Gynaecol 100:342–347

Williams K 1993 Amniotic fluid assessment. Obstet Gynaecol Surv 48:795–800

Wladimiroff JW, Tonge HM, Stewart PA 1986 Doppler ultrasound assessment of cerebral blood flow in the human fetus. Br J Obstet Gynaecol 93:471

Woerden EE van, Geijn HP van, Caron FJM, Mantel R, Swartjes JM, Arts NF Th 1989 Fetal hiccups; characteristics and relation to the fetal heart rate. Eur J Obstet Gynecol Reprod Biol 30:209–216

Wood C, Walker A, Yardley R 1979 Acceleration of the fetal heart rate. Am J Obstet Gynecol 86:186

Young BK, Katz M, Klein SA 1979 The relationship between heart rate patterns and tissue pH in the human fetus. Am J Obstet Gynecol 134:685

Young BK, Katz M, Wilson SJ 1980 Sinusoidal fetal heart rate. I. Clinical significance. Am J Obstet Gynecol 136:587

11

Assisted reproduction

Robert W. Shaw, Nazar N. Amso

The contribution of the author of the equivalent chapter in the second edition, on which this chapter draws extensively, is gratefully acknowledged.

INTRODUCTION

Assisted reproduction has witnessed considerable advances in the past few years, though it continues to be controversial. Often such developments raise ethical and moral dilemmas and the widespread provision of these treatments remains a hotly debated topic, socially, medically and politically. The introduction of clinical guidelines into clinical practice in general and in assisted reproduction in particular has led to an ever increasing role for an evidence-based approach to the provision of these services. The need for streamlined investigations and avoidance of unnecessary waste of resources has seen the publication of clinical guidelines for the management of infertility in primary and sec-

ondary care centres by the Royal College of Obstetricians and Gynaecologists, London, UK (RCOG 1998a, b). More recently, evidence-based clinical guidelines for the management of infertility in tertiary care centres were published (RCOG 1999). There is an increasing demand to introduce new technology into clinical practice, often before adequate scientific evidence has accumulated. Hence, it is essential that clinical practice evolves appropriately in order to protect both the public and the profession. Additionally, there may be consequences such as the high multiple pregnancy rate and its implications for the cost of neonatal services. These issues are the subject of regular discussions between the Human Fertilisation and Embryology Authority (HFEA), the regulatory authority for assisted reproduction treatments in the UK, and the relevant professional and ethical bodies.

In this chapter we will review the current status of conventional *in vitro* fertilisation treatment (IVF), intracytoplasmic sperm injection (ICSI), egg and sperm donation, embryo cryopreservation and their indications. The obstetric and neonatal consequences of these treatments, and in particular the impact of the number of embryos transferred, on the outcome will be discussed in detail.

Current status of assisted reproduction treatments

In 1998, more than 200 000 treatment IVF cycles were carried out in Europe. In the UK about 34 000 IVF/ICSI cycles were reported, resulting in over 8700 births, and accounting for about 1.2% of all births (HFEA 1999). The number of treatment cycles for IVF and ICSI have been steadily increasing since the introduction of these treatments (Fig. 11.1), while donor insemination (DI) cycles have decreased since the widespread introduction of ICSI into clinical practice. Live birth rates per treatment cycle for IVF, ICSI and DI have steadily improved over the past decade (Fig. 11.2).

The effectiveness of infertility treatments (IVF, ICSI, egg and sperm donation, and embryo donation) is dependent on a reasonable likelihood that embryos can be created *in vitro* and then placed in the uterus with a reasonable expectation that implantation will occur. Many factors determine the outcome of treatment, such as patient selection, age, cause and duration of infertility and the number of attempts that couples undergo. However, the decision to recommend assisted reproduction treatment should be based on: the likelihood that a pregnancy will occur without treatment, the possibility that a less invasive form of treatment might be effective, and the likely outcome of IVF treatment (RCOG 1999). The likelihood of treatment-independent pregnancy depends on the woman's age, cause and duration of infertility and history of previous pregnancy (Collins et al 1995, Eimers et al 1995, Vardon et al 1995). In a retrospective study (Vardon et al 1995) the incidence of spontaneous treatment-independent pregnancy in couples enlisted on an IVF programme was reported to be 11%. The main difference from those in whom pregnancy did not occur was a shorter duration of infertility.

Infertility, its investigations and treatments, may be the source of considerable psychological stress. Appropriate advice and counselling decreases this stress and thus should be made available at all stages, including after the treatment process is completed. Counselling will also help couples come to terms with ending treatment and adjusting to their inability to have children. The HFEA Code of Practice distinguishes between information giving, assessment of couples for treatment and counselling. Counsellors should be adequately trained and appropriately qualified to address the complex issues relating to assisted reproduction treatments and couples' needs.

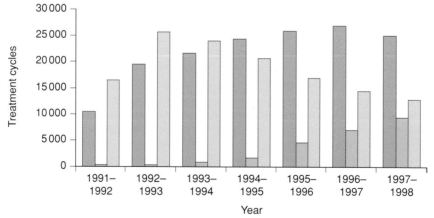

Fig. 11.1   Number of treatment cycles 1991–1998.
▓, IVF; ▨, micromanipulation; ▢, donor insemination. (HFEA 1999, with permission.)

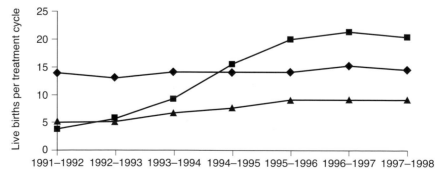

Fig. 11.2   Live birth rates per treatment cycle 1991–1998.
◆, IVF; ■, micromanipulation; ▲, DI. (HFEA 1999, with permission.)

FACTORS AFFECTING OUTCOME

Size of unit

Assisted reproduction treatment is not necessarily equally effective in all fertility units and success rates remain significantly dependent on where the provision of service takes place. It is clear from the HFEA annual reports that the outcome of treatment varies between small and large centres. When discussing the likelihood of birth following IVF treatment with any couple, it is essential to consider a number of factors that can significantly affect the outcome. These include female age, cause and duration of infertility, previous pregnancy history, number of embryos replaced, availability of surplus embryos for cryopreservation and the number of any previous treatment cycles. Such advice is particularly relevant and important in women over the age of 40 years, for whom success rates are considerably reduced and the risk of miscarriage is increased.

Female age

The woman's age at the time of treatment is an important prognostic factor when the success of IVF is discussed with any couple. The number of oocytes, and consequently the number of embryos, declines with age. However, the cleavage rate does not seem to alter in the same manner. The number of embryos replaced compounds the effect of age on embryo implantation rates and pregnancy rate. The total number of embryos available for replacement further influences this. When a larger number of embryos is available for replacement, the selection of the most appropriate embryos for transfer improves the implantation and pregnancy rates respectively.

Recent studies have reported that when women over the age of 40 had four or more embryos transferred, their pregnancy rate was not significantly different from that in younger women, whether following IVF (Widra et al 1996) or ICSI (Alrayyes et al 1997). Hence, it was concluded that older women with good ovarian response, producing three or more embryos suitable for transfer, had pregnancy rates similar to younger patients. It should be noted that these findings contradict early reports (Piette et al 1990). Increased preg-

nancy rates may reflect improvements in ovarian stimulation protocols and laboratory practices.

Fertilisation rates decrease with age. Women attempting pregnancy over the age of 40 have an approximately 50% lower fertility rate than with younger women (Toner & Flood 1993). Most reports have found significantly lower fertilisation rates in older women undergoing IVF or ICSI (Cordiero et al 1995, Tucker et al 1995, Ashkenazi et al 1996), although a few (Sharif et al 1998) reported that age had no significant association with fertilisation rates. Similarly, cumulative conception rates (Prietl et al 1998) and implantation rates appeared to decline significantly with age. However, maternal age alone was not found to be a useful predictor of embryo implantation or endometrial receptivity in IVF treatment cycles (Arthur et al 1994, Van Kooij et al 1996).

Age and pregnancy, miscarriage and live birth rates

Live birth rates per treatment cycle following IVF, ICSI and DI have increased consistently over the past decade (Fig. 11.2). However, live birth rate declines with advancing age when women's own eggs are used (Fig. 11.3). A number of investigators have examined different age cut-offs for treatment, such as 40 years (Widra et al 1996, Sharif et al 1998) or 35 years (Preutthipan et al 1996). Mardesic et al (1994) reported that the cut-off point of effectiveness for an IVF programme was an age of 36–37 years, with a marked decline in pregnancy rate per embryo transfer in women over the age of 38.

Similarly, Tan et al (1992a) found that both conception and live birth rates per cycle declined with age. The cumulative conception and live birth rates after five treatment cycles were about 54% and 45%, respectively, at 20–34 years (compared with 38% and 29% at 35–39 years and 20.2% and 14.4% at 40 years or more). It is likely that pregnancy rates are related to the quality of the embryos: when adjustment was made for equal embryonic quality, maternal age did not interfere significantly with pregnancy rates (Parneix et al 1995). Thus, women over the age of 40 with good response to controlled ovarian hyperstimulation have better prognosis and success rates than those with poor response.

Miscarriage rates have been reported to be higher in all

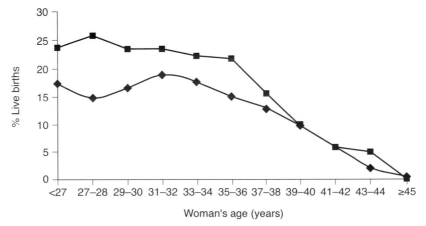

Fig. 11.3 Live birth rates by women's age.
◆, IVF; ■, micromanipulation (own eggs). (HFEA 1999, with permission.)

women following IVF than in spontaneous cycles and a risk of a 2–3-fold increase in the rate of spontaneous miscarriage in women aged 40 or more (Toner & Flood 1993). However, this has been disputed by others (Al Shawaf et al 1992, Mardesic et al 1994) who found no higher pregnancy loss in older women. It is likely that embryo quality is the main factor influencing the poor reproductive performance of women with advancing age rather than a defective response of uterine vasculature to steroids or uterine ageing. Increasing maternal age correlates with a higher risk of fetal chromosomal anomalies, which results in an increased miscarriage rate.

The live birth rate following IVF decreases with age (Fig. 11.3). In an attempt to identify factors that affect the outcome of treatment Templeton and colleagues (1996) analysed the HFEA database between 1991 and 1994. The authors reported that the overall live birth rate per cycle of treatment was 13.9%. The highest rates were in the age group 25–30 years; younger women (under 25 years) had lower rates and a sharp decline was noted in older women. At all ages over 30 years, the use of donor eggs was associated with significantly higher live birth rates than the use of a woman's own eggs, although there was also a downward trend in success rates with age. After adjustment for age, increasing duration of infertility was associated with a significant decrease in live birth rate. The indications for treatment had no significant effect on the outcome, while previous pregnancy and live birth significantly increased treatment success.

Cause of infertility

Reports have differed in their analysis of the impact of infertility factors on cumulative conception and live birth rates. While some have found significant differences, the lowest rates being in patients with male infertility or multiple infertility factors (Tan et al 1992a), others reported no significant effect on the outcome (Dor et al 1996, Templeton et al 1996). However, a history of previous pregnancy and live birth significantly increased treatment success (Templeton et al 1996, Prietl et al 1998). The IVF clinical pregnancy and live birth rates in the HFEA report of 1999 show similar results for tubal disease, endometriosis and unexplained infertility (Fig. 11.4).

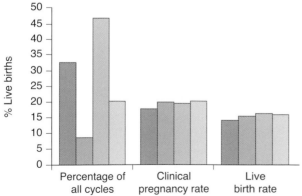

Fig. 11.4 IVF clinical pregnancy and live birth rates for female causes of infertility.
■, Tubal disease; ■, endometriosis; ■, unexplained; □, other. (HFEA 1999, with permission.)

ICSI was first successful in 1992 and since then the annual number of treatment cycles has increased steadily (Fig. 11.1). It enabled men who had been diagnosed with severe male factor infertility the chance to have their own genetic children. The sperm may be obtained by ejaculation, percutaneous extraction from the epididymis (PESE) or testicular extraction (TESE). Fertilisation rates are higher than with standard IVF, especially in men with borderline or very poor sperm quality. Recognised indications for treatment by ICSI include: very poor sperm quality, obstructive azoospermia, non-obstructive azoospermia, and previously failed or very poor fertilisation. Live birth rates following ICSI, overall and by age of women, are shown in Figs 11.2 and 11.3.

Duration of infertility

The duration of infertility remains one of the most important variables that influence the outcome of assisted reproduction, with lower pregnancy and live birth rates associated with a longer period of infertility. Analysis of the HFEA database between 1991 and 1994 showed that, even with adjustment for age, there was a significant decrease in live birth rate with increasing duration of infertility from 1 to 12 years (Templeton et al 1996).

Superovulation protocols

In most assisted reproduction centres superovulation protocols are employed to induce multiple follicular development to obtain a larger number of oocytes. The resulting embryos are evaluated and the best two or three are selected for replacement, usually on the second or third day after insemination. Superovulation protocols have varied considerably. In the early years, clomiphene citrate (alone, or in conjunction with human menopausal gonadotrophins) was the main drug used in superovulation protocols. The use of GnRH agonists (GnRH-a) in stimulation protocols has increased steadily since their introduction into clinical practice and has resulted in a reduction in the cancellation rates and an increase in the number of oocytes retrieved. A meta-analysis comparing the efficacy of GnRH-a in superovulation cycles for IVF (Hughes et al 1992) reported significantly improved clinical pregnancy rates and decreased cancellation rates in GnRH-a cycles compared with non-downregulated cycles.

More recently the long down-regulation protocol was found to be superior to the short or ultrashort regimens (Daya 1998), and the type of GnRH-a (short-acting or depot preparation) did not appear to affect pregnancy or miscarriage rates (Daya 1997, Dada et al 1999). The use of GnRH-a often prolongs the stimulation phase, and may be associated with poor response in some patients as well as introducing a higher risk of ovarian hyperstimulation syndrome. Some of the disadvantages can be obviated with the use of GnRH antagonists. However, some prospective studies showed lesser pregnancy rates in antagonist cycles, and the question remains whether this is inherent to the medication, due to adverse effects on the luteal phase, the type of patient population or limited experience with follicle stimulation in antagonist cycles (Devroey 2000).

Others (Van Os & Jansen 2000) have compared the antagonist Cetrorelix (ASTA Medica AG) in two groups of patients: previous poor responders (less than three oocytes retrieved in previous IVF/ICSI treatment) and normal responders. The Cetrorelix was started when the mean follicular diameter of the leading follicle was 14–15 mm, which corresponded to day 5 or 6 of gonadotrophin stimulation. The pregnancy rate and ongoing/delivery rate in the previously poor responders was poor and clearly showed that this group did not benefit from this new treatment strategy. In the normal responders, the results were more encouraging and overall pregnancy rate and implantation rates per embryo transfer were 45% and 22% respectively. However, these data should be interpreted with caution and further randomised controlled studies in predefined patient subgroups should be carried out to establish any further benefit from this new treatment.

Commercially available gonadotrophin preparations used in superovulation protocols were originally extracted from urine of menopausal women. They were of low purity, with the major protein components not being gonadotrophins! The repeated injection of non-gonadotrophin proteins may be the cause of unwanted effects, such as pain and allergic reactions. The desirability of high-purity preparations led to the development of an immunopurified FSH product of >95% purity. The introduction of high-purity gonadotrophins (high-purity FSH) was associated with a small but significant increase in pregnancy rate in comparison with conventional hMG preparations (Daya et al 1995).

Variations in bioactivity and continued dependence on human menopausal urine collection, however, remained as major obstacles in the production of these compounds. Recent progress in purification technology, genetic and molecular engineering led to the production of recombinant human FSH (rFSH) with high purity (>99%), high specific bioactivity (>10 000 IU/mg protein) and no intrinsic LH activity, which is suitable for intramuscular or subcutaneous administration (Mannaerts et al 1991). Its use produces results similar to those of high-purity FSH when fresh embryo replacement only is considered (Bergh et al 1997). It also results in the production of significantly more oocytes and, if pregnancies from frozen embryo replacement cycles are included, significantly more pregnancies (Out et al 1995).

Embryo transfer

The convention has been to replace embryos on the second day after insemination. It can be argued that there are advantages in delaying embryo transfer to allow selection of those embryos with greater potential for implantation and to replace them at a more physiological time into the uterine cavity. Some retrospective studies have failed to demonstrate any increase in the ongoing pregnancy rates whether embryos were replaced 2, 3 or 4 days post insemination (Huisman et al 1994, Dawson et al 1995) although others have demonstrated significantly higher pregnancy rates after day 3 transfers and even more so if the embryos replaced had eight or more blastomeres (Carrillo et al 1998). Significantly higher implantation rates (Dawson et al 1995, Carrillo et al 1998) and lower miscarriage rates

(Dawson et al 1995) were also reported following day 3 transfers.

Transfer of embryos at the blastocyst stage has potential advantages. It is a more physiological approach, allowing synchronisation of the embryo with the endometrium, and the selection of viable embryos for transfer will be more efficient. Furthermore, the reduction in the number of embryos transferred) and even if one only is transferred (leads to acceptable pregnancy rates while eliminating the risk of high-order multiple pregnancy rates (Gardner et al 1998). Assessment of blastocyst viability is mainly based on morphological appearance but this is a notoriously poor method. Early reports indicated that transfer of two or three blastocysts resulted in high viable pregnancy rates, 62% and 58% respectively. However, the advantage of two-blastocyst transfer is a lower multiple pregnancy rate of 39% (compared with 79% for three blastocysts) and the absence of triplet pregnancies (Milki et al 1999). Culture of human blastocysts in sequential media and the use of a systematic scoring and grading system can achieve much higher pregnancy and implantation rates when top-quality blastocyst(s) are transferred. This will be an important area of future research.

Endometrial thickness on its own is a poor predictor for pregnancy. However, no conception was recorded when endometrial thickness was below 5 mm on the day of transfer and hence it is recommended that consideration should be given to cryopreservation of all embryos and preparation of the endometrium with exogenous hormones at a subsequent cycle (Friedler et al 1996).

Variations in the technique of embryo transfer and the use of transabdominal ultrasound guidance to determine the precise depth of embryo placement within the uterus may also influence the pregnancy rate.

Tubal embryo transfer was the subject of considerable interest in the late 1980s, following reports of high pregnancy rates with gamete intrafallopian transfer (GIFT). Randomised controlled trials have failed to demonstrate any significant difference in the overall results between fresh tubal embryo transfer and uterine transfer (Fluker et al 1993, Amso 1996), although significantly higher pregnancy rates were reported after frozen tubal embryo transfers (Van Voorhis et al 1995). Interestingly, a randomised trial comparing transcervical tubal cannulation and embryo transfer with uterine embryo transfer reported higher pregnancy and implantation rates following uterine transfer (Scholtes et al 1998).

Luteal phase support

Pregnancy rates are higher when the luteal phase is supported in GnRH-a cycles. Human chorionic gonadotrophin is superior to progestogerone but is associated with a higher incidence of ovarian hyperstimulation syndrome (Soliman et al 1994). There is no evidence that any method of progesterone administration (oral, parenteral or vaginal) is better than another. Similarly, luteal phase support in non-downregulated GnRH-a cycles does not increase pregnancy rate.

Number of embryos transferred

Assisted reproduction treatment involving ovarian stimulation is associated with an increased multiple pregnancy rate. In England and Wales, the multiple birth rate increased from 9.9 per thousand pregnancies in 1975 to 13.6 in 1994. During the same period, an increase in the prescription of fertility drugs was reported, which led to the conclusion that fertility treatments were responsible for this increase in multiple pregnancies, especially triplet births. Unmonitored or poorly supervised ovulation induction treatment results in multiple pregnancy due to a surplus number of oocytes. However, with IVF treatment the multiple pregnancy rate is very much dependent on the number of embryos replaced.

Retrospective studies, as early as 1985, had suggested that multiple pregnancies and births increased with the increase in the number of embryos replaced (Wood et al 1985, Tucker et al 1991, Waterstone et al 1991). Randomised studies comparing two- three- (Staessen et al 1993) or four-embryo transfers (Vauthier-Brouzes et al 1994) reported similar pregnancy rates as long as there were sufficient morphologically normal embryos available for transfer. However, there were no higher-order multiple births when only two embryos were transferred. Analysis of the HFEA database involving more than 44 000 cycles (Templeton & Morris 1998) and the most recent HFEA report (1999) showed that when four or more fertilised eggs were available the transfer of three embryos did not improve pregnancy rates over the elective transfer of two embryos only. However, the incidence of triplets or higher-order multiple births decreased considerably when only two embryos were replaced (Fig. 11.5).

In contrast, when only two embryos are available for transfer in women at or above the age of 40 (e.g. due to the retrieval of few oocytes or poor fertilisation), the pregnancy rate is markedly reduced. Interestingly, the multiple pregnancy rate is only marginally reduced in women at or above the age of 40 when the best two instead of three embryos are electively replaced (Templeton & Morris 1998). Another study involving women aged over 40 years and undergoing

embryos than 1–3 only. However, there were no differences in the delivery, multiple pregnancy or spontaneous miscarriage rates between the two groups (Adonakis et al 1997).

The British Fertility Society (1997) advocates the transfer of a maximum of two embryos only in each treatment cycle as a standard of good practice. Additionally reduction in the number of embryos transferred from three to two also has economic implications. A clinical audit in Scotland (Liao et al 1997) demonstrated that the cost of neonatal intensive care was reduced by 85% when a two-embryo policy was adopted for most women.

Number of attempts of IVF procedures

The literature appears to be somewhat divided when the relation between pregnancy and live birth rates and number of IVF attempts are examined. In one study (Padilla & Garcia 1989), the pregnancy rate per embryo transfer was similar for at least seven attempts, while other studies (Tan et al 1992a, FIVNAT 1994, Templeton et al 1996) reported a decline in the chances of pregnancy and live birth with successive treatment cycles. The data from the HFEA 1998 annual report showed a steady decline after the fifth attempt, with both pregnancy rates and live birth rates per cycle being 11.1% and 8.6% respectively at the 10th and 11th attempts (Fig. 11.6).

When IVF cumulative pregnancy rates were estimated for a cohort of women, the rates showed a steady rise during the six initial IVF treatments and then reached a plateau subsequently (Dor et al 1996). The cumulative rates were reported to be as high as 80% after seven cycles, with a history of previous pregnancy significantly improving a couple's probability of conception (Croucher et al 1998).

Embryo cryopreservation

The ability to cryopreserve embryos enables any supernumeraries to be stored for some time before replacement when fresh embryo transfer has failed or if further children are desired. Cryopreservation has the added benefit of increasing the number of potential embryo replacement cycles without

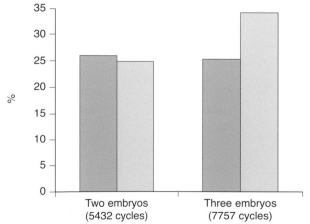

Fig. 11.5 Live and multiple births for two or three fresh embryos transferred in IVF.
▓, Live birth rate (percentage of cycles); ░, multiple birth rate (percentage of live births). (HFEA 1999, with permission.)

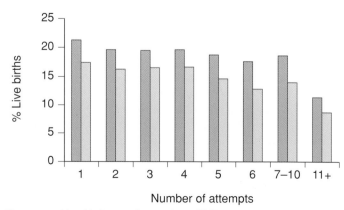

Fig. 11.6 Live birth rates by number of IVF attempts.
▓, Pregnancy rate per cycle; ░, live birth rate per cycle. (HFEA 1998, with permission.)

the need to undergo further superovulation and oocyte retrieval, hence reducing the risk of ovarian hyperstimulation syndrome. Embryo quality has the most significant impact on survival after thawing and ultimately pregnancy and implantation rates. As with fresh embryos, factors such as woman's age, the number of embryos transferred and whether a pregnancy resulted from the original stimulation cycle will affect the outcome of the frozen thawed embryo replacement (FER).

In 1999, the HFEA annual register reported a clinical pregnancy rate of 13.5% and a live birth rate of 10.4% per FER cycle in women using their own gametes. Over the past decade considerable improvement has taken place. The French register (FIVNAT 1996) reported an increase in the pregnancy rates per transfer from 11.5% to 16% between 1987 and 1995. It has been estimated that one FER cycle increases the take home baby rate by 5% (Kahn et al 1993) while treatment involving one fresh and two FER cycles achieves a cumulative viable pregnancy rate of 41% (Home et al 1997). Frozen thawed embryos can be replaced in natural or hormonally adjusted cycles utilising GnRH-a and oestrogen/progestagen preparations with comparable results. The use of GnRH-a is useful in anovulatory or irregular cycles and the use of different progestagens for luteal phase support is equally effective. The cost per delivery for FER cycle has been estimated to be between 25 and 45% of a fresh cycle. In view of these advantages, cryopreservation should be accessible and discussed with all couples where surplus good-quality embryos are available.

Sperm and oocyte donation

Donor insemination (DI) is an effective treatment for male factor infertility (azoospermia, severe oligo-astheno spermia), though pregnancies independent treatment may occur in some non-azoospermic couples while awaiting treatment. The success of DI depends on the availability of suitable semen donor with high fertilizing potential and the adequate investigation of women for factors that influence the probability of conception. Factors that may affect the success of DI include a woman's age, ovulatory status, fallopian tube patency, and the quality of frozen–thawed semen. The use of fresh semen in previous years resulted in cycle fecundity rates that approached natural conceptions (Peek et al 1984, Mackenna et al 1992). Pregnancy and live birth rates per cycle are similar in natural or stimulated cycles: 11.3% and 12.1% respectively (HFEA 1999). The multiple pregnancy rate is, however, considerably higher with stimulated than natural cycles (14% and 1.6% respectively), with a threefold and tenfold increase in the stillbirth and neonatal death rates per thousand births for twins and triplets compared with singleton births (HFEA 1999). Stillbirth and neonatal death rates are also higher in natural than stimulated DI cycles. It is recommended that, at first, a minimum of six cycles of insemination without ovarian stimulation should be carried out in regularly ovulating women (RCOG 1999). The use of donated sperm in IVF resulted in clinical pregnancy and live birth rates of 26.3% and 22.2% per treatment cycle for fresh replacements and 18.1% and 13.9% respectively for frozen embryo replacements (HFEA 1999).

Egg donation is an effective treatment for women with premature ovarian failure, gonadal dysgenesis such as Turner's syndrome, following oophorectomy, chemotherapy- or radiotherapy-related ovarian failure and where repeated failure of fertilisation is attributed to poor oocyte quality. High pregnancy rates have been reported following oocyte donation for women with Turner's syndrome (Khastgir et al 1997). However, women with Turner's syndrome were reported to have significantly higher biochemical pregnancy rates and early miscarriages, lower clinical pregnancy and delivery rates than other women with premature ovarian failure (Yaron et al 1996). An important factor in the establishment of pregnancy is an endometrial thickness of greater than 6.5 mm. Other factors include the number of previous natural conceptions and live births and the fertilisation rate (increasing female age does not affect the outcome) (Burton et al 1992). Oocyte donation has considerable emotional and social effects on both the donor and recipient, more so if the donor is undergoing IVF treatment herself. A comparison of pregnancy and live birth rates per treatment cycle following oocyte donation and other treatments is depicted in Figs 11.7, 11.8 (HFEA 1999).

Stress and infertility

Infertility and its treatment are associated with significant levels of stress. However, there is very little evidence to determine whether psychological distress is a consequence or cause of infertility (Brkovich & Fisher 1998). The precise effects of stress and anxiety on the outcome of treatment are not clear. Infertile women are more depressed and anxious than fertile ones (Van Balen & Trimbos-Kemper 1993) and the stress of IVF treatment may have important psychoendocrinological responses. Indeed, reduction of stress associated with IVF may even improve conception rates (Eugster & Vingerhoets 1999). The impact of infertility and IVF-related stress might be long term, with profound consequences for physical and mental health.

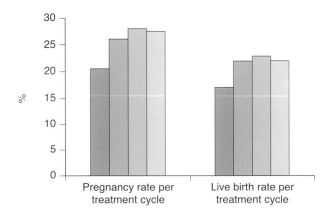

Fig. 11.7 Clinical pregnancy and live birth rates for IVF using fresh embryo transfer–stimulated cycles.
■, Own gametes; ■, donated sperm; ■, donated eggs; □, donated embryos. (HFEA 1999, with permission.)

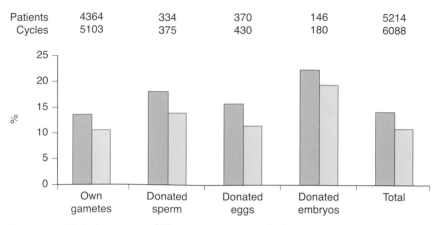

| Patients | 4364 | 334 | 370 | 146 | 5214 |
| Cycles | 5103 | 375 | 430 | 180 | 6088 |

Fig. 11.8 Clinical pregnancy (■) and live birth rates (□) for IVF using frozen embryo replacements. (HFEA 1999, with permission.)

OBSTETRIC OUTCOME OF ASSISTED REPRODUCTION TREATMENTS

The obstetric risks and outcome of assisted reproduction treatments have always been the subject of considerable debate—the first pregnancy reported following IVF was an ectopic pregnancy. The obstetric complications, the additional risks associated with multiple pregnancy and the perinatal complications will be discussed in the next two sections.

In the context of pregnancy outcomes, the aim of assisted reproduction treatments should be a healthy singleton delivery at term. However, infertile couples may not share this target (Goldfarb et al 1996, Murdoch 1997): they do not appreciate the risks associated with multiple pregnancy, and indeed 67–90% of couples may desire a twin birth (Gleicher et al 1995) while less than a third regard a single child as the ideal outcome. Increasing age or duration of infertility has been associated with a greater desire for multiple births (Murdoch 1997). The risk of multiple pregnancy is greater with superovulation with or without intrauterine insemination than IVF/ICSI treatments due to the overabundance of oocytes released from multiple follicles. IVF and ICSI allow greater control of the multiple pregnancy rate, as it is determined by the number of embryos replaced. Indeed, when there are more than four developing follicles with intrauterine insemination treatments, follicle reduction using transvaginal ultrasound guidance before insemination reduced the multiple pregnancy rate without compromising pregnancy rates (PS Bhal, personal communication 2000).

Antenatal and intrapartum complications following IVF

Many studies have examined obstetric outcome after fertility treatment. In early reports of IVF pregnancies, the miscarriage rate appeared to be higher in general (Australian *in vitro* Fertilisation Collaborative Group 1985) and more so when one or two embryos were transferred rather than three or four (Balen et al 1993). However, no increase in the spontaneous miscarriage rate was identified in a large series involving over 5000 cycles in more than 2391 women

(Alsalili et al 1995). Comparison of the obstetric outcome of IVF pregnancies with matched normally conceived pregnancies (Tan et al 1992b) showed a higher multiple pregnancy rate (25%), significantly increased incidence of vaginal bleeding and hypertension requiring hospitalisation, and caesarean births. Among IVF singleton pregnancies, there was a significantly increased incidence of intrauterine growth restriction, placenta praevia and preterm delivery.

The increased obstetric risks may reflect the women's history of infertility, a relatively high incidence of poor obstetric history and the lower threshold for intervention in these patients. A more recent retrospective cohort study in Sweden (Bergh et al 1999) compared the obstetric outcome of IVF babies born between 1982 and 1995 with all babies born in the general population during the same period. It reported an approximately fivefold increase in preterm birth and low birthweight rates in IVF babies over controls. The study concluded that high frequency of multiple births and maternal characteristics were the main factors leading to adverse outcome and not the IVF technique itself.

Others have also reported that IVF mothers may have a higher incidence of pregnancy-induced hypertension, premature labour, labour induction, and preterm delivery (Tallo et al 1995). Multiple pregnancies have a higher prevalence of pre-eclampsia; more so with triplets than with twins. A case-control study (Skupski et al 1996) concluded that fetal number, placental mass, or other factors unrelated to the success of implantation, are more important to the development of pre-eclampsia than is successful implantation alone. Comparison of singleton IVF pregnancies with matched controls showed a longer first stage of labour, greater intrapartum blood loss and a trend towards a higher caesarean delivery than controls (Howe et al 1990). The authors concluded that these differences probably do not arise from the physiology of IVF and are of minimal clinical significance; these pregnancies therefore should not be regarded as high risk in the absence of other predisposing factors.

The obstetric outcome of natural and IVF twin pregnancies was compared in a multicentre study. The mean gestational age was equal in the two groups, at 36 weeks, but the elective caesarean section rate was higher in the assisted conception group. Induction of labour rates did not differ and once labour commenced there was no difference in the mode of delivery or neonatal short-term morbidity between the two groups. Similarly, birthweight, gestational length and perinatal mortality rates by conventional and extended classification were not different (Agustsson et al 1997). Others have also reported comparable outcomes in the two groups in terms of mean duration of gestation, birthweight and incidence of congenital malformations (Dhont et al 1999) despite an earlier suggestion of a higher incidence of preterm deliveries (Dhont et al 1997). There was also no difference in the incidence of preterm labour, preterm premature rupture of membranes, pregnancy-induced hypertension or gestational diabetes (Fitzsimmons et al 1998).

Interestingly, for both singleton and twin IVF pregnancies the incidence of caesarean section is increased (Dhont et al 1999). In Agustssen's study (1997) it was noted that only the elective caesarean section rate was significantly higher. This may in part be a reflection of the generally held medical perception of assisted pregnancies being more precious but may also indicate a higher complication rate necessitating operative delivery.

Women who conceive following oocyte donation, especially those with a history of ovarian failure, should be considered as high risk. Analysis of 232 ovum donation pregnancies reported a higher risk of pregnancy-induced hypertension and postpartum haemorrhage, and an increased incidence of infants who were small for gestational age. Of the 151 babies born, the overall operative delivery rate was 85% and the caesarean section rate was 69% (Abdalla et al 1998).

Antenatal and intrapartum complications following ICSI

Pregnancy following ICSI has generated interest due to the additional complexity of technique and the tests involved with these pregnancies, namely the microinjection technique and the prenatal diagnostic tests often performed on the resulting pregnancies. The incidence of pregnancy loss in early observational reports ranged from 22% to 38% depending on the use of ejaculated, epididymal or testicular spermatozoa respectively (Wisanto et al 1996) and was no different from conventional IVF outcome in historical controls. Similarly, other complications such as prematurity and low birthweight were related to the multiplicity of the pregnancy. A national cohort study of all ICSI pregnancies in Denmark between 1994 and 1997 confirmed that ICSI pregnancy outcome was comparable with that of other studies except that no sex chromosome abnormalities were found (Loft et al 1999). In ICSI pregnancies where prenatal diagnosis (amniocentesis, chorion villus sampling) was carried out, the preterm delivery, low or very low birthweight rates were no higher than in cycles where no such tests were carried out. Furthermore, the fetal loss rates were comparable (Aytoz et al 1998). Retrospective comparison of ICSI pregnancies with matched IVF controls (Govaerts et al 1998) showed no differences in early pregnancy loss, congenital malformation, multiple pregnancy rates, singleton mean birthweight or

gestational age at birth. However, the last two parameters were significantly higher in ICSI twins than in IVF. Couples undergoing ICSI for severe male infertility (oligoastheno-terato-zoospermia) have slightly reduced fertilization rates but have pregnancy loss and delivery rates similar to other couples undergoing ICSI and IVF for non-male infertility (Mercan et al 1998).

Cryopreservation and obstetric outcome

Comparative retrospective studies of births resulting from cryopreserved embryos and conventional IVF reported a similar incidence of twins and triplet births, mean gestational age and birthweight for singletons, twins and triplets in the two groups (Wada et al 1994). More recently, pregnancies resulting from the transfer of fresh or frozen conventional IVF or ICSI embryos were compared (Aytoz et al 1999). The frozen ICSI group showed a significantly higher miscarriage rate than those receiving frozen conventional IVF. The incidence of preterm deliveries, very low birthweights, major malformations and intrauterine deaths were similar in all groups. However, the low birthweight rates in frozen IVF and ICSI were significantly lower than in the fresh groups.

PERINATAL AND PAEDIATRIC OUTCOME OF ASSISTED REPRODUCTION TREATMENTS

This section will address the impact of multiple pregnancy and prematurity on perinatal mortality and morbidity, the fears over a possible increase in congenital anomalies and whether there is an increase in the incidence of long-term or life-threatening illness in these children.

Multiple pregnancy and prematurity

An increase in twinning and triplet rates in developed countries such as England and Wales, Germany, the Netherlands and Switzerland has been attributed to the higher proportion of mothers treated with ovulation-inducing hormones and partially attributed to IVF (Imaizumi 1998). It is widely accepted that multiple pregnancies account for a disproportionately large share of adverse pregnancy outcomes (Powers & Kiely 1994) including an increased incidence of very low birthweight, low birthweight, perinatal and neonatal mortality and infant death. The increased incidence of death and morbidity in twin compared with singleton pregnancy has been attributed mainly to prematurity (Ho & Wu 1975) and to adverse outcomes associated with premature delivery such as hyaline membrane disease, hypocalcaemia, hypoglycaemia, hyperbilirubinaemia, small for dates, and low Apgar scores. In one recent study (Tough et al 2000), the contribution of IVF to changes in the incidence of low birthweight, preterm delivery and multiple birth over a 3-year period was substantial. The increased incidence of preterm delivery and low birthweight is partially related to multiple births, though an increase in preterm deliveries has also been seen in IVF singleton pregnancies (Dhont et al 1999). The high multiple pregnancy rate is related to the number of embryos transferred. The evidence supports the view that transferring two embryos instead of three does not compromise the chance of pregnancy but reduces the risk of triplets (Preutthipan et al 1996, Matson et al 1999). It results in an overall multiple pregnancy rate of 14.3% for double embryo transfers and 32.4% for triple embryo transfers, with no significant difference in the pregnancy rate if at least one good quality embryo was available for transfer (Tasdemir et al 1995).

In one report (Slotnick & Ortega 1996) it was suggested that monoamniotic multiple gestations may be increased in zona-manipulated cycles (ICSI, zona drilling, assisted hatching) and, although all resulting monoamniotic pregnancies ended in live births, there was high incidence of intrauterine discordance in fetal growth. Some early evidence suggested that assisted twin pregnancies have a higher incidence of preterm deliveries and need more neonatal intensive care than with matched control twin pregnancies (Dhont et al 1997).

Perinatal mortality/morbidity

Early reports (Tan et al 1992b) suggested that stillbirth and perinatal mortality rates following IVF were comparable with national maternal age-standardised rates. Twins conceived with IVF have perinatal mortality and morbidity rates comparable to those of spontaneously conceived controls (Dhont et al 1999). However, a retrospective cohort study (Fitzsimmons et al 1998) reported a significantly increased perinatal mortality in spontaneous twin gestations (but not in triplets) compared with those resulting from assisted therapies. Singleton IVF pregnancies were reported to have a significantly worse perinatal outcome than spontaneously conceived pregnancies, mainly due to the increased rate of preterm birth (Dhont et al 1999). Others (Ishii et al 1994) reported a doubling of the premature birth rate in singleton assisted pregnancy compared with normal controls, with an increased mortality rate.

Infants resulting from IVF may have a lower mean birthweight and shorter gestation. Additionally, these infants may require more days of oxygen therapy and continuous positive airway pressure and longer hospitalisation and may have increased prevalence of respiratory distress syndrome, patent ductus arteriosus and sepsis (Tallo et al 1995). The same authors concluded that couples who underwent IVF appear to be at increased risk of having low birthweight and preterm infants, but that multiple gestations accounted for most of the neonatal morbidity. ICSI treatment does not appear to differ from conventional IVF when the incidence of multiple pregnancies and perinatal outcome are compared (Bider et al 1999).

Retrospective comparison of births resulting from cryopreserved embryos with those after conventional IVF/fresh embryo transfer showed no difference in the perinatal mortality between the two groups (Wada et al 1994).

It is logical to assume that women with infertility problems are likely to have an increased incidence of pelvic or systemic pathology to account for their infertile status. It therefore follows that such women are likely to have an increase in their complication rate when pregnant. Indeed,

women with a medical history of infertility (whether treated or untreated) have a significantly increased risk of perinatal death (Draper et al 1999). In Draper's study, women with untreated infertility were at increased risk of perinatal death and any association with multiple births did not explain this finding. The same was true for women with treated infertility where the risks of associated multiple births explained some but not all of this excess. The authors advocated that at antenatal booking a history of infertility, irrespective of treatment, should be sought as these women have a significantly increased risk of perinatal death.

Congenital abnormalities

Tan et al (1992b) reported comparable malformation rates in children born following conventional IVF with matched normally conceived pregnancies. ICSI enabled men with severe oligospermia or azoospermia to pass their genes on to their own progeny, an event that may not have been possible just a few years ago. This raises questions about the genetic constitution of any resulting pregnancies: the quality of the sperm used for ICSI treatment may adversely affect the chromosome constitution of the resulting embryo (Obasaju et al 1999). This case report utilised fluorescence in situ hybridisation (FISH) to determine any chromosomal abnormalities in embryos before implantation. An infertile couple with severe male infertility and endometriosis underwent two ICSI cycles with the husband's sperm and one IVF cycle with donor sperm. Preimplantation genetic diagnosis with FISH showed that all the embryos derived from the cycle in which donor sperm was used were chromosomally normal, whereas 82% of the embryos derived from cycles in which the husband's sperm was used were chromosomally abnormal. It was concluded that paternal factors, thought to be derived from the paternal centrosome, could have contributed to numerical chromosomal abnormalities and may in turn have predisposed to implantation failure. It is possible that they would be manifested as congenital abnormalities that present to the paediatrician. The cycle in which donor sperm was used resulted in an ongoing pregnancy.

However, short and long-term follow-up data on children born by ICSI have thus far been encouraging. Bider et al (1999) did not note any major malformations or difference between children resulting from ICSI and conventional IVF. Similarly, a retrospective study comparing 132 children born after IVF and 120 after ICSI reported no differences between the two groups with regard to early embryonic development and obstetric outcome (Van Golde et al 1999). The congenital malformation rate was 3% after IVF and 1.7% after ICSI, though in both groups only 30% of women underwent prenatal chromosomal diagnosis. A long prospective follow-up study (Bonduelle et al 1999) of 1987 children born after ICSI, with subgroups depending on whether ejaculated, epididymal or testicular spermatozoa were used, reported no increase in the incidence of congenital malformations or abnormal karyotypes. Physical examination of these children was carried out at 2 months, 1 year and 2 years after birth and noted similar growth parameters and developmental milestones in all subgroup.

One condition that does appear to be directly associated with ICSI is hypospadias, a malformation of the penis. In one study (Wennerholm et al 2000) of over 1000 babies born after ICSI seven cases of hypospadias were identified, with an expectation in the general population of around two. Hypospadias appears to be associated with paternal subfertility so a link with ICSI is possible. The same study showed an increased risk of abnormalities in babies born after ICSI compared with babies born without the use of fertility treatments; however, this was mainly due to conditions associated with multiple or premature births rather than the ICSI treatment itself.

Couples requiring ICSI appear to have an increased incidence of chromosomal disorders, which appears to manifest itself in a low implantation rate (Scholtes et al 1998). This may increase the risk of transmitting chromosomal aberrations, though it can be minimised by karyotyping potential parents, preimplantation genetic diagnosis and prenatal fetal karyotyping. There is also a risk of transmitting fertility problems to the offspring. Overall, about 20 000 babies have been born worldwide through ICSI in the last decade and the vast majority of these are healthy normal children. However, since ICSI is still a relatively new procedure, the fertility potential of these children can not yet be determined and further follow-up studies are required. Potential parents may be reassured that generally there is no apparent increase in the incidence of major congenital malformations.

Retrospective comparison of births resulting from cryopreserved embryos with those after fresh replacement reported a significantly lower incidence of major congenital malformation (Wada et al 1994). However, in a study in which children born following FER were compared and matched for maternal age, parity, single or twin pregnancy and gestational age at birth with those born after fresh IVF and those conceived spontaneously (Wennerholm et al 1998) the authors reported similar growth rates, incidence of major malformations and prevalence of chronic disease at 18 months.

Risk of malignancy

It is important for potential parents undergoing assisted reproduction treatments to be counselled on the likely outcome of their unborn children—including any life-threatening illnesses such as cancer. Some case reports (Toren et al 1995) suggest a possible association between IVF and paediatric malignancies such as hepatoblastoma and clear cell carcinoma of the kidney. However, two recent studies (Bruinsma et al 2000, Lerner-Geva et al 2000) did not detect any significant increase in the incidence of cancer among cohorts of children born after IVF over the expected age-adjusted rates of the general population. Larger prospective studies are needed to provide the necessary power to reach definite conclusions.

CONCLUSIONS

For the obstetrician it is important to understand that the most significant factors affecting assisted reproduction pregnancies are those associated with multiple pregnancy and prematurity. Furthermore, multiple pregnancy is mostly iatrogenic and can be reduced by replacing two embryos only when there is a surplus, to permit the selection of those of highest quality. It is also reassuring that these procedures do not appear to increase the risks of major congenital abnormalities or of developing malignancies over the rates in the general population.

This field is constantly evolving, with new developments raising frequent ethical and moral dilemmas. Hence there is a constant need to implement the principles of evidence-based medicine in our daily practice and openly debate all controversial issues. Finally, as many of these procedures are relatively new, potential parents should be made aware of the possible unforeseen complications and the risks for any resulting children.

KEY POINTS

- A woman's age is an important prognostic factor for success of assisted reproduction treatment.
- Women over the age of 40 years have 50% lower fertility rates than younger women.
- Cumulative conception, live birth and implantation rates following IVF treatment decline significantly with age.
- The use of donor rather than own eggs in women over the age of 30 years significantly increases the live birth rate.
- IVF pregnancies are associated with: high multiple pregnancy rate; increased incidence of hypertension and vaginal bleeding; increased incidence of caesarean births; fivefold increase in preterm birth and low birthweight; increased incidence of IUGR.
- Rate of pregnancy complications following ICSI treatment is comparable with matched IVF controls.
- Hypospadias appears to be directly associated with ICSI treatment.
- Children born after IVF treatment do not show any increase in the incidence of cancer compared with age-adjusted controls.
- When sufficient morphologically normal embryos are available, the multiple pregnancy rate following the elective transfer of two embryos is similar to that following the transfer of three or four embryos.
- The incidence of high-order multiple pregnancy decreases considerably when two embryos only are transferred.
- There is a ninefold reduction in the cost of neonatal intensive care services when two embryos only are transferred.
- Singleton IVF pregnancies have significantly worse perinatal outcome than spontaneous ones.
- Past history of infertility significantly increases the risk of perinatal death.
- Previous pregnancy and live birth significantly increases the success rate of assisted reproduction treatments.
- Longer duration of infertility is associated with lower pregnancy and live birth rates.

- Egg donation is an effective treatment for women with ovarian failure, Turner's syndrome or following oophorectomy.
- Transfer of embryos on day 3 after insemination or at blastocyst stage results in higher pregnancy and implantation rates and lower miscarriage rate than for day 2 transfers.
- The pregnancy rate in GnRH-agonist cycles is higher when the luteal phase is supported with either hCG or progesterone.
- Cryopreservation of embryos increases the number of potential embryo replacement cycles without the risks of superovulation or egg retrieval and results in a live birth rate of about 10% per frozen embryo cycle.

REFERENCES

Abdalla HI, Billet A, Kan AK et al 1998 Obstetric outcome in 232 ovum donation pregnancies. Br J Obstet Gynaecol 105(3):332–337

Adonakis G, Camus M, Joris H, Vandervorst M, Van Streitegham A, Devroey P 1997 The role of the number of replaced embryos on intracytoplasmic sperm injection outcome in women over the age of 40. Hum Reprod 12(11):2542–2545

Agustsson T, Geirsson RT, Mires G 1997 Obstetric outcome of natural and assisted conception twin pregnancies is similar. Acta Obstet Gynecol Scand 76(1):45–49

Alrayyes S, Fakih H, Khan I 1997 Effect of age and cycle responsiveness in patients undergoing intracytoplasmic sperm injection. Fertil Steril 68(1):123–127

Alsalili M, Yuzpe A, Tummon I et al 1995 Cumulative pregnancy rates and pregnancy outcome after in-vitro fertilization. Hum Reprod 10:470–474

Al-Shawaf T, Nolan A, Guirgis R, Harper J, Santis M, Craft I 1992 The influence of ovarian response on gamete intra-Fallopian transfer outcome in older women. Hum Reprod 7(8):1106–1110

Amso NN 1996 Studies of the Fallopian tube environment and an assessment of its role in assisted reproduction. PhD thesis submitted to the Faculty of Medicine, University of London

Arthur ID, Anthony FW, Masson GM, Thomas EJ 1994 The selection criteria on an IVF program can remove the association between maternal age and implantation. Acta Obstet Gynecol Scand 73(3):562–566

Ashkenazi J, Orvieto R, Gold-Deutch R et al 1996 The impact of woman's age and sperm parameters on fertilization rates in IVF cycles. Eur J Obstet Gynecol Reprod Biol 66(2):155–159

Aytoz A, De Catte L, Camus M et al 1998 Obstetric outcome after prenatal diagnosis in pregnancies. Hum Reprod 13:2958–2961

Aytoz A, Van den Abbeel E, Bonduelle M et al 1999 Obstetric outcome of pregnancies after transfer of cryopreserved and fresh embryos obtained. Hum Reprod 14:2619–2624

Australian in vitro Fertilisation Collaborative Group 1985 High incidence of preterm births and early losses in pregnancy after in vitro fertilisation. BMJ 291(6503):1160–1163

Balen AH, MacDougall J, Tan SL 1993 The influence of the number of embryos transferred in 1060 in-vitro fertilization pregnancies on miscarriage rates and pregnancy outcome. Hum Reprod 8(8):1324–1328

Bergh C, Howels CM, Borg K et al 1997 Recombinant human follicle stimulating hormone (r-hFSH;Gonal-F) versus highly purified urinary FSH (Metrodin HP) results of a randomized comparative study in women undergoing assisted reproductive techniques. Hum Reprod 12:2133–2139

Bergh T, Ericson A, Hillensjo T, Nygren KG, Wennerholm UB 1999 Deliveries and children born after in-vitro fertilisation in Sweden 1982–95: a retrospective cohort study. Lancet 354(9190):1579–1585

Bider D, Livshitz A, Tur Kaspa I, Shulman A, Levron J, Dor J 1999 Incidence and perinatal outcome of multiple pregnancies after intracytoplasmic sperm injection compared to standard in vitro fertilization. J Assisted Reprod Genet 16(5):221–226

Bonduelle M, Camus M, De Vos A et al 1999 Seven years of intracytoplasmic sperm injection and follow up of 1987 subsequent children. Hum Reprod 14 (suppl 1):243–264

British Fertility Society 1997 Human Reproduction 12 Natl Suppl. J Brit Fertil Soc 2(2):88–92

Brkovich AM and Fisher WA 1998 Psychological distress and infertility: forty years of research. J Psych Obstet Gynaecol 19:218–228

Bruinsma F, Venn A, Lancaster P, Speirs A, Healy D 2000 Incidence of cancer in children born after in-vitro fertilization. Hum Reprod 15(3):604–607

Burton G, Abdalla HI, Kirkland A, Studd JWW 1992 The role of oocyte donation in women who are unsuccessful with in-vitro fertilization treatment. Hum Reprod 7(8):1103–1105

Carrillo AJ, Lane B, Pridman DD et al 1998 Improved clinical outcomes for in-vitro fertilisation with delay of embryo transfer from 48 to 72 hours after oocyte retrieval: use of glucose and phosphate-free media. Fertil Steril 69:329–334

Collins JA, Burrows EA, Willan AR 1995 The prognosis for live birth among untreated infertile couples. Fertil Steril 64(1):22–28

Cordiero I, Calhaz-Jorge C, Barata M, Leal F, Proenca H, Coelho AM 1995 Repercussao da idade da mulher da taxa de clivagem e da qualidad e embrionaria, na obtencao de gravidez por fertilizacao in vitro. Acta Med Port 8(3):145–150

Croucher CA, Lass A, Margara R, Winston RM 1998 Predictive value of the results of a first in-vitro fertilization cycle on the outcome of subsequent cycles. Hum Reprod 13(2):403–408

Dada T, Salha O, Baillie HS, Sharma V 1999 A comparison of three gonadotrophin-releasing hormone analogues in an in-vitro fertilisation programme: a prospective randomised study. Hum Reprod 14(2):288–293

Dawson KJ, Conaghan J, Ostera RM, Winston RM, Hardy Y 1995 Delaying transfer to the third day post-insemination, to select non-arrested embryos, increases development to the fetal heart stage. Hum Reprod 10:177–182

Daya S 1997 Optimal agonist protocol for GnRH agonists. J Assisted Reprod Genet 14:39S

Daya S 1998 Comparison of gonadotrophin releasing hormone agonist (GnRHa) protocols for pituitary desensitization in in vitro fertilization (IVF) and gamete intrafallopian transfer (GIFT) cycles (Cochrane Review). In: The Cochrane Library, Issue 4. Update Software, Oxford

Daya S, Gunby J, Hughes EG, Collins JA, Sagle MA 1995 Follicle-stimulating hormone versus human menopausal gonadotrophin for in vitro fertilization cycles: a meta-analysis. Fertil Steril 64(2):347–354

Devroey P 2000 GnRH antagonists. Fertil Steril 73:15–17

Dhont M, De Neubourg F, Van der Elst J, De Sutter P 1997 Perinatal outcome of pregnancies after assisted reproduction: a case-control study. J Assisted Reprod Genet 10:575–580

Dhont M, De Sutter P, Ruyssinck G, Martens G, Bekaert A 1999 Perinatal outcome of pregnancies after assisted reproduction: a case-control study. Am J Obstet Gynecol 3:688–695

Dor J, Seidman DS, Ben-Shlomo I, Levran D, Ben-Rafael Z, Maschiach S 1996 Cumulative pregnancy rate following in-vitro fertilization: the significance of age and infertility aetiology. Hum Reprod 11(2):425–428

Draper ES, Kurinczuk JJ, Abrams KR, Clarke M 1999 Assessment of separate contributions to perinatal mortality of infertility history and treatment: a case-control analysis. Lancet 353(9166):1746–1749

Eimers JM, Te-Velde ER, Gerritse R, Vogelzang ET, Looman CWN, Habbema JDF 1995 The prediction of the chance to conceive in subfertile couples. Fertil Steril 61(1):44–52

Eugster A, Vingerhoets AJJM 1999 Psychological aspects of in vitro fertilization: a review. Soc Sci Med 48:575–589

Fitzsimmons BP, Bebbington MW, Fluker MR 1998 Perinatal and neonatal outcomes in multiple gestations: assisted reproduction. Am J Obstet Gynecol 179:1162–1167

FIVNAT 1994 Evolutions des criteres pronostiques de fecondation in vitro selon le rang de la tentative. Contracept Fert Sex 22(5):282–286

FIVNAT 1996 Evaluation of frozen embryo transfers from 1987 to 1994. Contracept Fertil Sex 24:700–705

Fluker MR, Zouves CG, Bebbington MW 1993 A prospective randomised comparison of zygote intrafallopian transfer and in vitro fertilisation-embryo transfer for non-tubal factor infertility. Fertil Steril 60:515–519

Friedler S, Schenker JG, Herman A, Lewin A 1996 The role of ultrasonography in the evaluation of endometrial receptivity following assisted reproductive treatments: a critical review. Hum Reprod Update 2:323–335

Gardner DK, Vella P, Lane M, Wagley L, Schlenker T, Schoolcraft WB 1998 Culture and transfer of human blastocysts increases implantation rates and reduces the need for multiple embryo transfers. Fertil Steril 69(1):84–88

Gleicher N, Campbell DP, Chan CL et al 1995 The desire for multiple births in couples with infertility problems contradicts present practice patterns. Hum Reprod 10:1079–1084

Goldfarb J, Kinzer DJ, Boyle M, Kurit D 1996 Attitudes of in vitro fertilization and intrauterine insemination couples toward multiple gestation pregnancy and multifetal pregnancy reduction. Fertil Steril 65:815–820

Govaerts I, Devreker F, Koenig I, Place I, Van den Bergh M, Englert Y 1998 Comparison of pregnancy outcome after intracyoplasmic sperm injection and in vitro fertilization. Hum Reprod 13:1514–1518

Ho SK, Wu PY 1975 Perinatal factors and neonatal morbidity in twin pregnancy. Am J Obstet Gynecol 122(8):979–987

Home G, Critchlow JD, Newman MC, Edozien L, Matson PL, Lieberman BA 1997 A prospective evaluation of cryopreservation strategies in a two-embryo transfer programme. Hum Reprod 12:542–547

Howe RS, Sayegh RA, Durinzi KL, Tureck RW 1990 Perinatal outcome of singleton pregnancies conceived by in vitro fertilization: a controlled study. J Perinatol 10(3):261–266

Hughes EG, Fedorkow DM, Daya S, Sagle MA, van de Koppel P, Collins JA 1992 The routine use of gonadotrophin-releasing agonists prior to in vitro fertilisation and gamete intrafallopian transfer: a meta-analysis of randomised controlled trials. Fertil Steril 58(5):888–896

Huisman GJ, Alberda AT, Leerenveld RA, Verhoeff A, Zellmaker GH 1994 A comparison of in vitro fertilisation results after embryo transfer after 2, 3 and 4 days of embryo culture. Fertil Steril 61:970–971

Human Fertilisation and Embryology Authority 1998 Seventh Annual Report & Accounts. London, The Stationery Office

Human Fertilisation and Embryology Authority 1999 Eighth Annual Report & Accounts. London, The Stationery Office

Imaizumi Y 1998 A comparative study of twinning and triplet rates in 17 countries, 1972–1996. Acta Genet Med Gemellol (Roma) 47(2):101–114

Ishii S, Tanaka K, Okai T et al 1994 Perinatal outcome of pregnancies following therapy of infertility. Nippon Sanka Fujinka Gakkai Zasshi. Acta Obstet Gynecol Jap 46(12):1305–1310

Kahn JA, von During V, Sunde A, Sordal T, Molne K 1993 The efficacy and efficiency of an in-vitro fertilization programme including embryo cryopreservation: A cohort study. Hum Reprod 8:247–252

Khastgir G, Abdalla H, Thomas A, Korea L, Latarche L, Studd J 1997 Oocyte donation in Turner's syndrome: an analysis of the factors in recipients with or without premature ovarian failure. Hum Reprod 12(2):279–285

Liao XH, de Crestecker L, Gemmell J, Lees A, McIlwaine G, Yates R 1997 The neonatal consequences and neonatal cost of reducing the number of embryos transferred following IVF. Scot Med J 42:76–78

Lerner-Geva L, Toren A, Chetrit A et al 2000 The risk of cancer among children of women who underwent in vitro fertilization. Cancer 88(12):2845–2847

Loft A, Petersen K, Erb K et al 1999 A Danish national cohort of 730 infants born after intracytoplasmic sperm injection (ICSI) 1994–1997. Hum Reprod 14:2143–2148

Mackenna A, Zegers-Hochild F, Fernandez EO, Fabres CV, Huidobro CA, Guadarrama AR 1992 Intrauterine insemination: critical analysis of a therapeutic procedure. Hum Reprod 7:351–354

Mannaerts B, De Leeuw R, Geelen J et al 1991 Comparative in vitro and in vivo studies on the biological characteristics of recombinant human follicle stimulating hormone. Endocrinology 129:2623–2630

Mardesic T, Muller P, Zetova L, Mikova M 1994 Faktory ovlivnujici vysledky in vitro fertilizace-1. Vliv veku. Cesk Gynekol 59(5):259–261

Matson PL, Browne J, Deakin R, Bellinge B 1999 The transfer of two embryos instead of three to reduce the risk of multiple pregnancy: a retrospective analysis. J Assisted Reprod Genet 16(1):1–5

Mercan R, Lanzendorf SE, Mayer J Jr, Nassar A, Muasher SJ, Oehninger S 1998 The outcome of clinical pregnancies following intracytoplasmic sperm injection is not affected by semen quality. Andrologia 30(2):91–95

Milki AA, Fisch JD, Behr B 1999 Two-blastocyst transfer has similar pregnancy rates and a decreased multiple gestation rate compared with three-blastocyst transfer. Fertil Steril 72(2):225–228

Murdoch A 1997 Triplets and embryo transfer policy. Hum Reprod 12 (natl suppl), J Brit Fertil Soc 2:88–92

Obasaju M, Kadam A, Sultan K, Fateh M, Munne S 1999 Sperm quality may adversely affect the chromosome constitution of embryos that result from intracytoplasmic sperm injection. Fertil Steril 72(6):1113–1115

Out HJ, Mannaerts BM, Driessen SG, Bennink HJ 1995 A prospective, randomised, assessor-blind multicentre study comparing recombinant and urinary follicle stimulating hormone (Puregon versus Metrodin) in in-vitro fertilization. Hum Reprod 10:2534–2540

Padilla SL, Garcia JE 1989 Effect of maternal age and number of in vitro fertilization procedures on pregnancy outcome. Fertil Steril 52(2):270–273

Parneix I, Jayot S, Verdaguer S, Discamps G, Audebert A, Emperaire JC 1995 Age et fertilite: apport des cocultures sur cellules endometriales. Contracept Fertil Sex 23(11):667–669

Peek JC, Godfrey B, Matthews CD 1984 Estimation of fertility and fecundity in women receiving artificial insemination by donor semen and in normal fertile women. Br J Obstet Gynaecol 91:1019–1024

Piette C, de-Mouzon J, Bachelot A, Spira A 1990 In-vitro fertilization: influence of women's age on pregnancy rates. Hum Reprod 5(1):56–59

Powers WF, Kiely JL 1994 The risks confronting twins: a national perspective. Am J Obstet Gynecol 170(2):456–461

Preutthipan S, Amso N, Curtis P, Shaw RW 1996 The influence of number of embryos transferred on pregnancy outcome in women undergoing in vitro fertilization and embryo transfer (IVF-ET). J Med Assoc Thailand 79(10):613–617

Prietl G, Engleberts U, Maslanka M, van-der-Ven HH, Krebs D 1998 Kumulative Schwangerschaftsraten Der Konventionellen In Vitro Fertilisation In Abhangigkeit Der Diagnose Und Des Alters Der Patientinnen: Ergebnisse Des Bonner Ivf-Programms. Geburt Frauenheil 58(8):433–439

Royal College of Obstetricians and Gynaecologists 1998a The Initial Management of the Infertile Couple. Evidence-based Guideline No 2. RCOG Press, London

Royal College of Obstetricians and Gynaecologists 1998b The Management of Infertility in Secondary Care. Evidence-based Guideline No 3. RCOG Press, London

Royal College of Obstetricians and Gynaecologists 1999 Guidelines for the Management of Infertility in Tertiary Care. Evidence-based Guideline No 6. RCOG Press, London

Scholtes MC, Behrend C, Dietzel-Dahmen J et al 1998 Chromosome aberrations in couples undergoing intracytoplasmic sperm injection: influence on the implantation and ongoing pregnancy rates. Fertil Steril 70(5):933–937

Sharif K, Elgendy M, Lashen H, Afnan M 1998 Age and basal follicle stimulating hormone as predictors of in vitro fertilisation outcome. Br J Obstet Gynaecol 105(1):107–112

Skupski DW, Nelson S, Kowalik A et al 1996 Multiple gestations from in vitro fertilization: successful implantation alone is not associated with subsequent pre-eclampsia. Am J Obstet Gynecol 175:1029–1032

Slotnick RN, Ortega JE 1996 Monoamniotic twinning and zona manipulation: A survey of U.S. IVF centers correlating zona manipulation and high risk twinning frequency. J Assisted Reprod Genet 13(5):381–385

Soliman S, Daya S, Collins J, Hughes EG 1994 The role of luteal phase support in infertility treatment: a meta-analysis of randomized trials. Fertil Steril 61(6):1068–1076

Staessen C, Janssenswillen C, van den Abbeel E, Devroey P, van Streitegham AC 1993 Avoidance of triplet pregnancies by elective transfer of two good quality embryos. Hum Reprod 8(10):1650–1653

Tallo CP, Vohr B, Oh W, Rubin LP, Seifer DB, Haning RV Jr 1995 Maternal and neonatal morbidity associated with in vitro fertilization. J Ped 127(5):794–800

Tasdemir M, Tasdemir I, Kodama H, Fukuda J, Tanaka T 1995 Two instead of three embryo transfer in in vitro fertilisation. Hum Reprod 10(8):2155–2158

Tan SL, Royston P, Campbell S et al 1992a Cumulative conception and livebirth rates after in-vitro fertilisation [see comments]. Lancet 339(8806):1390–1394. Comment in Lancet 340(8811):116

Tan SL, Doyle P, Campbell S et al 1992b Obstetric outcome of in vitro fertilization pregnancies compared with normally conceived pregnancies. A J Obstet Gynecol 167(3):778–784

Templeton AA, Morris JK 1998 Reducing the risk of multiple births by transfer of two embryos after in-vitro fertilization. N Engl J Med 339:573–577

Templeton AA, Morris JK, Parslow W 1996 Factors that affect outcome of in-vitro fertilisation treatment. Lancet 348(9039):1402–1406

Tough SC, Greene CA, Svenson LW, Belik J 2000 Effects of in vitro fertilisation on low birth weight, preterm delivery, and multiple birth. J Ped 136(5):618–622

Toren A, Sharon N, Mandel M et al 1995 Two embryonal cancers after in vitro fertilisation. Cancer 76(11):2372–2374

Toner JP, Flood JT 1993 Fertility after the age of 40. Obstet Gynecol Clin N Am 20(2):261–272

Tucker M, Kost HI, Massey JB 1991 How many IVF embryos to transfer. Lancet 337:1482

Tucker MJ, Morton PC, Wright G, Ingargiola PE, Jones AE, Sweitzer CL 1995 Factors affecting success with intracytoplasmic sperm injection. Reprod Fertil Dev 7(2):229–236

Van Balen F, Trimbos-Kemper TCM 1993 Long-term infertile couples: a study of their well-being. J Psychosom Obstet Gynaecol (special issue):53–60

Van Golde R, Boada M, Veiga A, Evers J, Geraedts J, Barri P 1999 A retrospective follow-up study on intracytoplasmic sperm injection. J Assisted Reprod Genet 16(5):227–232

Van Kooij RJ, Looman CW, Habbema JD, Dorland M, te-Velde ER 1996 Age-dependent decrease in embryo implantation rate after in vitro fertilization. Fertil Steril 66(5):769–775

Van Os HC, Jansen CAM 2000 The use of GnRH antagonist for COH as a second line strategy in IVF or ICSI. In: proceedings of the 16th annual meeting of the European Society of Human Reproduction and Embryology. Hum Reprod 15 (abstr Book 1):134(P-089)

Van Voorhis BJ, Syrop CH, Vincent RD Jr, Chestnut DH, Sparks AE, Chapler FK 1995 Tubal versus uterine transfer of cryopreserved embryos: a prospective randomised trial. Fertil Steril 63:578–583

Vardon D, Burban C, Collomb J, Stolla V, Emy R 1995 Spontaneous pregnancies in couples after failed or successful in vitro fertilization. J Gynecol Obstet Biol Reprod 24(8):811–815

Vauthier-Brouzes D, lefebvre G, Lesourd S, Gonzales J, Darbois Y 1994 How many embryos should be transferred in in vitro fertilization? A prospective randomised study. Fertil Steril 62(2):339–342

Wada I, Macnamee MC, Wick K, Bradfield JM, Brinsden PR 1994 Birth characteristics and perinatal outcome of babies conceived from cryopreserved embryos. Hum Reprod 9:543–546

Waterstone J, Parsons J, Bolton V 1991 Embryo transfer of two embryos. Lancet 337:975–976

Wennerholm UB, Albertsson Wiklund K et al 1998 Postnatal growth and health in children born after cryopreservation as embryos. Lancet 351:1085–1090

Wennerholm UB, Bergh C, Hamberger L et al 2000 Incidence of congenital malformations in children born after ICSI. Hum Reprod 15(4):944–948

Widra EA, Gindoff PR, Smotrich DB, Stillman RJ 1996 Achieving multiple-order embryo transfer identifies women over 40 years of age with improved in vitro fertilization outcome. Fertil Steril 65(1):103–108

Wisanto A, Bonduelle M, Camus M et al 1996 Obstetric outcome of 904 pregnancies after intracytoplasmic sperm injection. Hum Reprod 11(suppl 4):121–129

Wood C, McMaster R, Rennie G 1985 Factors influencing pregnancy rates following in vitro fertilization and embryo transfer. Fertil Steril 43:245–250

Yaron Y, Ochshorn Y, Amit A, Yovel I, Kogosowski A, Lessing JB 1996 Patients with Turner's syndrome may have an inherent endometrial abnormality affecting receptivity in oocyte donation. Fertil Steril 65(6):1249–1252

12

Prenatal diagnosis of fetal abnormalities

Charles H. Rodeck, Pranav P. Pandya

The contribution of the author of the equivalent chapter in the second edition, on which this chapter draws extensively, is gratefully acknowledged.

INTRODUCTION

The aims of prenatal screening for fetal abnormality are:

1. To reassure parents by reducing the likelihood of undiagnosed fetal abnormality
2. To ensure that parents have full information about their options if fetal abnormality is diagnosed
3. To prevent the birth of handicapped children
4. To enable couples at risk of inherited disease to have healthy children by diagnosis of abnormality and selective termination of pregnancy
5. Preparation of the parents for the birth of an abnormal child if an abnormality is detected
6. To enable more rational perinatal management
7. To identify correctly the need for intrauterine treatment.

In order to achieve these aims, certain criteria must be met; these will be dealt with in this chapter. The population at risk must be identified and appropriate tests performed after counselling. There are three main groups of conditions that can be diagnosed:

- Structural malformations
- Chromosomal abnormalities
- Genetic (Mendelian) diseases.

It is vital to understand that tests fall into two broad groups, screening and diagnostic. The critical factors in a screening test are the ability to discriminate between affected and unaffected individuals and this is expressed in terms of the detection rate (sensitivity) and the false-positive rate (I-specificity) (Table 12.1). Screening tests are not diagnostic: their objective is to enable selection of pregnancies to which diagnostic tests can be applied, enabling early detection of a disease or defects whose treatment is more effective when undertaken at an earlier point in time (Cuckle & Wald 1984). Patients who are classified as at increased risk following a

Table 12.1 Performance of a screening test

	Test positive	Test negative
Affected	True positive (TP)	False negative (FN)
Unaffected	False positive (FP)	True negative (TN)

Detection rate = TP/TP + FN
False-positive rate = FP/FP + TN
Positive predictive value = TP/TP + FP

positive screening test are subsequently offered a diagnostic test.

- *Detection rate* (or *sensitivity*) is the ability of a test to give a positive result in individuals who have the condition for which they are being screened.
- *False-positive rate* is the proportion of unaffected individuals yielding a positive result.
- *Specificity* is the ability of a test to give a negative result in individuals who do not have the condition being screened for. This is the equivalent of 1-false positive rate.

Sensitivity, specificity and false-positive rate are independent of the frequency of the condition.

- *Positive predictive value* is the likelihood that the condition is present given a positive result. The predictive value is dependent on the prevalence of the disorder. As the prevalence decreases, the proportion of individuals with a positive test result who actually have the condition will fall and the proportion falsely identified as being at risk will rise.

It is with the introduction of prenatal screening tests that prenatal diagnosis has become applicable to all pregnant women and is now a major part of antenatal care.

SCREENING FOR STRUCTURAL MALFORMATIONS: ULTRASOUND

Since Donald introduced ultrasound into obstetrics in the late 1950s vast improvements have been made in ultrasound technology.

The information obtained from antenatal obstetric ultrasound includes the following.

- Confirmation of fetal viability.
- Accurate dating of the pregnancy.
- Diagnosis of multiple pregnancies and the determination of chorionicity.
- Detection of fetal anomalies.
- Monitoring of fetal growth.
- Assessment of fetal well-being.
- Localisation of the placenta and its margins.
- Real-time continuous monitoring for invasive fetal procedures.
- Detection of uterine and adnexal abnormalities.

Routine use of ultrasound has become an integral part of obstetric practice in the UK in the last 10–15 years. Unfortunately, few randomised trials were undertaken to evaluate its clinical effectiveness before widespread introduction. Studies performed to date are inconclusive about the value of routine ultrasound examination.

The RADIUS study from the USA initially registered 55 744 pregnancies, of which only 15 530 were subsequently randomised to ultrasound at 15–22 weeks and 31–35 weeks or to scanning on clinical indication only (Ewigman et al 1993). Of concern is the large number (60%) of women who were excluded or ineligible. Most were excluded because they had a clinical reason for an ultrasound examination and the remainder were lost to follow-up or refused to participate. The authors concluded that amongst the randomised women the detection of congenital abnormalities had no effect on perinatal outcome and no significant effect on the frequency of termination of pregnancy for fetal anomalies. However, only 16% of fetal abnormalities were detected in the screened group (before 24 weeks), which may say more about the quality of scanning than the value of ultrasound itself. Compare this with the 60–80% of major and 35% of minor malformations detected in other studies on routine screening in low-risk pregnancies (Chitty et al 1991, Luck 1992).

A South African study also failed to demonstrate any effect of routine ultrasound on perinatal outcome (Geerts et al 1996). More abnormalities were detected in the screened group (four of nine) than in the group scanned if clinically indicated (one of three); however, there was no difference in the number of therapeutic terminations of pregnancy, one in each group.

A meta-analysis including four randomised trials concluded that routine ultrasound did not improve the outcome of pregnancy, except in the detection of fetal malformations (Bucher et al 1993). However, in the Helsinki Ultrasound Trial the detection rate was 41% and the perinatal mortality rate was significantly lower in women undergoing routine ultrasound screening, half of the reduction arising from termination of abnormal fetuses (Saari-Kemppainen et al 1990). It should be borne in mind that these studies were performed more than 10 years ago, when both understanding and technology was not as advanced as today.

Table 12.2 summarises the studies reporting the detection of fetal abnormalities before 24 weeks using routine ultrasound, including trials that were not randomised. The specificities of these studies are very similar (99.8 to 100%); however, the sensitivities vary considerably (from 21 to 85% in the descriptive studies, compared with 16.6–76.9% in the randomised studies. Reasons for such variations include the skill and experience of the sonographers, the gestational age at which screening is performed and the definition of abnormality. In addition, care needs to be taken when interpreting these studies because of the small number of patients recruited in some trials and the different objectives and screening policies.

The Cochrane review suggested that routine ultrasound in early pregnancy (less than 24 weeks) appears to enable better assessment of gestational age and thereby reduce rates of induction of labour for post-term pregnancy (odds ratio 0.61; 95% confidence interval 0.52–0.72), earlier detection of multiple pregnancies (twins undiagnosed at 26 weeks odds ratio 0.08; 95% confidence interval 0.04–0.16) and earlier detection of clinically unsuspected fetal malformation at a time when termination of pregnancy is possible. However, the benefits for other substantive outcomes are less clear

Table 12.2 Summary of studies reporting the detection of fetal abnormalities before 24 weeks using routine ultrasound

Study	Number of fetuses	Gestational age (weeks)	Prevalence of abnormality (%)	Sensitivity (%)	Specificity (%)	Termination of pregnancy (%)
Rosendahl & Kivinen 1989	9012	18	1.03	39.4	99.9	0.16
Saari-Kemppainen et al 1990	4691	16–20	0.43	36–76.9	99.8	0.23
Chitty et al 1991	8785	18–20	1.5	74.4	99.98	0.6
Shirley et al 1991	6412	19	1.4	60.7	99.98	0.45
Luck 1992	8844	19	1.9	85	99.9	0.28
Ewigman et al 1990	7617	15–22	2.46	16.6	–	0.11
Levi et al 1995	9392	16–20	2.45	41	99.9	?
Geerts et al 1996	496	18–24	1.8	44.4	–	0.2

(Neilson 2000). In addition, based on existing evidence, routine ultrasound after 24 weeks in low-risk or unselected populations does not confer benefit on mother or baby (Bricker & Neilson 2000).

Safety of ultrasound

There is no substantive evidence of adverse effects from obstetric ultrasound. However, few studies have formally evaluated this issue. A Norwegian study followed children to the age of 8–9 years and found no difference, except a possible association with non-right-handedness (Salvesen et al 1993). In an Australian study fetuses exposed to repeated ultrasound and Doppler examination tended to have slightly lower birthweights (Newnham et al 1993). Thus, continued vigilance and caution are essential.

The RCOG (1997) has made a number of recommendations about ultrasound (see Table 12.3) including:

1. Universal screening rather than selective scanning is the only reliable way to identify fetal abnormalities. The regime adopted will depend on financial resource and screening objectives (Grade A).
2. Screening for fetal abnormalities does reduce the contribution they make to perinatal mortality rates through the identification and termination of affected pregnancies (Grade A, Grade B).
3. On current evidence a scan undertaken between 18 and 20 weeks is the most effective available method to detect a wide range of fetal abnormalities (Grade B).
4. Although the formal signing of consent before a scan seems unnecessary, women should positively opt for the scan to be performed. Written and spoken information

should be available before the scan. Provision for adequate counselling and information giving should be an integral part of any screening programme (Grade C).
5. When an abnormality is detected a full discussion of its implications should ensue. The parents will benefit from discussion with a multidisciplinary group comprising paediatrician, geneticist and paediatric surgeon, in addition to the ultrasonographer and obstetrician (Grade C).
6. Ultrasound examinations should be conducted only by appropriately trained personnel. A routine screening examination should be conducted using an agreed protocol or checklist (Grade C).

Diagnosis of structural malformations

The diagnosis of fetal abnormalities is made in one of three ways:

1. By direct visualisation of a structural defect, for example the absence of the fetal skull vault in anencephaly.
2. By demonstrating disproportionate size or growth of a particular fetal part, for example, the short limbs in cases of dwarfism.
3. By recognition of the effect of an anomaly on an adjacent structure, for example the presence of posterior urethral valves which may be diagnosed by the consequent dilatation of the renal tract.

The RCOG has recommended a two-stage scan programme: an initial scan at booking and a second scan at or around 20 weeks' gestation (RCOG Working Party 2000). A minimum standard was set for the 20-week scan (Table 12.4).

If an abnormality is suspected on a routine ultrasound examination the patient should be referred to appropriately trained personnel for detailed ultrasound examination and further management as required. The value of identifying fetal abnormalities at this stage is that it offers parents options. The decision as to which line of management to adopt is often difficult and should be made with appropriate input from a multidisciplinary team, including a fetal medicine specialist, geneticist, neonatologist and paediatric surgeon. The parents should obviously be fully involved and give informed consent.

If a lethal abnormality is detected the parents may elect to terminate the pregnancy. For non-lethal abnormalities or in

Table 12.3 RCOG Classification of evidence

Grade A: *Very strong evidence* derived from randomised controlled trials or systematic reviews from randomised trials [A].

Grade B: *Fairly strong evidence* from non-randomised controlled trials, other robust experimental evidence or good observational studies [B].

Grade C: *More limited evidence* from observational studies with poorer methodology or case reports, or the evidence relies on consensus among professional groups [C].

Table 12.4 RCOG Standards for 20-week ultrasound scan

Gestational age
By measurement of biparietal diameter:
  head circumference
  femur length.

Fetal normality
Head shape and internal structures:
  midline echo
  cavum pellucidum
  cerebellum
  ventricular size at atrium (<10 mm)
Spine: longitudinal and transverse
Abdominal shape and content (at level of stomach)
Abdominal shape and content (at level of umbilicus)
Renal pelvis (anterior–posterior distance <5 mm)
Longitudinal axis–abdominal–thoracic appearance (diaphragm/bladder)
Thorax at level of 4-chamber cardiac view
Arms—three bones and hand (not counting fingers)
Legs—three bones and foot (not counting toes)
Optional—cardiac outflow tracts, face and lips

(The use of ultrasound markers to screen for aneuploidy is discussed on p. 179)

Table 12.5 The chances of a fetus having congenital heart disease, according to the congenital anomaly in the mother

Congenital anomaly	Approximate risk of recurrence (%)
Transposition of the great arteries	0
Tetralogy of Fallot	3
Atrial septal defect	10
Coarctation of the aorta	14
Aortic stenosis	15
Ventricular septal defect	16

Data from: Burn J et al (1998), with permission

situations where the parents choose to continue with the pregnancy, the couple have the opportunity to prepare themselves through discussions with health care personnel and self-help groups. In addition medical staff can ensure appropriate arrangements are made for the remaining pregnancy and delivery.

With the widespread use of ultrasound, pregnant women and their attendants are coming to expect to deliver babies free from any structural abnormalities. With increasing litigation against health care practitioners it is important to realise what can reasonably be expected in routine clinical practice. Only the main areas of ultrasound diagnosis are summarised below. For more extensive reviews the reader should consult Rodeck and Whittle (1999).

Cardiac abnormalities

Congenital heart disease is the most common severe congenital anomaly found in live-born infants, occurring in 4–12 per 1000 live births. Cardiac defects are the cause of approximately one-fifth of perinatal deaths due to congenital malformations and are a major cause of death from congenital anomalies in childhood. Families having a previously affected child, in the absence of a recognised genetic syndrome, have a 2–3% risk of recurrence in subsequent pregnancies. Mothers with congenital heart disease have an increased risk of delivering a child with a cardiac anomaly of up to 16%. The recurrence risk varies with the nature of the anomaly – see Table 12.5. There are a number of other conditions associated with an increased risk of cardiac anomaly including maternal diabetes mellitus and certain drugs e.g. phenytoin and lithium.

Screening for cardiac defects has been introduced on the basis of the four-chamber view (Fig. 12.1). The sensitivity of this test for the detection of severe congenital heart disease during a routine 18–20-week scan is approximately 26% (Tegnander et al 1996). This view is abnormal, showing major defects such as hypoplastic ventricles, atrioventricular canal defects and tricuspid atresia, although many moderate or minor lesions such as septal defects may be missed. Visualisation of the outflow tracts enables the diagnosis of ductal-dependent lesions such as transposition of the great vessels. Fetuses with such abnormalities benefit from delivery in a tertiary referral centre with immediate referral to paediatric cardiology and often to cardiac surgery. If visualisation of the outflow tracts is included in the four-chamber view, the detection of major anomalies may be as high as 50–80% (Achiron et al 1992).

There is considerable controversy regarding the significance of isolated echogenic intracardiac foci (golf balls). Recent evidence from an unselected population suggests that the prevalence at 18–23 weeks is 0.9% and that their detection does not suggest an increased risk for Down's syndrome in women who have a prior low risk based on fetal nuchal translucency or maternal serum screening (Thiliganathan et al 1999).

Extracardiac malformations are found in approximately 30% of fetuses with a cardiac anomaly and therefore detailed ultrasound examination of the rest of the fetus is essential if a

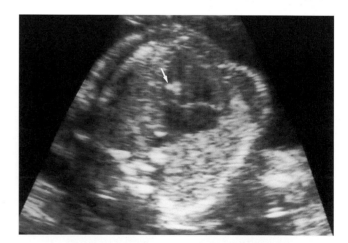

Fig. 12.1 Four-chamber view of the fetal heart, showing an echogenic intracardiac focus (arrow) in the left ventricle. (From Rodeck & Whittle 1999, with permission.)

cardiac defect is found. In addition, the incidence of chromosomal abnormalities is approximately 20% in fetuses with a cardiac anomaly and the option of fetal karyotyping should be discussed with the parents. In particular, microdeletions of the long arm of chromosome 22 (22q11.2) have been described in fetuses with conotruncal abnormalities (Wilson et al 1992).

Gastrointestinal anomalies

Bowel obstruction. Bowel obstruction above the ileum in the fetus usually results in polyhydramnios due to failure of absorption or regurgitation of swallowed amniotic fluid. Duodenal atresia presents with polyhydramnios and a characteristic 'double-bubble' sign (Fig. 12.2), which may not be apparent until the third trimester. These lesions are readily amenable to surgery but as only about 50% are isolated and up to one-third are associated with Down's syndrome, detailed ultrasound and karyotyping should be considered before a prognosis is given. Oesophageal atresia may be suspected because of the presence of polyhydramnios and the absence of a stomach bubble on repeated examinations. However, these signs are not present in the majority (95%) of cases due to the presence of a tracheo-oesophageal fistula. Large bowel obstruction, for example in Hirschsprung's disease or anal atresia, does not usually present until the third trimester and may be detected by the presence of distended loops of descending colon. Bowel perforation is associated with ascites and intra-abdominal calcification as a result of meconium peritonitis. Isolated hyperechogenicity of the gut may be secondary to cystic fibrosis, aneuploidy, fetal infection or fetal growth restriction, but it may also occur in normal fetuses.

Abdominal wall defects. Omphalocoeles are due to a midline defect in the abdominal wall, through which the peri-

toneal sac herniates, containing varying amounts of abdominal contents including small bowel and liver (Fig. 12.3). More severe abnormalities may also occur and are associated with midline defects involving the bladder (ectopia vesicae) or the thorax and heart (ectopia cordis). Approximately half of all fetuses with an omphalocoele will have associated cardiac or chromosome abnormalities. Karyotyping and detailed cardiac ultrasound are therefore important for assessment of the prognosis. As a general guideline the outlook for a fetus that has both an omphalocoele and a cardiac abnormality is poor, whereas if the omphalocoele is an isolated defect, surgical repair after birth carries an excellent prognosis, in the region of 90%. In most cases the optimal mode of delivery is vaginal birth in a tertiary referral centre with appropriate neonatology facilities, in particular paediatric surgery.

Gastroschisis used to be less common than omphalocoele, but its incidence is increasing in Western societies, which may in part be related to smoking and drug abuse. The insertion of the umbilical cord is intact and there are free loops of bowel in the amniotic cavity (Fig. 12.4). In about 95% of cases the anomaly is isolated, and there is no increased incidence of chromosomal abnormalities. Counselling of parents is best done in conjunction with a paediatric surgeon, but in general an encouraging prognosis can be given. The abdominal wall defect is usually small and the bowel can be readily replaced. The only caveat, however, is that the extruded small bowel does not have a peritoneal covering and may therefore become oedematous, matted and stenosed at the site of the extrusion. This may necessitate extensive resection of bowel with concomitant long-term intravenous feeding and malabsorption syndromes. To avoid this, induction of

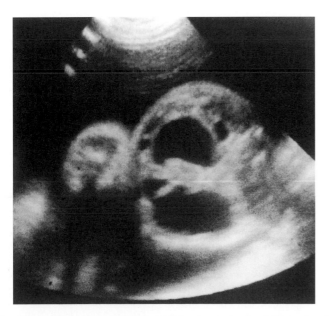

Fig. 12.2 Ultrasound appearance of duodenal atresia at 24 weeks of gestation—'double bubble'. (From Rodeck & Whittle 1999, with permission.)

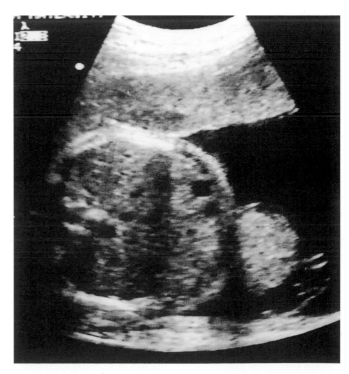

Fig. 12.3 Ultrasound appearance of an omphalocoele at 20 weeks' gestation. (From Rodeck & Whittle 1999, with permission.)

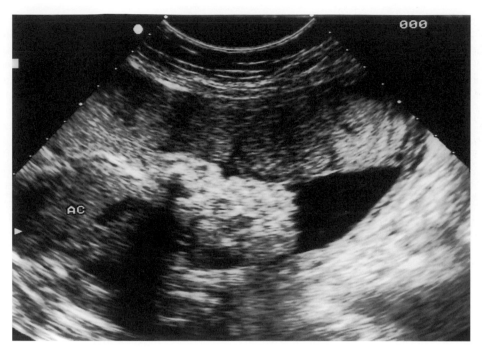

Fig. 12.4 Ultrasound appearance of a gastroschisis at 20 weeks' gestation. (From Rodeck & Whittle 1999, with permission.)

labour and early vaginal delivery are usually planned for 37 weeks.

Raised second trimester maternal serum alpha-fetoprotein is present in about two-thirds of all cases of omphalocoele and in almost all cases of gastroschisis.

Diaphragmatic hernia. Diaphragmatic hernia can be diagnosed by routine ultrasound in the second trimester. The findings vary, depending on the location of the hernia, and include the presence of the stomach on the same plane as the four-chamber view of the heart, mediastinal shift, presence of bowel in the thorax and the absence of the normal integrity of the diaphragm. In about 50% of affected fetuses there are associated chromosomal abnormalities, genetic syndromes or other structural defects. In those with isolated diaphragmatic hernia survival after postnatal surgery is about 60%; the remainder die from pulmonary hypoplasia and pulmonary hypertension. As yet there are no well recognised ultrasound findings to predict neonatal outcome.

Renal tract abnormalities

Normal fetal kidneys and bladder are clearly seen at the second trimester ultrasound examination. Major anomalies such as renal agenesis and lower urethral tract obstruction will be detected on a routine scan at 18–20 weeks due to the presence of severe oligohydramnios.

Polycystic kidneys. Polycystic disease of the kidneys is divided into infantile and adult types. The infantile variety shows an autosomal recessive pattern of inheritance and the gene for the disorder has been mapped to chromosome 6p21-cen. In utero, the expression of the disease is variable. Some fetuses will have sonographically normal kidneys and will present with renal failure in the second decade of life. At the other end of the spectrum, the fetus may present with anhy-

dramnios and enlarged echogenic kidneys in the second trimester. The cysts are microscopic and are therefore seen as echogenic enlarged kidneys on scan. Adult polycystic kidney disease is autosomal dominant which can present in utero with enlarged hyperechogenic kidneys. The diagnosis is aided by the fact that renal cysts are usually present in one of the parents.

Renal pelvic dilatation. The significance of mild pelvicalyceal dilatation (anteroposterior pelvic diameter exceeding 5 mm), found in about 2% of fetuses in the second trimester, is controversial (Fig. 12.5). As an isolated finding it may be physiological: however, it may also be the result of mild reflux or pelviureteric junction obstruction. Mild pyelectasis is considered a marker of chromosomal abnormality and the risk for trisomy 21 is about 1.5 times the maternal age-related risk (Snijders et al 1995b). If there is no antenatal progression, postnatal renal sonography is performed after the third day to establish whether the condition has resolved or progressed. If it has not resolved, the infant must be considered to be at an increased risk for urinary tract infections.

Craniospinal and central nervous system defects

Modern ultrasound has allowed detailed imaging with increased definition of craniospinal and central nervous system defects. However, the effect of specific anomalies on pregnancy outcome can be difficult to predict and therefore counselling the parents is often challenging. Both computed tomography (CT) and magnetic resonance imaging (MRI) are imaging modalities that can be used to delineate specific pathologies (Hubbard & Harty 2000).

Ventriculomegaly. Ventriculomegaly is diagnosed by elevated ratios of the widths of the anterior and posterior horns of the lateral ventricle to the hemispheric width in

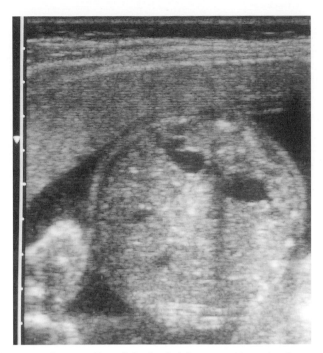

Fig. 12.5 Cross-section of the fetal abdomen at 23 weeks of gestation, showing mild bilateral renal pelvic dilatation. (From Rodeck & Whittle 1999, with permission.)

the transverse plane (Fig. 12.6). Ventriculomegaly does not usually increase the biparietal diameter or the head circumference measurement, but in hydrocephalus there is ventricular dilatation in conjunction with an enlarged head circumference. The level of obstruction to the passage of CSF is determined by examining the third and fourth ventricles and the aqueduct of Sylvius. Ventriculomegaly can be caused by a number of conditions including spina bifida or other CNS pathology, chromosomal abnormalities, congenital infection with cytomegalovirus or toxoplasmosis and genetic syndromes. Isolated ventriculomegaly is

uncommon, being found in approximately 20% of cases. The prognosis depends primarily on the cause of the ventriculomegaly and does not necessarily correlate with the severity of the condition. Approximately 80% of fetuses with isolated mild ventriculomegaly develop normally, while 50% of fetuses with mild ventriculomegaly and other congenital defects are developmentally impaired (Bromley et al 1991). Serial assessment is important to determine whether the condition is stable or progressive or has resolved spontaneously.

Holoprosencephaly is the presence of a single centrally placed cerebral ventricle and may be associated with midline abnormalities of the fetal face. It is a rare abnormality, occurring in about 1 in 16 000 births. When found in fetuses with multiple anomalies it is associated with trisomy 13 and, less commonly, trisomy 18, trisomy 21 and triploidy.

Choroid plexus cysts. While examining the fetal head, the cerebral ventricles should be further examined for the presence of cysts. Choroid plexus cysts (CPC) are detected in approximately 1% of mid-trimester scans as sonolucent areas within the echogenic choroids (Fig. 12.7). Controversy has centred on whether karyotyping should be offered routinely to all fetuses with CPCs, in view of the reported association with trisomy 18. The size, shape, laterality and persistence after 24 weeks are not helpful in predicting aneuploidy. Most CPCs are now believed to be benign structures which usually resolve by 24 weeks. Current opinion is that, if there are isolated CPCs on detailed anomaly scan, the risk of trisomy 18 is increased marginally (relative risk 1.5) over that from maternal age alone (Snijders et al 1994). Because very few babies with trisomy 18 survive long term, the risk to a normal pregnancy even of amniocentesis may not be considered justified.

Dandy Walker malformation. The Dandy Walker malformation is a rare anomaly which is manifest by cystic dilatation of the fourth ventricle, enlarged cisterna magna and absent or small cerebellar vermis. The Dandy Walker

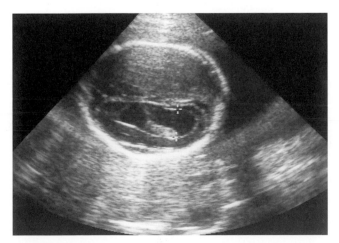

Fig. 12.6 Ultrasound appearance of moderate ventriculomegaly, in the absence of hydrocephalus (i.e. a head circumference within the normal range). (From Rodeck & Whittle 1999, with permission.)

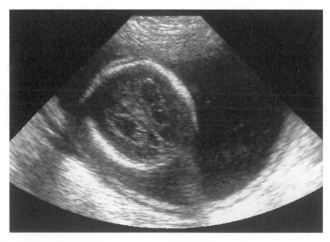

Fig. 12.7 Fetal head showing large bilateral choroid plexus cysts. (From Rodeck & Whittle 1999, with permission.)

malformation can be an isolated finding or it may be associated with chromosomal abnormalities, single-gene disorders or congenital infections (e.g. cytomegalovirus).

Microcephaly. Diagnosis of microcephaly by ultrasound should only be made in the presence of serial measurements of head circumference 3–4 standard deviations below the mean, so as to exclude growth restriction or incorrect dating. The diagnosis is frequently not possible before 24 weeks. The primary defect in microcephaly is in brain growth but, as brain growth determines head growth, the skull is also small. Microcephalic infants are nearly always severely abnormal intellectually. Amongst the better known causes for microcephaly are rubella infection in the first trimester, cytomegalovirus and toxoplasmosis infections, severe irradiation and maternal addiction to heroin. A few cases are associated with an autosomal mode of inheritance.

Neural tube defects. In the UK the birth prevalence of neural tube defect (NTD) in the absence of antenatal diagnosis and selective abortion is about 3–4 per 1000 live births. However, the prevalence in different communities has ranged from about 0.5 to 6 per 1000 births. This variation in birth prevalence in conjunction with a tenfold increase among women who have had an affected child suggests both environmental and genetic causes. Other known risk factors for NTDs include women with diabetes mellitus and use of certain anti-epileptic medication in the first trimester of pregnancy (e.g. sodium valproate and carbamazepine). It should be borne in mind that 95% of cases of NTD occur in women who have not had a previously affected pregnancy.

Anencephaly was the first fetal anomaly that was diagnosed with antenatal ultrasound and for which the pregnancy was terminated (Campbell et al 1972). The ultrasound diagnosis is straightforward as the cranial vault cannot be visualised in the standard view for biparietal diameter measurement. Encephalocoeles are rare lesions and constitute less than 1% of all NTD. They range in size from a small bony defect without brain tissue in the herniated meninges to a major vault defect in which there are large amounts of brain in the herniated sac, usually called exencephaly. Encephalocoeles may be occipital, parietal or frontal in origin although occipital encephalocoeles are by far the most common. They may be associated with Meckel–Gruber syndrome or autosomal recessive conditions.

The detection of open spina bifida is more complex. Figure 12.8 illustrates the abnormality seen in cases of spina bifida. The term spina bifida refers to the bony abnormality and Figure 12.9 illustrates the correct terminology for other abnormalities. In closed spina bifida the lesion is one in which neural tissue is completely covered by skin or a thick opaque membrane. This condition has a better prognosis than open NTD and may not be detected during routine screening, which is aimed at open NTD.

Screening for spina bifida has been greatly facilitated by two cranial signs found in almost all fetuses with myelomeningocoele. Scalloping of the frontal bones gives the head a lemon-shaped appearance, whereas the normally dumbbell-shaped cerebellum appears banana shaped (Nicolaides et al 1986) (Fig. 12.10). The latter results from

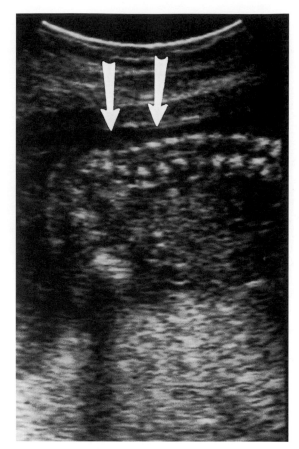

(a)

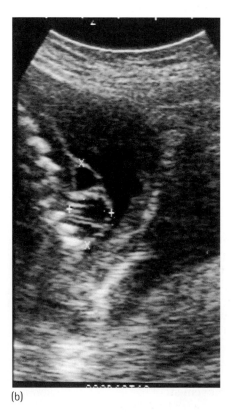

(b)

Fig. 12.8 Transverse view of the fetal spine. There is splaying of the lower thoracic vertebra with a meningocoele. (From Rodeck & Whittle 1999, with permission.)

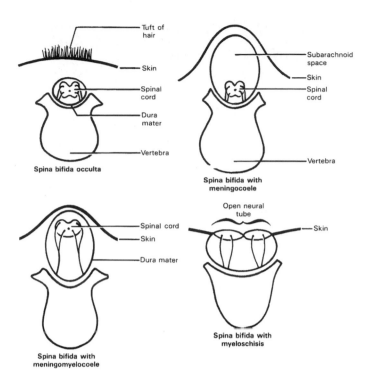

Fig. 12.9   Diagrams and terminology of different types of spina bifida.

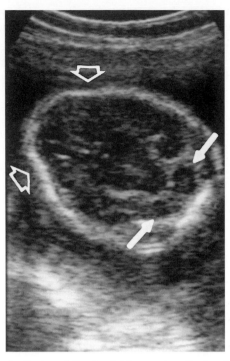

Fig. 12.10   Scalloping of the frontal bones gives the head a lemon-shaped appearance ('lemon' sign), whereas the normally dumbbell-shaped cerebellum appears banana shaped ('banana' sign). (From Rodeck & Whittle 1999, with permission.)

downward herniation of posterior fossa contents (Arnold-Chiari malformation) and the former from the subsequent reduction in intracranial volume.

The initial approach to screening for NTD comprised maternal serum AFP estimation at 16 weeks, with investigation of positive results (>2.5 MoM) by amniocentesis for amniotic fluid alpha-fetoprotein and acetylcholinesterase. However, only 88% of fetuses with anencephaly and 79% with myelomeningocoele were so identified (UK collaborative study 1982). Ultrasound became the preferred investigation for the screen-positive pregnancies in view of the parents' reluctance to terminate a pregnancy on the basis of amniotic fluid biochemistry alone. Although the accuracy of maternal serum alpha-fetoprotein versus ultrasound has not been addressed in comparative trials, reports indicate that the detection rates for myelomeningocoele of 80–100% with ultrasound exceed those with alpha-fetoprotein alone (Van den Hof et al 1990). Many centres have dispensed with alpha-fetoprotein screening for NTD, although others have retained it as a component of Down's syndrome serum screening. With few exceptions open spina bifida is now essentially an ultrasound diagnosis.

The severity of the neurological deficit is dependent upon the level of the spinal lesion: paralysis of the lower extremities and loss of bladder and bowel control are common. Individuals with an isolated sacral lesion may walk independently; an L5 lesion will result in paralysis of the muscles involving movement of the feet. Knee flexion and hip abduction is affected with L4 defects, requiring leg braces for ambulation. Patients with a defect extending to L2 usually require a wheelchair (McLaughlin & Shurtleff 1984).

It has been shown that about three-quarters of NTD can be prevented by folic acid supplementation before pregnancy (MRC Vitamin Study Research Group 1991). The UK Health Education Authority recommends that all women planning a pregnancy should be advised to take a daily 0.4 mg supplement of folic acid until the twelfth week of pregnancy and those women who have had a previously affected pregnancy are advised to take 4 or 5 mg folic acid.

Skeletal defects

Isolated malformations detected on routine ultrasound include kyphoscoliosis, hemivertebrae, limb reductions, sacral agenesis, polydactyly and flexion deformities. In addition over 100 distinct skeletal dysplasias are amenable to prenatal diagnosis, both by serial measurement of long bones and by detection of abnormal skeletal shape or mineralisation. However, the determination of the exact type of skeletal dysplasia is often difficult in the absence of a previous history, and requires detailed evaluation of hands and feet, thoracic dimensions, face and cranium, and measurement of all long bones.

Lethal forms of dwarfism (e.g. thanatophoric achondrogenesis) are often associated with early shortening of the limb bones, readily recognisable before 22 weeks of gestation. Non-lethal conditions (e.g. heterozygous achondroplasia) commonly result in slow growth of the long bones, which may not be apparent until the third trimester. Achondroplasia is inherited as an autosomal dominant condition. If it is suspected, amniocentesis can be performed for DNA testing on fibroblasts to detect or exclude the causative fibroblast growth factor (FGR3) receptor mutation known to cause achondroplasia (Bonaventure et al 1996).

In addition to dwarfism, hypomineralisation due to conditions such as achondrogenesis, hypophosphatasia and osteogenesis imperfecta can be recognised on ultrasound. Osteogenesis imperfecta is a heterogeneous group of collagen disorders with autosomal dominant, recessive and sporadic inheritances described. There is a wide clinical spectrum: in the most severe form multiple intrauterine fractures can be diagnosed, with short limbs and a soft deformed skull.

Soft-tissue abnormalities

Cleft lip, whether isolated or associated with cleft palate, can be detected by imaging the fetal face in coronal and transverse views. The diagnosis of an isolated cleft palate is extremely difficult and the lesion is usually detected only in those patients who have a previous history.

Cystic hygromata are developmental abnormalities of the lymphatic system. Prenatal diagnosis by ultrasonography is based on the demonstration of a bilateral, septated, cystic structure, located in the occipitocervical region. They may be associated with hydrops fetalis and fetal demise. The prevalence of chromosomal defects is high (46–90%) with Turner's syndrome accounting for the majority.

Hydrops fetalis is characterised by generalised skin oedema and pericardial, pleural, or ascitic effusions (Fig. 12.11). Hydrops is a non-specific finding in a wide variety of fetal, maternal and placental disorders, including fetomaternal blood group alloimmunisation (immune hydrops), chromosomal, cardiovascular, pulmonary, haematological, metabolic abnormalities and congenital infection, neoplasms and malformations of the placenta or umbilical cord (non-immune hydrops). Although in many instances the underlying cause may be determined by detailed ultrasound scanning including echocardiography, tests on maternal

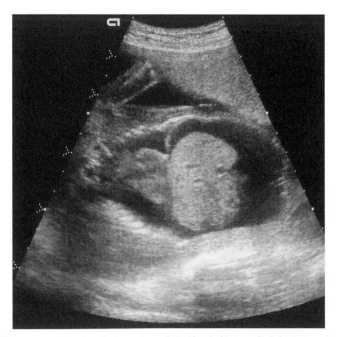

Fig. 12.11 Longitudinal section of the fetal chest and abdomen showing bilateral pleural effusions and ascites. (From Rodeck & Whittle 1999, with permission.)

blood and invasive fetal testing, in about 20–40% of cases the abnormality remains unexplained even after expert post-mortem examination. The overall mortality rate is high, ranging from 80 to 96% depending on the cause of the hydrops.

First-trimester fetal anomaly scanning

In addition to the improvement in the resolution of ultrasound machines, the development of transvaginal probes has made it possible to examine fetal anatomy in detail in the late first trimester. In some conditions, the sonographic features are similar to those described in the second and third trimesters, but in others there are characteristic sonographic features confined to the first trimester (Blaas & Eik-Nes 1999). At present most of the studies reported are from high-risk pregnancies. Economides found in a study of 1632 low-risk pregnancies that, of the fetal abnormalities diagnosed antenatally, 78% were diagnosed at 12–14 weeks (Economides & Braithwaite 1998). Larger studies are required to establish the clinical value of routine fetal anomaly scanning in the first trimester.

CHROMOSOME ABNORMALITIES

Human cytogenetics originated from the work of Tijo and Levan (1956) establishing that the normal diploid chromosome number was 46. Clinical cytogenetics is the study of chromosome structure and behaviour in relationship to clinical syndromes. Application of this knowledge for the diagnosis and screening of chromosome disease has been made possible by improvements in tissue culture, chromosome preparation, staining techniques to obtain banded chromosomes and advances in DNA technology including in situ hybridisation. Traditional chromosome analysis is performed on cells in metaphase after they have undergone hypotonic treatment, fixation and staining. Improvement in the banding techniques with in situ hybridisation using probes that paint entire chromosomes has enabled the diagnosis of small abnormalities (e.g. microdeletions) and is helpful in the assessment of structural rearrangements. In addition, in situ hybridisation is applicable to cells in interphase (i.e. uncultured cells) and this has enabled the rapid prenatal diagnosis of the major aneuploidies (21, 18, 13, X and Y) (Fig. 12.12).

Numerical chromosome abnormalities (aneuploidies)

Numerical chromosome abnormalities consist of monosomies (absence of one chromosome of a pair or of one sex chromosome) and trisomies (three copies of a specific chromosome). In triploidy, each chromosome in the complement is represented three times instead of two, the total chromosome number being 69. Most monosomies and trisomies are lethal early in pregnancy. Trisomies 21, 18, 13 and sex chromosome abnormalities are the most common aberrations found at birth (Fig. 12.13). Non-disjunction or anaphase lag are the

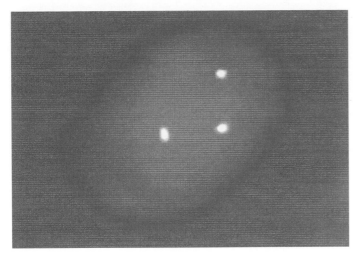

Fig. 12.12 Fluorescence *in-situ* hybridisation on interphase blood cells from a newborn child with trisomy 18. The hybridisation was performed with a locus-specific probe for chromosome 18. (From Rodeck & Whittle 1999, with permission.)

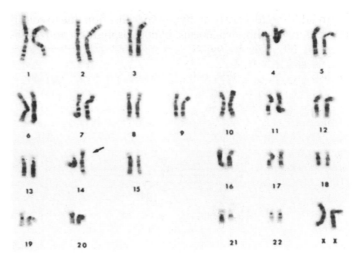

Fig. 12.14 G-banded karyotype of a patient with Down's syndrome with a Robertsian translocation between chromosomes 14 and 21, resulting in effective trisomy for chromosome 21.

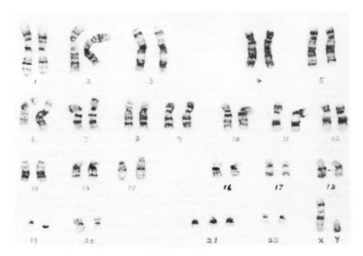

Fig. 12.13 G-banded karyotype of a male patient with Down's syndrome with standard trisomy 21.

mechanisms usually responsible for numerical abnormalities; they occur more frequently with advanced maternal age.

Structural chromosome abnormalities

A translocation involves transfer of genetic material between two chromosomes. As a consequence genetic material can be lost or gained, or simply exchanged. Translocations may therefore be unbalanced or balanced. Unbalanced translocations cause partial trisomies or monosomies of the involved chromosomes. Balanced translocations frequently involve the acrocentric chromosomes 13, 14, 15, 21 and 22 and are termed Robertsonian translocations (Fig. 12.14). If the balanced translocation involves chromosomes other than the acrocentric chromosomes it is termed reciprocal. Balanced translocations that are familial do not appear to have obvious clinical consequences to the individual but can result in

unbalanced translocations in the offspring. However, *de novo* balanced translocations may actually be submicroscopically unbalanced, resulting in congenital malformations. In a study based on 377 357 pregnancies undergoing amniocentesis, physical abnormalities associated with *de novo* chromosomal abnormalities were found in 6.1% of reciprocal translocations, 3.7% of Robertsonian translocations and 9.4% of inversions (Warburton 1991). The risk of mental handicap among carriers of *de novo* translocations is not known. However, among the mentally handicapped, the frequency of *de novo* translocations is two to three times higher than among clinically normal children.

The aneuploidies

Down's syndrome

J. Langdon Down (1866) made the observation of a subgroup of patients with particular facial features and mental handicap at the outpatient department of the London Hospital. In 1876 Fraser and Mitchell noted an association between Down's syndrome and advanced maternal age at the time of delivery. However, advanced maternal age could not be the only factor because in some cases there appeared to be a hereditary factor. Dizygotic twins were unequally, monozygotic twins equally, affected. The condition could be transmitted from mother to baby, and when more than one member of a family was affected the dependence on the mother's age was weakened. In the late 1950s it was demonstrated that an extra acrocentric chromosome was present in persons with Down's syndrome, resulting in a diploid chromosome number of 47 (Fig. 12.13). It is now known that Down's syndrome occurs when either the whole or a segment of the long arm of chromosome 21 is present in three copies instead of two. This can occur as a result of three separate mechanisms: non-disjunction (94% of cases), Robertsonian translocation (3.6%) and mosaicism (2.4%). The region that codes for most of the Down's syndrome phenotype is bands q22.2, q22.3 and the distal portion of band q21.1. This region determines the facial features, heart defects, mental retardation and probably the dermatoglyphic changes (Korenberg 1993).

If a fetus had a non-inherited form of Down's syndrome the risk in a subsequent pregnancy would be the maternal age-related risk plus an additive component of 0.75% (Snijders et al 1999). The risk to the offspring when the parent carries a translocation is about 12% if the mother is the carrier and 3% if the father is the carrier. However, carriers of a balanced 21:21 translocation cannot have a normal child; all will be either monosomic or trisomic for chromosome 21.

Natural history. Approximately 30% of Down's syndrome fetuses are miscarried between 12 weeks of gestation and term, while the estimated rate from 16 weeks to term is about 20% (Snijders et al 1995a). Infants with Down's syndrome are usually severely mentally handicapped and may have associated physical congenital abnormalities affecting the heart (about 35%), gastrointestinal tract, eyes and ears. About 20% die by the age of 5 years (mostly from cardiac disease), but over half are expected to survive into their 50s. The main burden of care arises from the fact that people with Down's syndrome are dependent on others and require considerable personal supervision throughout their lives. Most adults with Down's syndrome develop neurological changes in their brain typical of Alzheimer's disease. The amyloid polypeptide of Alzheimer's disease is coded by a gene on chromosome 21.

Trisomy 18 (Edward's syndrome)

Trisomy 18 is the second most common trisomy at birth, with a prevalence of 0.16 per 1000 live births. Approximately 85% of trisomy 18 fetuses that are alive at 12 weeks are destined to miscarry. Of live-born infants 50% die within 2 months; only 10% survive the first year and are usually severely mentally handicapped.

Trisomy 13 (Patau syndrome)

Trisomy 13 is a rare autosomal trisomy with a prevalence of 0.08 per 1000 live births. Approximately 80% of trisomy 13 fetuses that are alive at 12 weeks are destined to miscarry. Of live-born infants 70% die by 6 months; only 20% survive the first year, and these are usually severely mentally handicapped.

Triploidy

Polyploidy caused by fertilisation with multiple sperm or by failure of cell cleavage in the first mitotic division of the fertilised egg affects about 2% of recognised conceptions. Triploidy is highly lethal and is very rarely observed in live births. When the extra set of chromosomes is paternally derived triploidy is associated with a molar placenta and the pregnancy rarely persists beyond 20 weeks. When there is a double maternal chromosome contribution, the pregnancy may persist into the third trimester. The placenta is of normal consistency and the fetus demonstrates severe asymmetrical growth restriction.

Turner's syndrome

Turner's syndrome was initially described as a clinical entity with streak ovaries, stunted growth, webbing of the neck and cubitus valgus. In live births, the prevalence of Turner's syndrome is 0.2 per 1000 and the condition is not associated with increased postnatal mortality. Cognitive development is normal. In contrast to live births there is a high frequency of Turner's syndrome in spontaneous miscarriages and at prenatal diagnosis. Therefore the syndrome may have different phenotypes, some of which are associated with a high lethality at an early stage of pregnancy. These cases usually present with hydrops fetalis, cystic hygromata, cardiac abnormalities (in particular coarctation of the aorta) and horseshoe kidney.

Other sex chromosome defects

The main sex chromosome defects, other than Turner's syndrome, are 47,XXX, 47,XXY and 47,XYY. In infants with 47,XYY physical appearance, mental development and fertility are normal. However, compared with normal infants they have an increased incidence of mild impairments in language and reading, hyperactivity, impulsivity and a tendency for more aggressive behaviour. In Klinefelter syndrome (47,XXY) and in 47,XXX females mental retardation is unlikely and, although intelligence tends to be lower than that of siblings, there is a large individual variation. Adults with 47,XXY tend to be tall but their head circumference is generally reduced. In 47,XXX fertility is usually normal, whereas 47,XXY individuals are infertile. Adults with 47,XXY have increased susceptibility to autoimmune disease, malignancy and cerebrovascular disease.

Screening for chromosomal defects by maternal age

The risks for trisomies 21, 18 and 13 increase with advancing maternal age. Therefore screening is based on the detection of all three trisomies, even though trisomy 21 has the highest birth prevalence. The prevalence of trisomy 21 in the UK is estimated at 1.4 per 1000 live births. However, the incidence of chromosomal abnormalities in a fetus increases with maternal age and decreases with gestational age at birth.

This knowledge could not be utilised until prenatal diagnosis became available in the late 1960s (Valenti et al 1968). Amniocentesis is associated with a risk of miscarriage and this, in conjunction with the cost implications, meant that prenatal diagnosis was offered only to women aged 35 or above. This high-risk group constituted 5% of the pregnant population. As the average maternal age has increased, the oldest 5% of the pregnant population in the 1990s rose to age 37 years and above (OPCS 1994). Because finding for amniocentesis is limited, many health authorities therefore changed their age cutoff entitling women to free testing from 35 to 37 years. This meant that the average risk of Down's syndrome in the fetuses of women being tested increased.

Twenty years of screening by maternal age did not have a notable effect on the birth incidence of Down's syndrome

(Cuckle et al 1991). There are three major reasons for this failure:

- The great majority of affected babies are born to women under 35 years, by virtue of the much larger number of babies born to women of this age. Women who are 35 years and over contribute only 20–30% of the babies with Down's syndrome.
- The uptake of invasive fetal karyotyping in the high-risk group is generally less than 50%.
- An expected fall in the birth prevalence of Down's syndrome may have been reversed by the mean maternal age increasing from 26.1 years in 1970 to 29 years in 2000.

The poor performance of screening for Down's syndrome on the basis of advanced maternal age is now universally accepted and this has necessitated the introduction of newer screening policies.

Screening for chromosomal defects by serum biochemistry

Second trimester

In 1984 Merkatz retrospectively analysed the maternal serum alpha-fetoprotein (AFP) in 44 pregnancies diagnosed following amniocentesis as having Down's syndrome, and noted that the AFP was low in affected pregnancies (Merkatz et al 1984). Subsequently, Bogart found elevated levels of human chorionic gonadotrophin (hCG) in second-trimester maternal serum from Down's syndrome pregnancies (Bogart et al 1987). Low levels of unconjugated oestriol (uE₃) in maternal serum were found in association with Down's syndrome pregnancies by Canick et al (1988). The reason for these biochemical changes is not yet understood, but it may relate to functional immaturity, producing a delay in the normal gestational rise or fall.

In 1988, Wald analysed maternal serum samples at 16 weeks of gestation from 77 Down's syndrome pregnancies and 385 normal controls (Wald et al 1988). Screening for Down's syndrome by maternal age alone would have identified 30% of affected pregnancies for a 5% invasive testing rate; however, with the addition of maternal serum AFP, uE₃ and hCG tests the detection rate would be 35%, 41% and 48% respectively for the same false-positive rate (5%). When all metabolites were combined, in conjunction with maternal age, the detection increased to 59% (Wald et al 1988).

Subsequently other serum markers including free α-hCG, free β-hCG, inhibin A and neutrophil alkaline phosphatase have been found to be associated with Down's syndrome (Wald et al 1997). However, the most effective combination of serum markers still remains contentious. Screening performance varies according to the choice of markers used and whether ultrasound is used to estimate gestational age. The optimal gestation appears to be at 15–18 weeks, although screening can be performed up to 22 weeks. In addition to maternal age and the serum markers other factors need to be taken into account, including maternal weight, the presence of type 1 diabetes, multiple pregnancy,

ethnic origin, previous Down's syndrome pregnancy, smoking and vaginal bleeding. On the basis of results from prospective screening studies (demonstration projects) it appears that for a screen-positive rate of 5% the detection rate for Down's syndrome after revision of gestation by ultrasound is about 60% and is similar for the combination of maternal age with AFP, uE₃ and hCG, and that of maternal age with AFP and β-hCG (Wald et al 1997). The estimated detection rate for screening by maternal age and the quadruple test (AFP, uE₃, hCG and inhibin A) is about 76%, with a 5% screen-positive rate (Wald et al 1997). However, these predictions have not so far been established in a prospective screening study.

Analysis of performance in different age groups has shown a detection rate of about 40% in women under the age of 37 years and 70% in women who are 37 years or over. In the prospective screening studies the overall uptake of screening was about 80%, uptake of amniocentesis in screen-positive women was about 80% and acceptance of termination about 90% (Wald et al 1997).

Maternal serum markers and adverse pregnancy outcome

Pregnancies associated with abnormal maternal serum levels of AFP, hCG and uE₃ are associated with adverse pregnancy outcome. In addition to chromosomal abnormalities and structural defects, the pregnancy is also at an increased risk of miscarriage, intrauterine growth restriction, pre-eclampsia, preterm delivery, stillbirth and placental complications (Table 12.6). Once a high-risk pregnancy has been identified, it should be managed by Doppler examination of the uterine arteries at 20–24 weeks, serial ultrasound to assess fetal growth velocity and timely intervention (Jauniaux et al 1996). Unfortunately, there is little evidence to suggest that increased surveillance with currently available methods will improve pregnancy outcome.

First trimester

Since the 1990s the emphasis of biochemical markers has moved to the first trimester of pregnancy. Two markers, pregnancy-associated plasma protein-A (PAPP-A), which is lower in Down's syndrome, and β-hCG (which is elevated), are particularly useful. It is estimated that the combination of these markers with maternal age would identify about 60% of Down's syndrome pregnancies for a screen-positive rate of 5% (Wald & Hackshaw 1997), which is similar to that with second-trimester biochemical screening.

Risks of other aneuploidies

The primary purpose of serum screening is the detection of Down's syndrome. Results that are diametrically opposite (raised AFP and low hCG) to Down's syndrome or show very low levels of the biochemical markers may be suggestive of an increased risk of trisomy 18. There is some evidence that specific trisomy 18 screening detects 45% of trisomy 18 fetuses for a 0.5% false-positive rate (Reynolds 1997). No data are available on the performance of serum screening for other chromosomal abnormalities.

Table 12.6 Maternal serum markers and adverse pregnancy outcome

Serum marker	Increased (≥ 2.5 MoM)	Decreased (≤ 0.75 MoM)
Alpha-fetoprotein	Triploidy (or low)	Trisomy 21
	Neural tube defects	Trisomy 18
	Anterior abdominal wall defects	Triploidy (or high)
	Congenital nephrosis	Turner's syndrome
	Miscarriage	
	Pre-eclampsia	
	Intrauterine growth restriction	
	Preterm labour	
	Stillbirth	
Human chorionic gonadotrophin	Trisomy 21	Trisomy 18
	Triploidy (or low)	Triploidy (or high)
	Turner's syndrome (or low)	Turner's syndrome (or low)
	Miscarriage	
	Placental abnormalities including placental abruption and placenta praevia	
	Pregnancy-induced hypertension	
	Preterm delivery	
	Stillbirth	
	Multiple pregnancy	
Unconjugated oestriol		Trisomy 21
		Trisomy 18
		Triploidy
		Turner's syndrome
		Miscarriage
		Intrauterine growth restriction
		Stillbirth
		Placental sulphatase deficiency
		Congenital ichthyosis

Screening for chromosomal defects by ultrasonography

Second and third trimesters

Most fetuses with major chromosomal defects have either external or internal abnormalities that can be recognised by detailed ultrasonographic examination. Several studies have reported on the prevalence of chromosomal defects for a wide range of anatomical and biometrical abnormalities detected by ultrasound examination during the second and third trimesters of pregnancy (Benacerraf et al 1987, Nicolaides et al 1992). The studies were mostly from referral centres and therefore the patients examined were pre-selected. Consequently, no conclusions can be drawn from these studies as to the true prevalence of chromosomal defects for a given fetal abnormality in the general population. In reality, if many of the subtle deviations from normality ('soft markers') are taken as an indication for fetal karyotyping the

invasive testing rate would increase by at least 5%. Despite these limitations, the data are useful because they draw attention to the types of chromosomal defects that can be expected with any given abnormality or group of abnormalities (Table 12.7).

In cases where a lethal anomaly or an anomaly associated with severe handicap (e.g. holoprosencephaly, severe hydrops) is found, fetal karyotyping may help to determine the cause and the risk of recurrence. In addition, in cases where the defect is potentially amenable to intrauterine or postnatal surgery (e.g. pleural effusion, diaphragmatic hernia), it may be logical to exclude an underlying chromosomal abnormality. However, following the detection of a 'soft marker' (e.g. choroid plexus cysts, mild hydronephrosis) it is important to perform a detailed ultrasound examination to exclude additional anomalies. The risk of fetal aneuploidy rises with increasing number of sonographic defects detected (Nicolaides et al 1992). The adjusted risk for fetal aneuploidy should be based on the maternal age and the presence of single or multiple markers, as well as the type of marker or anomaly (Snijders et al 1996, Nyberg et al 1998). If no defects are found on detailed ultrasound examination the maternal age-related risk for Down's syndrome is reduced by about half. This is based on the assumption that approximately 50% of fetuses with Down's syndrome will have an anomaly or marker detectable by detailed ultrasound. Thus, for example, if a woman has a Down's syndrome risk for her fetus of 1 in 250 by serum screening, the risk will be 1 in 500 after a normal anomaly scan.

Abnormalities detected by ultrasound in common chromosomal defects

Many of the more common chromosomal abnormalities are associated with structural abnormalities, which are amenable to prenatal detection with ultrasound (Table 12.7). Studies from tertiary referral centres have found that 33–55% of fetuses with trisomy 21, 77–100% of fetuses with trisomy 18 and nearly all fetuses with trisomy 13 have defects detectable by detailed ultrasound examination (Ogle 2000). Unfortunately, there is little information from studies in low-risk populations. In the UK, in two studies of routine second-trimester ultrasound examination where detection of chromosomal abnormalities was reported, 26% of fetuses with an abnormal karyotype (four of 24 cases with trisomy 21, all four fetuses with trisomy 18 and one of two fetuses with trisomy 13) were detected (Chitty et al 1991, Shirley et al 1991).

Trisomy 21. This is associated with brachycephaly, mild ventriculomegaly, flattening of the face, nuchal oedema, atrioventricular septal defects, duodenal atresia and echogenic bowel, mild hydronephrosis, shortening of the limbs, sandal gap and clinodactyly or mid-phalanx hypoplasia of the fifth finger.

Trisomy 18. The sonographic anomalies associated with trisomy 18 include fetal growth restriction, strawberry-shaped head, choroid plexus cysts, absent corpus callosum, enlarged cisterna magna, facial cleft, micrognathia, nuchal oedema, heart defects, diaphragmatic hernia, oesophageal atresia, exomphalos, renal defects, myelomeningocoele,

Table 12.7   Abnormalities detected by ultrasound in common chromosomal defects

Fetal abnormality	Trisomy 21	Trisomy 18	Trisomy 13	Triploidy	Turner's syndrome
Skull/brain:					
Strawberry-shaped head	–	+++	–	–	–
Brachycephaly	++	++	++	+	++
Microcephaly	–	+	++	–	+
Ventriculomegaly	++	++	+	++	–
Holoprosencephaly	–	+	+++	–	–
Choroid plexus cysts	+	++	+	–	–
Absent corpus callosum	–	+	–	–	–
Posterior fossa cyst	+	++	++	+	–
Enlarged cisterna magna	+	++	++	–	–
Face/neck:					
Facial cleft	+	+	+++	+	–
Micrognathia	+	+++	+	+++	–
Nuchal oedema	+++	+	++	+	+
Cystic hygromata	+	+	–	–	+++
Chest:					
Diaphragmatic hernia	–	+	+	–	–
Cardiac abnormality	++	+++	+++	++	+++
Echogenic chordae tendeni	++	–	+	–	–
Abdomen:					
Exomphalos	–	++	+	–	–
Duodenal atresia	+	–	+	–	–
Absent stomach	+	++	+	+	–
Echogenic bowel	++	++	–	–	–
Mild hydronephrosis	++	++	++	+	+
Other renal abnormalities	+	++	++	+	+
Other:					
Hydrops	++	+	+	+	+++
Small for gestational age	++	+++	+++	+++	+++
Relatively short femur	++	++	+	+++	+++
Abnormal hands/feet	++	+++	+++	+++	+
Talipes	+	++	+	+	–

+++ = Common association; ++ = less common; + = uncommon; – no association.

growth retardation and shortening of the limbs, radial aplasia, overlapping fingers and talipes.

Trisomy 13.   The common defects include holoprosencephaly and associated facial abnormalities (facial cleft, severe hypotelorism, cyclopia and proboscis) microcephaly, cardiac and renal abnormalities (often enlarged and echogenic kidneys), exomphalos and postaxial polydactyly.

First trimester

With improved technology it has become feasible to examine the fetal anatomy in the first trimester of pregnancy. In particular, at 10–14 weeks of gestation there is a subcutaneous collection of fluid in the fetal nuchal region that can be visualised by ultrasonography as nuchal translucency (NT) (Fig. 12.15) (Szabo & Gellen 1990). Since the 1990s a series of studies have reported that increased NT is associated with chromosomal defects and a wide range of fetal abnormalities and genetic syndromes.

Studies from high-risk pregnancies (e.g. women undergo-

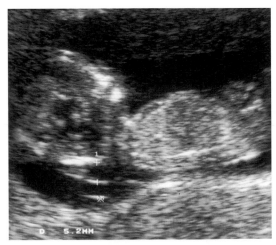

Fig. 12.15   Ultrasound picture of a 12-week fetus demonstrating increased nuchal translucency. (From Rodeck & Whittle 1999, with permission.)

ing fetal karyotyping for advanced maternal age) reported a mean prevalence of chromosomal defects of 29% (range 11–88%) (Pandya 1999) in fetuses with increased NT. In an unselected population of 20 804 pregnancies, the risk for fetal trisomies (21, 18 and 13) was derived by multiplying the maternal age-related risk by a likelihood ratio, which depended on the degree of deviation in NT from the normal median for crown–rump length (Pandya et al 1995). The detection rate was 77% for trisomy 21, and 78% for the other chromosomal defects, with a false-positive rate of 5%. The same observers found similar detection and false-positive rates in a multicentre screening study that examined a total of 100 311 pregnancies (Snijders et al 1998). The only other study with sufficient numbers to allow assessment of effectiveness of screening by nuchal translucency is that of Taipale et al, with 10 010 pregnancies. The sensitivity of screening at 10–14 weeks was 66% for a screen-positive rate of 0.9 (Taipale et al 1997). There is, however, considerable variation in the detection rate reported in different series in routine screening, from 29 to 91% (Pandya 1999).

Recent interest has focused on the combination of fetal NT and maternal serum biochemistry at 10–14 weeks of gestation. Two studies examining the potential value of combining maternal age, fetal NT, maternal β-hCG and PAPP-A have estimated that the sensitivity would be 80–90% for a screen-positive rate of 5% (Spencer et al 1999). Combining first-trimester and second-trimester screening (integrated screening) appears to improve the detection rate for a lower false-positive rate (94% for 5% or 85% for 1%) (Wald et al 1999). Confirmation of these figures is awaited in prospective studies.

Screening for Down's syndrome – which tests to use

It is widely accepted that maternal age alone has a low sensitivity and is no longer sufficient as a screening test alone. The introduction of second-trimester serum screening was a major advance in screening for Down's syndrome. It is a test

Table 12.8 Screening tests for Down's syndrome

Screening test	Advantages	Disadvantages
Maternal age	Simple, cheap	Low sensitivity
Nuchal translucency at 10–14 weeks	Early association with structural anomalies and genetic syndromes. Applicable in multiple pregnancies	Possible detection of fetuses that will miscarry spontaneously
Serum screening at 15–20 weeks	Screening for neural tube and anterior abdominal wall defects. Assessment of placental function	Second-trimester termination of pregnancy. Not applicable to multiple pregnancies
Anomaly ultrasound at 18–20 weeks	Detection of structural anomalies	Late. Poor sensitivity in routine practice

that can be applied to all pregnant women and achieves detection rates far superior to maternal age alone. However, second-trimester screening is unattractive to many women because of the late stage at which Down's syndrome is identified, when termination of pregnancy is less acceptable and more traumatic. This disadvantage also applies to the ultrasound examination at 18–20 weeks. However, ultrasound at this gestation has more value than just the detection of markers of chromosomal abnormality.

Screening in the first trimester has many theoretical advantages and is clearly the most acceptable time in pregnancy to perform screening. At present this optimally entails the measurement of fetal nuchal translucency in conjunction with β-hCG and PAPP-A. However, the role of NT in screening for chromosomal abnormalities is contentious. The major concern is that increased NT may detect fetuses that are destined to miscarry in any case, thus increasing intervention and cost unnecessarily. From a study involving over 100 000 pregnancies it would appear that, even after taking into account for the spontaneous loss of fetuses with Down's syn-

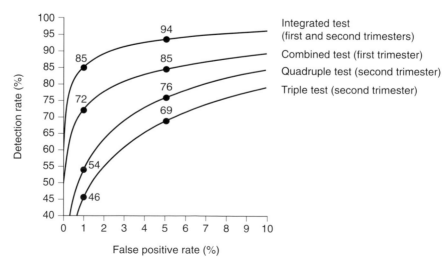

Fig. 12.16 Receiver operator curve for various screening tests for Down's syndrome.

drome, the detection rate for trisomy 21 was 78% (Snijders et al 1998).

However, earlier is not always better. It is important that parents do not feel rushed. The two-stage integrated test (e.g. 12 and 15 weeks) gives parents some time to assimilate information, allows spontaneous losses to occur naturally and thus avoids the need to make a decision about whether to terminate or not (Wald et al 1999). If the false-positive rate is kept down to 1–2% there will be fewer invasive tests and losses of healthy fetuses as well as considerable savings (Fig. 12.16). Crucially, this screening protocol must be linked to a rapid 48-hour diagnostic test on amniotic fluid such as FISH or PCR (see below) to capitalise on the advantage of early diagnosis, and to the prompt availability of surgical termination at 15–16 weeks.

Ultimately the decisions that parents make are based on intensely personal values. Some place a premium on early diagnosis enabling them to have the option of early termination of pregnancy. Others may decide that termination is not an option and may wish to wait to undergo either further screening tests or prenatal diagnosis in the second or third trimester to allow appropriate management of labour and referral to a tertiary paediatric unit. The role of those involved in antenatal care is to provide objective information and support to enable the parents to make their own choice.

Counselling

Counselling of patients is an integral part of any screening procedure. Women must be well informed before embarking on a screening programme; it is unethical if they are not. If a new screening test is introduced without adequate assessment and training of the relevant health care workers, many problems will arise. In addition to adequate information regarding the meaning of false-positive and negative results, those involved must have a mechanism whereby they can rapidly and sympathetically pass results of screening tests on to the patient, with a set protocol for managing those pregnancies with a positive screen result.

Management of a patient with an increased risk of fetal abnormality

A firm diagnosis of chromosomal abnormality can be made only by an invasive test to examine the fetal chromosomes. Women who are considered at increased risk should therefore be offered fetal karyotyping by invasive testing. Offering a second separate screening test (serum screening or anomaly ultrasound examination) to women who are screen positive can result in false reassurance (i.e. false negatives) and in an increased invasive testing rate (Kadir & Economides 1997).

GENETIC (MENDELIAN) DISORDERS

Inborn errors of metabolism

These disorders comprise conditions varying from slight deviations from the normal pattern to those incompatible with life. The inborn errors of metabolism are single-gene defects inherited according to Mendelian patterns. They are usually autosomal recessive or X linked. More than 5000 human disorders are caused by a single gene mutation (McKusick 1994). Mostly the defective gene product concerns an enzyme, but coenzymes, hormones, receptor and structural proteins are also involved. The primary metabolic defect has been established in about 400 disorders. Prenatal diagnosis is available for more than 200 inborn errors of metabolism, mostly by testing for the primary enzyme defect, sometimes by the demonstration of accumulating metabolites and increasingly by the detection of gene mutations. Tests are constantly being developed and refined, and it is important to seek advice from a genetics centre about the nature and availability of relevant investigations.

In most cases the realisation that a pregnancy is at risk will usually come from the recognition that a previous child of the parents was affected. Only in some conditions such as thalassaemia, where screening of the at-risk population is well established, can a couple be identified as at high risk of having an affected pregnancy before conception occurs.

Clearly it is preferable for maximum information to be available as soon as possible after an affected child is born, to allow full counselling of the parents and relatives before further pregnancies occur. A precise diagnosis may be difficult, either due to the overlapping clinical manifestations of different defects or due to the heterogeneity of individual metabolic defects. This needs to be borne in mind when undertaking prenatal diagnosis, which often relies upon assessing enzyme activity. In a homozygous affected individual enzyme activity is usually very low or absent. However, there may be overlap of enzyme activity between a heterozygous (carrier) fetus and homozygous (affected) fetus, and care must be taken. The standard techniques for diagnosing inborn errors of metabolism involve enzyme or metabolite analysis in amniotic fluid, cultured or uncultured chorionic villi or fetal fibroblasts (amniocytes). In a small number of cases the affected protein is not expressed in fibroblasts and a fetal liver biopsy (e.g. ornithine carbamyl transferase deficiency) or skin biopsy (e.g. junctional epidermolysis bullosa) may be more suitable. However, the molecular basis of many of these disorders has now been identified, so that DNA analysis of chorionic villi is preferred.

The list of inborn errors of metabolism for which prenatal diagnosis is suitable is long and constantly increasing (Kleijer 1999). *Online Mendelian Inheritance in Man (OMIM)* is an excellent database on the Internet (www3.ncbi.nlm.nih.gov/Omim/), providing up-to-date referenced information on genetic disorders.

Screening for inborn errors of metabolism

Population screening permits those who are carriers of the disease to adjust to the potential problems before embarking on pregnancy, which reduces anxiety and psychological morbidity. Screening of Ashkenazi Jews, of whom one in 30 is a carrier for Tay–Sachs disease, has been possible for over 20 years. This screening initially relied upon measurement of reduced enzyme activity of hexoaminidase A. Screening projects were introduced in the USA in 1970, and couples at risk were offered prenatal diagnosis and termination if the pregnancy was affected. By 1986 there had been an estimated fall of 70–85% in the incidence of babies being born with the disease (Chapple 1992).

Cystic fibrosis (CF) is the most common life-shortening Mendelian disorder found in children and in young adults of White European descent, with a birth prevalence of about 1 in 2500. Since the identification of the mutant gene responsible for cystic fibrosis on the long arm of chromosome 7, screening for carrier status has been possible, with an estimated heterozygote frequency of 1 in 22 (Brock 1996). However, it is not possible to screen for all the numerous cystic fibrosis alleles (over 600), and screening would therefore not identify all carriers. If prenatal diagnosis were performed in those identified to be at risk of the most common mutation (ΔF 508), found in 70–85% of CF chromosomes, up to a third of affected fetuses would be missed. Although this may be viewed as an insufficient detection rate to warrant population screening, many investigators suggest that the ability to reduce the birth incidence by two-thirds is a powerful argument for carefully constructed pilot trials.

Cascade screening, where the relatives of an affected individual are screened, offers a much more reliable pickup of carriers because the specific alleles involved are known. It is also the method of screening adopted in many of the much less common inborn errors of metabolism, although it obviously misses those at risk without an affected child. The most appropriate method of screening for CF has still not been established.

Haemoglobinopathies

The haemoglobinopathies are a diverse group of autosomal recessive disorders characterised either by the synthesis of a structurally abnormal globin chain (the haemoblobin variants) or the reduced synthesis of one or more globin chains (the thalassaemias). As a group they are the most common single-gene disorders in the world and are found at high frequencies in many populations as a result of positive selection pressure due to *Falciparum* malaria. Individuals with the carrier state are easily identifiable. Carrier screening enables parents to have informed choice, permitting appropriate counselling and prenatal diagnosis. The most important disorders for which prenatal diagnosis is considered are the α-thalassaemias, β-thalassaemias, sickle-cell anaemia and various compound heterozygous states that result in clinically significant disease.

For a detailed account of the haemoglobipathies, the reader shoulder consult Chapter 20.

Diagnosis

The prenatal diagnosis of haemoglobinopathies was introduced in 1974 by fetal blood sampling (FBS) and measuring globin chain synthesis at 18–23 weeks of gestation. With the advent of DNA technology, in particular the polymerase chain reaction (PCR), FBS was replaced by the analysis of fetal DNA, first obtained from amniotic fluid and later by chorionic villus sampling (CVS).

Invasive prenatal diagnosis has inherent risks to the fetus. Therefore non-invasive techniques are currently being evaluated. Prenatal diagnosis for haemoglobinopathies was performed on cervical mucus cells retrieved by aspiration from pregnant mothers at 10–12 weeks of gestation before CVS. A concordance between the results was observed in four of the six pregnancies tested. In addition, Cheung et al (1996) demonstrated the isolation of fetal nucleated red cells from the maternal circulation and the successful determination of the fetal globin genotypes in two pregnancies at risk for sickle cell anaemia and β-thalassaemia. This was the first example of the use of fetal cells in maternal blood for the non-invasive diagnosis of a single-gene disorder in pregnancy. However, further evaluation is required before introduction into routine clinical practice.

INVASIVE PROCEDURES

A number of techniques are available for the prenatal diagnosis of fetal disorders, including amniocentesis, CVS, fetal blood and tissue sampling and fetal endoscopy. The selection of the technique is dependent predominantly on the gestation of the pregnancy and the tissue sample required. Invasive procedures are also used in fetal therapy, for example fetal blood transfusion and intrauterine shunting. A prerequisite for any prenatal diagnosis programme is that the parents are accurately counselled before any procedure.

Counselling

No patient should undergo an invasive procedure without detailed counselling and informed consent. The counselling in certain conditions may be performed before the pregnancy, but in most cases it occurs during pregnancy. The parents should have access to written information and consultation with the appropriate specialists, including an obstetrician, a geneticist and a paediatrician. An interpreter should be present if English is not the parents' first language. Counselling should be non-directive, avoiding influencing or dictating the parents' decision and allowing them a sense of control over the pregnancy. More than one session may be required and couples should have the opportunity to go away to think about and discuss the problem. The parents should be given knowledge of the following areas.

- The disease or abnormality being investigated.
- The prognosis.
- The risk of occurrence and recurrence.
- The nature of the procedure, its risks and success rate.
- The possibility of other tests or options, including having nothing done.
- The diagnostic accuracy, and time taken for the result to be available.
- Termination of pregnancy, methods and complications.
- What to do in the event of complications.

Amniocentesis

Amniocentesis was first reported in the 1880s as a technique for amniotic fluid drainage in cases of polyhydramnios. Steele and Breg (1966) demonstrated the feasibility of karyotyping amniotic fluid cells, and trisomy 21 was first detected prenatally by Valenti (Valenti et al 1965). In the 1960s and early to mid 1970s amniocentesis was performed blindly without the use of ultrasound (amniocentesis should now be performed only with continuous ultrasound guidance). This technique has been adapted for more complex procedures including percutaneous fetal blood sampling, fetal catheterisation and fetoscopy (Rodeck 1980).

Technique

At 15 weeks' gestation the amniotic fluid volume is about 150–200 ml and the uterus can be reached transabdominally without major risks of traversing the bladder or bowel. After first scanning to confirm viability, gestational age, placental site and liquor volume, the skin is cleansed with antiseptic. Using aseptic technique, the ultrasound transducer is held in one hand while the needle is inserted into a pool of amniotic fluid, avoiding the placenta and fetus, under continuous ultrasound visualisation (Fig. 12.17). The needle most commonly used is a 22-gauge disposable spinal needle with a stylet. Once in place, the stylet is removed, a syringe attached to the hub of the needle and a small quantity of fluid aspirated. The fluid should be clear and a pale straw colour: if it is bloodstained, the initial sample must be discarded and a second syringe attached. A volume of 20 ml of fluid is then aspirated, watching for colour change all the time. Once the sample has been collected, the needle is withdrawn and the mother shown the fetal heart movement for reassurance. It is essential that the sample is placed in a sterile container labelled with the mother's name, age and hospital number or address, and that the mother checks the labelling with a member of staff. Anti-D-gammaglobulin should then be administered if the mother is rhesus negative. Following the procedure, many women prefer to rest for 20–30 minutes before going home and are advised to limit activity for 24–48 hours, although this is not of proven value.

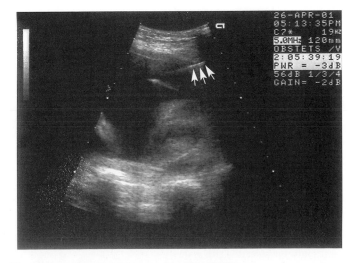

Fig. 12.17 Ultrasound image of amniocentesis.

Indications

In addition to fetal karyotyping and measurement of bilirubin (OD at 450 nm) in rhesus disease, the advent of new molecular biological techniques, including PCR and FISH, has increased the number of amniocenteses performed and reduced the need for fetal blood sampling with its inherent risks.

Risk of procedure

All invasive procedures carry a risk of pregnancy loss, by inducing miscarriage, preterm labour or intrauterine fetal death. The loss of a pregnancy may be due to bleeding, infection or preterm rupture of the membranes. The true risk of any invasive procedure used in prenatal diagnosis is difficult to establish, because the exact causation of pregnancy loss cannot always be established. Every pregnancy has a background rate of loss which is increased in pregnancies complicated by fetal abnormalities, whether structural, karyotypic, growth restriction or metabolic. Although a miscarriage within a few days of a procedure might be assumed to be a direct result of the procedure, it is much more difficult to be certain if the loss occurs 4 or more weeks later.

All operators learning a procedure should receive expert tuition, and ideally have the opportunity to develop their expertise on pregnancies undergoing termination. The Royal College of Obstetricians and Gynecologists has recommended that at least 30 procedures should be performed under direct supervision before the operator is deemed competent and that the operator should perform a minimum of 20 procedures each year. Careful audit of an individual centre's figures is essential to be able to assess the local risk of a procedure.

The only randomised controlled trial of amniocentesis has been performed in Denmark (Tabor et al 1986). In this study 4606 low-risk, healthy women aged 25–34 years old were randomly allocated at 14–20 weeks of gestation to amniocentesis or ultrasound examination alone. The total fetal loss rate in the patients undergoing amniocentesis was 1% higher than in the controls. There were significant associations between spontaneous fetal loss and puncture of the placenta, high maternal serum alpha-fetoprotein and discolored amniotic fluid. The Danish study also reported that amniocentesis was associated with an increased risk of respiratory distress syndrome (relative risk 2.1) and pneumonia in neonates (relative risk 2.9). Although some studies have reported an increased incidence of talipes and dislocation of the hip in the amniocentesis group (Medical Research Council 1978), this was not confirmed by the Danish study.

Cell culture and karyotype analysis generally takes 12–21 days following amniocentesis. With the use of FISH, results for chromosomes X, Y, 21, 18 and 13 are available from uncultured amniocytes within 48 hours. Approximately 0.5% of amniotic cell cultures fail to grow and maternal cell contamination leads to diagnostic difficulty in about 0.2%. Mosaicism occurs in 0.2% of amniotic fluid cultures and of these is confirmed in the fetus in 60% of cases. At present amniocentesis before 15 weeks of gestation needs further evaluation and should not be performed unless in the setting of a clinical trial.

Chorionic villus sampling

This was first attempted in the late 1960s by hysteroscopy (Hahnemann & Mohr 1968), but the technique was associated with low success in both sampling and karyotyping and was abandoned in favour of amniocentesis. In the 1970s the desire for early diagnosis led to the revival of chorionic villus sampling (CVS), which was initially carried out by aspiration via a cannula that was introduced blindly into the uterus through the cervix. The demonstration that villi could be used for gene analysis led to the development of further sampling methods. Ultrasound-guided insertion of transcervical catheters became the most widely used technique (Rodeck et al 1983). Curved biopsy forceps can be used similarly and their use is very successful (Fig. 12.18). Transabdominal CVS is now more widely used (Smidt-Jensen & Hahnemann 1984) (Fig. 12.19); its main advantage is that it can be used from the end of the first trimester to term, whereas transcervical CVS has a limit of 10–13 weeks. In the second and third trimester CVS (placental biopsy) can be performed for fetal karyotyping and DNA analysis in situations where amniocentesis or fetal blood sampling are considered inappropriate—e.g. anhydramnios.

The advantages of CVS are summarised in Table 12.9. Clearly the most important, particularly from the patient's point of view, is the possibility of first-trimester diagnosis. Chorionic villi provide two types of material (trophoblast and mesenchymal core) for examination of the fetal karyotype. The trophoblast cells in the villi are dividing rapidly and it is possible to obtain a direct karyotype result in 24–48 hours without the need for culture. However, direct preparations provide fewer metaphase spreads of poorer quality than those obtained from cultured cells. This limitation has resulted in some chromosomal rearrangements being undetected in direct analyses. Although the speed of obtaining a result from a direct preparation cannot be denied, many laboratories use

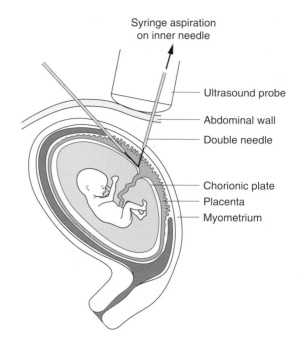

Fig. 12.19 Transabdominal needle aspiration of chorionic villi under ultrasound guidance.

cultures of the mesenchymal core as their primary technique, even though the results take about 2 weeks, considering the result to be more reliable.

Another disadvantage of CVS is confined placental mosaicism, which occurs in approximately 1% of cases. This is a condition where aneuploidy (mostly mosaic) may be confined to extraembryonic or extrafetal tissues while the fetus has a normal chromosomal constitution. It is more common in direct preparations than in cell culture. Confirmation of aneuploidy in the fetus should be detected by fetal blood

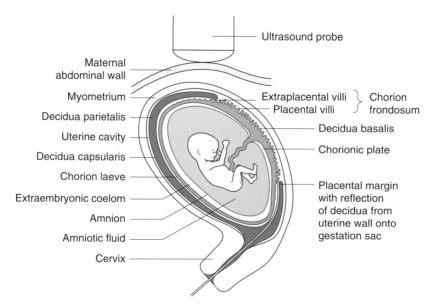

Fig. 12.18 Transcervical passage of biopsy forceps into the placental site under ultrasound guidance.

Table 12.9   Advantages of chorion villus biopsy

1. Enables first-trimester fetal diagnosis, i.e. early reassurance or early termination; avoidance of long delay and late termination
2. Villi are a good source of DNA
3. Villi are (nearly always) genetically, chromosomally and biochemically identical to the fetus
4. Villi can be sampled without perforating the membranes or fetus

sampling or amniocentesis. Confined placental mosaicism may be associated with intrauterine growth restriction and thus affect pregnancy outcome.

Indications

The indications for CVS are given in Table 12.10. Chorionic villi are an excellent source of DNA, supplying sufficient amounts for most molecular genetic techniques without prior culture.

Techniques

Before the procedure, the mother should be scanned to confirm viability, gestation and placental site. The preferred route can then be chosen.

All CVS is performed under continuous ultrasound guidance. For the transcervical approach, the woman lies on a couch in a modified lithotomy position (a colposcopy couch is ideal). After cleansing of the vulval area with antiseptic, a sterile bivalve speculum is introduced into the vagina and the cervix visualised. The cervix is then cleansed meticulously with antiseptic. The ultrasonographer or operator will then scan transabdominally to visualise the cervical canal, uterus and placental site. Either an aspiration catheter or biopsy for-

Table 12.10   Indications for chorion villus biopsy

DNA analysis
  Haemoglobinopathies—sickle cell disease, alpha-thalassaemia, most beta-thalassaemias
  Most haemophilias—A and B
  Duchenne muscular dystrophy (not all families)
  Cystic fibrosis (not all families)
  Alpha$_1$-antitrypsin deficiency
Chromosome abnormalities
Inborn errors of metabolism

ceps are then gently introduced through the cervix and guided into the placental tissue, from where a sample of villi is collected. Although there is some evidence to support the use of curved forceps for transcervical chorionic villus sampling (which is a technique that is very easy to learn), it is not strong enough to recommend a change in practice for clinicians who have become familiar with use of aspiration cannulas (Alfirevic 2000). No more than two passes should be attempted. The material obtained should be examined under a microscope to confirm the presence of villi, to allow removal of decidua if any is present and an assessment of the quantity obtained.

For transabdominal CVS, the patient lies supine on a couch and the preparation is similar to that for amniocentesis. However, many operators prefer to administer local unaesthetic into the skin and subcutaneous tissues before taking the sample. Under continuous ultrasound guidance, the chosen needle (single needle, double needle or forceps) is introduced into the placenta. The amniotic cavity should not be entered.

The route chosen depends on gestation, operator preference and site of the placenta. Under 12 weeks' gestation, many operators choose the transcervical route if the placenta is posterior and the transabdominal route for an anterior placenta.

Risks of procedure

Since the introduction of the current techniques there has been concern that the pregnancy losses after CVS are greater than after amniocentesis. Four randomised studies have compared the rate of fetal loss following first-trimester CVS with that of amniocentesis at 16 weeks of gestation (Table 12.11).

The result have demonstrated that in centres experienced in both procedures fetal loss is comparable with either technique (Firth et al 1991, CEMAT Group 1998). In the Medical Research Council study there was a significant increase in pregnancy loss following CVS, probably because many centres participated, some with little experience in CVS (MRC Working Party 1991). This is contentious and, unlike second-trimester amniocentesis, no randomised trial has been performed comparing CVS versus ultrasound alone in a low-risk population. In the UK CVS is used predominantly for those women at high risk of an affected pregnancy (i.e. those with single-gene defects where the risk of recurrence is 1:2 or 1:4) and in this group CVS has replaced amniocentesis and FBS.

Table 12.11   Total fetal loss rate in four randomised studies comparing first-trimester chorion villus sampling with second-trimester amniocentesis

Study	No. of samples	Fetal loss rate (%)	
		CVS	Amniocentesis
Canadian Collaborative CVS-Amniocentesis Clinical Trial Group 1989	2787	7.6	7.1
Smidt-Jensen et al 1992	3079	6.3	7.0
Ammala & Salonen 1995	800	6.3	6.4
MRC Working Party 1991	3248	14.0*	9.0

* $P < 0.01$

Three prospective studies to date have compared early amniocentesis (10–14 weeks) either with chorionic villus sampling (CVS) or with second-trimester amniocentesis. Both the Danish (Sundberg et al 1997) and Canadian (CEMAT Group 1998) studies found a significantly higher rate of talipes equinovarus after early amniocentesis than after CVS or second-trimester amniocentesis and the risk of pregnancy loss after early amniocentesis was higher in both the English (Nicolaides et al 1994) (4.9% v 2.1%) and Canadian (7.6% v 5.9%) studies.

In 1991 severe transverse limb abnormalities, micrognathia and microglossia were reported in five of 289 pregnancies in which single-needle transabdominal CVS had been performed at less than 9.5 weeks of gestation (Firth et al 1991). Subsequently, analysis of 75 cases demonstrated a strong association between the severity of the defect and the gestation at CVS (Firth et al 1994): median gestation at CVS was 8 weeks for those with amputation of the whole limb and 10 weeks for those with defects affecting the terminal phalanges. The background incidence of terminal transverse limb defects is about 1.8 per 10 000 live births, and the incidence following early CVS is estimated at one in 200–1000 cases. The limb reduction defects reported may be related to the trauma of the technique resulting in fetomaternal haemorrhage, release of vasoactive peptides or emboli (Rodeck 1993). Therefore CVS should be performed only after 10 weeks' gestation, by appropriately trained operators and as traumatically as possible. At present, if fetal karyotyping or DNA analysis is required in the first trimester of pregnancy CVS is the procedure of choice.

Fetal blood sampling

Fetal blood sampling (FBS) is a technique that permits direct vascular access to the fetus for diagnostic and therapeutic purposes. When a pure sample can be obtained, fetal blood provides the opportunity for numerous analyses, as do blood samples in postnatal medicine. Not only can lymphocytes be cultured for a rapid karyotyping, the result often being available in 48–72 hours, but also the full range of haematological, biochemical, pharmacological and immunological investigations can be performed.

Ultrasound-guided FBS

The first large series of ultrasound-guided FBS came from France, where the high incidence of toxoplasmosis was the stimulus for the development of a simple method for obtaining pure fetal blood (Daffos et al 1983). Most of the procedures performed today take blood from the placental insertion of the umbilical cord, although alternative sites include a free loop of cord, abdominal insertion, intrahepatic vein or fetal heart.

Technique

Fetal blood sampling is easiest to perform at 20–28 weeks' gestation. Before 20 weeks, it may be difficult to visualise the cord insertion, and there appears to be a higher risk of pregnancy loss. After 28 weeks, as the fetus increases in size, it may obscure the cord insertion and alternative sites may be more appropriate.

Indications

The indications for FBS, and therefore the frequency of the procedure are declining: in general, DNA analysis of fetal tissue obtained by CVS or amniocentesis has replaced FBS. Improvements in the non-invasive assessment of intrauterine growth restriction and fetal anaemia with Doppler blood flow studies have further reduced the need for FBS (Mari et al 2000). The main indications for FBS are now the assessment of potential anaemia or thrombocytopaenia. In the assessment of fetal hydrops, FBS remains invaluable in the investigation of the underlying cause. The groups of disorders that can be investigated with fetal blood sampling are shown in Table 12.12.

Risks of procedure

Operator technique and experience are obviously important factors that must be taken into account. The risk of pregnancy loss following ultrasound-guided FBS varies according the indication for the procedure—from 1% in normal fetuses to 9% in pregnancies affected by growth restriction and 13% in cases where multiple fetal anomalies are seen on ultrasound (Antsaklis et al 1998). The advantages of a rapid and reliable result of investigations by FBS must be balanced against an increased risk of losing the pregnancy.

Other sampling techniques

Aspiration of fluid collections, such as fetal urine from a dilated bladder or a pleural effusion, can easily be performed

Table 12.12 Indications for fetal blood sampling

Prenatal diagnosis
    Cytogenetic studies: failed amniocentesis, mosaicism in chorion or amniotic fluid
    Genetic disease amenable to DNA diagnosis
Fetal assessment
    Red-cell alloimmunisation: haematocrit, haemoglobin, transfusion
    Hydrops fetalis: karyotyping, haematology, virology
    Viral infections: PCR, IgM, haematology
    Platelet alloimmunisation: haematology, transfusion

Table 12.13 Summary of prenatal invasive procedures

Invasive procedure	Advantages	Disadvantages
Chorionic villus sampling	Early gestation. Rapid results—direct preparation. High DNA content for analysis	Increased risk of miscarriage. Confined placental mosaicism
Amniocentesis	Technically easy	Second-trimester termination
Fetal blood sampling	Rapid results. Suitable for haematology, immunology and biochemistry	Increased risk of fetal loss. Replaced by DNA analysis of chorionic villi

under ultrasound guidance. Assessment of the biochemistry of fetal urine is useful in the management of obstructive uropathy, and a raised white cell count in pleural fluid suggests the diagnosis of chylothorax. In addition fetal tissues including skin, liver and muscle can be taken for the diagnosis of specific disorders such as epidermolysis bullosa lethalis and ornithine carbamyl transferase deficiency.

MINIMALLY INVASIVE AND NON-INVASIVE TECHNIQUES

Transcervical flushing

In the early 1970s, studies examining the feasibility of isolating exfoliated placental cells from the cervical mucus using cotton swabs reported contradictory results. Recent studies have confirmed the presence of fetal cells in the endocervical canal and the possibility of performing *in vitro* cultures (Rodeck et al 1995). The technique of obtaining these samples varies from intrauterine lavage to aspiration of endocervical mucus. The former procedure is more invasive and may be associated with a higher risk of miscarriage.

Fetal cells can be obtained from endocervical mucus in approximately 50–70% of cases (Adinolfi et al 1995), although the result may be unreliable (Overton et al 1996). The initial sample obtained contains a mixture of both fetal and maternal cells and methods for separation and purification before analysis are not yet available. The safety of this test and the feasibility of producing reliable results remain to be established.

Detection of fetal cells in the maternal circulation

During the last 30 years extensive research has aimed at the development of a non-invasive method for prenatal diagnosis based on the isolation and examination of fetal cells found in the maternal circulation. A variety of nucleated fetal cells have been demonstrated in the maternal circulation, including erythrocytes, lymphocytes and trophoblasts. It is now believed that about one in 1 000 000 nucleated cells in maternal blood are fetal. Although complete separation of fetal from maternal cells is not yet possible, the proportion of fetal cells can be enriched by such techniques as magnetic cell sorting or fluorescence-activated cell sorting after attachment of magnetically labelled or fluorescent antibodies onto specific fetal cell-surface markers (Simpson & Elias 1994, Bianchi 1997).

The resulting sample is unsuitable for traditional cytogenetic analysis because it is still highly contaminated with maternal cells. With the use of chromosome specific DNA probes and fluorescent *in situ* hybridisation (FISH), it is possible to suspect fetal trisomy by the presence of three-signal nuclei in some of the cells of the maternal blood enriched for fetal cells. However, there is an overlap in the percentage of three-signal nuclei between normal and affected pregnancies, and it is therefore unlikely that this test will replace invasive testing in the near future—although it may provide another method of screening (Al-Mufti et al 1999). A possible clinical application of fetal cells in the maternal circulation is the pre-

diction of the fetal rhesus type when the mother is homozygous for the absence of RhD (Rh negative) and the father is heterozygous. The fetus has a 50% risk of being RhD positive and hence affected. In a study by Lo eight of the ten women carrying a RhD-positive fetus showed a RhD signal following PCR (Lo et al 1993). However, as fetal DNA has been found in maternal plasma, this may provide an easier and more direct way of rhesus genotyping the fetus.

NEW MOLECULAR ANALYTICAL TECHNIQUES

The last 20 years have seen major technological advances in molecular biology. Using techniques such as Southern blotting, PCR and FISH, many individual genes or specific mutations can be detected, permitting more sophisticated diagnosis of inherited disorders. All the modern techniques have applications that are expanding rapidly, and it is difficult to keep up to date with current advances. Referral to a genetics centre for advice concerning current diagnostic techniques permits the clinician to optimise the prenatal diagnosis service for every mother at risk.

Southern blotting

Southern blotting involves the cleavage of chromosomal DNA at specific sites using DNA nucleases of bacterial origin followed by gel electrophoretic separation of fragments and is used in the analysis of DNA from complex genomes.

Polymerase chain reaction

The PCR amplifies specific DNA or RNA fragments many millionfold, allowing further investigation (Saiki et al 1985). Once the sequence of nucleotides is known for a region of DNA strand either side of the area to be studied, complementary oligonucleotides and a polymerase are added to single-stranded DNA, which permits replication and therefore doubling of the DNA. This process is repeated up to 30 times until sufficient DNA is available. It requires very high-quality control to avoid contamination, which will also be amplified. PCR permits the identification of specific DNA sequences of gene mutations and allows the amplification of tiny quantities of DNA (a few cell nuclei) from sources as diverse as Egyptian mummies and the Guthrie spots from neonates. The need for only a small amount of starting template (e.g. a single cell) is the great advantage of PCR in modern prenatal diagnosis, and brings the possibility of prenatal diagnosis of inherited disorders being performed on a single cell taken from an embryo before transfer after IVF (preimplantation diagnosis) (Harper & Delhanty 1999).

Fluorescence *in situ* hybridisation

FISH allows the detection and localisation of specific DNA sequences directly in interphase (uncultured, non-dividing cells) or metaphase. It allows the rapid prenatal diagnosis of major aneuploidies and is useful in the analysis of intricate chromosome complements (e.g. translocations, insertions,

191

deletions and microdeletions). Under appropriate examination conditions, the presence of the probe in the nuclei of the cells confirms that the DNA sequence is present in the chromosomes.

The advantage of interphase FISH is that it is faster (results available in 24–48 hours) because cell culture is not needed, and it requires fewer cells than conventional cytogenetics. This may be of particular relevance in prenatal diagnosis following the ultrasound detection of fetal anomalies or abnormal serum screening. Traditional cytogenetic analysis of amniotic fluid would take 2–3 weeks and the alternative of FBS is associated with an increased risk of fetal loss. The disadvantage of interphase FISH is that it would fail to detect structural rearrangements or mosaics. However, it may identify up to 80% of clinically relevant chromosomal abnormalities (i.e. aneuploidies for chromosomes 21, 18, 13, X and Y) (Whiteman & Klinger 1991).

At present, cells are sent for routine cytogenetic analysis with cell culture in addition to FISH, which incurs additional expense.

Improvements in FISH technology include multicolour probes allowing the simultaneous detection of up to 24 chromosomes combined with automated analysis based on digital imaging microscopy.

Quantitative fluorescent multiplex PCR (QF–PCR)

This technique has been developed for the rapid detection of sex and autosomal aneuploides, enabling results to be available within 24 hours (Pertl et al 1997). The technique uses highly polymorphic small tandem repeat markers, which allows distinction between normal and trisomic DNA. In the future it is hoped that QF-PCR will cover the entire chromosomal complement but at present conventional cytogenetic analysis is still required to detect other chromosomal disorders.

Comparative genomic hybridisation

Comparative genomic hybridisation is a technique in which test DNA from a sample is compared with reference DNA (duManoir et al 1993). The test and reference DNA are labelled with two different colours (e.g. reference red and test green) in equal amounts. The hybridised metaphases are analysed by digital image microscopy and specific computer software, which measures ratios between colour intensities along the chromosomes. Where test and reference DNA are present in equal amounts the colour will be the result of the equimolar mixture; deletions and duplications will be detected by red or green fluorescence.

THE ORGANISATION OF PRENATAL DIAGNOSIS SERVICES

All obstetricians and midwives involved in antenatal care should have some knowledge of the conditions that can be diagnosed prenatally, how diagnosis is made and where the relevant investigations can be performed. However, the sophistication of the techniques involved means that expertise is generally concentrated in regional referral centres for fetal medicine and genetics. Referral across normal administrative boundaries must be smooth and swift, as delays in achieving prenatal diagnosis may deny a couple the opportunity of terminating an affected pregnancy, with the attendant problems. Referral centres must have counsellors trained in prenatal diagnosis and bereavement care. There should ideally be a dedicated perinatal pathology service.

Patient support groups are extremely valuable, and exist for mutual support of families affected by a variety of inherited disorders. In addition, organisations exist for the support of those parents who have lost affected pregnancies. Obstetricians should be aware of these groups, and enable their patients to contact the relevant ones.

Termination of pregnancy

The diagnosis of an inherited disorder in any pregnancy does not automatically mean that pregnancy will be terminated. Prenatal diagnosis is an exercise in information gathering that permits all those involved in an affected pregnancy to give the best management to that couple.

Counselling women for prenatal diagnosis must include non-directive discussion of the options available if an abnormality is confirmed, and this may include termination of an affected pregnancy. Details of the procedure of termination must be given before prenatal testing occurs, as some women faced with a mid-trimester termination would rather not undergo prenatal diagnosis at all.

The introduction of mifepristone (RU486) and misoprostol have been important advances in the methods available for medical termination in the second and third trimesters of pregnancy following prenatal diagnosis. Previous techniques of dilatation and evacuation or the use of intra-amniotic/extra-amniotic prostaglandin infusions were associated with higher morbidity and/or a longer interval from induction to abortion. Mifepristone is a 19 nor-steroid with a high affinity to the progesterone receptor (anti-progesterone). Clinically mifepristone increases the uterine response to exogenous prostaglandins and causes softening and dilatation of the cervix (Urquhart & Templeton 1990). In the UK since 1991, mifepristone can be administered orally as a single dose of 600 mg followed 36–48 hours later by a prostaglandin analogue such as gemeprost (Cervagem) or misoprostol. Misoprostol is a potent orally active prostaglandin E_1 analogue and has been shown to be at least as effective as gemeprost (El-Refaey et al 1993). One regimen is that 36–48 hours after oral mifepristone, 800 µg of misoprostol is given vaginally and followed by 400 µg orally every 3 hours up to a maximum of four doses. The advantage of misoprostol is that it is supplied in tablet form and is cheap compared with gemeprost, which requires refrigeration and is far more expensive. However, misoprostol is currently unlicensed for this application and a major side-effect is shivering, which in rare cases is associated with maternal hyperthermia.

Terminations performed after 22 weeks carry the risk of the fetus being born alive so fetocide by an invasive procedure such as the intracardiac injection of potassium chloride should be considered.

Consent should be sought for a postmortem examination, which should be performed by a trained perinatal pathologist. Although consent is legally required only if the fetus is more than 24 weeks of gestation, it must be remembered that the parents will still consider this fetus as a baby. The parents should also be given a chance to see and hold the baby after it has been suitably clothed.

The main focus of the postmortem is to provide a diagnosis; however, it also has important implications in auditing the results of prenatal screening, education and research. In addition, whether consent is given for postmortem or not, further appropriate investigations should be carried out.

- Fetal tissue (blood, skin or placenta) should be obtained for karyotyping.
- Swabs from the baby and placenta should be sent to microbiology and virology if indicated.
- The placenta and membranes should be sent for histology.
- The baby should be radiographed.
- The baby should be photographed (views of the whole body and of any obvious abnormalities). The parents should be offered a photograph of their baby suitably dressed. If they refuse the photograph should be filed in case they later change their minds.

After termination of a pregnancy for a fetal abnormality, the parents should return to discuss the results of the various investigations and to plan appropriate management in subsequent pregnancies.

ETHICAL CONSIDERATIONS

Prenatal diagnosis offers the potential for improvement of the health of future generations, by avoiding handicap and abnormality in the community. However, there are many areas of controversy and ethical difficulty, such as late termination of pregnancy for fetal abnormality (RCOG Ethics Committee 1998). An ethical discussion may be helpful to both parents and doctors in difficult cases without being prescriptive in the conclusions. The basic ethical principles that are essential for good medical practice are autonomy, confidentiality and beneficence.

Informed consent

Most couples attending for antenatal care do not consider themselves at risk of having a pregnancy affected by an inherited disorder. The approach to the routine ultrasound examination is generally that of confirming normality rather than exclusion of abnormality. Many women, when informed that their baby has an abnormality, will say that they were unaware that abnormalities were being looked for. It is essential that all women give informed consent to every aspect of prenatal diagnosis, including the routine scan. The introduction of serum screening for chromosomal abnormality has emphasised the fact that many health care workers do not understand the implications of the tests they

are offering, and thus cannot counsel the women appropriately.

CONCLUSIONS

Prenatal diagnosis can now be performed for a wide spectrum of fetal abnormalities. It is essential that health care providers are aware of the benefits and burdens of the tests performed and are able to counsel pregnant women appropriately.

A number of screening tests for the detection of pregnancies at risk of fetal abnormalities are routinely offered antenatally. These include ultrasound examination and the analysis of maternal blood (e.g. haemoglobin electrophoresis or maternal serum screening). Patients who are classified as being at increased risk following a positive screening test are offered the option of a diagnostic test. A screen positive result often raises anxiety in the parents; in addition, many of the diagnostic tests are invasive and associated with a risk of miscarriage. It is therefore essential that the screening tests have a low false-positive rate and a high detection rate.

When an abnormality is detected the parents will benefit from discussion with members of the multidisciplinary team, comprising a perinatal obstetrician, neonatologist, midwife, geneticist and paediatric surgeon.

KEY POINTS

- Screening tests are not diagnostic: their objective is early detection of a disease or defects whose management is more effective when undertaken early. Patients who are classified as at increased risk following a positive screening test are offered a diagnostic test.
- Routine ultrasound at less than 24 weeks enables better gestational age assessment, reducing rates of induction of labour for post-term pregnancy, earlier detection of multiple pregnancies and earlier detection of fetal malformation at a time when termination of pregnancy is possible.
- There is no substantive evidence of adverse effects from obstetric ultrasound.
- Screening for Down's syndrome is at present most effectively performed by the combination of fetal nuchal translucency and maternal serum biochemistry.
- Amniocentesis should be performed under continuous ultrasound guidance from 15 weeks of gestation.
- If fetal karyotyping or DNA analysis is required in the first trimester of pregnancy chorionic villus sampling is the procedure of choice and should be performed after 10 weeks of gestation.

REFERENCES

Achiron R, Glaser G, Gelernter I, Hegesh J, Yagel S 1992 Extended fetal echocardiolographic examination for detecting cardiac malformations in low risk pregnancies. BMJ 304:671–674

Adinolfi M, Sherlock J, Tutschek B, Halder A, Delhanty J 1995 Detection of fetal cells in transcervical samples and prenatal diagnosis of chromosomal abnormalities. Prenat Diagn 15:33–39

Alfirevic Z 2000 Instruments for transcervical chorionic villus sampling for prenatal diagnosis (Cochrane Review). In: The Cochrane Library 4. Update Software, Oxford

Al-Mufti R, Hambley H, Farzaneh F, Nicolaides KH 1999 Investigation of maternal blood enriched for fetal cells: Role in screening and diagnosis of fetal trisomies. Am J Med Genet 85:66–75

Ammala P, Salonen R 1995 First-trimester diagnosis of hydrolethalus syndrome. Ultrasound Obstet Gynecol 5:60–62

Antsaklis A, Daskalakis G, Papantoniou N, Michalas S 1998 Fetal blood bampling—indication related losses. Prenat Diagn 18:934–940

Benacerraf BR, Gelman R, Frigoletto FD 1987 Sonographic identification of second trimester fetuses with Down's syndrome. N Engl J Med 317:1371–1376

Bianchi DW 1997 Progress in genetic analysis of fetal cells in maternal blood. Curr Opin Obstet Gynecol 9:121–125

Blaas HG, Eik-Nes SH 1999 First trimester diagnosis of fetal malformations. In: Rodeck CH, Whittle MJ (eds) Fetal Medicine: Basic science and clinical practice. Churchill Livingstone, London, pp 581–597

Bogart M, Pandian MR, Jones OW 1987 Abnormal maternal serum chorionic gonadotrophin levels in pregnancies with fetal chromosomal abnormalities. Prenat Diagn 7:623–630

Bonaventure J, Rousseau F, Legeani-Mallet L, Le Merrer M, Munnieh A, Maroteaux P 1996 Common mutations in fibroblast growth factor 3 (FGR-3) gene account for achondroplasia, hypochondroplasia, and thanatophoric dwarfism. Am J Med Genet 63:143–154

Bricker L, Neilson JP 2000 Routine ultrasound in late pregnancy (after 24 weeks gestation) (Cochrane Review). In: The Cochrane Library, 4, 2000. Update Software, Oxford

Brock DJH 1996 Prenatal screening for cystic fibrosis: five years experience reviewed. Lancet 347:148–151

Bromley B, Frigoletto FD, Benacerraf BR 1991 Mild fetal lateral ventriculomegaly: clinical course and outcome. Am J Obstet Gynecol 164: 863–867

Bucher HC, Schmidt JD 1993 Does routine ultrasound scanning improve outcome in pregnancy? Meta-analysis of various outcome measures. BMJ 307:13–18

Burn J, Brennan P, Little J et al 1998 Recurrence risks in offspring of adults with major heart defects: results from first cohort of British Collaborative study. Lancet 351:311–316

Campbell S, Johnstone FD, Holt EM, May P 1972 Anencephaly: early ultrasonic diagnosis and active management. Lancet 2:122–126

Canadian Collaborative CVS–Amniocentesis Clinical Trial Group 1989 Multicentre randomized clinical trial of chorion villus sampling and amniocentesis. Lancet i:1–6

Canick J, Knight GJ, Palomaki GE, Haddow JE, Cuckle HS, Wald NJ 1988 Low second trimester maternal serum unconjugated oestriol in pregnancies with Down's syndrome. Br J Obstet Gynecol 95:330–333

CEMAT Group 1998 Randomised trial to assess safety and fetal outcome of early and midtrimester amniocentesis. Lancet 351:242–247

Chapple JC 1992 Genetic screening. In: Brock DJH, Rodeck CH, Ferguson-Smith MA (eds) Prenatal diagnosis and screening. Churchill Livingstone, Edinburgh, pp 579–593

Cheung MC, Goldberg JD, Kan YW 1996 Prenatal diagnosis of sickle cell anaemia and thalassemia by analysis of fetal cell maternal blood. Nature Genetics 14:264–268

Chitty LS, Hung GH, Moore J, Lobb MO 1991 Effectiveness of routine ultrasonography in detecting fetal structural abnormalities in a low risk population. BMJ 303:1165–1169

Cuckle HS, Wald NJ 1984 Principles of screening. In: Wald NJ (ed) Antenatal and Neonatal screening. Oxford University Press, Oxford

Cuckle HS, Nanchahal K, Wald NJ 1991 Birth prevalence of Down's syndrome in England and Wales. Prenat Diagn 11:29–34

Daffos F, Capella-Pavlovsky M, Forestier F 1983 Fetal blood sampling via the umbilical cord using a needle guided by ultrasound. Prenat Diagn 3:271–274

duManoir S, Speicher MR, Joos S et al 1993 Detection of complete and partial chromosome gains and losses by comparative genomic in situ hybridisation. Hum Genet 90:590–610

Economides DL, Braithwaite JM 1998 First trimester diagnosis of fetal structural abnormalities in a low risk population. Br J Obstet Gynaecol 105:53–57

El-Refaey H, Hinshaw K, Templeton AA 1993 The abortifacient effect of misoprostol in the second trimester. Hum Reprod 8:1744–1746

Ewigman BG, Crane JP, Frigoletto FD, LeFevre ML, Bain RP, McNellis D and the RADIUS Study Group 1993 Effect of prenatal ultrasound screening on perinatal outcome. N Engl J Med 329(12):821–827

Firth HV, Boyd PA, Chamberlain P, MacKenzie IZ, Lindenbaum RH, Huson SM 1991 Severe limb abnormalities after chorion villous sampling at 56–66 days' gestation. Lancet 337:762–763

Firth HV, Boyd PA, Chamberlain PF, MacKenzie IZ, Morriss-Kay GM, Huson SM 1994 Analysis of limb reduction defects in babies exposed to chorion villus sampling. Lancet 343:1069–1071

Fraser J, Mitchell A 1876 Kalmuc idiocy: report of a case with autopsy with notes on 62 cases by A. Mitchell. J Ment Sci 22:169–179

Geerts Lut TGM, Brand EJ, Theron GB 1996 Routine obstetric ultrasound examinations in South Africa: cost and effect on perinatal outcome—a prospective randomised controlled trial. Br J Obstet Gynaecol 103:501–507

Hahnemann N, Mohr J 1968 Genetic diagnosis in the embryo by means of biopsy from extra-embryonic membranes. Bull Eur Soc Hum Genet 2:23–29

Harper J, Delhanty J 1999 Preimplantation genetic diagnosis. In: Rodeck CH, Whittle MJ (eds) Fetal medicine: Basic science and clinical practice. Churchill Livingstone, London, pp 465–472

Hubbard AM, Harty MP 2000 MRI for the assessment of the malformed fetus. Baillières Best Pract Res Clin Obstet Gynaecol 14(4):629–650

Jauniaux ER, Gulbis B, Tunkel S, Ramsay B, Campbell S, Meuris S 1996 Maternal serum testing for alpha-fetoprotein and human chorionic gonadotrophin in high risk pregnancies. Prenat Diagn 16:1129–1135

Kadir RA, Economides DL 1997 The effect of nuchal translucency measurement on second trimester biochemical screening for Down's syndrome. Ultrasound Obstet Gynecol 9:244–247

Kleijer WJ 1999 Inborn errors of metabolism. In: Rodeck CH, Whittle MJ (eds) Fetal medicine: Basic science and clinical practice. Churchill Livingstone, London, pp 525–544

Korenberg JR 1993 Toward a molecular understanding of Down syndrome. Prog Clin Bio Res 384:87–115

Langdon Down J 1866 Observations on an ethnic classification of idiots. Clinical Lectures and Reports, London Hospital, 3:259–262

Levi S, Schaaps JP, De Havay P, Defoort P 1995 End-result of routine ultrasound screening for congenital anomalies: the Belgium multicentre study 1984–92. Ultrasound Obstet Gynecol 5:366–371

Lo YD, Bowell PJ, Selinger M et al 1993 Prenatal determination of fetal RhD status by analysis of peripheral blood of rhesus negative mothers. Lancet 342:54–55

Luck C 1992 Value of routine ultrasound scanning at 19 weeks: a four year study of 8849 deliveries. BMJ 304:1474–1478

Mari G, Deter RL, Carpenter RL et al 2000 Noninvasive diagnosis by Doppler ultrasonography of fetal anemia due to maternal red-cell alloimmunization. Collaborative Group for Doppler Assessment of the Blood Velocity in Anemic Fetuses. N Engl J Med 342(1):9–14

McKusick VA 1994 Mendelian inheritance in man. A catalog of human genes and genetic disorders, 11th edn. The John Hopkins University Press, Baltimore

McLaughlin JF, Shurtleff DB 1984 Management of the fetus and newborn with neural tube defects. J Perinatol 4:3–12

Medical Research Council 1978 An assessment of the hazards of amniocentesis. Br J Obstet Gynaecol 85 (suppl 2)

Merkatz IR, Nitowsky HM, Macri JN, Johnson WE 1984 An association between low maternal serum alpha-fetoprotein and fetal chromosomal abnormalities. Am J Obstet Gynecol 148:886–894

MRC Vitamin Study Research Group 1991 Prevention of neural tube defects: results of the MRC Vitamin Study. Lancet 338:132–137

MRC Working Party on the Evaluation of Chorion Villus Sampling 1991 Medical research council European trial of chorion villus sampling. Lancet 337:1491–1499

Neilson JP 2000 Ultrasound for fetal assessment in early pregnancy (Cochrane Review). In: The Cochrane Library, 4, 2000. Update Software, Oxford

Newnham JP, Evans SF, Michael CA, Stanley FJ, Landau L 1993 Effects of frequent ultrasound during pregnancy: a randomized controlled trial. Lancet 342: 887–891

Nicolaides KH, Campbell S, Gabbe S, Guidetti M 1986 Ultrasound screening for spina bifiba: cranial and cerebellar signs. Lancet 2:71–74

Nicolaides KH, Snijders RJM, Gosden CM, Berry C, Campbell S 1992 Ultrasonographically detectable markers of fetal chromosomal abnormalities. Lancet 340:704–707

Nicolaides KH, Brizot ML, Patel F, Snijders RJM 1994 Comparison of chorionic villus sampling and amniocentesis for fetal karyotyping at 10–13 week's gestation. Lancet 344:435–439

Nyberg DA, Luthy DA, Resta RG, Nyberg BC, Williams MA 1998 Age-adjusted ultrasound risk assessment for fetal Down's syndrome during the second trimester: description of the method and analysis of 142 cases. Ultrasound Obstet Gynecol 12:8–14

Ogle RF 2000 Second trimester markers of aneuploidy. Baillières Best Pract Res Clin Obstet Gynaecol 2000 14(4):595–610

Overton TG, Lighten AD, Fisk NM, Bennett PR 1996 Prenatal diagnosis by minimally invasive first trimester transcervical sampling is unreliable. Am J Obstet Gynecol 175:382–387

Pandya PP 1999 In: Nicolaides KH, Sebire NJ, Snijders RJM (eds) The 11–14 week scan: the diagnosis of fetal abnormalities. Diploma in Fetal Medicine Series. Parthenon Publishing, London, pp 3–33

Pandya PP, Snijders RJM, Johnson S, Brizot M, Nicolaides KH 1995 Screening for fetal trisomies by maternal age and fetal nuchal translucency thickness at 10–14 weeks of gestation. Br J Obstet Gynaecol 102:957–962

Pertl P, Kopp S, Kroisel PM et al 1997 Quantitative fluorescent PCR for the rapid prenatal detection of common aneuploides and fetal sex. Am J Obstet Gynecol 177:899–906

RCOG Ethics Committee 1998. A consideration of the law and ethics in relation to late termination of pregnancy for fetal abnormality. RCOG, London

RCOG Working Party 1997 Ultrasound screening for fetal abnormalities. RCOG, London.

RCOG Working Party 2000 Routine ultrasound screening in pregnancy. Protocols, standards and training. Supplement to ultrasound screening for fetal abnormalities. RCOG, London

Reynolds TM 1997 The Mahalanobis distance: should atypically be a feature of all Down syndrome screening programmes or would a specific screening test for trisomy 18 be better? In: Grudzinskas JG, Ward RHT (eds) Screening for Down Syndrome in the First Trimester. RCOG press, London, pp 54–66

Rodeck C 1980 Fetoscopy guided by real-time ultrasound for pure fetal blood samples, fetal skin samples and examination of the fetus in utero. Br J Obstet Gynaecol 87:449–456

Rodeck CH 1993 Fetal development after chorionic villus sampling. Lancet 341:468–469

Rodeck CH, Whittle MJ (eds) 1999 Fetal Medicine: Basic science and clinical practice. Churchill Livingstone, London

Rodeck CH, Morsman JM, Nicolaides KH, McKenzie C, Gosden CM, Gosden JR 1983 A single operator technique for first trimester chorion biopsy. Lancet ii:1340–1341

Rodeck CH, Tutschek B, Sherlock J, Kingdom J 1995 Methods for transcervical collection of fetal cells during the first trimester of pregnancy. Prenat Diagn 15:933–942

Rosendahl H, Kivinen S 1989 Antenatal detection of congenital malformations by routine ultrasonography. Obstet Gynecol 73(6):947–951

Saari-Kemppainen A, Karjalainen O, Ylostalo P, Heinonen OP 1990 Ultrasound screening and perinatal mortality: controlled trial of systematic one-stage screening in pregnancy. Lancet 336:387–391

Saiki RK, Scharf S, Faloona F et al 1985 Enzymatic amplification of beta-globin genomic sequences and restriction site analysis for diagnosis of sickle cell anaemia. Science 230(4732):1350–1354

Salvesen KA, Vatten LJ, Eik-Nes SH, Hugdahl K, Bakketeig LS 1993 Routine ultrasonography in utero and subsequent handedness and neurological development. BMJ 307:159–164

Shirley IM, Bottomley F, Robinson VP 1991 Routine radiographer screening for fetal abnormalities by ultrasound in an unselected low risk population. Br J Radiol 65:565–569

Simpson JL, Elias S 1994 Isolating fetal cells in maternal circulation for prenatal diagnosis. Prenat Diagn 14:1229–1242

Smidt-Jensen S, Hahnemann N 1984 Transabdominal fine needle biopsy from chorionic villi in the first trimester. Prenat Diagn 4:163–169

Smidt-Jensen S, Permin M, Philip J et al 1992 Randomised comparison of amniocentesis and transabdominal and transcervical chorionic villus sampling. Lancet 340:1238–1244

Snijders RJM, Nicolaides KH 1996 In: Nicolaides KH (ed) Ultrasound markers for fetal chromosomal defects. Frontiers in Fetal Medicine. Parthenon Publishing, London

Snijders RJM, Shawwa L, Nicolaides KH 1994 Fetal choroids plexus cysts and trisomy 18: assessment of risk based on ultrasound findings and maternal age. Prenat Diagn 14:1119–1127

Snijders RJ, Sebire NJ, Nicolaides KH 1995a Maternal age and gestation specific risk for chromosomal defects. Fetal Diagn Ther 10(6):356–367

Snijders RJM, Sebire NJ, Faria M, Patel F, Nicolaides KH 1995b Fetal mild hydronephrosis and chromosomal defects: relation to maternal age and gestational age. Fetal Diagn Ther 10:349–355

Snijders RJM, Noble P, Sebire NJ, Souka AP, Nicolaides KH 1998 UK multicentre project on the assessment of risk of trisomy 21 by maternal age and fetal nuchal translucency thickness at 10–14 weeks of gestation. Lancet 35:343–346

Snijders RJM, Sunderberg K, Holzgreve W, Henry G, Nicolaides KH 1999 Maternal age and gestation specific risk for trisomy 21. Ultrasound Obstet Gynecol 13:167–170

Spencer K, Souter V, Tul N, Snijders RJM, Nicolaides KH 1999 Screening program for trisomy 21 at 10–14 weeks using fetal nuchal translucency and maternal serum free β-hCG and PAPP-A. Ultrasound Obstet Gynecol 13:231–237

Steele MW, Breg WR 1966 Chromosome analysis of human amniotic-fluid cells. Lancet i:383–385

Sundberg K, Bang J, Smidt-Jensen S et al 1997 Randomised study of risk of fetal loss related to early amniocentesis versus chorionic villus sampling. Lancet 350:697–703

Szabo J, Gellen J 1990 Nuchal fluid accumulation in trisomy-21 detected by vaginosonography in first trimester. Lancet 336:1133

Tabor A, Philip J, Madsen M, Bang J, Obel EB, Norgaard-Pedersen B 1986 Randomised controlled trial of genetic amniocentesis in 4,606 low-risk women. Lancet i:1287–1293

Taipale P, Hiilesmaa V, Salonen R, Ylostalo P 1997 Increased nuchal translucency as a marker for fetal chromosomal. N Engl J Med 337:1654–1658

Tegnander E, Eik-Ness SH, Johansen OJ, Linker DT 1996 Prenatal detection of heart defects at the routine fetal examination at 18 weeks in a non-selected population. Ultrasound Obstet Gynecol 5:372–380

Thilaganathan B, Olowaiye A, Sairam S, Harrington K 1999 Isolated intraventricular echogenic focus or 'golf balls': is karyotyping for Down syndrome indicated? Br J Obstet Gynaecol 106:1294–1298

Tijo JH, Levan A 1956 The chromosome number of man. Hereditas 42:1–6

UK Collaborative Study on Alphafetoprotein in relation to neural tube defects 1982 Fourth report. Estimating an individual's chance of having an open spina bifida and the value of repeat AFP testing. J Epidemiol Community Health 36:87–92

Urquhart DR, Templeton AA 1990 The use of mifepristone prior to prostaglandin induced mid-trimester abortion. Hum Reprod 5:883–886

Valenti C, Schutta EJ, Kehaty T 1968 Prenatal diagnosis of Down's syndrome. Lancet ii:220

Van den Hof MC, Nicolaides KH, Campbell J, Campbell S 1990 Evaluation of the lemon and banana signs in one hundred and thirty fetuses with open spina bifida. Am J Obstet Gynecol 162:322–327

Wald NJ, Hackshaw AK 1997 Combining ultrasound and biochemistry in first-trimester screening for Down's syndrome. Prenat Diagn 17:821–829

Wald NJ, Kennard A, Hackshaw A, McGuire A 1997 Antenatal screening for Down's syndrome. J Med Screen 4:181–246

Wald NJ, Cuckle HS, Densem JW et al 1988 Maternal serum screening for Down's syndrome in early pregnancy. BMJ 297:883–888

Wald NJ, Watt HC, Hackshaw AK 1999 Integrated screening for Down's syndrome based on tests performed during the first and second trimester. N Engl J Med 341:461–467

Warburton D 1991 De novo balanced chromosome rearrangements and extra marker chromosomes identified at prenatal diagnosis: clinical significance and distribution of break points. Am J Hum Genet 46:995–1013

Whiteman DAH, Klinger K 1991 Efficiency of rapid in situ hybridisation methods for prenatal diagnosis of chromosome abnormalities causing birth defects. Am J Hum Genet 49 (suppl):A1279

Wilson DI, Goodship JA, Burn J, Cross IE, Scrambler PJ 1992 Deletions within chromosome 22q11 in familial congenital heart disease. Lancet 340:573–575

13

Fetal growth restriction; small for gestational age

Nicholas M. Fisk, Richard P. Smith

The contribution of the author of the equivalent chapter in the second edition, on which this chapter draws extensively, is gratefully acknowledged.

DEFINITION

Intrauterine growth restriction

The best definition of intrauterine growth restriction (IUGR) is failure of a fetus to reach its genetic growth potential (Steer 1998) (note that the term restriction rather than retardation is preferred to avoid parents associating retardation with mental handicap). Even this has limitations; e.g. chromosomally abnormal fetuses are difficult to fit into this definition.

Currently we do not have an accurate method of assessing the genetic growth potential of a fetus: the best guide is to establish fetal size early in gestation when the variation in size is least. Defining growth restriction as failure of a fetus to reach its genetic growth potential means that failure to grow along a consistent centile is more important than absolute size. In other words, a fetus with an abdominal circumference (AC) on the 90th centile at 28 weeks gestation and the 50th centile at 36 weeks is more likely to be growth restricted than a fetus which is on the 5th centile at 28 and again at 36 weeks. Other associations with growth restriction, such as decreased amniotic fluid volume, estimated fetal weight and abnormal umbilical artery waveforms, may also be incorporated into the definition. The fetal femur length can be used to estimate the crown–heel length (Vintzileos et al 1984), allowing calculation of an in utero ponderal index (PI). This provides an index of weight against length (weight (g)/crown–heel length (cm)^3 × 100), and may be used to identify fetuses which are growth restricted. This has failed to gain favour in clinical practice because it is less useful at predicting a malnourished fetus than the AC.

Estimated fetal weight

There are numerous formulae for calculating the estimated fetal weight (EFW) from ultrasound measurements. Two such examples are that devised by Warsoff, which uses the biparietal diameter and abdominal circumference (Shepard et al 1982), and that of Hadlock, which uses head circumference, abdominal circumference and femur length (Hadlock et al 1984). In growth restriction, inclusion of head and femur measurements will lead to an overestimation of fetal weight because growth of these parameters tends to be preserved, whereas the AC is affected early in growth restriction owing to decreased glycogen storage in the liver. Consequently, EFW is less sensitive than AC at identifying a malnourished fetus, but the positive predictive value is greater.

Neonatal indicators

As well as in utero definitions of growth restriction, neonatal factors can be used to make a retrospective diagnosis. These may include neonatal PI (defined above), more complex indices of fetal weight and size involving assessment of body fat, and metabolic markers, e.g. tendency to hypothermia or hypoglycaemia.

What definition should be used?

There is no absolute point when a fetus changes from a 'normal' to a 'growth-restricted' fetus; however, when a group of fetuses with more growth-restricted characteristics (e.g. AC <10th centile) are compared with a group of fetuses with more normal characteristics, they are more likely to exhibit the signs of dysfunction associated with growth restriction. A significant number of babies with no signs of dysfunction will also be included (i.e. the test is not very specific). If, instead, the 5th centile is used, a higher proportion will exhibit signs of dysfunction (i.e. the test will be more specific) but some dysfunctional babies with AC between the 10th and the 5th centile will have been excluded (i.e. it will be less sensitive). This sliding scale of sensitivity versus specificity can be expressed graphically as a receiver operator curve (Fig. 13.1). Any cut-off value for measurements such as the EFW, AC or in utero PI, will give a sensitivity and specificity for that cut-off value. These can be plotted against each other to give a receiver operator curve. Broadly speaking, the best cut-off is one that maximises the sum of the sensitivity and specificity, i.e. is nearest the top left-hand corner; however, in practice, the best cut-off will depend on the aim of the investigation (e.g. a cut-off for AC below which an umbilical artery Doppler was performed could have quite low specificity, whereas a cut-off below which a referral was made to a tertiary centre some distance away would need to be more specific).

Low birthweight and small for gestational age

Two other terms requiring clarification are low birthweight (LBW) and small for gestational age (SGA). LBW is defined by the WHO simply as birthweight <2.5 kg, so does not correct for gestation. SGA is used variably prenatally and postnatally by authors to describe a fetus or neonate with growth parameter(s) (e.g. EFW, AC, birthweight) below a given centile for gestational age. The centiles used are commonly the 10th, 5th and 3rd, but may be any centile as long as it is specified. Alternatively, the measurement may be described as below a certain standard deviation (Z score) from the mean. An appropriate definition will depend on the aim of defining a fetus as SGA: the same arguments can be applied as above regarding sensitivity and specificity. The terms IUGR, LBW and SGA are not synonymous but there is considerable overlap: some fetuses may meet the criteria for just one of these definitions, whereas others may meet all three (Fig. 13.2).

What is an appropriate reference population?

When describing a local population, the term small for gestational age can be used to compare the local population to a standard population (e.g. 'eight per cent of our babies have birthweights below the 10th centile of the Aberdeen charts'). Alternatively, it can be used to describe the local population (e.g. 'the 10th centile for birthweight of our population is 2.7 kg at 40 weeks'). This raises the question of whether it is appropriate to use 'normal' ranges for the local population, or whether it is better to use national charts. If the local population consists mainly of ethnic groups that tend to have smaller babies owing to genetic variation, then it would seem sensible to use local charts with lower centiles; however, if the local population tends to have smaller babies because it is deprived and has a higher incidence of malnutrition, then using local charts with lower centiles would mean that some fetuses and neonates would be classified as appropriate for gestational age (AGA) when they were in fact at risk of dysfunction. The same argument can be extended to fetuses and neonates of mothers with a low body mass index. These mothers will tend to have smaller babies, in part due to their genetic make-up but in part due to poor nutritional status. In summary, it seems sensible to correct for *physiological* variables, such as maternal height, booking weight, ethnic group, parity and sex of the fetus, which would increase the specificity of poor growth as a marker of dysfunction. Computer-generated customised growth charts (Gardosi et al 1992) have been used to correct for these variables (Fig. 13.3), but this facility is not available in most units; however, we must bear in mind that by doing so we may be inadvertently correcting for *pathological* variables (e.g. poor nutrition

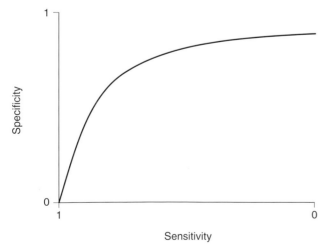

Fig. 13.1   Diagram of a receiver operator curve.

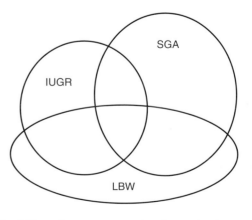

Fig. 13.2   A Venn diagram representing the overlap between intrauterine growth restriction (IUGR), small for gestational age (SGA) and low birthweight (LBW).

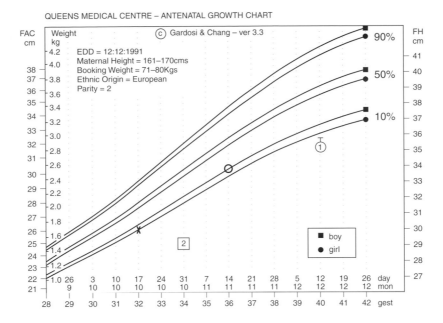

Fig. 13.3 A customised fetal growth chart (AC and EFW) with centiles adjusted for maternal weight, height, ethnic group and parity, and fetal sex. (Reproduced from Gardosi et al 1992, with the permission of the publisher.)

associated with certain ethnic groups or women of very low body mass index) and reducing the sensitivity.

Implications of growth restriction

Growth-restricted fetuses have a higher risk of stillbirth and mortality than appropriately grown fetuses of a similar gestation. They are more at risk of hypothermia, hypoglycaemia, pulmonary haemorrhage, infection, encephalopathy, and necrotising enterocolitis compared with normally grown babies of a similar gestation. The incidence of fetal heart rate abnormality in labour, and operative delivery is higher. Size at birth seems to be the better predictor of mortality, whereas gestation seems to be the better predictor of morbidity in survivors. When interpreting studies of growth restriction and outcome one must consider the criteria used to diagnose growth restriction, whether screening or diagnosis for chromosomal anomalies has been undertaken, the population studied, and what interventions if any were made. Many studies of 'growth-restricted' fetuses actually study fetuses that are SGA, and while there is a large overlap between these two groups (Fig. 13.2), some fetuses may be SGA that are not growth-restricted, and vice versa. Consequently, results from these studies must be applied to growth-restricted fetuses with caution. Epidemiological studies by Barker et al have suggested that a range of diseases may be associated with the fetal environment. Small infants, particularly those remaining small at 1 year, seem to be at increased risk from later cardiovascular and metabolic disease (Barker 1995). The mechanisms underlying this are not clear, and to address this, research in animal models is currently being undertaken. The suggestion that our predisposition to some of the most common diseases of later life can be programmed by events before birth may have profound implications for preventative health care in the future.

AETIOLOGY

Small fetuses are a heterogeneous group, with many diverse aetiologies, some of which remain obscure. There are a wide range of associations, some fetal, some maternal and some placental. These in turn may have a genetic or environmental basis. The term small is used in this chapter to refer to fetuses that may be SGA, growth-restricted, or both.

Fetal causes

Chromosomal abnormality

Since the incidence of fetal loss is much higher in fetuses with chromosomal abnormalities, the incidence of aneuploidy in a population of small fetuses depends on gestational age at the time of investigation. The incidence also depends on any prior screening test for chromosomal abnormality. Snijders et al studied over 400 patients from 17 to 40 weeks gestation referred with 'fetal growth retardation' (AC and subsequent birthweight below the 5th centile) with no known cause at the time of referral (Snijders et al 1993). The fetal karyotype was abnormal in 19%. In early pregnancy, the commonest chromosomal abnormality was triploidy (58%), whereas after 26 weeks it was trisomy 18 (46%). The karyotype was more likely to be abnormal in the presence of associated ultrasonographic malformations (40 versus 2%), normal or increased amniotic fluid volume (40 versus 8% with reduced amniotic fluid), or normal uterine and umbilical artery waveforms (44 versus 8%). Trisomy 13 is also associated with first trimester smallness, whereas trisomy 21 and Turner's syndrome are associated with a later onset (second trimester) and more variable degree of smallness.

The cause of SGA in aneuploid fetuses is not well understood but probably reflects a lack of cell division or cell growth in either the fetus or placenta. This may be primary, or secondary to other factors such as impaired placental perfusion or hormonal abnormality.

Structural anomalies

Virtually all major structural defects (central nervous system, cardiovascular, gastrointestinal, genitourinary and musculoskeletal) are associated with an increased risk of having a small fetus. It is not clear whether one predisposes to the other, or whether there is a common cause for both.

Infection

Fetal infection is thought to be an uncommon cause of smallness, but good studies are few, and are also limited by the difficulty in diagnosing infection in utero. Malaria is a major cause of growth restriction worldwide, and treatment of malaria reduces the incidence of growth restriction. Rubella, cytomegalovirus, toxoplasmosis and syphilis can affect cell division and growth and have all been implicated in fetal smallness. These are discussed further in the relevant chapters elsewhere in this book.

Genetic causes

Critics of the programming theory argue that the same genes that cause small thin babies also cause susceptibility to diabetes and heart disease, rather than the intrauterine environment causing both smallness and disease susceptibility (Hattersley et al 1998). Many genes are likely to play a role, and one example is the gene for glucokinase, which is the key component in the pancreatic β cell's glucose-sensing mechanism. Heterozygous mutations can alter the sensitivity of glucokinase such that adequate insulin secretion is only achieved with an increase in circulating glucose levels. Clinically, this causes maturity-onset diabetes of the young, which is dominantly inherited. Fetuses carrying such a mutation are approximately 500 g lighter at birth than their siblings, presumably due to a deficit of insulin and its growth-promoting effects. This weight discrepancy is only seen when the mutation is inherited from the father: the most likely reason for this is that if instead it is the mother who has the mutation, she will have elevated glucose levels which will cross the placenta and cause fetal insulin levels to approach normal.

Genomic imprinting

Genomic imprinting is the phenomenon whereby the expression of a gene depends on whether it is maternally or paternally inherited. An extreme example is triploidy. Triploid conceptuses with an extra paternally derived set of genes usually have a large overgrown placenta and fetal growth restriction, whereas those with two maternal sets abort early in gestation with an underdeveloped placenta. It is likely that the parental origin of genes in euploid pregnancies plays an important role in fetal growth. There are approximately 20–30 known imprinted genes, with an estimate of a further 50–100 likely to be discovered. Many of these genes are expressed in early development and can be linked to fetal growth, the insulin-like growth factor-2 gene which is paternally expressed (maternally imprinted) being a good example.

Uniparental disomy and confined placental mosaicism

Uniparental disomy (UPD) is implicated in causing fetal growth restriction. It occurs when a pair of homologous chromosomes is inherited from the same parent, a phenomenon well demonstrated in the mouse model (Fig. 13.4). It can result from fertilisation of a nullisomic by a disomic gamete, from chromosome duplication in a monosomic somatic cell, or from loss of a supernumerary chromosome from a trisomic cell (trisomic rescue). Aneuploidy rates of up to 50% in oocytes (compared with 5% in spermatozoa) suggest that maternal UPD may be more common, with trisomic rescue being the more likely mechanism. Detection requires DNA rather than cytogenetic analysis, as the karyotype will be normal. Trisomic rescue would account for the finding of confined placental mosaicism, where the karyotype in part (or all) of the placenta is different to the fetus. Trisomy 16 is the most common trisomy found as a confined placental mosaicism in IUGR, and consequently chromosome 16 was one of the first candidate chromosomes to be studied with respect to IUGR. Twenty cases of confined placental mosaicism for chromosome 16 with a normal fetal karyotype have been reported, and, of these, 12 had maternal UPD for 16. Eleven of the 12 were growth-restricted at birth. It is currently unclear whether UPD 16 is itself a cause of IUGR or whether the major determinant is the proportion of trisomy 16 cells within the placenta. There are several other phenotypes that have been found to result from UPD or deletions of one parental chromosome effectively withdrawing the expression from one or other parent's imprinted genes. In

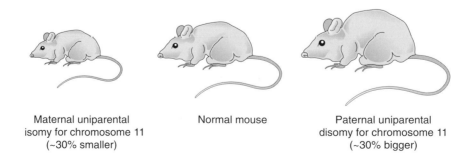

Maternal uniparental isomy for chromosome 11 (~30% smaller) Normal mouse Paternal uniparental disomy for chromosome 11 (~30% bigger)

Fig. 13.4 Diagram of the different effects of maternal and paternal uniparental disomy in mice. With thanks to Dr G Moore.

several cases, these phenotypes include growth-related problems; for example, the Silver–Russell syndrome, the main features of which are IUGR and lateral asymmetry, is associated with maternal UPD of chromosome 7.

Nutrient supply

Inadequate maternal nutrition can restrict growth in the third trimester, as reported after the Dutch famine and the Leningrad siege. Preconceptual nutritional status is important, as the degree of growth restriction was much greater after the protracted Leningrad siege than the shorter Dutch famine (approximately 700 versus 300 g). It is not clear whether it is lack of overall calories or a specific substrate that causes the IUGR. Glucose, amino acids and lactate are the major substrates for the fetus. Some growth-restricted fetuses are hypoglycaemic, and work in sheep has shown that placental utilisation of glucose is also reduced and fetal supply decreased. Growth-restricted fetuses have low serum amino acids, but some non-essential amino acids are increased, probably as a result of tissue breakdown. Growth restriction is also associated with high lactate concentrations in fetal blood. Paradoxically, malnutrition in the first trimester, with later restoration of food supply, can cause an increase in birthweight, perhaps by encouraging compensatory placental growth. It has been suggested that hyperemesis in the first trimester might be an adaptation to enhance fetal growth later in pregnancy.

Oxygen may also be an important factor, as babies born at altitude are smaller than those born at sea level; however, oxygen supplementation has not been shown to increase birthweight in IUGR compared with untreated IUGR pregnancies (Battaglia et al 1992).

Placental causes

The placenta is the sole channel of nutrition to the fetus from 6 weeks onwards. An adequate supply of oxygen and nutrients is essential for normal growth. Abnormalities of the fetal or maternal circulation can lead to IUGR. Although they are dealt with separately here, the concept of a primary placental pathology underlying growth restriction is often debated. This point is important because it underpins the logic behind attempts at treatment. Another pivotal concept is whether the placenta is primarily at fault, or whether some abnormality in the uterus is to blame.

Uteroplacental insufficiency

Endovascular trophoblast normally invades the spiral arteries of the uterus and converts them into uteroplacental arteries. This takes place in two stages. In the first and early second trimester, only the decidual part of the spiral arteries is converted. The so-called second wave of invasion occurs in the middle of the second trimester, and converts the myometrial part of the spiral arteries to create a low-resistance circulation which allows high blood flow to the placenta. In many pregnancies complicated by growth restriction and pre-eclampsia, this second wave of trophoblast invasion fails (Khong et al 1986). The arteries show changes of acute atherosis; thrombosis, haemorrhage and infarction may follow.

These pathological changes are consistent with a decrease in uterine blood flow and consequently a reduction in fetal nutrition; however, it is still not clear why this should occur in some pregnancies and not in others. These changes are probably the end-point of more than one disease process.

Fetoplacental insufficiency

In the first trimester, the umbilical arteries usually show no end-diastolic flow (as assessed using ultrasound to measure Doppler flow velocity waveforms), which suggests that the low-resistance circulation in the placenta is not formed by this stage. In normal pregnancies, end-diastolic flow is usually present by the early second trimester, and increases until term (Hendricks et al 1989). Growth-restricted fetuses often have absent or reversed end-diastolic flow in the umbilical artery, suggesting increased resistance in the fetoplacental circulation. This is compatible with a failure of trophoblast invasion and conversion of spiral arterioles to low-resistance vessels. Histological studies have suggested that the small muscular arteries in tertiary stem villi are obliterated in pregnancies with abnormal umbilical artery flow velocity (Giles et al 1985). Studies of terminal villi have shown increased syncytial nuclei, thickened basal lamina, increased stromal deposition of collagens and laminin, reduced proliferating cytotrophoblast, and increased capillary erythrocyte congestion within the terminal villous capillaries of the placentae (i.e. distal to the small muscular arteries) in growth-restricted fetuses compared with controls (Macara et al 1996).

Maternal causes

Smoking

Active and passive smoking is a major cause of IUGR (Roquer et al 1995), especially smoking during the third trimester (Lieberman et al 1994). Mothers who smoke during pregnancy generally deliver infants weighing 100–300 g less than children born to non-smoking mothers (Butler et al 1972, Sexton & Hebel 1984). This is influenced by the number of cigarettes smoked (particularly >10) and the sex of the fetus (male fetuses being more affected than females). The mechanism is not clear, but carboxyhaemoglobin levels in fetuses of smokers are almost double those of non-smokers (Soothill et al 1996). Other factors include vascular effects on the uteroplacental or fetoplacental circulation, and toxic metabolites in the fetus.

Alcohol

Alcohol crosses the placenta freely. Maternal reporting of alcohol consumption varies depending on the method of data collection, which makes studies difficult. One study found no reduction in mean birthweight with light alcohol consumption (1–3 drinks per month), a 120 g reduction with moderate alcohol consumption (1–13 drinks per week), and a 522 g reduction with heavy alcohol consumption (≥2 drinks per day) (Virji 1991).

Drugs

It is difficult to estimate the size of the effect due to concurrent use of alcohol and tobacco, undernutrition and unreliable reporting. Cocaine has been considered to be strongly associated with growth restriction, but new evidence suggests that once confounding variables are corrected for (especially tobacco), IUGR is not increased. Heroin and methadone use are associated with growth restriction. One meta-analysis found a mean reduction in birthweight of 489 g associated with heroin use, and 279 g associated with methadone use (Hulse et al 1997), but undernutrition may be a factor.

Chronic disease

Several maternal diseases may restrict fetal growth. Congenital heart disease is associated with an increased risk of having a small infant, especially if the woman is cyanotic. Maternal chest disease such as cystic fibrosis, bronchiectasis, kyphoscoliosis and asthma only reduce growth in severe cases where there is marked respiratory compromise. Chronic renal disease is associated with smallness, especially if there is associated hypertension, proteinuria and elevated serum creatinine levels. Diabetes mellitus is more often associated with large fetuses, but the incidence of IUGR is also increased, especially in the presence of renal disease (Reece et al 1998). Hyperthyroidism is also a risk factor for IUGR.

Thrombophilia

Maternal antiphospholipid antibodies are associated with smallness. In one study, a group of unselected women with anticardiolipin antibodies (one of the antiphospholipid antibodies) had a relative risk of 18 for having a small fetus (Katano et al 1996). The mechanism for this is not clear. Placental thrombosis is a common finding, but this is neither universal nor specific. Evidence from murine models suggests that antiphospholipid antibodies impair trophoblast function via mechanisms unrelated to thrombosis, by binding to surface phospholipids on the trophoblast, resulting in direct cellular injury, inhibition of syncytia formation, and defective invasion of the uterine decidua. There is also evidence that inherited thrombophilias are almost five times more common in women with small fetuses (Kupferminc et al 1999), but the precise risk of IUGR in women with genetic or acquired thrombophilia is unknown.

SCREENING

Clinical examination

Palpation has been reported as having a low sensitivity and positive predictive value respectively of 44% and 29% in predicting SGA fetuses (Villar & Belizan 1986). Symphyseal–fundal height (SFH) measurements are a somewhat better predictor of fetal size, with sensitivities of 64–86% and positive values of 29–79% (Villar & Belizan 1986).

Ultrasound

Ultrasound is generally considered to have a better detection rate for the SGA fetus than clinical examination. Several studies have assessed the effectiveness of ultrasound at detecting small fetuses in the low-risk population, with sensitivities varying from 43 to 94%, and positive predictive values from 20 to 70% (Villar & Belizan 1986).

In the UK, the human resource implications of scanning every low-risk woman even twice for growth during the third trimester would be huge, and even then IUGR may well occur before or after the time of scanning. Randomised controlled trials have failed to demonstrate any benefit in terms of morbidity or mortality (Villar & Belizan 1986), although some studies have shown an increase in admission and early induction in groups screened with ultrasound. Ultrasound screening for IUGR and/or SGA in low-risk populations is currently not justified.

Fetoplacental Doppler

There are several studies of umbilical artery Doppler waveform indices as a screening tool for IUGR, but it has not been shown to be of value. This is not surprising, as abnormalities in fetal blood flow are most often associated with fetal hypoxia, whereas the underlying cause of IUGR may involve many other factors, with hypoxia being a relatively late event, if it occurs at all.

Uteroplacental Doppler

Using abnormal uterine artery waveforms (defined as a resistance index >95th centile and/or the presence of an early diastolic notch) at 18–22 weeks to predict SGA babies at birth has a sensitivity of 14–47%, and a positive predictive value of 13–38% (Bower et al 1993, Harrington et al 1996, Mires et al 1998). No improvement in perinatal outcome has been demonstrated by screening the general obstetric population (Davies et al 1992), and its use as a screening tool is not justified.

PREVENTION

Because the commonest risk factor for IUGR is smoking, all women should be encouraged to stop, or reduce if they cannot. Even passive smoking is harmful, and partners should also be persuaded to give up. Women with previous growth-restricted fetuses are at risk of a recurrence, and there are several studies looking at the role of aspirin in prevention. Antiplatelet drugs would seem likely candidates for prophylaxis in view of the possible role of placental thrombosis in IUGR. Although individual studies have been inconclusive, meta-analysis (Fig. 13.5) showed that early aspirin treatment reduced the risk of IUGR (Leitich et al 1997). The effect was greatest if the dose of aspirin was 100–150 mg/day, and if started before 17 weeks. Those authors concluded, however, that low-dose aspirin should not be used routinely until those most likely to benefit from aspirin have been clearly identified.

MANAGEMENT

The terms symmetric and asymmetric growth restriction are descriptions, not diagnoses. Probably more relevant to the

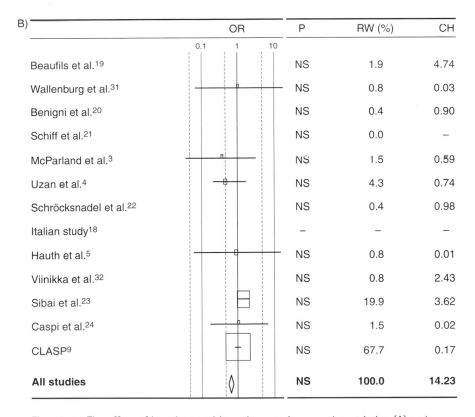

Fig. 13.5 The effect of low-dose aspirin on intrauterine growth restriction (A) and perinatal mortality (B). Odds ratios (OR), 95% confidence intervals, relative weights (RW) and contribution to heterogeneity (CH) of each study and all studies combined. (Reproduced from Leitich et al 1997, with permission of the publisher.)

aetiology is the timing of IUGR. Broadly speaking, growth deficiency detected at any gestation without associated anomaly is most likely to represent true growth restriction as a result of uteroplacental dysfunction, but the earlier the gestation, the more likely the fetus is to be aneuploid or infected.

Initial assessment

The gestational age should be checked using the last menstrual period, and any early scans. In patients in whom smallness is suspected, fetal size should be assessed ultrasonographically. Different charts (Fig. 13.6) are appropriate for deriving the likely gestation from fetal size and assessing size at a known gestation (Dewbury et al 1993). The diagnosis of mild and moderate degrees of impaired growth should only be made on serial scans, and measurements of fetal size should be performed no more frequently than every 2 weeks. This is because normal growth over 1 week is less than the accuracy of the measurement, and therefore failure of measurements to increase over 1 week cannot be relied upon as indicating growth restriction or failure. A thorough survey of the fetus for associated anomalies is undertaken, as these increase the likelihood of aneuploidy. The liquor volume should be quantified (preferably by amniotic fluid index), as a normal or increased volume increases the likelihood of aneuploidy. Doppler waveforms of the uterine and umbilical artery should be obtained, with normal waveforms once again increasing the likelihood of aneuploidy.

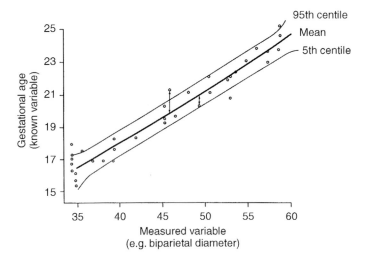

(A)

(B)

Fig. 13.6 The difference between a chart used to assess fetal size at a known gestation (A) and one used to assess gestation from fetal size (B). (Reproduced from Dewbury et al 1993.)

Early-onset growth restriction (<32 weeks)

The principle differential diagnoses are:

- chromosomal abnormality or some other genetic/syndromal problem
- congenital infection
- uteroplacental dysfunction.

Findings that would make a chromosomal problem more likely include normal uterine artery Doppler findings, normal liquor volume and presence of a structural abnormality. Such patients are counselled regarding the risk of aneuploidy and offered karyotyping by fetal blood sampling or amniocentesis. Even if an offer of termination of pregnancy is inappropriate, knowledge of an abnormal karyotype may be useful in planning the propriety of intervention during labour and at delivery. Nevertheless, it is important to remember that if the patient decides to forgo monitoring and intervention in labour on the basis of an abnormal karyotype, that the aneuploid fetus may be live born, and possibly further compromised by hypoxia. Parents must understand the limitations of karyotyping, in that it may not detect small deletions or rearrangements and will not detect genetic syndromes.

A history suggestive of an infection during pregnancy should be sought, but viral infections may be asymptomatic. The diagnosis of fetal viral infection is difficult, with prediction of damage even more so. The prevalence of pathogens varies in different countries and at different times. The frequency of maternal infection and the rate of transplacental passage are often not known. Fetal serological studies (for IgM) are unreliable before 20 weeks, and later in pregnancy may still be insensitive. Fetal IgG simply reflects maternal antibody levels. Polymerase chain reaction is more sensitive, but prone to false-positive results from contamination. Indirect tests for fetal infection include fetal haematological and biochemical indices. The commonest infection associated with IUGR is cytomegalovirus (CMV) and if the mother has a history of a flu-like illness, or the fetus has other sonographic findings compatible with CMV (e.g. microcephaly, cerebral calcification) then this possibility should be discussed with the mother. However, it is vital that she is aware of the limitations of diagnosing infection in the fetus, the lack of treatment and the difficulty of predicting outcome. This is discussed in detail in Chapter 22.

Uteroplacental dysfunction is really a diagnosis of exclusion. Factors supporting this are a history of growth restriction in a previous pregnancy, reduced liquor volume, or abnormal uterine or umbilical artery waveforms.

Late-onset growth restriction (>32 weeks)

The most likely cause is uteroplacental insufficiency, often associated with the development of pre-eclampsia. The assessment and monitoring is essentially the same as with early-onset growth restriction suspected of being due to uteroplacental insufficiency. It should be remembered that early- and late-onset growth restriction are merely descriptive categories that alter the most likely underlying cause; IUGR may be diagnosed at any stage.

Fetal monitoring

Monitoring the growth-restricted fetus involves serial fetal measurement (particularly AC), amniotic fluid index, cardiotocography and, more recently, Doppler ultrasound. Study of the fetal circulation may provide further clues as to fetal condition, but none of the vessels in the fetus have yet been evaluated with regard to clinical decision making.

Umbilical arterial flow

Absent end-diastolic flow (AEDF) in the umbilical artery has been shown to discriminate growth-restricted fetuses at high risk of perinatal death from those at low risk. Fetuses with AEDF are hypoxaemic. However, these changes may appear up to 5 weeks before demise, so they cannot be used alone as indicators for preterm delivery. Reversed end-diastolic flow (Fig. 13.7) is suggestive of preterminal compromise, and these fetuses usually die within 1–2 days if not delivered.

The Cochrane database has analysed 11 studies of over 7000 patients, looking at the use of umbilical artery Doppler in high risk pregnancy. In those whom the results were revealed to the clinician there was a trend to reduction in perinatal death (RR 0.71, 95% CI 0.50 to 1.01), a reduction in induction of labour (RR 0.83, 95% CI 0.74 to 0.93), a reduction in antenatal admissions (RR 0.56, 95% CI 0.43 to 0.72), but no demonstrable effect on the incidence of fetal distress in labour (RR 0.80, 95% CI 0.59 to 1.13) or caesarean section (RR 0.94, 95% CI 0.82 to 1.06). An earlier meta-analysis (Fig. 13.8), which included data from one group the authenticity of which has since been questioned, found a significant reduction in perinatal death (reduction of 38%, 95% CI 15 to 55%) (Alfirevic et al 1995).

Fetal cerebral flow

The fetus is able to redistribute its blood flow to the brain and heart at the expense of less vital organs in response to stresses such as hypoxia. This is can be demonstrated by increased flow velocity and decreased resistance in the middle cerebral artery (MCA).

The maximum reduction in PI is reached when the fetal P_{O_2} is 2–4 SD below the mean for gestation, after which the PI tends to rise, possibly due to development of brain oedema (Vyas et al 1990). Consequently a fetus with IUGR seen for the first time at a late stage in the disease process may have an MCA PI that is normal, or even raised. There is a wide range of normal values for MCA PI, and a trend in MCA PI, studied with the other parameters discussed, is a more useful indicator of fetal condition than a single measurement.

Fetal aortic flow

The descending thoracic aorta waveforms of growth-retarded fetuses show increased resistance compared with normal fetuses (Griffin et al 1984), and one group has correlated decreased peak systolic velocity with fetal hypoxia (Soothill et al 1986, Bilardo et al 1990).

Fetal venous flow

Cardiac decompensation with alterations in venous flow represents an end-stage response. There is correlation between venous Doppler indices (ductus venosus and inferior vena cava) and hypoxia (Rizzo et al 1996), with flow velocity waveforms in the ductus venosus showing reversal of flow at the time of atrial contraction (Fig. 13.9). Pulsatile flow in the umbilical vein is a sign of severe fetal compromise (Ozcan et al 1998).

Amniotic fluid index

Reduction in amniotic fluid index (the sum of the four deepest vertical pools in each quadrant) is associated with an increase in perinatal mortality (Chamberlain et al 1984). Fetal urine production is significantly lower in the SGA fetus than in the AGA fetus, and the degree of reduction in urine production correlates with both the degree of fetal hypoxaemia and the degree of fetal smallness (Nicolaides et al 1990). Oligohydramnios is associated with redistribution of fetal blood flow (Yoshimura et al 1997), so oliguria may be a consequence of decreased renal perfusion in favour of essential organs.

Biophysical profile

This scoring system for monitoring fetal well-being is not widely used in the UK. Firstly, it is time-consuming, requiring a 40 min observation of fetal breathing movements. Secondly, the most predictive components are the cardiotocography (CTG) and amniotic fluid volume, which are standard monitoring tests anyway. Thirdly, a persistently abnormal biophysical score was always associated with absence of end-diastolic flow in a study of 902 biophysical profile and Doppler assessments in 250 high-risk patients (Tyrrell et al 1990).

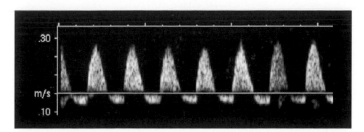

Fig. 13.7 Doppler flow velocity waveform of umbilical arterial flow showing reversed end-diastolic flow.

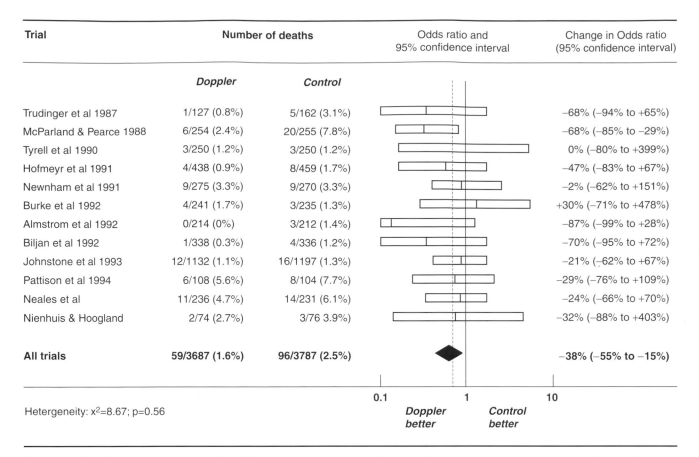

Trial	Number of deaths		Odds ratio and 95% confidence interval	Change in Odds ratio (95% confidence interval)
	Doppler	Control		
Trudinger et al 1987	1/127 (0.8%)	5/162 (3.1%)		−68% (−94% to +65%)
McParland & Pearce 1988	6/254 (2.4%)	20/255 (7.8%)		−68% (−85% to −29%)
Tyrell et al 1990	3/250 (1.2%)	3/250 (1.2%)		0% (−80% to +399%)
Hofmeyr et al 1991	4/438 (0.9%)	8/459 (1.7%)		−47% (−83% to +67%)
Newnham et al 1991	9/275 (3.3%)	9/270 (3.3%)		−2% (−62% to +151%)
Burke et al 1992	4/241 (1.7%)	3/235 (1.3%)		+30% (−71% to +478%)
Almstrom et al 1992	0/214 (0%)	3/212 (1.4%)		−87% (−99% to +28%)
Biljan et al 1992	1/338 (0.3%)	4/336 (1.2%)		−70% (−95% to +72%)
Johnstone et al 1993	12/1132 (1.1%)	16/1197 (1.3%)		−21% (−62% to +67%)
Pattison et al 1994	6/108 (5.6%)	8/104 (7.7%)		−29% (−76% to +109%)
Neales et al	11/236 (4.7%)	14/231 (6.1%)		−24% (−66% to +70%)
Nienhuis & Hoogland	2/74 (2.7%)	3/76 3.9%)		−32% (−88% to +403%)
All trials	**59/3687 (1.6%)**	**96/3787 (2.5%)**		**−38% (−55% to −15%)**

Hetergeneity: x^2=8.67; p=0.56

0.1   1   10

Doppler better   *Control better*

Fig. 13.8 The effect on perinatal mortality of Doppler ultrasonography of the umbilical artery in high-risk pregnancies. The death rates were 2.5% and 1.6% respectively in the control (no Doppler) and Doppler groups. (Reproduced from Alfirevic & Neilson 1995, with the permission of the publisher.)

Cardiotocography

The Cochrane database reports on four now quite old studies of 1588 patients using CTG for antepartum monitoring in high-risk patients. There was no significant reduction in perinatal mortality or morbidity; in fact there was a trend to an increased rate of perinatal death (odds ratio 2.85,95% CI 0.99 to 7.12). This may be due to false reassurance from normal CTG traces. Overview concluded that there is not enough evidence to justify antenatal cardiotocography for fetal assessment. Its role in conjunction with detailed fetal Doppler is not known, but it probably has a role once absent diastolic flow is noted in the umbilical artery. Whether the fetus is best delivered as soon as end-diastolic flow disappears, or whether it is better to wait until the CTG pattern becomes abnormal is currently being addressed by the GRIT study (Growth Restriction Intervention Trial). Interim results suggest a lower mortality and morbidity from IUGR if delivery is delayed until the CTG is abnormal than from the effects of premature delivery if the delivery is expedited as soon as the abnormal Doppler is discovered, but final conclusions must await the termination of the study.

Invasive assessment of fetal acid–base status

Fetal blood sampling has been advocated in IUGR for assessment of fetal well-being; however, the complex compensatory mechanisms make it unlikely that a single measurement of

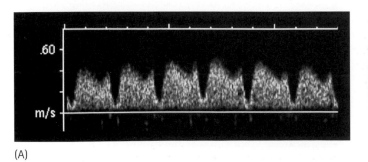

(A)

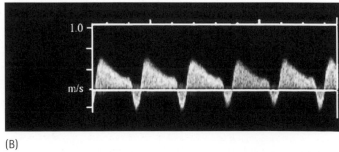

(B)

Fig. 13.9 Doppler flow velocity waveform of normal ductus venosus flow (A) and reversed flow at the time of atrial contraction (B).

pH could predict the stage at which decompensation occurs. In a study of 32 IUGR fetuses with AEDF there was no difference in pH, Po_2, Pco_2 or base excess between survivors and perinatal deaths (Nicolini et al 1990). The clinically useful finding was that hypoxia and/or acidaemia was rare amongst fetuses with EDF present (Fig. 13.10). The risks of fetal blood sampling are significantly increased in compromised fetuses. Most groups therefore do not now advocate fetal blood sampling to determine acid–base status in the growth-restricted fetus, in the absence of atypical features or a risk of aneuploidy.

Timing of fetal monitoring

Fetuses with IUGR should be monitored with Doppler ultrasound at least weekly, with growth measurements every 2 weeks. Assessment should include the liquor volume as well as the umbilical artery Doppler studies. If either are abnormal, surveillance should be increased to twice weekly or more, and assessment extended to the fetal circulation if facilities are available; daily or even twice daily CTG monitoring is also advisable.

Labour and delivery

The question of when to deliver a growth restricted fetus has no straightforward answer. Failure to deliver poses the risk of chronic hypoxia (including intrauterine death and adverse neurodevelopment), while delivery exposes the neonate to the risks of prematurity. Earlier intervention on the one hand may improve survival, but on the other may result in a severely handicapped survivor who might otherwise have died in utero. As gestation advances, the threshold for delivery becomes lower because the risks of prematurity decrease. Between 36 and 37 weeks, the authors would advocate delivery if there was absence of growth, or significant crossing of centiles (i.e. failure of abdominal growth) associated with oligohydramnios. Between 32 and 36 weeks, stronger evidence, such as severe oligohydramnios, AEDF in the umbilical artery, evidence of redistribution or abnormal venous Dopplers, would be required. Most fetuses will follow a decompensation cascade (Fig. 13.11), with AEDF preceding a decelerative CTG, which in turn precedes reversed EDF and fetal death. The basic principles within the limits of current knowledge involve delivery at about the time the CTG becomes abnormal, and before reversed EDF. Before 32 weeks, delivery should be considered on the same grounds, against the background of the estimated fetal weight, and gestation-specific morbidity and mortality rates. At the limits of viability the implications of delivery or non-intervention should be discussed with the parents and their wishes reflected.

The growth-restricted fetus, if not already hypoxic, is more likely to become hypoxic in labour. The fetus with evidence of acidaemia (absent or reversed end-diastolic flow in the umbilical artery, blood flow redistribution or abnormal

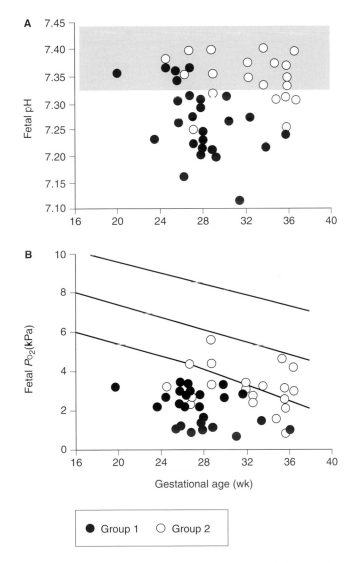

Fig. 13.10 The relationship between fetal pH (A), fetal Po_2 (B) and gestation in fetuses with absent (group 1) and present (group 2) end-diastolic flow in the umbilical arteries. This shows that pH and Po_2 are likely to be normal if EDF is present. (Reproduced from Nicolini et al 1990, with the permission of the publisher.)

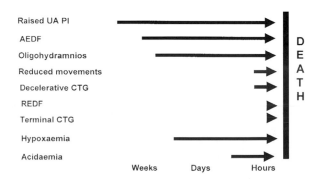

Fig. 13.11 Decompensation cascade in IUGR. The timing of different parameters of fetal monitoring hypoxia in the weeks from early fetal compromise, initially with only a raised umbilical artery pulsatility index (UA PI), through to reversed end-diastolic flow (REDF) and intrauterine death. AEDF, absent end-diastolic flow; CTG, cardiotocography.

venous Dopplers) should be delivered by caesarean section without a trial of labour because of the high incidence of intrapartum fetal compromise. In other fetuses a trial of labour is appropriate, subject to other obstetric considerations.

The importance of monitoring and timing of delivery has been highlighted by a recent study of 149 apparently unexplained stillbirths (Gardosi et al 1998). Forty-one per cent were found to be SGA. The authors suggest that many stillbirths classified as unexplained may be avoidable if slow fetal growth could be recognised as a warning sign.

KEY POINTS

- The aetiology of growth restriction remains poorly understood.
- Size is not the same as growth, and smallness is not the same as growth restriction.
- Early-onset growth restriction and associated abnormalities increase the risk of chromosomal abnormality.
- The mainstay of management revolves around biophysical fetal monitoring, with delivery indicated when the intrauterine risks outweigh the extrauterine risks.
- The use of umbilical artery Doppler decreases perinatal mortality in high-risk populations, such as those with suspected growth restriction.

REFERENCES

Alfirevic Z, Neilson JP 1995 Doppler ultrasonography in high-risk pregnancies: systematic review with meta-analysis. Am J Obstet Gynecol 172:1379–1387

Barker DJ 1995 Fetal origins of coronary heart disease. BMJ 311:171–174

Battaglia C, Artini PG, D'Ambrogio G, Galli PA, Segre A, Genazzani AR 1992 Maternal hyperoxygenation in the treatment of intrauterine growth retardation. Am J Obstet Gynecol 167:430–435

Bilardo CM, Nicolaides KH, Campbell S 1990 Doppler measurements of fetal and uteroplacental circulations: relationship with umbilical venous blood gases measured at cordocentesis. Am J Obstet Gynecol 162:115–120

Bower S, Schuchter K, Campbell S 1993 Doppler ultrasound screening as part of routine antenatal scanning: prediction of pre-eclampsia and intrauterine growth retardation. Br J Obstet Gynaecol 100:989–994

Butler NR, Goldstein H, Ross EM 1972 Cigarette smoking in pregnancy: its influence on birth weight and perinatal mortality. BMJ 2:127–130

Chamberlain PF, Manning FA, Morrison I, Harman CR, Lange IR 1984 Ultrasound evaluation of amniotic fluid volume. I. The relationship of marginal and decreased amniotic fluid volumes to perinatal outcome. Am J Obstet Gynecol 150:245–249

Davies JA, Gallivan S, Spencer JA 1992 Randomised controlled trial of Doppler ultrasound screening of placental perfusion during pregnancy. Lancet 340:1299–1303

Dewbury K, Meire H, Cosgrove D (eds) 1993 Ultrasound in obstetrics and gynaecology. Churchill Livingstone, London

Gardosi J, Chang A, Kalyan B, Sahota D, Symonds EM 1992 Customised antenatal growth charts. Lancet 339:283–287

Gardosi J, Mul T, Mongelli M, Fagan D 1998 Analysis of birthweight and gestational age in antepartum stillbirths. Br J Obstet Gynaecol 105:524–530

Giles WB, Trudinger BJ, Baird PJ 1985 Fetal umbilical artery flow velocity waveforms and placental resistance: pathological correlation. Br J Obstet Gynaecol 92:31–38

Griffin D, Bilardo K, Masini L et al 1984 Doppler blood flow waveforms in the descending thoracic aorta of the human fetus. Br J Obstet Gynaecol 91:997–1006

Hadlock FP, Harrist RB, Carpenter RJ, Deter RL, Park SK 1984 Sonographic estimation of fetal weight. The value of femur length in addition to head and abdomen measurements. Radiology 150:535–540

Harrington K, Cooper D, Lees C, Hecher K, Campbell S 1996 Doppler ultrasound of the uterine arteries: the importance of bilateral notching in the prediction of pre-eclampsia, placental abruption or delivery of a small-for-gestational-age baby. Ultrasound Obstet Gynecol 7:182–188

Hattersley AT, Beards F, Ballantyne E, Appleton M, Harvey R, Ellard S 1998 Mutations in the glucokinase gene of the fetus result in reduced birth weight. Nat Genet 19:268–270

Hendricks SK, Sorensen TK, Wang KY, Bushnell JM, Seguin EM, Zingheim RW 1989 Doppler umbilical artery waveform indices: normal values from fourteen to forty-two weeks. Am J Obstet Gynecol 161:761–765

Hulse GK, Milne E, English DR, Holman CD 1997 The relationship between maternal use of heroin and methadone and infant birth weight. Addiction 92:1571–1579

Jewell D, Sharp D, Saunders J, Peters T 2000 A randomised controlled trial of flexibility in routine antenatal care. Br J Obst Gynae 107:1241–1247

Katano K, Aoki A, Sasa H, Ogasawara M, Matsuura E, Yagami Y 1996 beta 2-Glycoprotein I-dependent anticardiolipin antibodies as a predictor of adverse pregnancy outcomes in healthy pregnant women. Hum Reprod 11:509–512

Khong TY, De Wolf F, Robertson WB, Brosens I 1986 Inadequate maternal vascular response to placentation in pregnancies complicated by pre-eclampsia and by small-for-gestational age infants. Br J Obstet Gynaecol 93:1049–1059

Kupferminc MJ, Eldor A, Steinman N et al 1999 Increased frequency of genetic thrombophilia in women with complications of pregnancy. N Engl J Med 340:9–13

Leitich H, Egarter C, Husslein P, Kaider A, Schemper M 1997 A meta-analysis of low dose aspirin for the prevention of intrauterine growth retardation. Br J Obstet Gynaecol 104:450–459

Lieberman E, Gremy I, Lang JM, Cohen AP 1994 Low birthweight at term and the timing of fetal exposure to maternal smoking. Am J Public Health 84:1127–1131

Macara L, Kingdom JC, Kaufmann P et al 1996 Structural analysis of placental terminal villi from growth-restricted pregnancies with abnormal umbilical artery Doppler waveforms. Placenta 17:37–48

Mires GJ, Williams FL, Leslie J, Howie PW 1998 Assessment of uterine arterial notching as a screening test for adverse pregnancy outcome. Am J Obstet Gynecol 179:1317–1323

Nicolaides KH, Peters MT, Vyas S, Rabinowitz R, Rosen DJ, Campbell S 1990 Relation of rate of urine production to oxygen tension in small-for-gestational-age fetuses. Am J Obstet Gynecol 162:387–391

Nicolini U, Nicolaidis P, Fisk NM et al 1990 Limited role of fetal blood sampling in prediction of outcome in intrauterine growth retardation. Lancet 336:768–772

Ozcan T, Sbracia M, d'Ancona RL, Copel JA, Mari G 1998 Arterial and venous Doppler velocimetry in the severely growth-restricted fetus and associations with adverse perinatal outcome. Ultrasound Obstet Gynecol 12:39–44

Reece EA, Leguizamon G, Homko C 1998 Pregnancy performance and outcomes associated with diabetic nephropathy. Am J Perinatol 15:413–421

Rizzo G, Capponi A, Talone PE, Arduini D, Romanini C 1996 Doppler indices from inferior vena cava and ductus venosus in predicting pH and oxygen tension in umbilical blood at cordocentesis in growth-retarded fetuses. Ultrasound Obstet Gynecol 7:401–410

Roquer JM, Figueras J, Botet F, Jimenez R 1995 Influence on fetal growth of exposure to tobacco smoke during pregnancy. Acta Paediatr 84:118–211.

Sexton M, Hebel JR 1984 A clinical trial of change in maternal smoking and its effect on birth weight. JAMA 251:911–915

Shepard MJ, Richards VA, Berkowitz RL, Warsof SL, Hobbins JC 1982 An evaluation of two equations for predicting fetal weight by ultrasound. Am J Obstet Gynecol 142:47–54

Snijders RJ, Sherrod C, Gosden CM, Nicolaides KH 1993 Fetal growth retardation: associated malformations and chromosomal abnormalities. Am J Obstet Gynecol 168:547–555

Soothill PW, Nicolaides KH, Bilardo CM, Campbell S 1986 Relation of fetal hypoxia in growth retardation to mean blood velocity in the fetal aorta. Lancet ii:1118–1120

Soothill PW, Morafa W, Ayida GA, Rodeck CH 1996 Maternal smoking and fetal carboxyhaemoglobin and blood gas levels. Br J Obstet Gynaecol 103:78–82

Steer P 1998 Fetal growth. Br J Obstet Gynaecol 105:1133–1135

Tyrrell SN, Lilford RJ, Macdonald HN, Nelson EJ, Porter J, Gupta JK 1990 Randomized comparison of routine vs highly selective use of Doppler ultrasound and biophysical scoring to investigate high risk pregnancies. Br J Obstet Gynaecol 97:909–916

Villar J, Belizan JM 1986 The evaluation of the methods used in the diagnosis of intrauterine growth retardation. Obstet Gynecol Surv 41:187–199

Vintzileos AM, Campbell WA, Neckles S, Pike CL, Nochimson DJ 1984 The ultrasound femur length as a predictor of fetal length. Obstet Gynecol 64:779–782

Virji SK 1991 The relationship between alcohol consumption during pregnancy and infant birthweight. An epidemiologic study. Acta Obstet Gynecol Scand 70:303–308

Vyas S, Nicolaides KH, Bower S, Campbell S 1990 Middle cerebral artery flow velocity waveforms in fetal hypoxaemia. Br J Obstet Gynaecol 97:797–803

Yoshimura S, Masuzaki H, Gotoh H, Ishimaru T 1997 Fetal redistribution of blood flow and amniotic fluid volume in growth-retarded fetuses. Early Hum Dev 47:297–304

14

Bleeding in pregnancy

James Drife

The contribution of the author of the equivalent chapter in the second edition, on which this chapter draws extensively, is gratefully acknowledged.

INTRODUCTION

The spectrum of bleeding in pregnancy ranges from a small show with little clinical significance to a catastrophic haemorrhage which quickly causes the death of mother or baby. Even slight vaginal bleeding can cause great anxiety to a pregnant woman.

Bleeding can occur at any stage of pregnancy or labour. Early pregnancy bleeding is discussed in the section on miscarriage in Chapter 9, and postpartum haemorrhage is discussed in Chapter 38. This chapter deals with ectopic pregnancy and with bleeding in late pregnancy.

Incidence

The British Births Survey of 1970 still gives useful data on the incidence of bleeding in pregnancy (Chamberlain et al 1978). There was a history of bleeding in one in ten among the 17 000 pregnancies in the survey. The bleeding varied from a small episode before 28 weeks in 4.2% of pregnancies, to placenta praevia in 0.5%. As Table 14.1 shows, it is often difficult to allocate cases to simple diagnostic categories, such as premature separation of placenta or placenta praevia.

Studies in Aberdeen have shown increased reporting of antepartum haemorrhage (APH) (MacGillivray & Campbell 1988). During the period 1951–1983 the overall incidence of APH was 4.1% among singleton pregnancies and 6% among twins, but the annual figures increased from less than 3% in 1951 to 8.5% among singleton and 12.6% among twin pregnancies in 1981–1983.

Table 14.1 Bleeding in pregnancy: frequency and perinatal mortality

Type of bleeding	Incidence (%)	Perinatal mortality rate (per 1000 births)
None	88.7	16.8
Placenta praevia	0.5	81.4
Accidental APH	1.2	143.6
Bleeding < 28 weeks	4.2	61.0
Other specified cause	2.2	39.7
Unspecified	2.4	32.6
No information	0.8	30.3
Total in survey	17005 (100%)	21.4

From Chamberlain et al 1978.
APH = antepartum haemorrhage.

ECTOPIC PREGNANCY

Ectopic pregnancy is the most common cause of maternal death in the first trimester of pregnancy (Department of Health 1998). In the UK in 1994–1996 it caused 12 maternal deaths, compared with nine in 1991–1993 and 15 in 1988–1990.

Incidence

The incidence rose in northern Europe from 11.2 per 1000 pregnancies in 1976 to 18.8 per 1000 in 1983. In the USA in 1992 the incidence was 19.7 per 1000, 2% of all pregnancies (Pisarska et al 1998, Tay et al 2000). In Britain the recorded incidence of ectopic pregnancy increased 3.8-fold between 1966 and 1996, from 3.25 to 12.4 per 1000 pregnancies (Rajkhowa et al 2000). This may be partly due to improved diagnosis but it is likely that the true incidence has increased, probably due to a sexually transmitted agent (Rajkhowa et al 2000).

Risk factors

The risk of ectopic pregnancy is increased by several factors (Table 14.2). Previous female sterilisation and current use of an intrauterine contraceptive device (IUD) are risk factors when patients with ectopic pregnancy are compared with pregnant controls but not when they are compared with non-pregnant women (Tay et al 2000). After female sterilisation the risk of ectopic pregnancy is up to 7.3 per 1000 within 10 years: if pregnancy does occur there is a high risk (up to 33%) that it will be ectopic, particularly if the sterilisation was by bipolar cautery. Intrauterine devices prevent intrauterine pregnancy more effectively than tubal pregnancy, and therefore pregnancy is more likely to be ectopic if it occurs in association with an IUD. The risk of ectopic pregnancy is not increased by the combined oral contraceptive pill, previous termination of pregnancy or previous caesarean section (Fylstra 1998).

After acute salpingitis the risk of an ectopic pregnancy is increased sevenfold. An important factor at present is *Chlamydia trachomatis*, the main cause of pelvic inflammatory disease in the UK. Reduction in the rates of chlamydial infection will reduce the rates of ectopic pregnancies.

Diagnosis

The most important factor in diagnosing ectopic pregnancy is to consider the diagnosis—i.e. 'think ectopic'. It is surprisingly easy to miss the condition if at the time of consultation an alternative diagnosis seems obvious—for example, if the case seems to be one of gastroenteritis (Department of Health 1998) or salpingitis. Any woman of reproductive age presenting with abdominal pain or vaginal bleeding should be screened for pregnancy.

Cases usually present with between five and nine weeks of amenorrhoea. The accompanying signs are variable (Table 14.3). The possible sites for an ectopic pregnancy are shown in Figure 14.1. Of them, the Fallopian tube is the most common. Even amenorrhoea may not be obvious, as the bleeding that often accompanies ectopic pregnancy may be mistaken for a normal period. Up to 9% of patients report no pain and 36% have no abdominal tenderness.

Modern pregnancy tests on urine or blood are very sensitive and the presence of chorionic tissue in the body can be

Table 14.2 Risk factors for ectopic pregnancy

Risk factor	Odds ratio
High risk	
Tubal surgery	21.9
Sterilisation	9.3
Previous ectopic pregnancy	8.3
In utero exposure to diethylstilboestrol	5.6
Use of IUD	4.2–45.0
Documented tubal pathology	3.8–21.0
Moderate risk	
Infertility	2.5–21.0
Previous genital infections	2.5–3.7
Multiple sexual partners	2.1
Slight risk	
Previous pelvic/abdominal surgery	0.9–3.8
Cigarette smoking	2.3–2.5
Vaginal douching	1.1–3.1
Early age at first intercourse (<18 years)	1.6

From Pisarska et al 1998, with permission.

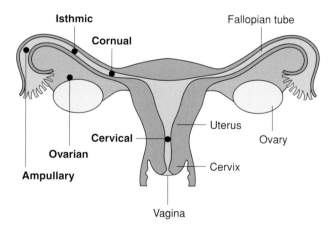

Fig. 14.1 Sites of ectopic pregnancies. (From Tay et al 2000, with permission.)

Table 14.3 Ectopic pregnancy: percentage of cases with symptoms or signs

Abdominal pain	97%
Vaginal bleeding	79%
Abdominal tenderness	91%
Adnexal tenderness	54%
History of infertility	15%
Use of an IUD	14%
Previous ectopic pregnancy	11%

Adapted from Tay et al 2000, with permission.

confirmed or excluded relatively easily—but (it should be emphasised again) only if the test is carried out. Screening by measurement of human chorionic gonadotrophin beta (β-hCG), and transvaginal ultrasound has a sensitivity of 84–88% and specificity of 100% (Pisarska et al 1998). If a fetal heartbeat is seen within the uterine cavity, this effectively rules out ectopic pregnancy, as the incidence of heterotopic pregnancy (combined intrauterine and extrauterine) is as low as 1 in approximately 4000 pregnancies (Fylstra 1998). Heterotopic pregnancy is, however, much more common (1–3%) after infertility treatment with superovulation.

If the scan shows fluid but no heartbeat within the uterus, a gestation sac has to be differentiated from a 'pseudosac'—a collection of fluid within the endometrial cavity. A true gestation sac is eccentrically placed within the uterus beneath the endometrial surface.

If no sac is seen within the uterus, the serum concentration of hCG should be measured. In these circumstances a concentration of 2000 IU or more per litre is diagnostic of ectopic pregnancy, but a lower concentration, 1500 IU/l, is diagnostic if there is an ectopic mass or if there is fluid within the pouch of Douglas. The level of hCG at which all intrauterine pregnancies should be visible on ultrasound is the discriminatory zone. Compared with transvaginal ultrasound, the discriminatory zone with abdominal ultrasound is much higher, at 6500 IU/l.

If the diagnosis remains in doubt, the serum hCG should be measured every 2 days. In a normal pregnancy the doubling time is every 2–3.5 days between the fourth and the eighth week of pregnancy, but with ectopic pregnancy the rate of increase is slower.

Treatment

The traditional treatment of ectopic pregnancy was salpingectomy through a transverse lower abdominal incision. Surgery was regarded as mandatory because of the risk that the pregnancy would rupture a blood vessel, leading to life-threatening intraperitoneal haemorrhage. Early diagnosis now makes expectant or medical management possible in selected cases, though surgery remains essential if the pregnancy has ruptured or if there is hypotension or anaemia.

Surgical

Surgery is the appropriate treatment if the diameter of the ectopic gestational sac is greater than 3 cm (Pisarska et al 1998) or 4 cm (Fylstra 1998) on ultrasonography, if the pregnancy has ruptured, or if pain persists beyond 24 hours (Pisarska et al 1998). Laparotomy and salpingectomy are indicated if the patient is haemodynamically unstable or if the surgeon is not trained in laparoscopic technique. Otherwise laparoscopic surgery is generally preferred.

Salpingectomy is carried out if the fallopian tube is extensively diseased or damaged. Attempts to preserve the tube in these circumstances may lead to recurrent ectopic pregnancy. For ampullary ectopic pregnancies, laparoscopic linear salpingostomy is recommended. A longitudinal incision is made on the antimesenteric surface of the tube and products of conception are removed with forceps or suction. Fimbrial

expression (by 'milking') may be appropriate if the pregnancy is aborting from the open end of the tube. Success rates (in terms of requiring no further therapy) of 93% have been reported for laparoscopic salpingostomy or fimbrial expression. Isthmic pregnancies are treated with excision of the affected segment. Follow up is by regular checks of hCG levels until there is complete resolution. Persistent ectopic pregnancy can be treated with methotrexate.

Medical

If the patient is haemodynamically stable and there is an unruptured ectopic pregnancy measuring less than 3–4 cm in diameter, medical treatment with methotrexate may be appropriate. Methotrexate is a folic acid antagonist which interferes with cell multiplication. It may be given intramuscularly or injected into the ectopic pregnancy itself under laparoscopic or ultrasound guidance, but local treatment is no more successful than systemic treatment. Success rates of up to 87% have been reported, although in 8% of cases more than one treatment is required.

Higher success rates have been reported with a 'variable dose' regimen, giving methotrexate on alternate days until the serum hCG concentration begins to fall. This is less convenient than a single-dose regimen but can be successful in up to 93% of cases. In one prospective study, 67 women with unruptured tubal pregnancy were treated with intramuscular methotrexate 0.5 mg/kg for up to 5 days, in combination with local application of 12.5 mg methotrexate via laparoscopy. In 90% of these women no further surgical intervention was required, and 81% experienced a subsequent intrauterine pregnancy. Forty of the women underwent hysterosalpingography after treatment and patency of the affected tube was observed in all but one (Debby et al 2000).

Close monitoring of the hCG response is essential with medical treatment. Patients may experience pain as the pregnancy aborts. Side-effects of methotrexate may occur but are infrequent.

Alternatives to methotrexate, including local injection of prostaglandins, hyperosmolar glucose or potassium chloride, have been tried. Prostaglandins caused side-effects and success rates with the other alternatives were poor, so these options remain unattractive at present (Pisarska et al 1998).

Expectant

Selection of patients for expectant management depends not so much on the size of the pregnancy on ultrasound scanning as on the initial serum concentration of hCG, which is an indication of the quantity of viable chorionic tissue present. If the serum hCG concentration is less than 1000 IU/l, there is an 88% chance of successful resolution. At least 14 studies of expectant management of ectopic pregnancy have been reported (Pisarska et al 1998), involving 628 pregnancies, of which 68% resolved without surgery. Close monitoring of hCG levels is essential, with recourse to medical or surgical treatment if the fall in hCG does not continue. In one study, complete resolution took an average of 31 days.

Sequelae

After ectopic pregnancy there are risks of infertility and of another ectopic pregnancy; with modern treatment these risks are lower than in the past. Overall fertility rates after conservative laparoscopic surgery or medical treatment are around 65%, and among those who conceive the rate of recurrent ectopic pregnancy is around 10%. After expectant management the figures are rather better, with fertility rates of around 87% and recurrent ectopic rates of less than 7%. In a French population-based study of 291 women attempting to conceive after ectopic pregnancy, 197 (66%) conceived again spontaneously and 22 by *in vitro* fertilisation: crude rates of spontaneous intrauterine pregnancy were 57% after salpingectomy, 73% after laparoscopic surgery and 80% after medical treatment. The 2-year rate of recurrent ectopic pregnancy was 27%, with no difference between treatments (Bouyer et al 2000).

BLEEDING IN THE SECOND TRIMESTER

Antepartum haemorrhage (APH) used to be defined as 'bleeding from the genital tract after the 28th week of pregnancy and before labour'. Recently, however, this 28-week dividing line (formerly the legal definition of fetal viability) has become less relevant. Pregnancy bleeding is a continuum and both abruption and placenta praevia can occur before 28 weeks' gestation. With improved paediatric care, babies born as early as 24 weeks' gestation now have a good chance of survival, and under the Stillbirth (Definition) Act of 1992, stillbirths are now registered in Britain from 24 instead of 28 weeks. It therefore seems reasonable that 24 weeks should also form the new boundary between the definition of APH and bleeding of early pregnancy.

As the demarcation between APH and early pregnancy bleeding faded, there was a keener interest in the effect of bleeding in the second trimester. In the early 1990s several authors reported that second-trimester bleeding carries a poor fetal prognosis. In a study of 101 women admitted with bleeding in the second trimester, 40 proved later to have had abruption with a fetal loss rate of 37%, 27 had placenta praevia (loss rate 7.4%), 11 appeared to have both praevia and abruption (fetal mortality 18.2%) and in 23 no cause was identified (17.4% fetal loss) (Nielson et al 1991). In a study of 65 women admitted with bleeding between 14 and 26 weeks' gestation, 39 went to term and 18 delivered before 26 weeks, and the overall fetal loss rate was 31.8% (Lipitz et al 1991).

PLACENTA PRAEVIA

Definition

Placenta praevia means the placenta is partly or wholly implanted in the lower uterine segment. Traditionally the condition has been divided into four numbered grades (I–IV; Fig. 14.2), but with modern management there is little point in distinguishing grade III from IV, and it is more usual to

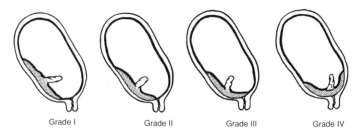

Fig. 14.2   Grades of placenta praevia.

describe only three degrees of severity—lateral, marginal and complete—or even two (minor and major).

- Lateral (grade I): the placenta just encroaches on the lower uterine segment.
- Marginal (grade II): the placenta reaches the margin of the cervical os.
- Complete (grade III): the placenta covers part of the os.
- Complete (grade IV): the placenta covers the os when dilated.

The placenta develops as a discoid condensation of trophoblast on the surface of the chorion at about 8–10 weeks' gestation and its position is determined by the site of implantation. A low-lying placenta identified in early pregnancy may seem to migrate upwards as pregnancy progresses, with formation of the lower segment and expansion of the upper segment. This phenomenon may be due in part to differential development of the placenta, possibly affected by previous scarring or changes in vascularisation. Adherence to a lower-segment scar may explain the increased incidence of placenta praevia following a previous caesarean section. Conditions in which the area of the placenta is increased, such as twins and placenta membranacea, have an increased incidence of placenta praevia (see below).

Incidence

It has been estimated that placenta praevia occurs in 0.4–0.8% of pregnancies, but with changes in risk factors such as parity these figures may no longer be reliable. In Aberdeen in 1981–1983 the incidence of placenta praevia was 0.48–0.56% among singleton pregnancies and 0.85% among twins with no relation to zygosity (MacGillivray & Campbell 1988). In a recent study of an unselected population in Finland the frequency was 0.16% (Taipale et al 1997). The current rise in the UK caesarean section rate may lead to an increase in incidence in future.

Risk factors

Age and parity
Increasing maternal age and parity are risk factors for placenta praevia (Rose & Chapman 1986) (Table 14.4).

Previous caesarean section
Numerous studies have found that a previous caesarean section increases the risk of placenta praevia (Hershkowitz et al

Table 14.4 The incidence of placenta praevia in relation to maternal age and parity (rates are per 100 pregnancies)

Reference	Maternal age (years)				
	< 20	20–24	25–29	30–34	35+
Chamberlain et al (1978)	0.1	0.3	0.5	0.6	1.5
Paintin (1962)	0.1	0.2	0.4	⊢— 0.7 —⊣	
Clark et al (1985)	0.1	0.2	0.3	0.4	0.9
Naeye (1980)					
Non-smokers	0.2	⊢— 0.4 —⊣		⊢— 0.8 —⊣	
Smokers	0.3	⊢— 0.7 —⊣		⊢— 1.8 —⊣	

	Pregnancy number			
	1	2	3–4	5+
Naeye (1980)				
Non-smokers	1.5	1.8	1.7	1.8
Smokers	1.8	1.9	2.2	2.9
Paintin (1962)	0.3	0.3	⊢— 0.7 —⊣	
Clark et al (1985)	0.1	0.2	0.4	0.6
Chamberlain et al (1978)	1.1	⊢— 1.4 —⊣		1.7

1995, Ananth et al 1997a, Macones et al 1997). For example, in a study of 97 799 deliveries, Clark et al (1985) found that the incidence of placenta praevia in those who had not had previous caesarean section was 0.25%; with one scar it was 0.65% and with three or more it was 2.2% (Table 14.5). Hershkowitz et al (1995) and Hemminki & Merilainen (1996) confirmed a significant association with one previous caesarean section but did not confirm that the risk increased with increasing numbers of previous caesareans. Ananth et al (1997a), however, did find that the risk increases with the number of previous caesarean deliveries.

Previous abortions

There has been some controversy about this risk factor. Rose and Chapman (1986) compared the gynaecological history of 80 women with placenta praevia with controls matched for age and parity. They found a significant relation to a history of dilatation and curettage, a less significant relation to evacuation of retained products of conception, but no relation to a previous induced abortion. Recent studies, however, have found a clear association with previous spontaneous or induced abortion (Ananth et al 1997a, Macones et al 1997) and a trend with increasing numbers of previous abortions (Hershkowitz et al 1995).

Table 14.5 Placenta praevia, placenta accreta and previous caesarean section

No. of caesarean sections	Patients (n)	Placenta praevia		Placenta accreta	
		n	%	n	%
0	92 917	238	0.26	12	5
1	3 820	25	0.65	6	24
2	850	15	1.8	7	47
3	183	5	3.0	2	40

From Clark et al 1985, with permission.

Ethnic origin

In a study in Washington State, USA, American women of Asian origin were 86% more likely to have a delivery complicated by placenta praevia than were White women, particularly primigravidae (Taylor et al 1995).

Smoking and drug abuse

A large US collaborative study showed that placenta praevia was more common in mothers who smoked during pregnancy than those who did not (Naeye 1980), though the relationship was not as strong as with placental abruption (see Table 14.4). The finding is difficult to explain but has been confirmed in more recent studies, which found that cigarette smoking is associated with a 2.6–4.4-fold increased risk of placenta praevia (Chelmow et al 1996). Placenta praevia is also associated with cocaine use (Macones et al 1997).

Hypertension

There is a reduced incidence of hypertension of pregnancy among women with placenta praevia, possibly because of abnormal placental perfusion (Ananth et al 1997b).

Diagnosis

With routine ultrasound scanning in early pregnancy, most cases of placenta praevia are suspected before there has been any bleeding. Indeed, there may be a problem of overdiagnosis and unnecessary anxiety.

Ultrasonography

Most British obstetric units now offer routine ultrasound scanning at 16–20 weeks' gestation. Such routine scanning can raise false fears, and placenta praevia should not be diagnosed on the basis of a single observation in the second trimester. The relationship between the placental site and the lower segment can change as pregnancy progresses, so that the placenta appears to migrate up the uterus. The later in pregnancy the scan is performed, the more accurate the prediction.

Comeau (Comeau et al 1983) found that of 222 cases of placenta praevia predicted by scan before 20 weeks, only five (2.2%) had significant bleeding or placenta praevia at term. Taipale, in a study of 6428 women scanned at 12–16 weeks' gestation, found that in 156 (2.4%) the placental edge extended 15 mm or more over the internal cervical os, but in only eight of these women was there placenta praevia at delivery (Taipale et al 1997). Two cases were missed, but among the 156 patients identified using this definition the likelihood of placenta praevia was 5.1%. Dawson and co-workers (Dawson et al 1996) concluded that transvaginal ultrasonography was superior to the transabdominal route in both the diagnosis and exclusion of placenta praevia. From 20 weeks' gestation onwards, an os–placenta distance of 3 cm or more excluded placenta praevia.

Symptoms

The characteristic clinical feature of placenta praevia is painless bleeding, usually in the third trimester. As pregnancy advances, Braxton Hicks contractions cause the lower segment to thin and in multiparae there is often some dilatation of the cervix. As a result, the abnormally inserted placenta separates from the decidua and bleeding results from the exposed uterine blood vessels. The bleeding is usually unprovoked, although there is occasionally a history of coitus just beforehand. Sometimes there is a history of bleeding in the second trimester but fortunately the first episode of bleeding is often minor. As the lower uterine segment has poor contractility, the bleeding from placenta praevia can be very severe, although it is unusual for it to be so before the 34th week of pregnancy. The most catastrophic cases of haemorrhage from placenta praevia occur from ill-advised attempts at vaginal examination.

Signs

The abdomen is soft with no tenderness. The presenting part is easily felt and the fetal heart rate should be normal. The low placenta displaces the presenting part, with a high incidence of malpresentation. The condition should be suspected if there is an unstable lie even without any bleeding. A deeply engaged presenting part is strong evidence that the praevia is of minor degree.

The clinical diagnosis can be difficult when bleeding occurs with the onset of labour, due to a grade I praevia. In these circumstances, the presenting part is engaged and the presence of labour contractions obscures the abdominal palpation.

Digital vaginal examination must not be undertaken in a case of suspected placenta praevia: it may provoke serious bleeding. Ultrasound examination should be arranged to identify the placental site. Transvaginal ultrasound is accurate, safe and well tolerated. It should rarely be necessary to have to confirm the diagnosis by vaginal examination, undertaken in an operating theatre with everything ready for an immediate caesarean section (see below), but this may be required if ultrasound is not available. If there is doubt about the cause of vaginal bleeding on admission, while digital vaginal examination is contraindicated, a speculum examination is often helpful before arranging a scan. For example, a heavy show is often associated with rapid cervical dilatation in early labour, and a speculum examination will reveal bulging membranes and cervical dilatation.

A speculum examination will also reveal whether the bleeding is coming from a local lesion of the vagina or cervix. The other reason for inserting a speculum is to collect a blood sample to test for fetal haemoglobin. Bleeding from vasa praevia is a rare cause of APH but unless it is recognised and the baby delivered by immediate caesarean section, fetal exsanguination will occur.

Magnetic resonance imaging (MRI)

This relatively new and expensive method of imaging is now available in most large centres. When a very powerful magnetic field is passed through the body the hydrogen atoms become polarised and the H$^+$ ions are aligned. The protons (the hydrogen atom nuclei) are displaced by radio pulses and in returning to their basal state give out a small radio signal. A series of images can be built up from the proton density maps of a section of the body. The sections may be at any

plane of the body and no ionising radiation is used. At present, the tissues need to be immobile for some seconds while the imaging is performed (hence clear fetal images are difficult to produce) but localisation of the placenta is excellent because both the placental edge and the cervical canal can be readily identified (Powell et al 1986). Ultrasound remains the method of choice because it is relatively cheap and readily available, but MRI offers the possibility of early diagnosis of some complications of placenta praevia (see below).

Clinical management

Most patients with placenta praevia present with a history of painless APH. There may have been more than one warning show of blood. The priority is to assess and deal with the blood loss and arrange for an adequate supply of blood should transfusion become necessary.

If routine ultrasound has been done in early pregnancy, the diagnosis should be easy and further localisation of the placenta may not be necessary, though one should bear in mind the high false-positive rate of early scans and the possibility of a false-negative result. Only in cases of serious haemorrhage is it necessary to make an immediate diagnosis; the important point is to distinguish placenta praevia from vasa praevia and placental abruption. In such circumstances ultrasound, if available, may be very helpful.

Real-time scanners can produce high-quality images (Fig. 14.3) and it is now possible to carry out ultrasound scanning within the delivery room. Once bleeding has occurred, however, diagnosis by ultrasound may be difficult because of the resemblance of placenta to blood clot and the indistinct appearance of the cervical os. This is particularly true close to term; in such circumstances, unless transvaginal ultrasound clarifies the diagnosis, clinical examination under controlled conditions as described below may be necessary.

Expectant management

Unless the bleeding is severe there is much to be gained by expectant management, with the aim of making a correct diagnosis and postponing delivery until about 37 weeks.

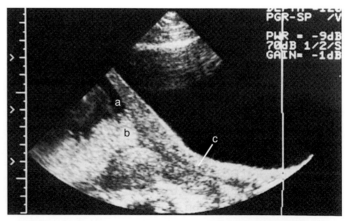

Fig. 14.3 Real-time ultrasonograph showing the edge of placenta overlying the cervical canal. a, Liquor; b, edge of placenta; c, cervical canal. Reproduced by kind permission of Dr P.G. Rose.

Conservative management was pioneered in Belfast by Macafee et al (1962) and rapidly adopted elsewhere. An expectant regimen was used, with bed rest, blood transfusion and more liberal use of caesarean section. The beneficial effects of this change in policy on maternal and fetal mortality are shown in Table 14.6. The advantage of adequate transfusion is self-evident; the advantages to the baby of avoiding premature delivery are less than they used to be, thanks to the improvements in neonatal paediatrics, but are still important.

Outpatient management. Until recently, 'conservative management' meant that the woman stayed in hospital, sometimes for weeks, so as to be close to an operating theatre if heavy bleeding occurred. With the advent of early diagnosis of placenta praevia by routine ultrasound this policy began to be questioned, and it was suggested that outpatient management may be safe, even for women who have experienced some bleeding. An Edinburgh study set out to identify women at higher risk of complications, who might need to stay in hospital. The study was based on 15 930 deliveries over a 3-year period, including 58 women with placenta praevia (Love & Wallace 1996), and concluded that the clinical outcomes are highly variable and cannot be predicted from antenatal events, and that 'in the majority of cases with or without bleeding and irrespective of the degree of praevia, outpatient management would appear to be safe and effective'.

Use of tocolytics. In general, haemorrhage is a contraindication to tocolytic treatment. Furthermore, these agents produce tachycardia and palpitations, neither of which is desirable in someone already suffering from hypovolaemia. Nevertheless, there have been several reports of the benefits of tocolysis when contractions occur in association with placenta praevia. Besinger et al (1995) reported that tocolytic intervention may be associated with significant prolongation of the pregnancy and increased birthweight and that it does not appear to have an impact on the frequency or severity of recurrent vaginal bleeding. Towers et al (1999) reported on the use of tocolysis in 76 patients with placenta praevia: the mean time from bleeding to delivery was 29 days and the neonatal mortality was as low as 39 deaths per 1000 live births. (In this report, tocolysis was also given to 93 women with abruption.)

Cervical cerclage does not appear to be an adequate intervention for the management of placenta praevia (Cobo et al 1998).

Vaginal delivery

In general, elective caesarean section should not be carried out before 39 weeks but with placenta praevia this has to be balanced against the possibility of spontaneous labour. One study of outcomes suggested that it may be safe to wait until the woman goes into labour, rather than planning elective caesarean section (Frederiksen et al 1999) but elective section makes it much easier for appropriate staff to be present. Many obstetricians feel there is little point in postponing delivery beyond 37 weeks' gestation except in women with minor degrees of praevia in whom the placenta is anterior and the head engaged. Such a situation may not be apparent until labour starts or an attempt is made to rupture the membranes. In such circumstances, the bleeding is usually controlled by amniotomy augmented by Syntocinon infusion.

Examination under anaesthesia and amniotomy. Vaginal examination should be carried out only under anaesthesia in an operating theatre, with everything prepared for an immediate transfusion and caesarean section should the examination provoke heavy bleeding. The instruments are laid out and the nursing staff scrubbed. The stage of gestation for delivery should be right; there is no point in carrying out an examination when conservative management would be more appropriate. It is a mistake to hurry the examination, which should be performed with the patient in the lithotomy position and using sterile drapes. After catheterising the bladder, two fingers are introduced into the vagina, avoiding the cervical os. Each vaginal fornix is palpated in turn, the object being to feel whether there is a placenta between the presenting head and the finger. If the four fornices are empty, then a finger can be introduced into the cervical os. If the cervical os is tightly closed and there is significant bleeding it is unwise to use force to dilate the cervix; instead a caesarean section should be performed.

The presence of clot may make it difficult to define the edge of the placenta, but if the membranes can be identified a forewater amniotomy is carried out. Heavily bloodstained liquor is suspicious of an abruption, but if the bleeding is separate from the liquor and it does not stop within a few minutes, it is best to proceed to caesarean section.

Examination under anaesthesia is also justified where clinical or ultrasound evidence suggests an anterior grade I placenta praevia. Vaginal delivery is therefore possible and amniotomy may be all that is necessary. Once the membranes are ruptured and the uterus is contracting, the presenting part compresses the lateral edge of the placenta against the back of the symphysis pubis and arrests the bleeding.

Caesarean section

With the exception already mentioned, delivery by caesarean section is the method of choice for most women with any severe degree of placenta praevia. The operation, however, can be hazardous. When the placenta is anterior the lower segment can be very vascular, with huge veins coursing across the potential site of incision. Once the lower segment has been opened, to reach the baby the placenta must be either incised or separated. Each method has its problems: incising the placenta may be speedy but can cause fetal exsanguination as it opens the fetal vessels; on the other hand, separating the placenta may be difficult, especially if it is adherent. Once placental separation has been started, the fetus is deprived of maternal oxygen and delivery becomes

Table 14.6 Maternal and fetal mortality in placenta praevia before and after introduction of conservative management in Belfast

Year	No. of cases	Maternal mortality (%)	Caesarean section (%)	Fetal mortality (%)
1932–1936	76	2.6	—	51
1937–1944	174	0.6	31	24
1945–1952	206	0.0	68	15

From Macafee 1945 and Macafee et al 1962, with permission.

urgent. Further difficulty can arise if there is a transverse lie—this is one of the few occasions in which it may be prudent to resort to an upper segment incision. An alternative to the classical incision is to convert the transverse lower segment incision into an inverted T, an approach which many obstetricians consider does not heal well, although there is no published evidence on this.

Much will depend on the exact circumstances, but our preference is for a lower segment approach, under-running the large vessels with a catgut suture before dividing them. The anterior placenta is then separated with the finger until the edge is reached and the amniotic sac can be opened. If necessary the incision is extended into an inverted T.

General anaesthesia has been preferred in the past because of fears that epidural anaesthesia may exacerbate hypotension, but a recent study showed that general anaesthesia was associated with increased intraoperative blood loss and the need for blood transfusion, and that regional anaesthesia appears to be a safe alternative (Frederiksen et al 1999).

Placenta accreta

In this condition the placenta is abnormally adherent to the uterine wall. It may even invade the uterine muscle (placenta increta) or penetrate through the uterus and into the bladder wall (placenta percreta). Attempts to remove the placenta lead to uncontrollable bleeding. Placenta accreta occurs in approximately 1 in 2500 deliveries but among women with placenta praevia the incidence is nearly 10%. In this high-risk group, maternal age and previous caesarean section are independent risk factors (Miller et al 1997). It is particularly liable to occur with anterior placenta praevia in a woman who has had one or more caesarean sections (Clark et al 1985). Not only does the risk of placenta praevia increase with the number of previous caesarean sections; so does the likelihood of placenta accreta (see Table 14.5). McShane et al (1985) reported that of the 22 women in their series with a previous caesarean section scar, six (27%) had placenta accreta.

Diagnosis

The diagnosis of placenta accreta can be made antenatally and ultrasound diagnosis is increasingly reliable. Women at high risk (i.e. those with placenta praevia or repeated caesarean sections, should be checked antenatally using Doppler ultrasound and, if necessary, MRI. Diagnosis at 28 weeks with power amplitude ultrasonographic angiography has been reported (Chou & Shih 1997) and placenta praevia percreta has been diagnosed in the first trimester with MRI after haemorrhage (Thorp et al 1998).

Management

Of women with placenta percreta 90% will lose more than 3000 ml of blood during the operation. Hysterectomy may be necessary. This is one of the reasons why caesarean section for placenta praevia should always be carried out under the supervision of an experienced obstetrician; it is not an operation for the tyro. The decision to proceed with definitive surgery needs to be carefully considered and a multidisciplinary approach is best (Leaphart et al 1997).

Increasingly cases are being diagnosed before labour, and maternal mortality and morbidity can be reduced by careful preparation (Hudon et al 1998). Prophylactic placement of arterial catheters allows rapid occlusion of these vessels if necessary (Hansch et al 1999), although the value of this has been questioned (see below). Other suggested measures include the use of antenatal erythropoietin to increase the haemoglobin concentration before surgery, or prophylactic uterine or hypogastric artery ligation (Hudon et al 1998).

Pelvic arterial embolisation. Arterial embolisation in obstetrics and gynaecology was first reported in 1979 for the treatment of postpartum haemorrhage and of bleeding after gynaecological surgery (Vedantham et al 1997). A recent report from Paris described its use in 12 cases of primary postpartum haemorrhage and four of late secondary postpartum haemorrhage (Merland et al 1996). It may have particular value in cervical ectopic pregnancy and in abdominal pregnancy.

After initial angiography, the procedure is performed by a vascular radiologist usually with Gelfoam (Merland et al 1996, Vedantham et al 1997). All cases reported so far have successfully avoided maternal death, but complications have included arterial perforation, low-grade fever, abscess formation, pelvic pain and buttock ischaemia (Vedantham et al 1997). Antibiotic cover is recommended. Pregnancy can occur subsequently and so far there have been no reports of infertility or intrauterine growth retardation.

The technique appears promising, but in a series of six cases in California bleeding could not be controlled in one and hysterectomy was performed (Hansch et al 1999); in a series of five cases of antenatally diagnosed placenta accreta in Philadelphia all but one required hysterectomy despite prophylactic preoperative pelvic artery balloon catheterisation. In this group the outcome was no different from that among patients with undiagnosed placenta accreta (Levine et al 1999).

Conservative management. Because of the risks of caesarean hysterectomy there is now increasing interest in conservative management of placenta increta. A recent report described two cases. In one, a firmly adherent placenta was left in place and monitored with ultrasound and MRI. At 8 months postpartum the patient passed a large piece of fleshy tissue and at 9 months she was menstruating normally, despite having a residual mass in the uterus measuring $22 \times 15 \times 15$ mm. In the second case, the placenta was left *in situ*; Doppler ultrasound showed persistent vascularity and she was given methotrexate 50 mg intravenously on alternate days and six doses of folinic acid (6 mg) in between. The woman's β-hCG dropped to <2U/L by day 52. The placenta calcified, measuring $50 \times 50 \times 50$ mm, but 12 months later she was menstruating regularly.

On the basis of these cases and other reports of subsequent conception and normal delivery after the placenta was left *in situ*, the authors recommend conservative management of placenta increta unless there is life-threatening haemorrhage. They suggest that methotrexate should probably be reserved for cases of placenta percreta, persistent vascularity or persistently raised β-hCG (Panoskaltsis et al 2000).

Maternal mortality

Haemorrhage is the leading cause of maternal death worldwide but in the UK the number of deaths from this cause has fallen steadily. In the first report on confidential enquiries into maternal deaths in England and Wales 1952–1954, there were 29 deaths due to placenta praevia, with avoidable factors present in 55% (Ministry of Health 1957). The numbers fell until 1985–1987 when, for the first time ever, no woman died from placenta praevia in the UK. Since then, however, there have been a small number of deaths from this cause in each triennium, with five in 1988–1990, four in 1991–1993 and three in 1994–1996 (Department of Health 1998).

The following conclusions were drawn from detailed examination of these cases, and are repeatedly stated in the triennial reports.

- Caesarean section for placenta praevia must be performed or directly supervised by an experienced obstetrician, normally a consultant.
- All units should have protocols for dealing with massive haemorrhage, and
- because haemorrhage is relatively infrequent there should be regular practice runs for all personnel.

An example of a protocol for massive haemorrhage is given in Figure 14.4.

Major Obstetric Haemorrhage

Definition Blood loss ≥1500 ml

If IV access available turn drip full on.

Call:
Obstetric registrar
Obstetric senior registrar
Anaesthetic registrar
Anaesthetic nurse/ODA

Two Brown venflons:
Crossmatch at least 6 units of blood
FBC/coagulation screen
Urea and electrolytes
- Give colloid as soon as possible with pressure bag.
- Identify cause and treat appropriately*.
- Transfuse as much as estimated loss as soon as possible.
- Catheterise.
- Monitor blood pressure, SAo_2 and consider central venous pressure +/– arterial line.
- Inform on-call consultant.
- Record all observations and fluid balance.
- Discuss management with haematology consultant.

NB Clear communication with Haematology MLSO and Blood Bank is essential

*Appropriate treatment of antepartum haemorrhage

Blood loss is always difficult to quantify, particularly in the case of abruption and thus it is not possible to be prescriptive about the management in every case scenario.

If haemodynamically stable
- Cardiotocohograph
- Ultrasound scan for placental site—to be performed on delivery suite

Placenta praevia with major ongoing bleeding—deliver by LSCS.

Consultant should be at lower-segment caesarean section (LSCS)
- >37 weeks deliver by LSCS when theatre available
- <34 weeks:
  - Give dexamethasone 12 mg IM (two doses)

— Inform neonatal intensive care unit
— Observe on delivery suite until bleeding subsides
— Further management will depend on extent of further blood loss and gestational age

Abruption
- >37 weeks; induction of labour if fetal well-being allows, LSCS if not.
- <34 weeks:
  - Give dexamethasone 12 mg IM (two doses)
  - Inform neonatal intensive care unit
  - May be transferred to the ward once satisfied that both maternal and fetal condition is stable
  - Will require close monitoring of both fetal and maternal condition until delivery
- 34–37 weeks gestation—discuss management with consultant and neonatal intensive care unit

If haemodynamically unstable
- Transfuse appropriately
- Ultrasound scan for placental site and fetal viability

Viable fetus
- Vaginal examination not fully dilated or nearly fully—deliver by LSCS.
- Nearly fully dilated—may be allowed to labour and deliver vaginally if the cardiotocohograph is of good quality and reassuring and is making rapid progress.
- Fully dilated—if delivery imminent, allow spontaneous vaginal delivery; if not imminent assist with forceps/ventouse.

Non-viable fetus
- Induction of labour.
- Maintain maternal circulation.
- Treat coagulopathy in consultation with haematologist.
- Only resort to caesarean section in extreme circumstances.

Note: Management in cases of major obstetric haemorrhage, whether before or after delivery, should always be discussed with the consultants on call (obstetric and anaesthetic).

Fig. 14.4 Protocol for massive obstetric haemorrhage.

Perinatal mortality

The fetal outlook following placenta praevia is more favourable than in placental abruption and has continued to improve over the past 50 years (Macafee et al 1962). In the 1960s perinatal mortality rates of around 126 per 1000 total births were reported but the figure has been reduced by a more active approach (McShane et al 1985) and better neonatal care. Scotland, with its system for detailed recording of every pregnancy, provides excellent epidemiological data. During the 2 years 1984 and 1985, there were 800 cases of placenta praevia with 19 perinatal deaths—a mortality of only 24 per 1000 (Scottish Health Service, personal communication). Unlike abruption, placenta praevia does not cause intrauterine hypoxia and premature delivery is the greatest cause of morbidity and mortality.

VASA PRAEVIA

The rare condition of vasa praevia is difficult to diagnose, but must always be borne in mind, particularly where the clinical picture is unusual. The diagnosis is made by testing the vaginal blood for fetal haemoglobin using the alkaline denaturation test.

With grey-scale ultrasonography, vasa praevia can be detected in asymptomatic women as early as the second trimester (Lee et al 2000). In a population of 93 874 women undergoing scans, 18 cases were suspected and the mean gestation at diagnosis was 26 weeks. Three of the women had normal scans in the third trimester and delivered normally, the other 15 underwent caesarean section, with generally favourable outcome. Over 50% of the women were asymptomatic in pregnancy: six had mild vaginal bleeding at a mean of 31 weeks. One case of vasa praevia was missed.

PLACENTAL ABRUPTION

Incidence

In the British Births study (Chamberlain et al 1970), placental abruption occurred in about 1% of pregnancies. Table 14.7 shows a good deal of variation in the recorded incidence, probably due to differences in definition and accuracy of diagnosis. In a study of births in Norway between 1967 and 1991, placental abruption occurred in 6.6 per 1000 births of a gestational age of 16 weeks or more, but there was a steady increase over time, from 5.3 per 1000 births in 1971 to 9.1 in 1990 (Rasmussen et al 1996a, b).

Mechanism

The word abruption (Latin: breaking away) describes the process by which the placental attachment to the uterus is disrupted by haemorrhage. The process begins with uterine vasospasm, followed by relaxation and subsequent venous engorgement and arteriolar rupture into the decidua (Egley & Cefalo 1985). The blood then attempts to escape by dissecting under the membranes, sometimes getting into the amniotic sac and producing bloodstained liquor—a common finding in cases of placental abruption. The alternative path is for the blood to dissect under the placenta, causing it to separate from its maternal attachment, and often extending into the uterine muscle itself (Fig. 14.5). The effect on the myometrium is to cause a tonic contraction, which makes the uterus feel woody and hard. The increase of intrauterine pressure embarrasses the placental circulation, adding to the hypoxia already caused by the separation of the placenta.

Examination of the placenta after birth typically shows an area of organising blood clot with an underlying compression of the maternal surface. Fox (1978) found evidence of retroplacental clot in 4.5% of placentas which he examined routinely, suggesting that small episodes are more common than is realised.

Aetiology

The aetiology remains an enigma. Although the cause is sometimes obvious, as in cases of direct trauma to the uterus, such cases are uncommon and in most cases the cause is obscure. Women who have an abruption are less likely than other women to have another pregnancy but among women who do have subsequent pregnancies placental abruption occurs significantly more frequently (odds ratio 7.1) (Rasmussen et al 1997). A woman who has suffered from the condition once has a recurrence rate with subsequent pregnancy of about 6%.

Abdominal trauma

A direct blow to the abdomen is a dramatic but infrequent cause of abruption. It can occur from assault or more commonly as a result of injury in a car collision. An incidence of 4% of placental abruption has been reported in women who survived a car crash while wearing a seat belt, suggesting that seat belts, although reducing fatal accidents, can also traumatise the pregnant uterus. This is not an argument against the use of seat belts, however, and it is important that women are instructed in their correct use in pregnancy (over and under the bump) (Department of Health 1998). Airbag

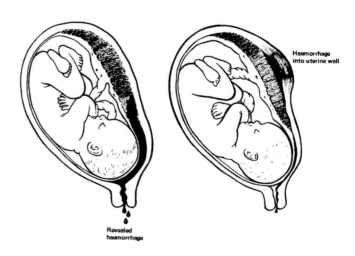

Fig. 14.5 Placental abruption.

deployment has also been described as a cause of abruption and fetal death (Schultze et al 1998).

Abruption was a well recognised complication of external cephalic version when it was performed under anaesthesia, with a reported incidence of 2–9%. The practice of external version is now being revived, with the addition of tocolytic drugs, but the complication rates are reported to be low.

Uterine decompression

Sudden decompression of the uterus occurs when the membranes rupture in the presence of polyhydramnios. The reduction of uterine volume causes a corresponding loss of surface area and as a result the placenta shears off. Nevertheless, this is an uncommon cause of abruption.

Prolonged rupture of the membranes

Pregnancies complicated by preterm premature rupture of the membranes (PPROM) that are managed expectantly are at significant risk of abruption. A meta-analysis suggested a threefold increase in risk compared with normal pregnancy (Ananth et al 1996). In such cases PPROM is more often preceded by bleeding (Major et al 1995).

Risk factors

Severe fetal growth restriction, prolonged rupture of the membranes, chorioamnionitis, hypertension (before pregnancy and pregnancy-induced), cigarette smoking, advanced maternal age, unmarried status, and male fetal gender are significant aetiological determinants of placental abruption (Kramer et al 1997).

Thrombophilia

There has been considerable interest in the role of the thrombophilias in adverse outcomes of pregnancy, including severe pre-eclampsia, intrauterine fetal growth retardation and abruption of the placenta (Sibai 1999). In one study of 110 women with these complications, thrombophilic mutations were found in 60% of women with an abruption, compared with 17% of women with normal pregnancies (Kupferminc et al 1999). Women with abruption had a 65% chance of having had, at 10 weeks' gestation, metabolic abnormalities such as protein S deficiency, hyperhomocysteinaemia or protein C deficiency (De Vries et al 1997).

The precise risk of serious obstetric complications in women with genetic or acquired thrombophilia is unknown (Sibai 1999) but it has been suggested that women whose pregnancies are complicated by placental abruption should be tested for thrombophilia, and that those with markers should be offered prophylactic treatment—heparin and low-dose aspirin for those with protein S deficiency, mutation in the factor V gene or anticardiolipin antibodies; prophylactic folic acid supplementation for those with mutations in the gene for methylenetetrahydrofolate reductase. The safety and efficacy of such prophylactic treatment in these cases, however, remain uncertain (Sibai 1999). Abruption is not reported as a risk of low-dose aspirin (Hauth et al 1995) or as a complication of anticoagulant therapy, but has been reported after snake bite.

Age and parity

The condition is more common with increasing age (Kramer et al 1997) and parity [20], although the data in Table 14.7 show that the rise with these parameters is consistent but not impressive. Rasmussen et al (1996a) found that the risk increased with age and that birth order two had the lowest proportion. The risk also increases with increasing gestation.

Maternal hypertension

In the past there has been controversy about whether maternal hypertension is a cause or a consequence of abruption. Early studies concluded that there was no evidence of pre-existing hypertension in most cases of placental abruption and that the hypertension and proteinuria happened as a consequence, not a cause, of the abruption. Naeye et al (1977) came to a similar conclusion from a study of 212 perinatal deaths following placental abruption; Abdella et al (1984) came to the opposite conclusion after examining 265 consecutive cases of placental abruption. The overall incidence in 24 258 deliveries was 1.2%, but it was 2.3% in those with pre-eclamptic toxaemia, 10% in those with chronic hypertension and 23.6% in those with eclampsia.

Evidence on the link between abruption and hypertensive disorders remains inconclusive. Ananth et al (1996), in a

Table 14.7 The incidence of placental abruption in relation to maternal age and parity (rates per 100 pregnancies)

Reference	Maternal age (years)				
	<20	20–24	25–29	30–34	35+
Hibbard & Hibbard (1963)	0.85	0.9	1.1	1.2	1.7
Chamberlain et al (1978)	1.4	1.2	1.0	1.2	1.8
Paintin (1962)	0.9	0.7	0.7	⊢ 0.8 ⊣	
Naeye (1980)					
Non-smokers	1.3	⊢ 1.7 ⊣		⊢ 2.3 ⊣	
Smokers	1.6	⊢ 2.1 ⊣		⊢ 3.3 ⊣	

	Pregnancy number			
	1	2	3–4	5+
Naeye (1980)				
Non-smokers	1.5	1.8	1.7	1.8
Smokers	1.8	1.9	2.2	2.9
Paintin (1962)	0.7	0.6	0.9	0.9
Hibbard & Hibbard (1963)	0.8	⊢ 1.0 ⊣		2.3
Chamberlain et al (1978)	1.1	⊢ 1.4 ⊣		1.7
Description of samples				
Hibbard & Hibbard (1963)	23 043 consecutive deliveries, Mill Road Hospital, Liverpool, UK			
Naeye (1980)	53 518 pregnancies in 12 university hospitals, USA, 1959–66 (collaborative perinatal project)			
Chamberlain et al (1978)	17 005 pregnancies born in UK during April 1970 (British births 1970 survey)			
Paintin (1962)	30 383 singleton pregnancies to married women resident in Aberdeen, UK, 1949–58			

meta-analysis, concluded that chronically hypertensive patients had a threefold increased risk of abruption compared with normotensive women, while the odds ratio for patients with pre-eclampsia was 1.73. He commented that the criteria for diagnosis of abruption and hypertensive disorders may have introduced variability among the results. In a retrospective cohort study of over 120 000 pregnancies, Ananth et al (1997c) found that chronically hypertensive women had no increased risk of abruption but that women with severe pre-eclampsia and those with chronic hypertension with superimposed pre-eclampsia had an approximately threefold increase in risk. (Uterine bleeding of unknown aetiology was not associated with hypertension, so may have a different aetiology.) Sibai et al (1998) found that women with chronic hypertension had no increased risk of abruption unless they had superimposed pre-eclampsia: the risk was not affected by aspirin therapy. Among women with severe pre-eclampsia, quantitative proteinuria and degree of blood pressure elevation were not predictive of either abruption or eclampsia (Witlin et al 1999).

Cigarette smoking

In the US collaborative study (Naeye 1980) the incidence of abruption was 1.69% in non-smokers, 2.46% in smokers and 1.87% in smokers who had given up in early pregnancy. These rates were independent of age and parity, and the fact that the effect of smoking was also found to be dose related suggests that the effect was pharmacological. Naeye found evidence of decidual necrosis at the edge of the placenta and thought this was ischaemic in origin. Cigarette smoking is known to affect uteroplacental blood flow. In a case-controlled study of 5727 patients in Denmark, cigarette smoking was twice as common in patients who suffered from abruption than in the control cases (Eriksen et al 1991).

Both cigarette smoking and hypertensive disorders carry an increased risk of placental abruption (Ananth et al 1999). Smoking was associated with reduced risks of mild and severe pre-eclampsia, but smokers in whom pre-eclampsia develops have very high risks of perinatal mortality, abruption and small-for-gestational-age infants (Cnattingius et al 1997).

Raised serum alpha-fetoprotein

Egley & Cefalo (1985) found that women who had an unexplained high level of serum alpha-fetoprotein on routine screening had an increased risk of placental abruption. They suggested that this was evidence of faulty implantation, but it could equally well be due to repeated small episodes of feto-maternal bleeding resulting from decidual necrosis. Yaron found that increased maternal serum alpha-fetoprotein levels (>2.5 MoM) were significantly associated with various complications including abruption (Yaron et al 1999).

Other factors

Lower social class is related to increasing perinatal mortality rates from APH. Placental abruption has also been reported in relation to cocaine abuse (Acker et al 1983). The suggestion that abruption is due to folate or vitamin deficiency has not been confirmed. Placental abruption was found to be the most common cause of fetal loss in an African city and was strongly associated with maternal poverty and malnutrition (Naeye et al 1979).

Diagnosis

Signs and symptoms

The presenting symptoms are bleeding and pain and usually the onset of premature labour. Hurd et al (1983) reported that 35% of women admitted with abruption were already in labour. About 10% give a history of previous small episodes of vaginal bleeding (Egley & Cefalo 1985). If the separation starts near the placental margin, vaginal bleeding occurs early and, because there is little concealed haemorrhage, pain is minimal. Here, the diagnosis may be less obvious. Tenderness over the placental site may not be apparent for several hours and, because the event may stimulate uterine contractions, the clinical presentation may resemble premature onset of labour with a heavy show. Cardiotocography can be diagnostic. There are characteristically frequent (one per minute) small contractions superimposed upon raised uterine tone. Evidence of fetal hypoxia (tachycardia, loss of variability, late decelerations) makes the diagnosis even more likely and indicates the necessity for urgent delivery, usually by caesarian section.

When bleeding occurs into the uterine muscle there is pain, increased uterine tone and a deceptive absence of vaginal bleeding. When seen at caesarean section, the Couvelaire uterus is deeply suffused with haematoma, looking like a huge bruise. On general examination the patient looks distressed and unwell, the abdomen is tender and the uterus has a woody consistency. If placental separation is extensive, fetal parts are difficult to identify and the fetal heartbeat may be very slow or absent. If the placenta is posterior, tenderness is less marked and the patient complains of backache. The blood pressure is a poor guide to the extent of bleeding. The coexistence of hypertension (whether it is cause or effect) confuses the usual association of haemorrhage with hypotension. Some cases are unsuspected (the silent abruption) and diagnosed only in retrospect.

With such a variation in clinical presentation, the division of placental abruption into three grades has much to commend it as a guide to management and comparison between centres (Sher & Statland 1985):

Grade I—not recognised clinically before delivery and usually diagnosed by the presence of a retroplacental clot.

Grade II—intermediate. The classical signs of abruption are present but the fetus is still alive.

Grade III—severe, the fetus is dead: IIIa without coagulopathy, or IIIb with coagulopathy.

Differential diagnosis

When vaginal bleeding, a tonically contracted tender uterus and fetal hypoxia occur together, there is little doubt about the diagnosis of placental abruption; however, a very similar picture is produced by a ruptured uterus. If the rupture is through a previous caesarean section scar, the tenderness tends to be localised to the suprapubic area, but real confusion can occur if the scar is from some other operation, such as a myomectomy, or is spontaneous.

In the absence of vaginal bleeding, other conditions causing acute abdominal pain and uterine tenderness in pregnancy that will have to be considered include:

- haematoma of the rectus sheath;
- retroperitoneal haemorrhage;
- rupture of an appendix abscess;
- acute degeneration or torsion in a uterine fibroid.

A more common problem occurs when there is a small amount of bleeding associated with uterine contractions and a slightly tender uterus. The difficulty is to distinguish a grade I placental abruption from spontaneous preterm labour with a heavy show, especially because a small abruption can itself provoke labour.

Bleeding without pain can also be confusing; it is important to make the distinction from placenta praevia. An ultrasound scan can be very helpful in diagnosing or excluding placenta praevia but is usually unhelpful in diagnosing abruption. With a good-quality machine and an experienced operator, however, it is possible to visualise the retroplacental clot or intraperitoneal bleeding. Previous knowledge of the placental site from routine examination in early pregnancy is, of course, very helpful in these circumstances.

Management

Initial assessment

Once placental abruption has been suspected, action should be swift and decisive because the prognosis for mother and fetus is worsened by delay. The first step is to set up an intravenous line and to correct blood loss as soon as possible. In severe cases, two lines should be set up in different veins. A central venous catheter is invaluable because it helps to prevent undertransfusion before delivery and overinfusion during the vital hours following delivery. In pre-eclampsia, the circulating blood volume is reduced and there is a risk of pulmonary oedema if too much fluid is infused. The temptation to overinfuse occurs during recovery when there is anxiety about the return of renal function; a good guide is to maintain the central venous pressure at about 4–8 cmH$_2$O. Blood is taken for cross-matching and to screen for clotting factors including a platelet count. Urinary output should be monitored by a self-retaining catheter in the bladder, using one of the calibrated collecting systems now available. Secretion of at least 30 ml/h indicates adequate renal perfusion; less raises the possibility of undertransfusion.

There are three practical options for management:

- Expectant—in the hope that the pregnancy will continue.
- Immediate caesarean section.
- Rupture the membranes and aim at vaginal delivery.

Expectant treatment

There is a place for conservative treatment when the diagnosis is in doubt or the abruption very minor, particularly if the gestation is very preterm. Such cases usually present with a small painless vaginal bleed, and a localised area of uterine tenderness appears only after several hours or an ultrasound shows a suspicious area of placental separation. In such circumstances there is something to be gained from allowing the pregnancy to continue, but the decision will depend on the length of gestation, whether there has been a previous episode, the state of the fetus and the extent of the placental separation. Abruption occurring in a posteriorly sited placenta can be treacherous because the only symptom may be backache and the site of tenderness is out of reach.

However innocuous the incident of abruption seems to have been, some damage is likely to have been done to the integrity and function of the placenta, and the fetus should be carefully monitored. It is a good principle to induce labour in all such patients at or before term.

Serial doppler measurements in uterine and fetal vessels may assist in deciding whether to deliver the baby immediately or to continue intense surveillance (Arabin et al 1998).

Caesarean section

If the baby is still alive (grade II abruption), electronic fetal monitoring should be continued and immediate preparations made for caesarean section, although the decision to proceed is not always easy. In the first place, the outlook for the fetus is poor, not only in terms of immediate survival but also because not all liveborn infants survive the neonatal period; Abdella et al (1984) reported a 15.4% neonatal mortality rate. Secondly, the presence of coagulopathy adds considerably to the risks of the operation; it can be difficult to achieve haemostasis when the myometrium is engorged by haematoma, even without the added problem of hypofibrinogenaemia. If the uterus is already contracting well and delivery appears to be imminent within a few hours, the membranes should be ruptured and the decision to operate postponed, as long as the fetal heart rate is satisfactory. In a series reported by Hurd et al (1983), the perinatal mortality following caesarean section was 3 in 20 (15%), compared with 6 of 30 (20%) for those delivered vaginally but the numbers are small.

Rupturing the membranes and hastening delivery

The main purpose of forewater amniotomy is to hasten the onset of labour and, by encouraging uterine contractions, to reduce uterine bleeding. In most cases it is effective but it also has dangers. If the uterus has become atonic, as happens rarely, the reduction of intrauterine pressure encourages further bleeding, which fills the space. Simple observation of the uterine outline gives warning of such continued bleeding. An intravenous infusion of Syntocinon should always be running before starting. The other disadvantage of rupturing the membranes is that a small premature breech baby may slip through a partially dilated cervical os. Rupture of the membranes should therefore be reserved for cases in which the fetus is already dead or labour is already well advanced.

Management of grade III placental abruption

When the baby is dead the only indication for caesarean section is uncontrollable bleeding or failure of conservative management. If labour has not already started, the membranes should be ruptured and an infusion of Syntocinon started. The outline of the uterus should be marked with a pen and the girth around the umbilicus measured at hourly intervals to detect bleeding that is not being expelled because the uterus has lost its ability to contract. This is fortunately rare, but if there is no response to Syntocinon and amniotomy and if bleeding, visible or concealed, continues, caesarean section may become necessary; though hazardous, it may be life-saving.

Complications

Hypovolaemic shock

The blood loss in cases of placental abruption is nearly always underestimated. This is partly because of the invisible bleeding behind the placenta and into the myometrium, but also because of the association with hypertension which tends to mask the signs of hypovolaemia.

Postpartum haemorrhage

High circulating levels of fibrin degradation products can have an inhibiting effect on the myometrium. Postpartum haemorrhage occurs in about 25% of cases and, coupled with the continuing coagulopathy and the heavy blood loss already sustained, severe postpartum haemorrhage can be a *coup de grâce*. Close liaison with a consultant haematologist is essential when coagulopathy occurs, and the use of aprotinin may be justified.

Renal failure

Ischaemic necrosis of the kidney is a serious complication of placental abruption. The most likely cause is inadequate perfusion during the phase of acute blood loss, but it can also occur from fibrin deposits resulting from disseminated intravascular clotting. Renal necrosis is the result of under-transfusion rather than anything to do with hypertension and should be preventable.

Oliguria during the first 12 hours following an abruption is common and does not necessarily imply permanent renal damage. Even when urinary output falls below the optimum of 30 ml/h, diuretics should be used only with the greatest caution, if at all. They cannot improve renal perfusion and may do harm (Sher & Statland 1985). If the oliguria persists after 12 hours and the central venous pressure indicates a normal circulating blood volume, the most important step is to prevent fluid and electrolyte overload by reducing the volume of the infusion to that of the urinary output. If the serum potassium, blood urea and creatinine levels start to rise, help is needed from a nephrologist; such experts prefer to be consulted early rather than too late.

Coagulopathy

In a woman already shocked by an abruption, coagulopathy adds considerably to the dangers to her and to the problems of management. Successful treatment requires the resources of a competent haematology laboratory and blood transfusion service, and liaison with a haematologist.

The sequence of events that lead to coagulopathy involves a cascade of changes affecting both thrombus formation and fibrinolysis and is considered in detail in Chapter 20. The consequences go beyond the loss of fibrinogen from the circulation because the peripheral deposition of fibrin may also affect the blood vessels in other organs such as kidney and liver. In addition there is sometimes a consumptive thrombocytopaenia. With the delivery of the placenta and the extrusion of old clot, the whole process reverts to normal and there is a dramatic improvement within a few hours. Rapid delivery is therefore the key to the treatment of coagulopathy.

Adequate blood transfusion is essential, not only to maintain the circulating haemoglobin, but also to replace platelets. If possible the blood should be fresh (although this is rarely available or used nowadays because of the risk of infection and transmission of Creutzfeld-Jakob disease) and supplemented by fresh platelet concentrate if the platelet count falls below 50 000 per ml. Although whole blood is preferable, an alternative will usually be necessary to start with. Packed red cells, with fresh or frozen plasma, can be used together with plasma-expanding agents such as degraded gelatin products. Dextrans are better avoided because they may inhibit blood clotting as well as interfering with cross-matching (see Chapter 20).

Replacement of fibrinogen is of doubtful value, because it is immediately deposited in peripheral veins, but may be of value in desperate circumstances such as to cover a caesarean section. An alternative is to use cryoprecipitate. The use of fibrinolytic inhibitors (such as aminocaproic acid or aprotinin) is controversial because it is said that they consolidate the intravascular clot, with serious consequences in the lungs or liver (Sher & Statland 1985). Heparin has also been advocated because of its effect in augmenting antithrombin III, but to most obstetricians its use seems illogical and dangerous.

Rhesus prophylaxis

Transplacental haemorrhage is likely to occur with any bleeding in pregnancy and can be quite extensive following placental abruption (Pritchard et al 1985). Anti-D immunoglobulin should therefore be given to every rhesus (D)-negative women within 48 hours of placental abruption. The usual dose in the UK is 500 IU, but this is inadequate if the volume of transplacental haemorrhage has exceeded 5 ml fetal blood. A Kleihauer test will give an estimate of the amount of transplacental haemorrhage, but the assessment is complicated by the effect of blood loss and replacement.

Management of a subsequent pregnancy

Abruption is a serious condition, with a high perinatal mortality and a risk of recurrence estimated at about 7% (Pritchard et al 1985). Although the causes are not known, there is an understandable desire to do something positive in the following pregnancy.

Prophylactic measures for women with thrombophilia have been discussed above.

The value of folate supplements during pregnancy has not been proven, but there is little to be lost from their use, preferably before conception. In spite of the uncertainty of the role of hypertension in the causation of abruption, hypertension discovered in such a patient should be investigated after the pregnancy is over and then treated accordingly, with antihypertensive treatment maintained during the next pregnancy.

The harmful effects of cigarette smoking are well documented and if smokers give up the habit, even during pregnancy, the risk of abruption is reduced by 23% (Naeye 1980). It is important to motivate the patient to give up smoking.

Admission to hospital around the time when the previous episode occurred has no proven value, but is reassuring to both patient and doctor. It also provides an opportunity to monitor fetal well-being, to treat any existing hypertension, to reinforce the non-smoking advice and to encourage early reporting of pregnancy bleeding.

Maternal mortality

Maternal mortality from placental abruption has fallen from 8% in 1917 to under 1% (Egley & Cefalo 1985). Although maternal mortality from haemorrhage in England and Wales fell steadily until 1985–1987, the small but continuing number of deaths since then is a reminder of the need to maintain high standards. The most recent report on confidential enquiries into maternal deaths in the UK (Department of Health 1998) registered four deaths from placental abruption (Table 14.8). Two were in the middle trimester of pregnancy. Despite the classic clinical picture of severe pain, the report describes one woman who seemed well enough to wait in a cubicle in an Accident and Emergency Department for 2 hours: when the doctor saw her at the end of this time she was dead. This tragic case underlines the fact that a fit woman may be able to compensate for severe haemorrhage until collapse occurs as a terminal event.

The report contains revised guidelines for the management of massive obstetric haemorrhage. Recommendations include the use of more than one intravenous line, and the use of a central venous catheter, to ensure adequate transfusion.

Perinatal mortality

Perinatal mortality is increased by any kind of bleeding in pregnancy, but is highest following placental abruption. The British Births 1970 Study (Chamberlain et al 1970) reported a perinatal mortality of 143.6 per thousand. Perinatal mortality due to abruption decreased over time in Norway from 2.5 per 1000 in 1967 to 0.9 per 1000 births in 1991. Case fatality rate decreased from 47% in 1967–1971 to 21.7% in 1987–1991, and decreased in all gestational age categories (Rasmussen et al 1996b).

In the US collaborative study abruption was the second

most frequent cause of perinatal mortality and accounted for 15% of all perinatal deaths (Naeye 1980). Population-based statistics from Scotland (Scottish Health Service 1986) reported 72 deaths from placental abruption (12.3% of the total); 81% of these weighed less than 2500 g. There were another 10 deaths among late abortions between 20 and 28 weeks' gestation, but these were not registered as stillbirths.

More than half of the perinatal deaths are stillborn. In a series of 274 admissions with abruption (Naeye et al 1977), 57 (23%) babies were stillborn, and of these 44 (16%) were dead before arrival in hospital. Of the remaining 217 live births, 35 (16%) died within 28 days, most of them weighing under 2500 g. As would be expected, the chances of survival depended on the gestation. For liveborn babies weighing 2500 g or more the survival rate is reported as 98%. According to Abdella et al (1984), the presence of chronic hypertension trebles the fetal mortality from abruption.

There is also concern about the quality of life for the survivors. The Apgar score and the incidence of respiratory distress syndrome are both worse in babies following abruption than would be expected in infants of equivalent birthweight.

OTHER CONDITIONS

Local disease of the cervix or vagina may cause APH. Benign cervical lesions such as polyps may be treated by removal during pregnancy. Cervical carcinoma may present during pregnancy, although this is now rare with routine cervical screening. The cervix should always be inspected, however, in a case of APH. Systemic diseases such as leukaemia are rare causes of APH.

UNEXPLAINED ANTEPARTUM HAEMORRHAGE

In the British Births 1970 Study (Chamberlain et al 1970), of 1079 cases of APH 406 (38%) had bleeding of unspecified cause. The fact that perinatal mortality was twice that of those with no history of bleeding (see Table 14.1) suggests that placental function was being compromised. Placental anomalies such as circumvallate placenta have been implicated.

Management

Once other causes of APH have been excluded, the possibility of a silent abruption must be constantly reviewed. Even when no uterine tenderness develops and there is no ultrasound evidence of retroplacental clot, fetal monitoring with car-

Table 14.8   Maternal deaths from antepartum haemorrhage in the UK

	1952–1954*	1985–1987	1988–1990	1991–1993	1994–1996
Placental abruption	78	4	6	3	4
Placenta praevia	29	0	5	4	3
Maternal mortality per million maternities	52.1	2.0	4.7	3.0	3.2

* England and Wales only
From Ministry of Health 1957 and Department of Health 1998, with permission

225

diotocography should be performed and the pregnancy should not be allowed to go beyond term.

It is not clear why perinatal mortality is increased in cases of unexplained APH. In some there will have been minor episodes of silent abruption or there may be anatomical anomalies of the placenta.

CONCLUSION

Bleeding in pregnancy remains an important cause of maternal death globally and of fetal loss in the UK. Ectopic pregnancy can nowadays be diagnosed relatively easily provided the condition is thought about in a woman of reproductive age with abdominal symptoms or vaginal bleeding. Laparoscopic surgery and medical treatment are associated with a better prognosis for future pregnancy.

Ultrasound has made the suspicion of placenta praevia possible in early pregnancy but the diagnosis must be confirmed in the third trimester. Caesarean section for placenta praevia is risky and requires an experienced obstetrician. The rising caesarean section rate may lead to an increase in the incidence of placenta praevia and of placenta accreta in future pregnancies.

Placental abruption still causes a small number of maternal deaths in the UK and is associated with high perinatal mortality, which is often unpreventable. The causes are still not understood and further research is needed into the roles of thrombophilias and abnormalities of the placental bed.

ACKNOWLEDGEMENTS

Material in this chapter contains contributions from the first and second editions and we are grateful to the previous authors for the work done.

KEY POINTS

Placenta praevia
- Occurs in 0.2–0.5% of pregnancies—increased by age, parity, previous caesarean section.
- High false-positive rate with ultrasound scans in early pregnancy.
- Diagnosed by ultrasound in late pregnancy (transvaginal scanning is safe).
- Characteristic symptom is painless bleeding.
- Vaginal examination contraindicated: EUA rarely necessary.
- Grade 1 praevia: amniotomy and induction of labour may be acceptable.
- Other grades: caesarean section by the most senior obstetrician available.
- Regional anaesthesia is safe for caesarean section.

Placenta accreta
- With placenta praevia risk of accreta increases to 10%.
- Previous caesarean section is an independent risk factor.
- Antenatal diagnosis can be made by ultrasound or, if necessary, MRI.

- Multidisciplinary preparation for caesarean.
- Catheters may be placed before caesarean for possible pelvic arterial embolisation.
- Experienced operator essential: hysterectomy may be necessary.

Abruption of placenta
- Occurs in about 1% of pregnancies.
- Risk factors: thrombophilia, pre-eclampsia, smoking, raised alpha-fetoprotein.
- Presents with abdominal pain and a hard uterus, with or without vaginal bleeding.
- Initial management: central venous pressure line and bladder catheter.
- If abruption minor and very preterm—expectant treatment.
- Otherwise if baby alive—caesarean section. If dead, induction of labour.
- Blood loss usually underestimated.
- Renal damage is preventable by prompt and adequate transfusion.
- Treatment of coagulopathy requires cooperation with haematologist.
- Risk of recurrence: 7%.

Maternal mortality: UK, 1994–1996
- Twelve deaths due to ectopic pregnancy.
- Three deaths from placenta praevia.
- Four deaths from abruption of placenta.

REFERENCES

Abdella TN, Sibai BM, Hays JM, Anderson GD 1984 Relationship of hypertensive disease to abruptio placentae. Obstet Gynecol 63:365–370

Acker D, Sachs BJ, Tracey KJ, Wise WE 1983 Abruptio placentae associated with cocaine use. Am J Obstet Gynecol 146:220–221

Ananth CV, Savitz DA, Williams MA 1996 Placental abruption and its association with hypertension and prolonged rupture of membranes: a methodologic review and meta-analysis. Obstet Gynecol 88:309–318

Ananth CV, Smulian JC, Vintzileos AM 1997a The association of placenta previa with history of cesarean section and abortion: a metaanalysis. Am J Obstet Gynecol 177:1071–1078

Ananth CV, Bowes WA, Savitz DA, Luther ER 1997b Relationship between pregnancy-induced hypertension and placenta previa: a population-based study. Am J Obstet Gynecol 177:997–1002

Ananth CV, Savitz DA, Bowes WA, Luther ER 1997c Influence of hypertensive disorders and cigarette smoking on placental abruption and uterine bleeding during pregnancy. Br J Obstet Gynaecol 104:572–578

Ananth CV, Smulian JC, Vintzileos AM 1999 Incidence of placental abruption in relation to cigarette smoking and hypertensive disorders during pregnancy: a meta-analysis of observational studies. Obstet Gynecol 93:622–628

Arabin B, van Eyck J, Laurini RN 1998 Hemodynamic changes with paradoxical blood flow in expectant management of abruptio placentae. Obstet Gynecol 91:796–798

Besinger RE, Moniak CW, Paskiewicz LS, Fisher SG, Tomich PG 1995 The effect of tocolytic use in the management of placenta praevia. Am J Obstet Gynaecol 172:1770–1778

Bouyer J, Job-Spira N, Pouly JL, Coste J, Germain E, Fernandez H 2000 Fertility following radical, conservative-surgical or medical treatment for tubal pregnancy: a population-based study. Br J Obstet Gynaecol 107:714–721

Chamberlain GVP, Philipp E, Howlett B, Masters K 1978 British births, 1970. Heinemann, London, pp 54–79

Chelmow D, Andrew DE, Baker ER 1996 Maternal cigarette smoking and placenta previa. Obstet Gynecol 87:703–706

Chou MM, Shih E 1997 Prenatal diagnosis of placenta previa accreta with power amplitude ultrasonic angiography. Am J Obstet Gynecol 177:1523–1525

Clark SL, Koonings PP, Phelan JP 1985 Placenta previa/accreta and prior cesarean section. Obstet Gynecol 66:89–92

Cnattingius S, Mills JL, Yuen J, Eriksson O, Ros HS 1997 The paradoxical effect of smoking in preeclamptic pregnancies: Smoking reduces the incidence but increases the rates of perinatal mortality, abruptio placentae, and intrauterine growth restriction. Am J Obstet Gynecol 177:156–161

Cobo E, Conde-Agudelo A, Delgado J, Canaval H, Congote A 1998 Cervical cerclage: an alternative for the management of placenta previa? Am J Obstet Gynecol 179:122–125

Comeau J, Shaw L, Marcell CC, Lavery JP 1983 Early placenta previa and delivery outcome. Obstet Gynecol 61:577–580

Dawson WB, Dumas MD, Romano WM, Gagnon R, Gratton RJ, Mowbray RD 1996 Translabial ultrasonography and placenta previa: does measurement of the os-placenta distance predict outcome? J Ultrasound Med 15:441–446

Debby A, Golan A, Sadan O, Zakut H, Glezerman M 2000 Fertility outcome following combined methotrexate treatment of unruptured extrauterine pregnancy. Br J Obstet Gynaecol 107:626–630

Department of Health 1998 Why mothers die: report on confidential enquiries into maternal deaths in the United Kingdom 1994–1996. The Stationery Office, London

deVries JIP, Dekker GA, Huijgens PC, Jakobs C, Blomberg BME, van Geijn HP 1997 Hyperhomocysteinaemia and protein S deficiency in complicated pregnancies. Br J Obstet Gynaecol 104:1248–1254

Egley C, Cefalo RC 1985 Abruptio placenta. In: Studd J (ed) Progress in obstetrics and gynaecology, vol 5. Churchill Livingstone, London, pp 108–120

Eriksen G, Wohlert M, Ersbak V, Hvidman L, Hedegaard M, Skajaa K 1991 Placental abruption. A case-control investigation. Br J Obstet Gynaecol 98:448–452

Fox H 1978 Pathology of the placenta. Saunders, London, pp 108–112

Frederiksen MC, Glassenberg R, Stika CS 1999 Placenta previa: a 22-year analysis. Am J Obstet Gynecol 180:1432–1437

Fylstra DL 1998 Tubal pregnancy: a review of current diagnosis and treatment. Obstet Gynecol Surv 53:320–328

Hansch E, Chitkara U, McAlpine J, El-Sayed Y, Dake MD, Razavi MK 1999 Pelvic arterial embolization for control of obstetric haemorrhage: a five-year experience. Am J Obstet Gynecol 180:1454–1460

Hauth JC, Goldenberg RL, Parker CR, Cutter GR, Cliver SP 1995 Low-dose aspirin: lack of association with an increase in abruptio placentae or perinatal mortality. Obstet Gynecol 85:1055–1058

Hemminki E, Merilainen J 1996 Long-term effects of cesarean sections: Ectopic pregnancies and placental problems. Am J Obstet Gynecol 174:1569–1574

Hershkowitz R, Fraser D, Mazor M, Leiberman JR 1995 One or multiple previous cesarean sections are associated with similar increased frequency of placenta praevia. Eur J Obstet Gynecol Reprod Biol 62:185–188

Hibbard BM, Hibbard ED 1963 Aetiological factors in abruptio placentae. BMJ 2:1430–1436

Hudon L, Belfort MA, Broome DR 1998 Diagnosis and management of placenta percreta: a review. Obstet Gynecol Surv 53:509–517

Hurd WW, Miodovnik M, Hertzberg V, Lavin JP 1983 Selective management of abruptio placentae: a prospective study. Obstet Gynecol 61:467–473

Kramer MS, Usher RH, Pollack R, Boyd M, Usher S 1997 Etiologic determinants of abruptio placentae. Obstet Gynecol 89:221–226

Kupferminc MJ, Eldor A, Steinman N et al 1999 Increased frequency of genetic thrombophilia in women with complications of pregnancy. N Engl J Med 340:9–13

Leaphart WL, Schapiro H, Broome J, Welander CE, Bernstein IM 1997 Placenta previa with bladder invasion. Obstet Gynecol 89:834–835

Lee W, Lee V, Kirk JS, Sloan CT, Smith RS, Comstock CH 2000 Vasa previa: prenatal diagnosis, natural evolution, and clinical outcome. Obstet Gynecol 95:572–576

Levine AB, Kuhlman K, Bonn J 1999 Placenta accreta: comparison of cases managed with and without pelvic artery balloon catheters. J Maternal-Fetal Med 8:173–176

Lipitz S, Admon D, Menczer J, Ben-Baruch G, Oelsner G 1991 Mid-trimester bleeding—variables which affect the outcome of pregnancy. Gynecol Obstet Invest 32:24–27

Love CDB, Wallace EM 1996 Pregnancies complicated by placenta praevia: what is appropriate management? Br J Obstet Gynaecol 103:864–867

Macafee CHG, Miller WG, Harley G 1962 Maternal and foetal morbidity resulting from placenta praevia. Obstet Gynecol 65:176–182

Macafee CHG 1945 Placenta praevia – a study of 174 cases. J Obs Gyn of the British Empire 52:313–324

MacGillivray I, Campbell DM 1988 Management of twin pregnancies. In: MacGillivray I, Campbell DM, Thompson B (eds) Twinning and twins. Wiley, Chichester, pp

Macones GA, Sehdev HM, Parry S, Morgan MA, Berlin JA 1997 The association between maternal cocaine use and placenta previa. Am J Obstet Gynecol 177:1097–1100

Major CA, de Veciana M, Lewis D, Morgan MA 1995 Preterm premature rupture of membranes and abruptio placentae: Is there an association between these pregnancy complications? Am J Obstet Gynecol 172:672–676

McShane PM, Heyl PS, Epstein MF 1985 Maternal and fetal morbidity resulting from placenta praevia. Obstet Gynecol 65:176–182

Merland JJ, Houdart E, Herbreteau D et al 1996 Place of emergency arterial embolisation in obstetric haemorrhage about 16 personal cases. Eur J Obstet Gynecol Reprod Biol 65:141–143

Miller DA, Chollet JA, Goodwin TM 1997 Clinical risk factors for placenta previa–placenta accreta. Am J Obstet Gynecol 177:210–214

Ministry of Health 1957 Report on confidential enquiries into maternal deaths in England and Wales 1952–1954. Her Majesty's Stationery Office, London

Naeye R 1980 Abruptio placentae and placenta previa: frequency, perinatal mortality and cigarette smoking. Obstet Gynecol 55:701–704

Naeye RL, Harkness WL, Utts J 1977 Abruptio placentae and perinatal death: a prospective study. Am J Obstet Gynecol 128:740–746

Naeye RL, Tafari N, Marboe CC 1979 Perinatal death due to abruptio placentae in an African city. Acta Obstet Gynecol Scand 58:37–40

Nielson EC, Varner MW, Scott JR 1991 The outcome of pregnancies complicated by bleeding during the second trimester. Surg Gynecol Obstet 173:371–374

Paintin D 1962 The epidemiology of ante-partum haemorrhage. J of Obs and Gyn of the British Commonwealth 69:614–624

Panoskaltsis TA, Ascarelli A, de Souza N, Sims CD, Edmonds KD 2000 Placenta increta: radiological investigations and therapeutic options of conservative management. Br J Obstet Gynaecol 107:802–806

Pisarska MD, Carson SA, Buster JE 1998 Ectopic pregnancy. Lancet 351:1115–1120

Powell MC, Buckley J, Price H, Worthington BS, Symonds EM 1986 Magnetic resonance imaging and placenta previa. Am J Obstet Gynecol 154:565–569

Pritchard JA, MacDonald PC, Gant NF 1985 Williams obstetrics, 17th edn. Appleton-Century-Croft, Norwalk, p 399

Rajkhowa M, Glass MR, Rutherford AJ, Balen AH, Sharma V, Cuckle HS 2000 Trends in the incidence of ectopic pregnancy in England and Wales from 1966 to 1996. Br J Obstet Gynaecol 107:369–374

Rasmussen S, Irgens LM, Bergsjo P, Dalaker K 1996a The occurrence of placental abruption in Norway 1967–91. Acta Obstet Gynecol Scand 75:222–228

Rasmussen S, Irgens LM, Bergsjo P, Dalaker K 1996b Perinatal mortality and case fatality after placental abruption in Norway 1967–91. Acta Obstet Gynecol Scand 75:229–234

Rasmussen S, Irgens LM, Dalaker K 1997 The effect on the likelihood of further pregnancy of placental abruption and the rate of its recurrence. Br J Obstet Gynaecol 104:1292–1295 [and comment, 105:1125]

Rose GL, Chapman MG 1986 Aetiological factors in placenta praevia. Br J Obstet Gynaecol 93:586–589

Schultze PM, Stamm CA, Roger J 1998 Placental abruption and fetal death with airbag deployment in a motor vehicle accident. Obstet Gynecol 92:719

Scottish Health Service, Information Services Division 1986 Perinatal mortality survey, Scotland 1985. Common Services Agency, Edinburgh

Sher G, Statland BE 1985 Abruptio placentae with coagulopathy: a rational basis for management. Clin Obstet Gynecol 28:15–23

Sibai BM 1999 Thrombophilias and adverse outcomes of pregnancy—what should a clinician do? N Engl J Med 340:50–52

Sibai BM, Lindheimer M, Hauth J et al, for the National Institute of Child Health and Human Development Network of Maternal-Fetal Medicine Units 1998 Risk factors for preeclampsia, abruptio placenta, and adverse neonatal outcomes among women with chronic hypertension. N Engl J Med 339:667–671

Taipale P, Hiilesmaa V, Ylostalo P 1997 Diagnosis of placenta previa by transvaginal sonographic screening at 12–16 weeks in a nonselected population. Obstet Gynecol 89:364–367

Tay JI, Moore J, Walker JJ 2000 Ectopic pregnancy. BMJ 320:916–919

Taylor VM, Peacock S, Kramer MD, Vaughan TL 1995 Increased risk of placenta praevia among women of Asian origin. Obstet Gynecol 86:805–808

Thorp JM, Wells SR, Wiest HH, Jeffries L, Lyles E 1998 First-trimester diagnosis of placenta previa percreta by magnetic resonance imaging. Am J Obstet Gynecol 178:616–618

Towers CV, Pircon RA, Heppard M 1999 Is tocolysis safe in the management of third-trimester bleeding? Am J Obstet Gynecol 180:1572–1578

Vedantham S, Goodwin SC, McLucas B, Mohr G 1997 Uterine artery embolization: An underused method of controlling pelvic haemorrhage. Am J Obstet Gynecol 176:938–948

Witlin AG, Saade GR, Mattar F, Sibai BM 1999 Risk factors for abruptio placentae and eclampsia: analysis of 445 consecutively managed women with severe preeclampsia and eclampsia. Am J Obstet Gynecol 180:1322–1329

Yaron Y, Cherry M, Kramer RL et al 1999 Second-trimester maternal serum marker screening: maternal serum alpha-fetoprotein, beta-human chorionic gonadotrophin, estriol, and their various combinations as predictors of pregnancy outcome. Am J Obstet Gynecol 181:968–974

15

Multiple pregnancy

James P. Neilson, Rekha Bajoria

The contribution of the author of the equivalent chapter in the second edition, on which this chapter draws extensively, is gratefully acknowledged.

INTRODUCTION

Recent advances in the diagnostic and therapeutic techniques of fetal medicine have altered many aspects of antenatal care in multiple pregnancies. Assisted conception has increased the incidence of multiple pregnancy and fetal reduction has created a new category of twin pregnancy. More babies from multiple births survive the perinatal period but multiple gestations still contribute disproportionately to perinatal mortality. Morbidity is also increased, with important associated long-term sequelae, including cerebral palsy. The high-risk nature of multiple pregnancy requires vigilant antepartum and intrapartum care.

TYPES OF TWIN PREGNANCY

There are two types of twins: monozygotic and dizygotic. Monozygotic twins arise from the splitting of a single fertilised ovum; dizygotic twins result from fertilisation of two ova by different spermatozoa. In White European populations, 30% of twin pregnancies are monozygotic. The rate of monozygotic twinning, at 3–5 per thousand births, is relatively constant throughout the world; the rate of dizygotic twinning varies between 4 and 50 per thousand births, and is influenced by such factors as ethnicity, age, height, weight, parity, and assisted reproduction. The highest twinning rates are seen in Nigeria (49 per thousand), and the lowest in Japan and China (2 per thousand) with intermediate incidence in Europe and USA (5.9–8.9 per thousand). The incidence of dizygotic twins increases with maternal age, with a peak occurring between the ages of 35 and 39. Tall women are more likely to have dizygotic twins than shorter women (Hollenbach & Hickok 1990).

Relationship between zygosity and chorionicity

Zygosity refers to the type of conception, while chorionicity denotes the type of placenta. Twin placentas can be divided into two categories according to the layers of membrane in the dividing septa that separate the amniotic cavities. The septa of monochorionic placentas consist of two layers of amnion alone; dichorionic placentas have two layers of both chorion and amnion. Monochorionic placentas can either be diamniotic (with two amniotic cavities) or, rarely, monoamniotic (with a single amniotic cavity). Dichorionic placentas may consist of two discrete masses or be fused because of the proximity of their implantation sites.

Dizygotic twins always have dichorionic placentas but the type of placentation in monozygotic conception depends on the time of splitting of the fertilised ovum (Benirschke & Kaufmann 1995). Dichorionic placentas occur in 25% of monozygotic pregnancies, and are found when cleavage occurs within 3 days of fertilisation. A monochorionic diamniotic placenta (75%) is formed when splitting occurs 4–7 days after fertilisation. In less than 1% of monozygotic conceptions, twinning occurs 8 days after fertilisation and a single placental mass is formed with no dividing amniotic membrane. Conjoined twinning, which is a rare variant of monochorionic monoamniotic placentation, occurs when splitting takes place more than 14 days after fertilisation (Fig. 15.1).

PERINATAL MORTALITY AND MORBIDITY

Perinatal mortality rates are six times higher in twin babies than in singletons. The risks increase with an increasing number of fetuses. Recent epidemiological work has revealed a substantial decline in the stillbirth rate in twins from

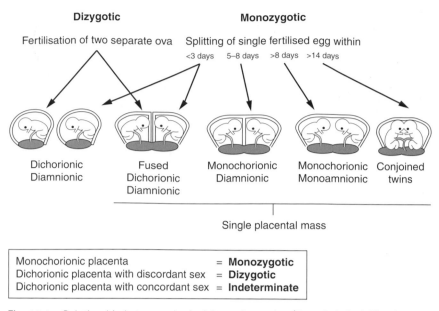

Fig. 15.1 Relationship between chorionicity and zygosity. (From Bajoria & Kingdom 1997, with permission.)

antepartum asphyxia and congenital malformations but the mortality rate from immaturity in twins remains sixfold higher than in singleton births (Glinianaia et al 2000).

Recent studies also suggest that, in monozygotic pregnancy, the risk of both twins dying *in utero* or of neonatal death of at least one twin is, respectively, 19 and 2.3 fold higher than dizygotic twins (West et al 1999). This is largely attributed to monochorionic placentation, where the presence of intertwin vascular shunts increases perinatal risks.

There may be differences in neurodevelopmental status and congnitive function between twins and singleton infants born before 33 weeks of gestation (Stewart 1995). Twins are more likely to suffer from brain lesions of cerebral atrophy (cystic periventricular leukomalacia) rather than ventricular dilatation type, indicating that twins may experience a different pattern of insult from singletons. Twins are more likely to have neurological impairments, lower IQ scores and require extra educational provisions than singletons. Deficits are more pronounced with verbal skills and may only emerge at the age of 8 years, when detailed cognitive testing is possible.

The incidence of cerebral palsy after multiple births is disproportionately higher than after singleton pregnancies, with an odds ratio of 4.94 (95% CI 4.24–5.33). Cerebral palsy in twins is more likely to be spastic hemiplegia or diplegia but the distribution of severity of motor impairment and of associated impairment such as epilepsy and intellectual disability is no different from that in singletons. The likelihood per pregnancy of cerebral palsy is eight times greater for twins and 47 times greater for triplets than singleton pregnancies (Petterson et al 1993). For a given low birthweight the risk of cerebral palsy in multiples is comparable with singletons. The risk of cerebral palsy is higher in multiples weighing below 2500 g than in singleton infants. Several antenatal factors have been associated with the increased risk of cerebral palsy in multiple gestation. The risk is higher in monozygotic twins because the splitting of the fertilised zygote may predispose to

some specific cerebral abnormality, and the presence of placental anastomoses linking twins' circulations. Fetal death of one twin after 20 weeks confers a risk of 20% for some form of cerebral impairment, and 29% for cerebral palsy (Pharoah & Adi 2000). The incidence of cerebral palsy is comparable between the first and second twin.

DETERMINATION OF CHORIONICITY

Prenatal determination of chorionicity is important in stratification of clinical risk, genetic counselling, and prenatal screening and diagnosis of structural and chromosomal abnormalities. Chorionicity can be established prenatally by ultrasound by one of the following (Bajoria & Kingdom 1997).

- Number of extraembryonic coeloms in early pregnancy. Dichorionic twins have two extraembryonic coeloms divided by a thick chorion laeve, monochorionic twins a single extraembryonic coelom, usually containing two yolk sacs.
- Number of placentas. Two placental masses indicate dichorionicity (although a single placental mass may be monochorionic or dichorionic).
- Fetal sex. Gender assignment early in the second trimester is feasible in more than 90% of cases with >99% accuracy, provided visualisation of the external genitalia is used to diagnose sex. Discordant genitalia indicate dichorionicity (although concordant sex does not, obviously, equate with monochorionicity).
- Assessment of the interfetal dividing membrane. Counting the number of layers in the dividing membrane by high-resolution ultrasound or assessing septal thickness can predict chorionicity with a substantial degree of accuracy. The twin peak or *lambda* sign is an ultrasound feature of dichorionic placentae representing echodense chorionic

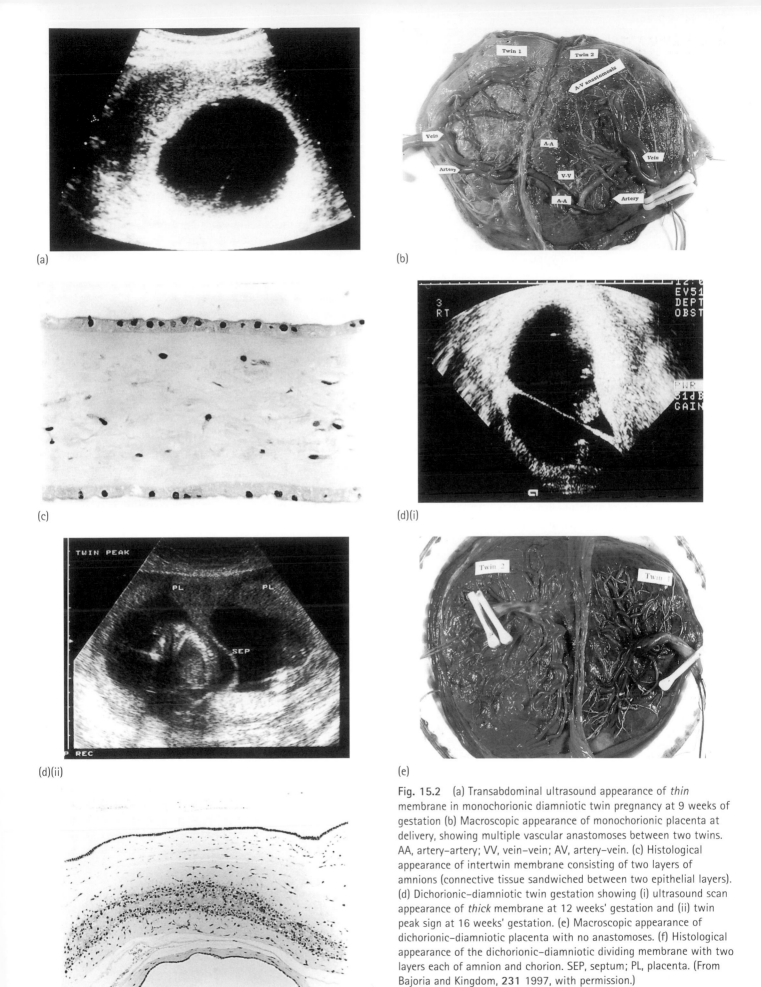

Fig. 15.2 (a) Transabdominal ultrasound appearance of *thin* membrane in monochorionic diamniotic twin pregnancy at 9 weeks of gestation (b) Macroscopic appearance of monochorionic placenta at delivery, showing multiple vascular anastomoses between two twins. AA, artery–artery; VV, vein–vein; AV, artery–vein. (c) Histological appearance of intertwin membrane consisting of two layers of amnions (connective tissue sandwiched between two epithelial layers). (d) Dichorionic–diamniotic twin gestation showing (i) ultrasound scan appearance of *thick* membrane at 12 weeks' gestation and (ii) twin peak sign at 16 weeks' gestation. (e) Macroscopic appearance of dichorionic–diamniotic placenta with no anastomoses. (f) Histological appearance of the dichorionic–diamniotic dividing membrane with two layers each of amnion and chorion. SEP, septum; PL, placenta. (From Bajoria and Kingdom, **231** 1997, with permission.)

villi between the two layers of intertwin membrane at its origin from the placenta. This is not seen in a monochorionic placenta (Fig. 15.2).

Chorionicity and amnionicity can be assessed accurately in 100% of cases when performed before 13 weeks. If this window of opportunity is missed, determination of chorionicity in late pregnancy is still feasible by using composite ultrasonographic criteria of fetal sex, number of placentas, membrane thickness and twin peak sign with a sensitivity and specificity of greater than 91% (Tables 15.1 and 15.2).

It is good practice to confirm chorionicity by examination of the placenta(s) after delivery. Much can be achieved by naked eye examination as separate placental discs represent dichorionic twinning. In a case of single placental mass, the presence of two layers of chorion and two layers of amnion in the septum indicates a dichorionic placenta, while presence of two amnions alone indicates monochorionicity. For research studies, dyes can be injected into vessels in monochorionic placentas to demonstrate anastomototic connections.

ANTENATAL ASSESSMENT

Before 20 weeks' gestation

Early diagnosis

A proven benefit of routine ultrasound in early pregnancy is the earlier diagnosis of multiple pregnancy although this has not been shown so far, in clinical trials, to improve perinatal outcome (Neilson 2000). Examination should include assessment of chorionicity and there are opportunities to screen for chromosomal abnormality by nuchal translucency thickness if the examination is performed around 11 weeks. Detailed examination for structural abnormalities may be performed around mid-pregnancy.

Fetal reduction

In pregnancies with four or more fetuses, there is evidence that embryo reduction to twins is associated with a decrease in the risk of miscarriage and perinatal death (Evans et al 1998). In triplet pregnancies, embryo reduction is not a routine practice as the overall survival of triplets reduced to twins is comparable with those managed expectantly. The procedure involves the injection of potassium chloride into the fetal thorax, either by the transabdominal or transvaginal route. The use of this technique creates major human and ethical dilemmas, is more usually carried out after IVF or stimulation of ovulation and is better avoided by the prudent use of assisted conception. The overall miscarriage rate following embryo reduction is about 2%, while extreme prematurity occurs in approximately 8% of pregnancies.

The vanishing twin

The vanishing twin syndrome describes the spontaneous cessation of cardiac activity in a previously viable fetus in a multiple pregnancy. Although the precise mechanisms and pathophysiology are obscure, the process of early pregnancy disappearance ultimately involves resorption. When fetal death occurs beyond the first trimester, a fetus papyraceus may develop (Landy & Keith 1998).

The true incidence is difficult to assess because of timing of ultrasonography, interpretative and artefactual errors. It has been estimated that the frequency of the vanishing twin syndrome ranges from 0 to 78%. The data collated from all pertinent studies published after 1990, evaluating the take-home baby rate in women with multiple pregnancies conceived by assisted reproduction, indicates that the visualisation of two and three or more sacs are associated with 43% and an 80% chance respectively of resorption of one fetus. In contrast, the overall probability for twin birth is 87% when two viable embryos are seen in the first trimester. Similarly, for spontaneous conception, if two sacs are identified on ultrasound scan the resorption rate is 40%, while the loss rate is 7% if two embryos are seen.

The biological significance of vanishing twins is being researched. It has been hypothesised that cerebral palsy in

Table 15.1 Positive predictive values* of ultrasonographic parameters in the prediction of chorionicity

Criterion	Monochorionicity	Dichorionicity
Placenta	Single (42%)	Separate (98%)
Fetal sex	Concordant (40%)	Discordant (100%)
Dividing membrane	Absent—monochorionic monoamniotic (100%)	
Number of layers	Two layers (94%)	Four layers (100%)
Thickness	<2 mm (39–82%)	>2 mm (95%)
Twin peak sign	Not present (44%)	Present (100%)
Use of all criteria	(92%)	(97%)

*Positive predictive values are given in parenthesis. For specific references see Bajoria and Kingdom 1997.

Table 15.2 Clinical implications of misdiagnosis of chorionicity in prenatal period

Ultrasound scan diagnosis	Histological diagnosis	Clinical consequences
Monochorionic	Dichorionic	Not serious; may lead to injudicious use of ultrasound scan
Monochorionic monoamniotic	Monochorionic diamniotic	Not serious
Monochorionic diamniotic	Monochorionic monoamniotic	May be serious; failure to appreciate cord complications; interlocking twins, conjoined twins and inappropriate intrapartum management
Dichorionic	Monochorionic	May be serious; failure in early diagnosis of chronic twin–twin transfusion syndrome; inappropriate management of discordant fetal anomalies, single intrauterine death

singleton children may be the result of unrecognised co-twin embryonic death, due to a mechanism similar to that described for single fetal death late in a monochorionic pregnancy. An argument against this interesting hypothesis, proposed by Pharoah and Cooke (1997), is that the vanishing twin syndrome is mainly seen by ultrasound scans in dichorionic placentas that are known to be devoid of anastomoses (Landy & Keith 1998). It is perhaps possible that small anastomoses may be present in the septal zone of dichorionic placentas early in gestation which may subsequently disappear.

Prenatal screening, diagnosis and management of fetal anomalies

Structural anomalies. Monochorionic twins have a higher incidence of structural anamolies than singletons. The increased incidence is confined to monochorionic twins and the incidence of malformations in dizygotic twins is similar to that in singleton pregnancies (Neilson 1992). The higher incidence in monochorionic twins is attributed to early splitting of the conceptus with consequent discordance in the two fetuses for differentiated cells or expression of certain genes (Burn 1995).

The structural defects in multiple pregnancy can be grouped as those unique to twins such as conjoined twins and acardiac twins and those that are not specific to twins but are more common in like-sex twin pairs. These include congenital heart defects, anencephaly, omphalocoele, hydrocephalus and atresia/stenosis of the gastrointestinal tract. Congenital heart defects are twice as prevalent in monozygotic as in dizygotic twins and singleton pregnancies. Anomalies not unique to twins, but observed with increased frequency because of mechanical and vascular factors, include talipes, skull asymmetry and congenital dislocation of the hip.

Most of the anomalies specifically associated with twinning can be diagnosed reliably by routine ultrasound in early gestation and usually affect one only of the twin pair. In an unselected series of 490 twins, 37 of 45 anomalies were detected among 21 of 24 affected fetuses for a sensitivity of 80%. The overall incidence of congenital anomalies was 24/490 (4.4%) with a mean gestational age at diagnosis of 22.3 (± 5.4) weeks (Edwards et al 1995). This detection rate compares favourably with previous studies of singletons, with detection rates of the order of 30–50%.

Chromosomal abnormalities

Incidence. With an increasing incidence of twinning and frequency of fetal aneuploidy with advancing maternal age, the risk and implications of aneuploidy for dizygotic twinning may differ from singleton gestation. In dizygotic conception, each embryo has an independent risk for nondisjunction leading to fetal aneuploidy and therefore the risk that at least one fetus is aneuploid will be twice the maternal age risk for a singleton. The probability of both fetuses being involved is, however, small. This is not true for monozygotic pregnancies, where both fetuses have the same karyotype, and hence the risk of an aneuploid fetus is the same as the maternal age risk for a singleton (although when an abnormality occurs, it will affect both babies rather than just one). The genetic risks are magnified in the event of a higher-order multifetal pregnancy. As the vast majority are the results of assisted reproductive techniques, and hence frequently polyzygotic, the risk of aneuploidy is three times the singleton maternal risk for triplets, and so on for higher-order multiple gestations. When considering prenatal diagnosis for family history of Mendelian disorders an even steeper increase in risk is present with twin gestation, a 3 in 8 risk of at least one affected fetus and 1 in 8 chance that both will be affected (Burn 1995).

Screening Biochemical screening for fetal aneuploidy based on maternal serum markers has a poor sensitivity (50%) and positive predictive value (5%) and therefore is not used in clinical practice.

The most promising method for screening for aneuploidy in twin pregnancies is the measurement of nuchal translucency at 10–14 weeks of gestation. Preliminary results on 392 twins are encouraging and suggest that detection of trisomy 21 has a similar sensitivity to that in singletons (Sebir et al 1996). However, the false-positive rate was higher in monochorionic than dichorionic twins; discordant nuchal translucency measurements in monochorionic twins may herald the development of chronic twin–twin transfusion syndrome.

Invasive procedures Determination of chorionicity is essential before undertaking any invasive procedure because the type of placentation influences the choice of technique and the interpretation of cytogenetic results. In monochorionic twins, it is usual practice to undertake karyotyping on one twin only, because monochorionic pregnancies are invariably monozygotic, and therefore unlikely to be cytogenetically discordant. However, in a small proportion of cases the genetic make-up of monochorionic twins may differ in terms of inheritance of certain X-linked diseases due to random inactivation of the maternal or paternal X-chromosome and mitotic accidents involving the sex chromosomes at the time of splitting of the fertilised ova. No such dilemma exists with dichorionic placentation, where each twin must be tested separately.

Despite the advantage of early diagnosis, chorionic villus sampling is not widely used in multiple pregnancies because of concern regarding an increased frequency of mosaicism, intertwin contamination (2–6%), and the difficulty of accurate interpretation of identical results with fused dichorionic placentas. Amniocentesis is often required to exclude the possibility of sampling error (Neilson 1992).

Mid-trimester amniocentesis is still, therefore, the gold standard invasive procedure. However, it is technically more demanding and precautions are necessary to avoid sampling the same sac twice. The use of various dyes to confirm separate sampling of each sac has been abandoned because of the increased risk of intestinal atresias. Sampling of both sacs through a single uterine entry and traversing the membrane, or separate sac puncture, are both satisfactory options.

Management of fetal abnormalities. It is important that women understand the implications of positive prenatal diagnoses (and especially the implications of discordant abnormality) before diagnostic tests are undertaken.

The option of selective termination in twins discordant for abnormality (aneuploidy or structural) is influenced by chorionicity. In dichorionic pregnancies, fetocide can be performed by the intracardiac injection of potassium chloride in the abnormal fetus without affecting the co-twin. Although previous studies observed a threefold increase in second- versus first-trimester losses, recent outcome data in 402 cases from eight centres suggests that selective termination for fetal anomalies is associated with successful outcomes in >90% of cases in all three trimesters (Evans et al 1999). Selective fetocide is not a viable option in monochorionic twins because of the risk of acute transfusion of the surviving twin into the dead fetus and the probability that potassium chloride may pass via placental vascular communications into the circulation of the normal cotwin. Therefore, recently, attempts have been made to achieve total occlusion of the umbilical cord of the abnormal twin by using potential occlusive agents (Deprest et al 2000).

Expectant management of twin pregnancies discordant for fetal abnormality has also been reviewed. In dichorionic twins discordant for anencephaly, good fetal outcome in a series of 14 cases has been reported with conservative management alone, with under half of the pregnancies developing polyhdramnios and none requiring amnioreduction. Similarly, expectant management was found to be as safe and effective as selective fetocide in twins discordant for lethal chromosomal abnormalities such as trisomies 13 and 18. However, the conservative approach in monochorionic twins discordant for certain lethal fetal malformations, may pose a potential risk of intrauterine death or neurological handicap of the normal co-twin in the event of death of the abnormal co-twin.

After 20 weeks' gestation

Maternal complications (Table 15.3)

Pre-eclampsia and antepartum haemorrhage. The overall incidence of hypertensive disorders in multiple pregnancy is 10–30%, with a 2–3.5-fold higher risk for pre-eclampsia and a sixfold higher risk for eclampsia. A retrospective study of 2473 twin pregnancies in Scotland suggested that, irrespective of parity, the relative risks for gestational hypertension, pre-eclampsia and eclampsia in twin pregnancies are all increased compared with singleton pregnancies (Campbell & MacGillivray 1999).

The cause of the higher incidence of hypertensive disease in twin pregnancies is not clear. Hyperplacentosis seems an unlikely mechanism, as placental mass is not increased in singleton pregnancies complicated by pre-eclampsia. Immunological differences between the mother and the fetuses also seems unlikely as the frequency of mild and severe pre-eclampsia between monozygotic and dizygotic twin gestations is comparable. Failure of successful implantation may be the most likely mechanism.

Twin pregnancy also confers an added risk of placenta praevia, with an incidence of 0.55% (compared with 0.31% in singleton pregnancies). The relatively higher incidence may be attributed to larger placental mass in multiple pregnancy. Abruption of the placenta is 2.8 times more frequent in twin gestations and may be due to the higher incidence of pre-eclampsia and/or a higher chance of sudden decompression of an over-distended uterus.

Preterm labour. Preterm delivery is the single most common cause of perinatal mortality in multiple pregnancies (Neilson & Crowther 1993). Compared with singletons, twins are 5.4 and 8.2 times more at risk to be born before 37 and 33 weeks of gestation respectively. Similarly, twins are 9.2 times more likely than singletons to weigh less than 1500 g.

Prediction of preterm birth

Various methods have been evaluated to predict preterm labour and thereby prompt preventive measures to try to improve adverse perinatal outcome. Risk scoring systems using factors such as previous preterm delivery, socioeconomic class, race, pregnancies after assisted reproduction, smoking, and maternal stress have only low predictive values.

A positive fetal fibronectin in a high vaginal swab at 28 weeks is predictive of birth before 35 weeks (odds ratio 11.5; 95% CI 3.4–38.6) and neonatal morbidity (odds ratio 11.3; 95% CI 2.4–46.9). However, the false-positive rate is relatively high.

Cervical assessment to identify women at risk of preterm delivery has also been evaluated. The cervix can be assessed either by digital examination or by ultrasound. Although earlier clinical work indicates that serial digital examination is useful to predict preterm birth (Neilson et al 1998a), variability between examiners makes this method subjective and less reproducible. Ultrasound provides a more objective assessment of the integrity of the internal os, funnel length and width. Transvaginal ultrasound is more effective than the transabdominal approach as it obviates the pressure effect from the maternal urinary bladder on the cervix. A prospective study of 219 twin pregnancies also suggests that monochorionic and dichorionic pregnancies had similar cervical length at 23 weeks. Cervical length of less than 25 mm at 23 weeks' gestation is associated with an 80% sensitivity for the prediction of spontaneous preterm delivery before 30 weeks of gestation and a 47% sensitivity for delivery before 32 weeks. The estimated risk for preterm delivery increases exponentially with decreasing cervical length—from about 2.9% at >46 mm to 4.3% at 36–45 mm, 31% at 16–25 mm, and 66% at 15 mm or less (Souka et al 1999). However, in order to have an impact on perinatal mortality, an effective strategy of cervical surveillance with a view to selective cerclage is necessary (Fig. 15.3).

Prevention of preterm birth

Interventions that have been studied in randomised trials include bed rest, beta-mimetics, elective cervical cerclage and progestins. There is no evidence that a policy of routine hos-

Table 15.3 Common prenatal maternal complications in twin and singleton pregnancies

Parameters	Twins (%) (n = 1253)	Singletons (%) (n = 5119)	Odds ratio	95% CI
Hypertension	12.9	5.6	2.5	2.1–3.1
Abruption	2.2	0.8	3.0	1.9–4.7
Anaemia	9.4	4.1	2.4	1.9–3.0
Urinary tract infection	8.7	6.7	1.4	1.1–1.7
Pyelonephritis	0.7	0.3	2.1	0.9–4.5
Post dates	1.2	3.1	2.6	1.6–4.4

After Spellacy et al 1990.

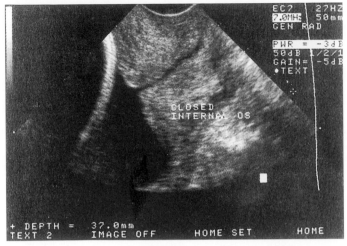

(a)

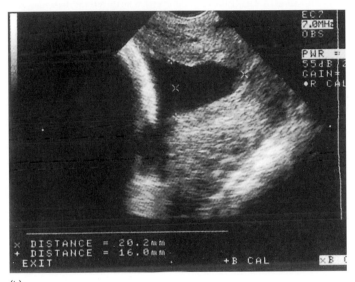

(b)

Fig. 15.3 Transvaginal ultrasound demonstration of the normal cervix and (b) herniation of the membranes through the 1.6 cm dilated internal os at 24 weeks of gestation. (From Kingdom and Bajoria 1998, with permission.)

pitalisation will reduce the risk of preterm birth or perinatal death. Instead, such policy may increase the risk of very preterm birth and very-low-birthweight infants. Selective hospitalisation of women with early cervical changes has also not been shown to be advantageous (Crowther et al 1989).

The prophylactic use of beta-mimetics has been evaluated in seven randomised controlled trials. Although treatment heterogeneity makes meaningful comparison difficult, meta-analysis shows no effect on the risk of preterm birth, birthweight or neonatal mortality from prophylaxis. Similarly, a meta-analysis of 15 published controlled trials on the use of progestational agents showed no advantage in terms of miscarriage, stillbirths and neonatal deaths.

Prophylactic routine cervical cerclage also failed to show any effect on the risk of preterm birth or perinatal mortality. Instead, this policy is associated with increased risk of mater-

nal infection and prelabour preterm rupture of membranes.

Management. In the absence of proven interventions to prevent preterm birth, it is important to ensure that infants destined to be born preterm are delivered in optimal conditions. The beneficial effects of maternal administration of corticosteroids to reduce the fetal risk of respiratory distress and intraventricular haemorrhage may be less in multiple than singleton pregnancies; perhaps higher doses are required. The use of tocolytic drugs to suppress active labour to permit the use of corticosteroids should be used with caution, as women with twin pregnancies have higher risks of pulmonary oedema.

Spontaneous delivery of the first fetus before 28 weeks of gestation does not necessarily imply a need to expedite delivery of the second. In the absence of overt chorioamnionitis, pre-eclampsia or fetal compromise, a combination of antibiotics, tocolysis and sometimes cervical cerclage can occasionally prolong the intertwin delivery interval.

Fetal complications

Fetal growth restriction. Intrauterine growth restriction (IUGR) is second only to prematurity as a major contributor to the increased perinatal morbidity and mortality seen in multiple pregnancy. The incidence of fetal growth restriction in twins ranges from 12 to 47% (as opposed to 5–7% in singleton gestations) and may affect either one or both the fetuses. Clinical examination is of very limited value in twin pregnancies in detecting small for gestational age fetuses (Neilson et al 1988b).

Normally, twin fetuses grow with the same velocity as singletons up to approximately 30–32 weeks. Thereafter, the femur length, head circumferences and biparietal diameter of twins are within the normal range for singletons but there is a reduction in the abdominal circumference after 32–34 weeks. Such a biometric profile is consistent with an asymmetric IUGR. Because of these observations, some investigators have proposed constructing ultrasound growth charts specifically for twins. It is our preference to use established singleton growth charts—there is no reason to think that twins have inherited different growth potentials than singletons.

Fetal growth in multiple pregnancies may also be expressed as growth discordance, which refers to the percentage difference of the estimated fetal weight of the smaller and larger of the twins. Perinatal risk, however, is not increased unless the smaller twin is small for gestational age, so the concept has limited practical value.

Poor growth has traditionally been attributed to the ill-defined concept of uterine overcrowding, which suggests that fetal competition for maternal nutrition inevitably results in an overall reduction of individual fetal growth. Poor placentation, unequal placental sharing, fetal structural and chromosomal anomalies may all be implicated (Matijevic & Bajoria 2000). Although the clinical phenotype may differ between monochorionic and dichorionic twins, the underlying cause for restricted growth is independent of chorionicity and placental vascular anastomoses (Bajoria 1998a). This is not surprising as our recent work provides evidence that intrauterine growth restriction is due to impaired placental transfer of certain essential amino acids (Bajoria et al 2000) and reduced fetal levels of growth promoting insulin-like growth factors (Bajoria et al 2001).

Fetal abdominal measurements are the best ultrasound indices of small-for-gestational-age twin fetuses (Neilson 1981) and of growth discordance. Umbilical artery Doppler studies can provide useful adjunctive evidence of placental dysfunction (Giles et al 1988). It is our practice to perform ultrasonographic surveillance for growth abnormalities by undertaking these measurements at 3 weekly intervals from 20 weeks in all twin pregnancies. However, recent data suggests that the positive predictive value for the finding of growth restriction at birth, after an abnormal growth finding on ultrasonography, is greatest (85%) when suspected growth restriction is first documented at 20–24 weeks of gestation and decreases with increasing gestational age. This finding thereby suggests that a routine 2- to 4-week interval between sonograms for all twin gestations may be unwarranted (Grobman & Parilla 1999).

Management of discordant IUGR needs to be individualised depending on the stage of pregnancy at which it is encountered. Discordant IUGR before 32 weeks can pose an especially difficult clinical problem, in which the growth-restricted fetus would benefit from early delivery while the normally grown cotwin would benefit from remaining in utero. As in singleton IUGR, the use of other tests of fetal well-being such as cardiotocography, measurement of amniotic fluid volume and Doppler velocimetry can fine tune decisions about the optimal timing of delivery. The timely administration of dexamethasone is important.

Single intrauterine death. Antepartum death of one fetus complicates 2.5–5% of twin pregnancies and may be associated with significant morbidity and mortality in the surviving co-twin. The cause of death of one twin remains undetermined in most cases. Death of a twin in monochorionic pregnancies is associated with 25% risk of cotwin death or 25% risk of neurological handicap in the survivor although no such risk exists in dichorionic twin pairs (Bajoria et al 1999b).

The mechanism of co-twin damage in monochorionic twins is not clear. Traditionally, passage of thrombotic materials from the dead twin along the placental vascular anastomoses with disseminated intravascular coagulopathy in the initially healthy surviving twin was considered to be the most likely mechanism (Benirschke & Kaufmann 1995) but recent demonstration of normal coagulation status following intrauterine death in the surviving monochorionic twin refutes this possibility (Bajoria & Kingdom 1997). The alternative theory to explain this phenomenon is based on the rapid and profound haemodynamic alteration that occurs at the time of death of one twin, with acute shift of blood from the surviving twin into the dead fetus along the superficial anastomotic channels. Demonstration of the severity of fetal anaemia *in utero* following intrauterine demise of one twin supports this hypothesis. Furthermore, configuration of vascular anastomoses in monochorionic placentas in relation to the outcome of the surviving twin suggests that passage of thrombotic material is virtually impossible because of the negative pressure gradient along the anastomoses (dead twin

with zero and alive twin with higher systemic pressure) (Bajoria et al 1999b).

Management of a twin pregnancy after a single intrauterine death is thus influenced by chorionicity. The death of the compromised twin in dichorionic pregnancies is seldom a risk factor for the surviving healthy co-twin and in general this complication does not influence obstetric management.

In monochorionic pregnancies, delivery soon after the death of one twin can prevent sudden demise of the co-twin, but is unlikely to reduce the neurological morbidity of the survivor. Therefore, in the absence of reliable parameters to predict which 50% of monochorionic twins will be compromised by the sequelae of an intrauterine death, there is a dilemma regarding management of patients between 24 to 28 weeks of gestation where one fetus is compromised. The preferred option, especially before 26 weeks, is to await spontaneous demise of the compromised twin, followed by close surveillance of the healthy co-twin using serial ultrasound scans or MRI to search for any signs of ischaemic cerebral damage. *In vivo* detection of artery–artery anastomoses by Doppler may also influence the clinical management of this unusual and difficult problem. The presence of such anastomoses is associated with an increased chance of cotwin death and neurological morbidity (Bajoria et al 1999b). However, absence of superficial anastomoses, which is commonly associated with chronic twin–twin transfusion syndrome, increases the risk of fetal demise (55%), severe anaemia (100%) and neurological morbidity (90%) only if the recipient twin dies first (Bajoria et al 1999b).

Monoamniotic pregnancy. Monoamniotic placentation, a rare variant of monozygotic conception, occurs in 1 in 10 000 pregnancies and is associated with perinatal loss rates of up to 50–70%. The most common cause of intrauterine death is cord entanglement within the single amniotic cavity. The presence of multiple anastomoses in monoamniotic placentas protects against chronic twin–twin transfusion syndrome (Bajoria 1988b). The perinatal loss rate is higher in early gestation (i.e. before 32 weeks) because there is relatively more amniotic fluid and greater fetal mobility, encouraging knot formation and cord entanglement (Dubecq et al 1996).

Early prenatal determination of monoamnionicity and close surveillance and timely intervention are prudent. Monoamniotic twins should be suspected in the presence of a single placental mass with same-sex twins, normal amniotic fluid volume, absence of a visible dividing membrane on two examinations at least 12 hours apart, and unrestricted fetal movement. The best gestational window for diagnosing monoamniotic twins ultrasonically is 9–12 weeks, examining the amniotic membranes and the number of yolk sacs.

The antenatal management of monoamniotic twins is controversial, and should include serial ultrasound scans to monitor fetal growth and the relationship between the cords. Cord entanglement can be visualised as a series of knots or as a braid of umbilical cords on real-time scanning, and on colour Doppler as free-floating intertwined vessels with apparent branching of the umbilical artery (Fig. 15.4). However, sonographic evidence of extensive knotting does not necessarily equate with compromised umbilical circula-

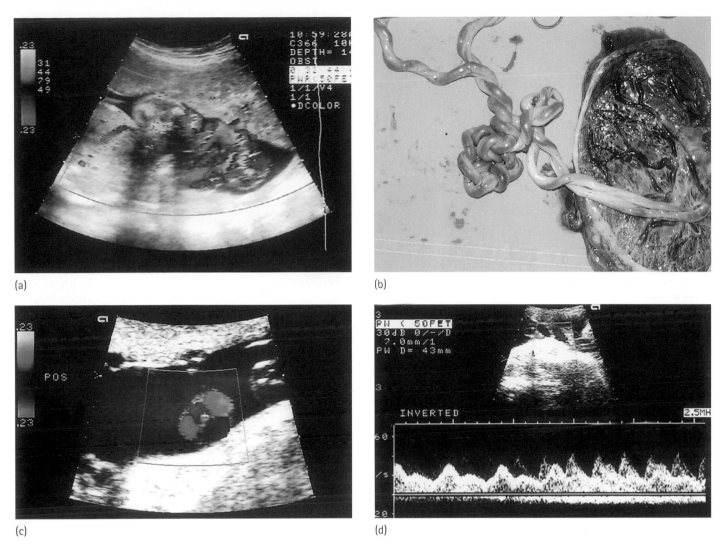

Fig. 15.4 (a) Monochorionic–monoamniotic twin pregnancy at 24 weeks' gestation. Colour Doppler revealed the entangled cords, which appeared as a braid of knots. (b) Both fetuses were delivered by elective caesarean section at 33 weeks of gestation after confirmation of lung maturity. The entangled cords can be seen forming a braid of cords. (c) Monochorionic monoamniotic conjoint twin pregnancy at 28 weeks' gestation. The colour Doppler shows a four-vessel cord. (d) Discordant umbilical artery Doppler waveform in the pregnancy shown in (c). (From Bajoria and Kingdom 1997, with permission.)

tion because this is seen in nearly all monoamniotic pregnancies. It has been suggested that the presence of a notch in the umbilical artery velocity waveform may suggest narrowing of the umbilical vessels due to cord entanglement.

Because of the worry about cord entanglement before labour, or confusion about which cord belongs to which twin during delivery, elective caesarean section before term is recommended.

Twin reversed arterial perfusion (TRAP) sequence. The most bizarre form of monochorionic twinning is acardiac or TRAP, and occurs in 1 in 35 000 pregnancies. Acardiac twinning results in the twin-reversed arterial perfusion (TRAP) sequence, where fetal tissue parts grow in tandem with the normal fetus and are perfused in the reverse direction, with deoxygenated blood entering the single umbilical artery. Hence the normally formed twin is referred to as the 'pump twin'. The risk to the pump twin from cardiac failure or preterm delivery from associated polyhydramnios is related

to the size and growth of the acardiac fetus. Overall perinatal mortality for the pump twin is 50% while the perfused fetus is never viable. Pregnancies complicated by an acardiac anomaly are most often twins, but cases of triplet, quadruplet and quintuplet pregnancies have been reported (Fig. 15.5). The acardiac and its co-twin are always of the same sex and the female gender predominates.

Acardiac twinning can occur due to primary failure of cardiac development early in embryogenesis from chromosomal abnormality, polar body twinning or other reasons. Alternatively, acardia results from an imbalance in the interfetal circulation, leading to atrophy of the heart. The early pressure flow in the placental artery of one of the twins exceeds that of the other and therefore results in a reversal of flow in the umbilical vessels of the other twin, causing a preferential development of the lower part of the body. The organs such as the head, heart, limbs, kidneys, and upper intestines commonly do not develop. A single umbilical

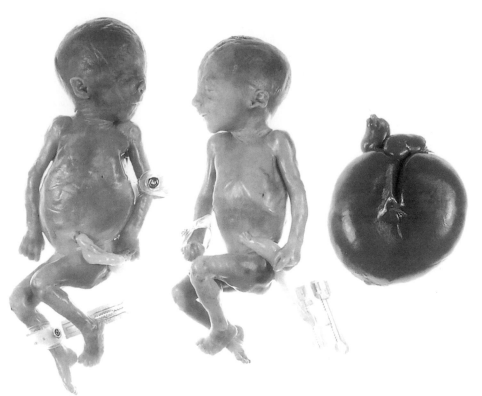

(a)

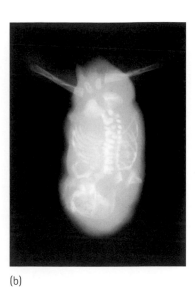

(b)

Fig. 15.5 A monochorionic tri-amniotic triplet pregnancy at 27 weeks of gestation: (a) triplets delivered by emergency caesarean section. Triplets 1 and 2 died early in the neonatal period as a consequence of chronic twin–twin transfusion syndrome, while triplet 3 was a non-viable acardiac. (b) Radiograph of the acardiac triplet.

artery is usually present. The external genitalia may be normal, deficient or absent.

The diagnosis of TRAP is made on ultrasound scan when a grossly malformed fetus with absence of cardiac pulsation, amorphous shape of the cephalic pole and poor definition of trunk and extremities is seen in a monochorionic twin pregnancy. However, the acardiac fetus may be mistaken for a single fetal death in a twin pregnancy and serial sonograms are often required to establish the correct diagnosis by documentation of growth in the twin suspected of being dead. The presence of a heartbeat in the malformed twin does not preclude the diagnosis as this may represent a rudimentary heart, or be the result of the normal twin's cardiac function. The diagnosis of acardiac twin can be made as early as the ninth week of gestation by transvaginal sonography. Demonstration of arterial flow towards rather than away from the affected fetus on colour Doppler is diagnostic of the TRAP syndrome (Brassard et al 1999). The dilemma in managing these cases is whether to perform an invasive therapeutic procedure, and thus risk the normal pump twin or to pursue conservative management, with the attendant risks of cardiac overload and polyhydramnios.

Conjoined twins. The term conjoined twins is used to describe those infants closely united at some point of their anatomy and the condition has been reported as 1 in 50 000–100 000 births. Conjoined twins are always monozygotic and result from division of the embryonic disk more than 13 days after conception. Although commonly associated with twin pregnancy, it may occur in triplet and quadruplet pregnancies. Female conjoined twins occur more frequently than males, in a ratio of 1.6 to 1.

Conjoined twins may be broadly classified as either equal or unequal. The equal form shows equal or near-equal duplication of structures. The unequal forms include the parasitic variety in which there is unequal duplication of structures. Classification is typically based on the fused anatomic region followed by the Greek suffix *pagus* to indicate fastened. The most frequent types of conjoined twins are thoraco-omphalopagus (28%), thoracopagus (18%), omphalopagus (10%), incomplete duplication (10%) and craniopagus (6%).

The prenatal diagnosis of conjoint twins is important for adequate planning of the site and type of delivery, preparation of the parents and counselling for pregnancy termination. The diagnosis is suspected on ultrasound scan early in pregnancy by the presence of a bifid appearance of the fetal pole, inability to separate the fetal bodies, four vessels in the umbilical cord, the heads at the same level, extended spine and no change in fetal position relative to one another with time or movement (see Fig. 15.4). Other diagnostic means such as radiography or MRI may be required for the detection of bony connection.

The surgical separation of conjoined twins is complex, and may pose major ethical and technical difficulties. With better prenatal assessment methods, lethal forms are frequently offered termination, while delivery and postnatal management of potentially separable pairs can be contemplated. Conjoined twins with minimal zones of coalescence can be surgically separated. In a small proportion, separation can only be achieved, often in stages, with the unequal allocation of organs between two separated twins. In cases where one twin is malformed and markedly growth restricted, management is aimed at saving the more completely formed twin.

Twin–twin transfusion syndrome. Placental vascular anastomoses are either superficial or deep, and are found in 83% of monochorionic placentas (Fig. 15.6). Superficial anastomoses may connect artery to artery or vein to vein, with the former being more common. Superficial anastomoses are functionally bidirectional depending on the relative pressure difference between the twins. In contrast, deep anastomoses are present within the substance of the placenta and receive arterial blood from one twin's circulation and drain into the venous system of the other; they are always unidirectional (Fig. 15.7).

Intertwin transfusion occurs in most monochorionic twins, and only if it is unbalanced do specific clinical sequelae

follow (Bajoria et al 1995, Bajoria 1998a). Severe twin–twin transfusion syndrome results when deep artery–vein anastomoses are uncompensated by superficial artery–artery and vein–vein anastomoses, with resultant net flow in one direction, causing associated hypovolaemia in one twin and volume overload in the other. Although the severity of the disease process in terms of intrauterine death, hydrops and acute twin–twin transfusion syndrome correlates with the presence of artery–artery, vein–vein anastomoses, severity of the growth restriction is independent of placental macroangioarchitecture. Computer modeling studies also support the anatomical data indicating the role of unidirectional arteriovenas anastomoses in the initiation of the chronic twin–twin transfusion syndrome (Talbert et al 1996).

Twin–twin transfusion syndrome can be classified as acute or chronic. The underlying pathology, clinical presentation and fetal morbidity and mortality associated with these two types are quite distinct. The high perinatal loss rate associated with twin–twin transfusion syndrome is predominantly due to the chronic form.

Acute. If an acute shift of blood from one twin to the other occurs it usually does so in the third trimester of pregnancy or during labour in an otherwise uncomplicated monochorionic pregnancy. The diagnosis is often made in the postnatal period based on the historical neonatal criteria of twin–twin transfusion syndrome (i.e. haemoglobin differences). Although usually not lethal, it may account for the sudden intrauterine death of one of the monochorionic twins in the third trimester, or during labour, in an otherwise uncomplicated pregnancy.

Chronic. Twin–twin transfusion syndrome complicates only 1–5 per 10 000 total pregnancies but accounts for 1% of the total perinatal loss rate and 20% of the overall perinatal mortality in twins. If untreated, the loss rate may approach 100%. The major cause of perinatal loss in chronic twin–twin transfusion syndrome is due to preterm labour secondary to severe polyhydramnios. If the pregnancy continues, both the fetuses are at risk. The recipient twin may develop pulmonary hypertension, right ventricular outflow obstruction and renal failure. The donor twin is at risk of the well described complications of severe intrauterine growth restriction.

The older diagnostic criterion of a haemoglobin discordance below 5 g/dl has not been substantiated by more recent studies as such differences have been demonstrated in dichorionic twins with discordant birthweight and in uncomplicated monochorionic twins with concordant birthweight (Danskin & Neilson 1989). Indeed, haematological discordance is uncommon in mid-trimester cases of twin–twin transfusion syndrome investigated by fetal blood sampling. Ultrasound diagnosis of chronic twin–twin transfusion syndrome is based on discordant fetal size with severe polyhydramnios around the larger twin and oligohydramnios around the smaller stuck twin. Chronic twin–twin transfusion syndrome presents in the early mid-trimester of pregnancy with clinical polyhydramnios. The donor becomes oliguric and the recipient polyuric. The polyuric recipient fetus may develop features suggestive of congestive cardiac failure, with cardiac dilatation, myocardial hypertrophy, tricuspid regurgitation and hydrops (Zosmer et al 1994). Ventricular afterload rather than volume over-

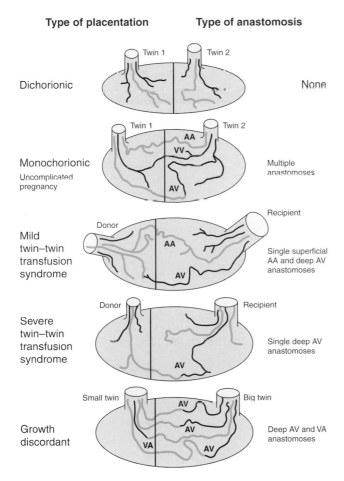

Type of placentation   **Type of anastomosis**

Dichorionic — None

Monochorionic, Uncomplicated pregnancy — Multiple anastomoses

Mild twin–twin transfusion syndrome — Single superficial AA and deep AV anastomoses

Severe twin–twin transfusion syndrome — Single deep AV anastomoses

Growth discordant — Deep AV and VA anastomoses

Fig. 15.6 Presence of different types of vascular anastomoses in monochorionic placenta in relation to the clinical outcome. Vascular shunts are absent in dichorionic placentas. Uncomplicated monochorionic placentas have multiple anastomoses of both superficial and deep type. Mild twin-twin transfusion syndrome has a single deep arteriovenous anastomosis and a superficial anastomosis, while the severe syndrome has a single unidirectional arteriovenous anastomosis. Monochorionic placenta with growth discordance has multiple deep anastomoses; number of deep anastomoses (AV) from smaller to larger twin nearly always exceeds those running in opposite direction (VA). Anastomoses: AA, arterial–arterial; VV, venous–venous; AV, arterial–venous; VA, venous–arterial. Dark and light lines represent arteries and veins respectively. (From Bajoria 1998a and 1998b with permission.)

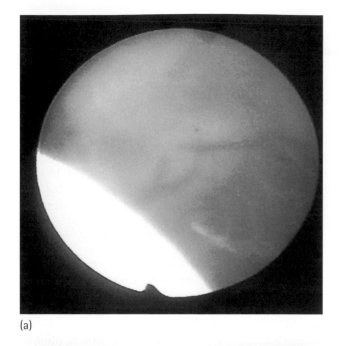

(a)

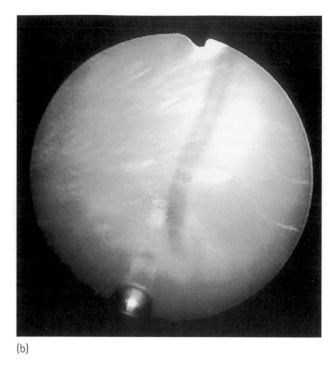

(b)

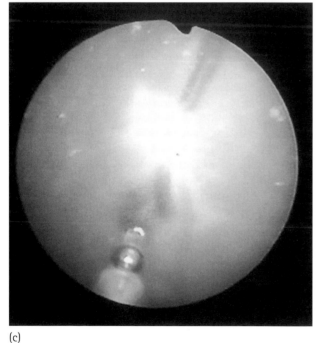

(c)

Fig. 15.7 Treatment of chronic twin–twin transfusion syndrome at 24 weeks' gestation by laser ablation of placental vascular anastomoses. (a) Endoscopic view of artery–vein anastomoses and dividing septum. (b) Initial targetting with 0.5 mm diameter HeNe pilot beam. (c) White spot represents coagulated tissue. (Courtesy of Professor Martin JC van Gemert, University of Amsterdam, Netherlands.)

load may be the underlying cause of cardiac dysfunction (Bajoria et al 1999a).

Early ultrasound demonstration of an unexplained increase of nuchal translucency thickness and fetal heart rate in one of monochorionic twins may predict later twin–twin transfusion syndrome. Similarly, infolding of the intertwin membrane between 15–17 weeks in monochorionic pregnancies suggests a 50% risk of subsequent twin–twin transfusion syndrome (Sebire et al 2000).

Treatment of chronic twin–twin transfusion syndrome. Much controversy surrounds the optimal treatment of chronic twin–twin transfusion syndrome. Various therapeutic options—such as transplacental digoxin therapy,

intrauterine venesection and exchange transfusion, selective fetocide and transplacental indomethacin—have been used either independently or in combination with mixed results (Filkins et al 1998).

Currently, most centres prefer serial amnioreduction for the treatment of twin–twin transfusion syndrome because it is a relatively simple technique, working on the principle that restoration of normal amniotic fluid volume should decrease the risk of preterm labour. Several groups have reported aggressive amnioreduction to be associated with a perinatal survival rate of 37–83%. The therapeutic efficacy of amnioreduction may be governed by the presence or absence of superficial anastomoses. In women with superficial anastomoses, the total number of amnioreductions required per pregnancy is likely to be 2.5-fold less than those who have only deep artery–vein anastomoses. Similarly, twin–twin transfusion syndrome without superficial anastomoses have a 3.5-times higher perinatal loss rate and markedly higher incidence of fetal morbidity in terms of hydrops, cardiomegaly and porenchaphalic cyst (Bajoria 1998c).

Recently, intentional puncture of the intervening membrane (septostomy) with or without attempts at amnioreduction for the treatment of the twin–twin transfusion syndrome has been proposed. Initial results based on 12 patients suggest that rapid accumulation of fluid around the stuck fetus occurred in all cases following a single procedure, with a combined survival of 83.3%. The septostomy to delivery interval ranged between 0.6 and 13 weeks (Kaufman et al 1998). However, more recent data, along with our own unpublished data ($n = 14$), failed to substantiate this promising outcome as the overall survival rate was only 36%. Further studies are required to assess its therapeutic value.

Because twin–twin transfusion syndrome has been attributed to net unidirectional flow along anastomoses, a simple hypothesis emerged that occluding the anastomoses would correct the underlying pathophysiology and treat the condition. Accordingly, attention has focused on fetoscopic laser ablation of placental anastomoses. Techniques for photocoagulating via a fetoscope were developed in animals and recently attempted in humans with mixed success. A published total of 343 patients from three centres suggests that success with this procedure is 53%–69%, which is comparable to serial amnioreduction. The main advantage of laser ablation is that the risk of white matter brain lesions in the survivor may be significantly less than after amnioreduction (0–6% compared with 18–30%). However, there has been a maternal death following this procedure.

HIGHER-ORDER MULTIPLE BIRTHS

Incidence

Higher-order multiple births are increasingly common as a result of assisted reproductive technologies in that 50–60% of all triplets, 75% of all quadruplets and virtually all quintuplet pregnancies now follow induced ovulation or assisted reproduction.

Perinatal mortality and morbidity

The principal determinant of successful outcome amongst higher-order births is gestational age at delivery, which is inversely related to the number of fetuses. Despite advances in neonatal care, mortality rates are considerably higher for triplets and higher multiple births. The perinatal mortality in a large cohort of triplet pregnancies was 121 per 1000 births, with no significant difference in outcome based on triplet birth order.

Triplets and higher-order births suffer significant perinatal morbidity due to prematurity and its consequences, low birthweight and growth retardation, and leave many survivors with long-term handicap. Triplets are also more likely to develop mild intraventricular haemorrhage and retinopathy of prematurity than singletons. When stratified by gestational age, triplet babies delivered at 24–34 weeks' gestation have similar outcomes to twins, with the only clinically significant difference being a sixfold increased incidence of retinopathy of prematurity in triplets (Kaufman et al 1998). One-year follow-up data on 38 triplets weighing less than 1500 g suggested severe neurological disability, including spastic diplegia and quadriplegia and marked developmental delay in 11% of the infants, while milder developmental problems were noted in 20%. The incidence of neurodevelopmental abnormalities was 30% in 11 higher-order multiples (more than three fetuses).

Maternal and fetal complications

Antenatal care is essentially similar to that for twin pregnancies, with vigilant surveillance for maternal and fetal complications. The role of ultrasonography for early diagnosis, viability, accurate dating and determining amnionicity and chorionicity is important, as is detailed scanning of fetal anatomy (Malone et al 1999).

Although antenatal complications are similar to those in twin pregnancies, the risk increases with increasing number of fetuses. The most common complications are preterm labour and fetal growth abnormalities. Preterm labour occurs in 75% of triplets and 100% of quadruplets. The mean gestational age at delivery in triplets is 34.5 weeks and that in quadruplets approximately 32 weeks. Prophylactic cerclage in high-order multiples has not been shown to improve pregnancy outcome. Because of the propensity for premature cervical dilatation, close monitoring of cervical length on ultrasound scan may provide an opportunity for cerclage (although there is no evidence that cerclage prolongs pregnancy in such cases). It is not our practice to admit women with triplet pregnancies routinely to the antenatal ward.

Sonographic data generated on fetal growth in triplets suggest that there is a mean difference of 2 weeks delay between 25–36 weeks' gestation in the growth patterns compared with twin fetuses. It is estimated that the incidence of growth discordance in triplet gestation is approximately double that occurring in twin pregnancies. Ultrasound scans every 2–3 weeks until delivery are essential to detect growth abnormalities. A quarter of triplets and quadruplets show IUGR by 32–34 weeks, and more than 60% by 35–36 weeks.

The incidence of pre-eclampsia is approximately 25% in triplet pregnancies. As antenatal and postnatal maternal complications occur in almost all triplet gestations, such pregnancies should be managed at centres that have appropriate multidisciplinary expertise available.

INTRAPARTUM CARE

The increased incidence of fetal malpresentation, preterm labour, IUGR and placental abnormalities, together with the need for skilled obstetrical manoeuvres, suggest that appropriate intrapartum management is as important as intensive antenatal care to improve overall neonatal morbidity and mortality (Houlihan & Knuppel 1996).

Mode of delivery

Twins are delivered by one of three ways: vaginal, abdominal or combined delivery (i.e. caesarean section for the second twin after vaginal delivery of the first twin).

Caesarean section

The incidence of caesarean section in twins is steadily increasing and appears to be related to the decreasing experience of obstetricians in the management of vaginal birth, especially internal podalic version. This increased risk of emergency caesarean section during labour, including caesarean section for the second twin, has led to a rising trend in favour of elective caesarean section for twin gestation. Caesarean section rates in twins are 2–3 times higher than for singleton pregnancy, thereby exposing more mothers to the risk of surgery, anaesthesia and postpartum thrombosis and infectious morbidity, with a three-fold increase risk of endometriosis and doubled risk of wound infection.

The obstetric indications for elective caesarean section, together with their relative importance, in twin gestation are shown in Table 15.4. The two common indications for elective caesarean section are non-vertex presentation of twin 1 and maternal request. The latter indication is related to a high proportion of twins are a consequence of infertility treatment in older couples.

In the absence of a clear indication for delivery, caesarean section should not be performed until after 38 weeks' gestation. This is important as neonatal respiratory disorders are more common in twin pregnancies where caesarean section is performed before labour or before 38 weeks' gestation (Chasen et al 1999).

Technique. Epidural anaesthesia is commonly employed for caesarean section in the absence of placenta praevia. This method results in preservation of uterine tone, which may in turn cause problems with delivery of the second twin in certain special circumstances such as IUGR of the second twin, chronic twin–twin transfusion syndrome resulting in a stuck twin in the fundus or uterine distortion by fibroids. Under these circumstances the second twin may become entrapped in the fundus, especially if the membranes are ruptured early to attempt a breech extraction. Administration of intravenous bolus of nitroglycerin (100–150 µg) to temporarily relax the uterus for delivery of the second twin should be considered. Reduction in maternal blood pressure is reported to be minimal.

Vaginal delivery and management of labour

It is usual to aim for the vaginal delivery of vertex/vertex twins as long as there are no obstetric or maternal contraindications (see Fig. 15.8). There is no increase in neonatal morbidity or mortality when twins are delivered vaginally compared with caesarean section. In the group where the first twin presents as a vertex and the second twin is in non-vertex presentation, most British obstetricians would attempt vaginal delivery under epidural with the provision for external version, internal podalic version, breech delivery or caesarean section if required. A considerable body of evidence supports this line of management when estimated birthweight is over 1500 g, with no increased perinatal morbidity and mortality in the second twin delivered vaginally. Caesarean section seems preferable for non-vertex/vertex or non-vertex/non-vertex fetuses.

Induction of labour. Induction of labour in twin pregnancies with a cephalic presentation of the first twin is common practice by 38 weeks of gestation. This is based on the assumption that the optimal length of gestation in twins is shorter than singletons because 30–50% of twins are small for gestational age at birth. Perhaps more importantly, many women find the discomforts and insomnia of late twin pregnancy hard to bear. Induction of labour is not necessarily a straightforward intervention, but a recent trial failed to find any significant differences in neonatal outcome, birthweight and caesarean section rate between induction of labour and expectant management policy at 37 weeks (Suzuki et al 2000).

Management of labour. On admission the woman should be reviewed to re-evaluate the safety of attempted vaginal delivery since the last clinic visit. Routine serial ultrasound reports will alert the birth attendants to the problems of discordant growth or malpresentation.

Intravenous access should be achieved and a blood sample sent to the laboratory for group and save or crossmatch depending on the perceived risk of subsequent blood loss.

Epidural anaesthesia can be advantageous for twin delivery, so as to facilitate either external or internal manipulation of twin 2 into a longitudinal lie or perform breech extraction where indicated. Where epidural anaesthesia is contraindicated or declined by the woman, then an anaesthetist should be present throughout the second and third stages of labour, because any need for general anaesthesia is likely to be immediate.

Labour should ideally be managed in a large room that can be converted for caesarean section and which can accommodate staff and equipment. Continuous electronic monitoring is desirable. In the first stage a scalp clip is recommended for twin 1 to simplify abdominal ultrasound monitoring for twin 2. Management of the second stage of labour is the same as for a singleton gestation, but delivery should be conducted in the presence of obstetric and anaesthetic staff.

Table 15.4 Obstetric indications for caesarean section in twin gestation

Accepted indications
Non-cephalic presentation of twin 1
Estimated birthweight of twin 2 greater than 500 g than twin 1
Placenta praevia
Congenital malformation of one twin
Chronic TTTS in monochorionic twins
Monoamniotic twins
IUGR in dichorionic twins
Antepartum death of first twin
Conjoined twins
Contentious indications
Maternal request
Death of co-twin
Uncomplicated monochorionic twins
Previous caesarean section

Houlihan & Knuppel 1996

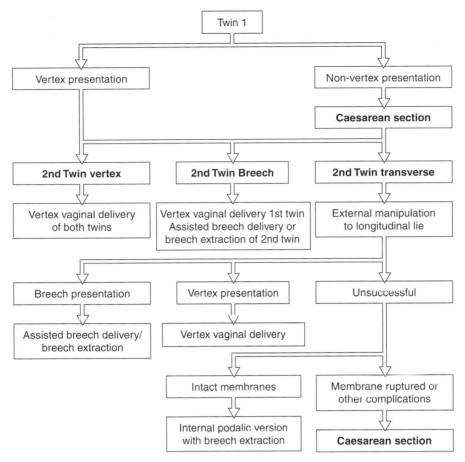

Fig. 15.8 Proposed intrapartum management of mature twin gestation according to presentation of the fetuses.

Immediately after the delivery of the first twin, its umbilical cord should be tightly clamped at both fetal and placental ends. This practice prevents acute intrapartum fetoplacental transfusion, which can be disastrous to the second twin in monochorionic gestation.

An obstetrician should palpate the abdomen immediately following delivery of twin 1 to ensure that the lie of twin 2 is longitudinal. Ultrasound should be readily available, if required, to assess the presentation and heart rate of twin 2.

External cephalic version for a breech presentation of the second twin is not common practice in UK because it confers little advantage to the fetus and may result in complications such as rupture of the membranes while the lie is transverse, bradycardia, failed version, and non engagement of the head; all may necessitate caesarean section.

Where rapid delivery of the second twin is indicated, for example due to a bradycardia, vaginal bleeding or cord prolapse, the fastest (and therefore safest) method is normally by breech extraction. This is why skilled obstetricians are comfortable with the second twin presenting as a breech, which exposes the weakness of the argument in favour of routine external cephalic version for the second twin presenting as a breech.

Immediate augmentation using oxytocin can shorten the intertwin delivery interval by preventing the commonly observed quiescence in uterine activity following delivery of twin 1. As such, efficient descent of the presenting part, sur-

rounded by intact forewaters, is achieved, thereby preventing the cervix from closing. Some obstetricians rupture the membranes once the presenting part is in the pelvis and complete the delivery. Others prefer to leave the membranes intact to ensure that the cervix remains fully dilated. It should be noted that syntocinon should not be restarted until the obstetrician is absolutely confident that the lie of twin 2 is longitudinal, otherwise an impacted transverse lie may result.

Where operative delivery is required for the cephalic second twin, this is commonly associated with malposition and a high station. For this reason the ventouse is far safer than forceps delivery. A smaller cap is preferred, so that application at a higher station than in a singleton delivery will not include maternal soft tissue. In the unlikely event of a failed attempt at delivery by vacuum, forceps delivery may be attempted provided descent has been achieved.

The acceptable interval between vaginal delivery of twins remains actively debated. Before epidural analgesia and widespread electronic fetal heart rate monitoring, it was common to perform amniotomy, resorting to operative vaginal delivery after a further 10 minutes if spontaneous delivery was not imminent. These arguments do not apply in modern obstetrics when epidural analgesia and continuous fetal heart rate monitoring is the norm. Early routine recourse to oxytocin to achieve descent of the second twin will result in few women remaining undelivered after 30 minutes. Delay beyond this time is still acceptable provided progress is being made towards successful vaginal delivery, bleeding is minimal, and the cardiotocograph tracing is normal. The observation that 5-minute Apgar scores do not correlate with the time interval between the twin deliveries supports this practice.

In the third stage of labour the risk of atonic primary postpartum haemorrhage is considerably increased with twin delivery. Upon delivery of the second twin the oxytocin infusion should be accelerated and intramuscular syntometrine given. The oxytocin infusion may need to be continued for some time. Following delivery the placenta should be inspected for completeness and to ascertain chorionicity.

Combined delivery

Caesarean section for the second twin after successful vaginal delivery of the first twin used to be an infrequent and unusual occurrence but the incidence steadily increased from 0.33% to 11% over 15 years. This appears to be related to the reducing experience of obstetricians and the increasing rate of caesarean section for twins in many maternity units. In those units with low elective caesarean rates in twins, combined deliveries are infrequent and occur due to unexpected and unfortunate intrapartum events, for example the use of syntocinon in the presence of an undiagnosed transverse lie.

Caesarean section delivery for the second twin is most commonly associated with a vertex presentation of the first twin because it is these cases that are generally allowed to be delivered vaginally until an untoward event complicates the delivery of second twin. The prime reason caesarean delivery of the second twin with the safest configuration (vertex/vertex) is cord prolapse, while inability to perform version and extraction is most common for a vertex/transverse lie with back down. The other reasons for caesarean are fetal distress, abruption, compound vertex presentation and mentoposterior face presentation.

In order to diminish the number of combined deliveries, a preplanned protocol for vaginal twin deliveries should be followed in each unit. Evidence suggests that vaginal delivery of the non-vertex second twin is a safe intrapartum management option, with no evidence of excessive morbidity or mortality associated with total breech extraction of the second twin. Correction of the lie can be attempted either manually or by gentle pressure with the ultrasound transducer to breech or vertex presentation according to the ease and the proximity of the presenting part to the pelvic brim. Breech delivery or extraction of the malpresenting second twin is preferable to external cephalic version because it is associated with a significantly lower incidence of fetal distress and abdominal delivery with comparable neonatal outcome (Suzuki et al 2000). In the even of unsuccessful version, internal podalic version followed by breech extraction is safe in skilled hands, particularly in presence of intact membranes.

Special considerations

Caesarean section for preterm labour with a non-vertex second twin remains controversial for the fetus with an estimated fetal weight of under 1500 g. The largest modern series of 416 pairs from deliveries between 1985 and 1990 do not support caesarean for non-vertex second twins weighing over 500 g and suggest that applicability of external cephalic version or breech extraction is safe (Chauhan et al 1995).

The management of women with multiple pregnancies with previous caesarean section is also controversial. A retrospective study of 210 twin gestations with previous caesarean deliveries (39 with two previous operations) suggest that there is 70% chance of successful vaginal delivery of both twins with a 14% risk of having to deliver the second twin by caesarean section. This policy was not associated with uterine rupture in this series. Vaginal delivery reduced overall maternal morbidity and hospital stay. These figures are in keeping with those expected for singletons delivering vaginally after caesarean section and indicate that a trial of scar is suitable for women with twins (Miller et al 1996). Trial of scar is usually restricted to those women with a first twin with a cephalic presentation. The use of judicious external or internal manipulations is not contraindicated for the second twin.

The management of a pregnancy in which one fetus has died *in utero* includes delivery after 34 weeks, once lung maturity is documented. The method of delivery is usually determined by other obstetric indications, and also if the presenting fetus is the dead twin.

Locked twins represents a potentially catastrophic intrapartum situation and occurs when the after-coming head of the first twin, presenting by the breech, is prevented from entering the pelvis by the presenting head of the second twin. Occurrence of locked twins is more common in monoamniotic twin pregnancies, and in preterm twins where the amniotic sac of the second twin has ruptured. Usually the diagnosis is made in the second stage of labour. In these circumstances manually pushing the head of the second twin out of the maternal pelvis, thereby allowing the after-coming head of the first twin to enter the pelvis and be delivered by the Mauriceau–Smellie–Veit procedure or by forceps extraction is usually the only course of action. Thereafter, the second twin can be delivered normally or with the assistance of forceps. Alternatively the Zavanelli manoeuvre may be applied to return the first infant into the vagina, and both twins can be safely delivered by emergency caesarean section. Alternatively, where the Zavanelli manoeuvre is not feasible or has failed, an emergency caesarean section to unlock the heads of the twin by open manipulation followed by delivery of the second twin from the uterine incision can be considered. The head of the first twin then can be pushed into the vaginal canal to allow successful vaginal delivery. In the rare instance where the first twin dies of asphyxia, decapitation of this fetus would allow its body to be delivered vaginally, followed by delivery of the living second twin and lastly retrieval of the head of the first twin. However, most obstetricians have no experience of decapitation and it might be safer for the mother under these circumstances if caesarean section is performed.

In quadruplets and higher-order multiples the prevailing management option is routine caesarean section. This practice is based on sporadic case reports and the absence of large series concerning the preferred route of delivery.

In triplet pregnancy the preferred route of delivery in most centres is by planned caesarean section as it allows the relevant neonatal staff and equipment to be gathered and obviates the difficulties associated with intrapartum surveillance. However, studies suggest that vaginal delivery can be contemplated if the following criteria are fulfilled:

- non contracted pelvis;
- cephalic presentation of the first triplet;
- unscarred uterus;
- onset of labour at >32 weeks;
- no triplet with fetal compromise or severe growth restriction.

Neonatal outcome in terms of Apgar scores and stay in special care unit are better in the vaginally delivered than the caesarean section group. Similarly, duration of maternal hospital stay and requirement of blood transfusion are shorter in those delivered vaginally. Nevertheless, adequate neonatal resuscitation facilities and the presence of an obstetrician experienced in performing intrauterine manoeuvres at delivery is an essential prerequisite (Dommergues et al 1998).

NEONATAL CARE AND SUPPORT

Twins and higher-order multiples have increased neonatal morbidity, mainly as a result of prematurity, growth restriction and monochorionicity. Severe birth asphyxia related to delay in delivery of the second twin is now less common with the use of fetal monitoring. With the exception of complications related to monochorionicity, most neonatal problems encountered in twins also occur in singletons and their management is essentially similar. Major neonatal complications of prematurity such as intracranial haemorrhage, retinopathy of prematurity, persistent ductus arteriosus, necrotising enterocolitis or chronic lung disease are more common in twins, because gestational age at birth is shorter. Data from the Mersey regional neonatal unit suggest that, compared at each week of gestational age, there are no significant differences in the incidence of neonatal complications in twins and singletons. However, below 28 weeks' gestation, singletons had better survival rates than twins (odds ratio 0.49).

Monochorionic twins, in addition, can encounter neonatal problems due to chronic twin–twin transfusion syndrome, malformations and damage to surviving twins from the death of a cotwin. The recipient twin is at a greater risk and may have respiratory distress related to their high haematocrit, high serum protein and increased blood viscosity. Pronounced hyperbilirubinaemia may also occur on the second and third days. Venous thrombosis with cerebral or gut infarction is more likely in the recipient than the donor twin.

SUPPORT FOR PARENTS

The support for parents is perhaps the most challenging aspect of the management of multiple births, which often results in premature or abnormal birth. Parents often need specific information and support to help them prepare for caring for their babies. Prenatal preparation should be started early in pregnancy and should encompass discussion regarding mode of delivery, premature birth, higher chance of being admitted to the neonatal unit, increased risk of complications (particularly in monochorionic conception), requirement for frequent monitoring and possible admission to hospital. Parents of twins need special understanding and support, particularly if the babies are in a neonatal unit. These problems become more acute when one infant is dying or has a major morbidity.

Experienced parents of twins are one of the best sources of support and advice for others in a similar situation. Joining a local twin club offers many opportunities and support to families. Greater professional awareness of the needs of multiple-birth families should allow individual children to reach their full potential and parents and children alike to enjoy their very special relationships to the full.

CONCLUSIONS

Multiple pregnancies are at higher risk of perinatal mortality and morbidity. Despite this challenge, the care of women with multiple pregnancies has not been met with the same commitment as for, say, women with diabetes during pregnancy. In keeping with the Royal College of Obstetricians and Gynaecologists' Study Group recommendations, women with multiple pregnancies should, ideally, receive antenatal care in special twin clinics to meet their special needs. The multidisciplinary team should be led by an obstetrician and should include midwives, ultrasonographers, neonatologists, social workers and anaesthetists. Such a service would provide a structured plan that will enable early detection, appropriate management and effective use of the resources for the antenatal, intrapartum and postnatal needs of the parents. The twin clinic would focus on education about prevention of preterm birth, intensive maternal surveillance and, more importantly, the provision of a consistent care provider— some feel that this could reduce the frequency of very-low-birthweight deliveries due to preterm labour and associated perinatal mortality (Ellings et al 1993). Twin clinics can also provide a base for what has been an under-researched aspect of obstetrics.

REFERENCES

Bajoria R 1998a Vascular anatomy of monochorionic placenta in relation to discordant growth and amniotic fluid volume. Hum Reprod 13:2933–2940

Bajoria R 1998b Abundant vascular anastomoses in monoamniotic compared to diamniotic monochorial placentae: a controlled study. Am J Obstet Gynecol 179:788–793

Bajoria R 1998c Chorionic plate vascular anatomy determines the efficacy of amnioreduction in twin-twin transfusion syndrome. Hum Reprod 13:1709–1713

Bajoria R, Kingdom JCP 1997 A case for routine determination of chorionicity in multiple pregnancy. Prenat Diagn 17:1207–1225

Bajoria R, Wigglesworth J, Fisk NM 1995 Angioarchitecture of monochorionic placentas in relation to the twin-twin transfusion syndrome. Am J Obstet Gynecol 172:856–863

Bajoria R, Sullivan M, Fisk NM 1999a Endothelin in association with cardiac dysfunction in the recipient fetus of twin–twin transfusion syndrome. Hum Reprod 14:1614–1618

Bajoria R, Wee LY, Anwer S, Ward S 1999b Outcome of twin pregnancies complicated by single intrauterine death in relation to vascular anatomy of the monochorionic placenta. Hum Reprod 14:2124–2130

Bajoria R, Hancock M, Ward B, D'Souza SW, Sooranna SR 2000 Discordant amino acid profiles in monochorionic twins with twin-twin transfusion syndrome. Pediatr Res, 16:567–573

Bajoria R, Gibson MJ, Ward S, Sooranna SR, Neilson JP, Westwood M 2001 Placental regulation of IGF axis in monochorionic twins with chronic twin-twin transfusion syndrome. J Clin Endocrinol Metabol, 86:3150–3156

Benirschke K, Kaufmann P 1995 Multiple pregnancy. In: Pathology of the human placenta, 2nd edn. Springer-Verlag, New York

Brassard M, Fouron JC, Leduc L, Grignon A, Proulx F 1999 Prognostic markers in twin pregnancies with an acardiac fetus. Obstet Gynecol 94:409–414

Burn J 1995 The spectrum of genetic disorders in twins. In: Ward RH, Whittle M (eds). Multiple pregnancy. RCOG Press, London, pp 74–83

Campbell DM, MacGillivray I 1999 Preeclampsia in twin pregnancies: incidence and outcome. Hypertens Pregnancy 18:197–207

Chasen ST, Madden A, Chervenak FA 1999 Cesarean delivery of twins and neonatal respiratory disorders. Am J Obstet Gynecol 181:1052–1056

Chauhan SP, Roberts WE, McLaren RA, Roach-H, Morrison JC, Martin JN Jr 1995 Delivery of the nonvertex second twin: breech extraction versus external cephalic version. Am J Obstet Gynecol 173:1015–1020

Crowther CA, Neilson JP, Verkuyl DAA, Bannerman C, Ashurst HM 1989 Preterm labour in twin pregnancies: can it be prevented by hospital admission? Br J Obstet Gynaecol 96:850–853

Danskin FH, Neilson JP 1989 The twin to twin transfusion syndrome: What are suitable diagnostic criteria? Am J Obstet Gynecol 161:365–369

Deprest JA, Audibert F, Van Schoubroeck D, Hecher K, Mahieu-Caputo D 2000 Bipolar coagulation of the umbilical cord in complicated monochorionic twin pregnancy. Am J Obstet Gynecol 182:340–345

Dommergues M, Mahieu-Caputo D, Dumez Y 1998 Is the route of delivery a meaningful issue in triplets and higher order multiples? Clin Obstet Gynecol 41:24–29

Dubecq F, Dufour P, Vinatier D et al 1996 Monoamniotic twin pregnancies. Review of the literature, and a case report with vaginal delivery. Eur J Obstet Gynecol Reprod Biol 66:183–186

Edwards MS, Ellings JM, Newman RB, Menard MK 1995 Predictive value of antepartum ultrasound examination for anomalies in twin gestations. Ultrasound Obstet Gynecol 6:43–49

Ellings JM, Newman RB, Hulsey TC, Bivins HA Jr, Keenan A 1993 Reduction in very low birth weight deliveries and perinatal mortality in a specialized, multidisciplinary twin clinic. Obstet Gynecol 81:387–391

Evans MI, Hume RF Jr, Yaron Y, Kramer RL, Johnson MP 1998 Multifetal pregnancy reduction. Baillières Clin Obstet Gynaecol 12:147–159

Evans MI, Goldberg JD, Horenstein J et al 1999 Selective termination for structural, chromosomal, and mendelian anomalies: international experience. Am J Obstet Gynecol 181:893–897

Giles WB, Trudinger BJ, Cook CM, Connelly A 1988 Umbilical artery flow velocity waveforms and twin pregnancy outcome. Obstet Gynecol 72:894–897

Glinianaia SV, Pharoah P, Sturgiss SN 2000 Comparative trends in cause-specific fetal and neonatal mortality in twin and singleton births in the North of England, 1982–1994. Br J Obstet Gynaecol 107:452–460

Grobman WA, Parilla BV 1999 Positive predictive value of suspected growth aberration in twin gestations. Am J Obstet Gynecol 181:1139–1141

Hollenbach KA, Hickok DE 1990 Epidemiology and diagnosis of twin gestation. Clin Obstet Gynecol 33:3–9

Houlihan C, Knuppel RA 1996 Intrapartum management of multiple gestations. Clin Perinatol 23:91–116

Kaufman GE, Malone FD, Harvey-Wilkes KB, Chelmow D, Penzias AS,

D'Alton ME 1998 Neonatal morbidity and mortality associated with triplet pregnancy. Obstet Gynecol 91:342–348

Kingdom JCP, Bajoria R 1998 In: Bonnar J (ed) Recent advances in obstetrics and Gynaecology. Churchill Livingstone, Edinburgh, Gynaecol 103:999–1003

Landy HJ, Keith LG 1998 The vanishing twin: a review. Hum Reprod Update 4:177–183

Malone FD, Kaufman GE, Chelmow D, Athanassiou A, Nores JA, D'Alton ME 1999 Maternal morbidity associated with triplet pregnancy. Am J Perinatol 15:73–77

Matijevic R, Bajoria R 2000 Non-invasive method of evaluation of trophoblast invasion of spiral arteries in monochorionic placenta with twin-twin transfusion. J Soc Gyn Invest 7:7A

Miller DA, Mullin P, Hou D, Paul RH 1996 Vaginal birth after cesarean section in twin gestation. Am J Obstet Gynecol 175:194–198

Neilson JP 1981 Detection of the small-for-dates twin fetus by ultrasound. Br J Obstet Gynaecol 88:27–32

Neilson JP 1992 Prenatal diagnosis in multiple pregnancy. Curr Opin Obstet Gynecol 4:280–285

Neilson JP 2000 Routine ultrasound in early pregnancy < 24 weeks. (Cochrane review) In: The Cochrane Library, Issue 2. Update Software, Oxford

Neilson JP, Crowther CA 1993 Preterm labour in multiple pregnancies. Fetal Maternal Med Rev 5:105–119

Neilson JP, Verkuyl DAA, Crowther CA, Bannerman C 1998a Preterm labor in twin pregnancies: prediction by cervical assessment. Obstet Gynecol 72:719–723

Neilson JP, Verkuyl DAA, Bannerman C 1988b Tape measurement of symphysis-fundal height in twin pregnancies. Br J Obstet Gynaecol 95:1054–1059

Petterson B, Nelson KB, Watson L, Stanley F 1993 Twins, triplets, and cerebral palsy in births in Western Australia in the 1980s. BMJ 307:1239–1243

Pharoah PO, Adi Y 2000 Consequences of in-utero death in a twin pregnancy. Lancet 355:1597–1602

Pharoah PO, Cooke RW 1997 A hypothesis for the aetiology of spastic cerebral palsy—the vanishing twin. Dev Med Child Neurol 39:292–296

Saade GR, Belfort MA, Berry DL et al 1998 Amniotic septostomy for the treatment of twin oligohydramnios–polyhydramnios sequence. Fetal Diagn Ther 13:86–93

Sebir NJ, Snijders RJM, Hughes K, Sepulveda W, Nicolaides KH 1996 Screening for trisomy 21 in twin pregnancies by maternal age and nuchal translucency thickness at 10–14 weeks of gestation. Br J Obstet Gynaecol 103:999–1003

Sebire NJ, Souka A, Skentou H, Geerts L, Nicolaides KH 2000 Early prediction of severe twin-to-twin transfusion syndrome. Hum Reprod 15:2008–2010

Souka AP, Heath V, Flint S, Sevastopoulou I, Nicolaides KH 1999 Cervical length at 23 weeks in twins in predicting spontaneous preterm delivery. Obstet Gynecol 94:450–454

Stewart AL 1995 Does the infant neurodevelopment of multiple births differ from singleton? In: Ward RH, Whittle M (eds) Multiple pregnancy. RCOG press, London, pp 297–308

Suzuki S, Otsubo Y, Sawa R, Yoneyama Y, Araki T 2000 Clinical trial of induction of labor versus expectant management in twin pregnancy. Gynecol Obstet Invest 49:24–27

Talbert D, Bajoria R, Sepulveda W, Bower S, Fisk N 1996 Hydrostatic and osmotic pressure gradients produce manifestations of fetofetal transfusion syndrome in a computerised model of monochorial twin pregnancy. Am J Obstet Gynecol 174:598–608

West CR, Adi Y, Pharoah PO 1999 Fetal and infant death in mono- and dizygotic twins in England and Wales 1982–91. Arch Dis Child Fetal Neonatal Edn 80:F217–220

Zosmer N, Bajoria R, Weiner E, Rigby M, Vaughan J, Fisk NM 1994 Clinical and echographic features of in utero cardiac dysfunction in the recipient twin in twin-twin transfusion syndrome. Br Heart J 72:74–79

16

Alloimmunisation in pregnancy: rhesus and other red cell antigens

Charles H. Rodeck, Anna P. Cockell

The contribution of the author of the equivalent chapter in the second edition, on which this chapter draws extensively, is gratefully acknowledged.

INTRODUCTION

Severe haemolytic disease of the fetus and newborn (HDFN) is now a relatively rare event in modern obstetric practice. It occurs as a result of paternally derived red-blood cell (RBC) antigens, which the mother lacks, presenting on fetal RBCs. Alloimmunisation by the Rhesus (D) (Rh(D)) antigen remains the most prevalent cause of HDFN, but its incidence has dramatically fallen over the last 30 years with the introduction of anti-D immunoglobulin (IgG) prophylaxis, use of which began in 1969 and reduced the perinatal deaths associated from this disorder from 460 per million before 1969 to 16 per million in 1990 (Mollison et al 1997). There is consequently an increasing proportion of alloimmunised pregnancies attributable to rhesus antigens other than D (in particular c and E) and non-rhesus antigens such as Kell, Duffy and Kidd. Management of affected pregnancies is now focused in regional units where the level of expertise in non-invasive and invasive care is maintained. Management has improved as our understanding of the pathophysiology of RBC alloimmunisation has been increased by the development of molecular techniques for fetal genotyping and by better ultrasound technology that has enabled safer non-invasive and invasive management. Simultaneously, significant advances have been made in neonatal care, thus facilitating earlier safe delivery of the affected fetus.

HISTORICAL BACKGROUND

The first description of the birth of a hydropic fetus has been attributed to Hippocrates in about 400 BC. It was Jakesch in Prague in 1878 who reported the birth of a stillborn hydropic baby with marked splenomegaly, yellow amniotic fluid and placental oedema. On microscopy there was 'a leukaemic diathesis and corresponding findings in the spleen and liver' later shown to be extramedullary haemopoiesis. The term 'erythroblastosis fetalis', characterised by the triad of hydrops fetalis, icterus gravis and severe anaemia of the newborn (Diamond et al 1932), is used to describe the typical features of what we now know to be due to alloimmunisation.

The basic aetiology of red-cell alloimmunisation in erythroblastosis fetalis was unravelled during the late 1930s. Levine & Stetson (1939) reported a severe transfusion reaction in a woman following stillbirth and leading to the development of antibodies in her blood, which agglutinated RBCs from her husband and from most of a large number of blood group O subjects. They suggested that the mother was immunised to a fetal antigen from her husband. Landsteiner & Wiener (1940) then identified an antigen present in blood from rhesus monkeys which stimulated the production of an antibody when injected into rabbits. Once a rabbit was sensitised, the rabbit serum containing rhesus antibodies was found to agglutinate human blood in about 80% of cases (i.e. about 80% of humans are Rh-positive). Levine et al (1941) provided the final serological proof that erythroblastosis fetalis is due to maternal rhesus immunisation by demonstrating that the father of the stillborn baby reported in 1939 was Rh-positive and the mother Rh-negative. It remained to be proved that fetal red cells could cross the placental barrier into the mother's circulation.

As early as 1932 it was noted that erythroblastosis fetalis did not occur in Rh(D)-positive fetuses born to Rh(D)-negative mothers when the ABO blood group differed in mother and fetus. This suggested a protective affect of ABO incompatibility in these pregnancies (Mollison et al 1997). It was this that led Finn (1960) to reason that nature might be mimicked effectively by injecting anti-D antibodies, to give a temporary passive immunity to mothers that would neutralise the D-positive red cells entering her circulation before they could induce a lasting active immunisation. Following a series of investigations in Liverpool and New York, experimental studies of Rh(D) immunoprophylaxis in male volunteers (Finn et al 1961) led to the demonstration that anti-D IgG could prevent immunisation of RhD-negative women after delivery. Since then, there has been ample evidence that when anti-D IgG is given within 72 hours after delivery by intramuscular injection, immunisation of the mother is prevented if she has not already been sensitised.

PATHOPHYSIOLOGY

Red blood cell membranes have surface antigens in a combination specific to each individual. The various antigens are of differing potency in their ability to stimulate an antibody response when presented to an individual recognising them as non-self. In practice it is the ABO, Rhesus and Kell groups that should be considered as the antigens most likely to cause moderate to severe HDFN. About 75% of pregnant women have fetal RBCs circulating at some time during their pregnancy and delivery, thus stimulating the maternal immune response. This maternal response is the production of RBC antigen-specific antibodies. After a latent period of some weeks, the initial exposure to fetal (non-self) RBC antigens causes a primary IgM response. IgM does not cross the placenta and therefore cannot cause HDFN. On subsequent exposure of the mother to the antigen, as in her second pregnancy, her previously primed B cells act swiftly to produce IgG. With only a small exposure to fetal antigen substantial amounts of maternal IgG are produced and are actively transported across the placenta to the fetal circulation. Maternal IgG binds to the antigen expressed on the fetal RBCs, causing sequestration and destruction of these cells. Transfer of maternal IgG across the placenta does not appear to be clinically significant until the second trimester. Before this, despite very high levels of maternal IgG, the risk of severe fetal haemolysis is small; we have never seen a hydropic fetus or an intrauterine death before 16–17 weeks' gestation.

Rhesus blood group system

The rhesus blood group antigens constitute at least three very similar transmembrane proteins: D, C and E. Two of the transmembrane proteins have an immunologically distinct isoform (C or c and E or e). There is no evidence that an isoform of the major rhesus antigen D exists (d). A woman's rhesus genotype is inherited following Mendelian principles and the individual is either homozygous or heterozygous for each antigen represented in the genotype. The parental genotype is therefore described as, for example, CDe/cde, one set being inherited from each parent, with d indicating the absence of the Rh(D) antigen. This nomenclature was adopted by Fisher and Race in 1946 and has been universally accepted, replacing previous systems due to its distinctive symbols and logical pairs of alleles. The Rh(D) and Rh(CE) proteins are coded for by the *RH* gene (encompassing *RHD* and *RHCE*) at chromosome 1p34–36 (Cherif-Zahar et al 1991). *RHD* codes for the Rh30 protein carrying the Rh(D) antigen and *RHCE* codes for Rh30 polypeptides coexpressing the Ce, ce and cE antigens. Both genes comprise 10 exons of 69kb of DNA. They are expressed in the erythrocyte envelope before the red cell loses its nucleus.

There are at least 40 rhesus antigens other than D, C and E, but the Rh(D) epitophe is the most immunogenic, followed by Rh(c) which is 20 times less potent. The order of immunogenicity of the most potent antigens of the rhesus system is D > c > E > e > C. Certain antigen combinations are more prevalent and these vary between different ethnic groups.

- In White European populations CDe, cde and cDE are the most common (in decreasing frequency).
- The cDe combination is the most common genotype in Black Afro-Caribbeans though it is very unusual in White Europeans.
- About 15% of White Europeans are homozygous Rh(D) negative, 7–8% of Black Afro-Caribbeans and only 1% of Chinese and Japanese ethnic groups.
- 56% of Rh(D) positive White Europeans are heterozygous for the Rh(D) antigen and therefore there is only an approximately 50% chance of an Rh(D)-positive offspring

when a woman is Rh(D) negative (the male may be Rh(D) negative, and even when positive, in 56% of cases has only a 50% chance of contributing the gene for Rh(D) positivity).

Other RBC antigens

There are numerous antigens on the surface of RBCs other than the rhesus system. Antigens that are particularly immunogenic, though causing less severe HDFN than that from the Rh antigens, include Kell, Fy^a (Duffy) and Kidd (Jk^a, Jk^b). Maternal antibody production to these antigens can usually be attributed to a prior blood transfusion. In some cases a number of different antibodies can occur simultaneously and in combination with Rh(D). When a maternal antibody is detected its clinical significance must be evaluated in liaison with the Regional Blood Transfusion Centre in the UK. For example, the presence of anti-Fy^a (Duffy), which rarely causes more than mild HDFN, would suggest the induction of slightly early delivery (38 weeks' gestation) rather than invasive testing.

About 90% of the Caucasian population are Kell-negative. Maternal anti-Kell antibodies most frequently occur following transfusion of Kell-positive blood to a Kell-negative woman. Anti-Kell antibodies can cause severe HDFN. It has been suggested that Kell alloimmunisation causes fetal anaemia by antibody-induced erythroid suppression rather than direct fetal RBC haemolysis as in other causes of alloimmunisation (Vaughan et al 1995). In Kell-induced fetal anaemia, the amniotic fluid bilirubin concentration correlates poorly with fetal haematocrit, which would be consistent with reduced erythroblastosis rather than RBC breakdown. Amniocentesis to assess haemolysis is therefore not helpful in determining the severity of HDFN in Kell disease. In the management of these patients the paternal genotype should be obtained and if the father is Kell negative the fetus is not at risk, even if maternal Kell antibodies are very raised. If the father is Kell positive, he is likely to be heterozygous as only 3% of people are homozygous Kell positive, so the fetus may still be Kell negative. Early fetal genotyping is advisable (see below) so that plans can be made regarding the degree of prenatal surveillance that will be required.

Some women form IgG antibodies and not the typical IgM antibodies to the ABO blood group antigens. Anti-A and B IgG are capable of crossing the placenta. Fortunately these antigens are poorly expressed on fetal RBCs in utero and therefore maternal IgG to ABO RBC antigens is unlikely to cause severe disease. In this situation there is probably no advantage to early delivery but the neonate requires close observation and early resort to phototherapy if indicated. A second pregnancy is not always affected.

DEVELOPMENT OF RHESUS (D) ANTIBODIES

About 75% of pregnant women have fetal RBCs circulating at some time during pregnancy and delivery. However, transplacental fetomaternal haemorrhage from a Rh(D)-positive fetus to a Rh(D)-negative mother does not always lead to alloimmunisation. The maternal response to circulating fetal RBC depends on several factors.

- Maternal inborn responsiveness: about one-third of women are unresponsive to the stimulus.
- Strength of the antigenic stimulus. Rh(D) is the most potent Rh antigen, especially when CDe/cde is the fetal genotype.
- The volume of fetomaternal haemorrhage (Whitfield 1976).
- ABO blood group compatibility of mother and fetus.

ABO incompatibility between mother and fetus provides substantial protection against Rh(D) immunisation. A mother with blood group O carrying a group A or B fetus reduces her incidence of Rh(D)-induced HDFN to about one-tenth of that when there is ABO compatibility (Levine 1958). When ABO-incompatible fetal RBCs enter the mother's bloodstream, they quickly combine with her naturally occurring anti-A and/or anti-B agglutinins and are neutralised by sequestration in her liver. In contrast, ABO-compatible fetal RBC will persist in the maternal circulation for their normal lifespan, facilitating stimulation of the maternal immune response. Only about 1% of Rh(D)-negative mothers will have detectable Rh(D) antibodies before delivery of their first Rh(D)-positive baby. When antibodies become detectable during or shortly after her first Rh(D)-positive pregnancy, the mother is probably a strong responder and her next Rh(D)-positive pregnancy may become severely affected. Presumably, primary immunisation will occur before birth in the same proportion (1%) during each subsequent Rh(D)-positive pregnancy. As most fetomaternal haemorrhages occur during labour, immunisation is more likely to occur after birth, and antibodies can be detected in about 8% of at-risk mothers 6 months after delivery.

Once a woman has developed Rh(D) antibodies, even if they have declined below the sensitivity of laboratory tests, they will almost always become detectable from an early stage in a further pregnancy, especially when the pregnancy is again Rh(D) positive, but sometimes even if it is Rh(D) negative. By the end of the second Rh(D)-positive pregnancy, in the absence of anti-D prophylaxis, 17% of Rh(D)-negative mothers will have detectable antibodies, most of which will have resulted from primary immunisation in the first pregnancy (Mollison et al 1997).

FETAL AND NEONATAL EFFECTS OF RED BLOOD CELL ALLOIMMUNISATION

Maternal IgG antibodies to fetal RBC antigens cross the placenta and attach to the fetal RBCs. This causes early destruction of RBC by the reticuloendothelial system and an abnormally high level of bilirubin is present in the fetal circulation. The rate of haemolysis is dependent on the amount of IgG entering the fetal circulation and the ability of the fetal reticuloendothelial system to remove antibody-coated RBCs. The rapidity and severity of fetal anaemia is then dependent on compensatory fetal erythropoiesis in bone marrow, spleen and liver. In the most severely affected cases the fetal liver and spleen enlarge and may even reach the iliac crests. There may also be a compensatory placental hyperplasia to increase oxygen transfer. Immature nucleated erythroblasts are present in the circulation as a result of the extramedullary erythropoiesis. Increased haemopoiesis cannot always compensate for the excessive destruction of RBCs and anaemia ensues. Before birth the fetal bilirubin is cleared through the placenta into the mother's circulation but some reaches the amniotic fluid, where it provides a useful marker of the severity of RBC breakdown (see below).

In an affected fetus the anaemia may be so severe that there is tissue hypoxia and acidosis, circulatory failure with generalised oedema including scalp oedema, ascites and often pleural and pericardial effusions. These are the features of hydrops fetalis and are the cardinal signs of fetal anaemia on sonographic assessment. Initially, to maintain tissue oxygenation, cardiac output rather than heart rate is increased as a consequence of the fall in peripheral resistance and decreased blood viscosity (Huikeshoven et al 1988). The pathophysiology of fetal hydrops in RBC alloimmunisation has yet to be fully elucidated but various mechanisms have been proposed (Rodeck and Deans (1999). These include hypoproteinaemia from protein loss into the body cavity spaces, infiltration of the liver by erythropoietic tissue disturbing liver function and compression of the portal and umbilical veins by hepatic infiltrate. In normal fetal development the haemoglobin concentration rises with gestational age and therefore hydrops tends to occur at higher fetal haemoglobin levels later in pregnancy than in early gestation (Nicolaides et al 1988b). Critical anaemia can therefore be defined only by reference to the gestation-dependent haemoglobin levels but is usually a deficit if more than 7 g/dl.

Following birth, bilirubin is no longer being cleared across the placenta into the mother's circulation so jaundice develops rapidly and the anaemia increases. Some of these babies require prolonged assisted ventilation, parenteral nutrition and other intensive neonatal support. They are also prone to serious complications such as disseminated intravascular coagulation, severe thrombocytopenia, necrotising enterocolitis and bronchopulmonary dysplasia. At birth the baby will need a blood transfusion. Rh(D)-negative blood is used until maternal anti-Rh(D) IgG falls to a minimal level. A particular risk for the baby is kernicterus, a permanently crippling disorder caused by high levels of unconjugated bilirubin crossing the blood–brain barrier and damaging the basal ganglia. This occurs when fetal unconjugated bilirubin levels reach above 310 μmol/l; preterm infants are more susceptible and therefore levels requiring urgent treatment are gestation dependent. Neonatal prevention of kernicterus includes adequate hydration, phototherapy and/or exchange transfusion.

PREVENTION OF RHESUS (D) ALLOIMMUNISATION

The train of events leading to and resulting from RBC alloimmunisation is similar whichever antigen/antibody is involved, and is initiated by entry into the maternal circulation of erythrocytes carrying an antigen which the mother lacks. It is now extremely rare for this to follow a Rh(D)-incompatible blood transfusion, but it still can occur from transfusion of blood containing one of the rhesus antigens other than D, or more frequently a non-rhesus antigen such as Kell. Alloimmunisation of a Rh(D)-negative woman is therefore usually as a result of fetomaternal haemorrhage in the presence of a Rh(D)-positive fetus in the antenatal or peripartum period.

As the Rh(D) antigen is the most immunogenic antigen of the rhesus system and therefore the most clinically significant of all the other relevant antigens, the reduction of fetal disease attributable to this antigen was very important. The work of Clarke and Finn on anti-D prophylaxis in the early 1960s (Finn 1960, Finn et al 1961) has allowed a significant reduction in the incidence of severe Rh(D) alloimmunisation to be achieved (see above). Without a programme of anti-D prophylaxis, approximately 1% of Rh(D)-negative women will have detectable anti-D in their serum by the end of their first pregnancy with a Rh(D)-positive fetus. A further 7–9% of these women will develop antibodies in the 6 months following delivery, and roughly the same number again will develop antibodies during a second Rh(D)-positive pregnancy. Thus around 17% of Rh(D)-negative women are immunised by a single Rh(D)-positive pregnancy (1). Maternal administration of anti-D IgG at the time of, or shortly after, fetomaternal haemorrhage has been shown to reduce the likelihood of alloimmunisation. The amount of anti-D administered must be calculated in accordance with the estimated volume of circulating fetal RBCs in the maternal circulation.

Evaluating fetomaternal haemorrhage

The frequency of fetomaternal haemorrhage became well recognised when the Kleihauer–Betke test came into general use after 1957 (Kleihauer et al 1957). Following acid or alkaline denaturation of a maternal blood sample, maternal RBCs appear 'ghost like' as the adult haemoglobin has been eluted out leaving only the RBC membrane. Fetal haemoglobin is more resistant to elution, and therefore fetal RBCs maintain their colour. By counting the number of filled cells per unit volume before and after elution, the amount of fetomaternal haemorrhage can be approximated.

Woodrow and Finn (1966) extensively studied fetomaternal haemorrhage using the Kleihauer acid elution test in their work to prevent Rh(D) alloimmunisation. They found that fetal RBCs were present in the blood of about 3% of women during the third trimester and half of these women demonstrated at least 0.2–0.25 ml of circulating fetal blood, certainly sufficient to cause alloimmunisation. They also showed that after delivery more than 50% of mothers had fetal RBCs in their blood. This was equivalent to more than 0.2 ml of fetomaternal haemorrhage in 18% of women when there was ABO compatibility between mother and baby. Conversely, when there was ABO incompatibility, only 1.9% of women had significant numbers of circulating fetal RBCs.

Quantitative assessment of fetal cells in the maternal circulation following fetomaternal haemorrhage may be more accurately determined by tests other than the Kleihauer acid elution test. These tests include immunofluorescence differentiating Rh(D)-positive from Rh(D)-negative RBCs and flow cytometry. Regional blood centres (reference laboratories) offer the latter specialised technique. In most units in the UK Rh(D)-negative women who have delivered a Rh(D)-positive baby are assessed by a Kleihauer acid elution test. If this estimates a fetomaternal haemorrhage greater than 4 ml of fetal RBCs or an equivocal result, a maternal sample is sent to the regional reference laboratory for confirmation by flow cytometry. The clinician is then advised about the appropriate dose of anti-D IgG for the mother.

Tests to estimate the size of potential fetomaternal haemorrhage are recommended following delivery in many, but not all, countries. This is usually performed by the Kleihauer acid elution test, as in the UK and Canada, or by more specific tests, as in the USA. Some countries routinely administer 1000–1500 IU of anti-D without quantifying the size of haemorrhage and so therefore will potentially under-treat the 0.3% of women with a haemorrhage greater than 15 ml. This highlights the necessity for assessing potential fetomaternal haemorrhage, as advised by the recent Royal College of Obstetricians and Gynaecologists (RCOG) guidelines (RCOG 1999).

Fetomaternal haemorrhage is most common at the time of delivery, when placental separation occurs. Particular care should be taken to minimise the risk of maternal alloimmunisation in a Rh(D)-negative woman in the following circumstances:

- Caesarean delivery
- Instrumental delivery
- Stillbirth
- Abdominal trauma
- Multiple pregnancies (at delivery)
- Unexplained hydrops fetalis
- Manual removal of placenta

For example, following a caesarean birth, meticulous attention to remove blood from the mother's peritoneal cavity will reduce the amount of fetal RBCs absorbed into the maternal circulation.

Anti-D immunoglobulin preparations and administration

In the UK, until 1994 anti-D IgG was provided solely from the immune plasma of volunteers. With the increasing awareness of infection from blood products it is appropriate that before administration women are aware that anti-D poses a theoretical risk of hepatitis, other viral illnesses or new-variant Creutzfeld–Jakob Disease (CJD). In the case of CJD the risk is currently considered to be posed only by UK plasma and so, at the time of going to press, plasma from the USA is currently being used in preference. This has required the licensing of imported anti-D IgE. Anti-D is an intramuscular preparation (250–5000 IU), best administered in the deltoid muscle rather than the gluteus as injection into the latter may reach only the subcutaneous tissues, thus delaying absorption.

Since 1976, the UK guidelines on rhesus immunoprophy-laxis have been regularly updated. Despite this, there are still reports of failed implementation and unnecessary maternal alloimmunisation. The RCOG has updated their guidelines on the prevention of sensitisation in women (RCOG 1999) and these are based on the report from a joint working party of the British Blood Transfusion Society and RCOG. The following discussion on immunoprophylaxis is based on this document. Administration of anti-D IgG should be within 72 hours of the potentially sensitising event (Table 16.1), though even a delayed dose (up to 10 days) may provide some benefit. It is currently recommended that for every estimated 4 ml of fetal blood in the maternal circulation 500 IU of anti-D should be given. Thereafter, for each additional 1 ml of fetal RBCs, 125 IU anti-D is advised.

Sensitisation following early pregnancy loss

The RCOG guidelines (1999) recommend that below 24 weeks' gestation anti-D IgG should be given to all Rh(D)-negative women, who have not been sensitised previously, in the following circumstances (see Table 16.1):

- Therapeutic termination of pregnancy: anti-D should be given irrespective of whether medical or surgical methods are used.
- Ectopic pregnancy: anti-D IgG should be given irrespective of whether treated by medical or surgical methods.
- Spontaneous miscarriage: Anti-D IgG should be given if the miscarriage occurs after 12 weeks' gestation. Before 12 weeks, without surgical evacuation of the uterus, the risk of sensitisation is extremely small and therefore a spontaneous complete miscarriage before 12 weeks' gestation does not require immunoprophylaxis.
- Threatened miscarriage: immunoprophylaxis should be given to all Rh(D)-negative women who threaten to miscarry after 12 weeks' gestation. This should be repeated at 6-weekly intervals if bleeding continues. Before 12 weeks' gestation sensitisation is unlikely but immunoprophylaxis

Table 16.1 Indications for anti-D immunoprophylaxis in Rh(D)-negative women

First trimester
- Miscarriage
- Ectopic pregnancy
- Threatened miscarriage
- Surgical termination of pregnancy
- Medical termination of pregnancy
- Chorionic villous sampling

Second trimester
- Amniocentesis
- Chorionic villous sampling
- Fetal blood sampling
- Antepartum haemorrhage

Third trimester
- Routine prophylaxis
- Antepartum haemorrhage
- External cephalic version
- Delivery

should be considered before 12 weeks if the bleeding is heavy and/or associated with abdominal pain.

A dose of 250 IU anti-D IgG should be given before 20 weeks' gestation and 500 IU thereafter. A test for the size of fetomaternal haemorrhage should be performed (see above) after 20 weeks to establish that adequate anti-D has been given. Appropriate first-trimester and early second-trimester immunoprophylaxis is often complicated by inadequate knowledge of the gestational age of the pregnancy. An ultrasound assessment of crown–pump length determines fetal gestation though ultrasound dating is not always possible if products of conception have already been lost by the time of presentation. The risk of significant fetomaternal haemorrhage and alloimmunisation increases as the pregnancy grows, so the prudent course is to assume and act on the longest plausible gestational age.

Antenatal sensitisation

As sensitisation of Rh(D)-negative women has been associated with asymptomatic fetomaternal haemorrhage, particularly towards term, postnatal administration of anti-D IgG is too late to prevent some cases of sensitisation. It is practical to assume that all Rh(D)-negative pregnant women are at risk of Rh(D) immunisation, irrespective of their partner's rhesus genotype, and these women are considered to be carrying a Rh(D)-positive fetus until the postnatal confirmation of neonatal blood group. This avoids the assumption that the putative father is actually the true biological father, an assumption which is untrue in a significant number of cases. It is now recommended that all previously non-sensitised Rh(D)-negative women (primigravidas and multigravidas) receive two doses of anti-D IgG, one at 28 and a second at 34 weeks' gestation (RCOG 1999). The currently recommended IgG dose is at least 500 IU. A number of studies have shown that, provided sufficient anti-D IgG is administered, adoption of this policy will reduce sensitisation of Rh(D) mothers from 1.5% to 0.2% (Bowman 1988). At 28 weeks, routine RBC antibody testing is performed and anti-D IgG administered. Thereafter maternal serological evidence of sensitisation is difficult to determine as passively acquired anti-D IgG and immune IgG cannot be differentiated. Similarly, passive IgG may still be present after birth and should not prevent the administration of appropriate amounts of anti-D IgG if the baby is Rh(D) positive.

Other antenatal events requiring immunoprophylaxis

Fetomaternal haemorrhage can occur after antenatal invasive procedures such as chorionic villous sampling, amniocentesis or other events such as external cephalic version for breech presentation or after maternal abdominal trauma (Table 16.1). If such procedures are undertaken, a Kheihauer test and injection of an appropriate dose of anti-D should be performed.

Postpartum prophylaxis

At delivery of a baby born to a Rh(D)-negative woman, cord blood is sent to Rh(D) group the fetus (and for haemoglobin and bilirubin levels). Maternal blood is sent for RBC antibodies and the Kleihauer acid elution test to evaluate if there has been a significant fetomaternal haemorrhage. Routine postpartum prophylaxis of 500 IU anti-D IgG within 72 hours is recommended for all previously unimmunised Rh(D)-negative mothers following delivery of a Rh(D)-positive baby, irrespective of parity or ABO grouping. This is also irrespective of the presence of alloantibodies other than anti-Rh(D) (e.g. Kell, anti-c). The recommended dose varies between countries as discussed earlier. However, the MRC dosage trial reported in 1974 showed that 500 IU given intramuscularly, capable of suppressing the sensitisation effect of 4–5 ml of Rh(D)-positive fetal RBCs, is as effective as 1500 IU and 1000 IU.

MANAGEMENT OF RED BLOOD CELL ALLOIMMUNISATION

Aim of management

The aim of management of RBC alloimmunisation is to minimise the number of invasive procedures performed and thus reduce the incidence of iatrogenically elevated antibody levels. This is particularly relevant as a higher proportion of mild to moderately affected pregnancies are being seen since the introduction of routine anti-D prophylaxis. Non-invasive assessment of the fetus is now the mainstay of management of an affected pregnancy; amniocentesis and fetal blood sampling only performed when there is a strong likelihood that the fetus will be anaemic and require an intrauterine transfusion.

Initial screening

The first step in the management of RBC alloimmunisation is to identify all pregnancies at risk. At the first attendance in pregnancy the mother's blood group and Rh(D) status are assessed and a RBC antibody screen performed. Even when antibodies are not found initially screening should be repeated because they may develop later (even in a first pregnancy). Mothers already very weakly immunised may not have detectable antibody levels in the early months. Rh(D)-positive women, and Rh(D)-negative women in whom immunisation has not already been detected, should be screened again at 28 and 34 weeks' gestation (Fig. 16.1).

Regional centres in the UK

Pregnancies complicated by clinically relevant maternal RBC antibodies are managed in regional blood transfusion centres and fetal medicine units. These centres maintain expertise in the diverse clinical presentation of these cases, follow them non-invasively and perform invasive tests or therapy, as the case requires:

- Maternal antibody quantification
- Paternal blood group genotyping
- Fetal blood group genotyping
- Ultrasound assessment

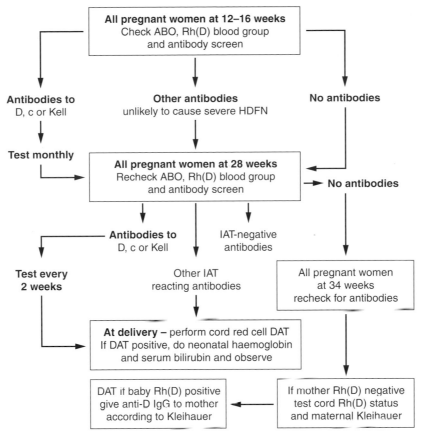

Fig. 16.1 Serological testing during pregnancy. DAT, Direct antiglobulin test; IAT, indirect antiglobulin test. (From British Committee for Standards in Haematology 1996, with permission.)

- Amniotic fluid spectrophotometry
- Fetal blood sampling
- Fetal blood transfusion

As the severely affected fetus is now relatively rare, referral of affected cases to regional units also maintains experience in the management of the affected baby or complications associated with the newborn that have been treated prenatally. Liaison with the obstetrician of the referring hospital can facilitate a shared care approach in most cases, but overall responsibility for further management must lie with the regional unit. In other countries these specialist tests and facilities are likely to be concentrated in the major university hospitals.

Previous obstetric history

When developing a management plan for RBC alloimmunised pregnancies, the previous obstetric history plays an important role. In the first sensitised pregnancy, the risk of fetal anaemia is very low. Following an affected pregnancy the risk to a subsequent fetus increases and may lead to fetal anaemia at an earlier gestation. If hydrops has occurred in a previous pregnancy, then it is likely to occur at an earlier stage in subsequent pregnancies carrying a Rh(D)-incompatible fetus if treatment is not undertaken.

Determining fetal genotype

Before fetal blood sampling (FBS) began in the late 1970s, serial amniocentesis and even serial intraperitoneal transfusion was sometimes performed on fetuses that were thought to be affected by Rh(D) alloimmunisation, and then found to be Rh(D) negative at birth. Fetal genotyping before 20 weeks' gestation rationalises surveillance and minimises invasive tests in at-risk pregnancies. Any invasive test will increase the likelihood of fetomaternal haemorrhage and risk serious aggravation of maternal antibody production. This risk is then carried over to all subsequent Rh(D)-positive fetuses. Fetal genotyping and determination of fetal blood group is now readily performed by molecular techniques on amniocytes or fetal blood, the polymerase chain reaction amplifying minute amounts of fetal DNA (Bennett et al 1993). This technique identifies the rhesus gene locus on chromosome 1 from the nucleated fetal cell, as opposed to investigating the expression of the Rh(D) antigen present on the RBC. As these techniques have developed, FBS or chorionic villous sampling (CVS) to determine fetal genotype has been replaced by amniocentesis with its inherently lower risk of miscarriage and fetomaternal haemorrhage. The potential for CVS to cause fetomaternal haemorrhage and aggravate sensitisation limits its use for determining fetal genotype. It is mainly reserved for couples where the father is heterozygous and there is a very severe history of alloimmunisation, who would opt to terminate a Rh(D)-positive fetus. The most recent development has been the discovery of free fetal DNA in maternal plasma (Lo et al 1998). This may enable fetal genotyping on a maternal blood sample without performing an invasive test.

Serological surveillance

Antibodies are detected in the maternal serum by an initial screening test before specific antibody testing (British Committee for Standards in Haematology 1996). RBC antibodies with a significant IgG component are detectable by the Coombs indirect antiglobulin test (IAT). The antibody (or antibodies) is identified and quantified by titration using IAT in both saline (for IgM) and in albumen (for IgG). If necessary, ultra-sensitive enzyme tests are available.

The management of RBC alloimmunisation is similar regardless of the inciting antigen, with the exception of Kell (which will be discussed later), but for the sake of clarity Rh(D) immunisation will be referred to here. When maternal RBC antibodies have been detected they are quantified. Traditionally quantification has been by a titration method that may be poorly reproducible. This has now been succeeded by an immunoassay measurement in IU/ml for Rh(D) antibodies. For anti-D quantification, samples are paired with previous samples to detect any significant change in level. Although automated immunoassay can be set up for antibodies other than Rh(D), this is not generally available and so these less-potent antibodies must still be quantified by titration. Serial quantification is performed at 2–4 weekly intervals. Once the patient has been reviewed at the regional unit to explain and plan the management, antibody testing can be performed at the referring hospital (Fig. 16.1).

Following the detection of maternal RBC antibodies, the paternal genotype is determined from a venous blood sample to assess if the fetus is at risk (see above). If the father is heterozygous for the relevant RBC antigen, amniocentesis is performed from 15 weeks onwards to genotype the fetus. It may be appropriate to delay amniocentesis until an invasive procedure is indicated to determine if the fetus is anaemic. It is likely that in the future fetal DNA testing from maternal plasma will supersede amniocentesis. This would prevent a pregnancy with a non-susceptible fetus being considered as high risk.

In conjunction with the previous history, the level of maternal antibody, its known antigenicity and its rate of change in level, a management plan for fetal surveillance can be provisionally prepared. For example, in a case where previous babies have not been affected by Rh(D) disease, a maternal anti-D concentration persistently less than 2.5 IU/ml suggests that a non-invasive approach, with delivery at 38 weeks, would be a safe approach (Fig. 16.1). However, if antibody concentrations exceed 10 IU/ml, the fetus may become affected. Antibody levels do not always correlate with fetal disease. A sharp increase—e.g. from below 5 to 20 IU/ml—should always suggest that haemolysis may be occurring in the fetus. This is an indication for immediate fetal surveillance and possibly invasive testing or delivery if gestation allows.

Management of non-Rh(D) RBC alloimmunisation

The management of pregnancies with non-Rh(D) antibodies of clinical significance to the fetus is similar to that of Rh(D) immunisation. The approach therefore includes determination of the paternal genotype, monitoring maternal RBC alloantibodies at regular intervals and identification of possible additional antibodies. Advice from the regional transfusion centre and fetal medicine unit is essential in planning care.

In alloimmunisation other than that attributed to Rh(D) disease, maternal antibody levels may be unreliable indicators of impending HDFN. Even in cases where titres of 1 in 16 for anti-c, anti-E and anti-Kell occur, only 4% of newborns require transfusion, compared with 20% when an equivalent titre is found with Rh(D) antibodies (van Dijk et al 1995). With anti-C levels below 7.5 IU/ml the fetus is unlikely to be seriously affected. Other aspects of non-Rh(D) alloimmunisation surveillance also require careful interpretation. Fetal hydrops has been reported with anti-Kell indirect Coombs titres as low as 1:4 (Bowman et al 1992). In those patients with anti-Kell antibodies, amniotic fluid $\Delta OD450$ values have also been reported to under-predict the severity of HDFN (Vaughan et al 1995)—i.e. to give false-negative results.

Ultrasound

Ultrasound of the fetus is initially used to date the pregnancy accurately in the first trimester. This is critical to the interpretation of gestation-dependent fetal assessments, invasive or non-invasive. Later in gestation, ultrasound is integral to fetal surveillance, for example when the antibody levels have risen or the previous obstetric history is predictive of fetal anaemia. Ultrasound assessment is on a 1–3 weekly basis, as the case dictates (Table 16.2).

The severely anaemic fetus is readily identifiable on scan by the detection of skin oedema, ascites, pleural or pericardial effusions, cardiomegaly and an oedematous placenta. However early detection of mild anaemia would be helpful. Ultrasonographic measurements of placental thickness, extrahepatic umbilical vein diameters, abdominal circumference, head/abdominal circumference ratio and intraperitoneal volume have not been shown to be reliable in the absence of ascites in the prediction of fetal anaemia (Nicolaides et al 1988a).

Doppler ultrasound is another non-invasive sonographic method that has been rigorously evaluated for the detection of fetal anaemia. Doppler velocity waveform studies have

Table 16.2 Role of ultrasound in the non-invasive management of alloimmunised pregnancies

- Gestational age
- Growth
- Identify hydrops or fetal ascites
- Non-invasive assessment:
  - liver length
  - spleen circumference
  - umbilical vein maximal velocity
  - middle cerebral artery peak systolic velocity

assessed various parts of the fetal circulation (e.g. cardiac outflow tracts, descending aorta), but in practice the prediction of fetal anaemia has not been consistent using this technique. This may be because the fetal haemodynamic response is variable and, as anaemia progresses, is poorly understood so that the relevant parameters may not have been evaluated. It is unclear, for example, how the fetal peripheral resistance responds with impending hydrops (Nicolaides et al 1988a). With the development of fetal anaemia the blood viscosity falls and cardiac output increases. This hyperdynamic circulation is identified by an increase in velocity of the fetal blood (Rightmire et al 1986), which can be assessed during fetal apnoea by measurement of the umbilical vein maximal velocity (UV Vmax), with an angle of insonation less than 30° (Fig. 16.2). The middle cerebral artery peak velocity of systolic blood flow can also identify the moderately and severely anaemic fetus (Mari et al 2000).

Other ultrasound measurements of the fetus that may be useful are the fetal liver length and spleen circumference (Oepkes 1993). These are both important sites of extramedullary erythropoietic activity and therefore an increase in size indicates fetal compensation for developing anaemia. The liver length is measured from the diaphragm to the tip of the right lobe of the liver in the parasagittal plane (Fig. 16.3) and the spleen circumference at the level of the fetal stomach in a transverse view (Fig. 16.4).

Our current practice at University College London Hospitals combines serial fetal growth measurements with liver length, spleen circumference and UV Vmax. Placental thickness and amniotic fluid volume are also assessed. These values are recorded on gestation-dependent charts, as shown in Figs 16.2(b), 16.3(b) and 16.4(b) (Oepkes 1993). While the measurements remain within the normal ranges, inva-

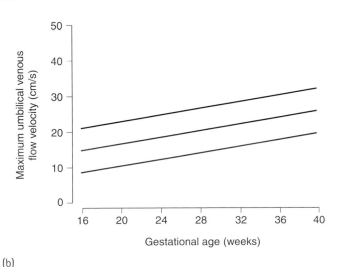

(a)

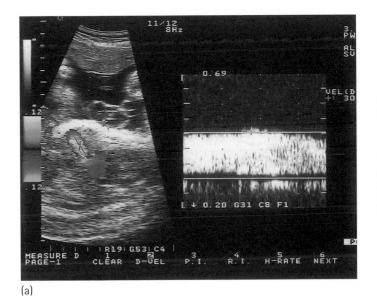

(b)

Fig. 16.2 (a) Longitudinal section of the fetal body, demonstrating measurement of the umbilical vein maximal flow velocity. (b) Normogram for the umbilical vein maximal flow velocity. (From Oepkes 1993, with permission.)

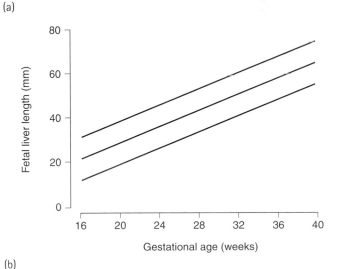

(a)

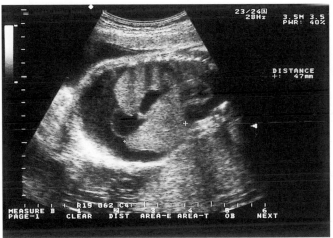

(b)

Fig. 16.3 (a) Ultrasound image of the fetal liver length measurement. The maximum fetal liver length is measured in a parasagittal plane of the fetal abdomen, from the diaphragm to the lower edge of the right lobe of the liver (calipers +—+). The fetus has hydrops. (b) Normogram for liver length. (From Oepkes 1993, with permission.)

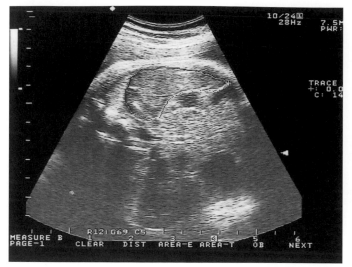

(a)

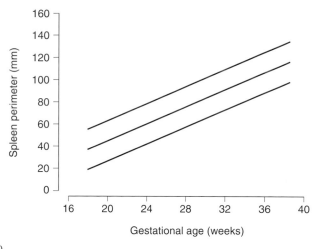

(b)

Fig. 16.4 (a) Ultrasound image of a transverse section of the fetal abdomen at the level of the stomach; behind it is the spleen with its perimeter outlined. (b) Nomogram for spleen perimeter. (From Oepkes 1993, with permission.)

sive assessment is avoided. Measurements above 2 standard deviations imply a high likelihood of fetal anaemia, but false positives may occur. However, if the maternal antibody level shows a significant rise, even with non-invasive assessment within the normal range, amniocentesis should be performed because of the possibility of a false-negative result. We have recently reported, in a prospective study, the successful use of non-invasive monitoring in RBC alloimmunisation and demonstrated a reduced need for invasive testing (Iskaros et al 1998). In women with a severe history, these observations may be commenced at 17–18 weeks' gestation.

Other non-invasive techniques for the assessment of fetal anaemia

Fetal heart rate changes have been noted with severe anaemia. A sinusoidal pattern with the loss of normal base-line variability of the cardiotocograph is highly suggestive of severe anaemia. A cardiotocograph can occasionally be a useful arbiter for or against immediate intervention. However, more subtle changes in fetal haematocrit are not easily detected by the technique. Biophysical profile assessment of at risk fetuses has also been found to be of no value.

Amniocentesis and amniotic fluid analysis

Bevis in 1952 first suggested the potential use of amniocentesis as an indirect assessment of fetal anaemia in HDFN. He showed a correlation between the severity of erythroblastosis fetalis and the amount of certain haemoglobin breakdown products, including bilirubin, in the amniotic fluid of affected pregnancies. The amniotic fluid becomes bright yellow from the bilirubin derived from fetal haemolysis. Liley in 1961 established that amniotic fluid bilirubin concentration could be quantified by spectrophometry by assessing the change in optical density at 450 nm (ΔOD450). Furthermore, he reported that the concentration of amniotic fluid bilirubin declines towards zero during the last trimester in non-anaemic pregnancies. In attempting to evaluate any excess of bilirubin present as a result of abnormal haemolysis, interpretation of the ΔOD450 therefore must be dependent on the gestation. Plotting the normal range on a logarithmic vertical scale, Liley implemented three prediction zones to give useful separation between pregnancies proceeding to stillbirth, the birth of babies with different degrees of anaemia and unaffected infants (Fig. 16.5). The original data from Liley's work has been modified by a number of authors (Whitfield (1970) and Freda (1965)) in an attempt to improve detection of the at-risk fetus. Amniocentesis for the investigation of fetal anaemia is considered to be reliable after 24 weeks, but may be less so at 18–24 weeks as the Liley zones cannot be extrapolated backwards to these earlier gestations. Queenan et al (1993) have devised a four-zone management method with ΔOD450 values from 14 weeks' gestation.

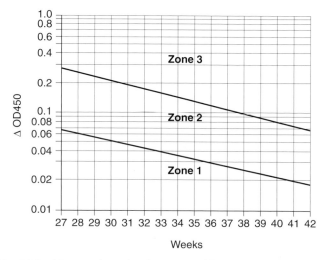

Fig. 16.5 Liley graph used to interpret Δ OD450 values in relation to gestation, to predict the likelihood of fetal anaemia. (From Liley 1961, with permission.)

Amniocentesis is performed under continuous ultrasound control, avoiding the placenta to minimise the risk of fetomaternal haemorrhage, withdrawing about 5 ml of amniotic fluid. The fluid is placed in an opaque bottle to avoid light degradation. Once the laboratory has reported on the sample, it is plotted on the ΔOD450 chart and a management plan made for the pregnancy. If the fetus is severely affected (Fig. 16.6), FBS (± intravascular transfusion) is scheduled within the next week (see below). If the ΔOD450 is satisfactory but there are high antibody levels or the non-invasive assessment is predictive of anaemia, the amniocentesis may be repeated in 1–2 weeks. A rising ΔOD450 may then lead to FBS (± intravascular transfusion) or if after 34 weeks, early delivery.

Fetal blood sampling

FBS has an established role in the management of RBC alloimmunisation (Fig. 16.6), for the determination of fetal haematocrit or haemoglobin. Early studies have established that haemoglobin concentration values rise from 11.5 to 13.5 g/dl between 20 and 30 weeks and haematocrit from 37% to 42% over the same period (Daffos et al 1985). A fetus with hydrops will be severely anaemic with a haematocrit below 15–20% and a haemoglobin deficit of 7 g/dl or more. However, a fetus may be this anaemic but not be hydropic, emphasising the importance of FBS to measure the fetal haematocrit. FBS is an outpatient procedure and well tolerated by mother and fetus. It is good practice to only perform FBS if there is a high likelihood that the fetus is anaemic and would require treatment. Blood for transfusion is therefore always prepared. FBS is performed under ultrasound guidance and full aseptic precautions. Tocolysis, antibiotic prophylaxis and fetal neuromuscular blockade are not used routinely. The site for sampling is determined by the fetal and placental position, bearing in mind that a transplacental approach will cause fetomaternal haemorrhage and increased antibody levels. The umbilical cord at the placental insertion is the most commonly used site. The intrahepatic portion of the umbilical vein is often a preferred site as it reliably yields a pure fetal venous sample, minimising risks of arterial spasm, cord tamponade and fetomaternal haemorrhage. The FBS (1–3 ml) is analysed immediately and later

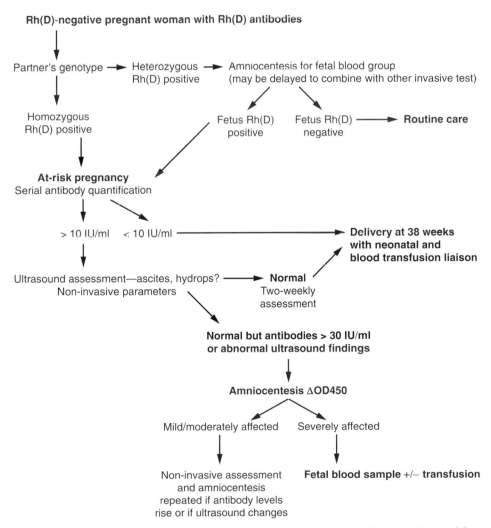

Fig. 16.6 Schematic representation of the management of pregnancies affected by Rhesus (D) alloimmunisation.

assessed for fetal reticulocyte count and blood group. Following sampling the mother and fetus are monitored to exclude bleeding, preterm labour or fetal distress.

Published fetal loss rates following antenatal FBS vary between 0% and 25%. Fetal loss rates have been shown to be related to the indication for the procedure, such as a loss rate of 12.7% with severe growth restriction and 1% for the diagnosis of fetal haemoglobinopathies (Antsaklis et al 1998). The complication rate falls as both fetal gestation and operator experience increase. The undoubted value of a precise measurement of haemoglobin or haematocrit should be balanced against the greater simplicity of amniocentesis, its lesser direct risk to the fetus, and much smaller risk of feto-maternal haemorrhage. However, FBS is the invasive test of first choice in a few circumstances: firstly, it should be used from 20 to 24 weeks in the few cases when the history or ultrasound suggests that fetal death may occur as early as this; secondly, if there is fetal ascites without oedema, suggesting that hydrops may soon develop FBS should be used; thirdly, FBS is indicated if there is obvious polyhydramnios with its diluting effect on bilirubin concentration. In these circumstances the fetal haematocrit or haemoglobin concentration is probably a more reliable guide than the ΔOD450 in the amniotic fluid. FBS should be avoided before 20 weeks, because of the greater risk of fetal death related to the procedure at early gestations.

Intravascular transfusion

The FBS technique was first adapted for intravascular transfusion (IVT) by Rodeck et al in 1981 using an umbilical vessel viewed at ultrasound-guided fetoscopy. Bang et al in 1982 demonstrated the feasibility of ultrasound-guided IVT into the intrahepatic part of the umbilical vein, usually seen dilated in severe anaemia. A modification of Daffos' technique for FBS (Daffos et al 1985) became widely adopted (Fig. 16.7) and we use both depending on ease of access to, and visualisation of, the target. There is some evidence (Rodeck & Deans 1999) that the intrahepatic umbilical vein may be the safer site because there are umbilical arteries in the proximity, the puncture of which can cause complications. Infusion of adult haemoglobin in an IVT increases the oxygen Daffos et al 1985 carrying capacity of the blood and therefore improves tissue hypoxia. An FBS is performed as described above and an immediate haematocrit obtained using a blood analyser within the clinic. Neuromuscular blockade may be required if the placenta is posterior and fetal paralysis is achieved using pancuronium (0.25 mg/kg estimated fetal weight). There is as yet no agreement on the haematological criteria for IVT. In most fetal medicine units a defined haematocrit value is taken as the indication, and is generally between 25% and 30%, with some account taken for the normal increase in fetal haematocrit as gestation proceeds (Nicolaides et al 1988b). The lower of these values (25%) leaves a clear margin of safety from the 15–20% haematocrit above which hydrops does not occur (Grannum et al 1988). At the first IVT, the aim is to raise the haematocrit a little above the physiological range—before 24 weeks to 35–40%, after 24 weeks to 45–50%, and after 28 weeks to 50–55%. Sudden

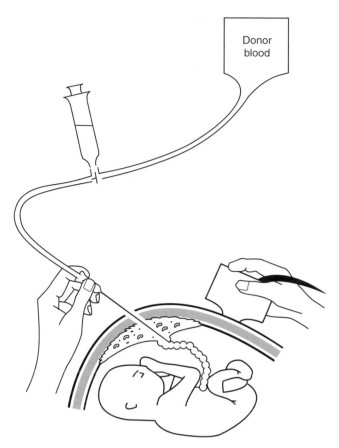

Fig. 16.7 Schematic representation of a fetal intravascular transfusion.

larger increases may elevate the fetal blood viscosity and compromise the circulation.

The method of calculating the volume of blood to be transfused to the fetus has been recently reviewed (Rodeck & Deans 1999), and is dependent on fetal gestation and donor haematocrit. During the procedure the fetal heart activity is checked intermittently and after Doppler ultrasound is performed to ensure circulatory stability. The interval between the first and second IVTs is kept short, at 1–2 weeks. The aim of IVT is to maintain fetal haematocrit with adult Rh(D)-negative RBCs at a physiological level and therefore suppress fetal Rh(D)-positive RBC production. However, the haematocrit falls between IVTs because fetal growth and plasma expansion dilute the Rh(D)-negative cells, and because of haemolysis of any remaining endogenous Rh(D)-positive cells. The rate of fall of haematocrit after the first IVT is uncertain but usually greater than or equal to 1% Hct/day. After the second IVT fetal erythopoietin is usually suppressed, the rate of fall in haematocrit is 0.8–1.2% per day, and subsequent IVTs can be performed at 3–4-week intervals, depending on the post-IVT haematocrit. This approach enables accurate planning of transfusions and delivery and reduces the number of unnecessary procedures (see Rodeck & Deans 1999).

Adult blood donors suitable for fetal IVT are registered with the regional blood centre and these volunteers are willing to provide blood on request. They are of blood group O, Rh(D)-negative, CMV-negative and have no atypical antibodies. The donor blood is cross-matched against the mother and leucocyte depleted, irradiated and packed to a haematocrit of about 80–85%. In some centres maternal blood is used for fetal IVT.

Intraperitoneal transfusion

Liley first described intraperitoneal transfusion (IPT) in 1963. Nowadays it is an alternative to IVT in some circumstances. Donor blood can be transfused into the intraperitoneal cavity, where it is absorbed over a period of time via the fetal lymphatics. IPT is the method of choice for transfusion below 18 weeks' gestation when the umbilical vein is too small for safe venepuncture and when venous access is inaccessible due to the fetus lying with its spine anterior overlying a posterior placenta. However, blood is not well absorbed from the abdominal cavity if the fetus is hydropic. A technique similar to FBS is used and a 20 G needle is inserted into the flank of the fetus. When transfusion is commenced, increasing sonolucency will be seen within the abdominal cavity. IPT is also used to supplement an IVT to prolong intervals between procedures, perhaps later in gestation or if the intravascular needle position becomes compromised and the IVT is thought to be inadequate.

Complications and outcome following intrauterine transfusion

Invasive procedures present risks to the pregnancy:

- Premature labour
- Prelabour ruptured membranes
- Fetal haemorrhage
- Fetal bradycardia
- Cardiac asystole
- Tamponade of umbilical cord
- Failure to obtain a sample
- Increase in maternal alloimmunisation by inducing feto-maternal haemorrhage

Instrumentation of the uterus may stimulate premature labour or cause premature rupture of membranes. The overall pregnancy loss for FBS without IVT is reported to be in the region of 1–2%, although severely affected fetuses or those at early gestations are at greater risk. The IVT itself presents further risk to the fetus due to the length of time the needle remains *in situ*, and additional risks are associated with administration blood products.

At UCLH we have reported a fetal loss rate per transfusion of 2.4% and an overall survival rate of 90% (92% for non-hydropic fetuses and 88% for hydropic fetuses). There were no losses in those fetuses having their first transfusion after 29 weeks' gestation (Rodeck & Deans 1999).

Delivery and paediatric care

Continued improvements in specialised neonatal care have also influenced the management of RBC alloimmunisation in recent years. Invasive procedures, with their inherent fetal risks, should be balanced against the increasing safety of early delivery. Even as early as 32 weeks the risks of delivery may be less than the risks of repeated IVT. However, for the severely anaemic fetus, especially if hydropic, an IVT will restore the circulation to a more normal oxygen-carrying capacity, correct acidosis and improve fetal well-being prior to delivery. A preterm infant or one expected to be anaemic may be most safely delivered by caesarean section, although with a fetus expected to be only mildly affected or following serial IVT, labour may be induced at 37–38 weeks and vaginal delivery expected. It is imperative that careful intrapartum monitoring is performed as these babies are at particular risk from intrapartum hypoxia and acidosis.

When delivery of a woman who is alloimmunised is planned or expected, preparation of the appropriate antigen-negative blood should be arranged for possible immediate transfusion of both mother and fetus. If the hospital for delivery is distant from the site of fetal management, prior liaison with the neonatal unit is essential. As HDFN is becoming rarer in modern clinical practice, so is the procedure of neonatal exchange transfusion. An exchange transfusion of one neonatal blood volume will replace approximately 75% of the infant's RBCs but carries the inherent intricacies of acid–base management (potassium and citrate) and fluid homeostasis. If a Rh(D)-positive baby has received Rh(D)-negative blood in utero, the neonatal circulation will contain virtually all Rh(D)-negative blood. Fetal erythropoiesis will be suppressed and will take a number of weeks to resume, during which the neonate may need top-up transfusions as the baby grows. Regular assessment of the haemoglobin level may be required up to 4 months of age.

Alternative management for RBC alloimmunisation

A number of alternative treatments have been tried in the management of alloimmunised pregnancies. These include repeated maternal plasma exchange from early pregnancy in an attempt to reduce circulating levels of anti-D, maternal immunosuppression with promezathine, corticosteroids alone or combined with azothioprine and high-dose immunoglobulin infusion (for review see Rodeck & Deans 1999).

Counselling

Some couples have experienced repeated fetal and neonatal losses from Rh(D) disease. Each pregnancy will have involved extensive medical surveillance and intervention. A fully informed and sympathetic discussion will be welcomed by the couple following a severely affected pregnancy or at the initial consultation in a subsequent one. Some couples may be apprehensive about trying again. However, as discussed, there is not only considerable individual variation in the course of RBC alloimmunisation in successive pregnancies, but new methods of treatment continue to be developed.

When there have been repeated fetal losses from severe alloimmunisation and the male partner is homozygous for the RBC antigen it may be appropriate to discuss donor insemination from an antigen-negative male donor. If the partner is heterozygous for the RBC antigen, the couple may opt for early fetal genotyping and termination of a pregnancy if the fetus is antigen positive. As a last resort, surrogate pregnancy may be considered.

SUMMARY

Since the introduction of Rh(D) immunoprophylaxis the incidence of Rh(D) HDFN has been significantly reduced. A greater proportion of HDFN is now from other RBC antigens such as anti-c or Kell. The management of RBC alloimmunisation is based in regional units where non-invasive and invasive expertise is maintained. The outcome of affected pregnancies has dramatically improved due to advances in both fetal and neonatal care.

KEY POINTS

- The RhD antigen is the most important; alloimmunisation is preventable by anti-D prophylaxis. Meticulous preventative care of the RhD-negative woman is the cornerstone of management.
- The molecular biology of the rhesus antigens has been worked out. The fetus can be genotyped by DNA analysis, which is now possible on free fetal DNA present in maternal plasma.
- Alloimmunisation will never completely disappear, but as cases become less common, management should be centralised in tertiary or even quaternary centres.
- The alloimmunised woman can be monitored non-invasively by serial antibody measurement and Doppler ultrasound. This greatly reduces the need for amniocentesis and fetal blood sampling.
- Intravascular transfusion is a precise and successful treatment which, in experienced centres, has a survival rate of more than 90%.

REFERENCES

Antsaklis A, Daskalakis G, Papantoniou N, Michalas S 1998 Fetal blood sampling—indication related losses. Prenat Diagn 18:934–940

Bang J, Bock JE, Trolle D 1982 Ultrasound-guided fetal transfusion for severe rhesus haemolytic disease. BMJ 284:373–374

Bennett PR, Le Van Kim C, Colin Y et al 1993 Prenatal determination of fetal RhD type by DNA amplification. N Engl J Med 329:607–610

Bevis DCA 1952 The antenatal prediction of haemolytic disease of the newborn. Lancet i:395–398

Bowman JM 1985 The prevention of Rh immunisation. Transfus Med Rev 2:129–150

Bowman JM, Pollock JM, Manning FA, Harman CR, Menticoglou S 1992 Maternal Kell blood group alloimmunization. Obstet Gynecol 79:239–244

British Committee for Standards in Haematology, Blood Transfusion Task Force 1996 Guidelines for blood grouping and red cell antibody testing during pregnancy. Transfus Med 6:71–74

Cherif-Zahar B, Mattei M, Le Van Kim C, Bailly P, Cartron JP, Coin Y 1991 Localization of the human Rh blood group gene structure to chromosome region 1p34–1p36 by in situ hybridization. Hum Genet 86:398–400

Daffos F, Capella-Pavlovsky M, Foriester F 1985 Fetal blood sampling during pregnancy with use of a needle guided by ultrasound: a study of 606 cases. Am J Obstet Gynecol 153:655–660

Diamond LK, Blackfan KD, Baty JM 1932 Erythroblastosis fetalis and its association with universal oedema of the fetus, icterus gravis neonatorum and anaemia of the newborn. J Pediatr 1:269–309

Finn R 1960 Erythroblastosis. Lancet i:526–527

Finn R, Clarke CA, Donohoe WTA et al 1961 Experimental studies on the prevention of Rh haemolytic disease. BMJ 1:1486–1490

Fisher RA, Race RR 1946 Rh gene frequencies in Britain. Nature 157:48–49

Freda VJ 1965 The Rh problem in obstetrics and a concept of its management using amniocentesis and spectrophotometric scanning of amniotic fluid. Am J Obstet Gynecol 92:341–374

Grannum PAT, Copel JA, Moya FR et al 1988 The reversal of hydrops fetalis by intravascular intrauterine transfusions in severe isoimmune fetal anaemia. Am J Obstet Gynecol 158:914–919

Huikeshoven FJ, Hope ID, Power GG, Gilbert RD, Longo LD 1988 A comparison of sheep and human fetal oxygen delivery systems with the use of a mathematical model. Am J Obstet Gynecol 151:449–455

Iskaros J, Kingdom J, Rodeck CH 1998 Prospective non-invasive monitoring of pregnancies complicated by red cell alloimmunization. Ultrasound Obstet Gynecol 11:432–437

Kleihauer E, Braun H, Betke K et al 1957 Demonstration of fetal haemoglobin in the circulating erythrocytes. Klin Wochenschr 35:637–642

Landsteiner K, Wiener AS 1940 An agglutinable factor in human blood recognised by immune sera for rhesus blood. Proc Soc Exp Biol Med 43:223

Levine P 1958 The influence of the ABO system on Rh haemolytic disease. Hum Biol 30:14–28

Levine P, Stetson RE 1939 Unusual cases of intra group agglutination. J Am Med Assoc 113:126–127

Levine P, Katzin EM, Burnham L 1941 Isoimmunisation in pregnancy: its bearing on the aetiology of erythroblastosis fetalis. J Am Med Assoc 116:817–825

Liley AW 1961 Liquor amnii analysis in the management of the pregnancy complicated by rhesus sensitization. Am J Obstet Gynecol 82:1359–1370

Liley AW 1963 Intrauterine transfusion of the foetus in haemolytic disease. BMJ 2:1107–1109

Lo YM, Hjelm NM, Fidler C et al 1998 Prenatal diagnosis of fetal Rh(D) status by molecular analysis of maternal plasma. N Engl J Med 339:1734–1848

Mari G, Carpenter RL, Rahman F et al 2000 Non-invasive diagnosis by Doppler ultrasonography of fetal anaemia due to maternal red cell alloimmunization. Collaborative Group for Doppler Assessment of the Blood Velocity in Anemic Fetuses. N Engl J Med 342:52–53

Mollison PL, Engelfriet CP, Contreras M 1997 Haemolytic disease of the newborn. In: blood transfusion in clinical medicine, 10th edn. Blackwell Science.

MRC 1974 Controlled trial of various anti-D dosages in suppression of Rh sensitization following pregnancy. Report to the Medical Research Council of a Working Party on the use of anti-D-immunoglobulin for the prevention of isoimmunization of Rh-negative women during pregnancy. BMJ 2:75–80

Nicolaides KH, Fontanarosa M, Gabbe SG, Rodeck CH 1988a Failure of ultrasonographic parameters to predict the severity of fetal anaemia in rhesus isoimmunization. Am J Obstet Gynecol 158:920–926

Nicolaides KH, Soothill PW, Clewell WH, Rodeck CH, Mibashan RS, Campbell S 1988b Fetal haemoglobin measurement in the assessment of red cell alloimmunisation. Lancet i:1073–1075

Oepkes D 1993 Ultrasonography and Doppler in the management of red cell alloimmunized pregnancies. MD Thesis, University of Leiden, The Netherlands

Queenan JT, Tomai TP, Ural SH, King JC 1993 Deviation in amniotic fluid optical density at a wavelength 450 nm in Rh-immunized pregnancies from 14–40 weeks' gestation: a proposal for clinical management. Am J Obstet Gynecol 168:1370–1374

RCOG 1999 Guideline No 22. Use of anti-D immunoglobulin for Rh prophylaxis. RCOG, London, p 22

Rightmire DA, Nicolaides KH, Rodeck CH, Campbell S 1986 Fetal blood velocities in Rh isoimmunization: relationship to gestational age and to fetal hematocrit. Obstet Gynecol 68:233–236

Rodeck CH, Deans A 1999 Red cell alloimmunisation. In: Rodeck CH, Whittle MJ (eds) Fetal Medicine: Basic science and clinical practice Churchill Livingstone, Edinburgh, pp 785–804

Rodeck CH, Holman CA, Karnicki J, Kemp JR, Whitmore DN, Austin MA 1981 Direct intravascular fetal blood transfusion by fetoscopy in severe rhesus isoimmunisation. Lancet i:625–627

van Dijk BA, Dororen MC, Overbeeke MA 1995 Red cell antibodies in pregnancy: there is no 'critical' titre. Transfus Med 5:199–202

Vaughan JL, Warwick R, Letsky E, Nicolini U, Rodeck CH, Fisk NM 1995 Erythropoietic suppression in fetal anaemia because of Kell alloimmunisation. Am J Obstet Gynecol 171:247–252

Whitfield CR 1970 A three-year assessment of an action-line method of timing intervention in Rhesus isoimmunization. Am J Obstet Gynecol 108:1239–1244

Whitfield CR 1976 Rhesus haemolytic disease. J Clin Pathol 29(suppl (RCP) 103):54–62

Woodrow JC, Finn R 1966 Transplacental haemorrhage. Br J Haematol 12:297–309

17

Cardiovascular problems in pregnancy

Michael de Swiet

Cardiovascular disease in pregnancy is a worrying condition for the obstetrician. Even excluding hypertensive disease (considered in Chapter 21), cardiovascular disease and specifically heart disease has an appreciable maternal mortality (1.8 per 100 000 in the most recent Report on Confidential Enquiries into Maternal Deaths Series (Department of Health and Social Security 1998)). Indeed there are now more deaths in the UK from heart disease than from hypertension, the second most common direct cause of maternal mortality.

If the presence of a heart murmur is considered indicative of heart disease, the majority of women are at risk, for as many as 90% have systolic murmurs in pregnancy. Yet the prevalence of heart disease in pregnancy in the West is probably no more than 1%.

In this chapter we will consider, with respect to pregnancy, the physiology of the cardiovascular system, the epidemiology of heart disease, the general management of patients with heart disease and certain specific conditions. For further reviews see de Swiet (1995), Oakley (1997).

THE PHYSIOLOGY OF THE CARDIOVASCULAR SYSTEM IN PREGNANCY

During pregnancy, oxygen consumption at rest increases by about 50 ml/min, i.e. from 300 to 350 ml/min. The oxygen is used by the fetus and other contents of the developing uterus, and to support the increased metabolic rate of the mother. Arterial blood is fully saturated. The only ways in which the mother can increase the supply of oxygen to peripheral tissues are either to increase the quantity of oxygen removed from the blood (increased arteriovenous oxygen difference) or to increase the delivery of oxygenated blood to the tissues (increased cardiac output). The pregnant woman takes the latter course and, as in so many other physiological adaptations to pregnancy, overcompensates for the increased load, so that cardiac output increases to such an extent that arteriovenous oxygen difference decreases from 100 ml/l in the non-pregnant state to 80 ml/l in pregnancy. Perhaps this is because the primary stimulus to increase cardiac output seems to be vasodilatation rather than hypoxaemia (see below).

The 40% increase in cardiac output from 3.5 to 6.0 l/min occurs early in pregnancy; at least two-thirds of the increase has occurred by the end of the first trimester. Although some studies have suggested that cardiac output falls at the end of pregnancy, even in patients in the left lateral position where the uterus does not obstruct venous return (Davies et al 1986), measurements made with pulsed Doppler have shown no consistent fall (Robson et al 1989) and this technique must be considered the most reliable.

It is not clear to what extent myocardial contractility increases in pregnancy independently of the increase in preload and decrease in afterload. However, echocardiographic studies show an increase in the speed of circumferential shortening (Rubler et al 1977), which would suggest some increase in contractility.

Most studies have been performed at rest. Cardiac output rises still further on exertion and in labour. Each uterine contraction will increase cardiac output by about 20% by increasing preload (increased venous return). The pain of contractions also increases cardiac output independently of any effect of increased preload. This emphasises the importance of effective analgesia in labouring patients with heart disease.

Cardiac output does increase on exercise in pregnancy, but as pregnancy progresses the increase gets smaller. Limitation of venous return is a probable reason. Although heart rate increases by about 10% in pregnancy, this is not sufficient to account for the 40% increase in cardiac output and so there is also an increase in stroke volume. Indeed an increase in resting heart above 100/min is an ominous sign in women with heart disease.

In normal pregnancy, blood pressure does not rise and, indeed, it usually falls in the second trimester. The increased cardiac output is, therefore, accommodated by a decrease in peripheral resistance. At one time it was thought that these effects were driven by increased oestrogen levels. Now it seems more likely that ecoisinoids and locally acting agents such as nitric oxide are more important.

Cardiac output also increases in pregnancy because of the increased preload caused by increased circulating blood volume. Blood volume rises very early in pregnancy; the total increase is about 40%, and this rise is maintained until delivery. The cardiac output has nearly returned to normal by two weeks after delivery, but it may take up to three months for the blood pressure to return to normal. The primary stimulus for the physiological changes in the circulation in pregnancy is decreased afterload (vasodilatation). This leads to:

- initial decrease in systemic arterial pressure
- increased circulating blood volume
- increased cardiac output
- increased drug volume
- increased heart rate.

The rise in cardiac output and associated vasodilatation in pregnancy cause changes in the circulation which may mimic heart disease. Heart rate increases and it is likely that arrhythmias are more common in pregnancy. Pulse volume is increased. Jugular venous pressure waves are more prominent, though the height of the venous pressure is not increased in pregnancy. Heart size increases and displacement of the apex beat by up to 1 cm from the mid-clavicular line should not be considered abnormal. The first heart sound is loud; there is often a very prominent third heart sound and an ejection systolic murmur up to grade 3/6 in intensity is heard over the whole precordium in up to 90% of pregnant women. Venous hums—continuous murmurs usually audible in the neck, which can be modified by stethoscope pressure—may also be heard in pregnancy.

In addition, peripheral oedema is very common in pregnancy, and rarely indicates heart disease.

NATURAL HISTORY

Prevalence of heart disease

The prevalence and incidence of all heart disease in pregnancy varies between 0.4% in a recent UK study (Tan & de Swiet 1998) and 1.5% in a similar study in Sri Lanka (Kaluarachchi & Seneviratne 1995). The figures vary because of differences in referral pattern and because of differences in the prevalence of heart disease in different communities at different times. In developed countries rheumatic heart disease is becoming less common while congenital heart disease and degenerative vascular disease are proportionately more important. There are also changes in the pattern of congenital heart disease in pregnancy following the increase in paediatric cardiac surgery, which occurred between 1965 and 1975. So specialist referral centres are seeing more women in pregnancy who have had surgery in childhood for congenital heart disease. However, this effect has been surprisingly slow considering how long ago the increase in surgery occurred; presumably and understandably many of these women are very wary of becoming pregnant.

In all series, the dominant lesion in rheumatic heart disease has been mitral stenosis. Out of 1048 patients with rheumatic heart disease reported from Newcastle, when rheumatic heart disease was common in the UK, Szekely et al (1973) found dominant mitral stenosis in 90%. In the more recent series from Sri Lanka (Kaluarachchi & Seneviratne 1995), mitral valve disease was present in all but 4% of 116 women with rheumatic heart disease and mitral stenosis was the only lesion in 61%.

The distribution of congenital heart disease in pregnancy in two series from the UK and Sri Lanka already considered is shown in Table 17.1. Other centres will inevitably see a different pattern and specialist centres' experience will very much depend on the surgical referral base that they serve.

Table 17.1 Congenital heart disease in London and Sri Lanka

	London[a]		Sri Lanka[b]	
	cases	%	cases	%
Mitral valve prolapse	17	35	0	0
Ventricular septal defect	11	22	6	12
Atrial septal defect	5	10	30	60
Pulmonary stenosis	4	8	0	0
Patent ductus arteriosus	3	6	3	6
Fallot's tetralogy	2	4	1	2
Bicuspid aortic valve	2	4	1	2
Coarctation of the aorta	2	4	1	2
Transposition of great vessels	1	2	1	2
Aortic stenosis	1	2	5	10
Anomalous pulmonary venous drainage	1	2	0	0
Congenital heart block	0	0	3	6
Total	49	100	51	100

[a] Tan & de Swiet 1998
[b] Kaluarachchi & Seneviratne 1995

Maternal mortality

Although sporadic fatalities will be seen in all forms of heart disease in pregnancy, maternal mortality is highest in those conditions where there is obstruction to blood flow and in particular to pulmonary blood flow. In the pulmonary circuit this occurs because of obstruction, either within the pulmonary blood vessels or at the mitral valve. The situation is documented clearly in Eisenmenger's syndrome, for which up to now there has been no effective treatment, and for which the maternal mortality is between 30 and 50% (Morgan Jones & Howitt 1965, Yentis et al 1998). An elevation in pulmonary vascular resistance is also seen in primary pulmonary hypertension in which the reported maternal mortality is 40–50% (Morgan Jones & Howitt 1965).

In contrast, in women with Fallot's tetralogy, in which pulmonary vascular resistance is normal, the reported maternal mortality varies between four and 20%. A series from Connecticut USA (Whittemore et al 1982) shows how good the results can be with obsessional care: in 482 pregnancies from 233 women, including eight mothers with Eisenmenger's syndrome, there were no maternal deaths.

The data from the Confidential Maternal Mortality series in the UK (Table 17.2) emphasise the risks of pulmonary vascular disease. Six out of 10 deaths from congenital heart disease and further one out of 25 deaths from acquired heart disease (Table 17.3) a total of 20%, resulted from pulmonary vascular disease. Yet in the two series quoted of heart disease complicating pregnancy (Table 17.1) there were no cases of pulmonary vascular disease: the risk of pulmonary vascular disease is out of all proportion to its prevalence.

In rheumatic heart disease, maternal mortality can now be very low. Szekely et al (1973) report 26 mortalities (about 1%) in 2856 pregnancies complicated by rheumatic heart disease between 1942 and 1969. Half of the deaths were caused by pulmonary oedema, which became much less common once mitral valvotomy was freely available. The authors reported no maternal deaths in approximately 1000 pregnancies occurring after 1960.

Table 17.3 shows that there were no deaths from rheumatic heart disease in the UK between 1994 and 1996. The pattern of death from acquired heart disease has changed completely. Women now die from degenerative vascular disease: myocardial infarction and dissecting aneurysm. Endocarditis remains a problem. Although there were no deaths from endocarditis in the UK between 1994 and 1996, overall about 10% of maternal mortality from heart disease in the UK in the last 15 years, relates to endocarditis. The major causes of maternal mortality from heart disease are:

- mitral stenosis in the developing world
- pulmonary vascular disease leading to pulmonary hypertension
- myocardial infarction
- dissecting aneurysm
- cardiomyopathy
- endocarditis.

There is no evidence that a well-managed pregnancy is detrimental to the long-term health of the woman with heart disease providing she survives pregnancy itself. Chesley (1980) has reported a group of 38 women with 51 pregnancies occurring after they were diagnosed as having severe heart disease. These were compared with a group of 96 women with equally severe rheumatic heart disease who did not have any pregnancies after diagnosis. The mean survival time (14 years) was greater in the group that did have further pregnancies compared with the group that did not (12 years).

Fetal outcome

The fetal outcome among those whose mothers have rheumatic heart disease in pregnancy is usually good and little different from that in those whose mothers do not have heart disease (Sugrue et al 1981). However, the babies are likely to be lighter at birth by about 200 g.

In most series of patients with congenital heart disease in pregnancy there is also no excess fetal mortality, except in the group with cyanotic congenital heart disease. Here the babies are generally growth-restricted and the fetal loss including abortion may be as high as 45%. This is hardly surprising in view of the inefficient mechanisms of placental exchange, which cannot compensate for maternal systemic hypoxaemia. It is likely that the fetus dies because of inadequate oxygen supply or because of prematurity, which may be iatrogenic.

Of great importance is the prevalence of congenital heart disease in the infants of mothers who themselves have congenital heart disease; this prevalence varies according to series from 3 to 14% (Nora 1977, Whittemore et al 1982). This compares with a prevalence of 1% in the general population (Nora 1977). The highest prevalence was in infants whose mothers had outflow obstruction, particularly left-sided. Most congenital abnormalities were represented in the infants; in about one-half, the child had the same abnormality as the mother.

Table 17.2 Confidential Enquiry into maternal deaths, 1994–1996: congenital heart disease (DHSS 1998)

• Aortic valve disease, endocarditis	2
• VSD, Eisenmenger's syndrome	3
• Primary pulmonary hypertension	3
• HOCM	1
• Anomalous coronary arteries	1
• Total	10

Table 17.3 Confidential Enquiry into maternal deaths, 1994–1996: acquired heart disease (DHSS 1998)

• Myocardial infarct	6
• Aneurysm of thoracic aorta and branches	7
• Puerperal cardiomyopathy	4
• Other cardiomyopathy	4
• Pericarditis	1
• Thrombosed MVR	1
• Secondary pulmonary hypertension	1
• Left ventricular hypertrophy	1
• Total	25

In a more recent UK study, the prevalence of heart disease was examined in 393 children who had either fathers or mothers with congenital heart disease (Burn et al 1998). The overall recurrence risk was 4.1%, more in the offspring of women with heart disease than in those from affected fathers.

MANAGEMENT

If possible, all women with heart disease attending one maternity hospital should be managed in a combined obstetric/cardiac clinic by one obstetrician and one cardiologist. In this way, the number of visits the patient makes to the hospital is kept to a minimum, and the obstetrician and cardiologist obtain the maximum experience in the management of relatively rare conditions. Granted the rarity of heart disease in pregnancy in the developed world, those who have haemodynamically significant disease should be reviewed in a tertiary referral centre even if they are not delivered there.

Patient history

As in all forms of medicine, the history is the most important single factor in the assessment of a patient who may have heart disease. In developed countries, most patients know whether they have heart disease. Even in developing countries it is very unusual though not unknown to have haemodynamically significant heart disease with no symptoms. For example, only four women were diagnosed with heart disease *de novo* in a cohort of 17 503 deliveries in London UK; and three of these were recent immigrants (Tan & de Swiet 1998).

The most frequent symptom of heart disease in pregnancy is breathlessness (Morley & Lim 1995). This can be difficult to assess because it is a variable feature of all pregnancies; it is, therefore, important to consider whether the woman was breathless before she became pregnant. Syncope occurs in severe aortic stenosis, hypertrophic cardiomyopathy, Fallot's tetralogy and Eisenmenger's syndrome; it is also a feature of normal pregnancy. Syncope, like chest pain, may occur because of dysrhythmias. The pregnant woman may also be aware of the dysrhythmia as a feeling of palpitations.

Chest pain is usually a feature of ischaemic disease, which is uncommon in pregnancy though an increasing cause of maternal mortality (Table 17.3). Chest pain may also occur in severe aortic stenosis, or, more commonly in pregnancy, in hypertrophic cardiomyopathy.

Physical signs

As noted above, the hyperdynamic circulation of pregnancy causes alterations in the cardiovascular system that mimic heart disease. Therefore, 20% of patients originally thought to have rheumatic heart disease may be found to have none at all following a reassessment performed up to 30 years later (Gleicher et al 1979). The changes that occur in the cardiovascular system in association with normal pregnancy have already been considered. Any other murmurs or additional heart sounds should be considered to be significant. Particular difficulty occurs with systolic murmurs, since they are so common in pregnancy (Tan & de Swiet 1998). Significant murmers are:

- pansystolic murmurs of ventricular septal defect, mitral regurgitation or tricuspid regurgitation
- late systolic murmurs of mitral regurgitation, mitral valve prolapse or hypertrophic cardiomyopathy
- ejection systolic murmurs louder than grade 3/6 of aortic stenosis
- ejection systolic murmurs that vary with respiration in pulmonary stenosis
- ejection systolic murmurs associated with other abnormalities, e.g. ejection clicks—valvar pulmonary and aortic stenosis.

In addition, an assessment of the patient's cardiac status should also include the signs of heart failure: whether the patient is cyanosed or has finger-clubbing, the presence of pulse deficits and other peripheral signs of endocarditis such as splinter haemorrhages.

Investigations

Chest radiography

The chest radiography is unhelpful in the diagnosis of minor degrees of heart disease but will, of course, show typical changes in those who have haemodynamically significant heart pathology. In pregnancy, women with normal hearts show slight cardiomegaly, increased pulmonary vascular markings and distension of the pulmonary veins. Pregnancy is not a contraindication to chest X-rays. The radiation exposure is trivial: less than that received in one transatlantic flight in a modern jetliner. The potential benefit of diagnosing serious and potentially fatal heart disease in pregnancy far outweighs any possible radiation risk.

Electrocardiography

In pregnancy, T wave inversion in lead III, S-T segment changes and Q waves, which would usually be considered pathological, occur frequently. In pregnancy, therefore, the electrocardiograph is more helpful in the diagnosis of dysrhythmias than in the demonstration of a structural abnormality of the heart.

Echocardiography

Recent studies have shown that the majority of structural cardiac abnormalities can be detected by echocardiography. This is the investigation of choice in pregnancy, since there is no radiation hazard, and because of the detailed information available in skilled hands. However, most murmurs can be evaluated by clinical criteria alone and echocardiography is only necessary when there is doubt about their significance.

Clinical management

The nature and severity of the heart lesion should first be assessed in the combined clinic. In practice, many patients will have no evidence of any lesion at all and no further follow-up will be required. Some may only have a mild lesion with no haemodynamic problems, such as congenital mitral valve prolapse which has such an excellent prognosis that again, no further follow-up is necessary. The remainder will have a condition with real or potential haemodynamic implications. These women must firstly be assessed about the need for termination, if seen early enough in pregnancy, and secondly, about the need for surgery. In patients with well managed heart disease, these assessments would have been made before the patient became pregnant.

Because of the mortality statistics indicated above, Eisenmenger's syndrome and primary pulmonary hypertension are absolute indications for termination of pregnancy. Very rarely, termination may also be indicated in patients with such severe pulmonary disease that this has caused pulmonary hypertension. In all other cases, the decision whether the pregnancy should continue depends on an individual assessment of the risk of pregnancy and the patient's desire to have children.

In general, the indications for surgery in pregnancy are similar to those in the non-pregnant state: failure of medical treatment with either intractable heart failure or intolerable symptoms. However, because of the bad reputation of severe mitral stenosis in pregnancy, mitral valvotomy or valvuloplasty is performed relatively commonly in patients with suitable heart valves, whereas open heart surgery is only performed with reluctance because of worries about the fetus. More recent studies suggest that these worries about fetal survival are not justifiable, at least in the short term (Becker 1983). Possible long-term effects on the development of the child are unknown.

Antenatal care

After the initial assessment of the pregnant woman, the remainder of medical management during pregnancy is associated with avoiding, if possible, those factors which increase the risk of heart failure, and the vigorous treatment of any heart failure if it occurs. Risk factors for heart failure in pregnancy include infections (particularly urinary tract infection), hypertension (both pregnancy-associated and pregnancy-induced), obesity, multiple pregnancy, anaemia, the development of arrhythmias and, very rarely, hyperthyroidism. The increase in cardiac output in twin pregnancy, which is about 30% greater than in singleton pregnancy, is achieved by increasing heart rate and contractility rather than by increasing venous return. This suggests that cardiac reserve is particularly compromised in multiple pregnancy.

Treatment of heart failure

The principles of treatment of heart failure in pregnancy are the same as in the non-pregnant state.

Digoxin. This is used to control the heart rate in atrial fibrillation and some other supraventricular tachycardias, and, when given acutely in heart failure, to increase the force of contraction. Dosage requirements of digoxin are the same in pregnancy as in the non-pregnant state. Both digoxin and digitoxin cross the placenta, producing similar drug levels in the fetus to those seen in the mother. Digoxin enters the umbilical circulation within five minutes of intravenous administration to the mother. In general, there is no evidence that therapeutic levels of digoxin in the mother affect the neonatal electrocardiograph or cause any harm to the fetus. However, although therapeutic drug levels in the mother do not harm the fetus, toxic levels do.

There may be a place for prophylactic digoxin therapy in selected women who are not in heart failure. This is most likely to be of value in those at risk from developing atrial fibrillation, i.e. those with rheumatic mitral valve disease with an enlarged left atrium, and possibly those who have paroxysmal atrial fibrillation or frequent atrial ectopic beats. However, this form of treatment has not been subjected to formal clinical trial, and there is certainly no case for digitalisation of all women with heart disease in pregnancy. Digoxin is also secreted in breast milk, but since the total daily excretion in the mother with therapeutic blood levels should not exceed 2 μg this too is unlikely to cause any harm to the baby, unless it suffers from some other disorder predisposing to digitalis toxicity, such as hypokalaemia.

Diuretic therapy. Frusemide is the most commonly used and rapidly acting loop diuretic for the treatment of pulmonary oedema. In congestive cardiac failure, where speed of action is not so important, oral thiazides are normally used in the first instance, although the extra potency of the loop diuretics may be necessary in a minority of cases. The use of thiazide in late pregnancy is not associated with any significant salt or water depletion in the baby.

There are no risks with the use of diuretics for the treatment of heart failure specific to pregnancy, but, as in the non-pregnant state, hypokalaemia is an important complication in the woman who may also be taking digoxin. Treatment of pulmonary oedema should also include opiates such as morphine, which reduces anxiety and decreases venous return by causing venodilatation. Angiotensin converting enzyme inhibitors should not be used in general in pregnancy because they may cause lethal renal failure in the newborn, but they may also be life saving in heart failure and in these circumstances should not be withheld. Life-threatening pulmonary oedema that does not respond to drug therapy may be helped by mechanical ventilation. If this is successful, and in other cases which do not respond to medical treatment, cardiac surgery should be considered in pregnancy if the patient has a potentially operable lesion.

Dysrhythmias

Most dysrhythmias that require treatment are a result of ischaemic heart disease, which usually presents in women after their childbearing years and is rare in pregnancy. Therefore, there is limited experience in the treatment of dysrhythmias during pregnancy. Nevertheless, the problem does exist, particularly in patients who have non-ischaemic abnormalities of cardiac-conducting tissue, such as are believed to occur in the Wolff–Parkinson–White, Lown–Ganong–Levine and Long Q-T syndromes. Furthermore, paroxysmal atrial tachycardia is said to occur more frequently in pregnancy than in non-pregnant women.

The antidysrhythmic drugs used most frequently in pregnancy are verapamil, digoxin, quinidine and beta-adrenergic blocking agents, in particular propranolol, oxprenolol, atenolol and sotalol. The indications for the use of these drugs are unaltered by pregnancy. Although there are isolated case reports of intrauterine growth restriction, acute fetal distress in labour and hypoglycaemia in the newborn in patients taking beta-adrenergic blocking agents, these have not been confirmed in clinical trials of oxprenolol used for treating hypertension in pregnancy. It would seem reasonable, therefore, to use propranolol, oxprenolol or sotalol in both the acute and long-term treatment of supraventricular and ventricular tachycardia in pregnancy. Atenolol is associated with growth restriction if given in the first half of pregnancy and probably is best avoided at this time.

Quinidine is used to maintain or induce sinus rhythm in patients either after DC conversion or when taking digoxin. It is well tolerated in pregnancy and has only minimal oxytocic effect. There is much less experience with other antidysrhythmic drugs such as verapamil, diltiazem, amiodarone or disopyramide. The use of disopyramide has been associated with hypertonic uterine activity, therefore, it should be used in pregnancy with caution. The long-term risks of phenytoin are well known. However, this drug is only likely to be used in the acute treatment of dysrhythmias, particularly those induced by digitalis intoxication. Procainamide has also been used successfully to abolish atrial fibrillation in pregnancy. Amiodarone has been used in several cases in pregnancy. The drug contains substantial quantities of iodine and may cause transient abnormalities in fetal thyroid function and temporary goitre in the fetus, but no long-term problems have been reported. At present it would seem reasonable to use amiodarone for resistant arrhythmias in late pregnancy that cannot be treated in any other way. Support for the use of amiodarone and verapamil in pregnancy comes from their use in the intrauterine treatment of fetal supraventricular tachycardia. However flecainamide is being used with increasing frequency for this indication and is probably now the drug of choice for the intrauterine treatment of fetal supraventricular tachycardia. Therefore, it would seem sensible to consider flecainamide after verapamil as first line therapy for maternal supraventricular tachycardia, notwithstanding concern about its effects in more elderly patients with ischaemic heart disease.

DC conversion for tachyarrhythmias is safe in pregnancy and does not harm the fetus. Intravenous adenosine (3–12 mg) is so effective in terminating supraventricular tachycardias that it is now the treatment of choice. It has been used safely in pregnancy and is most unlikely to affect the fetus since its half-life is less than two seconds.

The difficulty arises in considering long-term prophylactic treatment with antidysrhythmic drugs that have not been extensively used in pregnancy. Here each case must be considered on its own merits, paying particular attention to the frequency and severity of the attacks of dysrhythmia. A single short episode of supraventricular tachycardia associated with no other symptoms does not require prophylactic treatment. Frequent attacks of ventricular tachycardia associated with syncope would require prophylaxis whatever the outcome in the fetus.

Anticoagulant therapy is a major problem in the management of patients with heart disease in pregnancy, and it is considered in the section on artificial heart valves below.

Labour and delivery

Heart disease per se is not an indication for induction of labour; indeed, the risks of failed induction and of possible sepsis might be reasons to avoid it. Nevertheless, these risks are slight, and induction should not be withheld if it is necessary for obstetric reasons. Furthermore, in complicated cases requiring optimal medical support, induction near term may be justified to plan delivery in daylight hours.

Fluid balance necessitates careful and expert attention during labour in women with significant heart disease. Many women in labour are given copious quantities of intravenous fluid and, if they have normal hearts, can cope with the resultant increase in circulating blood volume. Patients with heart disease cannot, however, and they may easily develop pulmonary oedema. This effect is exacerbated by the tendency to use crystalloid intravenous fluids that decrease the colloid osmotic pressure of plasma by about 5 mmHg over the course of labour.

Some centres are gaining increasing experience in the use of elective central catheterisation (Swan–Ganz technique) to measure right atrial pressure, wedge pressure (indirect left atrial pressure) and cardiac output in labour in patients with heart disease. There is no doubt that this technique facilitates a more rational use of fluid therapy, diuretics and inotropes. Preliminary results also suggest that measurement of central venous pressure alone is so misleading as an index of left ventricular filling pressure that it should not be used for this purpose (although it is still invaluable in managing patients with bleeding problems). However the technique of Swan–Ganz catheterisation is quite difficult and it has a significant morbidity. Therefore, it should only be used in centres where there is sufficient experience.

Women with heart disease are also particularly sensitive to the effects of aortocaval compression by the gravid uterus when lying in the supine position. Marked hypotension can develop, causing maternal and fetal distress. The risk of this complication developing is even greater after epidural anaesthesia.

Most patients with heart disease do have quite rapid, uncomplicated labours. In the majority, analgesia is best given by epidural anaesthesia since it is an effective analgesic that also decreases cardiac output, by causing peripheral vasodilatation and decreasing venous return, and by reducing pain induced tachycardia. However, epidural anaesthesia is inadvisable in Eisenmenger's syndrome and contraindicated in hypertrophic cardiomyopathy (see chapter 28).

Most obstetric emergencies arising in labour, including the need for caesarean section, can be managed using epidural anaesthesia and in general this is commonly believed to be safer than general anaesthesia though not necessarily in cardiac patients. Epidural block causes less haemodynamic changes than does spinal block and in women without heart disease, it does not affect haemodynamics.

However, these observations may not be relevant to women with heart disease. In addition there are few adequate comparisons of these forms of anaesthesia in comparable patients, and much depends on the skill and preference of the anaesthetist who is present.

In women with heart disease, it seems sensible to keep the second stage of labour short in order to decrease maternal effort, but there is obviously no advantage in performing forceps delivery in a woman who would deliver easily by herself.

The use of oxytocic drugs in the third stage of labour is much debated. The theoretical disadvantage is that ergometrine and Syntocinon will cause a tonic contraction of the uterus, expressing about 500 ml of blood into a circulation whose capacitance has also been reduced by associated venoconstriction. The consequent rise in left atrial pressure (Fig. 17.1), which averages 10 mmHg in patients with mitral stenosis, may be quite sufficient to precipitate pulmonary oedema. However, the management of postpartum haemorrhage in a patient with heart disease is not easy. Syntocinon should be used in all patients in the third stage, unless they are in cardiac failure, since it has less effect on blood vessels than ergometrine and it can be given by intravenous infusion, which can be accompanied by intravenous frusemide.

It has been traditional to avoid caesarean section in women with heart disease because of concern about maternal mortality and because as noted these women often have quick easy labours. But what used to happen was that the woman would become sick because of heart failure and caesarean section was performed as a last resort to obtain a live baby; not surprisingly the women often died. By contrast, elective caesarean section has a lot to offer. It allows the delivery to be timed with precision. Anticoagulant drugs can be withheld for the minimum period and modern anaesthetic techniques allow the minimum of haemodynamic disturbance. There are no hard data from which to draw conclusions with regard to the route of delivery. Each case should be considered individually, and the preferences of the obstetrician, cardiologist, anaesthetist and patient should all be considered before making a final decision.

Endocarditis and its prevention in pregnancy

The Report on Confidential Enquiries into Maternal Deaths in England and Wales (Department of Health and Social Security 1998) shows that there were 11 deaths from endocarditis in the UK between 1988 and 1996: 11% of all cardiac deaths. However, the case for antibiotic prophylaxis in labour has not been proven. There are several large series of women with heart disease in pregnancy to whom no antibiotics were given and in whom no endocarditis was observed (Sugrue et al 1981). Yet, the data in the Confidential Enquiries into Maternal Deaths series suggest that women are at increased risk from endocarditis in pregnancy. What is not clear from these reports is whether the endocarditis was contracted during labour, and therefore potentially preventable by antibiotics, or whether it arose at some other time. Until more details are available, the author continues to use antibiotic prophylaxis. For patients not allergic to penicillin and who have not had penicillin more than once in the preceding month, amoxycillin 1 g i.v. plus gentamicin 120 mg i.v. at the onset of labour or induction followed by amoxycillin 500 mg i.v. six hours later. For patients who are allergic to penicillin or who have had a penicillin more than once in the preceding month, teicoplanin 400 mg i.v. and gentamicin 120 mg i.v. at the onset of labour or induction. Teicoplanin is easier to give and has lower side effects than vancomycin which was previously recommended though the use of teicoplanin may need sanction by the local infectious disease control team (Endocarditis Working Party of British Society for Antimicrobial Chemotherapy 1990).

SPECIFIC CONDITIONS OCCURRING DURING PREGNANCY

Chronic rheumatic heart disease

As already indicated, this form of heart disease has been commonest in pregnancy in the UK and still is in many parts of the world. By far the most important lesion is mitral stenosis, which may be the only lesion or the dominant abnormality amongst several others. Women with mitral stenosis are particularly likely to develop pulmonary oedema in pregnancy because of the increase in cardiac output, the increase in heart rate preventing ventricular filling and the increase in pulmonary blood volume. Mitral stenosis is the lesion that is most likely to require treatment for pulmonary oedema or heart failure and also to require surgery during pregnancy. The haemodynamic changes associated with labour in patients with mitral stenosis have been documented by Swan–Ganz catheterisation. Women entering labour with a wedge pressure (indirect left atrial pressure) less than 14 mmHg are unlikely to develop pulmonary oedema (Clark et al 1985).

Mitral regurgitation puts a volume load on the left atrium and left ventricle, but it does not cause pulmonary hyperten-

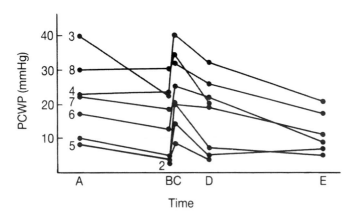

Fig. 17.1 Intrapartum alterations in pulmonary capillary wedge pressure (PCWP) in eight patients with mitral stenosis. A = First-stage labour; B = second-stage labour, 15–30 min before delivery; C = 5–15 min postpartum; D = 4–6 h postpartum; E = 18–20 h postpartum. From Clark et al (1985) with permission.

sion until late in the condition, and heart failure is rare in pregnancy; it occurs usually in older women. The major risk is the sudden development of atrial fibrillation.

Rheumatic aortic valve disease is much less common in women than in men and much less common than mitral valve disease in pregnancy. Severe aortic regurgitation causes pulmonary oedema; aortic stenosis may be associated with chest pain, syncope and sudden death, but aortic valve disease is usually not severe enough to be a problem in pregnancy. If aortic stenosis is severe it has a 17% maternal mortality (Ardias & Pineda 1978).

Disease of the tricuspid valve almost never occurs in isolation. Also, tricuspid valve disease rarely requires specific treatment; the patient improves when the rheumatic disease of the other valves is treated, either medically or surgically.

Pregnancy in women with artificial heart valves

Anticoagulation is the major problem in this group. Those who have successful isolated aortic or mitral valve replacements usually have near normal cardiac function and they do not incur haemodynamic problems in pregnancy. Even those with multiple valve replacements usually have sufficient cardiac reserve for a successful pregnancy.

The problem of anticoagulation is that warfarin is safest for the mother but dangerous for the fetus, whereas heparin, though safe for the fetus since it does not cross the placenta, may not give sufficient anticoagulation for the mother. In addition prolonged heparin therapy carries the risk of maternal bone demineralisation.

The fetal risks of warfarin are dose dependent. Vitale et al (1999) found only 12% full term healthy pregnancies in 25 women taking >5 mg warfarin per day; in those taking <5 mg warfarin per day the corresponding figures were 85% healthy babies from 33 pregnancies. The risks of warfarin include miscarriage, which occurs in up to 45% (Sadler et al 2000). Warfarin is teratogenic and in the first trimester causes a variety of abnormalities of which chondrodysplasia punctata, a cartilage defect, is the most specific. However, abnormalities of the central nervous system have also been described in women taking warfarin in the second trimester and these are serious: optic atrophy and microcephaly. Sudden intrauterine death is also a risk at this time. The cause of these problems is thought to be haemorrhagic; warfarin crosses the placenta freely and the fetus has a relatively immature clotting system. A level of warfarin that anticoagulates the mother appropriately is likely to overanticoagulate the fetus. Certainly gross fetal and retroplacental haemorrhage can be a problem in the third trimester and women should not deliver taking warfarin because of these fetal (and the maternal) risks. Nevertheless the fetal risks of maternal warfarin therapy should be kept in perspective. If the woman does not miscarry probably no more than 5% of fetuses will have birth defects.

Bioprosthetic valves usually do not require anticoagulation and would, therefore, appear to be the best choice for a woman requiring valve replacement before or during her reproductive life. Unfortunately these valves appear to deteriorate during pregnancy, particularly when inserted in the mitral position.

All these problems are well illustrated in a comprehensive study from Auckland, New Zealand (Sadler et al 2000). Pregnancy loss was 70% in pregnancies treated with warfarin compared with 25% for those who switched from warfarin to heparin. All four thromboembolic complications occurred in women treated with heparin throughout pregnancy. Structural valve deterioration occurred in 10% of 33 pregnancies where there was a bioprosthetic valve in the mitral position.

There is no ideal solution to this problem. Even though the risk of fetal defects persists after 16 weeks' gestation, warfarin should be used from before conception until about 37 weeks' gestation because subcutaneous heparin does not give adequate protection. The optimal INR with warfarin appears to be three times control. Any further prolongation does not decrease the thromboembolism risk but would further increase fetal risks.

Alternative approaches to management in early pregnancy are to use intravenous heparin given by a Hickman catheter or to use high-dose subcutaneous low molecular weight heparin. The aim should be to at least double the partial thromboplastin time (unfractionated heparin) or to achieve anti Xa levels four hours after dosing of 0.6–1.0 units/ml (low molecular weight heparin). Warfarin could then be restarted in the second trimester though some have attempted to continue anticoagulation throughout pregnancy with low molecular weight heparin.

Such treatment, which ideally should be given from before conception, must be considered experimental at present and it is unlikely to suit all women. In addition they must be warned of the risk of fracture from bone demineralisation which has been estimated to be 1–2% per pregnancy for unfractionated heparin, and 0.2% for low molecular weight heparin.

By 37 weeks the risks of fetal and maternal bleeding associated with labour and delivery in patients treated with warfarin are considerable. Therefore, the woman should be admitted to hospital and given continuous intravenous heparin to at least double the partial thromboplastin time. As indicated heparin does not cross the placenta and, therefore, it will not cause bleeding in the fetus. It is believed that the clotting system of the fetus will return to normal after warfarin has been withheld for one week. At that time maternal heparin therapy should be reduced to give a heparin level of less than 0.2 units/ml and a normal thrombin time. Under these circumstances the woman is not at risk of bleeding and labour should be induced. If the woman inadvertently goes into labour while taking warfarin, she should be given vitamin K to reverse the action of warfarin in the fetus, and started on heparin therapy as above. In extreme cases vitamin K has been given intramuscularly to the fetus in utero by transamniotic injection.

After delivery, because of the risk of maternal postpartum haemorrhage, the patient should continue to receive heparin alone for a few days aiming to achieve full anticoagulation with warfarin at about five days. Warfarin therapy is not a contraindication to breast feeding, since insignificant quantities of warfarin are secreted in breast milk. However, phenindione (Dindevan) is excreted in breast milk and women taking it should not breast feed.

Myocardial infarction

Myocardial infarction is rare in pregnancy (1 in 10 000 women or less) and in young women in general. However, it is an increasingly common cause of maternal mortality (Table 17.3). Often death is sudden and unexpected.

About 40% of women with acute myocardial infarction die in pregnancy or within one week of delivery. However, infarction occurring in the first two trimesters has a lower mortality (23%) than that occurring in the last trimester (45%) when the cause is often dissection of the coronary arteries or coronary thromboembolism unassociated with atheroma.

The diagnosis of myocardial infarction in pregnancy is made on the basis of chest pain, with possible pericardial friction rub and fever, supported by the typical changes in the electrocardiogram and enzyme changes. Moderate elevations of the white cell count and erythrocyte sedimentation rate are seen in normal pregnancy, when the level of lactic acid dehydrogenase may also be raised. The serum glutamine acid transaminase level may also be elevated because of contraction of the uterus and it is certainly elevated in the puerperium when the uterus is involuting. However, the creatine kinase MB isoenzyme is specific to heart muscle and is the test of choice for the diagnosis of myocardial infarction in pregnancy.

It is difficult to be dogmatic about management, for there is little experience and the pathology may be diverse. It would be sensible to treat the initial episode in a coronary care unit with aspirin, conventional opiate analgesics and medication for complications such as dysrhythmias. Because of the possibility of coronary spasm, nitroglycerine or other vasodilators should be used early in pregnant women with continuing pain. Once delivery has occurred, there is a good case for coronary arteriography. The angiographic demonstration of coronary embolus would be an indication for anticoagulation, but otherwise the benefits of anticoagulation in myocardial infarction associated with pregnancy do not seem great enough to justify the considerable extra risks imposed by warfarin on the pregnancy. High-dose subcutaneous low molecular weight heparin would remain a possible alternative. Streptokinase and other thrombolytic drugs are contraindicated because of the risk of bleeding. Spontaneous vaginal delivery should be allowed unless there are good obstetric reasons for interfering. Epidural anaesthesia should be used because of its efficacy as an analgesic and in reducing cardiac output by reducing pre-load. As in some other cases of heart disease, the second stage can be limited by forceps delivery. Syntocinon infusion should be used rather than ergometrine in the third stage, since ergometrine is more likely to cause coronary artery spasm.

There is no evidence that pregnancy specifically predisposes women to myocardial infarction. Unless it is thought that the woman has had a coronary embolus, pregnancy should not be discouraged in those who have had myocardial infarction in the past.

Cardiomyopathy in pregnancy

Cardiomyopathy may arise *de novo* during pregnancy, and there is probably at least one form of cardiomyopathy (peri-partum cardiomyopathy) that is specific to pregnancy. Alternatively, any form of cardiomyopathy from other causes may complicate pregnancy.

Hypertrophic obstructive cardiomyopathy

The most common of these other causes is hypertrophic obstructive cardiomyopathy, subaortic stenosis. The pathological features are hypertrophy and disorganisation of cardiac muscle, particularly that of the left ventricular outflow tract. Rapid advances are being made to understand the molecular and genetic basis of this disease. Patients present with chest pain, syncope, arrhythmias or the symptoms of heart failure. Diagnosis is based on echocardiographic features although within affected families electrocardiography is more sensitive in detecting those with the disorder.

Patients should not be allowed to become hypovolaemic, since this increases the risk of obstruction of the left ventricular outflow tract. Particular care should be taken to give adequate fluid replacement if there is antepartum haemorrhage and also in avoiding postpartum haemorrhage. During labour, those with hypertrophic obstructive cardiomyopathy should not have epidural anaesthesia, since this causes relative hypovolaemic by increasing venous capacitance in the lower limbs. Beta-blocking drugs are often used in women with symptoms and should be considered safe in pregnancy apart from the risk of intrauterine growth-restriction described with atenolol (see above).

Peripartum cardiomyopathy

The woman usually presents with heart failure either at the end of pregnancy or more commonly in the puerperium (Fig. 17.2). There is no predisposing cause for the heart failure and the heart is grossly dilated. The pathogenesis is unknown; immunological, nutritional and infective aetiologies have been proposed.

The diagnosis is made by excluding all other causes of right and left ventricular dysfunction. Patients tend to be

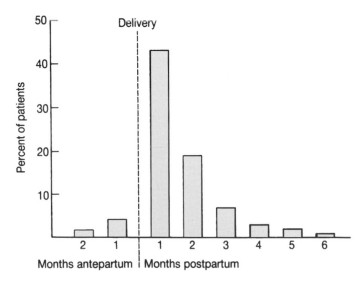

Fig. 17.2 Onset of peripartum cardiomyopathy in relation to time of delivery. From Homans (1985) with permission.

multiparous, black, relatively elderly and socially deprived. Pregnancy has often been complicated by hypertension. Pulmonary, peripheral and particularly cerebral embolisation are major causes of morbidity and mortality. Apart from conventional treatment for cardiac failure, these women should also receive anticoagulant therapy until heart size has returned to normal, and until they have no further dysrhythmias. Immunosuppressive therapy with prednisone and azathioprine has been used to improve left ventricular function. If they recover from the initial episode, the long-term prognosis is good, but the condition may recur in future pregnancies, particularly if there is evidence of even subclinical left ventricular dysfunction.

A specific form of peripartum cardiac failure occurs in the Hausa tribe in northern Nigeria. The peak incidence is four weeks postpartum. During this period, for up to 40 days after delivery, the Hausa woman spends 18 h/day lying on a mud bed, heated so that the ambient temperature reaches 40°C. She also increases her sodium intake to 450 mmol/day by eating *kanwa* salt from Lake Chad. Many are hypertensive, but the condition regresses rapidly with diuretic and digoxin therapy (Davidson & Parry 1978). The contribution of hypertension to the heart failure is debated but this would seem an extreme example of the instability of the cardiovascular system in the first few weeks of the puerperium interacting with the particular susceptibility of West Africans to dilated cardiomyopathy.

Eisenmenger's syndrome

Eisenmenger's syndrome has a very high maternal mortality, particularly if there is superimposed pre-eclampsia. The condition arises following a large left to right shunt (typically ASD, VSD, patent ductus) which reverses as a consequence of the subsequent increase in pulmonary vascular resistance. Only recently has there been any form of surgical treatment—heart and lung transplantation—and that must be considered experimental.

Most of those with Eisenmenger's syndrome who die do so in the puerperium. Although death may be occasionally sudden and caused by thromboembolism, this is unusual. More frequently, these women die because of a slowly falling systemic P_{O_2} with associated decrease in cardiac output. It is likely that this is caused by a change in the shunt ratio whereby pulmonary blood flow decreases at the expense of systemic blood flow (Fig. 17.3).

What can be offered to the pregnant woman with Eisenmenger's syndrome? Unfortunately, termination of pregnancy would appear to be the answer. The maternal mortality associated with this is only 7% in comparison to 30% for continuing pregnancy. However, if she decides to continue with pregnancy, prophylactic anticoagulation, probably with subcutaneous heparin, should be offered, because of the risk of systemic and pulmonary thromboembolism. Labour should not be induced unless there are good obstetric reasons. Induced labour carries a higher risk of caesarean section, which is associated with a particularly high maternal mortality in Eisenmenger's syndrome.

There is controversy concerning the place of epidural anaesthesia for the management of labour. Although epidural anaesthesia could decrease the shunt ratio by decreasing systemic vascular resistance, this is not invariable. On balance, an elective epidural anaesthetic carefully administered at the beginning of labour is probably preferable to emergency epidural or general anaesthesia, necessary if a sudden decision is made to perform instrumental delivery.

If the woman does become hypotensive with increasing cyanosis and decreasing cardiac output, high inspired oxygen concentrations will decrease pulmonary vascular resistance, increasing the pulmonary blood flow and increasing peripheral oxygen saturation. In addition, alpha-sympathomimetic agents, such as phenylephrine, methoxamine and noradrenaline, will increase systemic resistance and thus divert blood to the lungs. However, drugs such as tolazoline, phentolamine, nitroprusside and isoprenaline, which have been used to decrease pulmonary vascular resistance in other clinical situations, probably should not be given since they will also decrease the systemic vascular resistance. The same problem may occur with dopamine and beta-sympathomimetic drugs that have been given to increase cardiac output.

Intravenous prostacyclin and inhaled nitric oxide, which have been used successfully to reduce pulmonary vascular resistance in both newborn babies and adults with other conditions, have not been helpful in the majority of cases of deteriorating Eisenmenger's syndrome.

Coarctation of the aorta and Marfan's syndrome

In both these conditions, the maternal risk is of dissection of the aorta associated with the hyperdynamic circulation of pregnancy and possibly with an increased risk of medial degeneration as a result of the hormonal environment of pregnancy. Although earlier studies of coarctation indicated

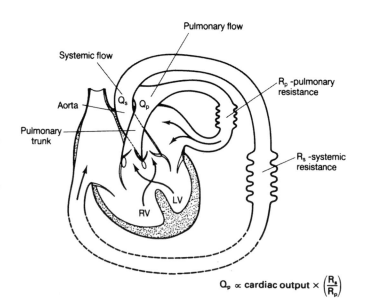

Fig. 17.3 Pulmonary (Q_p) and systemic (Q_s) blood flows and resistances (R_p, R_s) in Eisenmenger's syndrome associated with ventricular septal defect. From de Swiet & Fidler (1981) with permission.

a high maternal mortality, they date from the period before surgery was available for correction of severe cases.

Only those who already have evidence of dissection should have the coarctation repaired in pregnancy. Any upper limb hypertension should be treated aggressively with beta blocking antihypertensive drugs. If there is gross widening of the ascending aorta, suggesting intrinsic disease, the baby should be delivered by elective caesarean section to reduce the risk of dissection associated with labour.

In Marfan's syndrome there is also a risk of dissection of the aorta. In one series this occurred in four of 91 pregnancies in 36 women and was not necessarily proceeded by aortic root dilatation (Lipscomb et al 1997). Dilatation of the aorta to more than 40 mm (determined echocardiographically) is the limit at which pregnancy is contraindicated (Pyeritz 1981). As in coarctation of the aorta, any associated hypertension should be treated aggressively with beta blockade and delivery should be by caesarean section if there is evidence of aortic disease.

Congenital heart block

This usually presents no problem in pregnancy. Although part of the normal response to pregnancy includes an increase in heart rate to increase the cardiac output, this is not obligatory. There are many records of successful pregnancy among those with heart block. Presumably patients are able to increase stroke volume sufficiently to cope with the increased demands of pregnancy. A few are unable to increase cardiac output sufficiently at the end of pregnancy or during labour, therefore, women with heart block who are not paced, or those in whom there is any possibility of pacemaker failure, should be managed in obstetric units where there is access to pacing facilities.

CONCLUSIONS

Heart disease in pregnancy remains a worrying problem for the obstetrician because of those women (very much in the minority) who are at risk. Future advances will help us to define this minority with more precision and optimise management strategies for these patients.

KEY POINTS

- Heart disease is a significant cause of maternal mortality.
- It is best managed in a combined clinic attended by an obstetrician and a physician.
- Initial assessment can be clinical only, though echocardiography is pivotal to management of those with significant heart disease.
- Consider termination for Eisenmenger's syndrome and other causes of pulmonary hypertension.
- Anticoagulation is a major problem: warfarin is safest for the mother, heparin is safer for the fetus.
- Vaginal delivery is preferred but elective caesarean section may be best for selected cases.

REFERENCES

Ardias F, Pineda J 1978 Aortic stenosis and pregnancy. J Reprod Med 20:229–232

Becker RM 1983 Intracardiac surgery in pregnant women. An Thoracic Surgery 36:453–458

Burn J, Brennan P, Little J 1998 Recurrence risks in offspring of adults with major heart defects: results from first cohort of British collaborative study. Lancet 351:311–316

Chesley LC 1980 Severe rheumatic cardiac disease and pregnancy: the ultimate prognosis. Am J Obstet Gynecol 136:552–558

Clark SL, Phelan JP, Greenspoon J, Aldahl D, Horenstein J 1985 Labor and delivery in the presence of mitral stenosis: central hemodynamic observations. Am J Obstet Gynecol 152:984–1088

Davidson NMcD, Parry EHO 1978 Peripartum cardiac failure. Quart J Med 47:431–461

Davies P, Francis RI, Docker MF, Watt JM, Selwyn Crawford J 1986 Analysis of impedance cardiography longitudinally applied in pregnancy. Br J Obstet Gynaecol 93:717–720

Department of Health and Social Security 1998 Report on Confidential Enquiries into Maternal Deaths in England and Wales 1994–1996. HMSO, London

Endocarditis Working Party of British Society for Antimicrobial Chemotherapy 1990 Antibiotic prophylaxis of infective endocarditis. Recommendations from the Endocarditis Working Party of the British Society for Antimicrobial Chemotherapy. Lancet 335:88–89

Gleicher N, Midwall J, Hochberger D, Jaffin H 1979 Eisenmenger's syndrome and pregnancy. Obstet Gynecol Survey 34:721–741

Kaluarachchi A, Senviratne HR 1995 Heart disease in pregnancy-evaluation of disease pattern and outcome in Sri Lanka. J Obstet Gynaecol 15:9–14

Lipscomb KJ, Smith JC, Clarke B, Donnai P, Harris R 1997 Outcome of pregnancy in women with Marfan's syndrome. Br J Obstet Gynaecol 104:210–216

Morgan Jones A, Howitt G 1965 Eisenmenger syndrome in pregnancy. Br Med J 1:1627–1631

Morley CA, Lim BA 1995 The risks of delay in diagnosis of breathlessness in pregnancy. Br Med J 311:1083–1084

Nora JJ 1978 The evolution of specific genetic and environmental counselling in congenital heart disease. Circulation 57:205–213

Oakley CM 1997 Heart Disease in Pregnancy. BMJ Publishing Group, London

Pyeritz RE 1981 Maternal and fetal complications of pregnancy in the Marfan syndrome. Am J Med 71:784–790

Robson SC, Hunter S, Boys RJ, Dunlop W 1989 Serial study of factors influencing changes in cardiac output during human pregnancy. Am J Physiol 256:H1060–H1065

Rubler S, Prabod Kumar MD, Pinto ER 1977 Cardiac size and performance during pregnancy estimated with echocardiography. Am J Cardiol 40:534–540

Sadler L, McCowan L, White H, Stewart A, Bracken M, North R 2000 Pregnancy outcomes and cardiac complications in women with mechanical, bioprosthetic and homograft valves. Br J Obstet Gynaecol 107:245–253

Sugrue D, Blake S, MacDonald D 1981 Pregnancy complicated by maternal heart disease at the National Maternity Hospital, Dublin, Ireland, 1969 to 1978. Am J Obstet Gynecol 139:1–6

de Swiet M 1995 Heart disease in pregnancy in medical disorders in obstetric practice de Swiet (ed) Blackwell Science, Oxford pp 143–81

Szekely P, Turner R, Snaith L 1973 Pregnancy and the changing pattern of rheumatic heart disease. Br Heart J 35:1293–1303

Tan J, de Swiet M 1998 Prevalence of heart disease diagnosed de novo in pregnancy in a West London population. Br J Obstet Gynaecol 105:1185–1188

Vitale N, De Feo M, De Santo LS, Pollice A, Tedesco N, Cotrufo M 1999 Dose-dependant Fetal Complications of Warfarin in Pregnant Women with Mechanical Heart Valves. J Am Coll Cardiology 33:1637–41

Whittemore R, Hobbins JC, Engle MA 1982 Pregnancy and its outcome in women with and without surgical treatment of congenital heart disease. Am J Cardiol 50:641–651

Yentis SM, Steer PJ, Plaat F 1998 Eisenmenger's syndrome in pregnancy: maternal and fetal mortality in the 1990s. Br J Obstet Gynaecol 105:921–922

18

Medical disorders in pregnancy

Catherine Nelson-Piercy, Catherine Williamson

The contribution of the author of the equivalent chapter in the second edition, on which this chapter draws extensively, is gratefully acknowledged.

Most women of an age group who have babies in the UK are fit and have no underlying medical problems. This is not so all over the world. Pregnancy has an effect on the progress of such conditions, while they in their turn may affect the pregnancy and its management. The major ones are considered in this chapter.

DIABETES MELLITUS

Introduction

Diabetes mellitus occurs as a consequence of either insulin deficiency or peripheral resistance to the action of insulin resulting in hyperglycaemia. Symptoms of marked hyperglycaemia include polyuria, polydipsia, weight loss and blurred vision, and the life-threatening complication of ketoacidosis. Long-term consequences of diabetes mellitus include retinopathy, nephropathy, peripheral neuropathy and autonomic neuropathy. Outside pregnancy, the condition can be broadly divided into two major categories, insulin-dependent diabetes mellitus (IDDM, type 1 diabetes) and non-insulin dependent diabetes mellitus (NIDDM, type 2 diabetes). Individuals with IDDM have an absolute deficiency of insulin, and can often be identified by serological evidence of autoimmune destruction of the pancreatic islets and by genetic markers. NIDDM is much commoner and is caused by peripheral insulin resistance and an inability to compensate by increasing insulin secretion. Individuals with NIDDM can have hyperglycaemia for a long period of time without clinical symptoms. It is therefore important to screen for possible occult long-term complications of the condition at the time of diagnosis. Gestational diabetes mellitus (GDM) develops as a consequence of the increased insulin resistance of pregnancy, and resolves postpartum; however, there is considerable overlap with NIDDM, and women with GDM are at increased risk of developing NIDDM in later life.

There are different priorities in the management of pregnant women with IDDM, NIDDM and GDM, although there are considerable areas of overlap in the management strategies. Most established diabetics in the UK will have IDDM, although the prevalence of NIDDM in pregnancy is increasing, partly due to women having children at an older age. Also, NIDDM is commoner in women of Asian and Middle Eastern origin.

Carbohydrate and lipid metabolism in pregnancy

Normal pregnancy is associated with altered maternal glucose homeostasis and metabolism. Many of the changes are a result of the progressive rise in the levels of oestrogen, progesterone, human placental lactogen, cortisol and prolactin as pregnancy advances. Many of these hormones are insulin antagonists, causing insulin resistance in the mother, and this is most marked in the last trimester. This results in a doubling of insulin secretion from the end of the first trimester to the third trimester (Maresh et al 1995) to keep the maternal plasma glucose level stable. These changes are likely to underlie the increased insulin requirements of established diabetics, and the development of abnormal glucose tolerance in gestational diabetics, in whom there is insufficient insulin secretion to compensate for the insulin resistance.

Every aspect of lipid metabolism is affected by pregnancy, particularly free fatty acids, triglycerides, phospholipids and cholesterol. The plasma level of free fatty acids falls from early to mid-pregnancy and subsequently shows a significant rise. The same is true of the plasma level of glycerol. This is in keeping with the accumulation of body fat that occurs during the anabolic phase of pregnancy (first two trimesters). In the catabolic phase of pregnancy (last trimester), raised free fatty acid and glycerol level are available as fuel to the maternal tissues to offset the increasing diversion to the rapidly growing fetus of glucose and amino acids. Also, in normal pregnancy, starvation results in early breakdown of triglyceride, resulting in the liberation of fatty acids and ketone bodies. Free fatty acids and glycerol levels fall postpartum, followed by a rise during breast-feeding, presumably to allow similar diversion of the ingested maternal nutrients for the synthesis of breast milk. As with free fatty acids, glycerol and triglycerides, plasma levels of cholesterol and phospholipid are also increased in pregnancy.

Glycosuria

Glycosuria is common in pregnancy, starting within 6 weeks of the last menstrual period. This is due to a decreased renal tubular threshold for glucose. There is a tendency for glycosuria to increase as pregnancy advances but there is a great deal of diurnal and day-to-day variation in excretion rate. There is no constant relationship between urinary and blood glucose levels. Therefore, glycosuria is not a reliable diagnostic tool for impaired glucose tolerance or diabetes in pregnancy.

Fetomaternal blood glucose relationships

Glucose crosses the placenta by a process of facilitated diffusion, and therefore fetal plasma glucose levels are similar to those of the mother, usually being 0.5 mmol/l lower, providing the maternal plasma glucose is ≤13 mmol/l. The glucose transport mechanism becomes saturated above this level, so if there is more marked maternal hyperglycaemia, the fetal plasma glucose will not rise (Oakley et al 1972). Fetal insulin secretion occurs from 10 weeks' gestation, but in the fetus of a non-diabetic mother insulin does not play a significant role in glucose homeostasis; however, in diabetic pregnancy, there is a brisk fetal insulin response to raised plasma glucose levels and sustained fetal hyperglycaemia secondary to maternal hyperglycaemia can result in fetal β-cell hyperplasia (Maresh et al 1995).

Diagnostic criteria for IDDM, NIDDM and GDM

Most established diabetics will have been diagnosed before attendance at the antenatal clinic. New diagnostic criteria proposed by the Expert Committee on the Diagnosis and Classification of Diabetes Mellitus (Report 1997), are summarised in Table 18.1. New-onset IDDM rarely needs an oral glucose tolerance test (OGTT) for diagnosis in pregnancy. Because the maximum age of incidence is 11–14 years, most women have been diagnosed and are taking insulin before

Table 18.1 Criteria for the diagnosis of diabetes mellitus and impaired glucose tolerance

Diagnosis of diabetes mellitus
If one of these criteria is met, it must be confirmed on a subsequent day by any of the three criteria below:
- Symptoms of diabetes plus casual plasma glucose ≥ 11.1 mmol/l. Causal is defined as any time of the day without regard to time since last meal
- Fasting plasma glucose ≥ 7.0 mmol/l. Fasting is defined as no caloric intake for at least 8 h
- 2 h plasma glucose ≥ 11.1 mmol/l during an oral glucose tolerance test (OGTT). The test should be performed using a 75 g glucose load dissolved in water

Diagnosis of impaired glucose tolerance
- 2 h plasma glucose ≥ 7.8 mmol/l, and < 11.1 mmol/l during an OGTT, performed as described above

Diagnosis of impaired fasting glucose
- Fasting plasma glucose ≥ 6.1 mmol/l and < 7.0 mmol/l. Fasting is defined as described above

From Report of the Expert Committee on the Diagnosis and Classification of Diabetes Mellitus (1997).

they become pregnant. A few women develop IDDM in pregnancy; indeed it is more common to develop IDDM in pregnancy than in the non-pregnant state in women of childbearing age. The diagnosis is rarely in doubt for such women, as they are usually symptomatic at presentation with very high blood sugars and often keto-acidosis (Buschard et al 1990).

NIDDM is important because it carries risks for the fetus almost as great as those of IDDM. Since the patients are often not symptomatic, an OGTT is necessary for diagnosis and the possibility of diagnosing NIDDM is probably the only valid justification for a glycaemic screen in all patients. In White Europeans the prevalence of NIDDM in this age group is so low that such a universal screen is not justified. In Asians (Mather & Keen 1985) and Afro-Caribbeans (Dooley et al 1991) the prevalence is higher and such patients should probably be screened in pregnancy. A positive OGTT does not differentiate between NIDDM and GDM, and the differential diagnosis can only be made postpartum.

The plasma glucose level at which gestational diabetes GDM is diagnosed varies in different centres and in different countries (Nelson-Piercy & Gale 1994). It is generally accepted that GDM should be treated, but there is no consensus about the management, or the clinical relevance, of lesser degrees of gestational impaired glucose tolerance (IGT). Briefly, there have been two recent studies of whether intensive treatment alters the maternal and fetal prognosis in GDM; the larger study demonstrated no significant differences (Garner et al 1997), but the smaller study revealed that improved glycaemic control reduced the incidence of neonatal hypoglycaemia, macrosomia and caesarean section (de Veciana et al 1995). These studies are discussed in more detail on page 278.

Glycosylated haemoglobin and fructosamine

The level of HbA$_{1c}$ is raised in diabetes, reflecting diabetic control over the previous 2 or 3 months. HbA$_{1c}$ estimation has proved a valuable additional aid to good control and, when elevated in early pregnancy, serves as a warning to the obstetrician to be alert for major congenital abnormality.

Fructosamine is glycosylated albumin. It reflects the mean blood glucose over a period of 2 weeks rather than 3 months as in the case of glycosylated haemoglobin. Fructosamine levels are insensitive as a predictor of abnormal glucose tolerance in pregnancy (Comtois et al 1989, Roberts et al 1990) or of fetal hyperinsulinaemia (Hofmann 1990) but may be of use in the management of diabetes to confirm home blood glucose monitoring (Roberts et al 1988), particularly when short-term changes in mean blood glucose are anticipated.

Effect of pregnancy on established diabetes mellitus

Once an established diabetic is pregnant there is increased insulin requirement due to the insulin resistance of pregnancy. Most pregnant diabetics succeed in improving their control, and this can be associated with an increased risk of hypoglycaemia (Nelson-Piercy 1997). Diabetic nephropathy and retinopathy can deteriorate, but most changes are reversible postpartum. The altered carbohydrate metabolism of pregnancy can result in an increased risk of keto-acidosis. The management of these complications of diabetic pregnancy is discussed in more detail below.

Effect of diabetes mellitus on pregnancy

Diabetic pregnancy is associated with an increased risk of congenital malformation and this is directly related to the degree of diabetic control at conception and during the first trimester (Casson et al 1997, Hawthorne et al 1997). The congenital malformation rate is up to 10 times higher than non-diabetic pregnancy (Casson et al 1997), and the commonest abnormalities are cardiac and neural tube defects. Caudal regression syndrome is specific to diabetes, but rare.

Later pregnancy complications include macrosomia, polyhydramnios and unexplained stillbirth. Macrosomia can result in an increased risk of traumatic vaginal delivery, shoulder dystocia and caesarean section. In addition there is an approximately threefold increased incidence of preterm delivery (<37 weeks), but this is partly iatrogenic. Such late pregnancy complications are usually associated with poor glycaemic control and can affect women with GDM as well as established diabetics, although the level of risk in gestational IGT and GDM is controversial.

There is increased neonatal morbidity following diabetic pregnancy, including hypoglycaemia (Hod et al 1991), polycythemia (Mimouni et al 1986, Hod et al 1991), jaundice (Hod et al 1991), hypocalcaemia and hypomagnesaemia (Hod et al 1991). There is no large study to prove that respiratory distress syndrome (RDS) of the newborn is commoner in diabetic pregnancy; however, one study reported it more commonly in the babies of women with IDDM who were delivered by caesarean section (Midovnik et al 1987).

Medical management of diabetic pregnancy

Ideally diabetic women should receive prepregnancy counselling and be advised to optimise their glycaemic control before conception. At this time the presence of pre-existing diabetic complications can be assessed and any necessary treatment given. Women with NIDDM may be overweight and are more likely to have coexistent hypertension or dyslipidaemia, and if necessary these can be tackled at the same time.

Women with pre-existing diabetes should be counselled with regard to the maternal and fetal risks of diabetic pregnancy and the importance of good glycaemic control. Dietary advice should be given and they should start home capillary blood glucose monitoring, aiming for fasting levels <5.5 mmol/l and 2 hour postprandial levels of <7 mmol/l. Women with NIDDM who are taking oral hypoglycaemic drugs may be changed to insulin therapy. In women with IDDM or NIDDM a treatment regimen which allows optimal glycaemic control should be used, and for the majority this will mean using a pre-bedtime longer acting insulin, such as Insulatard, and three pre-meal injections of a fast acting insulin, such as

Human Actrapid. This allows maximal flexibility in altering the insulin dose to compensate for the increased requirements as pregnancy progresses, and the achievement of good glycaemic control. A recent study in which pregnant women with pre-existing diabetes and GDM were randomised to receive either a four-dose regimen, or twice-daily insulin (a mixed short- and medium-acting insulin), demonstrated that glycaemic control was better with the four times daily regimen (Nachum et al 1999).

Increasing numbers of women with IDDM are taking the recently introduced short-acting insulin analogue lispro instead of conventional fast acting preparations. Although there have been two case reports of congenital malformations in pregnancies where the mother was treated with lispro (Diamond & Kormas 1997), it should be remembered that IDDM is associated with an increased risk of congenital anomalies, and there have been no other reports of adverse maternal or fetal events associated with lispro. One study comparing lispro and regular insulin as part of a basal bolus regimen in 42 women with GDM found fewer hypoglycaemic episodes in women treated with lispro and no fetal or neonatal abnormalities in either group (Jovanovic et al 1999).

Most women with gestational diabetes are initially given dietary advice and taught capillary blood glucose monitoring. If their glycaemic control remains suboptimal they are started on insulin and managed in the same way as established diabetics. There is considerable debate about the need for and type of treatment in GDM. A randomised trial of 300 women with GDM compared strict glycaemic control and tertiary level obstetric care with routine obstetric care, and despite lower maternal glucose levels in the treatment group there was no significant difference in birthweight, birth trauma, neonatal hypoglycaemia or other fetal metabolic abnormality (Garner et al 1997). However, a randomised trial comparing preprandial and postprandial glucose measurement in 66 insulin-treated gestational diabetics demonstrated that the achievement of improved glycaemic control using postprandial glucose measurement reduces the incidence of neonatal hypoglycaemia, macrosomia and caesarean section (de Veciana et al 1995). In summary, there is no consensus on the optimal management of IGT/GDM at present, but it is hoped that the results of further large randomised controlled studies will be available soon.

Angiotensin-converting enzyme inhibitors

Angiotensin-converting enzyme inhibitors (ACEI) are commonly used for the treatment of hypertension and diabetic nephropathy, and women with established diabetes may conceive while taking these drugs. Use of ACEI in the second and third trimesters of pregnancy has been reported to cause a pattern of fetal defects termed ACEI fetopathy. The commonest feature of ACEI fetopathy is renal tubular dysplasia. It is also associated with intrauterine growth restriction (IUGR) and a patent ductus arteriosus with fetal hypocalvaria. Two recent studies have not demonstrated features of fetopathy in pregnancies where ACEIs were only used in the first trimester (Centers for Disease Control and Prevention 1997, Steffensen et al 1998). Therefore, most authors would not advise against the use of ACEIs in women of childbearing age, but recommend either changing treatment before conception, or cessation of treatment as soon as pregnancy is confirmed.

Diabetic complications

Established diabetics who become pregnant should be assessed for the presence of the complications of nephropathy, retinopathy and neuropathy. In women with nephropathy, renal function should be closely monitored using serum creatinine, creatinine clearance, 24 h urinary protein and the clinical features of proteinuria, hypertension and fluid retention. There may be a transient worsening of renal function, and there is usually an increase in pre-existing proteinuria, which subsequently improve in the postpartum period. Diabetic nephropathy is associated with IUGR, low birthweight, premature delivery and pre-eclampsia (Kitzmiller et al 1981, Landon & Gabbe 1996). The presence of either proteinuria (>3.0 g/24 h), serum creatinine >135 μmol/l, anaemia (haematocrit <25%), or hypertension (mean arterial pressure >107 mmHg) before 20 weeks' gestation are predictive of a poor perinatal outcome (Landon & Gabbe 1996). Several cases of diabetic pregnancy following renal transplantation have been reported (Penn et al 1980, Grenfell et al 1986). It should be borne in mind that the long-term prospects for patients with diabetic renal disease are not generally good and many will require renal transplantation or long-term dialysis when the disease has progressed.

Most women who have had diabetes for more than 15 years will have retinopathy. This will not be seriously affected by pregnancy in the majority of women, but in approximately 50% there will be some worsening of the retinopathy (Serup 1986), although most cases resolve postpartum. The risk is increased with bad metabolic control, diastolic hypertension, renal disease, anaemia, rapid reduction of HbA_{1c} and severity of baseline retinopathy. The progression of retinopathy is due to the rapid improvement of diabetic control, and to the increased retinal blood flow which may be secondary to abnormal autoregulation in diabetics (Nelson-Piercy 1997). Women should have ophthalmoscopy performed during each trimester and if sight-threatening retinopathy is detected urgent ophthalmological consultation should be requested.

Peripheral neuropathy is present in some pregnant women but rarely causes problems with the pregnancy. Conversely, those with autonomic neuropathy and gastric paresis often experience deterioration of their symptoms in pregnancy.

Diabetic keto-acidosis

In a recent series of 635 insulin treated diabetic pregnancies, the prevalence of diabetic keto-acidosis was estimated at 2% (Kilvert et al 1993). The majority of admissions with keto-acidosis occur in women who have had diabetes for over 5 years and who are ill with a problem other than their diabetes, e.g. influenza or another infection (Cousins 1988). Fetal mortality has been quoted as approximately 30%, with much higher rates in association with coma. In a recent series of 20 cases of keto-acidosis in women with IDDM, the fetal loss rate was 35%, and this was associated with later gestational age, poor glycaemic control, higher blood urea nitrogen and a longer duration of features of keto-acidosis (Montoro et al 1993). Treatment of keto-acidosis should be the same as in non-pregnant women. The risk of keto-acidosis is increased when diabetic women are treated with drugs which cause hyperglycaemia, such as dexamethasone to induce fetal lung maturity (Bedalov & Balasubramanyam 1997), or β-agonists for preterm labour (Kilvert et al 1993). Therefore, diabetic women receiving these treatments should increase the frequency of blood glucose monitoring and check for urinary ketones. Indeed, since dexamethasone and i.v. β-agonists may induce hyperglycaemia, the blood glucose should be measured in all women being treated in this way for preterm labour.

Hypoglycaemia

Women with IDDM are at increased risk of hypoglycaemia as a consequence of improving their glycaemic control, and should be given i.m. glucagon and counselled on its use. Women with NIDDM are less likely to have hypoglycaemic episodes as they will be more insulin-resistant. Severe hypoglycaemia can result in confusion, coma or seizures. If there is any clinical suspicion of hypoglycaemia, the capillary blood glucose should be checked immediately and a laboratory glucose sent for confirmation, in addition to a biochemical profile. Women should be treated with oral dextrose if they are able to eat and drink, and otherwise with 50 ml 50% dextrose and/or glucagon 1 mg i.v., i.m. or s.c. Hypoglycaemia rarely causes fetal distress and there have been no conclusive studies to prove that it is associated with fetal abnormality.

Obstetric management of diabetic pregnancy

It is important for all diabetic women to have an early scan to provide accurate gestational dating, as this will be required to assess fetal growth, and to ensure accurate timing of delivery. Dating is best performed in the first trimester; if available, this can be at the same time as the nuchal translucency scan for abnormalities. Detailed anomaly scans at 18–20 weeks' gestation and fetal echocardiograms should be offered because of the increased risk of congenital abnormalities. Serial scans should be performed regularly (every 4 weeks routinely and every 2 weeks if an abnormality is found) in the third trimester to assess growth and liquor volume. Blood pressure monitoring and urinalysis for protein should be performed regularly to screen for pre-eclampsia and/or renal dysfunction.

Management of labour and delivery in diabetic pregnancy

There should be close fetal monitoring throughout labour, even in mothers with good glycaemic control. Many units have a policy of delivering established diabetics by 38–39 weeks' gestation to reduce the risk of birth trauma and neonatal complications. In one study, women with uncomplicated insulin-treated diabetes and GDM were randomised

to have either expectant management or elective delivery by 38+5 weeks' gestation. Expectant management resulted in an increased prevalence of large-for-gestational-age infants (23 versus 10%) and shoulder dystocia (3% vs 0%) (Kjos et al 1993). The authors recommend that delivery should therefore be contemplated at 38 weeks and the pregnancy only be allowed to continue if fetal size appears normal (Kjos et al 1993). In an Irish report of conservative management of labour in 276 diabetic pregnancies (Rasmussen et al 1992), the mean gestation at delivery was 39 weeks, with 83% of deliveries occurring at ≥38 weeks and 41% at ≥40 weeks. There were 16 perinatal deaths in this series, including five deaths of normally formed infants after 38 weeks' gestation. All these five were preceded by clinically apparent polyhydramnios or macrosomia and poor glycaemic control. The authors of this study do not advocate elective delivery before 37 weeks' gestation, but emphasise the importance of good diabetic control and close fetal surveillance, with the use of polyhydramnios and macrosomia as indicators of risk approaching term in diabetic pregnancies.

The rate of caesarean section is considerably higher in diabetic women, occurring in up to 50% (Landon & Gabbe 1996). One factor that contributes to the high caesarean section rate is failed early induction of labour; however, there are no large studies to support delivery by caesarean simply because a woman has insulin-treated diabetes or GDM. One study compared the mode of delivery of 122 pregnancies in 100 women with IDDM to investigate whether this influenced the rate of neonatal polycythaemia, hyperbilirubinaemia, respiratory distress syndrome, or hypoglycaemia (Midovnik et al 1987). The women were divided into three groups according to whether they had a planned caesarean section, a caesarean section following spontaneous or induced labour, or a vaginal delivery. The rate of neonatal polycythemia was significantly lower in both caesarean section groups, and that of neonatal hyperbilirubinaemia was significantly lower in the planned caesarean section group; however, the risk of respiratory distress syndrome was significantly higher in this latter group, even when corrected for gestational age and Apgar scores.

Overall, there is little evidence from randomised controlled trials to support either elective delivery or expectant management at term in pregnant women with insulin-requiring diabetes (Boulvain et al 2000). Most units reserve caesarean section for cases with an obstetric indication.

Established diabetics and most insulin-requiring gestational diabetics are best managed with i.v. infusion of both insulin and glucose during labour given with two separate infusion sets. The infusion should provide 500 ml of fluid every 8 h. The woman's capillary blood glucose should be estimated hourly, and the insulin infusion rate altered accordingly. A standardised regimen, using i.v. infusions of dextrose and of insulin via a sliding scale, was evaluated in the management of labour and delivery in 25 insulin-treated diabetic women, and was found to be clinically reliable for both midwifery and medical staff (Lean et al

1990). Combined glucose, insulin and potassium (GIK) infusions are advocated by some authors in preference to separate i.v. infusions of dextrose and insulin via a sliding scale in diabetics undergoing surgical procedures. However, there are no studies evaluating GIK regimens in pregnancy, and given that the current regimens are used successfully and extensively, the authors recommend the use of separate i.v. infusions of both insulin and glucose. Established diabetics should have the rate of the i.v. insulin infusion halved at the time of delivery of the placenta. Women with diet-treated GDM should have their capillary blood glucose checked every 2 h and, if this rises above 10 mmol/l, they should be managed in the same way as insulin-requiring diabetics. The newborn is at risk of hypoglycaemia and should be closely monitored.

Once women with IDDM are eating normally, subcutaneous insulin should be recommended at either the prepregnancy dose, or at 25% lower dose than this if the women intend to breast-feed. Most established diabetics are capable of adjusting their own insulin doses and can be advised that tight glycaemic control is not as important during the postpartum period. Women with NIDDM can either continue insulin treatment until they finish breast-feeding or return to oral hypoglycaemics. There is a theoretical possibility that oral hypoglycaemics can pass to the neonate in breast milk but in clinical practice this appears to be insignificant. Women should be counselled with regard to the importance of good glycaemic control should they wish to conceive again, and it may be appropriate to continue to use insulin. Women with GDM should have an oral glucose tolerance test performed 6–12 weeks postpartum and should be advised that they have a risk of developing diabetes in later life of approximately 50% (Dornhurst et al 1990). This risk may be reduced by avoiding obesity. Women of Asian or Afro-Caribbean origin develop subsequent diabetes sooner than those of White european origin. The risk of developing GDM in a subsequent pregnancy is almost 100%.

Conclusions

Diabetic pregnancy is associated with increased maternal and fetal risks and these can be reduced by education and close surveillance of the diabetic mother from preconception until the postpartum period. There should be joint management of the pregnancy by a team including obstetricians, specialist physicians, midwives, diabetes specialist nurses and dieticians. Nephropathy and retinopathy can deteriorate during pregnancy, but this is usually reversible postpartum. If pregnancy in a woman with pre-existing diabetes is allowed to continue past 38 weeks' gestation, close surveillance for macrosomia and polyhydramnios is advised, but there is no consensus that women should be delivered by caesarean section solely because they are diabetic. Labour should be managed with i.v. insulin and a dextrose infusion, and women with GDM should be managed in a similar manner if their blood glucose rises above 10 mmol/l.

KEY POINTS: DIABETES

- Diabetic pregnancy should be jointly managed by a team including specialist obstetricians, physicians and anaesthetists.
- Women with pre-existing diabetes should aim for optimum control from the time of conception.
- There should be regular surveillance for the maternal and fetal complications of diabetic pregnancy.
- If pregnancy progresses past 38 weeks' gestation in an established diabetic, there should be close surveillance for macrosomia, polyhydramnios and pre-eclampsia.
- Most diabetics require an increased insulin dose as pregnancy progresses, and treatment with i.v. insulin and dextrose to cover labour. The insulin dose usually returns to the prepregnancy level immediately postpartum and may require further reduction with breast-feeding.

THYROID

Physiological changes

During pregnancy hepatic synthesis of thyroid-binding globulin (TBG) is increased, while total levels of thyroxine (T_4) and tri-iodothyronine (T_3) are increased to compensate for this rise. Levels of free T_4 are not substantially altered, although there is a small reduction in the third trimester. Normal ranges for free T_4 are: non-pregnant 9–23 pmol/l, first trimester 10–24 pmol/l, second trimester 9–19 pmol/l, third trimester 7–17 pmol/l (Parker 1985, Kotarba et al 1995). The normal ranges for free T_3 are similarly reduced (3–5 pmol/l at term compared to 4–9 pmol/l non-pregnant) (Kotarba et al 1995). Serum concentrations of thyroid-stimulating hormone (TSH) are less affected by pregnancy than total T_4 and T_3, but may rise or fall in the first trimester. This is because TSH has structural and immunological similarities to human chorionic gonadotrophin (hCG) (levels of which are substantially elevated in early pregnancy). Hyperemesis gravidarum may be associated with a biochemical thyrotoxicosis with high levels of free T_4 and a suppressed TSH in up to 60% of cases (Goodwin et al 1992). In the third trimester, TSH levels increase so the upper limit of the reference range is raised (7.0 mu/l) compared with the non-pregnant (4.0 mu/l) (Kotarba et al 1995).

Pregnancy is associated with a state of relative iodine deficiency. This is due to increasing maternal iodine requirements because of active transport to the fetoplacental unit and a twofold increase in iodine excretion in the urine secondary to increased glomerular filtration and decreased renal tubular reabsorption. Because the plasma level of iodine falls, the thyroid gland increases its uptake from the blood. If there is already dietary insufficiency of iodine, the thyroid gland hypertrophies in order to manufacture enough thyroid hormone; the physiological goitre of pregnancy. Biochemical assessment of thyroid function in pregnancy should include assays of free T_4 and, in some cases, free T_3. Immunoradiometric assays of TSH are useful, but should not be used in isolation because of the variable effects of gestation (Girling 1996).

Hyperthyroidism

Thyrotoxicosis complicates about 0.2% of pregnancies (Burrow 1993). Ninety-five per cent of cases of hyperthyroidism in pregnancy are due to Graves' disease, an autoimmune disorder caused by TSH receptor-stimulating antibodies (TSA). More rarely in women of childbearing age, hyperthyroidism may be due to toxic multinodular goitre or toxic adenoma, or occasionally subacute thyroiditis, iodine, amiodarone or lithium therapy. Most cases encountered in pregnancy have already been diagnosed and will already be on treatment. If thyrotoxicosis occurs for the first time in pregnancy it usually presents late in the first or early in the second trimester. Many of the typical features are common in normal pregnancy: heat intolerance, tachycardia, palpitations, palmar erythema, emotional lability, vomiting and goitre. The most discriminatory features in pregnancy are weight loss, tremor, lid lag or retraction and a persistent tachycardia. Exophthalmos does not correlate with thyroid activity. Eye signs are a marker for thyroid disease, either current or past. Thyroid-associated ophthalmopathy may occur before hyperthyroidism and is present in up to 50% of patients with Graves' disease. Clinical diagnosis of hyperthyroidism should be supported by elevated free T_4 or free T_3 levels with suppression of TSH.

Thyrotoxicosis often improves during pregnancy, especially in the second and third trimesters. As with some other autoimmune conditions, there is a state of relative immunosuppression in pregnancy and levels of TSA may fall, with consequent improvement in Graves' disease and a lower requirement for antithyroid treatment (O'Doherty et al 1999). Exacerbations may occur in the first trimester, possibly related to hCG production, and in the puerperium (especially if there has been improvement during pregnancy) related to a reversal of the fall in antibody levels seen during pregnancy. If thyrotoxicosis is severe and untreated it is associated with inhibition of ovulation and infertility. Those who do become pregnant and remain untreated have an increased rate of miscarriage, IUGR, premature labour and perinatal mortality (Burrow 1993, O'Doherty et al 1999). Poorly controlled thyrotoxicosis may lead to a thyroid crisis (storm) in the mother and heart failure particularly at the time of delivery. For those with good control on antithyroid drugs or with previously treated Graves' disease in remission, the maternal and fetal outcome is usually good and unaffected by the thyrotoxicosis (Wing et al 1994).

Carbimazole and propylthiouracil (PTU) are the most commonly used antithyroid drugs in the UK. Most cases are treated for 12–18 months after the initial presentation of Graves' disease, but relapse rates are high, and some women are managed with long-term antithyroid drugs. Both drugs cross the placenta, PTU less than carbimazole, and in high doses may cause fetal hypothyroidism and goitre (O'Doherty et al 1999). Several case reports have described a scalp defect, aplasia cutis, in the infants of women taking carbimazole or methimazole. The risk is low and no cases occurred in nearly 650 neonates born to mothers with Graves' disease (Ramsay et al 1983). The aim of treatment is to maintain optimal control of thyrotoxicosis with the lowest dose of antithyroid medication. The woman should be clinically euthyroid, with a free T_4 at the upper end of the normal range. There is no place for block and replace regimens in the management of thyrotoxicosis in pregnancy. The high doses of antithyroid drugs required may render the fetus hypothyroid, and the thyroxine replacement does not cross the placenta in sufficiently high doses to protect the fetus (O'Doherty et al 1999). Newly diagnosed thyrotoxicosis should be aggressively treated with high doses of carbimazole or PTU (40 mg or 400 mg daily, respectively) for 4–6 weeks, after which time gradual reduction in medication to the lowest dose that maintains euthyroidism is usually possible. A drug rash or urticaria occurs in 1–5% of patients on antithyroid drugs, and should prompt a switch to a different preparation. Women should be seen monthly in the case of newly diagnosed hyperthyroidism, but less frequent thyroid function tests may be appropriate in the case of those who are stable on long-term antithyroid drugs. PTU is probably preferable for newly diagnosed cases in pregnancy (less transfer across the placenta and to breast milk), but women already on maintenance carbimazole before pregnancy need not be switched to PTU in pregnancy (Drug and Therapeutics Bulletin 1995). Doses of PTU at or below 150 mg/day and carbimazole 15 mg/day are unlikely to cause problems in the fetus. Thyroid function should be checked in umbilical cord blood and at regular intervals in the neonate if the mother is breast-feeding and taking antithyroid drugs. Very little PTU is excreted in breast milk, and only 0.07% of the adult dose is consumed by the baby. It is therefore safe for mothers to breast-feed while taking doses of PTU at or below 150 mg/day and carbimazole 15 mg/day (0.5% of adult dose received by baby) (Lamberg et al 1984, O'Doherty et al 1999).

Beta blockers are often used in the early management of thyrotoxicosis, or during relapse to improve symptoms of tachycardia, sweating and tremor. They are discontinued once biochemical control is achieved. They are therefore unlikely to be required for more than a month in pregnancy, and doses of propranolol of 40 mg three times daily for such short periods of time are not harmful to the fetus.

Thyroidectomy is rarely indicated in pregnancy, but if required may safely be performed in the second trimester. It is usually reserved for those with dysphagia or stridor related to a large goitre, those with confirmed or suspected carcinoma, and those who have allergies to both antithyroid drugs. Between 25 and 50% of patients will become hypothyroid after thyroid surgery, and therefore close follow-up is required to ensure rapid diagnosis and treatment with replacement therapy.

Radioiodine therapy is contraindicated in pregnancy and breast-feeding as it is taken up by the fetal and neonatal thyroid (after 10–12 weeks), with resulting thyroid ablation and hypothyroidism. Diagnostic radioiodine scans (as opposed to treatment) are also contraindicated in pregnancy, but may be performed if a mother is breast-feeding, although mothers should stop breast-feeding for 24 h after the procedure. Pregnancy should be avoided for at least 4 months after treatment with radioiodine in view of the theoretical risk of chromosomal damage and genetic abnormalities (O'Doherty et al 1999).

Neonatal or fetal thyrotoxicosis results from transplacental passage of TSA. It occurs in about 1% of babies of mothers with a past or current history of Graves' disease, but is most common in those with active disease in the third trimester, especially if poorly controlled (Burrow 1993). It is possible to predict babies at risk by measuring the level of thyroid-stimulating antibodies, although the assay is not universally available. If the condition develops in utero, it may present with fetal tachycardia, IUGR or goitre (Pekonen et al 1984). Without treatment the mortality may reach 50%. In the newborn, the onset of the condition may be delayed for 1 day to 2 weeks (Zakarija et al 1986) while maternal antithyroid drugs are cleared. The late presentation of neonatal hyperthyroidism may also relate to blocking substances, analogous to alpha-fetoprotein in myasthenia gravis, which inhibit the action of TSA in utero. Features include weight loss, tachycardia, irritability, jitteriness, poor feeding, goitre, and in severe untreated cases, congestive cardiac failure. Without treatment mortality is about 15% (Hollingsworth 1985). Serial ultrasound to check fetal growth, heart rate and the fetal neck (for goitre) is advisable, especially in those mothers with poorly controlled or newly diagnosed thyrotoxicosis. Percutaneous fetal blood sampling for measurement of fetal thyroid function is accurate, but carries an inherent risk. In practice, a normal fetal heart rate makes both hypo- and hyperthyroidism in the fetus unlikely. Treatment is with antithyroid drugs. In the case of fetal thyrotoxicosis, these are given to the mother. If the woman is euthyroid, these are combined with replacement thyroxine. In the baby, treatment must begin promptly, but is only needed for a few weeks, after which time maternal TSAs disappear from the circulation.

Hypothyroidism

Hypothyroidism affects about 1% of pregnancies. Most cases encountered in pregnancy have already been diagnosed and will be on replacement therapy. Many of the typical features, including weight gain, lethargy and tiredness, hair loss, dry skin, constipation, carpal tunnel syndrome, fluid retention and goitre, are common in normal pregnancy. The most discriminatory features in pregnancy are cold intolerance, slow pulse rate and delayed relaxation of the tendon (particularly the ankle) reflexes. Hypothyroidism is associated with other autoimmune diseases, for example pernicious anaemia, vitiligo, and type I diabetes mellitus. Most cases are due to autoimmune destruction of the thyroid gland associated with microsomal autoantibodies. There are two principal subtypes: atrophic thyroiditis and Hashimoto's thyroiditis. The latter is the name given to the combination of autoimmune thyroiditis and goitre. Hypothyroidism may be iatrogenic following radioiodine therapy, thyroidectomy or related to drugs (amiodarone, lithium, iodine or antithyroid drugs). Transient hypothyroidism may be found in subacute (de Quervain's) thyroiditis and in postpartum thyroiditis (see later). Diagnosis is made by finding a low free T_4 and raised TSH. Normal pregnant ranges for each trimester must be used (see before). The finding of thyroid peroxidase (microsomal) antibodies may help confirm the diagnosis, but these are present in 10–20% of the normal population (Hall et al 1993) and should not be used in isolation.

If hypothyroidism is severe and untreated it is associated with inhibition of ovulation and infertility. Those who do become pregnant and remain untreated have an increased rate of miscarriage, fetal loss and gestational hypertension (Leung et al 1993). The fetus is dependent on maternal thyroid hormone until autonomous fetal thyroid function begins at around 12 weeks' gestation. Some have found an association between untreated hypothyroidism in the mother, as assessed by low free T_4 (Pop et al 1999) and raised TSH (Haddow et al 1999), and mild impaired neuropsychological development in the offspring. It is only maternal iodine deficiency that relates to severe permanent brain damage (neurological cretinism) in the child. For those women on adequate replacement therapy, who are euthyroid at the beginning of pregnancy, the maternal and fetal outcome is usually good and unaffected by the hypothyroidism (Mestman et al 1995). Only very small amounts of thyroxine cross the placenta and the fetus is not at risk of thyrotoxicosis from maternal T_4 replacement therapy. Thyroid function should be checked in all hypothyroid women, ideally before they are pregnant, or at least during the first trimester, to ensure adequate replacement. Although some believe that an increased dose of T_4 is required in pregnancy (Hall et al 1993), this is disputed (Girling & de Swiet 1992). If the dose does need to be increased in pregnancy, this is usually because of inadequate replacement before pregnancy (Girling 1996). For those with newly diagnosed hypothyroidism in pregnancy, replacement with thyroxine should begin immediately. Provided there is no history of heart disease, an appropriate starting dose is 100 μg daily. In women on adequate replacement, thyroid function should be checked once in each trimester. Following any adjustment in T_4 dose, thyroid function should be checked after 4–6 weeks.

Neonatal/fetal hypothyroidism is very rare (1 in 180 000), and thought to be due to the transplacental passage of TRA. These antibodies are more common in women with atrophic, rather than Hashimoto's, thyroiditis. The diagnosis may be suspected in the presence of a fetal goitre, or fetal tachycardia.

Postpartum thyroiditis

If active steps are taken to diagnose the condition, it has been found to affect up to 5–10% of all women (Girling 1996). It is more common in women with a family history of hypothyroidism and those with thyroid peroxidase antibodies (Hall et al 1993). Presentation is usually between 3 and 4 months postpartum with symptoms of hyper- or hypothyroidism (Girling 1996), but a high index of suspicion is needed. The condition is caused by a destructive autoimmune lymphocytic thyroiditis (Hall et al 1993). Most patients recover spontaneously and treatment is not always required. Postpartum thyroiditis is a significant predictor of future hypothyroidism (Girling 1996).

Thyroid nodules

The incidence of malignancy in thyroid nodules first discovered in pregnancy is higher than in the non-pregnant and in one series was almost 40% (Doherty et al 1995). If there is a long history, this is less likely, but it is impossible to exclude cancer clinically. Radioactive iodine cannot be used to differentiate inactive (cold) and active (hot) nodules, which are less likely to be cancerous. Ultrasound examination of the nodule and thyroid gland should be performed, and fine-needle aspiration is recommended for nodules in pregnancy if they are rapidly enlarging, associated with cervical lymphadenopathy, solid and >2 cm, or cystic and >4 cm (Doherty et al 1995). If there is any suspicion of tracheal compression, an X-ray should be taken of the thoracic inlet and the patient should be discussed with an anaesthetist.

KEY POINTS: THYROID

- Untreated thyrotoxicosis is dangerous for the mother and fetus.
- The lowest possible dose of antithyroid drug should be used.
- In hypothyroidism, doses of thyroxine rarely require adjustment in pregnancy.

EPILEPSY

Epilepsy is the commonest chronic neurological disorder to complicate pregnancy, affecting approximately 0.5% of pregnancies (O'Brien & Gilmour-White 1993). Epilepsy is classified according to the clinical type of seizure, of which the most common are grand mal (tonic-clonic seizure), petit mal (absence seizure) and temporal lobe seizures (complex partial seizure). The term petit mal should be reserved for typical absences occurring almost exclusively in children and associated with 3 Hz spike and wave discharge on the EEG. Absence attacks do occur in adulthood as a feature of partial seizures. Most cases of epilepsy are idiopathic and no underlying cause is found. Secondary epilepsy may be encountered in pregnancy in patients who have previously undergone surgery to the cerebral hemispheres or who have intracranial mass lesions. This should always be considered if the first fit occurs in pregnancy. Epilepsy may be a feature of the antiphospholipid syndrome. Other causes of seizures in pregnancy include eclampsia, cerebral vein thrombosis, thrombotic thrombocytopenic purpura, cerebral infarction, drug and alcohol withdrawal and hypoglycaemia (complicating insulin-treated diabetes). Most women with epilepsy in pregnancy have already been diagnosed, but when a first fit occurs in pregnancy, having excluded pre-eclampsia, imaging with CT or MRI of the brain is appropriate (Nelson-Piercy 1997).

Effect of pregnancy on epilepsy

In general, pregnancy does not affect the frequency of seizures. About 25% of women report improvement, and 10–30% of women experience an increased seizure frequency in pregnancy. Poorly controlled epileptics, especially those who fit more than once a month, are more likely to deterio-

rate in pregnancy (Crawford et al 1999). There is no relation to the seizure type or the course of epilepsy during previous pregnancies. Reasons for deterioration in seizure control during pregnancy include pregnancy itself, stress, poor compliance with anticonvulsant medication (due to fears about teratogenesis), decreased drug levels related to nausea and vomiting in early pregnancy, decreased drug levels related to increased volume of distribution and changes in protein binding and increased drug clearance, lack of sleep towards term and during labour, lack of absorption of anticonvulsant drugs from the gastrointestinal tract during labour and hyperventilation during labour. There is no difference in the change of seizure frequency between trimesters (Vidovic & Della Marina 1994), although the risk of seizures is greatest peripartum (see below).

Effect of epilepsy on pregnancy

The majority of women with epilepsy have uncomplicated pregnancies with normal deliveries and healthy children. The fetus is relatively resistant to short episodes of hypoxia, and there is no evidence of adverse effects of single seizures on the fetus. Some have documented fetal bradycardia during and after maternal convulsions, but cerebral damage in the long term is not a feature. Status epilepticus is dangerous for both mother and fetus and should be vigorously treated. Fortunately it affects only 1–2% of pregnancies in epileptics. In the Confidential Enquiry into Maternal Deaths in the UK (1994–1996) there were 19 deaths due to epilepsy (Department of Health et al 1998). Most occurred antenatally, with 10 in the third trimester. In 10 women the cause of death was aspiration, but epileptic seizures may be fatal in themselves. Only five women had poorly controlled epilepsy, and two women died not having had a fit for the previous 2 years. The problem with these data is that there is a risk of sudden unexplained death in epilepsy (SUDEP), even outside pregnancy, which has been estimated at 1 per 500 woman-years. Although some workers have suggested an increased risk of obstetric complications such as miscarriage, pre-eclampsia, premature labour, antepartum haemorrhage and caesarean section (Yerby 1994), most recent prospective studies have not indicated any increase in adverse pregnancy outcome (Crawford et al 1993).

The main concern in pregnancies complicated by epilepsy stems from the increased risk of congenital abnormalities. Even epileptics who are not taking any anticonvulsants have a slightly increased risk (4%) compared with the general population (3%) (Friis et al 1986). The risk to the child of developing epilepsy is also increased (4% compared with 1% background) if either parent has epilepsy. If there is a previously affected sibling the risk is 10%. If both parents have epilepsy the risk is 15–20%.

Teratogenic risks of anticonvulsants

Phenytoin, primidone, phenobarbitone, carbamezepine and sodium valproate all cross the placenta and are teratogenic. The major malformations caused by anticonvulsants are neural tube defects (10 times background incidence; particularly valproate [1–2%] and carbamezepine [0.5–1%]) (Lyons Jones et al 1989, Rosa 1991), orofacial clefts (particularly phenytoin) and congenital heart defects (particularly phenytoin and valproate). There is little difference in the level of risk for major malformations between individual drugs. The risk for any one drug is about 6–7% (i.e. double to three times the background level). The risk increases with the number of drugs, so for those taking two or more anticonvulsants the risk is 15%, and for those taking the combination of valproate, carbamezepine and phenytoin the risk is as high as 50% (Nakane et al 1980). One mechanism for teratogenesis is thought to be folate deficiency. Phenytoin and phenobarbitone particularly, but also carbamezepine and valproate, interfere with folate metabolism. The risk of defects (particularly those of the neural tube) can be decreased by the use of prepregnancy and first trimester folic acid (MRC Vitamin Research Study Group 1991). Minor malformations (fetal anticonvulsant syndrome) occur in 5–30% of infants exposed to anticonvulsants in pregnancy. These include dysmorphic features (V-shaped eyebrows, low-set ears, broad nasal bridge, irregular teeth), hypertelorism, and hypoplastic nails and distal digits (Ornoy & Cohen 1996). Although specific syndromes have been ascribed to phenytoin, carbamezepine and valproate, there is considerable overlap.

The newer anticonvulsant drugs vigabatrin, lamotrogine, topiramate and gabapentin are often prescribed in combination with other anticonvulsants and it is therefore difficult to ascertain the teratogenic risk of these drugs in isolation. Very few data of their use in human pregnancy exist, but in animal studies vigabatrin and topiramate demonstrate teratogenicity. The benzodiazepines (e.g. clonazepam) are not teratogenic. Lamotrogine and gabapentin are not teratogenic in animals and, although lamotrogine carries a theoretical risk because it may interfere with folate metabolism, in practice it seems to carry a low risk of teratogenesis. Whether this risk is low enough to justify replacement of an older anticonvulsant for lamotrogine prepregnancy is not yet known.

Management

Prepregnancy counselling

It should be assumed that all women of childbearing age may become pregnant, and therefore any opportunity to counsel such women should not be missed. Control of epilepsy should be maximised before pregnancy. For women still having seizures, the lowest dose of the most effective treatment which gives best control of seizures is appropriate. Polytherapy should be avoided if possible. Sodium valproate therapy should be changed to a thrice-daily regimen or modified-release preparation to lower peak concentrations and reduce the risk of neural tube defects (the neural tube closes at day 26 of biological life, 40 days after the mother's last normal menstrual period) (Cleland 1996). For valproate also there is evidence of a dose-dependent teratogenic effect. Thus offspring of mothers using >1 g per day are at sixfold increased risk of congenital malformations, particularly neural tube defects, compared to those exposed to 600 mg per day (Sauren et al 1997).

Women who have been fit-free for more than 2–3 years may wish to discontinue anticonvulsants, at least preconceptually and for the first trimester. This should be a fully informed decision after counselling concerning particularly the risk of losing a driver's licence in the event of a seizure. The current recommendations are to stop driving from the start of the period of drug withdrawal and for a period of 6 months after cessation of treatment, even if there is no recurrence of seizures (Crawford et al 1999). All women on anticonvulsant drugs should be advised to take folic acid (5 mg rather than 400 μg per day) for at least 12 weeks before conception.

Antenatal

Folic acid should be continued throughout pregnancy as there is also a small risk of folate-deficiency anaemia (Nelson-Piercy 1997). There is no need to change the anticonvulsant used in pregnancy if the woman is well controlled. Prenatal screening for congenital abnormalities with maternal serum screening or nuchal translucency testing, if available, and detailed ultrasound at 18–20 weeks should be offered. A repeat scan at 22 weeks is advisable if cardiac defects are suspected. The altered pharmocokinetics in pregnancy mean that drug levels are likely to change, and, for most drugs, concentration of the free drug falls. This is because of the increased plasma volume and the enhanced renal and hepatic drug clearance. These effects are partially offset by decreased protein binding. In practice it is useful to have a baseline blood level early in pregnancy to confirm compliance, and to guide any increases which may be necessary. If a woman is fit-free, there is no need to measure serial drug levels or adjust the dose. In women who have regular seizures, and who are dependent on critical drug levels, it is worth monitoring drug levels (preferably of the free drug), as they are likely to fall, and increasing dosages of anticonvulsants should be guided by serum concentrations. Anticonvulsant dosage should only be altered on clinical grounds. Vitamin K (10–20 mg orally) should be prescribed in the last 4 weeks of pregnancy (Deblay et al 1982). This is because, in the fetuses of women taking hepatic enzyme-inducing drugs, vitamin K-dependent clotting factors may be reduced, thus increasing the risk of haemorrhagic disease of the newborn.

Intrapartum

The risk of seizures increases around the time of delivery. Between 1 and 2% of women with epilepsy will have a seizure during labour, and 1–2% will fit in the first 24 h postpartum (Bardy 1982). Caesarean section is only required if there are recurrent generalised seizures in labour.

Postnatal

Epileptic patients require particular care in the immediate puerperium because of the increased risk of seizures. They should be supervised in the bath. Mothers with major seizures require advice regarding precautions such as bathing infants with somebody else around and changing nappies on the floor. The baby should also receive vitamin K. All women with epilepsy should be strongly encouraged to breast-feed (Crawford et al 1999). In some countries, mothers receiving anticonvulsants tend to choose formula feeding (Ito et al

1995). Although most anticonvulsants are secreted into breast milk, the dose that the baby receives is only a fraction of the therapeutic level for the newborn, and in any case is likely to be less than that received in utero. Babies whose mothers received phenobarbitone in pregnancy may experience withdrawal if they are not breast-fed, and although this is rare with the newer anticonvulsants, it provides a logical reason to encourage breast-feeding in all epileptic mothers. The ratio between breast milk and serum concentration is 0.36 for phenobarbitone, and doses received by the neonate may reach >50% of therapeutic. If the mother's dose of anticonvulsant was increased during pregnancy, it should be slowly decreased again during the puerperium. If a breast-fed baby of a mother taking anticonvulsants is unusually sleepy, or has to be woken for feeds, the mother should be encouraged to feed before rather than after taking her anticonvulsants. This should avoid peak serum and therefore breast milk levels.

Contraception

Women taking hepatic enzyme-inducing drugs (phenytoin, primidone, carbamezepine, phenobarbitone) require higher doses of oestrogen to achieve adequate contraception. They should be given a combined oral contraceptive pill containing at least 50 μg oestrogen or be advised to take two tablets daily of preparations containing 30 μg (O'Brien & Gilmour-White 1993). Higher doses of the progesterone-only pill are also required. Women should be advised to take two rather than one daily pill of norethisterone 350 μg (Micronor) or levonorgestrel 30 μg (Microval). An alternative is depot provera. This is entirely metabolised by first-pass effect in the liver and therefore a higher dose is not required. Valproate, clonazepam, vigabatrin, lamotrogine and gabapentin do not induce hepatic enzymes and therefore normal doses of oral contraception may be used. Alternatively, condoms may be used immediately, and after 6 weeks the intrauterine contraceptive device may be preferable.

KEY POINTS: EPILEPSY

- Women taking antiepileptic drugs should receive prepregnancy counselling regarding the teratogenic risks and be advised to take folic acid 5 mg preconceptually and throughout pregnancy.
- Vitamin K is prescribed from 36 weeks onwards to decrease the risk of haemorrhagic disease of the newborn.
- It is safe to breast-feed while taking anticonvulsant drugs.

ASTHMA

Asthma is the commonest chronic illness of young adulthood, and all those involved in the care of women during pregnancy and childbirth will encounter asthmatics. At least 3% of women of childbearing age have some degree of asthma and this prevalence is increasing.

Changes in respiratory function during pregnancy

During pregnancy, oxygen consumption increases by around 20% and the maternal metabolic rate by about 15%. This extra demand is met by a 40–50% increase in resting minute ventilation, resulting mainly from a rise in tidal volume rather than respiratory rate. This maternal hyperventilation causes a reduced partial pressure of arterial carbon dioxide (Pa_{CO_2}) to 4.0 kPa, and a compensatory fall in serum bicarbonate to 18–22 mmol/l. A mild respiratory alkalosis is therefore normal in pregnancy (arterial pH 7.44).

Up to 75% of women experience a subjective feeling of breathlessness at some time during pregnancy, possibly due to an increased awareness of the physiological hyperventilation. This dyspnoea of pregnancy is commonest in the 3rd trimester and may lead to diagnostic confusion.

Late in pregnancy, the diaphragmatic elevation caused by the enlarging uterus leads to a decrease in functional residual capacity, but diaphragm excursion is unaffected so vital capacity is unchanged.

Effect of pregnancy on asthma

Published evidence about the effect of pregnancy on asthma is conflicting, and there is no consistent trend to improvement or worsening of disease severity. A review of more than 1000 women reported in nine studies found a worsening of asthma in 22%, improvement in 29%, and no change in 49% (Gluck & Gluck 1976).

The course of asthma in pregnancy in individual patients is unpredictable. There may be some relationship to the severity of asthma before pregnancy, as women with only mild disease are unlikely to experience problems, whereas those with severe asthma are at greater risk of deterioration, particularly late in pregnancy (Gluck & Gluck 1976, White et al 1989). Many asthmatics experience worsening of their symptoms during pregnancy simply because they have stopped or reduced their usual medication due to either their fears, or those of their doctors, about its safety.

Effect of asthma on pregnancy and its outcome

In most women, asthma has no effect upon the outcome of pregnancy. However, severe, poorly controlled asthma could have an adverse effect on fetal outcome as a result of chronic or intermittent maternal hypoxaemia. Several large studies have suggested a slight increase in the risk of premature labour in asthmatic pregnancies (Schatz et al 1975, Fitzsimons et al 1986, Perlow et al 1992, Doucette & Bracken 1993, Demissie et al 1998), although two prospective case–control studies of over 600 pregnancies have not confirmed these findings (Stenius-Aarniala et al 1988, Schatz et al 1995). There is also some evidence of an association between asthma and babies of low birthweight (Gluck & Gluck 1976, Greenberger & Patterson 1988, Schatz et al 1990, Demissie et al 1998), but this was not found in all studies (Stenius-Aarniala et al 1988, Schatz et al 1995).

Some studies have reported an increased incidence of pregnancy-induced hypertension or pre-eclampsia in asthmatic women (Stenius-Aarniala et al 1988, Lehrer et al 1993, Demissie et al 1998). However, women with asthma are likely to be seen more frequently during the antenatal period than normal women, and therefore to have their blood pressure measured more often. The more frequent the measurements, the more likely it is that transient increases in blood pressure will be discovered. Similarly, a higher rate of caesarean section has been reported in some studies (Stenius-Aarniale et al 1988, Perlow et al 1992, Wendel et al 1996, Demissia et al 1998) but this may be a consequence of increased surveillance of asthmatic pregnancies, rather than a result of maternal asthma.

There have been reports of increased incidence of transient tachypnoea of the newborn (Schatz et al 1991), neonatal hypoglycaemia (Stenius-Aarniala et al 1988), neonatal seizures (Patterson et al 1989) and admission to the neonatal intensive care unit (Perlow et al 1992) in the babies of asthmatic women, but the magnitude of effect on any adverse perinatal outcome is small and related to the degree of control of the asthma. One retrospective study reported a higher incidence of congenital abnormalities in the children of asthmatic women (Demissie et al 1998), but this has not been shown to occur in two large prospective studies of over 650 pregnancies in asthmatic women (Stenius-Aarniala et al 1988, Schatz et al 1995), nor in one subsequent retrospective case–control study of 101 pregnancies (Minerbi-Codish et al 1998).

In conclusion, it seems that there may be a slight increased risk to the babies of asthmatic mothers, but this risk is small and may be minimised by maintaining good control of asthma throughout pregnancy.

Management of asthma in pregnancy

The successful management of asthma during pregnancy requires a cooperative approach between the obstetrician, the physician managing the asthma, and the woman. The aim of treatment is to achieve virtual total freedom from symptoms, such that the life style of the individual is not affected. The emphasis is on the prevention, rather than the treatment, of acute attacks. Regular inhaled anti-inflammatory medication

(usually a steroid such as betamethasome) is first-line maintenance treatment for all but those with infrequent symptoms (requiring ventolin less than once a day). If this does not control a woman's symptoms, high-dose inhaled steroids, or the long-acting inhaled β-agonist, salmeterol, are recommended. If this is insufficient, either a theophylline, inhaled ipratropium, or a course of regular steroid tablets can be tried (British Guidelines on Asthma Management 1997). The most sensitive indicator of inadequate control is breathlessness at night. Symptoms should be controlled by anti-inflammatory agents whenever possible, as regular use of bronchodilators has been linked to an increased incidence of sudden death in later life.

Home peak flow monitoring and personalised self-management plans have been shown to reduce morbidity in asthmatics. Peak flow meters can be prescribed to help women to monitor their asthma throughout pregnancy.

The drug treatment of asthma in pregnancy is, in essence, no different from the treatment of asthma in non-pregnant women. All the drugs commonly used to treat asthma, including systemic steroids, are safe. Table 18.2 summarises the major studies of the fetal effects of the commonly used treatments for asthma in pregnancy. Oral corticosteroids and leukotriene antagonists are not mentioned in the table and are considered in more detail below.

Corticosteroids

Systemic corticosteroids have serious and well-known side-effects when given frequently or in high doses for prolonged periods. Women and their doctors are therefore reluctant to use these drugs in pregnancy. This concern is misplaced, and steroids should be used to treat asthma in pregnancy in the same way and for the same reasons as outside pregnancy.

Prednisolone is metabolised by the placenta and very little (10%) active drug ever reaches the fetus. There is no evidence of increased risk of abortion, stillbirth, congenital malformations, adverse fetal effects or neonatal death attributable to treating the mother with steroids (Schatz et al 1975, 1997, Snyder & Snyder 1978, Fitzsimons et al 1986). There is a 46-year-old report of an increased incidence of cleft palate in the offspring of rabbits treated with cortisone early in gestation

Table 18.2 Studies of fetal complications following use of medication for asthma. (Oral corticosteroids and leukotriene antagonists are considered separately on page 287)

Drug	Route	No. cases	Congenital malformations (Y/N)	Reference
Salbutamol	Inhaled	259	Not increased	Schatz et al (1988)
Salbutamol	Inhaled	488	Not increased	Schatz et al (1997)
Salbutamol	Oral	130	Not increased	Schatz et al (1988)
Salmeterol	Inhaled	93	Not increased	Mann et al (1996)
Disodium cromoglycate	Inhaled	243	Not increased	Schatz et al (1997)
Theophylline	Oral	429	Not increased	Schatz et al (1997)
Theophylline	Oral	212	Not increased	Stenius-Aarniala et al (1995)
Beclomethasone	Inhaled	824	Not increased	Schatz et al (1997)
Beclomethasone	Inhaled	40	Not increased	Greenberger & Patterson (1983)
Budesonide	Inhaled	2014	Not increased	Kallen et al (1999)

(Fainstat 1954), and one recent retrospective study of 1184 cases of cleft lip suggested a possible association with oral corticosteroid treatment (Rodriguez-Pinilla & Martinez-Frias 1998). Of the five affected pregnancies in the latter study, two were complicated by multiple congenital abnormalities and in another case the mother was taking replacement steroids for Addison's disease. Therefore only two pregnancies (no greater than control) were complicated by isolated cleft lip in women taking therapeutic doses of corticosteroids. A larger case–control study of 20 830 cases of congenital abnormality revealed no association with corticosteroid treatment (Czeizel & Rockenbauer 1997).

Prolonged use of oral steroids increases the risk of infection and gestational diabetes, and deterioration in blood glucose control in women with established impairment of glucose tolerance in pregnancy. The blood glucose should be checked regularly, and hyperglycaemia should be managed as described on page 277. The development of hyperglycaemia is not an indication to discontinue or decrease the dose of oral steroids, the requirement for which must be determined by the asthma.

An increased risk of pregnancy induced hypertension (Wendel et al 1996) and pre-eclampsia (Schatz et al 1997) has been reported in oral corticosteroid-treated asthmatics; however, given the material and fetal consequences of severe asthma, the authors concluded that the use of oral corticosteroids remains clinically indicated. The rare, but important, psychiatric side-effects of oral glucocorticoids should be remembered, and all women who have been commenced on steroids should be reviewed within 1 week.

In summary, oral corticosteroids are safe in pregnancy, used as inhaled, nebulised or parenteral preparations. The addition of systemic corticosteroids to control exacerbations of asthma is appropriate, and these must not be withheld if current medications are inadequate.

Leukotriene antagonists

Leukotrienes are mediators of inflammation, and cause smooth muscle constriction and proliferation. Leukotriene antagonists are recently introduced drugs for asthma, and can be taken orally. At present there is insufficient information to establish whether they are safe in pregnancy. However, the manufacturer of zafirlucast is aware of the outcome of 43 pregnancies where this leukotriene antagonist was taken; there were 24 normal babies, 10 terminations, eight miscarriages and one baby was born with a heart murmur which was not believed to be due to the zafirlucast treatment (personal communication with the manufacturer).

Management of acute severe asthma

Acute severe attacks of asthma are dangerous and should be vigorously managed in hospital. In the last Confidential Enquiry into Maternal Deaths in the UK (Department of Health et al 1998), there were three deaths from asthma in 1994–1996, two of these occurring in the postpartum period. The treatment is no different from the emergency management of acute severe asthma outside pregnancy.

Oxygen, nebulised bronchodilators, oral or intravenous steroids, and in severe cases intravenous aminophylline or intravenous β_2-agonists should be used as indicated. Sudden severe deterioration or failure to respond to treatment should raise the possibility of a pneumothorax. The ionising radiation from a chest X-ray is approximately 0.002 Gy (less than 1/20th of the maximum recommended exposure in pregnancy (0.05 Gy)) and abdominal shielding will minimise the exposure to the fetus. If a chest X-ray is clinically indicated this investigation must not be withheld just because the patient is pregnant.

Management during labour and delivery

Acute attacks of asthma during labour and delivery are extremely rare, and women should be reassured accordingly. Women should continue their regular inhalers throughout labour. Those on maintenance oral steroids (>7.5 mg prednisolone daily), or who are being treated with steroids for more than 2 weeks before the onset of labour or delivery, should receive parenteral steroids (hydrocortisone 100 mg q.d.s.) during labour, and until they are able to restart their oral medication. Prostaglandin E_2 used to induce labour, to ripen the cervix, or for early termination of pregnancy is a bronchodilator and is safe to use. Prostaglandin $F_{2\alpha}$ given for obstetrical reasons should be used with caution as it may cause bronchospasm.

All forms of pain relief in labour, including epidural analgesia and Entonox may be safely used by asthmatic women, although, in the unlikely event of an acute asthmatic attack, opiates should be avoided. If anaesthesia is required, women with asthma should be encouraged to have epidural rather than general anaesthesia because of the increased risk of chest infection and associated atelectasis. Although ergometrine has been reported to cause bronchospasm, particularly in association with general anaesthesia, this does not seem to be a practical problem when syntometrine (oxytocin/ergometrine) is used to prevent postpartum haemorrhage.

Non-steroidal anti-inflammatory drugs (NSAID) are commonly used for pain relief after caesarian section. Women with asthma should be asked about any known aspirin, or NSAID, allergy before the use of these drugs.

Breast–feeding

Women with asthma should be encouraged to breast-feed their babies. The risk of atopic disease developing in the child of an asthmatic woman is about 1 in 10, or 1 in 3 if both parents are atopic, but this risk is probably reduced by exclusive breast-feeding. All inhaled preparations, oral steroids and methylxanthines are safe when breast-feeding.

Conclusions

Management of asthma in pregnancy does not differ significantly from management outside pregnancy. The priority should be effective control of the disease process, with the aim being total freedom from symptoms both day and night.

Great attention must, however, be given to explanation and reassurance about the safety, in pregnancy and during lactation, of the drugs used to treat asthma.

The small risk of harm to the fetus comes from poorly controlled severe asthma rather than from the drugs used to prevent or treat asthma.

KEY POINTS: ASTHMA

- All medication for the treatment of asthma is safe in pregnancy.
- Acute exacerbations should be treated in the same way as in non-pregnant women.
- Women treated with oral corticosteroids (>7.5 mg/day for several weeks) should have i.v. hydrocortisone 100 mg q.d.s. to cover labour.
- Prostaglandin $F_{2\alpha}$ and ergometrine can cause bronchospasm in asthmatic women.

SYSTEMIC LUPUS ERYTHEMATOSUS

Systemic lupus erythematosus (SLE) affects women much more than men, particularly during the childbearing years (ratio 15:1). The incidence is approximately 1 per 1000 women. The fundamental issues concerning SLE complicating pregnancy are the presence or absence of anti Ro/La and antiphospholipid antibodies (APA), the activity of the lupus, the drugs taken to control the disease, and the presence or absence of hypertension and renal involvement.

Effect of pregnancy on SLE

SLE flares may be difficult to diagnose during pregnancy because many features such as hairfall, oedema, facial erythema, fatigue, anaemia, raised ESR and musculoskeletal pain occur commonly in pregnancy. Whether pregnancy exacerbates SLE and increases the likelihood of flare, particularly postpartum, is controversial (Khamashta et al 1997). The percentage of women who flare during pregnancy ranges from 58 to 70%, compared with about 40% of non-pregnant women over a similar period (Ruiz-Irastoza et al 1996). Even in highly selected patients with mild controlled disease, one-third may be expected to flare (Khamashta et al 1997). In women with lupus nephritis, pregnancy does not seem to jeopardise renal function in the long term (Oviasu et al 1991), although SLE nephropathy may manifest for the first time in pregnancy. There is a greater risk of deterioration in patients with a higher baseline serum creatinine.

Effect of SLE on pregnancy

SLE is associated with increased risks of spontaneous miscarriage, fetal death, pre-eclampsia, preterm delivery and IUGR (Lima et al 1995). These risks may be attributed to the presence of APA, lupus nephritis or hypertension, and either active disease at the time of conception or first presentation of SLE during pregnancy. Pregnancy outcome is particularly affected by renal disease. Even quiescent renal lupus is associated with increased risk of fetal loss, pre-eclampsia and IUGR, particularly if there is hypertension or proteinuria predating the pregnancy. For women in remission, but without hypertension, renal involvement or APA, the risk of pregnancy loss and pre-eclampsia is probably no higher than in the general population.

Management of SLE in pregnancy

Ideally this should begin with counselling before pregnancy. Knowledge of the anti-Ro, antiphospholipid, renal and blood pressure status allows prediction of the risks to the woman and her baby. The outlook is probably better if conception occurs during remission. Pregnancy care is best undertaken in multidisciplinary combined clinics where physicians and obstetricians can monitor disease activity and the fetus regularly.

Disease flares must be actively managed. Corticosteroids are the drug of choice and these are not associated with adverse fetal outcome (see p. 286); however, in women with antiphospholipid syndrome (APS), treated with high doses of prednisolone throughout pregnancy, an increased frequency of premature rupture of the membranes has been reported (Cowchock et al 1992). Hydroxychloroquine should be continued, as stopping may precipitate flare. Furthermore, because it has a very long half-life, discontinuation in the first trimester is illogical because the fetus will remain exposed for several weeks afterwards (Buchanan et al 1996). Azathioprine, the commonest cytotoxic agent used in SLE, is also usually continued, as this reduces the need for steroids. Azathioprine appears to be safe, based on its successful use in large numbers of renal transplant mothers as well as women with SLE (Ostenson & Ramsey-Golman 1998); however, neonatal immunosuppression has been noted, and conflicting information exists regarding breast-feeding while taking azathioprine (Bermas & Hill 1995). Despite little or no drug being found in breast milk (Bermas & Hill 1995), most rheumatologists advise avoidance of azathioprine if possible, or would counsel against breast-feeding (Ostenson & Ramsey-Golman 1998).

Aspirin and non-steroidal anti-inflammatory drugs (NSAIDs) are not teratogenic, but NSAIDs may lead to oligohydramnios via effects on the fetal kidney (Ostenson & Ramsey-Golman 1998). As they are prostaglandin synthetase inhibitors, they may cause premature closure of the ductus arteriosus (because prostaglandin E_2 relaxation of pulmonary vessels is inhibited), with neonatal primary pulmonary hypertension, so they are usually avoided, especially in the last trimester. The alkylating agents cyclophosphamide and chlorambucil, and the folic acid antagonist methotrexate, are all teratogenic and fetotoxic and are contraindicated in pregnancy and lactation (Ostenson & Ramsey-Golman 1998).

Differentiation of active renal lupus from pre-eclampsia is notoriously difficult and the two conditions may be superimposed. Since hypertension, proteinuria, thrombocytopenia and even renal impairment are all features of pre-eclampsia, diagnosis of lupus flare requires other features, such as a rising anti-DNA antibody titre, the presence of red blood cells or cellular casts in the urinary sediment, or a fall in complement levels. Since steroids do not prevent flares, they are not routinely prescribed prophylactically or increased to cover the postpartum period.

Neonatal lupus syndromes

Anti-Ro is present in about 30% of patients with SLE. These autoantibodies, directed against cytoplasmic ribonucleoprotein, cross the placenta and may cause immune damage in the fetus. Several clinical syndromes have been described, of which cutaneous neonatal lupus is the most common (5% risk if anti-Ro positive) and congenital heart block is the most serious (2–3% risk if anti-Ro positive). The risk of neonatal lupus is increased if a previous child has been affected, rising to 25% with one affected child and 50% if two children are affected (McCune et al 1987) and subsequent infants tend to be affected in the same way as their sibling.

The cutaneous form of neonatal lupus usually manifests in the first 2 weeks of life. The infant develops typical geographical skin lesions, usually on the face and scalp, which appear after exposure to sun or UV light. The rash disappears spontaneously within 6 months and scarring is unusual. In contrast, congenital heart block appears in utero, is permanent, and may be fatal. The mechanism for damage is not fully understood. Congenital heart block is usually detected around 18–20 weeks. Perinatal mortality is increased with 20–30% of affected children dying in the early neonatal period, but most infants who survive this period do well (McCune et al 1987), although two-thirds (Waltuck & Buyon 1994) require pacemakers.

ANTIPHOSPHOLIPID SYNDROME

The combination of either anticardiolipin antibodies (aCL) or lupus anticoagulant (LA) with one or more characteristic clinical features such as thrombosis or recurrent pregnancy loss (Table 18.3) (Wilson et al 1999) is known as the antiphospholipid syndrome. It may complicate SLE, but many patients have primary APS with no features of SLE. Patients with primary APS should not be labelled as having SLE. The antibodies should be regarded as markers for a high-risk

pregnancy, and a previous poor obstetric history in addition is an important predictor of future fetal loss. Many of the adverse outcomes described (early-onset pre-eclampsia, IUGR, placental abruption, stillbirth) are the end-result of abnormal placentation, and this supports the concept that placental failure is the mechanism by which APA are associated with late loss. Studies on pregnancy outcome in women known to have APS show differing rates of obstetric complications, depending on the subgroup of women. Women found to have APS as a result of recurrent miscarriage (Granger & Farquharson 1997, Backos et al 1999) have lower rates of complications (Table 18.4) than those discovered because of late pregnancy losses, thrombosis or other systemic manifestations (Ware Branch et al 1992, Lima et al 1996).

The risk of recurrent thrombosis in patients with APS may reach 70% (Khamashta et al 1995). Women with APS and previous thromboembolism are at extremely high risk in pregnancy and the puerperium and should be given antenatal thromboprophylaxis with subcutaneous unfractionated (10 000 units b.d.) or low-molecular weight heparin (enoxaparin (Clexane) 40 mg o.d.; dalteparin (Fragmin) 5000 units/ml o.d.–b.d.) (Langford & Nelson-Piercy 1999). Many are on long-term warfarin and the change from warfarin to heparin should be achieved before 6 weeks' gestation to avoid

Table 18.3 Clinical criteria for antiphospholipid syndrome

Diagnostic criteria
One or more of:
    Thrombosis—venous/arterial
    Recurrent pregnancy loss
    Premature birth before 34 weeks due to pre-eclampsia or IUGR

Additional clinical features
Thrombocytopenia and haemolytic anaemia
Livedo reticularis
Cerebral involvement, particularly epilepsy, cerebral infarction, chorea and migraine
Heart valve disease, particularly mitral valve
Hypertension
Pulmonary hypertension
Leg ulcers

From Wilson et al (1999).

Table 18.4 Pregnancy complications in different populations of women with antiphospholipid syndrome

Study	Utah[a]	St. Thomas'[b]	Liverpool[c]	St. Mary's[d]
Pregnancies (*n*)	82	60	53	150
Population	Predominantly late loss/ thrombosis/SLE	Predominantly late loss/ thrombosis/SLE	Predominantly recurrent miscarriage	All recurrent miscarriage
Pre-eclampsia (%)	51 (severe 27%)	18	3	11
IUGR (%)	31	31	11	15
Preterm delivery (%)	92	43	8	24

[a] Ware Branch et al (1992).
[b] Lima et al (1996).
[c] Granger and Farquharson (1997).
[d] Backos et al (1999).

warfarin embryopathy. Heparin should be continued intrapartum and postpartum until the women are rewarfarinised. It is occasionally necessary to use warfarin in pregnancy in women with previous arterial thrombosis associated with APS if heparin proves inadequate to prevent further transient ischaemic events (Hunt et al 1998).

The management of pregnancy in women with APS and recurrent pregnancy loss, but without a history of thromboembolism, is debated. Most centres now advocate low-dose aspirin (75 mg) for all women, often before conception. Previously high-dose steroids (in the absence of active lupus) were used to suppress LA and aCL, in combination with aspirin. However, such high doses of prednisolone cause considerable maternal morbidity, and the use of subcutaneous heparin or low molecular weight heparin is now preferred (Cowchock et al 1992). Any additional benefit of heparin must be balanced against the risk of heparin-induced osteoporosis (Dahlman et al 1993). Many centres have traditionally reserved the addition of heparin for those women with previous late losses or intrauterine deaths (Ware Branch et al 1992, Lima et al 1996). Using such strategies, live-birth rates of 70–75% are achieved (Ware Branch et al 1992, Lima et al 1996, Granger & Farquharson 1997). However, two studies, in different populations of women, have both suggested that aspirin and heparin can improve the live-birth rate from about 40% to about 70–80% in women with recurrent miscarriage (Kutteh 1996, Rai et al 1997). A recent randomised study conversly found that asprin and heparin gave equivalent live birth rates (78%) to asprin alone (72%) (Forquharson et al 2001). Immunosuppression with intravenous immunoglobulin (IVIG) is extremely expensive, and its use in the UK is limited to occasional salvage therapy in women who develop complications despite aspirin and heparin (Gordon & Kilby 1998).

KEY POINTS: SYSTEMIC LUPUS ERYTHEMATOSUS AND ANTIPHOSPHOLIPID SYNDROME

- Adverse pregnancy outcome in SLE is related to the presence of antiphospholipid antibodies, hypertension, renal involvement and the activity of the disease.
- Disease flares should be activity managed with corticosteroids.
- Women with anti-Ro antibodies have a 2–5% risk of congenital heart block in the fetus/newborn.

Pregnancy complicated by SLE or APS requires expert care and a team approach by obstetricians, physicians and haematologists. Close monitoring of both mother and fetus is essential. Ultrasound monitoring of fetal growth and uteroplacental blood flow is crucial. This allows for timely delivery.

LIVER DISEASE IN PREGNANCY

The common presenting complaints of women with liver disease in pregnancy are pruritus and jaundice, and it is essential to investigate rapidly women with these symptoms to allow the diagnosis of conditions with potential serious complications. It is important to remember that certain stigmata of liver disease, such as spider naevi and palmar erythema, are normal signs in pregnancy and will disappear soon after delivery. Hepatic disorders specific to pregnancy are obstetric cholestasis (OC), acute fatty liver of pregnancy (AFLP) and the HELLP (haemolysis, elevated liver enzymes and low platelets) syndrome. We will consider OC and AFLP in this chapter. The HELLP syndrome is discussed on page 340. Other liver disorders may be incidental to pregnancy, such as viral hepatitis, autoimmune chronic active hepatitis and acute cholelithiasis and are beyond the scope of this chapter.

Changes in liver function tests during pregnancy

Physiological haemodilution results in reduced reference ranges for aspartate transaminase (AST), alanine transaminase (ALT), bilirubin and gamma-glutamyl transpeptidase (γ-GT) (Girling et al 1997). Serum alkaline phosphatase rises approximately two- to fourfold, primarily due to placental production. The hepatic and placental isoforms can be measured separately, but are not distinguished by routine laboratory tests. These changes are summarised in Table 18.5. Also, concentrations of fibrinogen, ceruloplasmin, transferrin, and of binding proteins, such as thyroid-binding globulin and cortisol-binding globulin, are increased. In addition, serum albumin reduces by 20–40% and this results in a reduced total serum protein concentration. It is clear that interpretation of liver function tests in pregnancy must be made by reference to appropriate gestational age-corrected normal ranges for pregnancy. Use of non-pregnant normal ranges will result in serious diagnostic errors.

Obstetric cholestasis

The prevalence of OC varies in different populations, with reported rates varying from 0.2% in France, to 1–1.5% in

Table 18.5 Normal ranges for liver function tests in pregnancy

Liver enzyme	Non-pregnant	1st trimester	2nd trimester	3rd trimester
Aspartate transaminase (units/l)	7–40	10–28	11–29	11–30
Alanine transaminase (units/l)	0–40	6–32	6–32	6–32
Bilirubin (μmol/l)	0–17	4–16	3–13	3–14
γ-GT (units/l)	11–50	5–37	5–43	3–41
Alkaline phosphatase (units/l)	30–130	32–100	43–135	133–418

From Fagan (1995) and Girling et al (1997).

Finland and 12% in Chile. The condition has a complex aetiology, with genetic and environmental factors playing a role. Approximately 35% of affected women have a family history, and the reported pedigrees show autosomal dominant sex-linked inheritance.

Genetic mutations have been reported in a subgroup of women with raised γ-GT (Jacquemin et al 1999). The pathogenesis is not clearly understood, but appears to relate to a predisposition to the cholestatic effect of increased circulating oestrogens (Bacq et al 1995), and progestogens may also play a role (Bacq et al 1997). The classical clinical feature of OC is generalised severe pruritus which commonly develops in the third trimester, becoming more severe with advancing gestation. It is usually most marked on the trunk, soles and palms and is not associated with any skin rash apart from dermatitis artefacta secondary to scratching. The severity of the pruritus is often sufficient to prevent sleep. Rarer symptoms include anorexia, malaise, abdominal discomfort, pale stools and dark urine. If jaundice does develop, it tends to follow the pruritus by 2–4 weeks and to plateau relatively quickly. There may also be malabsorption with steatorrhoea, and this can result in vitamin K deficiency, which can lead to prolongation of clotting times and an increased risk of postpartum haemorrhage (PPH).

While OC is associated with maternal morbidity, its most serious effect is to cause both perinatal morbidity and mortality. OC causes fetal distress (defined as either meconium staining of the amniotic fluid or fetal heart rate abnormalities), spontaneous preterm delivery and unexplained third-trimester intrauterine death (Reid et al 1976, Reyes 1982, Fisk & Storey 1988, Rioseco et al 1994). The perinatal mortality rate has reduced from 10–15% in older studies (Reid et al 1976, Reyes 1982) to 2.0–3.5% in more recent series in which women were delivered not later than 38 weeks' gestation (Fisk & Storey 1988, Rioseco et al 1994). The risk of stillbirth increases towards term but does not correlate with the severity of maternal symptoms.

Abnormal liver function tests (LFT) are necessary to make the diagnosis of OC. The serum total bile acid concentration is increased, and this is largely due to primary bile acids (Bacq et al 1995). The liver transaminases are also moderately raised (commonly two- to threefold), as are alkaline phosphatase (even more than in normal pregnancy) and, less commonly, bilirubin. γ-GT is raised in approximately 20% of cases. OC is a diagnosis of exclusion, and other causes of cholestasis, such as gallstones or extrahepatic obstruction, should be excluded by ultrasound examination. Investigations should also be performed to exclude infectious and autoimmune hepatitis. One large Italian study reported an increased prevalence of OC in women who are hepatitis C positive (Locatelli et al 1999).

The management of OC aims to avoid an adverse fetal outcome and reduce maternal morbidity. The mother should be counselled with regard to the fetal risks and the need for close surveillance. LFT, including prothrombin time, should be checked regularly and fetal well-being monitored at frequent intervals. There is accumulating evidence that the perinatal mortality is considerably reduced by induction of labour no later than 38 weeks' gestation (Reyes 1982, Fisk & Storey

1988, Rioseco et al 1994). Maternal vitamin K administration (10 mg o.d.) reduces the risk of PPH and fetal bleeding.

A variety of drug therapies have been used to reduce maternal pruritus. The two most commonly used drugs, ursodeoxycholic acid (UDCA) and dexamethasone, have been reported to improve both symptoms and LFTs. UDCA is a hydrophilic bile acid, which acts by altering the bile acid pool, and reducing the proportion of hydrophobic, and therefore hepatotoxic, bile acids. There have been several reports on the use of UDCA in OC in which patients are given approximately 1000 mg/day for periods of 7 days to 10 weeks, mainly during the third trimester (Palma et al 1992, 1997, Floreani et al 1996, Nicastri et al 1998). In all the studies the pruritus and LFTs were improved or normalised. All babies born to mothers given UDCA were delivered safely and no problems attributable to treatment were reported. However, UDCA is not yet licensed for use in pregnancy, and the drug should only be used following thorough counselling.

Dexamethasone can also be an effective therapy; a Finnish study reported reduced itching and lowered bile acids and transaminases following treatment with dexamethasone (Hirvioja et al 1992). S-adenosyl methionine has been reported to improve symptoms and LFTs in some studies (Frezza et al 1990, Nicastri et al 1998) but not in others (Floreani et al 1996). Cholestyramine has been used to treat the condition in the past, but few patients have been reported to respond to this treatment, which is in any case poorly tolerated.

Biochemical and clinical features of OC resolve following delivery, but recurrence in subsequent pregnancies is common. Some women may report pruritus associated with the use of oestrogen-containing oral contraceptives and these should either be avoided, or, if taken, the LFTs should be checked on a regular basis. In addition, gallstones are commoner in women with OC, and their relatives.

Acute fatty liver of pregnancy

AFLP is extremely rare but can be fatal for the mother and fetus. Maternal mortality rates (10–20%) are lower now that milder cases are recognised and appropriately treated, and perinatal mortality rates are 20–30%. In the 1994–1996 Confidential Enquiries into Maternal Deaths in the UK there was one death from AFLP (Department of Health et al 1998), compared with two between 1991 and 1993, and five in the previous triennium (1988–1990). AFLP is more common in first pregnancies and is associated with pre-eclampsia (30–60%), male fetuses (ratio 3:1), multiple pregnancy (9–25%) and maternal obesity (Fagan 1995).

Recent studies have demonstrated that a subgroup of women with AFLP and HELLP syndrome are heterozygous for mutations in the mitochondrial trifunctional protein (Wilcken et al 1993, Treem et al 1996, Ibdah et al 1999). These women may succumb to AFLP or HELLP when the fetus is homozygous for β-fatty acid oxidation disorders. The child may present several months after birth with severe hypoglycaemia and hepatic encephalopathy, which can be fatal. It has been suggested that the children of mothers with AFLP should be screened for these disorders (Ibdah et al 1999).

Women typically present in the third trimester with non-specific symptoms. Nausea, anorexia and malaise are common presenting symptoms, and severe vomiting and abdominal pain often develop. Jaundice usually appears within 2 weeks of the onset of symptoms, and women may have pruritus, fever or ascites. Hypertension and proteinuria can occur but are usually mild. An association with transient diabetes insipidus has been reported in some cases (Kennedy et al 1994). The serious complications of fulminant liver failure, disseminated intravascular coagulation (DIC) (see p. 313) and encephalopathy, are becoming less prevalent with prompt diagnosis and delivery.

The main differential diagnosis of AFLP is from other causes of acute liver failure, such as HELLP syndrome, severe pre-eclampsia, viral hepatitis, drug toxicity, paracetamol overdose and alcoholic hepatitis. Many biochemical features are shared between AFLP and HELLP, and the features which can be useful in distinguishing these conditions are shown in Table 18.6.

Classically, AFLP is associated with a three- to tenfold increase in transaminases, raised alkaline phosphatase (above the normal upper limit for pregnancy) and a marked neutrophil leucocytosis (often >15 000/mm^3. Distinctive features, which help to distinguish AFLP from HELLP, are profound hypoglycaemia and marked hyperuricaemia. In severe cases, there may be raised fibrin degradation products, reduced levels of antithrombin and haematological features consistent with DIC. While radiological investigations, such as MRI, CT or ultrasound have been advocated as non-invasive methods of diagnosing AFLP, abnormal liver appearances are not always demonstrated. In contrast, liver biopsy with specific fat stains (oil red O) demonstrates the classical histological features of microvesicular fatty infiltration of hepatocytes, most prominent in the central zone. However, not all units use radiological investigations or liver biopsy to make the diagnosis of AFLP, as diagnosis is possible using a combination of clinical and biochemical indices.

Once a diagnosis of AFLP is made, rapid delivery is essential. Severely ill patients require a multidisciplinary team approach in an intensive care setting. It is important to treat any hypoglycaemia and coagulopathy before delivery, as both can be severe and may require the use of 50% dextrose,

fresh frozen plasma (FFP) and albumin. Supportive therapy may be required for some time after delivery. If a woman has features of fulminant hepatic failure and encephalopathy she should be transferred to a specialist liver unit. Orthotopic liver transplantation should be considered in women who continue to deteriorate despite delivery.

Most women improve promptly after delivery, both clinically and biochemically, and if a woman survives, complete recovery without long-term damage is common. Recurrence of AFLP is rare but has been described, and is particularly likely in women who are heterozygous for disorders of β-fatty acid oxidation, so it is important to monitor subsequent pregnancies carefully.

KEY POINTS: LIVER DISEASE

- Women with jaundice or pruritus in pregnancy should be investigated promptly for liver disease.
- The upper end of the normal range for liver enzymes is reduced in pregnancy.
- Women with obstetric cholestasis should be delivered by 38 weeks' gestation to reduce the risk of fetal complications, including intrauterine death.
- Women with acute fatty liver of pregnancy should be delivered immediately after stabilisation and managed by a multidisciplinary team in an intensive care setting.

ANAEMIA

Physiological changes

Plasma volume increases progressively throughout normal pregnancy, and most of this 50% increase occurs by 34 weeks and is positively correlated with the birthweight of the baby. Because the expansion in plasma volume is greater than the increase in red cell mass, there is a fall in haemoglobin concentration, haematocrit and red cell count. Despite this haemodilution, there is usually no change in mean corpuscular volume (MCV) or mean corpuscular haemoglobin concentration (MCHC). Pregnancy causes a 2–3-fold increase in the requirement for iron, and a 10–20-fold increase in folate requirements. This is to meet the demands of the expanding red cell mass and the fetus and placenta. The increased demand for iron can only be met by a limited increase in absorption, and by mobilising iron stores.

The lower limit of normal for haemoglobin concentration in the non-pregnant female is taken as 11.5–12 g/dl. In the pregnant patient levels below 11 g/dl may be abnormal, although in certain situations, such as multiple pregnancy, associated with larger increases in plasma volume, the physiological dilution of haemoglobin may cause even lower concentrations of haemoglobin. If a haemoglobin level between 9.5 and 11 g/dl is associated with a well-grown fetus, an apparently normal pregnancy, and an MCV which is above 84 fl and which has not fallen more then 6 fl during the pregnancy, then it probably does not indicate anaemia (Steer et al 1995, Steer 2000).

Table 18.6 Differential diagnosis of AFLP and HELLP syndrome

	HELLP	AFLP
Epigastric pain	+	+
Hypertension	+++	+
Proteinuria	+++	+
Elevated liver enzymes	+	++
Hypoglycaemia	+/−	+++
Hyperuricaemia	+	++
Disseminated intravascular coagulation (DIC)	+	++
Thrombocytopenia without DIC	++	+/−
Raised white cell count	+	++
Primiparous	++	+
Male fetus	50%	70% (M:F = 3:1)

Iron-deficiency anaemia

The commonest haematological problem in pregnancy is anaemia, and in over 90% this is due to iron deficiency (Letsky 1995). Most cases present in the third trimester as this is when iron demands reach their peak (1–2 mg/day non-pregnant, 2.5 mg/day first trimester, 6.6 mg/day third trimester). Anaemia in pregnancy is usually diagnosed on routine testing, but may present with tiredness, lethargy, dyspnoea, dizziness or fainting. The adverse effects of chronic anaemia are well recognised, but when iron stores become depleted there are effects on iron-dependent enzymes present in every cell (Finch & Huebers 1982). These metabolic effects influence muscle and neurotransmitter activity, gastrointestinal absorption and epithelial changes. There are reports of an association between iron deficiency anaemia and preterm birth, low birthweight and increased blood loss at delivery (Scholl et al 1992).

Iron-deficiency anaemia is common because many women enter pregnancy with depleted iron stores. The reasons for this include menstrual loss, inadequate diet, or previous recent pregnancies (particularly with an interval of less than a year between delivery and conception). Blood loss at the time of delivery contributes to iron deficiency in the puerperium. Birth spacing and avoidance of teenage pregnancies allow deposition and normalisation of iron stores after pubertal growth or a previous pregnancy. Iron deficiency is more common in multiple pregnancy.

It is generally assumed that a woman who becomes anaemic in pregnancy is iron-deficient, but the diagnosis should be confirmed. The red cell indices give a good indication of iron deficiency. The MCV, mean cell haemoglobin (MCH) and MCHC are all reduced. The first to become abnormal is the MCV, but even this may still remain normal when stores first become depleted. Serum iron and total iron-binding capacity (TIBC) fall in normal pregnancy but levels of serum iron <12 µmol/l and TIBC saturation of <15% indicate iron deficiency. Serum ferritin probably provides an assessment of iron stores (although this has been disputed by some). Levels below 12 µg/l indicate iron deficiency and levels <50 µg/l in early pregnancy suggest the iron stores are inadequate to meet the demands of pregnancy and are therefore an indication for daily iron supplements. In a well-nourished population over 80% of pregnant women at 16 weeks had ferritin levels of 50 µg/l or below despite an Hb of 11 g/dl or above (Letsky 1995).

Many argue that the best approach to iron deficiency in pregnancy is prevention. The rationale for routine supplementation with oral iron is that the increased iron demand during pregnancy cannot be met by most diets and increased absorption alone, and that a high proportion of women in their reproductive years lack storage iron. It may be safer, more practical and more cost-effective to supplement all women rather than screen using a serum ferritin at booking. An Hb estimation alone is unreliable and the late diagnosis of iron-deficiency anaemia may necessitate blood transfusion before delivery. The World Health Organization, in conjunction with the International Nutritional Anemia Consultative Group and the United Nations Children's Fund (Stoltzfus & Dreyfuss 1998), have issued guidelines recommending routine supplements (60 mg iron and 400 µg folic acid daily) to all pregnant women for at least 6 months, extending to 3 months postpartum in areas with a high prevalence of anaemia (>40%). However, this recommendation may not be appropriate for well-nourished women in developed countries, and randomised trials of supplementation in such countries have consistently failed to demonstrate any benefits (Steer 2000). Many women develope significant side-effects from oral iron therapy and can probably safely avoid them if their haematological indices remain normal.

The standard oral preparations (Pregaday, Fefol) are combined with folic acid and are suitable for both prevention and treatment of iron deficiency in pregnancy. For those women who are unable to tolerate oral preparations, parenteral therapy (intramuscular, or more recently intravenous) is an option, but this does not provide more rapid correction of iron deficiency. Iron deficiency diagnosed late in pregnancy may necessitate blood transfusion as the maximum rise in haemoglobin achievable with either oral or parenteral iron is 0.8 g/dl a week.

Folate-deficiency anaemia

The normal dietary folate is inadequate to prevent megaloblastic changes in the bone marrow in about 25% of pregnant women. The incidence of megaloblastic anaemia is variable, depending on the socioeconomic status and nutrition of the population. Folate deficiency is more likely if the woman is taking anticonvulsant drugs. Haematological conditions such as haemolytic anaemia, thalassaemia and hereditary spherocytosis complicating pregnancy also increase the risk of folate deficiency.

Folate deficiency causes a macrocytic anaemia with megaloblastic change in the bone marrow. However, a raised MCV can be a feature of normal pregnancy. Diagnosis is confirmed by measurement of serum and red cell folate (it should be noted that the normal range in pregnancy is lower than in non-pregnant women). All women planning a pregnancy are now advised to take 400 µg/day folate periconceptually to lower the risk of neural tube defects and other fetal abnormalities (MRC Vitamin Study Research Group (1991).

In addition, women who have had a previous fetus with a neural tube defect and women taking anticonvulsants or sulphasolazine are advised to take 5 mg folate periconceptually, and in the case of anticonvulsants, throughout pregnancy. The 5 mg dose is also appropriate for those with other haematological problems and those with established folate deficiency. Routine folate supplementation in pregnancy is recommended by WHO (Stoltzfus & Dreyfuss 1998), as a normal diet is not sufficient to meet the increased requirement for folate in pregnancy, although studies have never demonstrated any adverse effects from folate deficiency after the first trimester.

Sickle cell disease

Sickle cell haemoglobin (HbS) is a variant of the β chain of haemoglobin. Sickling of the red cells occurs particularly in

293

response to hypoxia, cold, acidosis and dehydration. Intravascular sickling leads to vaso-occlusive symptoms and tissue infarction with severe pain. A number of variants of sickle cell disease exist, including homozygous sickle cell disease (HbSS), sickle cell/HbC (HbSC) and sickle cell thalassaemia. Sickle cell trait (HbAS) is the most common but, other than implications for genetic counselling, does not affect pregnancy in the same way as sickle cell disease. Sickle cell disease causes anaemia, painful crises and an increased risk of infections, partly due to loss of splenic function. The acute chest syndrome is characterised by fever, tachypnoea, pleuritic chest pain, leucocytosis and pulmonary infiltrates. It may be caused by pulmonary infection or infarction from intravascular sickling. Other features of sickle cell disease include splenic sequestration, retinopathy, leg ulcers, aseptic necrosis of bone, renal papillary necrosis and stroke. Women with HbSS have a chronic haemolytic anaemia, but are generally healthy except during periods of crisis, which are often precipitated by infection. A generalised vasculopathy or massive sickling leads to premature death at a mean age of under 50 years. Those with HbSC are not usually very anaemic, but are still at risk of sickling. They also have a reduced life expectancy (under 70 years).

Most women enter pregnancy with the diagnosis established, but if there is doubt, the diagnosis can be made by haemoglobin electrophoresis. Complications of sickle cell disease are more common in pregnancy. Recent data suggest crises complicate about 35% of pregnancies affected by sickle disease. Perinatal mortality is increased 4–6-fold. There is an increased incidence of miscarriage, IUGR, preterm labour, pre-eclampsia (which may have an early onset and an accelerated course), fetal distress and caesarean section (Howard 1996). Sickling infarcts in the placenta may be responsible for some of these factors, although maternal anaemia and increased blood viscosity also contribute to the high incidence of fetal growth restriction. There is an increased risk of pulmonary thrombosis, thromboembolism and bone marrow embolism. Maternal morbidity and mortality are increased and the latter has been estimated at 2.5%. There is also an increased risk of infection, particularly urinary tract infection, pneumonia and puerperal sepsis. This is due to the autosplenectomy resulting from sickle cell disease.

Antenatal care should be in combined clinics by haematologists, midwives and obstetricians with experience of these disorders. Folic acid (5 mg/day) should be given to all women. Electrophoresis will determine the level of HbF (the higher the level the better the outcome) and the % of HbS. If prepregnancy counselling and screening of the partner has not already been undertaken, this should be advised in order to determine the risk of the baby having HbSS (50% if the partner is sickle cell trait). Blood for haemoglobin estimation and MSU are sent at each visit. Prophylactic penicillin should be continued throughout pregnancy. Regular ultrasound assessment of fetal growth, with 2–4-weekly growth parameters and umbilical artery Dopplers from 24 weeks, should be performed. Crises are managed aggressively, as in the nonpregnant patient. This involves adequate pain relief with intravenous or subcutaneous infusions of morphine, adequate rehydration, and early use of antibiotics if infection is

suspected. Women should be kept warm and well oxygenated. Arterial blood gas measurement or pulse oximetry are mandatory, especially if high doses of opiates are being given. In the acute chest syndrome it may be necessary to use both intravenous heparin and antibiotics (Nelson-Piercy 1997). Blood transfusion may be required for severe anaemia or splenic sequestration, or in the acute chest syndrome. The role of routine exchange transfusion in pregnancy is controversial. Proponents claim a decrease in the number of crises, although there is little evidence for improved fetal outcome. The risks include delayed and immediate transfusion reactions, the precipitation of a crisis (particularly if the haematocrit is raised above 0.35), infection, red cell antibodies (because the donor blood is often from people of a different ethnic origin from the patient), and iron overload. Caesarean section should only be performed for obstetric indications and general anaesthesia should be avoided if possible, especially if the woman has not been transfused.

KEY POINTS: ANAEMIA

- Iron deficiency is very common in pregnancy and can be prevented with routine oral supplementation.
- In sickle cell disease, pregnancy is associated with an increased risk of crises, miscarriage, pre-eclampsia, IUGR and perinatal mortality
- Pregnant women with sickle cell disease should receive 5 mg folic acid and prophylactic penicillin.

REFERENCES

Backos M, Rai R, Baxter N et al 1999 Pregnancy complications in women with recurrent miscarriage associated with antiphospholipid antibodies treated with low dose aspirin and heparin. Br J Obstet Gynaecol 106:102–107

Bacq Y, Myara A, Brechot MC et al 1995 Serum conjugated bile acid profile during intrahepatic cholestasis of pregnancy. J Hepatol 22:66–70

Bacq Y, Sapey T, Brechot MC, Pierre F, Fignon A, Dubois F 1997 Intrahepatic cholestasis of pregnancy: a French prospective study. Hepatology 26:358–364

Bardy A 1982 Epilepsy and pregnancy: a prospective study of 154 pregnancies in epileptic women. University of Helsinki, Finland

Bedalov A, Balasubramanyam A 1997 Glucocorticoid-induced ketoacidosis in gestational diabetes: sequela of the acute treatment of preterm labour. Diabetes Care 6:922–924

Bermas BL, Hill JA 1995 Effects of immunosuppressive drugs during pregnancy. Arthritis Rheum 38:1722–1732

Boulvain M, Stan C, Irion O 2000 Elective delivery in diabetic pregnant women (Cochrane review). In: The Cochrane library, issue 3. Oxford: Update Software

British Guidelines on Asthma Management 1997 1995 review and position statement. Thorax 52 (suppl) S1–21

Buchanan NMM, Toubi E, Khamashta MA, Lima F, Kerslake S, Hughes G 1996 Hydroxychloroquine and lupus pregnancy: a review of a series of 36 cases. Ann Rheum Dis 55:486–488

Burrow GN 1993 Thyroid function and hyperfunction during gestation. Endocrinol Rev 14:194–202

Buschard K, Hougaard P, Molsted-Pedersen L, Kuhl C 1990 Type 1 (insulin dependent) diabetes mellitus diagnosed during pregnancy: a clinical and prognostic study. Diabetologia 33:31–35

Casson IF, Clarke CA, Howard CV et al 1997 Outcomes of pregnancy in insulin dependent diabetic women: results of a five year population cohort study. BMJ 315:275–278

Centers for Disease Control and Prevention 1997 Postmarketing surveillance for angiotensin-converting enzyme inhibitor use during the first trimester of pregnancy: United States, Canada and Israel 1987–1995. JAMA 277:1193–1194

Cleland PG 1996 Management of pre-existing disorders in pregnancy: epilepsy. Prescriber's J 36:102–109

Comtois R, Desjarlais F, Nguyen M, Beauregard H 1989 Clinical usefulness of estimation of serum fructosamine concentration as screening test for gestational diabetes. Am J Obstet Gynecol 160:651–654

Cousins L 1988 In: Reece EA, Coustan DR (eds) Diabetes mellitus in pregnancy: principles and practice. Churchill Livingstone, Edinburgh

Cowchock FS, Reece EA, Balaban D, Branch DW, Plouffe L 1992 Repeated fetal losses associated with antiphospholipid antibodies: a collaborative randomized trial comparing prednisone with low-dose heparin treatment. Am J Obstet Gynecol 166:1318–1323

Crawford P, Appleton R, Betts T et al 1999 Best practice guidelines for the management of women with epilepsy. Seizure 8:201–217

Czeizel AE, Rockenbauer M 1997 Population-based case–control study of teratogenic potential of corticosteroids. Teratology 56:335–340

Dahlman TC 1993 Osteoporotic fractures and the recurrence of thromboembolism during pregnancy and the puerperium in 184 women undergoing thromboprophylaxis with heparin. Am J Obstet Gynecol 168:1265–1270

Deblay MF, Vert P, Andre M, Marchal F 1982 Transplacental vitamin K prevents haemorrhagic disease of infant of epileptic mother. Lancet i:1247

Demissie K, Breckenridge MB, Rhoads GG 1998 Infant and maternal outcomes in the pregnancies of asthmatic women. Am J Respir Crit Care Med 158:1091–1095

Department of Health, Welsh Office, Scottish Home and Health Department and Department of Health and Social Services, Northern Ireland 1998 Confidential enquiries into maternal deaths in the United Kingdom 1994–96. HMSO, London

de Veciana M, Major CA, Morgan MA et al 1995 Postprandial versus preprandial blood glucose monitoring in women with gestational diabetes mellitus requiring insulin therapy. N Engl J Med 333:1237–1241

Diamond T, Kormas N 1997 Possible adverse fetal effect of insulin lispro. N Engl J Med 337:1009

Doherty CM, Shindo ML, Rice DH, Montero M, Mestman JH 1995 Management of thyroid nodules during pregnancy. Laryngoscope 105:251–255

Dooley SL, Metzger BE, Cho N, Liu K 1991 The influence of demographic and phenotypic heterogeneity on the prevalence of gestational diabetes mellitus. Int J Gynaecol Obstet 35: 13–18

Dornhurst A, Bailey PC, Anyaoku V, Elkeles RS, Johnston DG, Beard RW 1990 Abnormalities of glucose tolerance following gestational diabetes. Q J Med 77:1219–1228

Doucette JT, Bracken MB 1993 Possible role of asthma in the risk of preterm labor and delivery. Epidemiology 4:143–150

Drug and Therapeutics Bulletin 1995 The practical management of thyroid disease in pregnancy. Drug Ther Bull 33:75–77

Fagan EA 1995 Disorders of the liver, biliary system and pancreas. In: de Swiet M (ed) Medical disorders in obstetric practice, 3rd edn. Blackwell, Oxford, pp 321–378

Fainstat T 1954 Cortisone-induced congenital cleft palate in rabbits. Endocrinology 55:502

Farquharson RG, Quenby S, Greaves M (2001) J Obstet Gynaecol, 21:522

Finch LA, Huebers H 1982 Perspectives in iron metabolism. N Engl J Med 306:1520–1528

Fisk NM, Storey GNB 1988 Fetal outcome in obstetric cholestasis. Br J Obstet Gynaecol 95:1137–1143

Fitzsimons R, Greenberger PA, Patterson R 1986 Outcome of pregnancy in women requiring corticosteroids for severe asthma. J Allergy Clin Immunol 78:349–353

Floreani A, Paternoster D, Melis A, Grella PV 1996 S-adenosyl methionine versus ursodeoxycholic acid in the treatment of intrahepatic cholestasis of pregnancy: preliminary results of a controlled trial. Eur J Obstet Gynecol Reprod Biol 67:109–113

Frezza M, Centini G, Cammareri G, Le Grazie C, Di Padova C 1990 S-adenosyl methionine for the treatment of intrahepatic cholestasis of pregnancy. Results of a controlled clinical trial. Hepatogastroenterology 37(Suppl 2):122–125

Friis ML, Holm NV, Sindrup EH et al 1986 Facial clefts in sibs and children of epileptic patients. Neurology 36:346–350

Garner P, Okun N, Keely MD et al 1997 A randomised controlled trial of strict glycaemic control and tertiary level obstetric care versus routine obstetric care in the management of gestational diabetes: a pilot study. Am J Obstet Gynecol 177:190–195

Girling JC 1996 Thyroid disease and pregnancy. Br J Hosp Med 56:316–320

Girling JC, de Swiet M 1992 Thyroxine dosage during pregnancy in women with primary hypothyroidism. Br J Obstet Gynaecol 99:368–370

Girling JC, Dow E, Smith JH 1997 Liver function tests in pre-eclampsia: importance of comparison with a reference range derived for normal pregnancy. Br J Obstet Gynaecol 104:246–250

Gluck JC, Gluck P 1976 The effects of pregnancy on asthma: a prospective study. Ann Allergy 37:164–168

Goodwin TM, Montero M, Mestman JH 1992 Transient hyperthyroidism and hyperemesis gravidarum: clinical aspects. Am J Obstet Gynecol 167:648–652

Gordon C, Kilby MD 1998 Use of intravenous immunoglobulin therapy in pregnancy in systemic lupus erythematosus and antiphospholipid antibody syndrome. Lupus 7:429–433

Granger KA, Farquharson RG 1997 Obstetric outcome in antiphospholipid syndrome. Lupus 6:509–513

Greenberger P, Patterson R 1983 Beclomethasone dipropionate for severe asthma during pregnancy. Ann Intern Med 98:478–480

Greenberger PA, Patterson R 1988 The outcome of pregnancy complicated by severe asthma. Allergy Proc 9:539–543

Grenfell A, Bewick M, Brudenell M et al 1986 Diabetic pregnancy following renal transplantation. Diabet Med 3:177–179

Haddow JE, Palomaki GE, Allen WC et al 1999 Maternal thyroid deficiency during pregnancy and subsequent neuropsychological development in the child. N Engl J Med 341:549–555

Hall R, Richards CJ, Lazarus JH 1993 The thyroid and pregnancy. Br J Obstet Gynaecol 100:512–515

Hawthorne G, Robson S, Ryall EA, Sen D, Roberts SH, Ward Platt MP 1997 Prospective population based survey of outcome of pregnancy in diabetic women: results of the northern diabetic pregnancy audit, 1994. BMJ 315:279–281

Hirvioja ML, Tuimala R, Vuori J 1992 The treatment of intrahepatic cholestasis of pregnancy by dexamethasone. Br J Obstet Gynaecol 99:109–111

Hod M, Merlob P, Friedman S, Schoenfeld A, Ovadia J 1991 Gestational diabetes mellitus: a survey of perinatal complications in the early 1980s. Diabetes 40 (suppl 2):74–78

Hofmann HMH 1990 Fructosamine in relation to maternofetal glucose and insulin homeostasis in gestational diabetes. Arch Gynecol Obstet 247:173–185

Hollingsworth DR 1985 Neonatal hyperthyroidism. Paediatr Adolesc Endocrinol 14:210–222

Howard RJ 1996 Management of sickling conditions in pregnancy. Br J Hosp Med 56:7–10

Hunt B, Khamashta MA, Lakasing L et al 1998 Thromboprophylaxis in antiphospholipid syndrome pregnancies with previous cerebral arterial thrombotic events: is warfarin preferable? Thromb Haemost 79:1060–1061

Ibdah JA, Bennett MJ, Rinaldo P et al 1999 A fetal fatty-acid oxidation disorder as a cause of liver disease in pregnant women. N Engl J Med 340: 1723–1731

Ito S, Moretti M, Liau M, Koren G 1995 Initiation and duration of breast-feeding in women receiving antiepileptics. Am J Obstet Gynecol 172:881–886

Jacquemin E, Crestil D, Manouvier S, Boute O, Hadchouel M 1999 Heterozygous non-sense mutation in the MDR3 gene in familial intrahepatic cholestasis of pregnancy. Lancet 353: 210–211

Jovanovic L, Ilic S, Pettitt DJ et al 1999 Metabolic and immunologic effects of insulin lispro in gestational diabetes. Diabetes Care 22:1422–1427

Kallen B, Rydhstroem H, Aberg A 1999 Congenital malformations after the use of inhaled budesonide in early pregnancy. Obstet Gynecol 93:392–395

Kennedy S, Hall PM, Seymour AE, Hague WM 1994 Transient diabetes insipidus and acute fatty liver of pregnancy. Br J Obstet Gynaecol 101:387–391

Khamashta MA, Cuadrado MJ, Mujic F, Taub NA, Hunt BJ, Hughes GR 1995 The management of thrombosis in the antiphospholipid-antibody syndrome. N Engl J Med 332:993–997

Khamashta MA, Ruiz-Irastoza G, Hughes GRV 1997 Systemic lupus erythematosus flares during pregnancy. Rheum Dis Clin North Am 23:15–30

Kilvert JA, Nicholson HO, Wright AD 1993 Ketoacidosis in diabetic pregnancy. Diabet Med 10:278–281

Kitzmiller JL, Brown ER, Philippe M et al 1981 Diabetic nephropathy and perinatal outcome. Am J Obstet Gynecol 141:741–751

Kjos SL, Henry OA, Montoro M, Buchanan TA, Mestman JH 1993 Insulin-requiring diabetes in pregnancy: a randomised trial of active induction of labor and expectant management. Am J Obstet Gynecol 169:611–615

Kotarba DD, Garner P, Perkins SL 1995 Changes in serum free thyroxine, free tri-iodothyronine and thyroid stimulating hormone reference intervals in normal term pregnant women. J Obstet Gynaecol 15:5–8

Kutteh WH 1996 Antiphospholipid antibody-associated recurrent pregnancy loss: treatment with heparin and low-dose aspirin is superior to low-dose aspirin alone. Am J Obstet Gynecol 174:1574–1589

Lamberg BA, Ikonen E, Osterlund K et al 1984 Antithyroid treatment of maternal hyperthyroidism during lactation. Clin Endocrinol 21:81–87

Landon MB, Gabbe SG 1994 Diabetes mellitus. In: James DK, Steer PJ, Weiner CP, Gonik B (eds) High risk pregnancy: management options. WB Saunders, London, pp 277–297

Langford K, Nelson-Piercy C 1999 Antiphospholipid syndrome in pregnancy. Contemp Rev Obstet Gynaecol 11:93–98

Lean ME, Pearson DW, Sutherland HW 1990 Insulin management during labour and delivery in mothers with diabetes. Diabet Med 7:162–164

Lehrer S, Stone J, Lapinski R et al 1993 Association between pregnancy-induced hypertension and asthma. Am J Obstet Gynecol 168:1463–1466

Letsky EA 1995 Blood volume, haematinics, anaemia. In: de Swiet M (ed) Medical disorders in obstetric practice 3rd edn. Blackwell Science, Oxford, pp 33–70

Leung AS, Millar LK, Koonings PP, Montero M, Mestman JH 1993 Perinatal outcome in hypothyroid pregnancies. Obstet Gynecol 81:349–353

Lima F, Buchanan NMM, Khamastha MA, Kerslake S, Hughes GRV 1995 Obstetric outcome in systemic lupus erythematosus. Semin Arthritis Rheum 25:184–192

Lima F, Khamashta MA, Buchanan NMM, Kerslake S, Hunt BJ, Hughes GRV 1996 A study of sixty pregnacies in patients with the antiphospholipid syndrome. Clin Exp Rheumatol 14:131–136

Locatelli A, Roncaglia N, Arreghini A, Bellini P, Vergani P, Ghidini A 1999 Hepatitis C virus infection is associated with a higher incidence of cholestasis of pregnancy. Br J Obstet Gynaecol 106:498–500

Lyons Jones K, Lacro RV, Johnson KA, Adams J 1989 Pattern of malformations in the children of women treated with carbamazepine during pregnancy. N Engl J Med 320:1661–1666

McCune AB, Weston WL, Lee LA 1987 Maternal and fetal outcome in neonatal lupus erythematosus. Ann Intern Med 106:518–523

Mann RD, Kubota K, Pearce G, Wilton L 1996 Salmeterol: a study by prescription event monitoring in a UK cohort of 15 407 patients. J Clin Epidemiol 49:247–250

Maresh M, Beard R 1995 Diabetes. In: de Swiet M (ed) Medical disorders in obstetric practice. 3rd edn. Blackwell Science, Oxford

Mather HM, Keen H 1985 The Southall diabetes survey: prevalence of diabetes in Asians and Europeans. BMJ 291:1081–1084

Mestman JH, Goodwin TM, Montoro MN 1995 Thyroid disorders of pregnancy. Endocrinol Metab Clin North Am 24:41–71

Midovnik M, Mimouni F, Tsang RC et al 1987 Management of the insulin dependent diabetic during labor and delivery. Influences on neonatal outcome. Am J Perinatol 4:106–114

Mimouni F, Miodovnik M, Siddiqi TA, Butler JB, Holroyde J, Tsang RC 1986 Neonatal polycythemia in infants of insulin dependent diabetic mothers. Obstet Gynecol 68:370–372

Minerbi-Codish I, Fraser D, Avnun L, Glezerman M, Heimer D 1998 Influence of asthma in pregnancy on labor and the newborn. Respiration 65:130–135

Montero MN, Myers VP, Mestman JH, Yunhua X, Anderson BG, Golde SH 1993 Outcome of pregnancy in diabetic ketoacidosis. Am J Perinatol 10:17–20

MRC Vitamin Study Research Group 1991 Prevention of neural tube defects: results of the MRC vitamin study. Lancet 338:132–137

Nachum Z, Ben-Shlomo I, Weiner E, Shalev E 1999 Twice daily versus four times daily insulin dose regimens for diabetes in pregnancy: randomised controlled trial. BMJ 319:1223–1227

Nakane Y, Okuma T, Takahashi R et al 1980 Multi-institutional study on the teratogenicity and fetal toxicity of antiepileptic drugs: a report of a collaborative study in group in Japan. Epilepsia 21:663–680

Nelson-Piercy C 1997 Handbook of obstetric medicine. Isis Medical Media, Oxford

Nelson-Piercy C, Gale EAM 1994 Do we know how to screen for gestational diabetes? Current practice in one regional health authority. Diabet Med 11:493–498

Nicastri PL, Diaferia A, Tartagni M, Loizzi P, Fanelli M 1998 A randomised placebo-controlled trial of ursodeoxycholic acid and S-adenosylmethionine in the treatment of intrahepatic cholestasis of pregnancy. Br J Obstet Gynaecol 105:1205–1207

Oakley NW, Beard RW, Turner RC 1972 Effect of sustained maternal hyperglycaemia on the fetus in normal and diabetic pregnancies. BMJ 1:466–469

O'Brien MD, Gilmour-White S 1993 Epilepsy and pregnancy. BMJ 307:492–495

O'Doherty MJ, McElhatton PR, Thomas SHL 1999 Treating thyrotoxicosis in pregnant or potentially pregnant women. BMJ 318:5–6

Ornoy A, Cohen E 1996 Outcome of children born to epileptic mothers treated with carbamazepine during pregnancy. Arch Dis Child 75:517–520

Ostenson M, Ramsey-Golman R 1998 Treatment of inflammatory rheumatic disorders in pregnancy. Drug Safety 19:389–410

Oviasu E, Hicks J, Cameron JS 1991 The outcome of pregnancy in women with lupus nephritis. Lupus 1:19–25

Palma J, Reyes H, Ribalta J et al 1992 Effects of ursodeoxycholic acid in patients with intrahepatic cholestasis of pregnancy. Hepatology 15:1043–1047

Palma J, Reyes H, Ribalta J et al 1997 Ursodeoxycholic acid in the treatment of cholestasis of pregnancy: a randomized, double-blind study controlled with placebo. J Hepatol 27:1022–1028

Parker JH 1985 Amerlex free triiodothyronine and free thyroxine levels in normal pregnancy. Br J Obstet Gynaecol 92:1234–1238

Patterson CA, Graves WL, Bugg G, Sasso SC, Brann AW Jr 1989 Antenatal and intrapartum factors associated with the occurrence of seizures in term infant. Obstet Gynecol 74:361–365

Pekonen F, Teramo K, Makinen T, Ikonen E, Osterlund K, Lamberg BA 1984 Prenatal diagnosis and treatment of fetal thyrotoxicosis. Am J Obstet Gynecol 150:893–894

Penn K, Makowski EL, Harris P 1980 Parenthood following renal transplantation. Kidney Int 18:221–233

Perlow JH, Montgomery D, Morgan MA, Towers CV, Porto M 1992 Severity of asthma and perinatal outcome. Am J Obstet Gynecol 167:963–967

Pop VJ, Kuijpens JL, van Baar AL et al 1999 Low maternal free thyroxine concentrations during early pregnancy are associated with impaired psychomotor development in infancy. Clin Endocrinol 50:149–155

Rai R, Cohen H, Dave M, Regan L 1997 Randomized controlled trial of aspirin and aspirin plus heparin in pregnant women with recurrent miscarriage associated with phospholipid antibodies (or antiphospholipid antibodies). BMJ 314:253–257

Ramsay I, Kaur S, Krassas G 1983 Thyrotoxicosis in pregnancy: results of treatment by antithyroid drugs combined with T$_4$. Clin Endocrinol 18:73–85

Rasmussen MJ, Firth R, Foley M, Stronge JM 1992 The timing of delivery in pregnancy: a 10 year review. Aust N Z J Obstet Gynaecol 32:313–317

Reid R, Ivey KJ, Rencoret RH, Storey B 1976 Fetal complications of obstetric cholestasis. BMJ 1:870–872

Report of the Expert Committee on the Diagnosis and Classification of Diabetes Mellitus 1997 Diabetes Care 7:1183–1197

Reyes H 1982 The enigma of intrahepatic cholestasis of pregnancy: lessons from Chile. Hepatology 2:87–96

Rioseco AJ, Ivankovic MB, Manzur A et al 1994 Intrahepatic cholestasis of pregnancy: a retrospective case–control study of perinatal outcome. Am J Obstet Gynecol 170:890–895

Roberts AB, Baker JR, James AG, Henley P 1988 Fructosamine in the management of gestational diabetes. Am J Obstet Gynecol 159:66–71

Roberts AB, Baker JR, Metcalf P, Mullard C 1990 Fructosamine compared with a glucose load as a screening test for gestational diabetes. Obstet Gynecol 76:773–775

Rodriguez-Pinilla E, Martinez-Frias ML 1998 Corticosteroids during pregnancy and oral clefts: a case–control study. Teratology 58:2–5

Rosa FW 1991 Spina bifida in infants of women treated with carbamazepine during pregnancy. N Engl J Med 324:674–677

Ruiz-Irastoza G, Lima F, Alves J et al 1996 Increased rate of lupus flare during pregnancy and the puerperium: a prospective study of 78 pregnancies. Br J Rheumatol 35:133–138

Samren EB, van Duijn CM, Koch S et al 1997 Maternal use of antiepileptic drugs and the risk of major congenital malformations: a joint European prospective study of human teratogenesis associated with maternal epilepsy. Epilepsia 38: 981–990

Schatz M, Patterson R, Zeitz S, O'Rourke J, Melam H 1975 Corticosteroid therapy for the pregnant asthmatic patient. JAMA 233:804–807

Schatz M, Zeiger RS, Harden KM et al 1988 The safety of inhaled β-agonist bronchodilators during pregnancy. J Allergy Clin Immunol 82:686–695

Schatz M, Zeiger RS, Hoffman CP 1990 Intrauterine growth is related to gestational pulmonary function in pregnant asthmatic women. Kaiser-Permanente asthma and pregnancy study group. Chest 98:389–392

Schatz M, Zeiger RS, Hoffman CP, Saunders BS, Harden KM, Forsythe AB 1991 Increased transient tachypnoea of the newborn in infants of asthmatic mothers. Am J Dis Child 145: 156–158

Schatz M, Zeiger RS, Hoffman CP et al 1995 Perinatal outcomes in the pregnancies of asthmatic women: a prospective controlled analysis. Am J Respir Crit Care Med 151:1170–1174

Schatz M, Zeiger RS, Harden K, Hoffman CP, Chilingar L, Petitti D 1997 The safety of asthma and allergy medications during pregnancy. J Allergy Clin Immunol 100:301–306

Scholl TO, Hediger ML, Fischer RL, Shearer JW 1992 Anemia vs iron deficiency: increased risk of preterm delivery in a prospective study. Am J Clin Nutr 55:985–988

Serup L 1986 Influence of pregnancy on diabetic retinopathy. Acta Endocrinol Suppl Copenh 277:122–124

Snyder RD, Snyder D 1978 Corticosteroids for asthma during pregnancy. Ann Allergy 41:340–341

Steer P 2000 Maternal haemoglobin concentration and birth weight. Am J Clin Nutr 71 (suppl):12855–12875

Steer P, Alain AA, Wadsworth J, Welsh A 1995 Relation between maternal haemoglobin concentration and birth weight. BMJ 310:489–491

Steffensen FH, Nielsen GL, Sorensen HT, Olesen C, Olsen J 1998 Pregnancy outcome with ACE-inhibitor use in early pregnancy. Lancet 351:596

Stenius-Aarniala B, Piirila P, Teramo K 1988 Asthma and pregnancy: a prospective study of 198 pregnancies. Thorax 43:12–18

Stenius-Aarniala B, Riikonen S, Teramo K 1995 Slow-release theophylline in pregnant asthmatics. Chest 107:642–647

Stoltzfus RJ, Dreyfuss MI 1998 Guidelines for the use of iron supplements to prevent and treat iron deficiency anemia. International nutritional anemia consultative group, World Health Organization, United Nations Children's Fund. ILSI Press, Washington

Treem WR, Shoup ME, Hale DE et al 1996 Acute fatty liver of pregnancy, hemolysis, elevated liver enzymes, and low platelets syndrome, and long chain 3-hydroxyacyl-coenzyme A dehydrogenase deficiency. Am J Gastroenterol 91:2293–2300

Vidovic MI, Della Marina BM 1994 Trimestral changes of seizure frequency in pregnant epileptic women. Acta Med Croatica 48:85–87

Waltuck J, Buyon JP 1994 Autoantibody-associated congenital heart block: outcome in mothers and children. Ann Intern Med 120:544–551

Ware Branch D, Silver RM, Blackwell JL, Reading JC, Scott JR 1992 Outcome of treated pregnancies in women with antiphospholipid syndrome: an update of the Utah experience. Obstet Gynecol 80:614–620

Wendel PJ, Ramin SM, Barnett-Hamm C, Rowe TF, Cunningham FG 1996 Asthma treatment in pregnancy: a randomised controlled study. Am J Obstet Gynecol 175:150–154

White RJ, Coutts I, Gibbs CJ, MacIntyre C 1989 A prospective study of asthma during pregnancy and the puerperium. Respir Med 83:103–106

Wilcken B, Leung KC, Hammond J, Kamath R, Leonard JV 1993 Pregnancy and fetal long-chain 3-hydroxyacyl coenzyme A dehydrogenase deficiency. Lancet 341:407–408

Wilson WA, Gharavi AE, Koike T, Khamastha MA 1999 International consensus statement on preliminary classification criteria for antiphospholipid syndrome: report of an international workshop. Arthritis Rheum 42, 1309–1311

Wing DA, Millar LK, Koonings PP, Montoro MN, Mestman JH 1994 A comparison of propylthiouracil versus methimazole in the treatment of hyperthyroidism in pregnancy. Am J Obstet Gynecol 170:90–95

Yerby MS 1994 Pregnancy, teratogenesis, and epilepsy. Neurol Clin 12:749–771

Zakarija M, McKenzie JM, Hoffman WH 1986 Prediction and therapy of intrauterine and late-onset neonatal hyperthyroidism. J Clin Endocrinol Metab 62:368–371

19

Psychiatric problems in pregnancy and the puerperium

The late R. Kumar, Lorien O'Dowd

INTRODUCTION

Need for closer liaison between obstetricians and psychiatrists

Recognition and effective management of psychiatric disorders in childbearing women must become a clinical priority, not only because of undesirable consequences of such disorders for the mother, but also because of their potential adverse impact on the developing infant, as well as on the rest of the family. In this chapter it is argued that good and safe obstetric practice must include competence in recognising the major forms of mental illness and their associated complications. A proactive approach in liaison with a psychiatrist, where necessary, should not only improve obstetric and paediatric outcomes, but it should also reduce the burden of mental disorder.

A great deal has been achieved in developed nations in recent years to bring down rates of maternal and perinatal infant mortality and morbidity, but rates of maternal postnatal mental illness have not declined in parallel (Kumar 1994). Mortality rates are an index of underlying ill health and the fact that suicide is now one of the major causes of maternal death (Lewis & Drife 1998) highlights the need to confront the problem of mental illness in childbearing women. Similarly, in Britain the risk of being a victim of homicide is at least four times greater in the first year of life than it is in any other year and this risk is maximal in the first 3 months; the perpetrators are almost always parents (Marks & Kumar 1993). A recent catchment area survey in southwest England and Wales found the rate of subdural haemorrhage

to be 21/100 000 individuals at risk for 0–1-year-old children, the great majority being cases of non-accidental injury and less than 3 months old (Jayawant et al 1998). Not all parents who kill or harm their children are, however, mentally ill (Marks 1996) and most mentally ill adults are loving and caring parents. By the same token, only a tiny minority of mentally ill childbearing women commit suicide, and, in fact, having a baby is protective (Appleby 1996).

The challenge, therefore, is to identify the clusters of factors that confer increased risk of self-harm or of harming others and then of being able to do something about it. Ascertaining the presence or risk of mental disorder is crucial, but it is only a part of the process of enquiring about the personal, family and social context into which the child will be born.

There are other ways than physical harm in which parental mental illness exerts its adverse effects; for example, pregnant women who are severely ill may not comply with antenatal care. Psychotropic drugs, prescribed and non-prescribed, can affect fetal development and obstetric outcome. There is now compelling evidence that the psychological development of infants can be adversely affected if their mothers are depressed postnatally. Pregnancy and the puerperium are times when women see health professionals (obstetricians, midwives, general practitioners, health visitors, paediatricians) more than they will at any other time in their lives, yet there is little evidence of systematic protocols in antenatal clinics that are intended to identify women who are suffering from psychiatric disorders or those at risk (Kumar 1998).

Procedures that screen for mental health problems in

childbearing women cannot succeed without the full support and participation of obstetricians and midwives and, in order to be effective, they must be applied to everyone attending for maternity care. Mothers and clinicians may, however, argue that the primary purpose of a maternity service is to ensure a safe and healthy outcome to pregnancy and not to serve as an outpost for psychiatry. Furthermore, the majority of women having babies are mentally well and might regard questions about their psychological health as intrusive, as well as raising concerns about confidentiality. Thus, obstetricians and midwives have to be convinced about the benefits of a proactive approach to mental illness and that is one of the aims of this chapter.

Destigmatising mental illness in the population cannot be achieved unless there is openness and a positive attitude in professionals. Screening methods are based on the subject's consent and compliance, and sequential procedures avoid unnecessary questions. Professionals must adhere to strict rules concerning confidentiality, although important information must be permitted to be exchanged between professionals in a multidisciplinary setting. A mother's wishes as to whether or not she wants any particular intervention must be respected. Only in extreme circumstances, and then on an individual case basis, will it be necessary to proceed with an intervention against the mother's wishes, having first taken legal advice, by recourse to the Mental Health Act or Child Protection Legislation. On the other hand, it is also important not to delay a common-sense life-saving action, and, although the need for such decisions is rare, they are made easier by experience of risk assessment and by consultation with professional colleagues.

Psychological influences on obstetric outcome and impact of obstetric complications on mental health

Effects of psychosocial stress on pregnancy outcome

In a comprehensive review of the effects of psychosocial factors and pregnancy outcome, Paarlberg et al (1995) established the most consistent relationship to be between maternal exposure to taxing situations and preterm delivery. They suggested that there were both indirect mediating mechanisms, such as unhealthy coping and life style behaviours, and direct mechanisms, such as stress-dependent hormones and psychoimmunological factors. There was also an association between psychological stressors in pregnancy and low birthweight, and less consistent evidence for an association with spontaneous abortion and pre-eclampsia. Psychosocial stress in pregnancy is also associated with emotional disturbance in the mother (Bernazzani et al 1997) which, in turn may be linked with adverse perinatal outcome (Lou et al 1994, Bhagwanani et al 1997). One possible mediating mechanism may be impaired blood flow in the uterine artery (Teixeira et al 1999). Intervention studies have not yet demonstrated significant beneficial effects (Paarlberg et al 1995, Langer et al 1996).

Termination of pregnancy

About 20% of pregnancies in the UK end in therapeutic termination before 24 weeks' gestation, but it is unusual for a psychiatrist to be involved in the recommendation for termination. The great majority are carried out for psychosocial reasons, and thus, in this sense, psychological factors are the most important determinants of pregnancy outcome. Clare (1994) reviewed the psychiatric aspects of termination and, in line with other reviews, concluded that most studies show the psychiatric consequences to be mild and transient. Only 1.3% of women were reported as requiring treatment in the largest follow-up study of women after termination (Frank et al 1985). More psychological distress is experienced by women with a strong negative religious or cultural attitude to termination. Reported rates of termination being refused are low, and suicide is a rare complication of this. There is some evidence of negative effects in mothers (including deliberate self-harm) and in their offspring, following refusal of termination (Gilchrist et al 1995). Subsequent pregnancies may reactivate suppressed mourning from the previous termination (Kumar and Robson 1984). Women prefer to be given the opportunity to exercise choice in the method of termination used (Howie et al 1997). The relative risk of psychosis after termination in women without a previous history of psychosis is substantially less than the risk of postpartum psychosis (Clare 1994).

With respect to more recent developments in gynaecological practice, controlled retrospective research so far suggests that, although multifetal pregnancy reduction is experienced as highly stressful, it is relatively well tolerated, with grief resolution aided by the achievement of parenthood goals (McKinney et al 1995). However, terminations as a result of fetal anomalies resulted in similar reactions to those of women experiencing perinatal loss (Salveson et al 1997).

Spontaneous miscarriage

Spontaneous miscarriage is common, and knowledge of its psychological impact is, therefore, very important. In a review of this subject, Lee et al (1996) noted that the emotional consequences varied greatly between subjects. Psychologically, spontaneous miscarriage involves the experience of bereavement and grief, and also possibly the experience of a physically traumatic event. Many women feel dissatisfied with their care. Recurrent miscarriage is associated with increased psychological morbidity. Also, it is notable that the male partners of women who miscarry may experience significant levels of grief and stress; they may also deny their grief (Puddifoot and Johnson 1997). Couples may, therefore, benefit from professional follow-up, including discussion of emotional and physical aspects of the loss.

Stillbirth

Rådestad et al (1996) recently reported a population-based, controlled, follow-up study and reviewed the literature regarding perinatal loss. Previous research had suggested that 20–30% of women with perinatal loss had significant long-term psychiatric morbidity. Years ago, stillbirth used to be regarded as less important but a series of influential publications (Bourne 1958, Lewis 1976, 1978) gradually changed professional attitudes and management practices. Confrontation of parents with the reality of the loss, encouragement to keep mementos and to organise the funeral arrangements assisted the mourning process and resulted in reductions in levels of psychopathology. Rådestad et al (1996) also found raised levels of distress if there was an interval of 25 h or more between the diagnosis of death in utero and commencement of the delivery process. There was also increased risk associated with the mother not seeing the dead child for as long as she wished or not keeping any tokens of remembrance. They concluded that it was advisable to induce labour or arrange delivery as soon as possible after diagnosis of death in utero, to allow the mother to spend as much time as she wanted with the stillborn child, and to allow mementos to be collected, if desired. They describe how women may be in shock, but still feel a pride in their dead baby and how the process of meeting and parting at the same time is difficult but important, and should, therefore, be assisted by staff's supportive flexibility.

PSYCHIATRIC DISORDERS IN PREGNANCY AND THEIR TREATMENT

There are two main categories of psychiatric disorder that are likely to be of concern to obstetricians: the psychoses (schizophrenia and affective (manic depressive) psychosis); and a variety of non-psychotic disorders, the most common of which are reviewed below.

Psychosis

Schizophrenia is typically a lifelong condition, in one of its forms resulting in progressive personality, social and cognitive deterioration, or, alternatively, presenting as a florid illness with paranoid delusions, thought disorder and auditory hallucinations, which can substantially remit or be held in check with treatment. The two forms may overlap. Affective psychosis may be manic or depressive or mixed and often in puerperal subjects there are forms of affective illness that also contain schizophrenia-like symptoms, e.g. paranoid delusions and auditory hallucinations. The major difference, especially from the first form of schizophrenia, is the fact that women with puerperal affective psychosis usually make complete or near-complete recoveries, although the risk of future relapse, especially after childbirth, remains very high. Interested readers are referred to Brockington (1996) for a thorough review of the clinical features of mental illnesses in pregnancy and the puerperium.

Schizophrenia

There are no recent studies upon which to base reliable estimates of prevalence in childbearing populations and a suggested rate of 0.1% is derived from data from one maternity unit. The numbers of such women are likely to continue to increase as a result of the move from asylum to community care and the introduction of newer antipsychotic drugs that do not reduce fertility, as did the first generation of such drugs, which have powerful dopamine (D_2) receptor-blocking actions.

The subject of medication during pregnancy is discussed later; in addition to questions about hazards to the fetus through exposure to drugs and maternal life style, there is another important issue that should concern the obstetrician. Many schizophrenic mothers are single parents, often unsupported by their families and coping with considerable difficulty in the community. What will be best for the baby, to remain with its mother or to be placed elsewhere? The Children Act, 1989 requires that the child's welfare and safety are paramount, and there is therefore often a conflict between the mother's wishes and rights and the concerns held by responsible professionals about the infant's future welfare. The process of assessment, planning for the placement, whether with the mother or with others, is best begun in pregnancy and not as a crisis measure on a postnatal ward.

Affective (bipolar manic-depressive) and schizoaffective psychosis

On the basis of measures of contacts with psychiatric services and of admission rates, there appears to be a small but significant reduction in rates of affective and schizoaffective psychosis during pregnancy (Pugh et al 1963, Kendell et al 1981, 1987). The great majority of women with histories of such disorders are in remission and remain very well during pregnancy. They are therefore not even in contact with psychiatric services. The dramatically raised relative risk of recurrence in the first few weeks postnatally has already been mentioned in relation to effective screening and planning. Should the protocols include prophylactic medication, e.g. lithium (Stewart 1988, Stewart et al 1991), or antipsychotic drugs or hormonal preparations (Kumar et al 1998)? The small numbers of subjects that have been studied, and difficulties in controlling for confounding effects, limit conclusions that can be drawn about the relative efficacies of different types of pharmacological prophylaxis. This is an important subject for further research but sufficient subjects will eventually only be recruited through a multicentre trial. Keys to successful management must include effective professional liaison and full engagement of the mother during pregnancy in planning of any prophylactic procedures.

Clinical management of pregnant women who are severely mentally ill

Case history no. 1

A worried neonatal paediatrician telephoned for advice about the pharmacokinetics of various psychotropic drugs. The mother, who was in her late thirties and who was known to be dependent on alcohol, was discovered at the time of delivery to be taking anticonvulsants, antipsychotic drugs, antidepressants and benzodiazepine. There had been no liaison between the psychiatrist who was prescribing these drugs and the obstetrician, nor had the GP forewarned anyone. The mother had attended infrequently for antenatal care and there had been no real attempt by those responsible for her obstetric care to find out about her psychiatric health or her social situation. The baby was born 4 weeks early and was fitting, but there were no gross signs of stigmata associated with exposure to alcohol or anticonvulsants.

This extreme case raises questions about incompetence and negligence, but in lesser degree, variations on this theme can be found in the records of most obstetric services. Is it routine to enquire about past and current mental health and about the domestic and social situation of the mother? A history of affective psychosis confers a risk of recurrence after delivery of 25–50%, i.e. 250–500 times higher than in the general population (see section later, postpartum psychosis). Such women are typically entirely well and healthy when in remission, especially in pregnancy, and, unless there are proactive screening protocols in place, they may slip through the net and present a week or two after delivery as acute cases of florid psychosis for whom urgent psychiatric admission is needed. During the period of growing awareness that something is seriously amiss and the eventual hospitalisation of the mother (sometimes accompanied by her baby), much can go wrong for either or both of them (Kumar 1998).

The principles of the management of mothers who are severely ill with primary mood disorders during pregnancy are the same as for schizophrenia. Hospitalisation may be necessary and attendance at antenatal clinics can be organised from the psychiatric ward. Pregnancy is also a time to plan for the management of labour and delivery and for clinical management of mother and baby in the puerperium, when exacerbation of symptoms is probable. In the case of more severely mentally ill, hospitalised mothers, is it safe and sensible for them to be managed in disturbed, acute psychiatric admission wards, which often have a mixed-sex population just discernible through a haze of cigarette smoke? There are rules and regulations that prevent or restrict female staff who are pregnant from being exposed to risk, e.g. of violence in potentially disturbed environments. Should not female patients who are pregnant be similarly protected as of right?

Should labour be induced or is it all right to run the risk of delivery *in situ*? Sooner or later an infant will be delivered on a psychiatric ward by staff who are untrained in obstetrics and midwifery, and the baby will suffer some serious complications resulting in major handicap. Will the hospital be able to justify its *laissez-faire* management of a delivery that allegedly went disastrously wrong? Should one have to wait for a major legal case for compensation before doing something about establishing protocols for safe management of such cases? Should such protocols include active management of labour and planned delivery? Supposing the patient does not, or cannot, give informed consent – what then? If the mother is transferred from the psychiatric unit to the obstetric ward in good time, is there planning for psychiatric nursing cover during her stay in the obstetric wards and is it certain where the mother will go after delivery if the baby is to remain with her? If the baby is to be removed to foster-care, when is the best time to separate the mother from her baby, where and how? Some of these questions have no easy answers and, in general, more active participation by obstetricians will be essential in improving clinical practice in this very difficult area.

Non-psychotic disorders

Depressive disorder
Overall, the prevalence of depression in pregnancy is probably comparable with rates in matched non-gravid women (Kitamura et al 1996, Cohen and Rosenbaum 1998). The factors that are most powerfully associated with the presence of antenatal depression are a previous history of depression, conflict and lack of support in key relationships, especially with the baby's father, social adversity and ambivalence about proceeding with the pregnancy (Kitamura et al 1993, Llewellyn et al 1997). Diagnosis of depression in pregnancy may be difficult. Symptoms such as disturbances of sleep and appetite, fatigue and change in libido are common in non-depressed pregnant women. It is, therefore, necessary also to focus on other symptoms, such as lack of interest in the pregnancy, guilty ruminations, poor concentration, irritability, social withdrawal and profound anhedonia (not finding pleasure in anything). Notably, women during pregnancy (and in the first year after childbirth) have a low risk of suicide (Appleby 1991). The availability of therapeutic termination (Abortion Act, 1967; see Hall 1990) has coincided with a marked reduction in rates of suicide and parasuicide in pregnant women (Kendell 1991).

Anxiety disorders and obsessive compulsive disorder
Phobic states, panic disorder and obsessive compulsive disorders typically run a chronic course, and recent studies suggest persistence or worsening during pregnancy (see reviews by Shear and Oomen Mammen 1995, Cohen and Rosenbaum 1998). Specific anxiety symptoms (for example, fear of labour, fear of dying) are common in pregnancy, occurring in about 6% of pregnant women to a severe degree and in about 17% to a moderate degree (Shear and Oomen Mammen 1995).

Eating disorders
Although the prevalence of eating disorders in pregnant women is not known, the prevalence of bulimia nervosa in young women is about 1%, and of anorexia is between 0.25 and 0.5%. While fertility rates are low in anorexic women, bulimic women are less likely to be anovulatory and more likely to be sexually active. An increase in obstetric complications (including hypertension, difficult labour, spontaneous miscarriage, smallness for gestational age and increased perinatal mortality) in both anorexic and bulimic women has been reported; and babies may be born prematurely, be of low birthweight and have abnormal Apgar scores. Low birthweight is also associated with the mother being underweight at the time of conception and showing low weight gain during pregnancy (Fahy and Morrison 1993). The contribution of psychological factors to the aetiology of hyperemesis gravidarum remains very uncertain, and Kitamura et al (1996) report no association between nausea and vomiting and symptoms of antenatal depression. Lingam and McCluskey (1996) report on a patient of theirs, and five other patients, in whom an eating disorder appears to have been precipitated by hyperemesis in pregnancy.

Recreational drug use and alcohol
Substance abuse in pregnant women may be the most frequently missed diagnosis in all of obstetrics and paediatrics. Staff may be overtly critical and hostile towards pregnant drug or alcohol users, and this may act as a barrier to compliance with treatment or with research. Substance abuse is

linked with sexually transmitted diseases, prematurity, low birthweight, stillbirth, withdrawal syndromes in newborn babies, developmental problems and parenting problems generally (see review by Finkelstein 1993). Illicit drug use is notoriously difficult to assess and it is very difficult to separate the adverse effects of drugs from a wide range of confounding factors. Finkelstein (1993) reported that estimates of the prevalence of polydrug use in urban USA range between 0.4 and 27% (mean 11%).

Alcohol use is also often underreported; the incidence of fetal alcohol syndrome in the USA is reported as 1–3 per 1000 live births, while at least three times as many may be affected to a lesser degree by maternal alcohol use in pregnancy. Zukerman et al (1995) have drawn attention to methodological difficulties in research into the effects of drug and alcohol use during pregnancy. Maternal polydrug use and life style are major confounding factors in studies investigating the effects of prenatal exposure to illicit drugs (Kaltenbach 1994). Knowledge of dose-related effects and of differential sensitivity over time during pregnancy is incomplete. Accurate identification of use requires a combination of self-report and biological markers. Other problems include difficult in avoiding sample bias, and there is commonly a lack of blind assessment and outcome measures are crude.

Use of psychotropic medication in pregnancy

General issues

Knowledge about the risks associated with prescribed psychotropic drugs in pregnancy is sketchy. Women who are taking psychotropic drugs may discover that they are pregnant and are likely to seek advice about risks to the fetus. One of the best reference guides is by Briggs et al (1998) and it is regularly updated. Psychotropic drugs cross the placenta but relatively little is known about their pharmacokinetics in the fetus. Cohen and Rosenbaum (1998) describe three groups of risk occurring in association with psychopharmacotherapy: teratogenic effects, direct neonatal toxicity and behavioural teratogenicity or longer term neurobehavioural sequelae. It is necessary to weigh up the consequences of untreated psychiatric illness against risks of prenatal exposure to drugs. In every case, non-pharmacological alternatives should be considered. Additionally, in severe mood disorders electroconvulsive therapy is an option that is generally considered safe. Physiological changes in pregnancy, including changes in the glomerular filtration rate and in the activity of liver enzymes, may mean that a higher dosage of a psychotropic drug is required to produce the same effect in the mother. What happens in the fetus when maternal ingestion of a particular drug is discontinued? How long does it take for the drug to be cleared? Does it make sense to stop maternal ingestion of drugs such as antidepressants or antipsychotics a few weeks before delivery? Should this be done suddenly or slowly, and what are the differences between a fetus experiencing drug withdrawal as opposed to the newborn? We know something about sensitive periods of development when exposure to drugs such as lithium and anticonvulsants results in increased risk of teratogenicity, but what about more subtle adverse effects such as behavioural teratogenicity?

Schizophrenia

Cohen & Rosenbaum (1998) argue that in severe or chronic psychosis, particularly in patients who have previously been shown to deteriorate when medication is stopped, overall drug exposure may be less if maintenance therapy is continued rather than discontinued, because higher doses may be required to treat a relapse of illness. First onset of psychosis in pregnancy requires thoughtful assessment, as with any first-onset psychosis. The minimum possible medication should be used. Another question concerns the appropriateness of discontinuing medication before delivery (see above); although extrapyramidal side effects have been reported in the newborn, stopping medication could precipitate a severe puerperal relapse in the mother. In the review by Cohen & Rosenbaum (1998), a recent meta-analysis is reported to have shown a slightly higher risk of congenital malformations after first-trimester exposure to low-potency antipsychotics; however, several small and retrospective studies did not find any increased teratogenic risk with higher potency antipsychotics, hence a continuing degree of uncertainty exists. There is even greater uncertainty regarding the use of newer antipsychotics in pregnancy. With respect to possible toxic effects of antipsychotics, there are case reports of extrapyramidal side effects on newborn babies. Some early animal studies (see Goldberg & Nissim 1994) did suggest behavioural abnormalities but there is a lack of information regarding long-term neurodevelopmental effects in humans.

Affective psychosis (bipolar and schizoaffective disorder)

Llewellyn et al (1998) discuss the use of lithium in pregnancy and lactation and suggest that, if medication must be prescribed during early pregnancy, then lithium may be the safest first-line treatment. The importance of a careful and realistic risk–benefit assessment is emphasised. If a pregnant patient is withdrawn from stable lithium maintenance, the risk of relapse is related to the previous duration of illness and the number of episodes. It is possible to detect cardiac malformation or severe neural tube defects by ultrasound scanning before 20 weeks, and it is essential to have discussed options such as termination before the mother starts trying to conceive. In a planned pregnancy, lithium may be tapered down 7–10 days after onset of the last menses preceding the desired conception to minimise time without treatment, and only if the risk of stopping treatment appears to be less than its continuation. The medication could then be reintroduced after the first trimester and, if so, levels should be monitored weekly and thyroid investigations performed. If there has been first-trimester exposure level II ultrasonography is indicated. It is best to withdraw lithium 1–2 weeks before the expected date of delivery because changes in maternal plasma volume and in electrolyte balance around the time of delivery can result in toxicity at normal doses. The drug can be restarted 48 h after delivery; breast feeding is contraindicated.

Initial reports from the Register of Lithium Babies (for example, Schou et al 1973) which described increased rates of cardiovascular malformations, particularly Ebstein's anomaly, have been succeeded by more recent cohort and case–control studies (for example, Jacobsen et al 1992) which suggest that the risk of cardiovascular malformations is present but is less than was thought previously; for example, the increase in the relative risk of Ebstein's anomaly is of the order of 10–20 times, rather than of 400 times with first-trimester exposure. There are case reports of perinatal toxicity; including *floppy baby* syndrome with cyanosis and hypotonicity, cardiac arrhythmias, neonatal hypothyroidism and nephrogenic diabetes insipidus (Goldberg & Nissim 1994). Neurobehavioural follow-up data are limited but significant effects were not found in one 5 year follow-up study of offspring exposed to lithium in the second and third trimesters (see review by Altshuler et al 1998).

Some anticonvulsant drugs are effective mood stabilisers, e.g. carbamazepine and valproate, and these have significant teratogenic potential. Most of the data regarding anticonvulsants come from women suffering from epilepsy, as opposed to psychiatric illness. Women with epilepsy produce offspring with a higher rate of malformations than do women without epilepsy per se. If offspring of an epileptic mother are exposed to first-trimester carbamazepine, their risk of spina bifida is increased to about 1%. For valproic acid the risk is increased to about 3–5%. Polypharmacy appears to further increase this risk and malformations other than spina bifida may occur. Infants exposed to prenatal carbamazepine did not show IQ deficits when compared with non-exposed infants at 5 year follow-up (Llewellyn et al 1998).

Depressive disorders

Psychotherapies (cognitive behavioural and interpersonal therapies, in particular) are the first-line treatment for mild or mild-to-moderate depressive illness in pregnancy, particularly when mothers wish to discontinue medication that they were taking when they inadvertently become pregnant. There is a greater risk of relapse in all patients if antidepressant medication is suddenly discontinued. How quickly are these drugs cleared from the fetus, that is, what is the balance of risk to the fetus and benefit to the mother of stopping the medication slowly, for example over 2 weeks?

Despite reports in the 1970s of possible teratogenic risk with tricyclic exposure, numerous retrospective and some prospective studies have failed to find increased congenital malformations in association with first-trimester exposure. There are, at case report level only, reports of perinatal syndromes, with jitteriness, irritability and seizures in infants exposed to tricyclics in utero (see Cohen and Rosenbaum (1998) for a discussion, including reference to animal studies). If treatment is required during pregnancy, desipramine and nortriptyline are recommended as they have fewer anticholinergic side effects and are less likely to exacerbate the orthostatic hypotension of pregnancy.

Among the SSRI (selective serotonin reuptake inhibitors) antidepressants, most safety data exist about fluoxetine. Several prospective studies, a surveillance register and a retrospective study show no increase in minor malformations over that for the general population. The exception is a study by Chambers et al (1996) that found higher rates of minor malformation in association with fluoxetine exposure, but this research has been criticised on methodological grounds.

There are no prospective data regarding the other SSRIs. Perinatal toxicity with SSRIs remains uncertain. No differences in mean IQ and language scores were found in one study of children followed up to 4 years (Nulman et al 1997). Long-term follow-up studies of possible neurobehavioural problems have not been done. Such problems can also arise as a direct consequence of maternal postnatal depression (Sharp et al 1995) and any studies of postnatal adverse effects of drugs must incorporate assessments of underlying maternal mental disorders as well as documentation of other adverse influences, e.g. inadequate nutrition, smoking, drinking or the use of other recreational drugs.

The safety of monoamine oxidase inhibitor drugs in pregnancy is unknown, and they should be avoided if possible (Cohen & Rosenbaum 1998).

Anxiety disorders and obsessive compulsive disorder

Discontinuation or tapering of anxiolytic medication in pregnancy may contribute to risk of relapse. Slow tapering is recommended and cognitive behavioural therapy may help to support this and to maintain a patient drug-free. In the light of uncertainty surrounding the teratogenicity of benzodiazepines, Cohen & Rosenbaum (1998) suggest the use of tricyclics or fluoxetine as first-line drug treatment. Clomipramine may exaggerate orthostatic hypotension and has been linked, in a case report, to seizures. Behavioural therapy and cognitive behavioural therapy are already used as first-line treatment in obsessive compulsive disorders. Risk associated with benzodiazepines remains controversial due to methodological differences in studies. It is possible that malformations are increased, and one meta-analysis (Altshuler et al 1996) found the risk of oral clefts to be 0.7% after first-trimester exposure. It has been suggested that perinatal benzodiazepine exposure impairs temperature regulation, muscle tone and breathing but these reports were not confirmed in one small prospective study (reported in Cohen and Rosenbaum's review, 1998). Insufficient data exist on which to base firm conclusions regarding effects of perinatal benzodiazepines on neurodevelopment; so far no significant problems have been identified.

POSTNATAL PSYCHIATRIC DISORDERS AND THEIR TREATMENT

The disorders

Introduction

Traditionally, psychological problems in the postnatal period are divided into three groups: the maternity blues, postnatal depression and postpartum psychosis. As discussed later, the blues are not a disorder and, given their ubiquity, the challenge is to identify subtypes, which may assist in predicting who is likely to become depressed or psychotic and so lead on to prevention or early treatment. The widespread use of the terms 'postnatal depression' and 'puerperal or postpartum psychosis' implies that these conditions are recognised clinical entities, the pathological roots of which can be found in the physiological and psychological changes that accompany reproduction. This is an attractive working hypothesis but it is no more than that. One hindrance to the search for causes, especially of postnatal depression, has been a failure to distinguish between prevalence and incidence; secondly, in relation to incidence, there are no clear criteria for defining the temporal limit of the term 'postnatal'. Is it 4 weeks (American Psychiatric Association 1994), 6 weeks (the obstetric conventional length of the puerperium), 3, 6 or 12 months (Kumar & Robson 1984, Cooper et al 1988, Sharp et al 1995, respectively)?

In terms of prevalence, these questions are not vital because here the main emphasis is on identifying the size of the problem within a given time frame, irrespective of whether the cases are chronic, recurrent, have onsets in pregnancy or begin postnatally. There may be variations in responsiveness to particular therapies or in outcomes, but what matters is that large meta-analyses (for example, O'Hara & Swain 1996) clearly demonstrate that between 10 and 15% of mothers are clinically depressed in the 3 months following childbirth: that is the gross burden of disease. When it comes to studies of incidence and of causal pathways, however, it is very important to try to sort out the women with chronic, long-standing or recurrent depression who would have been present anyway even if there had been no pregnancy (Cooper & Murray 1995). It may turn out that less than half of all cases of depression identified postnatally (prevalence) have an onset or recurrence in pregnancy or postnatally (incidence). Recurrences meeting predetermined criteria can be included with first onset cases depending upon the questions being asked. At the present time, given that the great majority of women who become depressed during pregnancy remain thus postnatally, perhaps it is premature to distinguish between antenatal and postnatal depressions in searching for causes and effects.

Similar arguments apply to psychosis. In terms of service planning it is important to know that about 2 per 1000 mothers will need psychiatric admission (Oates 1996) on account of a psychotic illness (prevalence includes chronic schizophrenia and affective psychosis) but only half of them will be cases of first episodes of affective psychosis or of acute relapse following remission from a previous episode. It is in this latter group that studies of biological mechanisms related to incidence and acute recurrence are concentrated (Wieck et al 1991, Meakin et al 1995, Kumar et al 1998).

Maternity blues

The blues, because of their near universal prevalence, mildness and transience, fall within the range of normality and cannot be regarded as a disorder. They occur in 50–70% of women and Kendell et al (1981) reported a peak of symptomatology (on depression, tears and lability scales) on day 5 postpartum, with a more pronounced peak in women who became depressed later. Fossey et al (1997) found a relationship between postpartum blues on day 3 after delivery and severe postnatal depression evaluated 8 months later.

The blues may only be dysphoric in nature or there may also be mixed mild elation. If dysphoria is severe, or if there is mixed elation, there is a greater likelihood of postnatal depression (PND) (Kendell et al 1981, Hannah et al 1992). The most important differential diagnosis is puerperal psy-

chosis, as most cases of this condition develop in the first 2 weeks postnatally. One must differentiate between the tearfulness and dysphoria or mild elation that is characteristic of the blues and the more sinister signs (persistent insomnia, overactivity, overtalkativeness, wretchedness and guilt, agitation, retardation or other unusual behaviour) of puerperal psychosis. Midwives, general practitioners and health visitors are likely to be the first to detect that something is wrong but there may be delays because of lack of awareness or inexperience, given the relative rarity of such psychoses.

Postnatal depression

The incidence of women becoming depressed postnatally was first reported as 10% by Pitt in 1968, and this finding has been confirmed many times when onsets and recurrences are combined and cases of minor depression are included. As regards specificity of the condition, in a study of 232 women postdelivery versus matched controls, Cox et al (1993) found the rate of depression to be increased about threefold, but only in the first 5 weeks after childbirth; however, symptoms of depression after childbirth do not appear pathognomonic when compared with depression in the general population (Cox et al 1982). Nor is there any clear difference from depression in other settings in terms of major causal or contributory factors; these include early childhood stresses and traumas, a lack of social support, marital and family disharmony, social adversity and, possibly, genetic predisposition, which may be expressed through some kind of sensitivity to the physiological changes of childbirth. Very rarely, PND may follow anterior pituitary necrosis, and a small number of cases are related to thyroid dysfunction (Harris 1993), triggered by metabolic changes during pregnancy and at delivery. More recently, the risk of paternal PND has been identified. This appears more likely if the female partner is particularly depressed, if the relationship is unsupportive or if the man is unemployed (Ballard and Davies 1996).

Case history no. 2

A first-time mother, who was single and a health professional, had an unplanned but eventually wanted pregnancy. The father of the baby, although supportive in a limited way, both emotionally and practically, was already married and had four young children within his marriage, in which he intended to stay. The pregnancy was complicated towards the end by concerns about pre-eclampsia and the labour was induced (prostin gel, amniotomy, syntocinon), was very painful and prolonged and the baby, a boy, was delivered normally but needed some resuscitation. When the mother first held her son, she felt some dislike and revulsion, largely, she thought, because of his deformed looks following the labour. She tried breast feeding but found it painful and difficult and stopped after a week. At home it was a chore looking after her son. She was isolated from her workmates and she fended off attempts by her mother to help — partly because they had never got on well since her parents' divorce in her early teens and partly because her mother had disapproved of her pregnancy and relationship. There were no other close relatives. Throughout repeated contacts with her GP and her health visitor she put on a brave face and no one asked her directly about her mood. By 3 months, she was tearful, irritable, withdrawn, guilty about aggressive feelings towards her baby, sleeping poorly, feeling run down, concentrating poorly, becoming house-bound and sometimes wishing she were dead, at others that she had never had the baby. By 5 months, after a particularly difficult period when her baby had gone through repeated minor illnesses, and when there had been a major row with the baby's father, she asked a neighbour to look after the baby while she went shopping; instead, she went back to her flat and took 30 paracetamol tablets. After a period of intensive care she was admitted to a psychiatric mother and baby unit for a month and then followed up in outpatients, essentially to supervise her antidepressant medication and supports. She also began to attend for weekly counselling at her primary care centre. By the time the baby was 18 months old, she had found a childminder, was back at work, part-time, was in a new relationship and was off all treatment. Nevertheless, she still recalled the first six postnatal months as the blackest time of her life, and wondered if she had caused any lasting harm to her baby.

This case history illustrates many of the typical psychosocial antecedents of PND and it underlines the importance of early detection and intervention. The impact of this common disorder on the developing child is a subject of great importance. In a review of the literature, Murray and Cooper (1996) report that there is firm evidence for an association between PND and a number of indices of adverse cognitive and emotional child development; for example deficits in infant's early social interactions and cognitive function, an increase in insecure attachment and a longer term association with cognitive function (Sharp et al 1995). Observational studies reveal that maternal interaction with the baby is impaired when mothers are depressed, e.g. diminished sensitivity, lack of contingency in responding to cues from the baby, reduced proactive stimulation and warmth (see Murray & Cooper 1996). Such impairments of relationship and interaction with the baby may, through their presence at sensitive periods of the infant's development, stunt the child's psychological development, possibly irreversibly (Hay & Kumar 1995, Sharp et al 1995, Hay et al 2000). Fifty per cent or more of cases of PND still remain unrecognised by health visitors and by general practitioners, and the use of screening instruments such as the Edinburgh Postnatal Depression Scale (Cox et al 1987) may be beneficial, but only if it is checked by interview and the possibility of false-negative responses is borne in mind. The best form of screening is interested enquiry by someone who knows the mother and can evaluate the significance of changes in her psychological and social adjustment. Postnatal follow-up is mainly carried out by general practitioners and health visitors but obstetricians and midwives are also in a position to pick up early symptoms and signs of depression. Regular liaison meetings in obstetric clinics, involving midwives, obstetricians, health visitors, social workers and psychiatrists, provide an opportunity for following the progress of mentally ill mothers or those at risk of becoming ill, e.g. of developing PND. Non-directive counselling by health visitors (Holden et al 1989) is effective in the

short term. Similarly, brief cognitive behavioural psychotherapy is of benefit. For moderately severe depression, either drug treatment or combined drug and psychotherapy may be appropriate but nursing mothers do not want medication (Appleby et al 1997). With more severe depression a psychiatrist should be involved and admission may be considered (Kumar et al 1995).

Postpartum psychosis

The majority of schizophrenic mothers appear to have histories of pre-existing illness, and it is the general consensus that the puerperal psychoses are not of the schizophrenic type. In addition, the nature of schizophrenic illness appears to predict the risk of postnatal relapse: in a case-note study of a series of schizophrenic mothers, women who met restrictive criteria for schizophrenia showed no change in psychopathology after delivery, whereas about 40% of the sample meeting broader criteria showed clear evidence of relapse or illness exacerbation (Davies et al 1995). Such findings are relevant to the current debate about the classification of acute schizophrenia-like psychosis and its relationship to affective disorder. Here, however, it is only important to note that childbirth can trigger first episodes of bipolar and schizoaffective disorder but probably not first episodes of schizophrenia, although it can exacerbate or cause relapse of this illness if it is of the paranoid-hallucinatory type. The key issue for the obstetrician is to ascertain whether or not a pregnant woman has a history of psychosis, a crude but simple index for which is a history of mental hospital admission. Liaison with a psychiatrist can then sort out the niceties of diagnosis and prognosis and, most importantly, set in train the process of management during pregnancy and postnatally.

The incidence of affective psychotic illness postpartum in the general population is about 1 per 1000, but for women with a previous history of affective psychosis it is 25–50% (Marks et al 1992), and the risk appears to be greater the shorter the gap between last illness and current pregnancy. Most illnesses occur in the first 2 weeks postnatally and risk falls rapidly after the first month (Kendell et al 1987). There is cross-cultural consistency for the incidence of postpartum psychosis (Kumar 1994) and no good evidence has yet been found for separating these disorders from other affective psychoses (Platz and Kendell 1988), although prospective studies of pregnant women with histories of affective psychosis (puerperal and non-puerperal) testing for postpartum relapse and for associations between relapse and psychosocial as well as physiological factors may provide answers (cf. Wieck et al 1991, Marks et al 1992, Kumar et al 1998). Admission is almost always necessary in cases of acute affective or schizoaffective psychosis. Where possible this should be into a psychiatric mother and baby unit, but these services are sparse and they are not rationally distributed in response to need (Royal College of Psychiatrists 1992). Given the current practice of short stays in postnatal wards, most cases of psychosis occur after the mother has returned home, and the community midwife, health visitor and general practitioner are likely to be the first professionals to observe the onset of the illness. Early symptoms include persistent insomnia, perplexity, eccentricities of behaviour, unusual beliefs or perceptions. Whenever there is a concern a domiciliary visit by a psychiatrist should be urgently obtained. The psychiatrist will be aware of local facilities for admission. Pharmacotherapy of puerperal psychoses is based on the predominant clinical picture and can include antipsychotic drugs, mood stabilisers, antidepressants and, sometimes, ECT. Polypharmacy should be avoided (see Case history no. 1).

Case history no. 3

A woman in her second pregnancy rang one of the authors to seek advice. She had had a severe manic illness immediately after the birth of her first child 3 years ago and had been compulsorily hospitalised in an acute psychiatric admission ward while her parents had cared for her baby. The experience had been very frightening and she had repeatedly begged to be allowed to go home. She left the hospital as soon as the detention order ran out at about 6 weeks postnatally; there were no grounds for further detaining her. After this, she had become very depressed but had managed at home with a great deal of family support, buttressed by antidepressant medication and visits by her GP. The psychiatric nurse from the community mental health team had visited her two or three times these are not found to be helpful.

Now that she was pregnant again, she was terrified of recurrence of her illness, having read somewhere that it was likely. She had asked her GP, who had tried to reassure her, and her obstetrician had advised a psychiatric opinion. She did not want to return to the hospital where she had been admitted 3 years previously. At a consultation visit with her husband, the risks of recurrence were explained and a plan was formulated for prophylactic admission into a psychiatric mother and baby unit 2 days after delivery. Options for prophylaxis with lithium (cf. Stewart et al 1991) or oestrogen (Kumar et al 1998) were discussed. She was very relieved to know that a safety-net was in place even though it would mean temporary and partial separation from her 3-year-old child and from her husband. Her GP and her obstetrician were advised of the plan and were very supportive. She came into the mother and baby unit on the second day after delivery and decided not to start prophylactic medication because she wanted to breast feed. A week later there were signs of impending mania: treatment was started immediately and she improved rapidly. As before, she became depressed after she had gone home and, once again, treatment was started quickly and the whole episode was less severe and much less distressing. She had bonded well with her baby and had maintained regular contact through home visits with her older child and with her family.

This case history emphasises the importance of identifying mothers at risk of recurrence of affective psychosis after childbirth and of proactive management.

Psychotropic drugs and breast feeding

Yoshida et al (1999) discuss the two main groups of women for whom prescribing psychotropics during breast feeding is most likely: first, there are women who suffer from chronic schizophrenia and those with acute postpartum psychoses; these women almost always require psychotropic medication so the question is 'Is it safe to breast feed?' The second group consist of those women who suffer from non-psychotic depression and for them the primary question is 'Is it necessary to prescribe?' It may turn out to be so if support and psychotherapy are ineffective and the prescription of most common antidepressants in therapeutic doses is not a bar to breast feeding (Yoshida et al 1999). The main contraindications to breast feeding are premature birth or neonatal jaundice, when the infant may not be able to metabolise any drugs ingested in milk; or if the baby is unwell in any other way. All psychotropic drugs are lipophilic and are therefore present in breast milk in amounts that reflect their concentrations in plasma. The infant ingests relatively small doses—estimated in terms of volume of milk consumed to be between 1 and 3% of the maternal dose. The database upon which to base guidelines (British National Formulary 1999, Yoshida et al 1999) is pitifully small and certainly unreliable. Mothers who are taking lithium should not breast feed because the ion diffuses freely into milk and may be very dangerous if a breast fed baby becomes dehydrated, for whatever reason. Other psychotropic drugs are probably safe in therapeutic doses and the equation balances the known benefits of breast feeding against unknown hazards of exposing the developing baby to small doses of these drugs (see Yoshida et al 1999 for review).

Better services for mentally ill mothers and their babies

Figures for the prevalence and nature of mental illnesses in childbearing women are not in dispute. It is therefore relatively easy to estimate the need in relation to numbers of live births. Recent national surveys have not yet been reported but they will probably confirm earlier reports (Royal College of Psychiatrists 1992) that, at all levels (inpatient mother and baby units, day centres, psychiatric liaison for obstetrics and community support for mental health teams and for primary care), services for this particular group vary from none to sporadic. Ultimately, given limited resources, choices have to be made: for example, between costly new developments in assisted reproduction and the prevention of harm to babies who were born healthy. The challenge for obstetricians is to participate actively in local attempts to improve services by fostering psychiatric liaison in their clinics and by highlighting unmet needs. It does not make sense to make great efforts to promote better obstetrics and midwifery and then to do little to prevent the damage that is caused to mothers and babies by maternal mental illnesses that endure through pregnancy and after delivery or that begin postnatally.

CONCLUSIONS

The obstetric team needs to be alert both to possible interactions between psychological and obstetric factors, and to the range of psychiatric disorders that may occur during pregnancy and the puerperium. Despite increasing recognition of puerperal psychiatric disorders, there is relative neglect of pre-existing psychiatric disorders in pregnancy; with chronic, severe mental illness requiring particular focus. Knowledge and liaison regarding the use of psychotropic medication in pregnancy and the puerperium are vital, and the importance of a careful and realistic risk–benefit assessment in every patient is emphasised.

A more proactive approach to maternal mental health care is required as needs are currently unmet. This can be achieved by further training of professionals involved in obstetric care, and by closer liaison with focused psychiatric services. Combined use of antenatal and postnatal screening procedures, in the context of a less stigmatised, more open attitude to mental illness, is indicated. The availability of reliable maternal mental health statistics means service requirements can be relatively accurately predicted. We hope that obstetric and psychiatric teams can work together to improve their services locally and highlight the need for greater service provision everywhere.

KEY POINTS

- Birth rates and information about the prevalence and nature of psychiatric disorders are available. Despite frequent contacts with a variety of health professionals, existing services are not meeting the needs of mentally ill mothers.
- Early identification and effective management of mental illnesses in childbearing women will result in better obstetric outcome as well as better mental health and adjustment in the mother.
- In contrast with increasing recognition of postpartum psychiatric disorders (postnatal depression and postpartum psychosis) pre-existing, chronic and severe mental disorders that persist through pregnancy and after delivery have received scant attention.
- A greater emphasis on mental health promotion is needed in the training of obstetricians and midwives.

REFERENCES

Altshuler LL, Cohen L, Szuba MP, Burt VK, Sitlin M, Mintz 1996 Pharmacologic management of psychiatric illness during pregnancy: dilemmas and guidelines. Am J Psychiatry 153:592–606

Altshuler LL, Hendrick V, Cohen LS 1998 Course of mood and anxiety disorders during pregnancy and the postpartum period. J Clin Psychiatry 59:29–33

American Psychiatric Association 1994 DSM-IV: diagnostic and statistical manual of mental disorders, 4th edn. APA, Washington DC.

Appleby L 1991 Suicide during pregnancy and in the first postnatal year. BMJ 302:137–140

Appleby L 1996 Suicidal behaviour in childbearing women. Int Rev Psychiatry 8:107–115

Appleby L, Warner R, Whitton A, Faragher BA 1997 A controlled study of fluoxetine and cognitive-behavioural counselling in the treatment of postnatal depression. BM Journal 314:932–936

Ballard C, Davies R 1996 Postnatal depression in fathers. Int Rev Psychiatry 8:65–71

Bernazzani O, Saucier JF, David H, Borgeat F 1997 Psychosocial factors related to emotional disturbances during pregnancy. J Psychosom Res 42:391–402

Bhagwanni SG, Seagroves K, Kierker LJ et al 1997 Prenatal anxiety and perinatal outcome in nulliparous women: a prospective study. J Natl Med Assoc 89(2):93–98

Bourne S 1968 The psychological effects of stillbirth on women and their doctors. J R Coll Gen Pract 16:103–112

Briggs GG, Freeman RK, Yaffe SJ 1998 Drugs in pregnancy and lactation, 5th edn. Williams & Wilkins, Baltimore

British National Formulary 1999 British Medical Association and Royal Pharmaceutical Society of Great Britain, London

Brockington IF 1996 Motherhood and mental health. Oxford University Press, Oxford

Chambers CD, Johnson KA, Dick LM, Felix RJ, Lyons Jones K 1996 Birth outcomes in pregnant women taking fluoxetine. N Engl J Med 335:1010–1015

Clare AW (1994) Psychiatric aspects of abortion. I J Psychol Med 11(2):992–998

Cohen LS, Rosenbaum JF 1998 Psychotropic drug use during pregnancy: weighing the risks. J Clin Psychiatry 59 (suppl 2):18–28

Cooper PJ, Murray L 1995 The course and recurrence of postnatal depression. Br J Psychiatry 166:191–195

Cooper PJ, Campbell EA, Day A, Kennerley H, Bond A 1988 Non-psychiatric disorder after childbirth. A prospective study of prevalence, incidence, course and nature. Br J Psychiatry 152:799–806

Cox JL, Connor Y, Kendell RE 1982 Prospective study of the psychiatric disorders of childbirth. Br J Psychiatry 140:111–117

Cox JL, Holden JM, Sagovsky R 1987 Detection of postnatal depression. Development of the 10-item Edinburgh postnatal depression scale. Br J Psychiatry 150:782–786

Cox JL, Murray D, Chapman G 1993 A controlled study of the onset, duration and prevalence of postnatal depression. Br J Psychiatry 163:27–31

Davies RA, McIvor RJ, Kumar R 1995 Impact of childbirth on a series of schizophrenic mothers: a comment on possible influence of oestrogen on schizophrenia. Schizophr Res 16:25–31

Fahy TA, Morrison JJ 1993 Br J Obstet Gynaecol 100: 708–710

Finkelstein N 1993 Treatment programming for alcohol and drug dependent pregnant women. Int J Addict 28:1275–1309

Fossey L, Papiernik E, Bydlowski M 1997 Postpartum blues: a clinical syndrome and predictor of postnatal depression? J Psychosom Obstet Gynaecol 18:17–21

Frank PI, Kay CR, Wingrave BA, Lewis TLT, Osborne J, Newell C 1985 Induced abortion operations and their early sequelae. J R Coll Gen Pract 35:175–180

Gilchrist AC, Hannatard PC, Frank P, Kay GR 1995 Termination of pregnancy and psychiatric morbidity. Br J Psychiatry 167:243–248

Goldberg HL, Nissim R 1994 Psychotropic drugs in pregnancy and lactation. Int J Psychiatry Med 24:129–149

Hall MH 1990 Changes in the abortion law. BMJ 301:1109–1110

Hannah P, Adams D, Lee A, Glover V, Sandler M 1992 Links between early post-partum mood and post-natal depression. Br J Psychiatry 160:777–780

Harris B 1993 A hormonal component to postnatal depression. Br J Psychiatry 163:403–405

Hay DF, Kumar R 1995 Interpreting the effects of mothers' postnatal depression on children's intelligence: a critique and re-analysis. Child Psychiatry Hum Dev 25:165–181

Hay DF, Pawlby S, Asten P, Mills A, Sharp D, Kumar R 2000 Intellectual problems in 11 year olds whose mothers had postnatal depression: in preparation

Holden JM, Sagovsky R, Cox JL 1989 Counselling in a general practice setting: controlled study of health visitor intervention in treatment of postnatal depression. BMJ 298:223–226

Howie FL, Henshaw RC, Naji SA, Russell IT, Templeton AA 1997 Medical abortion or vacuum aspiration? Two year follow up of a patient preference trial. Br J Obstet Gynaecol 104:829–833

Jacobson SJ, Jones K, Johnson K et al 1992 Prospective multicentre study of pregnancy outcome after lithium exposure during first trimester. Lancet 339:530–533

Jayawant S, Rawlinson A, Gibbon F et al 1998 Subdural

haemorrhages in infants: population based study. BMJ 317:1558–1561

Kaltenback KA 1994 Effects of intrauterine opiate exposure: new paradigms for old questions. Meeting of the college on problems of drug dependence (Toronto, Canada). Drug Alcohol Depend 36:83–87

Kendell RE 1991 Suicide in pregnancy and the puerperium. BMJ Journal 802:126–127

Kendell RE, McGuire RJ, Connor Y, Cox JL 1981a Mood changes in the first three weeks after childbirth. J Affect Disord 3:317–326

Kendell RE, Rennie D, Clarke JA, Dean C 1981b The social and obstetric correlates of psychiatric admission in the puerperium. Psychol Med 11:341–350

Kendell RE, Chalmers JC, Platz C 1987 Epidemiology of puerperal psychoses. Br J Psychiatry 150:662–673

Kitamura T, Shima S, Sugawara M, Toda MA 1993 Psychological and social correlates of the onset of affective disorders among pregnant women. Psychol Med 23:967–975

Kitamura T, Shima S, Sugawara M, Toda MA 1996 Clinical and psychosocial correlates of antenatal depression: a review. Psychother Psychosom 65:117–123

Kumar R 1994 Postnatal mental illness: a transcultural perspective. Soc Psychiatry Psychiatr Epidemiol 29:250–264

Kumar R 1998 Deaths from psychiatric causes: suicide and substance abuse. In: Lewis G, Drife J (eds) Why mothers die: report on confidential enquiries into maternal deaths in the UK 1994–1996. TSO, London pp 140–153

Kumar R, Robson KM 1984 A prospective study of emotional disorders in childbearing women. Br J Psychiatry 144:35–47

Kumar R, Marks M, Jackson K 1995 Prevention and treatment of postnatal psychiatric disorders. Br J Midwifery 3:314–317

Kumar R, Marks MN, Wieck A et al 1998 Neuroendocrine treatments for postpartum psychosis and postnatal depression. Int J Neuropsychopharmacol 1 (suppl 1)S20

Langer A, Farnot U, Garcia C et al 1996 The Latin American trial of psychosocial support during pregnancy: effects of mother's wellbeing and satisfaction. Soc Sci Med 42:1589–1597

Lee C, Slade P, Lygo V 1996 The influence of psychosocial debriefing on emotional adaptation in women following early miscarriage: a preliminary study. Br J Med Psychol 69:47–58

Lewis E 1976 The management of stillbirth: coping with an unreality. Lancet ii:619–620

Lewis G, Drife J (eds) 1998 Confidential enquiries into maternal deaths in the UK 1994–1996. TSO, London

Lewis E, Page A 1978 Failure to mourn a stillbirth: an overlooked catastrophe. Br J Med Psychol 51:237–241

Lingam R, McCluskey S 1996 Eating disorders associated with hyperemesis gravidarum. J Psychosom Res 40:231–234

Llewellyn AM, Stowe ZN, Nemeroff CB 1997 Depression during pregnancy and the puerperium. J Clin Psychiatry 58:26–32

Llewellyn A, Stowe ZN, Strader JR 1998 The use of lithium and management of women with bipolar affective disorder during pregnancy and lactation. J Clin Psychiatry 59(suppl 6) 57–64

Lou HC, Hansen D, Nordentoft M et al 1994 Prenatal stressors of human life affects fetal brain developments. Dev Med Child Neurol 36:826–832

McKinney M, Downey J, Timor-Tritsch I 1995 The psychological effects of multifetal pregnancy reduction. Fertil Steril 64:51–61

Marks MN 1996 Characteristics and causes of infanticide in Britain. Int Rev Psychiatry 8:99–106

Marks M, Kumar R 1993 Infanticide in England and Wales. Med Sci Law 33:329–339

Marks M, Kumar R 1996 Infanticide in Scotland. Med Sci Law 36(4):299–305

Marks MN, Wieck A, Checkley SA, Kumar R 1992a Contribution of

psychological and social factors to psychiatric and non psychiatric relapse after childbirth in women with previous histories of affective disorder. J Affect Disord 29:253–264

Marks MN, Wieck A, Seymour A, Checkley SA, Kumar R 1992b Women whose mental illnesses recur after childbirth and partners' levels of expressed emotion during late pregnancy. Br J Psychiatry 161:211–216

Meakin CJ, Brockington IF, Lynch SE, Jones SR 1995 Dopamine supersensitivity and hormonal status in puerperal psychosis. Br J Psychiatry 166:73–79

Murray L, Cooper PJ 1996 The impact of postpartum depression on child development. Int Rev Psychiatry 8:55–63

Nulman I, Rovet J, Stewart D et al 1973 Neurodevelopment of children exposed in utero to antidepressant drugs. N Engl J Med 336:258–262

Oates M 1996 Psychiatric services for women following childbirth. Int Rev Psychiatry 8:87–98

O'Hara MW, Swain AM 1996 Rates and risk of postpartum depression: meta-analysis. Int Rev Psychiatry 8:37–54

Paarlberg K, Vingerhoets JJM, Passchier Y, Dekker GA, van Geijn HP 1995 Psychological factors and pregnancy outcome. A review with emphasis on methodological issues. J Psychosom Res 39:563–595

Pitt B 1968 Atypical depression following childbirth. Br J Psychiatry 136:339–346

Platz C, Kendell RE 1988 A matched control study and family study of puerperal psychosis. Br J Psychiatry 153:90–94

Puddifoot JE, Johnson MP 1997 The legitimacy of grieving: the partner's experience at miscarriage. Soc Sci Med 45:837–845

Pugh TF, Jerath BK, Schmidt WM, Reed RB 1963 Rates of mental disease related to childbearing. N Engl J Med 268:1224–1228

Rådested Steineck G, Nordin C, Sjogren B 1996 Psychological complications after stillbirth: influence of memories and immediate management. population based study. BMJ 312:1505–1508

Royal College of Psychiatrists 1992 Working party report on postnatal mental illness. Council report CR28. Rep, London

Salvesen KA, Oyen N, Schmidt N, Malt UF, Eik-Nes SH 1997 Comparison of long-term psychological responses of women after pregnancy termination due to fetal anomalies and after perinatal loss. Ultrasound Obstet Gynaecol 9:80–85

Schou M, Goldfield MD, Weinstein HR, Villeneuve A 1973 Lithium and pregnancy 1. Report from the register of lithium babies. BMJ 2:135–136

Sharp D, Hay DF, Pawlby S, Schmücker G, Allen H, Kumar R 1995 The impact of postnatal depression on boys' intellectual development. J Child Psychol Psychiatry 36(8):1315–1336

Shear MK, Oomen Mamen 1995 Anxiety disorders in pregnant and postpartum women. Psychopharmacol Bull 31:693–703

Stewart DE 1988 Prophylactic lithium in postpartum affective psychosis. J Nerv Ment Dis 176:485–489

Stewart DE, Klompenhouwer JL, Kendell RE, Van Hulst AM 1991 Prophylactic lithium in puerperal psychosis. The experience of three centres. Br J Psychiatry 158:393–397

Teixeira JMA, Fisk NM, Glover V 1999 Association between maternal anxiety in pregnancy and increased uterine artery resistance index: cohort based study. BMJ 318:153–157

Wieck A, Kumar R, Hirst AD, Marks MN, Campbell IC, Checkley SA 1991 Increased sensitivity of dopamine receptors and recurrence of affective psychosis after childbirth. BMJ 303:613–616

Yoshida K, Smith B, Kumar R 1999 Psychotropic drugs in mothers' milk: a comprehensive review of assay methods, pharmacokinetics and of safety in breast feeding. J Psychopharmacol 12:16–92

Zuckerman B, Frank D, Brown E 1995 Overview of the effects of abuse and drugs on pregnancy and offspring. NIDA Res Monogr 149.

20

Coagulation defects in pregnancy and the puerperium

Elizabeth A. Letsky

HAEMOSTASIS AND PREGNANCY

Healthy haemostasis depends on normal vasculature, platelets, coagulation factors and fibrinolysis. These act together to confine the circulating blood to the vascular bed and arrest bleeding after trauma. Normal pregnancy is accompanied by dramatic changes in all these systems (Letsky 1991). There is a marked increase in some of the coagulation factors, particularly fibrinogen. Fibrin is laid down in the uteroplacental vessel walls and fibrinolysis is suppressed. These changes, together with the increased blood volume, help to combat the hazard of haemorrhage at placental separation. They also produce a vulnerable state for intravascular clotting, and a whole spectrum of disorders involving coagulation occur in complications of pregnancy, falling into two main groups, thromboembolism (see Ch. 42) and bleeding, which may or may not be associated with disseminated intravascular coagulation (DIC). A short account follows of haemostasis during pregnancy and how it differs from that in the non-pregnant state.

Platelets and vascular integrity

It is not known how vascular integrity is normally maintained but it is clear that the platelets have a key role to play because conditions in which their number is depleted or their function is abnormal are characterised by widespread spontaneous capillary haemorrhages. Recent studies surveying large populations with the use of automated counting equipment suggest that if mean values for platelet concentration are analysed throughout pregnancy there is a downward trend, even though most values fall within the accepted non-pregnant ranges.

In a prospective study, of the 2263 women who delivered during 1 year at one centre (Burrows & Kelton 1988), 1357 were considered to be normal. One hundred and twelve (8.3%) had mild thrombocytopenia at term (platelet counts $97–150 \times 10^9$/l). The frequency of thrombocytopenia in their offspring was no greater than that of babies born to women with platelet counts in the normal accepted range and no infant had a platelet count $< 100 \times 10^9$/l. An extension of this study to include 6715 deliveries substantiates these original findings (Burrows & Kelton 1990).

It is not yet possible to propose with confidence a normal range for platelet count in pregnancy, but levels of 100×10^9 per litre or more are probably acceptable. Certain disease states specific to pregnancy have profound effects on platelet consumption lifespan and function. A decrease in platelet count and changes in platelet function have been observed in pregnancies with fetal growth restriction and the lifespan of platelets is shortened significantly even in mild pre-eclampsia (Ballegeer et al 1992).

Procoagulant system and pregnancy

The end-result of blood coagulation is the formation of an insoluble fibrin clot from the soluble precursor fibrinogen in the plasma. This involves a complex interaction of clotting factors and a sequential activation of a series of proenzymes, which has been termed the coagulation cascade (Fig. 20.1).

Normal pregnancy is accompanied by major changes in the coagulation system from the first trimester, with increases in levels of factors VII, VIII and X, and a particularly marked increase in the level of plasma fibrinogen. The amount of fibrinogen in late pregnancy is at least double that of the non-pregnant state (Forbes & Greer 1992).

Naturally occurring anticoagulants

Mechanisms that limit and localise the clotting process at sites of trauma are critically important to protect against generalised thrombosis, and also to prevent spontaneous activation of powerful procoagulant factors that circulate in normal plasma.

It is not appropriate to give an account of the complex interactions and biochemistry of all of these factors here. Only those of major importance in haemostasis and relevance to pregnancy will be mentioned.

Antithrombin

Antithrombin (AT) is considered to be the main physiological inhibitor of thrombin and factor Xa (Fig. 20.1). An inherited deficiency of AT is one of the few conditions in which a familial tendency to thrombosis has been described and is particularly hazardous in pregnancy (see Ch. 42).

AT is synthesised in the liver. Its activity is low in cirrhosis and other chronic diseases of the liver, as well as in protein-losing renal disease, DIC and hypercoagulable states. The commonest cause of a small reduction in AT is the use of oral contraceptives, related to the oestrogen content. During pregnancy there appears to be little change in AT levels but there is some decrease during parturition and an increase in the puerperium (Hellgren & Blomback 1981). There must presumably be increased synthesis in the antenatal period to maintain normal mean levels in the face of an increasing plasma volume.

Protein C, thrombomodulin, protein S

Protein C inactivates factors V and VIII in conjunction with its cofactors thrombomodulin and protein S. To exert its effect, protein C (a vitamin K-dependent anticoagulant synthesised in the liver) must be activated by an endothelial cell cofactor termed *thrombomodulin*.

Protein S, also a vitamin K-dependent glycoprotein, acts as a cofactor for activated protein C by promoting its binding to lipid and platelet surfaces, thus localising the reaction. Several families have been described with protein S deficiency and thromboembolic disease.

Data on normal protein C and protein S levels in healthy pregnancy are sparse. One study showed a significant reduction in functional protein S levels during pregnancy and the puerperium (Comp et al 1986). More recently, 14 patients

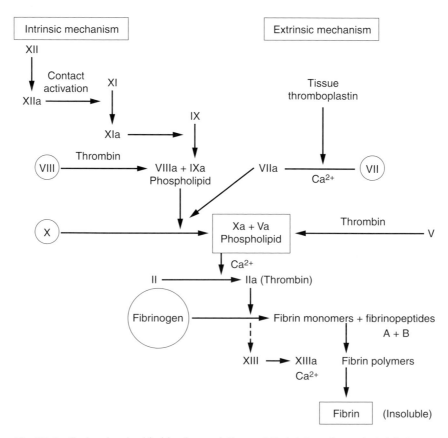

Fig. 20.1 Factors involved in blood coagulation and their interactions; circled factors show significant increases in pregnancy.

monitored longitudinally throughout gestation and postpartum showed a rise of protein C within the normal non-pregnant range during the second trimester. In contrast, free protein S fell from the second trimester onward but remained within the confines of the normal range (Warwick et al 1989). Another study supported these findings and the study was extended to women using oral contraception, in whom similar changes were noted (Malm et al 1988). A new factor, activated protein C resistance (APCR), has recently been identified and has a strong association with venous thromboembolic diseases. APCR is characterised by a poor anticoagulant response to activated protein C, resulting, in most cases, from a single mutation of the factor V gene, the mutation being known as factor V Leiden (Bertina et al 1994).

Two longitudinal studies of APCR in healthy pregnancy have shown an increase in resistance. In one study (Cumming et al 1995), a significant decrease in activated protein C (APC) activity was found throughout gestation. The other report (Peek et al 1997) showed a significant decrease in APC activity throughout gestation, the decrease being maximal in the 3rd trimester, but all values remained within the normal range for the non-pregnant population. One explanation of the increase in APCR (in the absence of factor V Leiden) could be the significant increase in factor VIII procoagulant activity that occurs in healthy pregnancy.

Knowledge of natural anticoagulants is now considerable and the picture is becoming increasingly complex. More components have been recognised as our ability to investigate objectively increases.

Fibrinolysis

Fibrinolytic activity is an essential part of the dynamic interacting haemostatic mechanism, and is dependent on plasminogen activator in the blood. Fibrin and fibrinogen are digested by plasmin, a proenzyme derived from an inactive plasma precursor plasminogen.

Increased amounts of activator are found in the plasma after strenuous exercise, emotional stress, surgical operations and other trauma. Tissue activator can be extracted from most human organs, with the exception of the placenta. Tissues especially rich in activator include the uterus, ovaries, prostate, heart, lungs, thyroid, adrenals and lymph nodes. Activity in tissues is concentrated mainly around blood vessels; veins show greater activity than arteries. Venous occlusion of the limbs will stimulate fibrinolytic activity, a fact which should be remembered if tourniquets are applied for any length of time before blood is drawn for measurement of fibrin degradation products (FDP).

The inhibitors of fibrinolytic activity are of two types: the antiactivators (antiplasminogens) and the antiplasmins. Inhibitors of plasminogen include epsilon amino caproic acid (EACA) and tranexamic acid. Aprotinin (Trasylol) is another antiplasminogen which is commercially prepared from bovine lung. When fibrinogen or fibrin is broken down by plasmin, FDP are formed (Fig. 20.2).

Plasma fibrinolytic activity is decreased during pregnancy, remains low during labour and delivery and returns to normal within 1 h of delivery of the placenta. This is

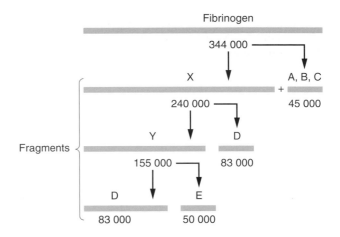

Fig. 20.2 Fibrin degradation products produced by degradation of fibrinogen by plasmin. Molecular weights are shown.

thought to be due to the effect of plasminogen activator inhibitor type II (PAI-2) derived from the placenta, which is present in abundance during pregnancy. In addition the activity in the fibrinolytic system in response to stimulation has been found to be significantly reduced in pregnancy (Ballegeer et al 1987).

Summary

The changes in the coagulation system in normal pregnancy are consistent with a continuing low-grade process of coagulant activity. Using electron microscopy, fibrin deposition can be demonstrated in the intervillous space of the placenta and in the walls of the spiral arteries supplying the placenta (Sheppard & Bannar 1974). As pregnancy advances, the elastic lamina and smooth muscle of these spiral arteries are replaced by a matrix containing fibrin. This allows expansion of the lumen to accommodate an increasing blood flow and reduces the vascular resistance of the placenta. At placental separation during normal childbirth, a blood flow of 500–800 ml/min has to be staunched within seconds, or serious haemorrhage will occur. Myometrial contraction plays a vital role in securing haemostasis by reducing the blood flow to the placental site. Rapid closure of the terminal part of the spiral artery is further facilitated by the structural changes within the walls. The placental site is rapidly covered by a fibrin mesh following delivery. The increased levels of fibrinogen and other coagulation factors help to meet the sudden demand for haemostatic components.

The changes also predispose to intravascular clotting, and a wide spectrum of disorders involving coagulation occurs in abnormal pregnancy.

DISSEMINATED INTRAVASCULAR COAGULATION

The changes in the haemostatic system and the local activation of the clotting system during parturition carry with them a risk not only of thromboembolism but also of DIC. This results in consumption of clotting factors and platelets, leading in some cases to severe (particularly uterine but sometimes generalised) bleeding.

DIC is never primary, but is always secondary to a general stimulation of coagulation activity by release of procoagulant substances into the blood (Fig. 20.3). Hypothetical triggers of this process in pregnancy include the leaking of placental tissue fragments, amniotic fluid, incompatible red cells or bacterial products into the maternal circulation. There is a broad spectrum of manifestations of the process of DIC (Table 20.1), ranging from a compensated state with no clinical manifestation but evidence of increased production and breakdown of coagulation factors, to the condition we all fear of massive uncontrollable haemorrhage with very low concentrations of plasma fibrinogen, pathological raised levels of fibrin degradation products and variable degrees of thrombocytopenia. Another confusing aspect is that there appears to be a transient state of intravascular coagulation during the whole of normal labour, maximal at the time of birth (Stirling et al 1984).

Fibrinolysis is stimulated by DIC, and the FDP resulting from the process interfere with the formation of firm fibrin clots. Thus a vicious circle is established, resulting in further disastrous bleeding (Fig. 20.4). FDP also interfere with myometrial function and possibly cardiac function and therefore aggravate shock as well as haemorrhage.

Obstetric conditions classically associated with DIC include abruptio placentae, amniotic fluid embolism, septic miscarriage and intrauterine infection, retained dead fetus, hydatidiform mole, placenta accreta, pre-eclampsia and eclampsia and prolonged shock from any cause (see Fig. 20.3).

Haematological management of the bleeding obstetric patient

The management of the bleeding obstetric patient is an acute and frightening problem. There is little time to think and in every unit there must be a planned practice and written protocol, agreed by haematologists, physicians, anaesthetists, obstetricians and nursing staff, to deal with this situation

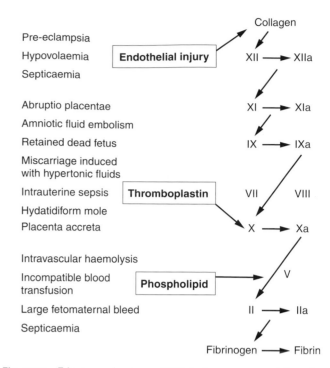

Fig. 20.3 Trigger mechanisms of DIC during pregnancy. Interactions occur in many of these obstetric complications.

whenever it arises. This should be read by all junior staff and attention should be drawn to it frequently, for when the emergency occurs there is little time for leisurely perusal. Good reliable communication between the various clinicians, nursing, paramedical and laboratory staff is essential. It is recommended that there should be regular rehearsals in dealing with this problem (Department of Health 1998). Portering services are an essential, often forgotten, component of dealing with this emergency.

It is imperative that the source of bleeding, often an unsuspected uterine or genital laceration, should be located and dealt with. Prolonged hypovolaemic shock, or indeed shock from any cause, may also trigger DIC and this may lead to haemostatic failure and further prolonged haemorrhage.

Table 20.1 Spectrum of severity of DIC: its relationship to specific complications in obstetrics

Severity of DIC[a]		In vitro findings	Obstetric conditions commonly associated
Stage 1	Low-grade compensated	FDP ↑ Soluble fibrin complexes ↑ vWF: factor VIIIC ratio ↓	Pre-eclampsia Retained dead fetus
Stage 2	Uncompensated but no haemostatic failure	As above, plus fibrinogen ↓ Platelets ↓ Factors V and VIII ↓	Small abruptio Severe pre-eclampsia
Stage 3	Rampant with haemostatic failure	Platelets ↓↓ Gross depletion of coagulation factors, particularly fibrinogen FDP ↑↑	Abruptio placentae Amniotic fluid embolism Eclampsia

FDP, fibrin degradation products; vWF, von Willebrand factor.
[a] Rapid progression from stage 1 to stage 3 is possible unless appropriate action is taken.

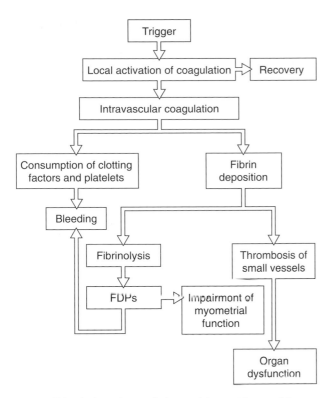

Fig. 20.4 Stimulation of coagulation activity and its possible consequences. FDPs, fibrin degradation products.

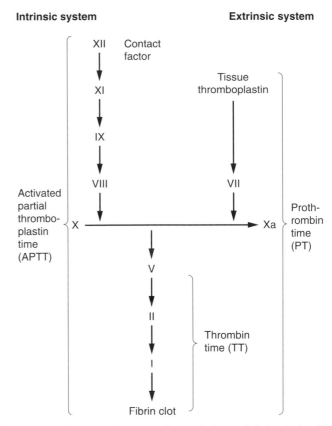

Fig. 20.5 *In vitro* screening tests of coagulation and their relationship to the systems involved.

In the author's experience, this is the most frequent cause of haemostatic failure associated with major obstetric haemorrhage.

The management of haemorrhage is the same whether the bleeding is caused or augmented by coagulation failure or not. The clinical condition usually demands urgent treatment and there is no time to wait for results of coagulation factor assays or sophisticated tests of the fibrinolytic system activity for precise definition of the extent of haemostatic failure, although blood can be taken for this purpose and analysed at leisure once the emergency is over.

Simple rapid tests, recommended below, will establish the competence or otherwise of the haemostatic system. In the vast majority of obstetric patients, coagulation failure results from a sudden transitory episode of DIC triggered by a variety of conditions (see Fig. 20.3). Useful rapid screening tests for haemostatic failure include the platelet count, partial thromboplastin time or accelerated whole-blood clotting time (which tests intrinsic coagulation), prothrombin time (which tests extrinsic coagulation), thrombin time and estimation of fibrinogen (Fig. 20.5).

Heparin characteristically prolongs the partial thromboplastin time and thrombin time out of proportion to the prothrombin time. As little as 0.05 units of heparin per millilitre will prolong the coagulation test times. It is customary, though not desirable, to take blood for coagulation tests from lines that have been washed through with fluids containing heparin to keep them patent. It is almost impossible to overcome the effect on the blood passing through such a line, however much blood is taken and discarded before obtaining

a sample for investigation. It is strongly recommended that blood is taken from another site not previously contaminated with heparin.

In obstetric practice the measurement of FDP is usually part of the investigation of suspected acute or chronic DIC. In the acute situation, raised FDP only confirm the presence of DIC, but are not diagnostic, and once the specimen is taken the laboratory measurement should be delayed until after the emergency is over, so that skilled laboratory workers can be performing a much more valuable service in providing results of coagulation screening tests and blood and blood products suitable for transfusion. Of the tests of coagulation, probably the thrombin time, an estimation of the thrombin clottable fibrinogen in a citrated sample of plasma is the most valuable overall rapid screen of haemostatic competence (Fig. 20.5).

Prolongation of the thrombin time is observed not only with depleted fibrinogen but in conditions where FDPs are increased, and even traces of heparin will significantly prolong the time it takes for a clot to be formed.

There is no point whatsoever in the obstetrician, anaesthetist or nursing staff wasting time trying in performing bedside whole-blood clotting tests. Whole-blood clotting normally takes up to 7 min and should be performed in clean tubes in a 37°C water bath with suitable controls. The alerted laboratory worker will be able to provide reliable results within half an hour of receiving the specimen in the laboratory.

The tests referred to above are straightforward and should

315

be available from any routine haematology laboratory. It is not necessary to have a high-powered coagulation laboratory to perform these simple screening tests to confirm or refute a diagnosis of DIC.

Treatment of severe haemorrhage must include prompt and adequate fluid replacement in order to avoid renal shutdown. If effective circulation is restored without too much delay, FDP will be cleared from the blood, mainly by the liver, which will further aid restoration of normal haemostasis. This is an aspect of management which is often not appropriately emphasised.

Plasma substitutes

There is much controversy about which plasma substitute to give to any bleeding patient. The remarks that follow are very much slanted towards the supportive laboratory management of acute haemorrhage from the placental site and should not be taken to apply to those situations in which hypovolaemia may be associated with severe hypoproteinaemia, such as occurs in septic peritonitis, burns and bowel infarction. The choice lies between simple crystalloids, such as Hartmann's solution or Ringer's lactate, and artificial colloids, such as dextran, hydroxyethyl starch and gelatin solution or the very expensive preparations of human albumin (albuminoids). If crystalloids are used, two or three times the volume of estimated blood loss should be administered because the crystalloid remains in the vascular compartment for a shorter time than colloids if renal function is maintained. The infusion of plasma substitutes, i.e. plasma protein, dextran, gelatin and starch solutions, may result in adverse reactions varying from allergic urticarial manifestations and mild fever to life-threatening anaphylactic reactions due to spasm of smooth muscle, with cardiac and respiratory arrest.

Dextrans adversely affect platelet function, may cause pseudo-agglutination and interfere with interpretation of subsequent blood grouping and cross-matching tests. They are, therefore, contraindicated in the woman who is bleeding as a result of a complication associated with pregnancy where there is a high chance of there being a serious haemostatic defect already. The anaphylactoid reactions accompanying infusion of dextrans are probably related to IgG and IgM antidextran antibodies, which are found in high concentrations in all patients with severe reactions. Acute fetal distress has been reported in mothers given dextran 70 who suffered anaphylactoid reactions (Barbier et al 1992). These dextran-induced anaphylactoid reactions have resulted in uterine hypertonia with subsequent severe fetal bradycardia even though immunoprophylaxis with dextran hapten has been administered (Berg et al 1991). There are many suitable superior alternatives for plasma expansion and dextran should be avoided in obstetric practice.

In many hospitals currently, the derivatives of gelatin (Haemaccel or Gelofusine) are the first-line fluids in resuscitation. They have a shelf-life of 8 years and can be stored at room temperature. They are iso-oncotic and do not interfere with platelet function or subsequent blood grouping or cross-matching. Renal function is improved when they are administered in hypovolaemic shock. They are generally considered to be non-immunogenic and do not trigger the production of

antibodies in humans, even on repeated challenge. The reactions associated with Haemaccel infusion are thought to be due to histamine release, the incidence and severity of reactions being proportional to the extent of histamine release. There have been a few rare reports of severe reactions with bronchospasm and circulatory collapse, and there has been one report of a fatality (Freeman 1979). Nevertheless, whatever substitute is used it is only a stopgap until suitable blood component therapy can be administered.

Use of blood and component therapy

Whole blood may be the treatment of choice in coagulation failure associated with obstetric disorders, but whole fresh blood is not available from regional centres in the UK. To release blood components earlier than the usual 18–24 h would increase the risk of serologically incompatible transfusions, viral hepatitis and human immunodeficiency virus (HIV) infection. Syphilis, cytomegalovirus and Epstein–Barr virus are examples of other infections that may be transmitted in fresh blood. Their viability diminishes rapidly on storage at 4°C. These infections, particularly in immunosuppressed or pregnant patients, can be particularly hazardous.

Fresh frozen plasma. Fresh frozen plasma (FFP) contains all the coagulation factors present in plasma obtained from whole blood within 6 h of donation. Frozen rapidly and stored at −30°C, the factors are well preserved for at least 1 year.

Cryoprecipitate. Although cryoprecipitate is richer in fibrinogen than FFP it lacks AT, which is rapidly consumed in obstetric bleeding associated with DIC. The use of cryoprecipitate also exposes the recipient to more donors and the potential associated hazards.

Platelets. Platelets, an essential haemostatic component, are not present in FFP and their functional activity rapidly deteriorates in stored blood. The platelet count reflects both the degree of intravascular coagulation and the amount of bank blood transfused. A patient with persistent bleeding and a very low platelet count (less than 20×10^9/l) may be given concentrated platelets, although they are seldom required in addition to FFP to achieve haemostasis in obstetric haemorrhage. A spontaneous recovery from the coagulation defect is to be expected once the uterus is empty and well contracted, provided that blood volume is maintained by adequate replacement monitored by central venous pressure and urinary output.

Problems arise when bleeding is difficult to control and the woman has a low haemoglobin before blood loss.

Red cell transfusion. Cross-matched blood should be available within 40 min of the maternal specimen reaching the laboratory. If the woman has had regular antenatal care her blood group will be documented. There is a good case for giving uncross-matched blood of her own group should the situation warrant it, provided that blood has been properly processed at the transfusion centre. If the blood group is unknown, uncross-matched group O Rh(D) negative blood may be given if necessary. By this time laboratory screening tests of haemostatic function should be available. If these prove to be normal, but vaginal bleeding continues, the cause is nearly always concealed trauma or bleeding from the placental site due to failure of the myometrium to contract. Prolonged hypovolaemic shock can lead to DIC and haemostatic failure with further prolonged haemorrhage.

If the blood loss is replaced only by stored bank blood, which is deficient in the labile clotting factors V and VIII and platelets, then the circulation will rapidly become depleted in these essential components of haemostasis, even if there is no DIC initially as the cause of haemorrhage. It is advisable to transfuse 2 units of FFP for every 4–6 units of bank red cells administered.

It seems sensible in any event, whatever the cause of bleeding, to change the initial plasma substitute and transfuse 2 units of FFP (plasma from two donations) once it has thawed, while waiting for compatible blood to be available.

A spontaneous recovery from the coagulation defect is to be expected once the uterus is empty and well contracted, provided that blood volume is maintained by adequate replacement monitored by central venous pressure and urinary output.

The single most important component of haemostasis at delivery in normal circumstances is contraction of the myometrium stemming the flow from the placental site. Transfused coagulation factors and platelets will not arrest haemorrhage if the uterus remains atonic. Vaginal delivery will make less severe demand on the haemostatic mechanism than delivery by caesarean section, which requires the same haemostatic competence as any other major surgical procedure. Should DIC be established with the fetus in utero, rather than to embark on heroic surgical delivery, it is better to wait for spontaneous delivery if possible, or to stimulate vaginal delivery, avoiding soft-tissue damage.

DIC in clinical conditions

In vitro detection of low-grade DIC

Rampant uncompensated DIC results in severe haemorrhage, with characteristic findings in vitro, are dealt with above; however, low-grade DIC does not usually give rise to any clinical manifestations, although the condition is potentially hazardous for both mother and fetus. Many in vitro tests have been claimed to detect low-grade compensated DIC and space does not allow an account of all of these.

Fibrin degradation products. Estimation of FDP will give some indication of low-grade DIC if these are significantly raised when fibrinogen, platelets and screening tests of haemostatic function appear to be within the normal range.

Soluble fibrin complexes. The action of thrombin on fibrinogen is crucial in DIC. Thrombin splits two molecules of fibrinopeptide A and two molecules of fibrinopeptide B from fibrinogen. The remaining molecule is called a fibrin monomer and polymerises rapidly to fibrin (see Fig. 20.1). Free fibrinopeptides in the blood are a specific measure of thrombin activity and high levels of fibrinopeptide A have been shown to be associated with compensated DIC in pregnancy.

Soluble fibrin complexes made up of fibrin–fibrinogen dimers are increased in conditions of low-grade DIC (Aznar et al 1982). These complexes are generated during the process of thrombin generation and the conversion of soluble fibrinogen to insoluble fibrin (see Fig. 20.1). Levels of soluble fibrin complexes are increased in patients with severe pre-eclampsia.

Factor VIII. During normal pregnancy the levels of both von Willebrand factor (vWF) and factor VIII coagulation activity (VIII:C) rise in parallel. An increase in the ratio of vWF to factor VIII:C has been observed in conditions accompanied by low-grade DIC, whether or not associated with pregnancy. An increase in the ratio has been observed in pregnancy with pre-eclampsia (Caires et al 1984) without any alteration in the simple screening tests of haemostatic function previously described.

The stages in the spectrum of severity of DIC (Table 20.1) are not strictly delineated and there may be rapid progression from low-grade compensated DIC, as diagnosed by paracoagulation tests described above, to the rampant form with haemostatic failure.

Abruptio placentae

Premature separation of the placenta, or abruptio placentae, is a well-known cause of coagulation failure in most obstetric units. The problems that confront the attendant in this situation are common to other conditions associated with DIC in pregnancy, therefore this will be used as the central focus of discussion of some of the controversial methods of management.

Abruptio placentae may occur in apparently healthy women with no clinical warning or may be in association with established pre-eclampsia. It is possible that clinically silent placental infarcts may predispose to placental separation by causing low-grade abnormalities of the haemostatic system, such as increased factor VIII consumption and raised FDP.

There is a great spectrum in the severity of the haemostatic failure in this condition which appears to be related to the degree of placental separation. Only 10% of patients overall with abruptio placentae show significant coagulation abnormalities. In some cases of a small abruptio, there is a minor degree of failure of haemostatic processes and the fetus does not succumb. When the uterus is tense and tender and no fetal heart can be heard, the separation and retroplacental bleeding are extensive. No guide to the severity of the haemorrhage or coagulation failure will be given by the amount of vaginal bleeding. Often there is no external vaginal blood loss, even when the placenta is completely separated, the fetus is dead, the circulating blood is incoagulable and there is up to 5 litres of concealed blood loss resulting in hypovolaemic shock.

Haemostatic failure may be suspected if there is persistent oozing at the site of venepuncture or bleeding from the mucous membranes of the mouth or nose. Simple, rapid screening tests will confirm the presence of DIC. There will be a low platelet count, greatly prolonged thrombin time, low fibrinogen and raised FDP due to secondary fibrinolysis stimulated by the intravascular deposition of fibrin. The mainstay of treatment is to maintain the circulating blood volume. This not only prevents renal shutdown and further haemostatic failure caused by hypovolaemic shock, it also helps clearance of FDP, which in themselves act as potent anticoagulants. It has also been suggested that FDP inhibit myometrial activity;

serious postpartum haemorrhage in women with abruptio placentae was found to be associated with high levels of fibrin degradation (Sher 1977).

If the fetus is dead the aim should be prompt vaginal delivery avoiding soft-tissue damage. Once correction of hypovolaemia is underway, measures to speed up delivery should be instituted. Amniotomy or, if this fails, prostaglandin or oxytocin stimulation can be used. There is no evidence that the use of oxytocic agents aggravates thromboplastin release from the uterus (Bonnar 1987). Following emptying of the uterus, myometrial contraction will greatly reduce bleeding from the placental site and spontaneous correction of the haemostatic defect usually occurs shortly after delivery if the measures recommended above have been taken. However, postpartum haemorrhage is a frequent complication and is the commonest cause of death in abruptio placentae (Department of Health 1998).

In cases where the abruptio is small and the fetus is still alive, prompt caesarean section may save the baby if vaginal delivery is not imminent. FFP, bank red cells and platelet concentrates should be available to correct the potentially severe coagulation defect in the maternal circulation. In rare situations where vaginal delivery cannot be stimulated and haemorrhage continues, caesarean section may be indicated even in the presence of a dead fetus. Despite extravasation of blood throughout the uterine muscle, its function is not impaired and good contraction will follow removal of fetus, placenta and retroperitoneal clot.

Heparin has been used to treat all kinds of DIC, whatever their cause. There is, however, no objective evidence to demonstrate that its use in abruptio placentae has decreased morbidity and mortality. Its use, with an intact circulation, would be sensible and logical to break the vicious circle of DIC but, in the presence of already defective haemostasis with a large bleeding placental site, it may prolong massive local and generalised haemorrhage.

Treatment with an antifibrinolytic agent such as tranexamic acid (Cyclokapron) or Trasylol can result in blockage with fibrin of small vessels in vital organs such as the kidney or brain. It is therefore contraindicated.

It has been suggested (Sher & Statland 1985) that aprotinin (Trasylol) may be helpful in the management of abruptio placentae, particularly in those cases with uterine inertia associated with high levels of FDP. There is a high incidence (1.5%) of abruptio placentae in the obstetric admissions (18 000 per annum) at the Groote Schuur Obstetric Unit, Cape Town, South Africa, where the study was carried out. In the past decade there has been a resurgence of usage of Trasylol, particularly in cardiac surgery (Bidstrup et al 1989) where significant reduction in blood loss has been shown following cardiac bypass operations. This is thought to be due predominantly to platelet sparing. However, it is doubtful whether Trasylol has any place in the current management of obstetric DIC. In recent years, obstetricians appear unconvinced of the benefits of Trasylol in the treatment of DIC and abruptio placentae, judging by many published reports.

Prompt supportive measures alone, maintaining central venous pressure and replacing blood loss together with essential coagulation factors, will result in reduction in FDP. This will improve myometrial function and contribute to the return of healthy haemostasis.

A report on reducing the frequency of severe abruptio placentae from Dallas, Texas (Pritchard et al 1991) noted that the 50% reduction in fetal death associated with abruptio over more than 30 years (1958–1990) could be accounted for by the decrease in women of very high parity and an increase in the proportion of Latin American as opposed to black women in the population served. With modern supportive measures, maternal death due directly to abruptio placentae is now extremely rare.

Amniotic fluid embolism

Amniotic fluid embolism (AFE) is very rare but is one of the most dangerous conditions in obstetrics because it is so difficult to treat. The incidence has been estimated as between 1 in 8000 and 1 in 80 000 in various reports (Morgan 1979) but the latter figure is probably nearer the true incidence. During the triennium 1994–1996 in the UK, 10 histologically confirmed cases occurred associated with 2 197 300 maternities; in seven cases the AFE was considered responsible for the fatality. Seventeen direct deaths in total were attributed to AFE (including those where the diagnosis was only clinical), giving a rate of 7.7 per million maternities. The maternal mortality of AFE is very high—over 80% in most reports. An excellent review of 272 cases in the English literature reported that only 39 survived, giving a mortality rate of 86% (Morgan 1979). AFE is the most common cause of death in the immediate postpartum period. (It is, however, possible that minor degrees of AFE may remain clinically unidentified, and therefore that the process occurs more commonly than is apparent from studies of maternal death.)

AFE is said to occur most frequently in elderly multiparous patients with large babies at or near term, following a short tumultuous labour associated with the use of uterine stimulants. However, the review quoted (Morgan 1979) and the most recent report on Confidential Enquiries into Maternal Deaths (Department of Health 1998) do not substantiate this statement.

There have been some reports of AFE occurring in young primiparous women during the second trimester, after evacuation of a missed abortion and in women undergoing legally induced terminations.

The clinical features associated with AFE are respiratory distress, cyanosis, cardiovascular collapse, haemorrhage and coma. Although coagulation failure occurs rapidly, the presenting clinical feature is sudden extreme shock with cyanosis due to an almost complete shutdown of the pulmonary circulation. The coagulation abnormalities are ascribed to the thromboplastic activity of amniotic fluid. Massive intravascular coagulation occurs and consumption of the clotting factors can be almost total. There is a high mortality from a combination of respiratory and cardiac failure; if the mother survives long enough, the effect of massive intravascular coagulation will invariably follow, with bleeding from venepuncture sites and severe haemorrhage from the placental site after delivery.

Confirmation of diagnosis in the past was only accepted by finding histological evidence of amniotic fluid and fetal tissue within the substance of the maternal lungs at autopsy. However, more recent techniques of diagnosis include detection of squamous cells and lanugo hair on cytological examination of blood aspirated through a Swan–Ganz catheter and detection of squamous cells in maternal sputum (although fetal tissue has also been found in pulmonary arterial blood in some women who have not apparently suffered AFE).

The management of cardiorespiratory failure associated with AFE must be carefully planned. The condition is similar to pulmonary embolism in its manifestations but there is also profound haemorrhage. Vigorous attempts at maintenance of the circulation, as recommended for other conditions associated with DIC, may result in cardiac failure due to resistance to flow in the pulmonary circulation. There should be careful monitoring of the central venous pressure to avoid cardiac overload; the object is to sustain the circulation while the intravascular thrombin in the lungs is cleared by the naturally stimulated intense fibrinolytic response of the endothelium of the pulmonary vessels.

If bleeding from the placental site can be controlled by stimulation of uterine contraction, the logical treatment is carefully monitored transfusion of FFP and packed red cells, with heparin administration and, if indicated, positive pressure ventilation. It is obviously essential that a competent intensive care unit should be immediately available for any obstetric service to deal promptly with this rare but often lethal complication of pregnancy. Use of steroids to suppress the inflammatory reaction in the lungs has also been suggested.

Retention of dead fetus

The question of intrauterine fetal death and haemostatic failure has been reviewed in the past (Romero et al 1985). There is a gradual depletion of maternal coagulation factors after intrauterine fetal death but the changes are not usually detectable, even *in vitro*, until after 3–4 weeks. Thromboplastic substances released from the dead tissues in the uterus into the maternal circulation are thought to be the trigger of DIC in this situation, which occurs in about one-third of patients who retain the dead fetus for more than 4–5 weeks. Problems arising from defective haemostasis are not observed in modern western obstetric practice because a dead fetus is almost always delivered before clinically significant coagulation changes have developed.

Retained dead fetus and living twin. The occurrence of single fetal death in a preterm multiple pregnancy poses unique therapeutic dilemmas. On occasion, selective termination of the life of one twin is being offered where it has been shown to be affected with a genetic disorder or involved in twin–twin transfusion syndrome. Haemostatic failure (particularly thrombosis and embolism) appears to be a hazard for the remaining fetus rather than for the mother.

Termination of pregnancy

Changes in haemostatic components consistent with DIC have been demonstrated in patients undergoing termination of pregnancy induced with hypertonic solutions of saline and urea.

The stimulus appears to be the release of tissue factor into the maternal circulation from the placenta, which is damaged by the hypertonic solutions. DIC has also been described in association with late dilatation and evacuation procedures especially when this is done by the two-stage method where an artificial rupture of membranes (ARM) with cord clamping is performed 24 h before dilatation and evacuation (which makes removal of the fetus easier and makes sure it is not born alive). It can also occur in association with termination using prostaglandins and oxytocin (Savage 1982). The haemorrhage may be massive and has resulted in maternal deaths. Prompt restoration of blood volume and transfusions with red cells and FFP, as described above, should resolve the situation which, once the uterus is empty, is self-limiting. Intravenous antibiotic therapy is also essential if there is any sign of sepsis.

Intrauterine infection

Endotoxic shock associated with septic abortion and antepartum or postpartum intrauterine infection can trigger DIC in pregnancy and the puerperium. Infection with Gram-negative microorganisms is the usual finding. Fibrin is deposited in the microvasculature because of endothelial damage by the endotoxin, and secondary red cell intravascular haemolysis with characteristic fragmentation, so-called microangiopathic haemolysis, is characteristic of the condition.

The patient is usually alert and flushed, with a rapid pulse and low blood pressure. Transfusion, unlike in other obstetric emergencies complicated by DIC, has little or no effect on the hypotension. A few centres in Europe have used heparinisation in the management of septic abortion and have claimed a decrease in mortality (Graeff & Kuhn 1980). Elimination of the uterine infection remains the most important aspect of management; claims that therapy with heparin has significantly decreased maternal mortality in septic abortions are in doubt and the use of heparin remains controversial.

Purpura fulminans

This rare complication of the puerperium is precipitated by Gram-negative septicaemia. Extensive haemorrhage occurs into the skin in association with DIC. The underlying mechanism is unknown but there appears to be an acute activation of the clotting system, resulting in the deposition of fibrin thrombi within blood vessels of the skin and other organs. The extremities and face are usually involved first; the purpuric patches have a jagged and erythematous border, which can be shown histologically to be the site of a leucocytoclastic vasculitis. Rapid enlargement of the lesions, which become necrotic and gangrenous, is associated with shock, tachycardia and fever. Without treatment the mortality rate is high, and, among those who survive, digit or limb amputation may be necessary. The laboratory findings are those of DIC with leucocytosis. In this situation treatment with heparin should be started as soon as the diagnosis is apparent, to prevent further consumption of platelets and coagulation factors. It should always be remembered, however, that bleeding from any site in the presence of the defective coagulation factors will be aggravated by the use of heparin.

Survival in purpura fulminans is currently much improved because of better supportive treatment for the shocked patient and effective control of the triggering infection, together with heparin therapy.

Low-grade DIC, pre-eclampsia and related syndromes

Platelets in pre-eclampsia. There have been many reports and reviews showing that the circulating platelet count is reduced in pre-eclampsia (Romero et al 1989, Baker & Cunningham 1999). The platelet count can be used to monitor severity of the disease process as well as for initial screening if there is concern about significant coagulation abnormalities (Leduc et al 1992). A fall in the platelet count may precede any detectable rise in serum FDP in women subsequently developing pre-eclampsia. The combination of a reduced platelet lifespan and a fall in the platelet count without platelet-associated antibodies (see later) indicates a low-grade coagulopathy. Platelets may either be consumed in thrombus formation or may suffer membrane damage from contact with abnormal surfaces and be prematurely removed from the circulation. Rarely, in very severe pre-eclampsia, the patient develops microangiopathic haemolytic anaemia. These patients have profound thrombocytopenia and this leads to confusion in the differential diagnosis between pre-eclampsia, haemolysis, elevated liver enzymes, low platelet count syndrome (HELLP) and thrombotic thrombocytopenic purpura (TTP).

Activation of the haemostatic mechanisms in normal pregnancy has led to the view that the haematological manifestations of pre-eclampsia merely represent augmentation of the hypercoagulable state which accompanies normal pregnancy. In this respect many studies have been carried out of the levels of individual coagulation factors. No clear pattern emerges but there appear to be some significant correlations of severity of the disease process with both the factor VIII complex (Redman et al 1977) and AT (Weiner et al 1985).

A readily available and sensitive indicator of activation of the coagulation system is assay of fibrinopeptide A concentration in the plasma. Although in mild pre-eclampsia, patients may have a normal or only slight increase in fibrinopeptide A levels, marked increases occur in patients with severe pre-eclampsia (Wallmo et al 1984).

Most studies in pre-eclampsia have shown increased levels of FDP in serum and urine. Plasma levels of soluble fibrinogen–fibrin complexes are also raised compared with normal pregnancies. Once the disease process is established, the most relevant coagulation abnormalities appear to be the platelet count, factor VIII and FDP. Those women with the most marked abnormalities in these parameters suffer the greatest perinatal loss (Thornton et al 1989). Following the reported association between thrombophilia factors, severe pre-eclampsia, and intrauterine growth restriction (IUGR) (Kupferminc et al 1999), it has been suggested that investigation of pre-eclampsia should also include a search for defects in the naturally occurring anticoagulants so that future pregnancies can be managed appropriately.

Many investigators now believe that gestational hypertension with or without proteinuria, IUGR, HELLP syndrome, acute fatty liver of pregnancy (AFLP) and eclampsia are part of the same disease process, which presents with the related signs and symptoms depending on the organ targeted by small vessel coagulopathy and varying degrees of DIC.

Summary

As emphasised, DIC is always a secondary phenomenon and the mainstay of management is therefore to remove the initiating stimulus if possible.

With rampant DIC and haemorrhage, recovery will usually follow emptying of the uterus provided the blood volume is maintained, and shock due to hypovolaemia is prevented. An efficiently acting myometrium after delivery will stem haemorrhage from the placental site. Measures to achieve a firm contracted uterus are the key to preventing continuing massive blood loss.

It is of interest that the maternal mortality of DIC associated with placental abruption is less than 1%, whereas that associated with infection and shock is 50–80%. The mortality rate reported in series of patients with DIC of various aetiologies is 50–85% and the wide variation probably reflects the mortality rate of the underlying disorder, not of DIC per se (Feinstein 1982). The major determinant of survival is our ability to identify the underlying trigger and manage it successfully.

ACQUIRED PRIMARY DEFECTS OF HAEMOSTASIS

Thrombocytopenia

The commonest platelet abnormality encountered in clinical practice is thrombocytopenia. Maternal thrombocytopenia remains a difficult management problem during pregnancy and can occasionally have profound effects on fetal and neonatal well-being. The causes and management of maternal and fetal thrombocytopenia have been reviewed (Letsky & Greaves 1996).

A low platelet count is seen most frequently in association with DIC, as already described. Sometimes severe megaloblastic anaemia of pregnancy is accompanied by thrombocytopenia, but the platelet count rapidly returns to normal after therapy with folic acid. Toxic depression of bone marrow megakaryocytes in pregnancy can occur in association with infection, certain drugs and alcoholism. Neoplastic infiltration may also result in thrombocytopenia. Probably the single most important cause of isolated thrombocytopenia in pregnancy is autoimmune thrombocytopenic purpura.

Autoimmune thrombocytopenic purpura

Autoimmune thrombocytopenic purpura (ITP) is relatively common in women of childbearing age, with an incidence of 1–2 per 10 000 pregnancies. Cases may present with skin bruising, and platelet counts between 30 and $80 \times 10^9/1$, but it is rare to see severe bleeding associated with low platelet counts in the chronic form.

With the screening of pregnant women, very mild thrombocytopenia may be discovered as an incidental finding and is not associated with risk to the mother or infant (Burrows & Kelton 1988). It may be that it represents very mild ITP, but even if it does, it is not associated with any adverse effects. ITP must be distinguished from cases of alloimmune thrombocytopenia, which results in infants affected with severe neonatal thrombocytopenia and the hazard of intracranial haemorrhage. There are no serological tests or clinical guidelines that reliably predict the hazard of thrombocytopenia in an individual fetus when their mothers have ITP, and correlation between maternal and neonatal counts is poor. (The diagnosis of alloimmune thrombocytopenia is nearly always on the basis of the birth of a first affected child, as the mother has no signs or symptoms.) It has been assumed that caesarean section delivery is less traumatic to the fetus than vaginal delivery and, while that premise could be debated, recognising and investigating the minority of pregnancies at risk of significant fetal thrombocytopenia would avoid many unnecessary fetal blood samples and caesarean sections.

Diagnosis. ITP is a diagnosis of exclusion, with peripheral thrombocytopenia and normal or increased megakaryocytes in the bone marrow, and the documented absence of other diseases. The red and white cells are essentially normal unless there is secondary anaemia. The diagnosis of ITP requires the exclusion of systemic lupus erythematosis (SLE), the antiphospholipid syndrome and HIV-associated thrombocytopenia.

There have been a number of analyses of outcome of cases of maternal ITP from the 1950s onwards. The findings may not be entirely applicable to current management because some of the documented poor fetal outcomes may have been associated with unrecognised maternal lupus, pre-eclampsia or alloimmune thrombocytopenia. Only symptomatic women and newborn babies were investigated because there was no general screening of the platelet count in healthy women. This resulted in an exaggerated view both of the incidence of neonatal thrombocytopenia and the rates of morbidity and mortality arising from it. In fact, the majority of thrombocytopenic patients are asymptomatic, and tests to estimate the bleeding risk in these patients and their infants are essential if overtreatment is not to occur.

In chronic platelet consumption disorders, a population of younger, larger platelets is established which have enhanced function. Measurement of the mean platelet volume (MPV) or, if not available, examination of the stained blood film will detect the presence of these large platelets. The risk of bleeding at any given platelet count is less in those patients with younger large platelets. The bleeding time, which has been severely criticised (Lind 1991) as a predictor of bleeding at surgery, still has a place in this context according to some respected workers (Burrows & Kelton 1992, Vandermeulen et al 1993). While some cases of ITP have normal or increased amounts of immunoglobulin coating the platelets or in the plasma, 10–35% of patients have no demonstrable platelet-associated IgG (PAIgG). The presence of IgG rather than IgM antibodies (Hegde et al 1985) has relevance to the pregnant patient because only IgG antibodies can be transported across the placenta and cause thrombocytopenia in the fetus.

The absence of a history of ITP before the index pregnancy is a low-risk indicator for neonatal thrombocytopenia. A review of the literature of ITP in pregnancy (Burrows & Kelton 1992) shows a neonatal mortality rate of 6 per 1000 ITP patients, about the same as the overall perinatal mortality rate. All the deaths in this survey occurred in babies delivered by caesarean section, unlike other reports, and all events appeared more than 24–48 h after delivery, the time of the nadir of platelet count in the newborn.

Management in pregnancy. Management of pregnancy associated with ITP is directed at three aspects: antenatal care of the mother, management of the mother and fetus during delivery and, lastly, the management of the neonate from the time of delivery.

The most important decision to make is whether the mother requires treatment at all. Many patients have significant thrombocytopenia (platelet count $<100 \times 10^9$/l) but no evidence of an *in vivo* haemostatic disorder. In general the platelet count must be $<50 \times 10^9$/l for capillary bleeding and purpura to occur.

There is no need to treat asymptomatic women with mild to moderate thrombocytopenia (count above 50×10^9/l) and a normal bleeding time. However, the maternal platelet count should be monitored at every clinic visit and signs of haemostatic impairment looked for. The platelet count will show a downward trend during pregnancy, with a nadir in the third trimester, and active treatment may have to be instituted to achieve a safe haemostatic concentration of platelets for delivery at term. If the woman wishes to have epidural anaesthesia for delivery, then treatment will be necessary to bring the platelet count above $70–80 \times 10^9$ per litre, as below this level there is a small but real risk of epidural haematoma which most anaesthetists consider contraindicates the procedure. The incidence of antepartum haemorrhage is not increased in maternal ITP but there is a small increased risk of postpartum haemorrhagic complications, not from the placental bed but from surgical incisions such as episiotomy and from soft-tissue lacerations.

Intervention in the antenatal period is based on clinical manifestations. The woman with bruising or petechiae requires measures to raise the platelet count but the woman with mucous membrane bleeding which may be life threatening requires urgent treatment with platelet transfusions and i.v. IgG and, occasionally, emergency splenectomy. The real dilemma in the pregnant woman with ITP is that nearly all patients have chronic disease. The long-term effects of treatment have to be considered in the light of the possible complications on the progress of pregnancy in the mother and of any effects on the fetus. The hazard for the mother who is monitored carefully and where appropriate measures have been taken is negligible. Most of her management is orientated towards what are thought to be optimal conditions for the delivery of the fetus, who in turn may or may not be thrombocytopenic.

Corticosteroids. The use of corticosteroids is a satisfactory short-term therapy but is unacceptable as long-term support unless the maintenance dose is very small. Side effects for the mother include weight gain, subcutaneous fat redistribution and hypertension, which are undesirable during pregnancy. In addition, the prevalence of pre-eclampsia, gestational diabetes, postpartum psychosis and osteoporosis are all increased with the use of corticosteroids. Nevertheless, they are often used but should be reserved as short-term therapy for patients with obvious risk of bleeding or to raise the platelet count of an asymptomatic woman at term, allowing her to have epidural or spinal analgesia for delivery if desired or indicated.

It has been suggested (Hegde 1985) that high doses of corticosteroids given to elevate platelet counts at or near term should be avoided because they may increase the transplacental passage of IgG antibody and thus expose the fetus to greater risk of severe thrombocytopenia. In the author's experience this is a theoretical hazard not seen in practice.

Intravenous IgG. The introduction of a highly successful treatment for ITP has altered the management options dramatically. It is thought that a prolongation of clearance of IgG-coated platelets in ITP results in an increase in the number of circulating platelets but the mechanism remains unknown. Used in the original recommended doses of 0.4 g/kg for 5 days by i.v. infusion, a persistent and predictable response was obtained in more than 80% of reported cases. More recently, alternative dosage regimens of this very expensive treatment have been suggested; these are just as effective but easier to manage and use less total immunoglobulin (Burrows & Kelton 1992). A typical dose is 1 g/kg over 8 h on one day. This dose will raise the platelet count to normal or safe levels in approximately half of the patients. In those in whom the platelet count does not rise, a similar dose can be repeated 2 days later. The advantages of this treatment are that it is safe, has very few side effects and the response to therapy is more rapid than with corticosteroids. The response usually occurs within 48 h and is maintained for 2–3 weeks. The main disadvantage is that it is very expensive (up to £1000 for each infusion) and seldom produces a long-term cure.

It has been suggested that IgG given intravenously can cross the placenta and should provoke an identical response in the fetus at risk, but this has never been proved. There is no doubt about the value of IgG in selected cases of severe maternal thrombocytopenia where a rapid response is required, but its use needs to be justified on a case by case basis because of the high cost.

Splenectomy will produce a cure or long-term drug-free remission in 60–80% of all patients with ITP. This is because the main site of antibody production is often the spleen and because many of the IgG-coated platelets are sequestered there. All patients should receive pneumovax before splenectomy and twice daily oral penicillin for life following surgery, to protect against pneumococcal infection. Older reviews of the management of ITP have associated splenectomy during pregnancy with high fetal loss rates; however, removal of the spleen remains an option if all other attempts to increase the platelet count fail (Gottlieb et al 1999). Surgery performed in the second trimester of pregnancy is best tolerated, when the size of the uterus does not make the operation technically difficult. Although transfused platelets will have a short life in the maternal circulation, they may help to achieve haemostasis at surgery. Platelet concentrates should be available but given only if abnormal bleeding occurs.

Other therapy. There are a number of other medications which have been used in ITP but most of them are contraindicated in pregnancy and only have moderate success rates. Danazol, an attenuated anabolic steroid, has been used with moderate success in a few patients. Vincristine has a transient beneficial effect in many patients but it is not rec-

ommended in pregnancy and long-term associated neurotoxicity limits its usefulness.

Very occasionally immunosuppressives, such as azothiaprine and cyclophosphamide, have to be used in severe intractable thrombocytopenia that does not respond to any other measures. Cyclophosphamide should be avoided in pregnancy. However, experience with relatively low doses of azathioprine in the increasing numbers of transplant patients who have now negotiated a subsequent pregnancy suggests that this drug is not associated with increased fetal or maternal morbidity. The most contentious issue in the management of ITP in pregnancy is the mode of delivery given that the fetus may also be thrombocytopenic and may bleed from trauma during the birth process.

Assessment of the fetal platelet count. The incidence of neonatal thrombocytopenia in retrospective analyses was distorted because only symptomatic women were likely to have been investigated and reported. More recent reports (Samuels et al 1990, Burrows & Kelton 1992) show the overall incidence of thrombocytopenia in the offspring of women with ITP much lower, at approximately 11%, compared with the earlier reported incidence of approximately 50% (Hegde 1985).

In one study only 4.9% of infants had a cord blood platelet count of $<50 \times 10^9/l$ and none suffered morbidity or mortality as a result. Two-thirds of the infants had a further fall in platelet count in the first 2 or 3 days after birth but in all the thrombocytopenia could easily be corrected (Burrows & Kelton 1992).

Some investigators have suggested that maternal splenectomy increases the probability of neonatal thrombocytopenia. Closer scrutiny of published reports (Burrows & Kelton 1992) shows that it is only in those women with splenectomy and persistent thrombocytopenia ($<100 \times 10^9/l$) that the risk of neonatal thrombocytopenia is increased. What has become clear over the years is that analysis of the older literature gave an exaggerated incidence of neonatal thrombocytopenia and of the morbidity and mortality arising from it.

Fetal blood sampling. A method for direct measurement of the fetal platelet count in scalp blood obtained transcervically before or early in labour has been described (Tchernia 1988). The authors recommend that caesarean section be performed in all cases where the fetal platelet count is less than $50 \times 10^9/l$. This approach is more logical than any other decision about the mode of delivery, such as is made on the basis of maternal platelet count, concentration of IgG or splenectomy status. It is not without risk of significant haemorrhage in the truly thrombocytopenic fetus and often gives false-positive results (Burrows & Kelton 1992). The cervix must be sufficiently dilated to allow the fetal scalp to be sampled; the uterine contraction to achieve this may have caused the fetus to descend so far in the birth canal that caesarean section is technically difficult and also traumatic for the fetus.

The only way a reliable fetal platelet count can be obtained so that a decision concerning the optimal mode of delivery can be taken is by percutaneous fetal cord blood sampling (FBS) before term. This gives time for discussion with obstetrician, paediatrician, haematologist, anaesthetist and the mother concerning delivery. FBS should be performed at 37–38 weeks' gestation under ultrasound guidance as the transfer of IgG increases in the last weeks of pregnancy and an earlier sample may give a higher fetal platelet count than one taken nearer term. There is no need for sampling earlier in gestation because the fetus is not at risk from spontaneous intracranial haemorrhage in utero (cf. fetus with alloimmune thrombocytopenia).

There is a risk associated with the sampling but in skilled hands this is no more than 1%. A caesarean section may be precipitated because of fetal distress during the procedure even if the platelet count proves to be normal. This is another good reason for performing a fetal blood sample as late as possible in gestation if it is thought to be necessary. There is a Catch 22 situation here, in that the risk of cordocentesis is low if the fetal platelet count is normal, but if the count is low, there may be persistent bleeding from the cord, resulting in fetal distress and the need for urgent delivery, which in itself causes a risk. Given that the risk of complications in utero and during delivery are very low, fetal blood sampling can hardly ever be justified in an ITP pregnancy, unless there is a history of a previously affected fetus.

Mode of delivery. There is little risk to the mother whatever the mode of delivery. In most cases the maternal platelet count can be raised to haemostatic levels to cover the event. Even if the mother has to deliver in the face of a low platelet count, she is unlikely to bleed from the placental site once the uterus is empty but she is at risk of bleeding from any surgical incisions, soft-tissue injuries or tears. Platelets should be available but not given prophylactically. It should be remembered that the unnecessary transfusion of platelet concentrates in the absence of haemostatic failure may stimulate more autoantibody formation synthesis and thus increase maternal thrombocytopenia. Most anaesthetists require that the platelet count is at least 80×10^9/l, and preferably over 100×10^9/l, before they will administer an epidural anaesthetic, but there is no good evidence that counts above 50×10^9/l are not sufficient to achieve haemostasis in ITP.

The major risk at delivery is to the fetus with thrombocytopenia who, as the result of birth trauma, may suffer intracranial haemorrhage. If there is any question that a vaginal delivery will be difficult because of cephalopelvic disproportion, premature labour or a history of previous delivery problems, elective caesarean section should be carried out.

For many centres the availability of planned or emergency transabdominal FBS is severely limited or non-existent and so decisions concerning the mode of delivery will have to be taken without knowing the fetal platelet count.

The incidence of *severe* thrombocytopenia in the fetus of a woman with proven ITP is not more than 10%. Even if caesarean section is the optimum mode of delivery for the thrombocytopenic fetus, this does not justify this mode of delivery for the nine out of 10 fetuses without thrombocytopenia.

It is not now thought to be optimum management to deliver all fetuses with potential or identified thrombocytopenia by caesarean section. Caesarean section should be performed for the usual obstetric reasons.

In the author's hospital there is considerable expertise in intrauterine fetal blood sampling but we only recommend this procedure:

1. where the women enter pregnancy with a history of ITP together with currently identifiable platelet-associated IgG antibodies, or
2. in those women who have to be treated for ITP during the index pregnancy.

Our obstetricians, like many others, prefer to deliver a fetus with significant thrombocytopenia (platelet count < 50 $\times 10^9$/l) by caesarean section; however, individual units may need different policies depending on local expertise and practice. Given the low risk of identifying a problem and of associated complications in utero, FBS cannot be justified in most ITP pregnancies. Some perinatologists, particularly in the USA, still consider FBS important and necessary in managing ITP pregnancies. However, as of 1999, a survey from the USA shows an increasing number of obstetricians are abandoning FBS and will allow a trial of labour without a procedure to determine fetal platelet count. Most clinicians surveyed did not consider caesarean section to be protective against intracranial haemorrhage (Peleg & Hunter 1999).

Management of the newborn. An immediate cord platelet count should be performed following delivery in all babies of mothers with ITP, whenever or however diagnosed. The vast majority will have platelet counts well above 50×10^9/l and will be symptom-free. For those with low platelet counts, with petechiae or purpura, steroids or preferably i.v. IgG should be administered. If there is mucous membrane bleeding, platelet concentrates should also be administered.

It should be borne in mind that the neonatal platelet count will fall further in the first few days of life and it is at the nadir that most complications occur, rather than at delivery. Measures should be taken to prevent the fall if the cord blood platelet count warrants this. The platelet count should be repeated daily for the first week in those neonates with thrombocytopenia at delivery.

At the time of writing, the emphasis of overall management of ITP is to return to a non-interventional policy (Fisk & Bower 1993, Peleg & Hunter 1999) of sensible monitoring, supportive therapy, and a mode of delivery determined mainly by obstetric indications and not primarily on either the maternal or fetal platelet count.

ITP associated with HIV infection

Thrombocytopenia is a well-recognised complications of HIV infection and may be due to drugs and severe infection. However, patients with HIV may have thrombocytopenia otherwise indistinguishable from ITP. This may be due to immune platelet destruction resulting from cross-reaction between the virus and the platelet glycoproteins IIb/IIIa (Bettaieb et al 1992) which may explain AIDS-free, HIV-associated ITP. It has also been suggested that disturbances in the B-cell subset, CD5, in HIV-infected patients may cause immunological changes correlating with the platelet count (Kouri et al 1992) and that non-specific deposition of complement and immune complexes on platelets leads to their removal from the circulation.

Young pregnant women in a high-risk group for HIV with thrombocytopenia should be considered for HIV testing (which in any case should be recommended for all pregnant women).

Thrombocytopenia and systemic lupus erythematosus

Systemic lupus erythematosus (SLE) is frequently complicated by thrombocytopenia but this is seldom severe: less than 5% of cases have platelet counts below $30 \times 10^9/1$ during the course of the disease (Hughes 1987). Thrombocytopenia is often the first presenting feature and may antedate any other manifestations by months or even years. Such patients are often labelled as suffering from ITP, unless appropriate additional tests are carried out. Platelet-associated IgG is often found on testing but it is not clear whether this is due to antiplatelet antibody, immune complexes or both. The management of isolated thrombocytopenia associated with SLE in pregnancy does not differ substantially from that of ITP but immunosuppressive therapy should not be reduced or discontinued during pregnancy. However, the main management problem of SLE and pregnancy is the complication of the variably present *in vitro* lupus anticoagulant and its paradoxical association with *in vivo* thromboembolism and recurrent mid-trimester abortion (see Ch. 9).

Alloimmune thrombocytopenia

Severe alloimmune thrombocytopenia is a rare but important cause of fetal death and long-term neurological morbidity. The vast majority of clinically significant cases arise from fetomaternal incompatibility for the human platelet antigen HPA-la.

Diagnosis and screening. It is important to identify fetomaternal alloimmune thrombocytopenia as a cause of fetal or neonatal thrombocytopenia because of the high risk of recurrence and of intracranial haemorrhage (ICH) in subsequent pregnancies.

Routine antenatal screening has been suggested as a perinatal health policy but has not been put into practice. Pilot studies have confirmed an incidence of 1 in 1000–2000 pregnancies (Williamson et al 1998), more common than some other conditions for which screening is carried out. However, HPA typing of platelets is not a routine hospital transfusion laboratory commitment and would require recently developed primer pairs for rapid HPA identification with allele-specific polymerase chain reaction.

Currently, the diagnosis of the maternal condition in the overwhelming majority of cases is made after the birth of a thrombocytopenic infant or identification of a fetus (or newborn) with unexplained ICH. Serological testing of both parents is enough to establish the diagnosis. The importance of using one of a limited number of laboratories with the full range of capabilities required (including DNA-based typing) is emphasised.

Female relatives of the affected mother should be tested for HPA status in order to identify potential cases before the birth of a first affected infant.

Antenatal management. Unlike Rh(D) haemolytic disease of the newborn, first pregnancies may be severely affected and the maternal alloimmune platelet antibody has not proved useful in identifying or monitoring severity of the condition in the fetus.

The primary goal of antenatal management is to prevent in utero or perinatal intracranial haemorrhage. In the UK, weekly fetal transfusions of compatible platelets from as early as 22–24 weeks' gestation until 32 weeks or more are usual in many fetal centres (Murphy et al 1994). The cumulative risk of fetal loss during a potential 15 procedures (20–34 weeks) could be as high as 13–23% and must be considered against the risk to the fetus from the disease (Burrows & Kelton 1995). The apparent success of weekly maternal infusions of i.v. IgG in preventing fetal ICH reported by many groups in the USA has therefore been welcomed (Bussel et al 1996a), but is still regarded with scepticism in the UK and Europe (Kaplan et al 1998).

There is a consensus that FBS and a platelet count is the only certain way to identify an affected fetus. Suitable platelet concentrates should be available to cover the procedure. The risk of exsanguination at FBS appears to be higher than in other conditions when cordocentesis is performed (Paidas et al 1995). It has been suggested that function is disturbed by the antibody binding to a platelet membrane site involved in fibrinogen binding and aggregation and also to HPA-1a sites on the vascular endothelium.

Discrepancies between management approaches in North American and European centres reflect uncertainties regarding non-invasive monitoring and the hazards associated with invasive procedures. Optimal management is in the process of evolution and the appropriate therapy in any individual case is uncertain. All approaches have drawbacks. Interventions are based on the balance of the assessed risk of the disease in the fetus exceeding the risk of the invasive procedures involved (Bussel et al 1996b).

Thrombotic thrombocytopenic purpura and haemolytic–uraemic syndrome

These conditions, extremely rare in pregnancy, share so many features that they have been considered as one disease, with pathological effects confined largely to the kidney in haemolytic–uraemic syndrome (HUS) and being more generalised in thrombotic thrombocytopenic purpura (TTP). Both are due to the presence of platelet thrombi in the microcirculation, causing ischaemic dysfunction and microangiopathic haemolysis.

In TTP, the focus shifts to multisystem disease, often with neurological involvement and fever. It has been associated with pregnancy and the postpartum period and with the platelet antiaggregating agent, ticlopidine (Page et al 1991). It is also associated with abnormal patterns of multimers of vWF in the plasma.

In the past few years the mechanisms of processing of vWF multimers have been clarified. A proteolytic enzyme present in normal plasma cleaves peptide bonds in monomeric subunits of vWF, thus degrading the large multimers. This proteolytic enzyme prevents the unusually large multimers from causing vWF-mediated adhesion of platelets to subendothelium after vascular damage (Moake 1998).

Exciting new research by two groups of investigators has elucidated the role of vWF-cleaving protease activity in TTP

(Furlan et al 1998, Tsai & Lian 1998). In all the patients studied with acute, single-episode TTP, there was little or no vWF-cleaving protease activity associated with an IgG autoantibody during the illness but the activity returned to normal following recovery (Tsai & Lian 1998). However, in patients with chronic, relapsing TTP unusually large multimers of vWF are found in the plasma even between acute episodes, together with absence or low levels of vWF cleaving-protease activity (Furlan et al 1998). What are the implications of these exciting new findings? First of all, the response of patients in the past to FFP component infusions which contain the vWF-cleaving protease activity is explained. The fact that plasmapheresis is often required in the acute phase to achieve a response is also clarified, as this will remove autoantibodies as well as the abnormal large vWF multimers. Secondly, the diagnosis of TTP, which has been confused with severe pre-eclampsia and HELLP syndrome, may be clarified by a single laboratory test measuring the vWF-cleaving protease activity in the plasma and its inhibitor. This test will also help clinicians to distinguish between TTP and HUS, thought in the past to be a spectrum of clinical expression of the same disease. In HUS, the levels of vWF-cleaving protease are normal or approaching normal, and it also explains why plasma exchange has disappointing results in HUS. The possible role of microbial infections and steroid therapy in acute TTP remain unexplained but provide areas of research to explore the triggering of this condition in patients who do not have a genetic lack of vWF-cleaving protease activity.

The pentad of fever, normal coagulation tests with low platelets, haemolytic anemia, neurologic disorders, and renal dysfunction are virtually pathognomonic of TTP. The thrombocytopenia may range from 50 to 100×10^9/l. The clinical picture is severe, with a high maternal mortality. A crucial problem when dealing with TTP is to establish the correct diagnosis, because this condition can be confused with severe pre-eclampsia and placental abruption, especially if DIC (very uncommon in TTP) is triggered.

Unlike cases of severe pre-eclampsia, HELLP and AFLP, there is no evidence that prompt delivery affects the course of HUS or TTP favourably. Most clinicians would recommend delivery if these conditions are present in late pregnancy so that the mother can be treated vigorously without fear of harming the fetus. Therapeutic strategies hinge on intensive plasma exchange or replacement.

In summary, objective diagnosis of TTP should now be facilitated by measurement of vWF-cleaving protease and its inhibitor. The basis of treatment depends on supplying the defective missing enzyme by infusion of plasma or cryosupernatant, preferably, in severe cases, by exchange transfusion. It is reassuring that the vWF-cleaving protease is still present in all virally inactivated plasma products, whatever method is used for inactivation.

Factor VIII antibody

An inhibitor of antihaemophilic factor is a rare cause of haemorrhage in previously healthy postpartum women (Reece et al 1982). There are fewer than 50 documented cases in the literature. Women who may have had this type of haemorrhagic disorder were first reported in the late 1930s and the nature of the defect was first reported in 1946, when the plasma of two such patients was shown not only to resemble haemophilic plasma but to have an inhibitory effect on normal clotting. In the late 1960s it was demonstrated that these inhibitors of factor VIII were immunoglobulins, as are the factor VIII antibodies found in treated haemophiliacs. Of the postpartum coagulation defects of this type reported, nearly all were found on *in vitro* testing to be directed against factor VIII. Only two were found to be anti-factor IX antibodies.

Aetiology. The aetiology of antibodies to factor VIII is complex. The appearance of anti-VIIIC in non-haemophilic individuals is usually attributed to an autoimmune process, or in postpartum women, to alloimmunisation; however, no difference between maternal and fetal factor VIII has been demonstrated and neutralisation of both maternal and fetal factor VIII by the antibody is similar.

There is at present no definite experimental evidence that factor VIII antigen allotypes exist. If the bleeding tendency is to be explained, the antibody formed by stimulation of the maternal immune system by fetal factor VIII has to cross-react with maternal factor VIII. One would expect such an antibody to reappear after some of the subsequent pregnancies (by analogy with Rh sensitisation), but relapses have not been reported. Assuming that these inhibitors are IgG antibodies, they are likely to cross the placenta and persist for several weeks in the newborn, as do anti-rhesus or antiviral antibodies. However, although factor VIII antibody and low levels of factor VIIIC have been found in babies born to mothers with antibody, there have been no case reports of haemorrhagic problems in their offspring.

The variable nature of this disorder argues in favour of a more complex pathogenesis. There is an association between factor VIII antibodies and autoimmune disorders, such as rheumatoid arthritis and systemic lupus erythematosus. There is also a well known alteration of immune reactivity in normal pregnancy. These observations suggest that a likely explanation of postpartum factor VIII antibodies is that of a temporary breakdown in the mother's tolerance to her own factor VIII (or factor IX). This rare disorder resembles other autoimmune states in its variable onset and is still a mystery.

Clinical manifestations. The patient usually presents within 3 months of delivery with severe bleeding, extensive painful bruising, bleeding from the gastrointestinal or genitourinary tract and occasional haemarthroses. The reported confirmed cases presented in a period of 3 days to 17 months postpartum. The factor VIII antibody is associated with life-threatening haemorrhage at various sites, not necessarily related to parturition.

Diagnosis. The diagnosis is established on the basis of characteristic laboratory findings. The prothrombin time and thrombin time are normal but the partial thromboplastin time is very long. The partial thromboplastin time is not corrected by the addition of normal plasma or factor VIII.

Management. Any woman who develops such an antibody should be under the care of an expert coagulation unit. Treatment of the acute bleeding episode is difficult because conventional amounts of factor VIII may merely enhance antibody formation and fail to control the bleeding. Immunosuppressive agents in combination with corticosteroid have been used, in some cases, resulting in a decrease or disappearance of the antibody in response to treatment.

The natural history is for the antibody to disappear gradually, usually within 2 years. Women should be advised to avoid further pregnancy until coagulation is back to normal, although in the one documented case where conception occurred in the presence of clinically active antibody, the antibody disappeared during the course of the pregnancy (Voke & Letsky 1977).

GENETIC DISORDERS OF HAEMOSTASIS

It is important to recognise these uncommon conditions, not only because the morbidity and mortality they cause in the sufferer is almost completely preventable by correct diagnosis and treatment but also because carriers of the most devastating of these conditions, particularly the X-linked haemophilias, can be identified and prenatal diagnosis offered if couples at risk so desire.

However, because of the profound changes in haemostasis during normal pregnancy it is desirable to establish a correct diagnosis with appropriate family studies and DNA analysis where relevant, before conception, so that appropriate management, and in conditions where DNA prenatal diagnosis is feasible, appropriate fetal tissue sampling can be planned in advance.

Severe congenital disorders of haemostasis are nearly always apparent early in life so that they will have been diagnosed before the obstetrician has to deal with the patient. Milder forms may go unrecognised until adult life and are more of a diagnostic challenge.

Patients with thrombocytopenia or platelet function abnormalities suffer primarily from mucosal bleeding with epistaxes, gingival and gastrointestinal bleeding and menorrhagia. Bleeding occurs immediately after surgery or trauma and may not occur at all if primary haemostasis can be achieved with suturing.

In contrast, patients with coagulation disorders typically suffer deep muscle haematomas and haemarthroses. Bleeding after trauma or surgery may be immediate or delayed. A history of previous vaginal deliveries without undue bleeding does not exclude a significant coagulopathy because of the increase in coagulation factors, particularly factor VIII, which occurs during normal pregnancy and the fact that powerful uterine contractility is the most important haemostatic factor at parturition.

Complete laboratory evaluation of a patient giving a history of easy bleeding or bruising is time-consuming and expensive and a history of significant previous haemostatic challenges should be obtained. For example, a patient who has undergone tonsillectomy without transfusion or special treatment and lived to tell the tale cannot possibly have an inherited haemostatic disorder.

Of more relevance perhaps is any history of dental extractions where haemorrhage can occur with both platelet disorders and coagulopathies. If prolonged bleeding has occurred, and particularly if blood transfusion has been required, then a high index of suspicion of a congenital haemorrhagic dis-

order is justified. In such cases, even if initial laboratory screening tests (partial thromboplastin time, prothrombin time, platelet count and bleeding time) are normal, the diagnosis should be vigorously pursued in consultation with an expert haematologist.

The most common congenital coagulation disorders are von Willebrand's disease, factor VIII deficiency (haemophilia A) and factor IX deficiency (haemophilia B). Less common disorders include factor XI deficiency, abnormal or deficient fibrinogen and deficiency of factor XIII (fibrin-stabilising factor). All other coagulation factor disorders are extremely rare (Kadir 1999). The most frequent disorders of platelet function are von Willebrand's disease and storage pool disease (How et al 1991).

Inherited platelet defects

Qualitative platelet abnormalities

Serious bleeding disorders due to genetic abnormalities of platelet function are rare, the inheritance being autosomal recessive. Clinically, the signs and symptoms are similar to those of von Willebrand's disease, with skin and mucosal haemorrhages. Spontaneous bruises are common but haemarthroses are not. Although these disorders can lead to life-threatening haemorrhage, particularly after surgery or trauma, the bleeding tendency is usually mild. The essential defect is intrinsic to the platelet. Bleeding time is prolonged and platelet function tests are abnormal, showing reduced aggregation and/or adhesion. In thrombasthenia (Glanzmann's disease), the platelets appear morphologically normal but they fail to aggregate with collagen, adenosine diphosphate (ADP) or ristocetin. There is a risk of intracranial haemorrhage in utero in the affected fetus (cf. alloimmune thrombocytopenia). In the very rare Bernard–Soulier syndrome, the aggregation defect is similar but the platelets have a characteristically abnormal giant appearance. Serious bleeding episodes in pregnancy have been treated with plasmapheresis and fresh platelet concentrate infusions (Peacemen et al 1989).

Thrombocytopenia

Genetically determined thrombocytopenia may be associated with aplastic anaemia or isolated megakaryocytic aplasia. The thrombocytopenia–absent radius (TAR) syndrome is thought to be an autosomal recessive defect and has been successfully diagnosed prenatally by examination of a fetal blood sample. The May–Heggelin anomaly is an autosomal dominant condition with variable thrombocytopenia and giant platelets. The condition is usually benign but patients may need platelet concentrates to achieve haemostasis at delivery and can be offered prenatal diagnosis.

von Willebrand's disease

Von Willebrand's disease is the most frequent of all inherited haemostatic disorders, with an overt disease incidence of more than 1 in 10 000, similar to that of haemophilia A. Because subclinical forms of the disorder are common, the total incidence of von Willebrand's disease is actually greater than that of haemophilia. In contrast to haemophilia (an X-linked condition), von Willebrand's disease has an autosomal inheritance and equal incidence in males and females and therefore is the most frequent genetic haemostatic disorder encountered in obstetric practice (Caldwell et al 1985).

Nature of the defect

Von Willebrand's disease is a disorder of the vWF portion of the human factor VIII complex. Factor VIII circulates as a complex of two proteins of unequal size. There is a low molecular weight portion (VIIIC), which promotes coagulation, linked to a large multimer known as von Willebrand factor (vWF). The larger vWF, under autosomal control, serves as a carrier for VIIIC, coded for on the X-chromosome. The complex is found in the circulation as polymers of varying size. vWF is the major protein in plasma which promotes platelet adhesion by forming a bridge between the subendothelial collagen and a specific receptor on the platelet membrane. Reduction in vWF usually leads to comparable decrease in VIIIC activity.

There are subgroups of von Willebrand's disease based on qualitative and quantitative changes in the multimers of the factor VIII complex (Caldwell et al 1985).

Clinical features

Clinical manifestations of the disease are primarily those of a platelet defect, namely spontaneous mucous membrane or skin bleeding and prolonged bleeding after trauma or surgery. There are also manifestations of a coagulation defect due to VIIIC activity reduction. The most frequent problem encountered in the non-pregnant female is menorrhagia, which may be quite severe. Patients with mild abnormalities may be asymptomatic, with the diagnosis made only after excessive haemorrhage related to trauma or surgery. The severity of the disorder does not run true within families and fluctuates from time to time in the same individual.

Treatment

Several treatments in von Willebrand's disease are in current use, the choice depending on the severity and type of disease, and on the clinical setting. The aim is to correct the platelet and coagulation disorder by achieving normal levels of factor VIII coagulant activity and a bleeding time within the normal range. The key feature in treatment is substitution with plasma concentrates containing functional vWF and VIIIC. In less severe cases the vasopressin analogue 1-desamino-8-arginine-vasopressin (DDAVP) has been used with success. Contraceptive hormones have been used with success in the treatment of menorrhagia in von Willebrand's disease. Aspirin and related anti-inflammatory drugs should not be used in the disorder as they will further compromise platelet function.

The main treatment in von Willebrand's disease in the past was replacement therapy with cryoprecipitate or FFP. Newer preparations of factor VIII concentrate retain some platelet-promoting activity and have the added advantage of being heat-treated and therefore sterile. They no longer carry the hazard of transmitting HIV and other viral infections. The use of cryoprecipitate and FFP is now contraindicated and cannot be recommended.

DDAVP has been shown to cause release of vWF from endothelial cells where it is synthesised and stored. It is particularly effective in mildly affected patients and may in some cases replace the use or need for blood products in patients undergoing surgery. Toxicity associated with use of this product has been trivial. Occasional patients experience flushing and dizziness. The theoretical risk of water intoxication and hyponatraemia due to a vasopressive effect has not been observed using the current dosage schedules. The recommended dose is an intravenous infusion of 0.3 µg/kg DDAVP given over 30 min, up to a total dose of 15–25 µg. This may be repeated every 12–24 h. In patients with severe von Willebrand's disease, DDAVP has no effect and replacement therapy must be used.

von Willebrand's disease and pregnancy

A rise in both factor VIIIC and vWF is observed in normal pregnancy. Patients with all but the severest forms of von Willebrand's disease show a similar but variable rise in both these factors, although there may not be a reduction in the bleeding time (How et al 1991).

After delivery, normal women maintain an elevated factor VIIIC level for at least 5 days. This is followed by a slow fall to baseline levels over 4–6 weeks. The duration of factor VIII activity postpartum in women with von Willebrand's disease seems to be related to the severity of the disorder. Women with more severe forms of the condition may have a rapid fall in factor VIII procoagulant and platelet haemostatic activity. They are then at risk of quite severe secondary postpartum haemorrhage.

Published reports of 33 pregnancies in 22 women showed abnormal bleeding in 27% at the time of abortion, delivery or postpartum (Conti et al 1986). The general consensus is that the most important determinant for abnormal haemorrhage at delivery is a low factor VIIIC plasma level. The vast majority of women will have increased their factor VIIIC production to within the normal range (50–150%) by late gestation, and, although factor VIII concentrate should be standing by at delivery, it will probably not be needed to achieve haemostasis (Milaskiewicz et al 1990).

While there is virtually no place for DDAVP in obstetric practice it is valuable in the management of women with von Willebrand's disease undergoing gynaecological surgery.

The haemophilias

The haemophilias are inherited disorders associated with reduced or absent coagulation factors VIII or IX, with an incidence of around 1 in 10 000 in developed countries. The most common is haemophilia A, which is associated with deficiency of factor VIII; about one-sixth of the 3000–4000 cases in Britain today have a condition known as Christmas disease, which is due to a lack of coagulation factor IX (haemophilia B). Clinical manifestations of the two conditions are indistinguishable; symptoms and signs are variable and depend on the degree of the lack of the coagulation factors concerned. Severe disease with frequent spontaneous bleeding (particularly haemarthroses) is associated with clotting factor levels of 0–1%. Less severe disease is found in subjects with clotting factors of 1–4%. Spontaneous bleeding and severe bleeding after minor trauma are rare even in cases with coagulation factor levels between 5 and 30%; the danger is that the condition may be clinically silent but, during the course of major surgery or following trauma, such subjects behave as those with the severest forms of haemophilia. Unless the defect is recognised and replacement of the lacking coagulation factor replaced, such patients will continue to bleed. The inheritance of both haemophilias is X-linked recessive, being expressed in the male and carried by the female.

The risks in pregnancy for a female carrier of haemophilia are twofold:

1. Those women with a very low factor VIII or IX level may be at risk of excessive bleeding after a traumatic or surgical delivery. Women possess two X chromosomes but in each cell only one of these two is utilised and the other is largely inactivated. This process is essentially random and varies over a normal distribution. As a result, some carriers may have an entirely normal level of factor VIII or IX and others may be significantly deficient. This chromosome inactivation is sometimes referred to as 'Lyonisation' after Mary Lyon, by whom it was first described.
2. Fifty per cent of her sons will inherit haemophilia and 50% of her daughters will be carriers like herself.

This has important implications now that prenatal diagnosis of these conditions is possible.

Management of haemophilia in pregnancy

Female carriers of haemophilia do not generally have clinical manifestations but, in rare individuals in whom the factor VIIIC or IX levels are unusually low (10–30% of normal), abnormal bleeding may occur after trauma or surgery. It is important to identify carriers before pregnancy, not only to provide genetic counselling (Peake et al 1993) but so that appropriate provision can be made for those cases with pathologically low coagulation factor activity. Fortunately, the level of the deficient factor tends to increase during the course of pregnancy, as in normal women. There have been anecdotal reports of female homozygotes for haemophilia A who have negotiated pregnancy successfully. Haemorrhage postpartum does not appear to be a consistent feature, particularly if delivery is by the vaginal route at term with little or no soft-tissue damage. The effect of pregnancy on factor VIIIC levels in these rare cases has not been studied.

If the factor VIII level remains low in carriers of haemophilia, heat-treated factor VIII concentrates should be given to cover delivery.

DDAVP has been shown to be of benefit in patients with mild haemophilia, as with von Willebrand's disease (see above). However, the storage pools of factor VIII released during treatment may become exhausted and tachyphylaxis does occur. There are no controlled studies concerning the use of DDAVP during pregnancy and its safety and efficacy in obstetric practice remain to be determined.

The effects of DDAVP on uterine contractability could limit its use, although it has been employed in the management of diabetes insipidus in pregnancy with no harm to the fetus (Caldwell et al 1985). However, as pointed out previously, if the stimulus of pregnancy has not raised the level of factor VIII as expected in mild haemophilia, it is unlikely that DDAVP will do so.

A clinical problem is more likely in carriers of factor IX deficiency (Christmas disease) than in women with factor VIII deficiency. In the exceptionally rare situations where factor IX level is very low and remains low during pregnancy, the patient should be managed with high-purity factor IX concentrates to cover delivery and for 3–4 days postpartum. Low-purity factor IX concentrates (prothrombin concentrate) contain factors II, VII and X, as well as factor IX, and therefore carry a much greater thrombogenic hazard, adding to the innate risk of thromboembolism in pregnancy. Now that plasma is treated, FFP does not carry the remote hazard (in the UK) of transmitting HIV infection (Williamson et al 1996). The product of choice is high-purity factor IX concentrate. These patients should be managed in a unit with access to expert advice, 24 h laboratory coagulation service and immediate access to the appropriate plasma components required for replacement therapy.

Factor XI deficiency (plasma thromboplastin antecedent (PTA) deficiency)

This is a rare coagulation disorder that is less common than the haemophilias but more common than the very rare inherited deficiencies of the remaining coagulation factors. It is inherited as an autosomal recessive, predominantly in Ashkenazi Jews, and both men and women may be affected. Usually only the homozygotes have clinical evidence of a coagulation disorder, although occasionally carriers may have a bleeding tendency. It is a mild condition in which spontaneous haemorrhages and haemarthroses are rare but the danger lies in the fact that profuse bleeding may follow major trauma or surgery if no prophylactic factor XI concentrate is given. Indeed it is often diagnosed late in life after surgery in an individual who was unaware of a serious haemostatic defect. The diagnosis is made by finding a prolonged partial thromboplastin time, with a low factor XI level in a coagulation assay system but in which all other coagulation tests are normal. Management consists of replacement with factor XI concentrates as prophylaxis for surgery or to treat bleeding and to cover operative delivery.

The effective haemostatic level of factor XI has a half-life of around 2 days. To cover surgery or delivery, women can be treated with one infusion of factor XI concentrate to raise the level to 80–100% and until primary healing is established.

Fortunately, the condition rarely causes problems either during pregnancy and labour or in the offspring; in particular, prolonged bleeding at ritual circumcision is not usual. There is, therefore, no justification in screening routinely for this condition in the mother, fetus or newborn.

Genetic disorders of fibrinogen (factor I)

Fibrinogen is synthesised in the liver, has a molecular weight of 340 000 and circulates in plasma at a concentration of

300 mg/dl. Both quantitative and qualitative genetic abnormalities are described.

Afibrinogenaemia or hypofibrinogenaemia

These are rare autosomal recessive disorders resulting from reduced fibrinogen synthesis. Most patients with hypofibrinogenaemia are heterozygous.

Congenital hypofibrinogenaemia has been associated with recurrent early miscarriages and with recurrent placental abruption (Ness et al 1983).

Afibrinogenaemia is characterised by a lifelong bleeding tendency of variable severity. Prolonged bleeding after minor injury and easy bruising are frequent symptoms. Menorrhagia can be very severe. Spontaneous deep tissue bleeding and haemarthroses are rare, but severe bleeding can occur after trauma or surgery and several patients have suffered intracerebral haemorrhages. In afibrinogenaemia all screening tests of coagulation are prolonged, but corrected by addition of normal plasma or fibrinogen. A prolonged bleeding time may be present. The final diagnosis is made by quantifying the concentration of circulating fibrinogen.

There are no fibrinogen concentrates available and plasma or cryoprecipitate have to be used as replacement therapy to treat bleeding, cover surgery or delivery. The *in vivo* half-life of fibrinogen is between 3 and 5 days. Initial replacement should be achieved with 25 ml plasma/kg and daily maintenance with 5–10 ml/kg for 7 days.

Dysfibrinogenaemia. Congenital dysfibrinogenaemia is an autosomal dominant disorder. In contrast to patients with afibrinogenaemia, patients with this disorder are often symptom-free. Some have a bleeding tendency; others have been shown to have thromboembolic disease. The diagnosis is made by demonstrating a prolonged thrombin time with a normal immunological fibrinogen level.

Affected women like those with hypofibrinogenaemia may have recurrent spontaneous abortion or repeated placental abruption (Ness et al 1983).

Factor XIII deficiency (fibrin–stabilising factor deficiency)

This is an autosomal recessive disorder classically characterised by bleeding from the umbilical cord during the first few days of life and later by ecchymoses, prolonged post-traumatic haemorrhage and poor wound healing. Bleeding is usually delayed and characteristically of a slow, oozing nature. Cases of intracranial haemorrhage have been described in a significant proportion of reported cases. Spontaneous recurrent abortion with excessive bleeding occurs in association with factor XIII deficiency (Kitchens & Newcomb 1979). All standard coagulation tests are normal. Diagnosis of severe factor XIII deficiency is made by the clot solubility test. Normal fibrin clots will not dissolve when incubated overnight in 5 mol/l urea solutions, whereas the unstable clots formed in the absence of factor XIII will be dissolved.

Since factor XIII has a half-life of between 6 days and 2 weeks, and only 5% of normal factor XIII levels is needed for effective haemostasis, patients can be treated with FFP in doses of 5 ml/kg repeated every 3 weeks. Using this therapy, pregnancy has progressed safely to term in a woman who had previously suffered repeated abortions. Because of the high incidence of intracranial haemorrhage, replacement therapy is recommended for all individuals known to have factor XIII deficiency (Kitchens & Newcomb 1979).

Other plasma factor disorders

Congenital deficiencies of factors II, V, VII and X are extremely rare and the reader is referred to Caldwell et al's review of hereditary coagulopathies in pregnancy for an account of their diagnosis and special management problems (Caldwell et al 1985). Of more current interest are the inherited defects of the naturally-occurring anticoagulants and their relationship to thromboembolism and adverse pregnancy outcome (see Ch. 42) (Lockwood 1999).

Genetic collagen vascular disease

Ehlers–Danlos syndrome

It is often forgotten that an essential part of the haemostatic system is healthy vasculature. The Ehlers–Danlos syndrome (EDS) may be associated with bleeding because of increased fragility of vessels due to defects in collagen synthesis. It is also associated with hyperextensible joints and cutis hyperelastica as a result of connective tissue disorders. The disease has an autosomal dominant inheritance and has been subdivided into 10 subtypes, of which type IV is the most severe and may have lethal complications. The bleeding symptoms include ease of bruising, gastrointestinal bleeding, haemoptysis and, most important of all, rupture of the long arteries. The diagnosis may be suspected if the patient has papyraceous scars and pseudo-tumours over bony prominences. There may be calcified subcutaneous nodules. EDS IV is associated with an abnormality of collagen type III as a result of mutations in the corresponding gene COL3A1, but this abnormality can also be detected in milder subtypes of EDS. Attention is drawn to a recent review of the spectrum of severity of this condition (Hamel et al 1998).

Surgical procedures should be avoided unless essential because the tissues are friable and massive bleeding may occur and the healing of incisions may be delayed. Pregnancy and delivery will be involved, with obvious potential hazards. This is drawn to the attention of readers because the diagnosis of this condition may be missed, especially in an obstetric situation where many women complain of easy bruising, which is one of the main presenting symptoms. To further confuse the situation, platelet and coagulation screening tests will all yield results within the normal range.

REFERENCES

Aznar J, Gilabert J, Estelles A et al 1982 Evaluation of the soluble fibrin monomer complexes and other coagulation parameters in obstetric patients. Thromb Res 27:691–701

Baker P, Cunningham F 1999 Platelet and coagulation abnormalities. In: Lindheimer M, Roberts J, Cunningham F (eds) Chesley's hypertensive disorders in pregnancy. Appleton & Lange, Stamford, CT, pp 349–373

Ballegeer V, Mombaerts P, Declerck PJ et al 1987 Fibrinolytic response to venous occlusion and fibrin fragment D-dimer levels in normal and complicated pregnancy. Thromb Haemost 58:1030–1032

Ballegeer VC, Spitz B, De Baene LA et al 1992 Platelet activation and vascular damage in gestational hypertension. Am J Obstet Gynecol 166:629–633

Barbier P, Jonville AP, Autret E et al 1992 Fetal risks with dextrans during delivery. Drug Safety 7:71–73

Berg EM, Fasting S, Sellevold OF 1991 Serious complications with dextran-70 despite hapten prophylaxis. Is it best avoided prior to delivery? Anaesthesia 46:1033–1035

Bertina RM, Koeleman RPC, Koster T et al 1994 Mutation in blood coagulation factor V associated with resistance to activated protein C. Nature 369:64–67

Bettaieb A, Fromont P, Louache F et al 1992 Presence of cross-reactive antibody between human immunodeficiency virus (HIV) and platelet glycoproteins in HIV-related immune thrombocytopenic purpura. Blood 80:162–169

Bidstrup BP, Royston D, Sapsford RN et al 1989 Reduction in blood loss and blood use after cardiopulmonary bypass with high dose aprotinin (Trasylol). J Thorac Cardiovasc Surg 97:364–372

Bonnar J 1987 Haemostasis and coagulation disorders in pregnancy. In: Bloom AL, Thomas DP (eds) Haemostasis and thrombosis, 2nd edn. Churchill Livingstone, Edinburgh, pp 570–584

Burrows RF, Kelton JG 1988 Incidentally detected thrombocytopenia in healthy mothers and their infants. N Eng J Med 319:142–145

Burrows RF, Kelton JG 1990 Thrombocytopenia at delivery: a prospective survey of 6715 deliveries. Am J Obstet Gynecol 162:731–734

Burrows RF, Kelton JG 1992 Thrombocytopenia during pregnancy. In: Greer IA, Turpie AG, and Forbes CD (eds) Haemostatis and thrombosis in obstetrics and gynaecology. Chapman & Hall, London, pp 407–429

Burrows RF, Kelton JG 1995 Perinatal thrombocytopenia. Clin Perinatol 22:779–801

Bussel JB, Berkowitz RL, Lynch L et al 1996a Antenatal management of alloimmune thrombocytopenia with intravenous γ-globulin: a randomized trial of the addition of low-dose steroid to intravenous γ-globulin. Am J Obstet Gynecol 174:1414–1423

Bussel JB, Skupski DW, MacFarland JG 1996b Fetal alloimmune thrombocytopenia: consensus and controversy. J Matern Fetal Med 5:281–292

Caires D, Arocha-Piñango CL, Rodriguez S et al 1984 Factor VIIIR:Ag/factor VIII:C and their ratio in obstetrical cases. Acta Obstet Gynecol Scand 63:411–416

Caldwell DC, Williamson RA, Goldsmith JC 1985 Hereditary coagulopathies in pregnancy. Clin Obstet Gynecol 28:53–72

Comp PC, Thurnau GR, Welsh J et al 1986 Functional and immunologic protein S levels are decreased during pregnancy. Blood 68:881–885

Conti M, Mari D, Conti E et al 1986 Pregnancy in women with different types of von Willebrand disease. Obstet Gynecol 68:282–285

Cumming AM, Tait RC, Fildes S et al 1995 Development of resistance to activated protein C during pregnancy. Br J Haematol 90:725–727

Department of Health 1998 Why mothers die. Report on confidential enquiries into maternal deaths in the United Kingdom 1994–1996. HMSO, London

Feinstein DI 1982 Diagnosis and management of disseminated intravascular coagulation: the role of heparin therapy. Blood 60:284–287

Fisk NM, Bower S 1993 Fetal blood sampling in retreat. BMJ 307:143–144

Forbes CD, Greer IA 1992 Physiology of haemostasis and the effect of pregnancy. In: Greer IA, Turpie AGG, Forbes CD (eds) Haemostasis and thrombosis in obstetrics and gynaecology. Chapman & Hall, London, pp 1–25

Freeman M 1979 Fatal reaction to haemaccel. Anaesthesia 34:341–343

Furlan M, Robles R, Galbusera M et al 1998 Von Willebrand Factor-cleaving protease in thrombotic thrombocytopenic purpura and the hemolytic–uremic syndrome. N Engl J Med 339:1578–1584

Gottlieb P, Axelsson O, Bakos O et al 1999 Splenectomy during pregnancy: an option in the treatment of autoimmune thrombocytopenic purpura. Br J Obstet Gynaecol 106:373–375

Graeff H, Kuhn W 1980 Coagulation disorders in obstetrics: pathobiochemistry, pathophysiology, diagnosis, treatment. In: Friedman EA (ed) Major problems in obstetrics and gynecology. Saunders, Philadelphia, p 86

Hamel BCJ, Pals G, Engels CHAM et al 1998 Ehlers–Danlos syndrome and type III collagen abnormalities: a variable clinical spectrum. Clin Genet 53:440–446

Hedge UM 1985 Immune thrombocytopenia in pregnancy and the newborn (editorial). Br J Obstet Gynaecol 92:657–659

Hedge UM, Ball S, Zuiable A et al 1985 Platelet associated immunoglobulins (PAIgG and PAIgM) in autoimmune thrombocytopenia. Br J Haematol 59:221–226

Hellgren M, Blomback M 1981 Studies on blood coagulation and fibrinolysis in pregnancy, during delivery and in the puerperium. I. Normal condition. Gynecol Obstet Invest 12:141–154

How HY, Bergmann F, Koshy M et al 1991 Quantitative and qualitative platelet abnormalities during pregnancy. Am J Obstet Gynecol 164:92–98

Hughes GRV 1987 Systemic lupus erythematosus. In: Hughes GRV (ed) Connective tissue diseases, 3 edn. Blackwell Scientific, Oxford, pp 3–71

Kadir RA 1999 Women and inherited bleeding disorders: pregnancy and delivery. Semin Hematol 36 (3 suppl 4):28–35

Kaplan C, Murphy MF, Kroll H et al 1998 Feto-maternal alloimmune thrombocytopenia: antenatal therapy with IvIgG and steroids: more questions than answers. Br J Haematol 100:62–65

Kitchens CS, Newcomb TF 1979 Factor XIII. Medicine (Baltimore) 658:413–429

Kouri YH, Basch RS, Karpatkin S 1992 B-cell subsets and platelet counts in HIV-1 seropositive subjects. Lancet 339:1445–1446

Kupferminc MJ, Eldor A, Steinman N et al 1999 Increased frequency of genetic thrombophilia in women with complications of pregnancy. N Engl J Med 340:9–13

Leduc L, Wheeler JM, Kirshon B et al 1992 Coagulation profile in severe preeclampsia. Obstet Gynecol 79:14–18

Letsky EA 1991 Mechanisms of coagulation and the changes induced by pregnancy. Curr Obstet Gynaecol 1:203–209

Letsky EA, Greaves M 1996 Guidelines on the investigation and management of thrombocytopenia in pregnancy and neonatal alloimmune thrombocytopenia. Br J Haematol 95:21–26

Lind SE 1991 The bleeding time does not predict surgical bleeding. Blood 77:2547–2552

Lockwood CJ 1999 Heritable coagulopathies in pregnancy. Obstet Gynecol Surv 54:754–765

Malm J, Laurell M, Dahlback B 1988 Changes in the plasma levels of vitamin K-dependent proteins C and S and of C4b-binding protein during pregnancy and oral contraception. Br J Haematol 68:437–443

Milaskiewicz RM, Holdcroft A, Letsky E 1990 Epidural anaesthesia and von Willebrand's disease. Anaesthesia 45:462–464

Moake JL 1998 Moschcowitz, multimers, and metalloprotease (editorial). N Engl J Med 339:1629–1631

Morgan M 1979 Amniotic fluid embolism. Anaesthesia 34:20–32

Murphy MF, Waters AH, Doughty HA et al 1994 Antenatal management of fetomaternal alloimmune thrombocytopenia (FMAIT): report of 15 affected pregnancies. Transfus Med 4:281–292

Ness PM, Budzynski AZ, Olexa SA et al 1983 Congenital hypofibrinogenemia and recurrent placental abruption. Obstet Gynecol 61:519–523

Page Y, Tardy B, Zeni F et al 1991 Thrombotic thrombocytopenic purpura related to ticlopidine (see comments). Lancet 337:774–776

Paidas MJ, Berkowitz RL, Lynch L et al 1995 Alloimmune thrombocytopenia: fetal and neonatal losses related to cordocentesis. Am J Obstet Gynecol 172:475–479

Peaceman AM, Katz AR, Laville M 1989 Bernard–Soulier syndrome complicating pregnancy: a case report. Obstet Gynecol 73:457–459

Peake IR, Lillicrap DP, Boulyjenkov V et al 1993 Report of a joint WHO/WFH meeting on the control of haemophilia: carrier detection and prenatal diagnosis. (Published erratum appears in Blood Coagul Fibrinolysis 1994:148)

Peek MJ, Nelson-Piercy C, Manning RA et al 1997 Activated protein C resistance in normal pregnancy. Br J Obstet Gynaecol 104:1084–1086

Peleg D, Hunter SK 1999 Perinatal management of women with immune thrombocytopenic purpura: survey of United States perinatologists. Am J Obstet Gynecol 180:645–649

Pritchard JA, Cunningham FG, Pritchard SA et al 1991 On reducing the frequency of severe abruptio placentae. Am J Obstet Gynecol 165:1345–1351

Redman CW, Denson KW, Beilin LJ et al 1977 Factor-VIII consumption in pre-eclampsia. Lancet ii:1249–1252

Reece EA, Fox HE, Rapoport F 1982 Factor VIII inhibitor: a cause of severe postpartum hemorrhage. Am J Obstet Gynecol 144:985–987

Romero R, Copel JA, Hobbins JC 1985 Intrauterine fetal demise and hemostatic failure: the fetal death syndrome. Clin Obstet Gynecol 28:24–31

Romero R, Mazor M, Lockwood CJ et al 1989 Clinical significance, prevalence, and natural history of thrombocytopenia in pregnancy-induced hypertension. Am J Perinatol 6:32–38

Samuels P, Bussel JB, Braitman LE et al 1990 Estimation of the risk of thrombocytopenia in the offspring of pregnant women with presumed immune thrombocytopenic purpura (see comments). N Engl J Med 323:229–235

Savage W 1982 Abortion: methods and sequelae. Br J Hosp Med 27:364–384

Sheppard BL, Bonnar J 1974 The ultrastructure of the arterial supply of the human placenta in early and late pregnancy. J Obstet Gynaecol Br Commonw 81:497–511

Sher G 1977 Pathogenesis and management of uterine inertia complicating abruptio placentae with consumption coagulopathy. Am J Obstet Gynecol 129:164–170

Sher GI, Statland BE 1985 Abruptio placentae with coagulopathy: a rational basis for management. Clin Obstet Gynecol 28:15–23

Stirling Y, Woolf L, North WR et al 1984 Haemostasis in normal pregnancy. Thromb Haemost 52:176–182

Tchernia G 1988 Immune thrombocytopenic purpura and pregnancy. Curr Stud Hematol Blood Transfus 55:81–89

Thornton JG, Molloy BJ, Vinall PS et al 1989 A prospective study of haemostatic tests at 28 weeks gestation as predictors of pre-eclampsia and growth retardation. Thromb Haemost 61:243–245

Tsai H, Lian E-Y 1998 Antibodies to von Willebrand factor-cleaving protease in acute thrombotic thrombocytopenic purpura. N Engl J Med 339:1585–1594

Vandermeulen EPE, Vermylen J, Van Aken H 1993 Epidural and spinal anaesthesia in patients receiving anticoagulant therapy. Baillière's Clin Anaesthesiol 7:663–689

Voke J, Letsky E 1977 Pregnancy and antibody to factor VIII. J Clin Pathol 30:928–932

Wallmo L, Karlsson K, Teger Nilsson AC 1984 Fibrinopeptide A and intravascular coagulation in normotensive and hypertensive pregnancy and parturition. Acta Obstet Gynecol Scand 63:637–640

Warwick R, Hutton RA, Goff L et al 1989 Changes in protein C and free protein S during pregnancy and following hysterectomy. J R S Med 82:591–594

Weiner CP, Kwaan HC, Xu C et al 1985 Antithrombin III activity in women with hypertension during pregnancy. Obstet Gynecol 65:301–306

Williamson L, Heptonstall J, Soldan K 1996 A SHOT in the arm for safer blood transfusion. BMJ 313:1221–1222

Williamson LM, Hackett G, Rennie J et al 1998 The natural history of fetomaternal alloimmunization to the platelet-specific antigen HPA-1a (PL^{A1}, Zw^a) as determined by antenatal screening. Blood 92:2280–2287

21

Pregnancy induced hypertension

Ian A. Greer

The contribution of the author of the equivalent chapter in the second edition, on which this chapter draws extensively, is gratefully acknowledged.

INTRODUCTION

Hypertension in pregnancy is a major cause of maternal death in the United Kingdom (Department of Health et al 1998) and also a major source of maternal and perinatal morbidity and perinatal mortality. Many of the problems relating to maternal mortality arise from a failure by clinicians to appreciate the varied presentations of pre-eclampsia and its severity or from inappropriate or inadequate treatment. Thus it is critical that obstetricians appreciate fully the protean nature of this condition and avoid complacency in its management. Pre-eclampsia is not simply hypertension arising in pregnancy but is a disorder that can affect virtually every organ and body system; hypertension represents but one facet of a complex disease process. The common pathological feature of the disease, whether in the placental bed or in the renal microcirculation, is endothelial damage and dysfunction.

DEFINITIONS AND DIAGNOSIS

The classification of hypertension in pregnancy is confused. Several conditions of various aetiologies make up the hyper-

tensive disorders of pregnancy. There is also a lack of agreement on their nomenclature and classification. To confuse the situation further, the true diagnosis, and therefore the classification, can only be confirmed after the pregnancy is over. Hypertension in pregnancy may present in one of three forms. Firstly, there are women who enter pregnancy with hypertension, the majority of whom will have essential hypertension, although some women with chronic hypertension will have an underlying problem, such as renal or connective tissue disease. Secondly, hypertension in pregnancy may arise from the coincidental development of a medical problem in pregnancy, such as phaeochromocytoma. Although such problems are rare, they must not be forgotten in assessing patients, particularly in severe or unusual cases. Thirdly, there are women who are normotensive before pregnancy and in early pregnancy but who develop hypertension during pregnancy, which remits within a few months of delivery; these women have pregnancy-induced hypertension. Classification of these pregnancy-related disorders is based on two clinical features: hypertension and proteinuria. The classification of the International Society for the Study of Hypertension in Pregnancy (ISSHP) (Davey & MacGillivray 1988) (Table 21.1) is a useful and widely used system. Pre-eclampsia is often loosely applied to patients, regardless of the

Table 21.1 Summary of the ISSHP classification

Hypertension
Diastolic BP of ≥110 mmHg on any one occasion
or
Diastolic BP of ≥90 mmHg on any two or more consecutive occasions ≥4 h apart

Severe hypertension
Diastolic BP ≥120 mmHg on any one occasion
or
Diastolic BP ≥110 mmHg on two or more consecutive occasions ≥4 h apart

Proteinuria
One 24 h urine collection with a total protein excretion of ≥300 mg/24 h
or
Two midstream or catheter specimens of urine (collected ≥4 h apart) with ≥ ++ protein on reagent strip testing
or
3 '+' protein (if urine SG <1.030 and pH ≤8)

From Davey & MacGillivray (1988).

severity of their hypertension or degree of proteinuria, but should be reserved for severe (proteinuric) pregnancy-induced hypertension. Gestational hypertension without proteinuria should be termed pregnancy-induced hypertension. The absence of proteinuria does not guarantee a lack of risk, as eclampsia, the most severe form of the disorder, can occur without proteinuria.

Hypertension

During normal pregnancy blood pressure starts to fall in the first trimester, reaching a nadir in mid-pregnancy, before increasing during the third trimester to values comparable with those in the non-pregnant state. As cardiac output increases by around 40% in the first trimester and is maintained through pregnancy, the fall in blood pressure must be due to a reduction in peripheral resistance. Hypertension results from an increase in systemic vascular resistance in the face of an unchanged cardiac output. Thus, blood pressure is an indirect measure of one of the pathological features of pregnancy-induced hypertension, namely vasoconstriction.

In pregnancy, just as in the non-pregnant population, blood pressure is continuously distributed and the dividing line between normotension and hypertension is arbitrary and artificial. A diastolic blood pressure of 90 mmHg after 20 weeks of pregnancy is usually considered the threshold for diagnosis. There is merit in this as the perinatal mortality rate increases when the maternal diastolic blood pressure exceeds this level. In mid-pregnancy, it also is in line with statistical descriptions of the distribution of blood pressure in the population. A diastolic pressure of 90 mmHg is 3 SD greater than the mean for mid-pregnancy and 2 SD above the mean for 34 weeks' gestation; however, it is only 1.5 SD above the mean at term, reflecting the physiological increase in blood pressure towards term (MacGillivray et al 1969). In late pregnancy

this can lead to overdiagnosis of the problem and may precipitate unnecessary intervention, indeed over 20% of pregnant women will have a blood pressure of 140/90 mmHg at least once in pregnancy (Redman 1995). In contrast, in the late second trimester a 90 mmHg threshold may lead to underdiagnosis. The 90 mmHg threshold also excludes women who have a substantial increase in blood pressure (over the preconception or early pregnancy measurement), but where the diastolic pressure does not exceed 90 mmHg, and yet includes some women with mild chronic hypertension who have a minimal increase in blood pressure (Redman & Jeffries 1988). It has been proposed that a threshold of 90 mmHg together with an increase of 25 mmHg should be used, as this will improve the diagnosis when compared with either measurement alone (Redman & Jeffries 1988). Repeated measures of blood pressure should be made to obtain an accurate diagnosis. The ISSHP definitions require that a value of >90 mmHg be recorded on two measurements at least 4 h apart or a single value >110 mmHg. It was customary to use Korotkoff phase IV (K4) (muffling) as the measure of diastolic pressure because Korotkoff phase V (K5) (disappearance) was thought not always to occur in pregnancy; however, it is now accepted that in most cases K5 is a more accurate, reproducible and reliable measure of diastolic pressure, which corresponds more closely to the true mean arterial pressure. Use of K5 does not have any adverse impact on the association between diastolic pressure and maternal or fetal outcome (Brown & de Swiet 1999). The use of K5 has recently been endorsed by the ISSHP. It is also important to use the correct technique and appropriate cuff size (arm circumference over 33 cm requires a large adult (15 cm) cuff) (Table 21.2). The systolic blood pressure is con-

Table 21.2 Measurement of blood pressure

- Use a bell stethoscope as it better amplifies the Korotkoff (K) sounds.
- Use a well-maintained sphygmomanometer
- A range of sphygmomanometer cuff sizes must be available. Too small a cuff will overestimate blood pressure; too large a cuff will underestimate it. (Ideally, bladder length should encompass 80% of the arm circumference and bladder width should be 40% of the arm circumference)
- Measurements should be taken with the woman sitting after a period of rest with the arm supported at heart level. Measurements are not significantly altered if the woman is lying with lateral tilt, provided that the arm is at heart level
- When the cuff is first inflated an approximation of systolic pressure should be taken by palpation of the radial pulse
- During auscultation, the cuff should initially be inflated to a pressure 20 mmHg higher than the estimated systolic pressure determined by palpation
- Systolic pressure is recorded as the level where repetitive sounds are first heard (K1) (rounded, upwards, to the nearest 2 mmHg)
- The diastolic pressure is recorded at the point of disappearance of these sounds (K5) rounded to the nearest 2 mmHg
- If K4 and K5 are markedly different, it can prevent confusion if both are recorded. Then, if another observer measures K4 rather than K5, they can compare like with like

sidered abnormal if it exceeds 140 mmHg but has not been widely used in classifications as it is considered more variable; however, it does correlate with perinatal mortality and inversely with birthweight (Tervila et al 1973).

Measurement of blood pressure is fraught with sampling errors of various forms, such as interobserver and intraobserver variation, digit preference, threshold avoidance and poor technique. Automated and ambulatory blood pressure measurement may be of value in overcoming sampling errors and factors such as *white coat hypertension* (Bellomo et al 1999), and also taking account of the diurnal rhythm of blood pressure in pregnancy, so avoiding many of the problems associated with conventional blood pressure measurement. It is important that such devices are appropriately validated in pregnancy, as has been carried out with the Spacelabs 90207 device (Greer 1993, Halligan et al 1995). In particular, it should be noted that some automated systems will significantly underestimate blood pressure in pre-eclampsia, particularly at extremes of blood pressure (Natarajan et al 1999); thus, when managing women with severe hypertension it is useful to check automated readings with traditional manual techniques.

Proteinuria

Proteinuria is easier to quantify than hypertension and is indicative of severe disease. The degree of proteinuria shows a correlation with perinatal mortality (Naeye & Friedman 1979) and incidence of growth restriction (Tervila et al 1973); proteinuria is even more strongly associated with perinatal mortality in women with eclampsia. The accepted threshold for significant proteinuria in pregnancy is 0.3 g/24 h (Davey & MacGillivray 1988). Although dipstick testing is satisfactory for screening for proteinuria, it is best to quantify proteinuria formally either by a 24 h collection or by measuring the urine protein:creatinine ratio. A value of >30 mg protein/mmol creatinine reflects quantitative proteinuria of >0.3 g/24 h (Saudan et al 1997). The protein:creatinine ratio has greater clinical utility than the 24 h assessment. Random urine samples assessed by dipstick may produce false-positive results due to contamination of the urine by vaginal discharge, chlorhexidine preparations, or if the urine is highly alkaline or very concentrated (specific gravity >1.030). False-negative results may occur if the urine is very dilute (specific gravity <1.010). However, in the clinical situation most management decisions are made on dipstick testing of urine, as the evolution of the disease, particularly the severe proteinuric form, may occur at a speed at which formal laboratory quantification of proteinuria may be unable to keep pace. The proteinuria can be severe enough to result in nephrotic syndrome.

While proteinuria is indicative of severe disease, the absence of proteinuria does not preclude a severe form of pregnancy-induced hypertension. Eclampsia and severe hypertension can occur without proteinuria (Sibai et al 1981). Further, proteinuria in the absence of significant hypertension can still be a manifestion of pre-eclampsia and is often associated with severe growth restriction. In addition, microalbuminuria is present in many women with milder forms of the disease (Thong et al 1991), suggesting that there is a spectrum of renal dysfunction ranging from an absence of proteinuria through microalbuminuria to gross proteinuria.

Additional diagnostic features

Oedema is part of the classical definition of pre-eclampsia and has been used as a diagnostic feature. Such use should be abandoned. While pathological oedema, associated with a rapid increase in weight, occurs commonly in pre-eclampsia, severe pre-eclampsia and eclampsia can occur without oedema. Perinatal mortality has been shown to be greater in pre-eclampsia without oedema compared to pre-eclampsia with oedema. Furthermore, significant oedema occurs in around 70% of normal pregnancies. Although rapid weight gain has been employed to identify women developing pre-eclampsia, this can occur without pre-eclampsia. In one series, only 10% of patients with eclampsia had rapid weight gain (Chesley 1978). Thus, oedema is of little value as an objective diagnostic sign.

Hyperuricaemia is a useful diagnostic feature as it precedes proteinuria and is of value in distinguishing women with pregnancy-induced hypertension from those with chronic hypertension. Elevated plasma urate together with hypertension is associated with a substantial increase in perinatal mortality compared with pregnancies with the same degree of hypertension, but with normal plasma urate values (Redman et al 1976a). Elevated plasma urate is not specific to pregnancy-induced hypertension, and normal pregnancy values increase with gestational age: Redman (1989) showed that plasma urate concentrations 2 SD above the mean at 16, 28, 32 and 36 weeks were 0.28, 0.29, 0.34 and 0.39 mmol/l, respectively. Urea increases along with uric acid, but both urea and creatinine generally stay within the normal non-pregnant range in mild/moderate disease, while with severe disease associated with renal compromise urea can be expected to be >7 mmol/l and creatinine >100 mmol/l.

Platelet consumption occurs in pregnancy-induced hypertension. It is often an early feature, present in the second trimester. Since there is a wide range of platelet counts in normal pregnancy, the absolute count is not usually of diagnostic value unless combined with other features, although serial counts are more helpful. It is also an inconsistent feature of the disease.

CLINICAL PRESENTATION

Hypertensive disorders in pregnancy are difficult to diagnose and classify, reflecting the problem of using signs of the disorder to define the problem. Despite this, the clinician must make management decisions based on the prognostic implications of the suspected problem. The diagnosis made during pregnancy is always provisional and may be modified on longer term follow-up. Clinical practice is, however, essentially concerned with only a few diagnostic groups.

Chronic hypertension

Chronic hypertension is found in around 1–1.5% of pregnancies and is associated with a persistently elevated blood pressure (>90 mmHg diastolic) occurring in the first or early second trimester (rare causes of early-onset pre-eclampsia such as hydatidiform mole must be excluded). It may be present before pregnancy but diagnosed for the first time in pregnancy. In over 95% of cases women with chronic hypertension have essential hypertension. In women with chronic hypertension, blood pressure shows the same physiological changes as in normal pregnancy. This may not be apparent if the woman is not seen until later in pregnancy. This can confuse the diagnosis when her blood pressure exhibits the normal physiological increase in the third trimester. Plasma urate is useful in helping to distinguish chronic from pregnancy-induced hypertension. An assessment of underlying medical conditions should be made, including the exclusion of renal and connective tissue disease. It must be remembered that such women have an increased risk of developing superimposed pregnancy-induced hypertension or pre-eclampsia (where proteinuria and/or increased plasma uric acid will be present) and also intrauterine growth restriction (IUGR). It is often possible to discontinue antihypertensive therapy in the first half of pregnancy in these women, although it may be required in the third trimester.

Pregnancy-induced hypertension and pre-eclampsia

Pregnancy-induced hypertension is the diagnosis applied to women who are normotensive in the first 20 weeks of pregnancy, but who develop hypertension in the second half of pregnancy. In association with significant proteinuria, it is pre-eclampsia. Proteinuria is not a constant feature of severe disease and a persistent diastolic blood pressure of >110 mmHg should also be considered severe pregnancy-induced hypertension (Davey & MacGillivray 1988). It is associated with variable systemic upset, including disturbance of coagulation and renal and hepatic function.

Eclampsia

Eclampsia can be regarded as the inevitable consequence of disease progression in pregnancy-induced hypertension; however, it can be the first clinical manifestation of the condition. It is characterised by grand mal seizures, which cannot be attributed to epilepsy or any other problem. It arises without any obvious symptoms in 15–20% of cases (Villar & Sibai 1988). A UK survey reported that almost 40% of cases occurred before hypertension or proteinuria was documented (Douglas & Redman 1994). In the UK survey, 38% of cases occurred antepartum, 44% of cases occurred postpartum, and the rest intrapartum (Douglas & Redman 1994). This is similar to North American reports where approximately 50% of cases occur before labour, 25% during labour and 25% postpartum (Villar & Sibai 1988). Postpartum eclampsia usually occurs, within the first 48 h but may occur up to 2–3 weeks later (Villar & Sibai 1988).

Eclampsia is usually accompanied by hypertension, although not always severe, and proteinuria is absent in 20–40% of cases (Villar & Sibai 1988). Where prodromal symptoms occur, those most commonly encountered are headache, epigastric pain and visual disturbance. Hyperuricaemia,

deranged liver function tests, thrombocytopenia and coagulation disturbances can also be seen. An awareness of the diverse presentations is important. Women with headache, epigastric pain and vomiting in pregnancy should be considered to have fulminating pre-eclampsia until proven otherwise. Hypertension and proteinuria in pregnancy must be treated seriously. Routine laboratory testing, including plasma urate and liver function tests, a platelet count and blood film should help resolve the diagnosis and allow suitable therapeutic measures to be taken. It is noteworthy that most cases of eclampsia in the UK occur despite the patient having antenatal care, with 75% occurring in hospital. The majority did not have liver function assessed before the seizure, and only two-thirds after the seizure (Douglas & Redman 1994), suggesting that investigation of such patients is often inadequate. This is in keeping with the findings of the Confidential Enquiries into Maternal Deaths in the UK (Department of Health et al 1998).

EPIDEMIOLOGY

Incidence and risk factors (Table 21.3)

The incidence of pregnancy-induced hypertension and pre-eclampsia has been difficult to establish owing to differences in various definitions and classification systems but, using ISSHP definitions, it is considered to be around 5% and 1–2%, respectively, in the UK. Pregnancy-induced hypertension is traditionally regarded as a disorder of the primigravida; previous pregnancies offer some protection, although it has become clear that primipaternity is a more accurate description, with the length of sexual cohabitation being inversely related to the risk (Robillard & Hulsey 1996). A first-trimester miscarriage or termination of pregnancy does not protect against pre-eclampsia in a second pregnancy. A late miscarriage reduces the risk of pre-eclampsia in a subsequent pregnancy by around 75%. If the first pregnancy reaches

Table 21.3 Risk factors

Positive risk factors	Negative risk factors
First pregnancy	Previous pregnancy reaching the second trimester and not complicated by pre-eclampsia
Previous pre-eclampsia	Long period of sexual cohabitation
Central obesity	Smoking
Migraine	
Age <20 and >35 years	
Maternal family history of pre-eclampsia	
Diabetes	
Congenital and acquired thrombophilia	
Renal and connective tissue disease	
Essential hypertension	
Multiple pregnancy	
Hydrops and molar pregnancy	
Fetal trisomy	

term without any hypertensive complication, the risk of pre-eclampsia in the subsequent pregnancy is reduced by almost 90%. However, if the first pregnancy is complicated by pre-eclampsia, then the incidence in the second pregnancy is similar to the average risk for all first pregnancies, and the risk is increased if the first pregnancy was also complicated by a low birthweight baby (<2.5 kg) (Campbell & MacGillivray 1985). Thus, while the incidence of pre-eclampsia is reduced overall in a second pregnancy, the protective effect is modified by the presence of hypertensive complications, gestation at delivery and birthweight of the first baby. Essential hypertension is associated with a risk of around 15% that the woman will develop pre-echampsia.

The risk of pre-eclampsia is increased in women aged under 20 years and over 35 years; the former may be associated with primiparity and the latter may be related to an increased prevalence of underlying chronic hypertensive problems which increase the risk of, or may be misdiagnosed as, pregnancy-induced hypertension. There does not appear to be an association with social class. Obese women are more likely to have both pre-eclampsia and chronic hypertension. Diabetes mellitus increases the risk of pregnancy-induced hypertension (although the risk is difficult to quantify accurately as such patients are predisposed to chronic hypertension and diabetic nephropathy, so confusing the diagnosis), with the incidence estimated at 12% in both established and gestational diabetes (Howy & Beard 1982). A history of migraine is another maternal risk factor, as is a family history of pre-eclampsia on the maternal side due to the genetic component of the process (see below). Fetal factors such as twin pregnancy, fetal hydrops, hydatidiform mole, triploidy and trisomy 13 are all associated with an increased risk of pregnancy-induced hypertension.

Eclampsia is uncommon in the UK, occurring in 4.9/10 000 (95% CI 4.5–5.4) maternities (Douglas & Redman 1994). This is similar to the incidence in North America. The risk of eclampsia is threefold higher in women under 19 years of age, but in contrast to pregnancy-induced hypertension there is no increase in risk in women aged 35 and over (Douglas & Redman 1994). Multiple pregnancy enhances the risk sixfold (Douglas & Redman 1994). Around 25% of women with eclampsia are parous and only about 25% have a past history of pre-eclampsia. Thus, it is important appropriately to assess parous women with any symptoms or signs that might be related to pre-eclampsia. Around 2% of cases will be associated with maternal death, and over a third will have serious complications such as disseminated intravascular coagulation (DIC), adult respiratory distress syndrome (ARDS) and renal failure. In addition, there is a high level of perinatal morbidity and mortality related independently to both the pre-eclampsia–eclampsia disease process and preterm delivery. Following eclampsia, the risk of problems in future pregnancies has been estimated at around 20% for pre-eclampsia, and around 2% each for recurrent eclampsia, abruption and perinatal death.

Maternal outcome

We have accurate data on the incidence and nature of deaths from pre-eclampsia and eclampsia in the UK from the Reports on Confidential Enquiries into Maternal Deaths in England and Wales. Although there has been a dramatic improvement in deaths from pre-eclampsia/eclampsia since the 1950s, there has been little improvement in the last decade or so (Department of Health et al 1998) (Fig. 21.1). The most frequent cause of death is related to the development of ARDS (Fig. 21.2). ARDS is rare in pre-eclampsia unless other complications are present, such as DIC, pulmonary oedema, fluid overload or overtransfusion (Mabie et al 1992, Catanzarite & Willms 1997). Pulmonary oedema can easily arise as a result of fluid overload, especially as vascular permeability is increased due to the endothelial damage. Cerebral haemorrhage is now less common as a cause of death (Fig. 21.3), perhaps suggesting that there is better control of blood pressure in women with severe disease than in the past. Other major causes of mortality and morbidity are cerebral oedema, cerebral infarction, DIC, renal failure and liver damage, including hepatic necrosis and liver rupture.

Women who suffer from pre-eclampsia and eclampsia used to be considered to have a prevalence of hypertension in later life similar to that of the general population (Chesley et al 1976, Fisher et al 1981); however, this is now considered

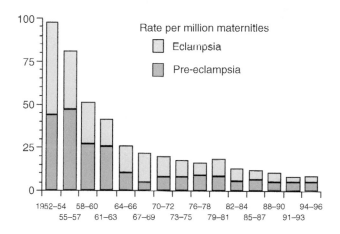

Fig. 21.1 Number of deaths from pre-eclampsia/eclampsia in England and Wales 1952–1984 and UK 1985–1996 (numbers of cases in each triennium). Data derived from Confidential Enquiries into Maternal Deaths in the UK.

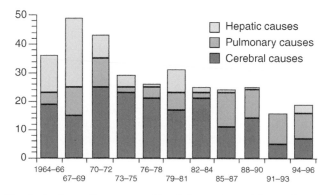

Fig. 21.2 Immediate cause of death from eclampsia/pre-eclampsia in the UK (total number of cases in each triennium). Data derived from Confidential Enquiries into Maternal Deaths in the UK.

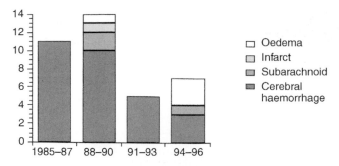

Fig. 21.3 Cerebral causes of death from eclampsia and pre-eclampsia in the UK (total number of cases in each triennium). Data derived from Confidential Enquiries into Maternal Deaths in the UK.

questionable. Where the hypertensive problem arises before 30 weeks' of gestation, or when there is recurrent hypertension in pregnancy, there is an increased incidence of subsequent chronic hypertension (Sibai et al 1986). Since both early-onset disease and recurrent disease are associated with an increased prevalence of chronic hypertension or renal problems, it is likely that this finding simply reflects this association. The prevalence of hypertension in later life is much lower in women who have had normotensive pregnancies than in the general population (Fisher et al 1981), suggesting that pregnancy may act as a hypertensive stress test. Women with a mild degree of hypertension in pregnancy have an increased risk of subsequent hypertension (Sibai et al 1986). This mild hypertension in pregnancy may simply be underlying chronic hypertension which is manifest due to the stress of pregnancy. Furthermore, data are accumulating to suggest that if the mother experiences pre-eclampsia, then she has a greater risk of vascular disease in later life.

The metabolic changes associated with pre-eclampsia (insulin resistance and hypertriglyceridacmia) provoke substantial stresses on carbohydrate and lipid metabolism and vascular endothelial function. Recent data show that women with a history of pre-eclampsia demonstrate higher circulating fasting insulin, lipid and clotting factors postpartum relative to body mass index (BMI)-matched controls (Laivuori et al 1996, He et al 1999). Such findings are consistent with reports of a significantly higher relative risk of ischaemic heart disease in formerly pre-eclamptic women in case–control studies (Jonsdottir et al 1995, Humphries et al 1999). Thus, the maternal response to pregnancy may identify women at risk of vascular disease in later life.

Fetal outcome

Pre-eclampsia and eclampsia are associated with intrauterine growth restriction (IUGR), intrauterine asphyxia and iatrogenic prematurity. The British Births Survey of 1970 (Chamberlain et al 1978) showed a perinatal mortality rate in severe pregnancy-induced hypertension (and eclampsia) of 33.7/1000, compared with the rate of 19.2/1000 in normotensive pregnancies. The perinatal mortality rate was not increased in mild/moderate disease and was 15.6/1000 in chronic hypertension. When chronic hypertension was com-

plicated by superimposed pre-eclampsia, the perinatal mortality rate rose to 30.7/1000. Thus, the severity of hypertension is important. Modern maternal and neonatal care has substantially improved these figures, and perinatal mortality is no longer a useful measure of the fetal effects of pre-eclampsia. A more recent Australian report reflecting practice in the 1990s found a rate of small for gestational age (SGA) infants of 24% in pre-eclampsia and a perinatal mortality rate of 38/1000; this fell to 17% for SGA infants and 6/1000 perinatal mortality rate for gestational hypertension using the ISSHP criteria (Brown & Buddle 1997). With regard to eclampsia, the British Eclampsia Survey (Douglas & Redman 1994) found a stillbirth rate of 22.2/1000 and a neonatal death rate of 34.1/1000. The presence of IUGR is important, as it is associated with a reduced risk of survival independently of other variables, such as gestation and severity of maternal disease (Witlin et al 2000). There is an association between severe disease and neurodevelopmental disability in childhood. In the longer term, the fetus with IUGR is at increased risk of developing cardiovascular disease and diabetes in later life, thus emphasising the importance of intrauterine well-being to adult health.

PATHOLOGY AND PATHOPHYSIOLOGY

The placental bed

In normal pregnancy, the spiral arteries of the placental bed undergo a series of physiological changes. They are invaded by the cytotrophoblast (Robertson & Khong 1987) which breaks down the endothelium, internal elastic lamina and muscular coat of the vessel, which are largely replaced by fibrinoid. Virtually every spiral artery in the decidua basalis will have undergone these physiological changes by the end of the first trimester (Brosens & Dixon 1966). Early in the second trimester, a second wave of cytotrophoblast invasion occurs and transforms the myometrial segments of the spiral arteries, and occasionally the distal segments of the radial arteries. These physiological changes convert the vessels supplying the placenta from muscular end-arteries to wide-mouthed sinusoids. The vascular supply is thus transformed from a high pressure–low flow system to a low pressure–high flow system to meet the needs of the fetus and placenta. Loss of the endothelial and muscular layers render these vessels unable to respond to vasomotor stimuli.

In pre-eclampsia, only about one-half to two-thirds of the decidual spiral arteries undergo these physiological changes (Khong et al 1986), and the conversion of myometrial components of the spiral arteries fails to occur, even in vessels where the decidual segments have undergone physiological change (Sheppard & Bonnar 1981). Thus, the primary invasion of trophoblast is partially impaired, and the second wave fails to occur, or is limited. This qualitative and quantitative restriction of normal physiological changes results in restricted placental blood flow, which becomes more critical with advancing gestation as the demands of the conceptus increases. In addition, the vessels maintain their muscular coats, and so remain sensitive to vasomotor stimuli (Fig. 21.4). These changes are not specific to pre-eclampsia and also occur in IUGR without pre-eclampsia.

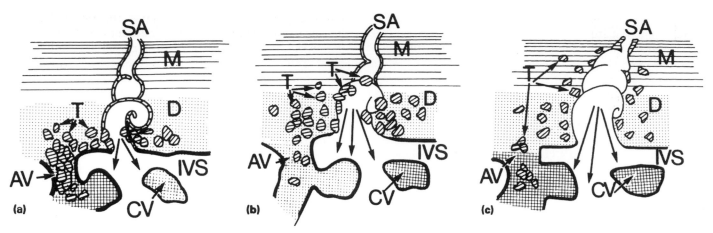

Fig. 21.4 Placentation and pre-eclampsia. Trophoblast (T) from an anchoring villus (AV) invades the decidua (D) and the distal end of a spiral artery (SA)—a process well established by 6 weeks after the last menstrual period ((a) left). At this stage the spiral artery is thick-walled but the action of the trophoblast breaks down the arterial structure so that the vessel becomes thin-walled and dilated, at first in its decidual segment (b) extending, by 18 weeks, into the myometrial (M) segment ((c) right). The effect is to allow the blood flow into the intervillous space (IVS) to increase. A chorionic villus (CV) is also shown. In pre-eclampsia this process fails to extend beyond the normal stage for 12 weeks so that the ability of the spiral artery to deliver an adequate flow of blood is impaired (Robertson et al 1967).

The typical, though non-specific, vascular lesion found in the placental bed in pregnancy-induced hypertension has been termed acute atherosis because of the presence of foam cells in the damaged vessel wall (Labarrere 1988). This can be seen in the intramyometrial segments of the spiral arteries in the placental bed, the basal arteries and the decidua parietalis, but is not seen in the intradecidual vessels of the placental bed which have undergone physiological change. Acute atherosis is a necrotising arteriopathy characterised by fibrinoid necrosis, accumulation of lipid-laden macrophages and damaged cells, fibroblast proliferation and a mononuclear cell perivascular infiltrate. Again, it is not specific to pre-eclampsia, also being present in IUGR. In the early stages, this lesion is characterised by endothelial damage. Evidence of endothelial damage can be seen ultrastructurally in the decidua at sites outside the placental bed throughout the maternal fetal boundary (Shanklin & Sibai 1989) and this correlates with the degree of maternal hypertension. Plasma urate, a marker of disease severity, also correlates with these vascular changes in the placental bed (McFadyen et al 1986). Ischaemia of the fetal placenta will occur because of the restricted blood flow and leads to infarcts, patchy necrosis and intracellular damage of the syncytiotrophoblast, an increase in villous cytotrophoblastic cells and an obliterative endarteritis of the fetal stem arteries (Fox 1988). More recently, it has been suggested that there is incomplete development of the fetal placental microvasculature in pre-eclampsia associated with IUGR, which could account for reduced perfusion of the fetal placenta seen in this condition (Macara et al 1995).

The kidney

The glomeruli enlarge and sometimes bulge, protruding into the proximal tubule due to swelling and lipid vacuolation of the cytoplasm of the glomerular endothelial cells in the capillary loops. This swelling narrows the lumen. The glomerular changes are termed glomerular endotheliosis. The epithelial cells of the glomerulus and their foot processes appear normal except for a few intracytoplasmic hyaline droplets. The mesangium, however, widens and shows an increase in mesangial matrix, with expansion of the mesangial cell cytoplasmic foot processes, which can grow round the capillary between the endothelium and the basement membrane (Tribe et al 1979). This interposition is associated with deposition of mesangial matrix in the area between the basement membrane and the endothelium, which may be mistaken for apparent thickening of the basement membrane (Fox 1987). Deposits of IgM and fibrin may also be found, but there is no evidence of deposition of any other immunoglobulin or of complement (Fox 1987). Again, these changes are characteristic of, but not specific to, pre-eclampsia, as similar changes can be seen in abruption. They may be related to low-grade DIC and fibrin deposition, which can occur in both conditions. There is no major tubular damage in pregnancy-induced hypertension, although dilatation and epithelial thinning of the proximal tubules, hyaline deposition related to protein reabsorption and tubular necrosis have been noted. The renal damage can be severe enough to produce acute renal failure, through either tubular or cortical necrosis (Lindheimer & Katz 1986). Although uncommon, this is more likely when there is further circulatory compromise, such as when abruption complicates pre-eclampsia.

This damage results in a reduced glomerular filtration rate. Although creatinine clearance is reduced, the serum creatinine does not usually increase noticeably, because of the geometric relationship between clearance and serum creatinine. Plasma urea increases, again usually modestly. The most obvious evidence of glomerular dysfunction is proteinuria, which reflects disease severity. It may be severe enough to lead to nephrotic syndrome. The mechanism underlying proteinuria is unclear, but it may be related to loss of the strong negative charge that normally repels proteins from the glomerular basement membrane. In addition, hypocalciuria is seen (Thong et al 1991). While glomerular dysfunction is manifest as proteinuria, tubular dysfunction is associated with hyperuricaemia (Chesley & Williams 1945) due to increased resorbtion of uric acid, which is coupled with tubular sodium reabsorption. It has been proposed that the hyperuricaemia is of benefit as it acts as an antioxidant (Moran & Davison 1999). This reduction in uric acid clearance precedes the proteinuria and the decline in glomerular filtration rate and is indicative of glomerular damage (Moran & Davison 1999). Tubular, red cell, hyaline and granular casts are also seen within the urine consistent with both tubular and glomerular damage (Leduc et al 1991).

The liver

The hepatic lesions seen in pre-eclampsia include haemorrhages, periportal fibrin deposition, and areas of infarction and necrosis (Sheehan & Lynch 1973). Thrombosis of the capillaries of the portal tract and small branches of the hepatic arteries is seen. These haemorrhages are thought to arise in the arteries of the portal tract, which show evidence of vascular damage similar to that seen in other sites. The hepatic lesions are likely to be secondary to activation of the coagulation system, endothelial damage and vasoconstriction. The lesions are not specific to pre-eclampsia, as similar changes can be seen in obstetric haemorrhage.

Liver enzymes (transaminases and gamma-glutamyl transferase) and plasma bilirubin are elevated. Clinical jaundice occasionally occurs, and may progress to hepatic failure. Subcapsular haematoma or hepatic rupture can also occur. Clinically, these changes may produce vomiting and epigastric pain and tenderness, usually indicative of a fulminating disease process; however, they may be absent, and screening for hepatic dysfunction should, therefore, be performed. The epigastric pain and tenderness is thought to be caused by stretching of Glisson's capsule. Shoulder-tip pain can occur with hepatic rupture and internal bleeding. Deranged liver function tests occur in around 20% of cases, and are associated with severe disease and an increased risk of premature delivery and of IUGR (Romero et al 1988). As associated neonatal morbidity is independent of the severity of hypertension and the presence of proteinuria, hepatic dysfunction may be an independent risk factor for both the mother and the fetus (Romero et al 1988).

HELLP syndrome

Haemolysis, abnormalities of liver function and thrombocytopenia have long been recognized as complications of pre-eclampsia, although they may exist without severe hypertension or gross coagulation disturbance. Weinstein (1982) described 29 cases of severe pre-eclampsia or eclampsia complicated by microangiopathic haemolytic anaemia, elevated liver enzymes and low platelet count. He derived the acronym HELLP: haemolysis (characteristic red cell morphology and lactate dehydrogenase >600 units/l), elevated liver enzymes (aspartate aminotransferase >70 units/l), and low platelets (<100×10⁹/l). This is not a distinct entity, but rather a well-recognised constellation of features associated with pre-eclampsia. The recognition of this syndrome is of value because it draws the clinician's attention to the wider ramifications of the disease process, which may be present even when blood pressure is not grossly elevated. These patients, regardless of blood pressure, must be considered as having severe disease. They have a high incidence of further complications, including DIC (although there will be underlying activation of the coagulation system which is not apparent on basic coagulation screening (Greer et al 1985)). There is also a high risk of neonatal morbidity and mortality, although this may not be higher than for women with pre-eclampsia when gestation at delivery is taken into account (Abramovici et al 1999).

The most common symptoms are epigastric or right hypochondrial pain, nausea and vomiting and visual disturbance, and all pregnant women presenting with such symptoms should have this syndrome excluded, regardless of blood pressure, as up to 50% may be normotensive by conventional criteria. Full blood count and a blood film is essential for diagnosis: a platelet count must be obtained and red cell fragmentation looked for. Biochemical tests are required: increased urate and elevated transaminases and bilirubin are present. A coagulation screen should be performed, as DIC can occur. In clinical practice, this is frequently misdiagnosed as viral hepatitis, cholestasis of pregnancy, cholecystitis, hyperemesis or acute fatty liver of pregnancy.

Management of such patients usually requires urgent delivery in the maternal interest, although conservative management has been used and is associated with an improved neonatal outcome. Conservative management must be balanced against the high risk of serious maternal morbidity, and delivery is often the safest option for the mother. Blood pressure control and careful maternal and fetal monitoring is required, and supportive therapy for coagulation disorders may be needed. High-dose steroid therapy may hasten the resolution of the problem postpartum.

In subsequent pregnancies, these women are at increased risk of pre-eclampsia (19%) and IUGR (12%), but the risk of recurrent HELLP syndrome is low (3%) (Sibai et al 1995). There is no evidence to suggest that these women are at increased risk of chronic hypertension and no evidence to contraindicate the subsequent use of oral contraceptives. However, if the woman has underlying chronic hypertension with superimposed HELLP syndrome, then the risk of recurrence is 75% for pre-eclampsia and 5% for HELLP, as well as the increased risk of other complications, such as IUGR and abruption associated with chronic hypertension (Sibai et al 1995).

The brain

Eclampsia is an extreme clinical manifestation of pre-eclampsia. It is associated with cerebral vasospasm. A significant increase in cerebrovascular resistance occurs, but subsequent loss of cerebral autoregulation is associated with a fall in resistance and overperfusion similar to hypertensive encephalopathy (Williams and Wilson 1999). This can persist for several days after the seizure. This alteration in perfusion contrasts with pre-eclampsia, where there is increased perfusion pressure and increased cerebral resistance with no change in blood flow. The pathological features include cerebral oedema, cerebral haemorrhage, petechial haemorrhages, thrombotic lesions and fibrinoid necrosis, secondary to endothelial dysfunction and vascular damage. Cerebral oedema is not a constant feature but may be seen on computed tomography of the brain in eclamptic patients (Richards et al 1988). This correlates with the duration of intermittent seizures, suggesting that oedema is not the primary cause of the symptoms and signs of eclampsia or the cause of the seizures, but it is a secondary feature occurring after seizures (Richards et al 1988). Cortical blindness can occur, which may be due to oedema or petechial haemorrhages, again resulting from vasospasm in the posterior cerebral circulation.

Vasomotor function

In contrast to the normal pregnant situation, a contracted plasma volume occurs in pre-eclampsia. This is associated with an increase in systemic vascular resistance, a normal or reduced cardiac output and reduced cardiac preload (Clarke & Cotton 1988, Wallenburg 1988). This reflects increased peripheral resistance due to vasoconstriction.

Despite increases in plasma renin concentration, renin substrate and angiotensin II (A II) in normal pregnancy, blood pressure falls. This is due to acquired vascular insensitivity to A II, which is maximal in the second trimester, after which it slowly returns towards the non-pregnant situation (Gant et al 1974) and is associated with downregulation of A II receptors (Baker et al 1991). In pre-eclampsia, there is a loss of the acquired insensitivity to A II, which antedates clinical disease, and an increase in A II receptors (Gant et al 1974, Baker et al 1991). The insensitivity is not specific to A II and is found with other agonists such as noradrenaline. *Ex vivo* studies suggest that endothelium-dependent vascular relaxation is reduced, so implicating the endothelium in the increased vasomotor activity of pre-eclampsia (Ashworth et al 1997). Furthermore, circulating plasma factors may be involved in altering the endothelial response (Ashworth et al 1997). The mechanism may be due to disturbance of or damage to key processes relating to vasomotor control.

Reduced production of endothelial-derived vasodilator prostaglandins, particularly prostacyclin, has been proposed, although the evidence is conflicting. Deficiency of the vasodilator nitric oxide, which is produced by the endothelium, has been evaluated, but results are again inconsistent. Similar inconsistent results have been obtained when the highly potent vasoconstrictor peptide endothelin has been measured in pre-eclampsia. Accurate measurement of these substances or their metabolites, to reflect accurately the *in vivo* situation, is difficult and the conflicting evidence may represent methodological difficulties. However, taken together, these results, assessing a variety of vasomotor agonists, are consistent with endothelial damage and/or dysfunction in pre-eclampsia which is responsible for vasoconstriction and the increased peripheral resistance.

Coagulation, fibrinolysis and platelets

The endothelium is intimately associated with the regulation of haemostasis and thrombosis, thus its dysfunction will trigger activation of the haemostatic system as well as disturbance of the vasomotor system (see above). Platelet consumption in pre-eclampsia is pivotal in identifying that endothelial dysfunction, the key underlying pathophysiological mechanism in the disorder, is present. The coagulation disturbance ranges from subclinical disturbance to DIC.

In normal pregnancy, there are significant changes to the coagulation system (Clark et al 2000). Coagulation factors such as fibrinogen, Factor VIII and von Willebrand factor (vWF) increase. Fibrinolysis is reduced as there is an increase in inhibitors of fibrinolysis, particularly plasminogen activator inhibitor type 2 (PAI-2), which is produced by the placenta. There is a reduction in the activity of the endogenous anticoagulant system as resistance to protein C is acquired and protein S levels fall (Clark et al 2000). Despite increased procoagulant potential, there is only a minor degree of activation of the coagulation and fibrinolytic systems, with generation of fibrin and subsequent fibrinolysis resulting in increased fibrin degradation products (FDPs), and there is no evidence of endothelial damage.

In pre-eclampsia, the widespread deposition of fibrin associated with vascular damage, such as acute atherosis, has long been known to be a pathological feature indicating that the coagulation system is activated, activation which is more marked in the uteroplacental circulation (Higgins et al 1998). There are also increases in coagulation factors, such as Factor VIII and vWF, that exceed the changes seen in normal pregnancy. Platelet activation and consumption occur and progresses as the disorder advances; markers of platelet activation correlate with disease severity. Coagulation activation is unlikely to be a primary phenomenon in the disorder, and probably represents a secondary event consequent upon endothelial activation or damage. Nonetheless, it will still contribute to this damage, promoting positive feedback through further endothelial damage. Increased levels of thrombomodulin and fibronectin reflect endothelial damage and correlate with disease severity. The possibility has been raised that fibronectin and thrombomodulin levels in early pregnancy may be a predictive marker for the development of pre-eclampsia (Halligan et al 1994, Boffa et al 1998). Antithrombin, which binds to and inactivates thrombin, is reduced, in keeping with the thrombin generation, and correlates with maternal and perinatal outcome. In particular, there is evidence that antithrombin levels correlate inversely with the level of both proteinuria and fibronectin, linking the consumption of antithrombin to endothelial damage and subsequent renal dysfunction (Clark et al 2000).

The key trigger to coagulation disturbance may be tissue factor expression on endothelial cells. Tissue factor, which is now recognised as the major activation step of coagulation, is increased in pre-eclampsia (Bellart et al 1999). Interestingly, tissue factor expression is stimulated by cytokines such as tumour necrosis factor (TNF). This links coagulation activation to increased cytokine production and a proinflammatory state, which are now recognised to be present in pre-eclampsia. Concentrations of specific markers of fibrinolysis such as D-dimer are increased, indicating that the fibrinolytic system is activated. There is an increase in the endothelial-derived tissue plasminogen activator (tPA) in plasma, reflecting endothelial activation. This increase in tPA is accompanied by an increase in plasminogen activator inhibitor PAI-1, again reflecting endothelial activation, and a reduction in PAI-2, reflecting impaired placental function and/or mass (Halligan et al 1994, Clark et al 2000). Routine coagulation tests are essentially normal, unless pre-eclampsia is complicated by DIC. The normal prothrombin time and activated partial thromboplastin time and slightly prolonged thrombin time do not imply that significant coagulation activation is not occurring, as these tests are relatively insensitive.

Thrombophilia and pre-eclampsia

It is already appreciated that acquired thrombophilia, in the form of antiphospholipid antibody syndrome, is associated with pre-eclampsia. Recent studies have shown that such an association occurs with several of the congenital thrombophilias, namely Factor V Leiden, the prothrombin gene variant and hyperhomocysteinaemia found in MTHFR (methylene tetrahydrofolate reductase) C677T homozygotes (Greer 1999). These conditions are prevalent in around 2–7%, 2% and 10% of Western populations, respectively. A cohort study of women with a history of pre-eclampsia found underlying activated protein C resistance in 15% (Dekker et al 1996). Activated protein C resistance can reflect underlying Factor V Leiden (a molecular variant of Factor V which is not susceptible to cleavage and inactivation by the endogenous anticoagulant protein C, so leading to a hypercoagulable state). Activated protein C resistance has also been reported in pregnancies complicated by HELLP syndrome. These data are supported by case–control studies where Factor V Leiden was associated with an odds ratio of 4.9 (95% CI, 1.3–18.3) (Grandone et al 1997) for pre-eclampsia. Normal pregnancy is associated with an acquired resistance to protein C (Clark et al 1998a) and is associated with an increased risk of pre-eclampsia, possibly related to increased thrombin generation, which may influence birthweight (Clark et al 1999, Clark et al 2000).

The underlying presence of homozygosity for the C677T variant of MTHFR has been found to have an odds ratio of 1.8 (95% CI, 1.0–3.5) for pre-eclampsia (Grandone et al 1997). This suggests that hyperhomocysteinaemia is a risk factor for pre-eclampsia, presumably due to the toxic effects that homocysteine has on the endothelium. It may therefore be of value to check folic acid and vitamin B6 and B12 status in women with adverse pregnancy outcome, as deficiency of these vitamins can lead to acquired hyperhomocysteinaemia. Treatment of hyperhomocysteinaemia with folic acid and vitamin B6 supplements will correct the abnormal methionine load test (Leeda et al 1998). Kupferminc et al (1999) have confirmed the association with Factor V Leiden and hyperhomocysteinaemia and extended the association with pregnancy complications to include the prothrombin gene variant, which is known to be associated with higher prothrombin levels and increased risk of venous thrombosis. These associations are not specific to pre-eclampsia and include other pregnancy complications, namely IUGR, abruption and stillbirth. Although there is no evidence, at present,

to support routine screening of all pregnant women for underlying congenital thrombophilia, patients with severe or recurrent IUGR or pre-eclampsia or stillbirth should be considered for screening.

If, however, we do establish that a patient with a history of pre-eclampsia has an underlying thrombophilia, management is uncertain. Some extrapolation can be made from the benefits of the combination of aspirin and heparin in women with antiphospholipid antibody syndrome and recurrent miscarriage, but we have no evidence that such intervention, although logical, is effective in patients at risk of pre-eclampsia. Thus, if such screening is to be employed, it is important that we develop appropriate trials to determine the effectiveness of the intervention. Only when such evidence becomes available can we weigh the advantages, disadvantages and cost-effectiveness of screening and intervention for thrombophilia in pre-eclampsia.

Metabolic factors

High body mass index is an established risk factor for pre-eclampsia, in particular central obesity, which is in turn associated with insulin resistance. Pre-eclampsia is associated with insulin resistance and a dramatic increase in free fatty acids (antedating clinical expression of the disorder) and plasma triglycerides, well above that seen in normal pregnancy (Lorentzen et al 1995). These changes are compatible with those seen in patients with coronary artery disease, in terms of the pattern of lipoprotein subfractions (Kaaja et al 1995, Sattar et al 1997). The dramatic increase in triglycerides results in an increase in very low density lipoprotein (VLDL), small changes in low density lipoprotein (LDL3) and decreased high density lipoprotein. Such hyperlipidaemia can induce vascular damage and dysfunction directly, and indirectly through enhanced oxidative stress, and also by potentiating insulin resistance (Hayman et al 1999, Sattar & Greer 1999). For example VLDL so VLDL can stimulate endothelial expression of proinflammatory adhesion molecules such as VCAM-1, which in turn is involved with monocyte activation and transformation into macrophages. These macrophages may then take up lipid and so lead to the characteristic vascular lesion acute atherosis. The disturbance in lipoproteins is likely to be triggered or contributed to by a placentally derived factor such as increased cytokine expression, for example the proinflammatory cytokine IL-6, which is elevated in pre-eclampsia (Greer et al 1995, Clark et al 1998b) and which enhances lipolysis. Alternatively or additionally there may be reduced hepatic beta-oxidation, as there is a link between defects in maternal beta-oxidation and HELLP syndrome, and pre-eclampsia (Sattar et al 1996).

Thus, pre-eclampsia may be the pregnancy-associated maternal expression of an underlying metabolic syndrome. This response is revealed in pregnancy by a change in insulin resistance with subsequent enhanced free fatty acid flux, hypertriglyceridaemia and subsequent endothelial dysfunction. Acute atherosis seen in the placental bed, similar to that seen in atherosclerosis in the non-pregnant, and the lipid accumulation in the glomerular endothelial cells noted above, would be in keeping with such a metabolic disturbance. Recently, pre-eclampsia has been identified as a potential risk factor for cardiovascular disease (Hannaford et al 1997). This might be due to similar pathological features or predispositions, such as genetic polymorphism for key steps in the lipid metabolism pathway or cytokine function.

Inflammatory changes and oxidative stress

There is substantial evidence of inflammatory changes in pre-eclampsia. Neutrophil activation, confined to the maternal circulation (Redman et al 1999), occurs (Greer et al 1989a, 1991b, Barden et al 1997) and may be an early part of the disease process. Neutrophils have also been localised to the placental bed in women with pre-eclampsia and this correlates with disease severity (Butterworth et al 1991). Neutrophil activation results in the release of a variety of substances capable of mediating vascular damage, including proteases, oxygen radicals and leukotrienes. Neutrophil activation markers correlate with von Willebrand factor levels (Greer et al 1991a), so linking neutrophil activation to vascular damage. Monocyte activation is also present (Oian et al 1985, Sacks et al 1998). These inflammatory changes are over and above those associated with normal pregnancy (Sacks et al 1998).

The leucocyte activation may be related to increased expression of cell adhesion molecules, which control leucocyte capture and activation, on the endothelium, as increased E-selectin and VCAM-1 have been found in pre-eclampsia (Clark et al 1998b). VCAM-1 is important in monocyte activation. As monocytes transform into macrophages, which in turn can take up lipid, particularly where hypertriglyceridaemia is present, and become the lipid-laden macrophages characteristic of acute atherosis, this may be a critical process in the vascular lesion of pre-eclampsia. There is an increase in proinflammatory cytokines in pre-eclampsia (Greer et al 1995, Vince et al 1995), which can stimulate adhesion molecule expression and leucocyte activation. As discussed previously, these cytokines may also influence the metabolic changes of pre-eclampsia. The associated increase in oxidative stress in pre-eclampsia is accompanied by a reduced antioxidant potential, so allowing the antioxidants potentially to provoke a greater degree of damage to the vessel wall, which is relevent to endothelial dysfunction.

The endothelium

The endothelium, as evident from the above discussion, is the victim of activation of many of the disease mechanisms in pre-eclampsia; increased free fatty acids, deranged lipoproteins, increased oxidative stress, increased cytokine production, coagulation activation and leucocyte activation. It is not an innocent bystander, however, as such damage will trigger expression of adhesion molecules and promote coagulation activity, so amplifying the response. The endothelium is consequently responsible for the wide diversity of presentations of this condition, as endothelial damage accounts for all aspects of the pathophysiology (Roberts et al 1989). Evidence of endothelial activation and damage include increased endothelin production, elevated levels of fibronectin, increased concentrations of von Willebrand's factor and plasminogen activator inhibitors.

Genetics of pregnancy-induced hypertension

Susceptibility to pre-eclampsia has an inherited maternal component, although its precise nature is unclear. Indeed, there is likely to be a variety of genetic predispositions that can influence the maternal response to pregnancy of defective trophoblast invasion and lead to the clinical expression of pre-eclampsia. Segregation analysis had suggested that a single autosomal recessive gene model is consistent with pre-eclampsia (Chesley & Cooper 1986, Arngrimsson et al 1990). However, a recent cohort study of monozygotic and dizygotic twin mothers was not consistent with a simple mendelian inheritance pattern. This suggests that the genetic component may be smaller or more varied and complex than previously thought (Thornton & MacDonald 1999) An association between eclampsia and miscarriage has been found (Cooper et al 1988), suggesting that there may be a genetic basis for disturbance of the normal fetomaternal interaction in the placental bed.

A variety of hypotheses about the genetic aetiology or associations with pre-eclampsia have been proposed over the last decade or so, in addition to the single recessive gene model noted above (Broughton Pipkin 1999). These include the following:

- Genetic linkage and chromosome exclusion studies have suggested that genes on chromosome 1, 3, 9 or 18 may play a role.
- A major dominant gene model with reduced penetrance or multifactorial inheritance.
- Thrombophilia: pre-eclampsia is associated with Factor V Leiden, the prothrombin gene variant 20210G and hyperhomocysteinaemia associated with MTHFR C677T homozygotes.
- The angiotensin gene variant M235T is found in greater frequency on pre-eclampsia but is also found more commonly in women with essential hypertension and cornary artery disease. It is associated with higher levels of angiotensinogen.
- The major histocompatibility complex HLA DR4 has been associated with pre-eclampsia in women and their babies, along with a higher incidence of HLA DR4 sharing with their partner. However, studies of exclusion mapping have found no evidence of linkage to the HLA region on chromosome 6.

Thus, there are a wide variety of possible genetic aetiologies and associations. This reflects the multifactorial nature of pre-eclampsia. Pre-eclampsia is likely to represent a maternal response to abnormal placentation rather than a single disease entity. The various genetic components will contribute to a maternal phenotype, which, when challenged with the appropriate placental trigger, will result in the clinical expression of the pre-eclampsia syndrome. The nature of this trigger is unknown at present, but could involve the paternal or fetal genotype possibly influencing the immunological response to placentation.

The pathophysiological process

Pre-eclampsia has a complex pathophysiology. What we see clinically as pre-eclampsia is a variety of manifestations of an abnormal (or possibly simply exaggerated) maternal response to pregnancy. The primary pathology in the placenta is not unique to pre-eclampsia. Nonetheless, there is clearly a placental trigger, as the disorder is dependent on the presence of trophoblast. The trigger may be a signal which is important for the normal physiological response to pregnancy, but which is overexpressed in situations of placental damage or abnormality. Such a situation is seen in classic cases of pre-eclampsia where a small, infarcted placenta that has not adequately invaded the maternal circulation is present. The signal may also be overexpressed in situations of increased placental mass, such as twins or molar pregnancy, which are associated with pre-eclampsia. Candidate triggers include placental cytokine production.

It is not simply the placental trigger that is important, as IUGR shares the same placental pathology, yet often occurs without accompanying pre-eclampsia. Thus, the mother's response to the trigger is critical. Her response may depend on her genotype and/or phenotype; for example, women with central obesity and insulin resistance may be more at risk, with an exaggerated metabolic response. Women with congenital thrombophilia have an exaggerated coagulation response, and women with an underlying inflammatory condition such as systemic lupus erythematosus have an exaggerated inflammatory response. On first impressions, these mechanisms seem too diverse to explain pre-eclampsia; however, as discussed above, they are all interrelated. An exaggerated metabolic response in terms of increased small dense LDL can trigger endothelial dysfunction, with expression of adhesion molecules, coagulation activation and leucocyte activation leading to further vascular damage. An enhanced procoagulant response to the placental trigger can similarly lead to endothelial damage with proinflammatory changes, which may trigger metabolic change. An enhanced inflammatory response to pregnancy will result in similar endothelial responses. As all these mechanisms are interrelated and provide positive feedback loops leading to further vascular damage, a vicious circle is established. The vicious circle can be triggered from any point as the interrelations will ensure that the other processes are activated, with the extent of each component dependent on the particular maternal genotype or phenotype.

Those women who do not have a susceptible phenotype for pre-eclampsia might develop IUGR alone. This model, dependent on both a trophoblast trigger, which could be of varying magnitude, and maternal genetic and phenotypic susceptibility, can provide the wide spectrum of pathology seen in pre-eclampsia, with gross multiorgan dysfunction through to IUGR without secondary maternal pathology. One might ask why such responses occur. It is possible that pre-eclampsia is an attempt by the fetus to provoke the mother to compensate for poor placentation by increasing blood pressure to improve perfusion (this would be in line with the association between chronic antihypertensive therapy and low birthweight) and increase lipids in an attempt to provide the fetus with a better supply of nutrients. These changes are at the mother's expense as they lead to vascular damage. Other women may develop pre-eclampsia not because of an abnormal placenta but rather a greater placental mass and/or maternal sensitivity. In this situation there may be no disturbance of fetal growth. In contrast, in IUGR alone, the mother fails to compensate for abnormal placentation and shows no increase in blood pressure, and fails to show even the normal lipid response seen in pregnancy (Sattar et al 1999). Thus, her genotype or phenotype allows her to neglect the growth-restricted fetus.

MANAGEMENT

Prediction and prevention

Although we can identify many risk factors for pre-eclampsia, such as obesity, family history, and high blood pressure in early pregnancy, none are specific or sensitive enough as a test to determine pregnancies at high risk. Even when a variety of clinical and biochemical markers are combined, sensitivity and specificity remain too low to provide useful screening (Stamilio et al 2000). Difficulty in identifying women at risk hampers assessment of possible interventions. Perhaps the best test available at present is the use of Doppler ultrasound of the uterine arteries. The presence of a persistent notching pattern at 22 weeks' gestation, thought to reflect failure of the second wave of trophoblast invasion, has a sensitivity of 75% and a specificity of 96%, although the positive predictive value is only 28% (Bower et al 1993).

Numerous interventions, including sodium restriction, prophylactic diuretics, calcium and magnesium supplements and supplementation of dietary Ω-3 unsaturated fatty acids, have been considered in the prevention or treatment of pre-eclampsia. None of these interventions has consistently shown any influence on the disease incidence. The use of low-dose aspirin (60–75 mg/day) to prevent pre-eclampsia was based upon the rationale that pre-eclampsia is associated with alterations in the production of prostacyclin and thromboxane, secondary to activation of the clotting system and changes in platelet function. Randomised controlled trials in over 20 000 women have failed to support the routine prophylactic or therapeutic administration of low-dose aspirin. Aspirin may have a prophylactic role in the management of women with a history of severe pre-eclampsia before 30–32 weeks' gestation: it seems likely that these women should begin prophylactic treatment early in the second trimester. It is clear from the randomised controlled trials that low-dose aspirin is not associated with adverse maternal or fetal outcome, and in particular is not associated with an increased risk of abruption (which was suggested in one study). Thus, it should be considered only for women with a history of severe early-onset disease or additional pathology, such as antiphospholipid antibody syndrome.

Most interest at present is focused on antioxidant vitamin supplements, which may be of value because of the oxidative stress and reduced antioxidant capacity associated with the disorder. A recent study identified almost 300 women at risk of pre-eclampsia using uterine artery Doppler ultrasound in mid-pregnancy and a previous history of pre-eclampsia. The women were randomised to vitamin C and vitamin E supplements or placebos. Vitamin supplementation was associated with an adjusted odds ratio of 0.24 for pre-eclampsia in the treated group (Chappell et al 1999). Although encouraging, this work urgently requires to be re-examined in a large-scale clinical trial. Of particular concern is the possibility that therapeutic measures to prevent pre-eclampsia might also abolish the beneficial effects of maternal hypertension on placental perfusion, thus increasing the incidence of IUGR (see above). Such an effect has been observed following the use of 100 mg aspirin daily in the ERASME study from northern France and southern Belgium (reported at the ISSHP meeting in Paris, June 2000).

Assessment

There is no clear pattern relating the timing of antenatal visits to the development of pre-eclampsia. Many cases develop rapidly and can progress to a severe form within days of a normal antenatal assessment. The Confidential Enquiries into Maternal Deaths found that the median time between the last antenatal attendance and severe pre-eclampsia, or eclampsia, was 6 days (range 0–28 days) in those attending for care. The median gestational age at presentation was 32 weeks (range 26–40 weeks). In view of the rapid development of some cases, even with regular antenatal assessment, it is important to ensure that antenatal education makes women aware of the symptoms associated with pre-eclampsia, their importance, and the need to obtain formal assessment if they occur. There is also a need for continued education of medical and midwifery staff, particularly in the community, with regard to the implications of pre-eclampsia and the need for accurate diagnosis, assessment and prompt referral, especially when proteinuria or severe hypertension is present.

It is clearly important to make a correct diagnosis, being constantly aware of the multiplicity of possible presentations of this disorder. The severity of the disease and rate of progression must also be assessed, necessitating not only a blood pressure profile and assessment and quantification of proteinuria, but also a full blood count (including platelets) along with biochemical assessment of urea and electrolytes, plasma urate and liver function. Patients with fulminating disease will also require a coagulation screen.

The fetus should also be assessed, using methods appropriate for gestational age and the clinical problem. Ultrasound assessment of growth will be required in pregnancies where growth restriction is suspected. Regular assessment of fetal well-being by cardiotocography or biophysical profile is also required. Doppler ultrasound assessment of the umbilical artery flow velocity waveform is helpful in identifying fetuses at high risk and has been shown to improve perinatal outcome.

The initial assessment can often be carried out in a day assessment unit, especially in patients whose mild/moderate hypertension is picked up at a routine antenatal visit. Those who are symptomatic or severely hypertensive require immediate admission and treatment, as do those with significant proteinuria or evidence of gross systemic disturbances. Patients with mild/moderate hypertension can usually be monitored as outpatients. The frequency and type of monitoring tests require to be tailored to the patients' needs, determined by the severity of the disease and presence of fetal growth restriction. These investigations will provide information about the rate of progression of the disease. They will allow the obstetrician to make informed management decisions, including when to admit outpatients to hospital, how frequently maternal and fetal monitoring is required, whether antihypertensive therapy is required, the need for antenatal steroids to reduce the risk of respiratory distress syndrome, and when and by what route the baby should be delivered.

The aim of treatment is to protect the mother and fetus from the consequences of hypertension and to prolong the pregnancy to avoid the problems of prematurity. There is no doubt that substantial prolongation of pregnancy, even in severe cases remote from term, can be obtained by conservative management, with antihypertensive therapy and careful monitoring, in a significant number of cases. This will require a constant evaluation of the risks to mother and fetus of continuing the pregnancy against those of delivery, to optimise the situation for both patients. Eclampsia, symptomatic disease, pulmonary oedema, gross hepatic dysfunction, coagulopathy and renal compromise are usually indications for immediate delivery.

Antihypertensive therapy

Pregnancy-induced hypertension and pre-eclampsia are curable: delivery of the fetus will abolish the disease. The philosophy of treatment is to protect the mother from the effects of severe hypertension (such as cerebrovascular haemorrhage) and eclampsia, and to attempt to reduce the disease progression and prolong the pregnancy, where this is desirable, reducing the risks of iatrogenic prematurity. The earlier in pregnancy the woman presents, the greater the justification in attempting conservative management, even in those with severe hypertension.

Antihypertensive treatment is essential in severe hypertension. At blood pressures over 170/110 mmHg, antihypertensive treatment is required to protect the mother from cerebral haemorrhage, cardiac failure and placental abruption. Treatment should aim to reduce the blood pressure to <160/110 mmHg or a mean arterial pressure <125 mmHg.

The value of antihypertensives in mild or moderate disease is unclear. There may be a reduction in the development of proteinuria, severe hypertension and ARDS, but there is no benefit in terms of gestation at eventual delivery, or reduced obstetric intervention (Duley 1994, Magee et al 1999). Nor is there compelling evidence to suggest that any one drug is better than another (Magee et al 1999). Recently, a meta-analysis has shown that reduction in blood pressure is associated with an increased risk of IUGR (von Dadelszen et al 2000). Thus, the risk:benefit profile in mild and moderate disease needs to be re-examined.

A stepwise approach to the use of antihypertensive therapy is required with first-line, second-line and third-line agents. First-line therapy is either methyldopa or an adrenoceptor antagonist, such as labetalol, atenolol or oxprenolol. Second-line therapy is usually a vasodilator, such as nifedipine. Third-line therapy will be either an adrenoceptor antagonist or methyldopa, depending on which of these agents was employed as first-line therapy. A suitable regimen is labetalol 200 mg thrice daily, increasing to 300 mg four times daily as required. If blood pressure is not controlled then nifedipine is added, using long-acting preparations such as nifedipine LA 30–60 mg once daily. Such therapy is usually sufficient; if blood pressure is not adequately controlled on this combination, the disease is usually sufficiently advanced to warrant delivery. However, occasionally a third-line agent is required and in this situation methyldopa is added, at a dose of 0.25 g two to three times daily, increasing up to 1.0 g three times a day. Where an adrenoceptor antagonist is contraindicated, methyldopa is used as first-line therapy. ACE inhibitors must not be used antenatally.

Methyldopa

Methyldopa is the most extensively studied drug used for the treatment of hypertension in pregnancy. Although now little used in the non-pregnant, its safety profile and efficacy allow it to maintain its position in pregnancy. It is the preferred agent for chronic therapy in pregnancy as there is some evidence that beta-blockers are associated with reduced fetal growth. However, this phenomenon appears, on the basis of a meta-analysis, to be related more to reduction in blood pressure rather than to an effect of any one class of drug (von Dadelszen et al 2000). This might be due to reduced placental perfusion and would fit with the hypothesis that increased blood pressure is an attempt by the fetus to induce the mother to enhance placental perfusion and compensate for the failure of adequate implantation.

Although effective in blood pressure control, one drawback to the use of methyldopa is the frequency of side effects, reported to be about 15% of patients in one study (Redman et al 1976b, 1977). Symptoms included tiredness, loss of energy, dizziness, depression, flushes, headache, vomiting and palpitations; however, only the incidence of loss of energy and dizziness were significantly different between the treatment and control groups. Long-term follow-up on the children from this study (Cockburn et al 1982) has confirmed that there is no long-term adverse effect.

Adrenoceptor antagonists

There is a wide range of adrenoceptor antagonists, with varying receptor specificity and varying degrees of intrinsic sympathomimetic activity. Only atenolol, labetalol and oxprenolol have been studied to any great extent in pregnancy (Rubin et al 1983, Gallery et al 1985, Pickles et al 1989). These agents are often preferred by clinicians, due to the low incidence of side effects associated with their use compared with methyldopa. They are highly effective as first-line antihypertensives and do not appear adversely to affect fetal monitoring tests, in particular cardiotocography (Rubin et al 1984). Long-term use of adrenoceptor antagonists has been subject to several reports of an association with growth restriction, particularly atenolol (Butters et al 1990), although labetalol has also been implicated (Sibai et al 1987). As discussed above, this is likely to be related to reduction of blood pressure rather than an effect confined to a single class of drugs.

Infants exposed to atenolol in utero (Rubin et al 1983) have been followed up after 1 year, and no harmful effects of treatment have been found (Reynolds et al 1984). Thus, at least in the short term, these agents appear to be safe for the fetus, although they have not yet been subject to the same extent of long-term paediatric assessment as methyldopa.

Both methyldopa and adrenoceptor antagonists are, therefore, suitable agents for the treatment of hypertension in pregnancy. The adrenoceptor antagonists cause fewer side effects than methyldopa, and within the adrenoceptor antagonist group, labetalol has several theoretical advantages (such as an alpha-adrenoceptor antagonist function) over atenolol, although these are of unproven value in the clinical setting. Atenolol does, however, have a slower onset of action and a flatter dose–response curve than labetalol. It is probably best for the clinician to use the agent that he or she is most familiar with to obtain good control of hypertension.

Hydralazine

Hydralazine is used for severe and acute hypertension, and may be given by intramuscular injection, intravenous boluses, or continuous intravenous infusions; it is also administered orally in the chronic situation as a second-line antihypertensive agent. It acts by inhibiting contraction of vascular smooth muscle, although precisely how it does this is not clear. It has a delay in onset of action of 20–30 min, even when given intravenously, and is associated with tachycardia brought about by two mechanisms: a baroreceptor-mediated reflex tachycardia, and prolonged stimulation of noradrenaline release. The stimulation of noradrenaline release may account for symptoms such as the anxiety and restlessness, as well as tachycardia, seen following administration. Headache is a significant side effect and may be due to dilatation of the cerebral venous circulation. These side effects are unwelcome in the management of severe pre-eclampsia: the headache and noradrenaline-related effects may mimic the prodromal symptoms of eclampsia, confusing the situation. These side effects can be reduced if hydralazine is used in conjunction with methyldopa or an adrenoceptor antagonist, which will inhibit the sympathetic effects and reflex tachycardia.

Hydralazine, although effective in reducing blood pressure, is far from ideal as a parenteral first-line antihypertensive, and labetalol and nifedipine are superior in terms of episodes of maternal hypertension, incidence of abruption, and caesarean section (Magee et al 1999) and side effects.

Calcium-channel blocking agents

Calcium-channel blocking agents such as nifedipine are established as first- and second-line agents in hypertension in the non-pregnant and pregnant (Allen et al 1987, Constantine et al 1987, Greer et al 1989b). These drugs are potent vasodilators with a rapid onset of action when given orally (or sublingually). They act by blocking calcium influx into smooth muscle cells, so interfering with excitation-contraction coupling. A useful attribute of these agents is that the degree of reduction in blood pressure that they produce appears to be directly proportional to the pretreatment pressure. They have been shown to reduce vascular sensitivity to A II infusions in pregnant sheep (Lawrence & Broughton Pipkin 1986) and also produce cerebral vasodilatation, which may reduce cerebral ischaemia in eclampsia or severe disease.

These agents have no major maternal or fetal adverse effects. Despite their vasodilator effects, there appears to be little problem with tachycardia. Transient facial flushing, headache and warm, sweaty extremities appear to be the most common side effects. The action of nifedipine is potentiated by magnesium sulphate, producing profound hypotension, muscle weakness and fetal distress, thus caution must be exercised in their concomitant use, although the risk of serious interaction appears small. The use of sublingual nifedipine can produce a rapid and profound drop in maternal blood pressure, leading to fetal hypoxia. This route of administration is probably best avoided in pregnancy.

Mild or moderate hypertension

Mild or moderate hypertension is usually picked up as a diastolic blood pressure between 90 and 110 mmHg with no proteinuria at an antenatal check. These women should have a repeat blood pressure measurement ≥4 h later. If hypertension is confirmed, basic surveillance of twice weekly monitoring of blood pressure, urine and clinical assessment of maternal and fetal well-being is required. Full blood count, urea and electrolytes and urate should be measured. Enhanced surveillance is required if:

- the diastolic blood pressure is greater than 100 mmHg at gestations less than 37 weeks
- the blood pressure increment is greater than 25 mmHg
- there is clinical suspicion of IUGR
- there is concern about maternal or fetal well-being
- biochemistry is abnormal.

This can take the form of thrice weekly assessment of blood pressure, urine and full blood count, urea and electrolytes and urate, and liver function tests. An assessment of the fetus should also be made including ultrasound assessment of fetal growth, and cardiotocography or biophysical profile (SOGAP 1997). There is no indication for admission or bed-rest for these women unless further abnormalities are found, such as evidence of fetal compromise or abnormal biochemistry, for example deranged liver function tests or HELLP syndrome. Thus in most cases care can be managed effectively, both clinically and in terms of cost, through a day care unit and/or in the community (Twaddle and Harper 1992, Duley 1993). The value of antihypertensive therapy in these women is uncertain. Meta-analyses suggest that it leads to a reduction in the development of proteinuric disease, severe hypertension and ARDS, but there is no benefit in terms of more advanced gestation at delivery or reduced obstetric intervention (Duley 1994, Magee et al 1999). Thus, perhaps antihypertensive therapy should be reserved for early onset disease

(<32 weeks) or diastolic blood pressure >100 mmHg, although the reduction in proteinuria and severe hypertension may be of value in reducing the perceived need for intervention. The usual first-line antihypertensive agents are methyldopa or labetalol. As these women are at increased risk of chronic hypertension in later life, persistent hypertension 6 weeks after delivery will require investigation.

Severe hypertension and the fulminating pre-eclamptic patient

Severe disease usually requires admission to hospital for careful assessment. The mother's blood pressure should be recorded at least 4-hourly, proteinuria should be quantified and regular enquiry made for symptoms. Investigations should include urea, urate and electrolytes, liver function and full blood count. A coagulation screen should be performed if there is clinical concern or there are significantly abnormal or deteriorating laboratory parameters. The chest should be auscultated if there is suspicion of pulmonary oedema, and a chest X-ray performed. Fetal growth and well-being should be assessed.

Drug treatment is required and a target blood pressure set. Stepwise therapy with methyldopa or labetalol or atenolol as first line followed by nifedipine, which is best given as a long-acting form. As severe disease is often of early onset, the key objective is to prolong pregnancy without risk to the mother. An average prolongation of 2 weeks can be achieved, with associated reduction in neonatal morbidity (Magee et al 1999), but careful maternal surveillance is required, with delivery if there is significant maternal compromise. In view of the risks to the mother, conservative management is rarely if ever indicated in severe disease beyond 34–36 weeks' getation. These patients are also at risk of venous thromboembolism and prophylaxis with elasticated stockings and low molecular weight heparin should be considered both antepartum and postpartum.

Fulminating pre-eclampsia, where the woman is symptomatic, blood pressure is uncontrolled and haematological and biochemical investigations are rapidly deteriorating, requires urgent, usually operative, delivery. The woman will be in high dependency care in a labour ward equipped and staffed for such patients. Management is best carried out by experienced obstetricians, midwives and an anaesthetist. The patient must be rapidly assessed, treated and monitored: monitoring, in addition to emergency biochemistry and coagulation status, will require automated blood pressure measurement, central venous pressure monitoring, and hourly urine output. Although venous access is essential, minimal fluids (maximum 500 ml over 6 h) should be given to maintain access, as these patients are overloaded with extracellular fluid although they have a contracted intravascular volume. Excessive administration of fluids, such as dilute drug solutions, can easily result in fluid overload, which is a serious complication of treatment as it can be followed by pulmonary oedema or ARDS, which may be fatal. It is important to appreciate that oliguria is a common feature postpartum in severe pre-eclampsia. Fluid management can be extremely difficult in these cases and requires input from experienced senior staff, and optimal assessment of fluid balance, circulatory status and, in particular, assessment for possible pulmonary oedema. Fluid management needs to be coordinated because a wide variety of infusions may be given, such as blood products for coagulation failure and dilute drug solutions to control blood pressure and prevent seizures. One member of staff should, therefore, take responsibility for the overall fluid management. If a coagulopathy complicates the situation, it is best corrected by delivery combined with supportive administration of blood products, such as platelet concentrate and fresh-frozen plasma, as required. Similarly, as discussed earlier, HELLP syndrome is usually best managed by delivery and supportive therapy, including steroids, to aid resolution of the syndrome.

The central haemodynamics of pregnancy-induced hypertension have been explored through central venous pressure lines and Swan–Ganz catheters employed in the management of severely ill patients (Clark & Cotton 1988). Such monitoring has shown that cardiac output and heart rate remain normal, while the systemic vascular resistance and arterial pressure are increased. The left ventricle is usually hyperdynamic and the pulmonary capillary wedge pressures are normal to low. The central venous pressure is also usually normal or low but does not always correlate with the wedge pressure. The wedge pressures are sometimes high due to an excessive after load, producing depressed left ventricular function due to fluid overload. Pulmonary oedema can occur due to depressed left ventricular function, capillary leakage and reduced colloid osmotic pressure due to hypoalbuminaemia. These multiple possible mechanisms mean that pulmonary oedema can occur without any significant elevation in central venous pressure.

Prophylactic anticonvulsant therapy (magnesium sulphate) should be administered if considered necessary, and blood pressure should be controlled. Hydralazine has been the main therapy employed in the past, but intravenous labetalol is highly effective and has several advantages, including a more rapid onset and fewer side effects. The dose should be titrated to control the patient's blood pressure. A suitable regimen is a loading dose of 50 mg labetalol i.v., with a continued infusion of 60 mg/h, doubling the dose every 15–30 min (maximum 480 mg/h) until control is achieved. When good control is not obtained by labetalol or hydralazine, sodium nitroprusside infusions are highly effective but potentially toxic to the fetus: they are best used following delivery or immediately prepartum. Calcium-channel blockers can also be given orally or sublingually in this situation, the latter providing rapid onset. This can be used in addition to, or as an alternative to, labetalol or hydralazine. Caution should be exercised as mentioned previously, to ensure that blood pressure is not reduced too much, too quickly, as this can produce fetal hypoxia.

Volume expansion and oliguria

As pre-eclampsia is associated with a contracted intravascular volume, volume expansion has been explored in severe disease in an attempt to lower blood pressure and increase renal and placental blood flow. The mechanism underlying the hypotensive effect of volume expansion with plasma protein solutions is not clear and appears not to be related to plasma volume expansion per se (Gallery et al 1984). Although volume expansion has been reported as being of value, there are insufficient data to provide any reliable estimate of its effectiveness (Duley 1992, Magee et al 1999). It is potentially dangerous, as it may provoke circulatory overload and pulmonary oedema. If it is to be employed, then central monitoring with at least a central venous pressure line is mandatory to guide therapy. Volume expansion is usually combined with vasodilator therapy to facilitate the administration of volume expansion to an already contracted vascular compartment under high pressure.

As discussed above, the usual haemodynamic status of women with severe pre-eclampsia is an increased systemic vascular resistance, a hyperdynamic left ventricle and normal pulmonary vascular resistance (Clark & Cotton 1988): this will usually be improved by volume expansion coupled with a vasodilator. If, however, left ventricular function is impaired, due to the increased systemic vascular resistance, and pulmonary artery pressures are increased, as sometimes occurs, then volume expansion can potentially worsen the situation. Similarly, if there is increased pulmonary capillary permeability (diagnosed by pulmonary oedema on chest radiographs, with normal left ventricular function and pulmonary artery pressure), then again volume expansion with plasma protein solutions will worsen the pulmonary oedema by increasing the extravascular colloid osmotic pressure, hence, the need for central monitoring.

Oliguria is common in severe disease due to reduced intravascular volume, vasospasm and sometimes the effect of antihypertensive therapy. Prerenal failure can occur, especially if there is a sudden reduction in blood volume, such as with major obstetric haemorrhage. This may tip the patient into renal failure and acute tubular necrosis, particularly if DIC occurs with haemoglobinuria. In the woman wth pre-eclampsia where urinary output is <25 ml/h for 4 h, the situation should initially be managed expectantly. If oliguria persists over a further 4 h, a fluid challenge should be considered. Recurrent fluid challenges require central venous pressure monitoring. If the central venous pressure (CVP) is less than 4 mmHg and oliguria persists, a further fluid challenge can be given. If the CVP is >8 mmHg, a careful assessment for pulmonary oedema (basal crepitations and oxygen saturation <92% plus signs on chest X-ray) should be made. If pulmonary oedema is present it should be treated with frusemide 20 mg i.v.; if no response give a further dose of 40 mg frusemide. With a CVP >4 mmHg and no pulmonary oedema, the initial management is expectant but a further fluid challenge should be considered. A dopamine infusion (1 µg/kg per minute increasing up to 5 µg/kg/per minute) to enhance renal blood flow should be used in persistent oliguria unresponsive to volume expansion. Clearly, the urea and creatinine must be monitored in all cases and where there is any suspicion of renal failure developing a renal physician should be involved.

Delivery

Delivery must be expedited by the most suitable route, decided upon by the obstetrician, who must assess the relative risks of abdominal and vaginal delivery, taking into account both the maternal and fetal state and length of gestation. In the absence of a coagulopathy, epidural analgesia is ideal for both abdominal and vaginal delivery. It will aid blood pressure control by reducing catecholamine release in response to pain, but should not be considered a primary treatment for hypertension. General anaesthesia can be hazardous in these patients: not only will they often have laryngeal oedema, making intubation difficult, but laryngoscopy may provoke extreme hypertension, with the risk of cerebral complications. This response can be ameliorated effectively by pretreatment with intravenous labetalol. Ergometrine-containing preparations should be avoided, if possible, in the management of the third stage of labour, as this will substantially worsen the hypertension.

Pulmonary oedema and ARDS

Pulmonary oedema may complicate up to 3% of severe cases, with a mortality less than 10%; around 70% of cases occur postpartum. It is uncommon in well-managed cases. The pre-eclamptic mother is at risk of pulmonary oedema because of increased capillary permeability and reduced oncotic pressure. When hypertension is severe, the high afterload may also precipitate pulmonary oedema. It can occur with a normal CVP. It is unusual without other complications, such as excess fluid or colloid administration, massive transfusion, sepsis, anaemia or DIC. Dyspnoea and difficulty maintaining adequate oxygen saturation on pulse oximetry will usually raise suspicion, although other complications such as pulmonary embolism must be considered. It will require oxygen and diuretic therapy along with vasodilator and antihypertensive therapy for hypertension and associated high afterload. ARDS can complicate pre-eclampsia and is more common postpartum. Again it is very unusal without the presence of additional complications, such as fluid overload, HELLP syndrome, aspiration, eclampsia or underlying medical problem. Management is supportive therapy in an intensive therapy unit, with ventilation, maintenance of cardiac and renal function, and treatment of DIC and any infection. Mortality is around 50%, usually due to multiorgan failure.

Management of eclampsia

Eclampsia may be asymptomatic or may be preceded by the classical prodrome of headache, visual disturbance and epigastric pain. Hypertension and proteinuria may not previously have been noted. It is important to be aware of the possible presentations to allow prompt and adequate treatment to be provided, especially in view of the limited experience that obstetricians now have of this uncommon condition. Our inadequacies in diagnosis of patients at risk are highlighted by the finding that most women have their first seizure while in hospital, and have inadequate investigation before the seizure and, in many cases, afterwards as well (Douglas & Redman 1994). The need for support from regional teams with special knowledge of the problem has been highlighted in the past (Department of Health et al 1998). The differential diagnosis will include epilepsy, coincidental cerebrovascular accident, a space-occupying lesion, infection or metabolic disturbance, and such conditions may need to be considered and excluded, especially in patients with atypical or late-onset presentation.

Guidelines for the management of eclampsia have been produced (Royal College of Obstetricians and Gynaecologists 1996). The objectives are to control convulsions and blood pressure, stabilise the situation and effect delivery. The patient should be placed in the left lateral position, the airway secured and oxygen given. Senior medical and midwifery staff should be alerted immediately. Intravenous access should be secured and intravenous magnesium sulphate given to treat the seizures (Table 21.4). An alternative to halt seizures is diazemuls 10–20 mg i.v. bolus, followed by magnesium sulphate to prevent further seizures. Secondary prophylaxis should be continued for at least 24 h after the last seizure.

Hypertension should be controlled with intravenous labetalol or hydralazine. A urinary catheter should be inserted and strict recording and control of fluid balance maintained. Pulse oximetry should be employed. A chest X-ray and arterial blood gases should be performed if pulmonary oedema is suspected. Frequent monitoring of full blood count (to pick up red cell fragmentation indicative of microangiopathic haemolytic anaemia, which can occur), a coagulation screen, liver function tests and urea and creatinine tests should be performed. Once seizures and hypertension are controlled, fetal well-being can be assessed and arrangements made for delivery. Caesarean section is usually required, especially in nulliparous women remote from term with an unfavourable cervix. Cerebral imaging is required to exclude haemorrhage in women with focal neurological signs or prolonged coma. After delivery, high-dependency care should be given for at least 24 h.

In the past, agents such as phenytoin and diazepam were preferred to control seizures. However, following the Eclampsia Trial Collaborative Group (1995) report demonstrating the superiority of magnesium sulphate over diazepam and phenytoin for the secondary prevention of eclampsia, magnesium sulphate has become the first and preferred choice for treatment and prevention of seizures. This study found that the incidence of recurrent seizure was reduced by 52% and 67% when magnesium sulphate was

Table 21.4 Magnesium sulphate for treatment and prophylaxis of eclamptic seizures

Regimen for the intravenous administration of magnesium sulphate
- loading dose of 4 g given slowly over 5–10 min
- maintenance i.v. infusion of 1 g/h
- recurrent seizures should be treated with a further i.v. bolus of 2 g
- serum magnesium levels can be monitored (therapeutic range 2–4 mmol/l)

Features of magnesium toxicity
- double vision
- slurred speech
- loss of deep tendon reflexes
- respiratory depression and respiratory arrest (treat with 10 ml of 10% calcium gluconate)

compared with diazepam and phenytoin, respectively. There were no problems with magnesium toxicity, despite no monitoring of magnesium levels being performed.

Magnesium sulphate does not cause maternal or neonatal sedation. Although its precise mechanism of action is unclear, it appears to have a peripheral site of action at the neuromuscular junction and does not cross the intact blood–brain barrier. It may, however, relax the constricted cerebral circulation in eclampsia.

The use of anticonvulsants for primary prevention of eclampsia in women with severe disease is controversial and obstetricians vary in the anticonvulsant they employ (Gülmezoglu & Duley 1998). The value of such treatment in pre-eclampsia is uncertain (Duley et al 1998) and is currently the subject to a large clinical trial with magnesium sulphate (the MAGPIE trial).

Care following delivery

After delivery, pre-eclampsia will resolve, although the hypertension and proteinuria may take several weeks to return to normal. In the immediate postpartum period, pre-eclampsia may initially worsen (indeed many cases of eclampsia occur at this time) before resolving, and intensive monitoring should continue for at least 24–48 h. Thus, hypertension frequently worsens in the first week postpartum, often reaching a peak 3–4 days after delivery. The antihypertensive regimen used antenatally can be continued and dose-adjusted, and second- and third-line agents introduced as required to control blood pressure. Where there is a poor response, agents such as ACE inhibitors can be employed alone or in combination. As blood pressure settles, therapy can be withdrawn under supervision and monitoring, usually as an outpatient at the day care unit. When possible, methyldopa is best avoided in the postnatal period, as a side effect is depression. Antihypertensive medications, including the ACE inhibitors, are not contraindicated in breast feeding. However, some cases of neonatal bradycardia have been reported in women breast feeding while on medication with atenolol, and newer agents such as metoprolol have been suggested as safer in this regard. Women with a history of essential hypertension can recommence their prepregnancy antihypertensive therapy postnatally. Oliguria can be managed as discussed above.

Where the blood pressure remains elevated or severe disease has occurred, the patient should be investigated to exclude an underlying medical condition, such as connective tissue disease, thrombophilia or renal disease. This is usually organised around 6 weeks after delivery and counselling about future pregnancies and contraception will also be required at this time.

CONCLUSIONS

Pre-eclampsia is a multisystem disorder that usually manifests clinically as hypertension, proteinuria and placental insufficiency, although its protean nature allows a wide variety of presentations. Pathophysiologically, these features result from vascular endothelial damage and dysfunction.

The trigger originates in the uteroplacental bed, due to defective trophoblast invasion and placental ischaemia; this is amplified by metabolic, inflammatory and coagulation disturbances, with these responses related to the maternal genotype and phenotype, such as congenital thrombophilia or central obesity. It is essential to appreciate the widespread nature of the potential clinical problem to diagnose it accurately and determine the extent of the problem.

Management at present focuses on controlling blood pressure and monitoring mother and fetus to optimise the timing and mode of delivery; however, antihypertensive therapy is not aimed primarily at the disease process, but rather at one of its manifestations. There is no established prophylactic therapy, although several areas, including antioxidant vitamin supplementation, are under investigation. The development and application of primary preventive therapy is hampered by our lack of a reliable means of identifying women at risk.

Much research is required to further unravel the enigma of pre-eclampsia, research which will require wide collaboration on a large scale if we want to address the problem in a coordinated and systematic way, to examine pathophysiological hypotheses, and to perform the necessary randomised controlled trials that no one centre is likely to be able to perform alone. This contention is not new; the need for such undertakings was highlighted over 70 years ago:

> "Would it not be right for us obstetricians to undertake the study of this problem collectively? Or shall we leave the matter to develop its natural course and wait for another 10 to 20 years and allow another 100 000 human lives to be lost? . . . this test cannot be postponed for long."

> Stroganoff 1930

We have postponed such coordination far too long; although collaborative trials have been conducted in the last decade or so with good effect, there is a need for further coordination to make the best use of resources and improve the rate of progress if we wish to protect our patients from the continued threat of pre-eclampsia.

REFERENCES

Abramovici D, Friedman S, Mercer BM, Audibert F, Kao L, Sibai B 1999 Neonatal outcome in severe preeclampsia at 24–36 weeks gestation: does the HELLP syndrome matter? Am J Obstet Gynecol 180:221–225

Allen J, Maigaard S, Forman A et al 1987 Acute effects of nitrendipine in pregnancy-induced hypertension. Br J Obstet Gynaecol 94:222–226

Arngrimsson R, Bjornsson S, Geirsson RT, Bjornsson H, Walker JJ, Snaedel G 1990 Familial and genetic predisposition to eclampsia and preeclampsia in a defined island population. Br J Obstet Gynaecol 97:762–770

Ashworth J, Warren AY, Baker PN, Johnson IR 1997 Loss of endothelium dependent relaxation in myometrial resistance arteries in preeclampsia. Br J Obstet Gynaecol 104:1152–1159

Baker PN, Broughton Pipkin F, Symonds EM 1991 Platelet angiotensin II binding sites in normotensive and hypertensive pregnancy. Br J Obstet Gynaecol 98:436–440

Barden A, Graham D, Beilin LJ et al 1997 Neutrophil CD11b

expression and neutrophil activation in preeclampsia. Clin Sci 92:37–44

Bellart J, Gilabert R, Anglès A et al 1999 Tissue factor levels and high ratio of fibrinopeptide A: D-dimer as a measure of endothelial procoagulant disorder in preeclampsia. Br J Obstet Gynaecol 106:594–597

Bellomo G, Narducci PL, Rondoni F et al 1999 Prognostic value of 24 hour blood pressure in pregnancy. JAMA 282:1447–1452

Boffa MC, Valsecchi L, Fausto A et al 1998 Predictive value of plasma thrombomodulin in pre-eclampsia and gestational hypertension. Thromb Haemost 79:1092–1095

Bower S, Bewley S, Campbell S 1993 Improved prediction of preeclampsia by two stage screening of the uterine arteries using the early diastolic notch as colour Doppler imaging. Br J Obstet Gynaecol 82:78–83

Brosens I, Dixon HG 1966 The anatomy of the maternal side of the placenta. J Obstet Gynaecol Br Commonw 73:357–363

Broughton Pipkin F 1999 Genetics of preeclampsia: ideas at the turn of the millennium. Curr Obstet Gynaecol 9: 178–182

Brown MA, Buddle ML 1997 What's in a name? Problems with the classification of hypertension in pregnancy. J Hypertens 15:1049–1054

Brown MA, De Swiet M 1999 Classification of hypertension in pregnancy. Baillieres Clin Obstet Gynaecol 13:27–39

Butters L, Kennedy S, Rubin PC 1990 Atenolol in essential hypertension in pregnancy. BMJ 301:587–589

Butterworth B, Greer IA, Liston WA, Haddad NG, Johnston TA 1991 Immunolocalisation of neutrophil elastase in term decidua and myometrium in pregnancy-induced hypertension. Br J Obstet Gynaecol 98:929–923

Campbell DM, MacGillivray I 1985 Pre-eclampsia in second pregnancy. Br J Obstet Gynaecol 92:131–140

Catanzarite VA, Willms D 1997 Adult respiratory distress syndrome in pregnancy: report of three cases and review of the literature. Obstet Gynecol Surv 52:381–392

Chamberlain G, Phillipp E, Howlett B, Masters K 1978 British births 1970, vol 2, obstetric care, 7. Heinemann, London, pp 80–100

Chappell C, Seed P, Briley AL et al 1999 Effect of antioxidants of preeclampsia in women at increased risk: a randomized trial. Lancet 354:810–816

Chesley LC 1978 Hypertensive disorders in pregnancy. Appleton-Century-Crofts, New York

Chesley LC, Cooper DW 1986 Genetics of hypertension in pregnancy: possible single gene control of pre-eclampsia and eclampsia in the descendents of eclamptic women. Br J Obstet Gynaecol 93:898–908

Chesley LC, Williams LO 1945 Renal glomerular and tubular functions in relation to the hyperuricemia of preeclampsia and eclampsia. Am J Obstet Gynecol 50:367–367

Chesley LC, Annitto JE, Cosgrove RA 1976 The remote prognosis of eclamptic women: sixth periodic report. Am J Obstet Gynaecol 124:446–459

Clark P, Brennand J, Conkie JA, McCall F, Greer IA, Walker ID 1998a Activated protein C sensitivity, protein C, protein S and coagulation in normal pregnancy. Thromb Haemost 79:1166–1170

Clark P, Boswell F, Greer IA 1998b The neutrophil and pre-eclampsia. In: Walsh S (ed) The endocrinology of pre-eclampsia. Semin Reprod Endocrinol 16:57–64

Clark P, Walker ID, Greer IA 1999 The acquired activated protein C resistance of pregnancy is associated with an increase in thrombin generation and is inversely associated with fetal weight. Lancet 353:292–293

Clark P, Sattar N, Walker ID, Greer IA 2001 The Glasgow Outcome, APCR and Lipid (GOAL) pregnancy study: significance of pregnancy associated activated protein C resistance. Thromb Haemost B5:1–6

Clarke SL, Cotton DB 1988 Clinical indications for pulmonary artery catheterisation in the patient with severe preeclampsia. Am J Obstet Gynecol 158:453–458

Cockburn J, Moar VA, Ounsted M, Redman CWG 1982 Final report of study on hypertension during pregnancy: the effects of specific treatment on the growth and development of the children. Lancet i:647–649

Constantine G, Beevers DG, Reynolds AL, Luesley DM 1987 Nifedipine

as a second line antihypertensive drug in pregnancy. Br J Obstet Gynaecol 94:1136–1142

Cooper DW, Hill JA, Chesley LC, Iverson Bryans C 1988 Genetic control of susceptibility to eclampsia and miscarriage. Br J Obstet Gynaecol 95:644–653

Davey DA, MacGillivray I 1988 The classification and definition of the hypertensive disorders of pregnancy. Am J Obstet Gynecol 158:892–898

Dekker GA, de Vries JIP, Doelitzsch PM et al 1996 Underlying disorders associated with severe early onset of pre-eclampsia. Am J Obstet Gynecol 173:104–145

Department of Health, Welsh Office, Scottish Home and Health Department and Department of Health and Social Services Northern Ireland 1998 Confidential enquiries into maternal deaths in the United Kingdom 1994–1996. TSO, London

Douglas K, Redman CWG 1994 Eclampsia in the United Kingdom. BMJ 309:1395–1400

Duley L 1992 Plasma volume expansion in pregnancy-induced hypertension. In: Enkin MW, Keirse MJNC, Neilson JP (eds) Pregnancy and childbirth module Cochrane database of systematic reviews, review no. 05734. Cochrane updates on disc, 1994, issue 1. Update Software, Oxford

Duley L 1993 Hospitalisation for non-proteinuric pregnancy hypertension. The pregnancy and childbirth module. The Cochrane collaboration, issue 2. Update Software, Oxford

Duley L 1994 Any hypertensive therapy for pregnancy hypertension. The pregnancy and childbirth module. The Cochrane collaboration, issue 2. Update Software, Oxford

Duley L, Gulmezoglu AM, Henderson-Smart D 1998 Anticonvulsants for women with preeclampsia (Cochrane review). In: The Cochrane library, issue 1. Update Software, Oxford

Eclampsia Trial Collaborative Group 1995 Which anticonvulsant for women with eclampsia? Evidence from the collaborative eclampsia trial. Lancet 345:1455–1463

Fisher KA, Luger A, Spargo BH, Lindheimer MD 1981 Hypertension in pregnancy, clinical-pathological correlations and remote prognosis. Medicine 60:267–276

Fox H 1987 Histopathology of pre-eclampsia and eclampsia. In: Sharp F, Symonds EM (eds) Hypertension in pregnancy. Perinatology Press, Ithaca, NY, pp 119–130

Fox H 1988 The placenta in pregnancy hypertension. In: Rubin PC (ed) Handbook of hypertension, vol 10: hypertension in pregnancy. Elsevier Science, Amsterdam, pp 16–37

Gallery EDM, Mitchell MDM, Redman CWG 1984 Fall in blood pressure in response to volume expansion in pregnancy associated hypertension (preeclampsia): why does it occur? J Hypertens 2:117–182

Gallery EDM, Ross MR, Gyory AZ 1985 Anti-hypertensive treatment in pregnancy: analysis of different responses to oxprenolol and methyldopa. BMJ 291:563–566

Gant NF, Chand S, Worley RJ, Whalley PJ, Crosby UD, Macdonald PC 1974 A clinical test useful for predicting the development of acute hypertension in pregnancy. Am J Obstet Gynecol 120:1–7

Grandone E, Margagilione M, Colazzo D et al 1997 Factor V Leiden. C>T MTHFR polymorphism and genetic susceptibility to pre-eclampsia. Thromb Haemost 77:1052–1054

Greer IA 1993 Ambulatory blood pressure in pregnancy: measurements and machines. Br J Obstet Gynaecol 100:887–889

Greer IA 1999 Thrombosis in pregnancy: maternal and fetal issues. Lancet 353:1258–1265

Greer IA, Cameron AD, Walker JJ 1985 HELLP syndrome: pathologic entity or technical inadequacy? Am J Obstet Gynecol 152:113–114

Greer IA, Haddad NG, Dawes J, Johnstone FD, Calder AA 1989a Neutrophil activation in pregnancy induced hypertension. Br J Obstet Gynaecol 96:978–982

Greer IA, Walker JJ, Bjornsson S, Calder AA 1989b Second line therapy with nifedipine in severe pregnancy induced hypertension. Clin Exp Hypertens B8:277–292

Greer IA, Leask R, Hodson BA, Dawes J, Kirkpatrick D, Liston WA 1991a Endothelin elastase and endothelial dysfunction in pregnancy induced hypertension. Lancet 337:558–558

Greer IA, Dawes J, Johnston TA, Calder AA 1991b Neutrophil

activation is confined to the maternal circulation in pregnancy induced hypertension. Obstet Gynecol 78:28–32

Greer IA, Lyall F, Perera T, Boswell F, Macara LM 1995 Increased concentrations of cytokines Il-6 and Il-1ra in plasma of women with preeclampsia: a mechanism for endothelial dysfunction. Obstet Gynecol 84:937–940

Gülmezoglu AM, Duley L 1998 Use of anticonvulsants in eclampsia and preeclampsia: survey of obstetricians in the United Kingdom and Republic of Ireland. BMJ 316:975–976

Halligan A, Bonnar J, Sheppard B, Darling M, Walshe J 1994 Haemostatic, fibrinolytic and endothelial variables in normal pregnancies and preeclampsia. Br J Obstet Gynaecol 101:488–488

Halligan A, Shennan A, Thurston H, de Swiet M, Taylor D 1995 Ambulatory blood pressure measurement in pregnancy: the current state of the art. Hypertens Pregnancy 14:1–16

Hannaford P, Ferry S, Hirsch S 1997 Cardiovascular sequelae of toxaemia of pregnancy. Heart 77(2):154–158

Harlan JD 1987 Neutrophil-mediated vascular injury. Acta Med Scand (suppl) 715:123–129

Hayman RG, Sattar N, Warren AY, Greer IA, Johnson IR, Baker PN 1999 Relationship between myometrial resistance artery behaviour and circulating lipid composition. Am J Obstet Gynecol 180:381–386

He S, Silveira A, Hamsten A, Blomback M, Bremme K 1999 Haemostatic, endothelial and lipoprotein parameters and blood pressure levels in women with a history of pre-eclampsia. Thromb Haemost 81:538–542

Higgins JR, Walshe JJ, Darling MRN, Norris L, Bonnar J 1998 Hemostasis in the uteroplacental and peripheral circulations in normotensive and preeclamptic pregnancies. Am J Obstet Gynecol 179:520–526

Howy C, Beard RW 1982 Report to the meeting on the results of the UK survey of diabetic pregnancies. Royal College of Obstetricians and Gynaecologists, London

Humphries KH, Westendorp I, Spinelli JJ, Carere RG, Hofman A, Witteman JCM 1999 Parity is associated with carotid artery plaques and reduced HDL-cholesterol levels: results from the Rotterdam study. Circulation 99:1111

Jonsdottir LS, Arngrimsson R, Geirsson RT, Sigvaldason H, Sigfusson N 1995 Death rates from ischaemic heart disease in women with a history of hypertension in pregnancy. Acta Obstet Gynecol Scand 74:772–776

Kaaja R, Tikkanen MJ, Viinikka L, Ylikorkala O 1995 Serum lipoproteins, insulin and urinary prostanoid metabolites in normal and hypertensive pregnant women. Obstet Gynecol 85:353–356

Khong TY, de Wolf F, Robertson WB, Brosens I 1986 Inadequate maternal vascular response to placentation in pregnancies complicated by preeclampsia and by small-for-gestational-age infants. Br J Obstet Gynaecol 93:1049–1059

Kupferminc MJ, Eldor A, Steinman N et al 1999 Increased frequency of genetic thrombophilia in women with complications of pregnancy. N Engl J Med 340:9–13

Labarrere CA 1988 Acute atherosis: a histopathological hallmark of immune aggression. Placenta 9:95–108

Laivuori H, Tikkanen MJ, Ylikorkala O 1996 Hyperinsulinaemia 17 years after pre-eclamptic first pregnancy. J Clin Endocrinol Metab 81:2908–2911

Lawrence MR, Broughton Pipkin F 1986 Effects of nitrendipine on cardiovascular parameters in conscious pregnant sheep. Abstracts of the 5th international congress of the international society for the study of hypertension in pregnancy, Nottingham

Leduc L, Lederer E, Lee W, Cotton DB 1991 Urinary sediment changes in severe preeclampsia. Obstet Gynecol 77:186–189

Leeda M, Riyazi N, de Vries JIP, Jakobs C, van Geijn HP, Dekker GA 1998 Effects of folic acid and vitamin B6 supplementation on women with hyperhomocysteinemia and a history of pre-eclampsia or fetal growth restriction. Am J Obstet Gynecol 179:136–139

Lindheimer MD, Katz AI 1986 The kidney in pregnancy. In: Brenner BM, Rector FC (eds) The kidney. WB Saunders, Philadelphia, pp 1253–1295

Lorentzen B, Drevon CA, Endresen MJ, Henriksen T 1995 Fatty acid pattern of esterified and free fatty acids in sera of women with

normal and pre-eclamptic pregnancy. Br J Obstet Gynaecol 102:530–537

Mabie WC, Barton JR, Sibai BM 1992 Adult respiratory distress syndrome in pregnancy. Am J Obstet Gynecol 167:950–957

Macara L, Kingdom JCP, Kohnen G, Bowman AW, Greer IA, Kaufman P 1995 Elaboration of stem villous vessels in growth restricted pregnancies with abnormal umbilical artery Doppler waveforms. Br J Obstet Gynaecol 102:807–812

McFadyen IR, Greenhouse P, Price AB, Geirsson RT 1986 The relation between plasma urate and placental bed vascular adaptation to pregnancy. Br J Obstet Gynaecol 93:482–487

MacGillivray I, Rose GA, Rowe D 1969 Blood pressure survey in pregnancy. Clinical Science 37:395–395

Magee LA, Ornstein MP, van Dadelszen P 1999 Management of hypertension in pregnancy. BMJ 318:1322–1336

Moran P, Davison JM 1999 The kidney and the pathogenesis of preeclampsia. Curr Obstet Gynaecol 9:196–202

Naeye RL, Friedman EA 1979 Causes of perinatal death associated with gestational hypertension and proteinuria. Am J Obstet Gynecol 133:8–10

Natarajan P, Shennan AH, Penny J, Halligan AW, de Swiet M, Anthony J 1999 Comparison of auscultatory and oscillometric automated blood pressure monitors in the setting of preeclampsia. Am J Obstet Gynecol 181:1203–1210

Oian P, Omsjo I, Maltau JM, Osterud B 1985 Increased sensitivity to thromboplastin synthesis in blood monocytes from preeclamptic patients. Br J Obstet Gynaecol 92:511–517

Pickles CJ, Symonds EM, Broughton Pipkin F 1989 The fetal outcome in a randomised double blind controlled trial of labetalol versus placebo in pregnancy-induced hypertension. Br J Obstet Gynaecol 96:38–43

Redman CWG 1989 Hypertension in pregnancy. In: de Swiet M (ed) Medical disorders in obstetric practice. Blackwell Scientific Publications, Oxford, pp 249–305

Redman CWG 1995 Hypertension in pregnancy. In: Chamberlain G (ed) Turnbull's obstetrics. Churchill Livingstone, Edinburgh, ch 24, p 441

Redman CWG, Jeffries M 1988 Revised definition of pre-eclampsia. Lancet i:809–812

Redman CWG, Beilin LJ, Bonnar J, Ounsted MK 1976a Plasma urate measurements in predicting fetal death in hypertensive pregnancy. Lancet i:1370–1373

Redman CWG, Beilin LJ, Bonnar J, Ounsted MK 1976b Fetal outcome in trial of antihypertensive treatment in pregnancy. Lancet ii:753–756

Redman CWG, Beilin LJ, Bonnar J 1977 Treatment of hypertension in pregnancy with methyldopa: blood pressure control and side effects. Br J Obstet Gynaecol 84:419–426

Redman CWG, Sacks GP, Sargent IL 1999 Preeclampsia: an excessive maternal inflammatory response to pregnancy. Am J Obstetrics and Gynecol 180:499–506

Reynolds B, Butters L, Evans J, Adams T, Rubin PC 1984 First year of life after the use of atenolol in pregnancy associated hypertension. Arch Dis Child 59:1061–1063

Richards A, Graham D, Bullock R 1988 Clinicopathological study of neurological complications due to hypertensive disorders of pregnancy. J Neurol Neurosurg Psychiatry 51:416–421

Roberts JM, Taylor RN, Musci TJ, Rodgers GM, Hubel CA, McLaughlin MK 1989 Preeclampsia: an endothelial cell disorder. Am J Obstet Gynecol 161:1200–1204

Robertson WB, Brosens IA, Dixon HG 1967 The pathological response of the vessels of the placental bed to hypertensive pregnancy. Journal of Pathology and Bacteriology 93:581–592

Robertson WB, Khong TY 1987 Pathology of the uteroplacental bed. In: Sharp F, Symonds EM (eds) Hypertension in pregnancy. Perinatology Press, Ithaca, NY, pp 101–113

Robillard PY, Hulsey TC 1996 Association of pregnancy-induced hypertension, preeclampsia and eclampsia with duration of sexual cohabitation before conception. Lancet 374:619–619

Romero R, Vizoso J, Emamian M et al 1988 Clinical significance of liver dysfunction in pregnancy-induced hypertension. Am J Perinatol 5:146–151

Royal College of Obstetricians and Gynaecologists 1996 Management of eclampsia. RCOG guideline number 10. RCOG Press, London

Rubin PC, Butters L, Clark DM et al 1983 Placebo controlled trial of atenolol in treatment of pregnancy associated hypertension. Lancet i:431–434.

Rubin PC, Butters L, Clark DM et al 1984 Obstetric aspects of the use in pregnancy-associated hypertension of the beta-adrenoceptor antagonist atenolol. Am J Obstet Gynecol 150:389–392

Sacks GP, Studena K, Sargent IL, Redman CW 1998 Normal pregnancy and preeclampsia both produce inflammatory changes in peripheral blood leukocytes akin to those of sepsis. Am J Obstet Gynaecol 179:80–86

Sattar N, Greer IA 1999 Lipids and the pathogenesis of pre-eclampsia. Curr Obstet Gynaecol 190–195

Sattar N, Gaw A, Packard CJ, Greer IA 1996 Potential pathogenic roles of aberrant lipoprotein and fatty acid metabolism in pre-eclampsia. Br J Obstet Gynaecol 103:614–620

Sattar N, Bendomir A, Berry C et al 1997 Lipoprotein subfraction concentrations in pre-eclampsia: pathogenic parallels to atherosclerosis. Obstet Gynecol 89:403–408

Sattar N, Greer IA, Packard CJ, Kelly T, Mathers AM 1999 A failure of LDL-cholesterol rise in pregnancies complicated by intrauterine growth restriction. J Clin Endocrinol Metab 84:128–130

Saudan PJ, Brown MA, Farrel T, Shaw L 1997 Improved methods of assessing proteinuria in hypertensive pregnancy. Br J Obstet Gynaecol 104:159–164

Shanklin DR, Sibai BM 1989 Ultrastructural aspects of pre-eclampsia. Am J Obstet Gynaecol 161:735–741

Sheehan HL, Lynch JB 1973 Pathology of toxaemia of pregnancy. Churchill Livingstone, London

Sheppard BL, Bonnar J 1981 An ultrastructural study of uteroplacental spiral arteries in hypertensive and normotensive pregnancy and fetal growth retardation. Br J Obstet Gynaecol 88:695–705

Sibai BM, McCubbin JH, Anderson GD, Lipschitz J, Dilts PV 1981 Eclampsia: observations from 67 recent cases. Obstet Gynecol 58:609–613

Sibai BM, El-Nazer A, Gonzalez-Ruiz A 1986 Severe pre-eclampsia–eclampsia in young primigravid women: subsequent pregnancy outcome and remote prognosis. Am J Obstet Gynecol 155:1011–1016

Sibai BM, Gonzalez AR, Mabie WC, Moretti M 1987 A comparison of labetalol plus hospitalisation alone in the management of pre-eclampsia remote from term. Obstet Gynecol 70:323–327

Sibai BM, Ramadan MK, Chari RS, Friedman SA 1995 Pregnancies complicated by HELLP syndrome: subsequent pregnancy outcome and long term prognosis. Am J Obstet Gynecol 172:125–129

SOGAP 1997 The management of mild, non-proteinuric hypertension in pregnancy. A clinical practice guideline for professionals involved in maternity care in Scotland. Scottish obstetric guidelines and audit project. Scottish programme for clinical effectiveness in reproductive health.

Stamilio DM, Sehdev HM, Morgan M, Propert K, Macones G 2000 Can antenatal clinical and biochemical markers predict the development of severe preeclampsia? Am J Obstet Gynecol 182:589–594

Tervila L, Groecke C, Timonen S 1973 Estimation of gestosis of pregnancy (EPH-gestosis). Acta Obstet Gynecol Scand 52:235–235

Thong J, Howie F, Smith AF, Greer IA, Johnstone FD 1991 Microalbuminuria in random daytime specimens in pregnancy induced hypertension. J Obstet Gynaecol 11:324–327

Thornton JG, Macdonald AM 1999 Twin mothers, pregnancy hypertension and preeclampsia. Br J Obstet Gynaecol 106:570–570

Tribe CR, Smart GE, Davies DR, Mackenzie JC 1979 A renal biopsy study in toxaemia of pregnancy using light microscopy linked with immunofluorescence and immuno-electron microscopy. J Clin Pathol 32:681–692

Twaddle S, Harper V 1992 Day care and pregnancy hypertension. Lancet 339:813–814

Villar MA, Sibai BM 1988 Eclampsia. Obstet Gynecol Clin North Am 15:355–377

Vince GS, Starkey PM, Austgulen R, Kwiatkowski D, Redman CWG 1995 Interleukin-6, tumour necrosis factor and soluble tumour necrosis factor receptors in women with pre-eclampsia. Br J Obstet Gynaecol 102:20–25

Von Dadelszen P, Ornstein MP, Bull SB, Logan AG, Koren G, Magee LA 2000 Fall in mean arterial pressure and fetal growth restriction in pregnancy hypertension: a meta-analysis. Lancet 355:87–92

Wallenburg HCS 1988 Hemodynamics in hypertensive pregnancy. In: Rubin R (ed) Hypertension in pregnancy. Elsevier, New York, pp 66–101

Weinstein L 1982 Syndrome of hemolysis, elevated liver enzymes and low platelet count: severe consequences of hypertension in pregnancy. Am J Obstet Gynecol 142:159–167

Williams KP, Wilson S 1999 Persistence of cerebral hemodynamic changes in patients with eclampsia: a report of three cases. Am J Obstet Gynecol 181:1162–1165

Witlin AG, Saade GR, Mattar F, Sibai BM 2000 Predictors of neonatal outcome in women with severe preeclampsia or eclampsia between 24 and 33 weeks' gestation. Am J Obstet Gynecol 182:607–611

22

Infections in pregnancy

Phillip E. Hay, Mike Sharland, Austin H.N. Ugwumadu

The contribution of the author of the equivalent chapter in the second edition, on which this chapter draws extensively, is gratefully acknowledged.

INTRODUCTION

Traditionally, obstetricians screen pregnant women for infections, which are recognised to cause fetal loss or damage during pregnancy or produce specific congenital syndromes in the newborn. Such infections include syphilis, rubella, cytomegalovirus and toxoplasmosis. The specific diseases screened for, varied widely depending on local prevalence and available resources. In recent years, however, the focus has shifted from the classical congenital infections to the role of subclinical intrauterine infection in the pathogenesis of adverse perinatal outcome. Intrauterine infection elicits a robust, albeit subclinical, fetomaternal host inflammatory response with the release of inflammatory mediators and cytokines. These agents mediate the process of preterm birth and are now also recognised to play a central role in the pathogenesis of fetal cerebral white matter damage and bronchopulmonary dysplasia—precursors of cerebral palsy and chronic lung disease respectively. The underlying disease mechanisms and pathogenic pathways are still unravelling and intervention trials are underway aimed at reducing the long-term sequelae. The relatively recent emergence of the retroviruses, HIV-1 and 2, and their vertical transmission to the fetus during the perinatal period, poses a major challenge to all perinatal care providers worldwide.

During the nineteenth and the early decades of the twentieth centuries, maternal mortality and morbidity caused by hospital acquired Group A streptococcus was very high. Today, advances in infection control measures and the availability of antibiotics have markedly reduced these complications and maternal death secondary to puerperal sepsis is now very rare. Unfortunately, neonatal deaths still occur from Group B streptococcal sepsis and viral infections such as herpes encephalitis. In developing countries, where optimal antenatal care is lacking, these infections continue to contribute significantly to perinatal complications.

INFECTION AND PRETERM LABOUR OR PRETERM DELIVERY

A large body of evidence has accumulated suggesting that as much as 25–40% of preterm births may be attributable to genital tract infections. Studies based on amniocentesis and histopathological examination of the placenta of infants delivered prematurely indicate that over 70% of cases are associated with infection (Lettieri et al 1993). The commonest organisms involved are the Mycoplasmas (*M. hominis* and *Ureaplasma urealyticum*) (Cassell et al 1983, 1993), which are atypical, non-pyrogenic and evade routine clinical and microbiological detection. Endometrial infection from cervico-vaginal organisms such as the Group B streptococcus and organisms associated with bacterial vaginosis may lead to decidual inflammation and chorio-amnionitis, which may progress to amniotic fluid infection and fetal sepsis (Fig. 22.1). There is good epidemiological, clinical and experimental data suggesting a causal relationship between infection and preterm delivery.

In experimental animal models, administration of microorganisms (*Shigella*) and microbial products (*Salmonella* and *Escherichia coli* endotoxins) to pregnant mice, rabbits and other species induced preterm labour and delivery (Zahl & Bjerknes 1943, Bang 1962, Kullander 1977). Prior immunisation of these animals with antiendotoxin antibodies prevented the biologic effect of the endotoxin (Rioux-Darrieulat et al 1978). Recently, a model of ascending intrauterine infection using the hysteroscope to place bacteria in the uterine cavity of rabbits has been developed (Dombroski et al 1990), and used to produce infection-driven preterm delivery in Rhesus monkeys (Gravett et al 1996).

In humans, severe untreated maternal systemic infections such as pneumonia, pyelonephritis, typhoid fever and malaria are strongly associated with preterm labour and delivery (Gilles et al 1969, Cunningham et al 1973, Benedetti et al 1982, Madinger et al 1989). Periodontal infection has been associated with increased risk of preterm delivery and low birthweight (Offenbacher et al 1996). These conditions are now rare in pregnancy in the UK while subclinical intrauterine infection has emerged as a major risk factor for preterm delivery.

The commonest pathway of intrauterine infection is through the ascent of lower genital tract microorganisms from the vagina and cervix (Blanc 1964, Benirschke 1965, Romero et al 1989a). Other routes include the transplacental or haematogenous, retrograde seeding through the fallopian tube from the peritoneal cavity and iatrogenic introduction of organisms during amniocentesis, cordocentesis and chorionic villous sampling. The amniotic cavity is normally sterile. Therefore, isolation of any microorganism from the amniotic fluid is evidence of microbial invasion of the cavity, provided that the amniotic fluid was sampled through the transabdominal route. Transcervical amniocentesis is associated with a high risk of contamination. Intrauterine infection limited to the decidua may elicit factors that mediate preterm labour (Vince et al 1992, Steinborn et al 1996) but will remain undetected because it is difficult to obtain this tissue for microbiological culture. Therefore, studies of patients in preterm labour which focus on microbial invasion of the amniotic fluid, overlook the extra-amniotic intrauterine infections, and thus underestimate the frequency of microbial colonisation of the uterine cavity.

Cellular and biochemical mechanisms

Macrophages activated by bacteria or lipopolysaccharide, respond by secreting a variety of pro-inflammatory cytokines, including interleukin-1 (IL-1), interleukin-6 (IL-6) and tumour necrosis factor (TNF). These endogenous host prod-

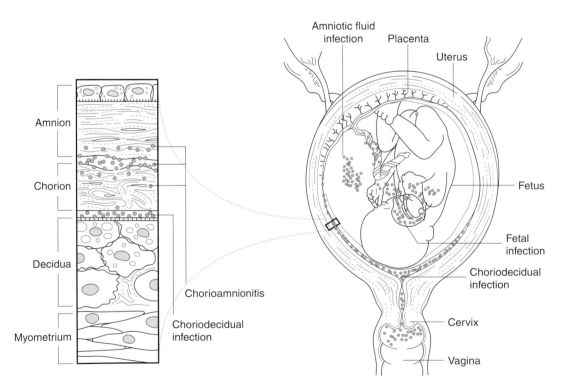

Fig. 22.1 Potential sites of bacterial infection within the uterus.

ucts play a pivotal role in the host response to infection and may also mediate the process of preterm labour and delivery. Human decidua produces IL-1 in response to bacterial products (Romero et al 1989b, Vince et al 1992) and IL-1 stimulates the production of prostaglandin (PG) by the amnion, decidua and myometrium (Hillier et al 1993). Placental tissue obtained from patients with chorio-amnionitis in labour produces larger amounts of IL-1 than that from women not in labour (Taniguchi et al 1991). Furthermore, the bioactivity and concentration of IL-1 is higher in the amniotic fluid and in fetal plasma during preterm labour with evidence of intra-amniotic infection compared to preterm labour without evidence of infection (Romero et al 1989c, 1992, Gomez et al 1998a and b).

Tumour Necrosis Factor alpha is produced by the human decidua in response to bacterial products. It has similar biologic properties to IL-1 (Romero et al 1991) and may act synergistically with IL-1 to increase PG production by intrauterine tissues (Romero et al 1989c, Bry & Hallman 1991). In human pregnancies, the amniotic fluid concentration of TNF-α is higher in patients with preterm labour and infection than in those in preterm labour but without infection (Romero et al 1989c).

Interleukin-6 expression is induced by the pro-inflammatory cytokines IL-1 and TNF and by bacterial products. It induces the production of acute phase proteins such as C-reactive protein by liver cells and the activation of T cells, natural killer cells, and immunoglobin producing B cells (Elder et al 1997). Like IL-1, IL-6 stimulates PG production by amnion and decidual cells, and its concentration and bioactivity are elevated in women with preterm labour and intra-amniotic infection. Amniotic fluid IL-6 measurement is currently the most sensitive and specific test for the detection of microbial invasion of the amniotic cavity (Romero et al 1993a, 1993b) and for the prediction of fetuses at risk of significant neonatal morbidity (Yoon et al 1995, 1996). It may also be a better marker than culture for intrauterine infections, since it may reflect inflammation in intrauterine compartments other than the amniotic cavity (Sebire et al 1996). A growing list of other cytokines with modulatory effects on the parturition process includes IL-6 Soluble Receptor, Colony Stimulating Factors, IL-8 and the inhibitory cytokines IL-1 Receptor Antagonist IL-1ra, Transforming Growth Factor-β, IL-10 and fetal Platelet Activating Factor (Elder et al 1997).

Bacterial phospholipase A_2 and C may stimulate PG output by the human amnion (Bejar et al 1981, Bennett et al 1987) chorion and decidua (Gomez et al 1995). Prostaglandins induce myometrial contractility (Wiqvist et al 1983) and extra-cellular matrix changes in the cervix associated with cervical ripening (Rajabi et al 1991). Amnion obtained from patients with chorio-amnionitis produce higher amounts of PG than amnion from patients without chorio-amnionitis (Lopez et al 1987).

Gestational tissues express both cyclooxygenase-1 (COX-1) and cyclooxygenase-2 (COX-2). COX-1 is constitutive, widely distributed in tissues and it is synthesised in response to physiological stimuli (Vane 1994). COX-2 is inducible and produced by macrophages in response to inflammatory stimuli (Jones et al 1993). Induction and upregulation of intrauterine COX-2 directly increases prostaglandin production, uterine activity and cervical effacement. In amnion tissue, COX-2 may be induced by treatment with IL-1β, TNF-α, and bacterial products (Zakar et al 1994) while IL-1β mediated COX-2 expression and PG biosynthesis may be abolished by the IL-1 receptor antagonist (IL1$_{ra}$) (MacDonald et al 1991).

The enzyme 15-OH prostaglandin dehydrogenase (PGDH) is located in the chorionic trophoblastic cells and rapidly degrades PG produced by amnion and chorion, thus preventing its passage towards the myometrium. It is plausible that excessive production of PG by amnion, chorion and decidua in response to intrauterine infection may overwhelm the PGDH barrier by exhausting its metabolic capacity. Several investigators have found significantly lower quantities of immunoreactive chorionic PGDH in patients with preterm labour and chorio-amnionitis than in patients in preterm labour but without chorio-amnionitis. (Sangha et al 1994, van Meir et al 1997). In addition, cortisol, which is increased in the amniotic fluid of patients in labour (term and preterm) may downregulate the expression of chorionic PGDH and up-regulate the expression of COX-2 through CRH (Jones et al 1990) thus increasing the availability of bioactive PG reaching the myometrium.

Management

Preterm labour or delivery is a syndrome produced by a variety of conditions operating through different pathways and mechanisms. Consequently, none of the currently available interventions such as tocolysis, antibiotic therapy, bed rest and cervical cerclage have definitively been proven to halt the process of preterm labour, prevent preterm delivery and reduce neonatal morbidity and mortality. Women at risk of infection related preterm delivery may present with silent dilatation of the cervix, contractions with intact membranes or with preterm prelabour rupture of membranes.

Studies in which amniotic fluid culture was performed in women with preterm labour and intact membranes suggest an average positive culture rate of approximately 12%. Women with positive cultures did not usually present with clinical evidence of infection, but they were more likely to develop clinical chorio-amnionitis, to be refractory to tocolysis and to rupture their membranes spontaneously than women with negative amniotic fluid cultures (Garite et al 1979, Cotton et al 1984a and b, Romero et al 1988, 1993c, Carroll et al 1996). The use of antibiotic therapy in women in preterm labour with intact membranes has not been shown to be beneficial and is currently not recommended (the results of the Oracle trial are awaited). Women in preterm labour should be transferred to units with neonatal intensive care facilities if these are not available locally. The diagnosis of preterm labour and accurate timing of such transfers is, however, difficult. Whereas uterine activity alone does not indicate labour, the opportunity for intervention may be missed if the clinician delays until the appearance of progressive cervical change. Assessment for other risk factors such as previous preterm birth (Mercer et al 1996), late miscarriages, polyhydramnios or multifetal gestation, may be helpful. However, over 50% of women who deliver prematurely have no identifiable risk factors. Ultrasound examination of the cervix has suggested that between 24 and 28 weeks' gestation, cervical length less than 2.5 cm is associated with a 6–10 fold increase in the risk of preterm delivery (Iams et al 1996). This tool should be employed in the clinical assessment of women in suspected preterm labour if the facilities and expertise exist. Steroid injection up until 34 weeks' gestation is associated with a 60% reduction in the risk of respiratory distress syndrome, 30–40% reduction in the risk of major intraventricular bleeding and necrotising enterocolitis with substantial overall improvement in neonatal morbidity and mortality. In the absence of apparent signs of infection, tocolytics may be administered to delay delivery by 24–48 hours to enable steroids to take effect. Clinical chorio-amnionitis, defined as tender and irritable uterus, associated with maternal pyrexia, tachycardia, leucocytosis and purulent or offensive vaginal discharge, however, is diagnosed in only 12% of women with microbiologically proven intra-amniotic infections (Romero et al 1989).

PRETERM PRELABOUR RUPTURE OF MEMBRANES

Fetal membranes consist of the amniotic epithelium, the extracellular matrix (made up of the amniotic basement membrane and the underlying connective tissue), chorion and decidua. The connective tissue provides the tensile strength of the membranes and is composed mainly of types I and III collagen (Klima & Schmidt 1988, Schmidt & Klima 1989). The membranes become thinner towards term because of apoptosis and a decrease in collagen content (Skinner et al 1981). Degradation of the extracellular matrix (ECM) by excessive matrix metalloprotease (MMP) activity has been proposed as a cause of a leak of amniotic fluid (French & McGregor 1996, Vandillo-Ortega et al 1996). Their natural inhibitors, tissue inhibitors of metalloproteases (TIMPs), regulate the activity of MMPs *in vivo*. Studies on cultured human fetal membranes show that, in response to bacterial polysaccharide, an imbalance in the levels of MMPs and TIMPs may occur, leading to increased MMP activity and ECM degradation (Fortunato et al 2000). Raised levels of MMPs and reduced concentrations of TIMPs have also been demonstrated in women with preterm prelabour rupture of the membranes (pPROM) (Fortunato 1999). In addition, lower genital tract organisms may elicit a host inflammatory response, elaborate proteases (McGregor et al 1986, 1987) or activate fibroblasts with a subsequent increase in collagenase activity, all of which can damage the fetal membranes (Vadillo-Ortega et al 1991).

It is now acknowledged that pPROM is nearly always the result of, and only rarely a predisposing factor for, infection. Clinical diagnosis of pPROM is made by visualisation of a pool of amniotic fluid in the vagina, with or without a positive nitrazine or ferning test and continually wet sanitary pads. The nitrazine test is based on pH changes and may give a false-positive result secondary to vaginitis, recent sexual intercourse, contamination with blood, or bacterial vaginosis.

The ferning phenomenon is absent in very early gestations and unreliable as the time from pPROM increases. Ultrasound scan may show diminished amniotic fluid volume, confirm fetal presentation, exclude fetal anomalies, provide estimated fetal weight and exclude placental insufficiency. Digital vaginal examination should be avoided as this is associated with a decreased latency period. An initial vaginal swab for microbiology may detect colonisation with group B streptococcus. In general, there is a discrepancy between the organisms isolated from the lower genital tract and those isolated from the amniotic fluid or fetal circulation. Repeated vaginal swabs do not enhance the rate of isolation of organisms and may introduce lower gut organisms. Head down tilt to prevent the leakage of amniotic fluid may provide a rich culture medium for organisms to flourish in the posterior fornix of the vagina. Maternal pyrexia, tachycardia, leucocytosis and raised CRP have variable and unreliable test characteristics as predictors of intrauterine infection in pregnancies complicated by pPROM, and correlate poorly with histologic chorio-amnionitis. This is probably because studies evaluating these indices used different end points for the diagnosis of infection. Histologic chorio-amnionitis is also an insensitive and non-specific marker of intrauterine infection. It is absent in approximately 30% of culture positive placentae and present also in about 30% of culture negative placentae (Hiller et al 1988, Zlatnik et al 1990). More importantly, chorio-amnionitis is a fetal rather than maternal disease, and it is the fetal inflammatory response syndrome (FIRS) that correlates with adverse neonatal outcome rather than abnormal maternal indices.

The aim of the clinical management of pPROM is to distinguish those cases without infection that can be managed expectantly from those with infection where early delivery is indicated. The current indiscriminate use of expectant management, corticosteroid and empiric antibiotic therapy without knowledge of the presence or absence of infection, may enhance the likelihood of occurrence of the complications that we seek to prevent. Clinical detection of intrauterine infection is exceedingly poor while there is strong and persuasive evidence that antenatal exposure of the fetus to infection and pro-inflammatory cytokines is a major risk factor for long-term neurologic and pulmonary damage (Gomez et al 1995, Yoon et al 1995, Watterberg et al 1996, Yoon et al 1996, 1997, 2000).

Management by amniocentesis

Subclinical intrauterine infection is demonstrated to be present in 30–40% of cases of pPROM (Romero et al 1988, Carroll et al 1996). This might be found to be even higher if more sensitive detection techniques such as polymerase chain reaction were used. Subclinical intrauterine infection is associated with a shorter latency period, faster progression to clinical chorio-amnionitis, less (or no) response to tocolysis, and greater risk of neonatal sepsis with long-term sequelae. The use of amniocentesis to demonstrate markers of infection in the amniotic fluid, however, remains controversial. This may reflect fears of procedure-related complications such as fetal injury and a general bias against invasive procedures in pregnancy. The resolution of modern ultrasound scan machines has improved remarkably since amniocentesis was first used to diagnose intrauterine infection in 1979 (Garite et al 1979). The risk of fetal death from exsanguination or trauma from the needle used to perform amniocentesis is very low indeed, albeit finite. These concerns should be balanced against the benefits of establishing or excluding infection when pPROM occurs. Amniocentesis has the potential to detect subclinical infection before the onset of FIRS (Gomez et al 1998) and permit targeted and selective interventions. Detection of intrauterine infection will select out babies that require expeditious delivery and prevent inappropriate use of high doses of tocolytics with the attendant risks of maternal and perinatal morbidity and mortality. If infection is excluded, conservative management can be pursued more confidently and without incurring extra costs and morbidity from hospitalisation and monitoring.

In spite of the apparent potential benefits, there is no evidence at present that the use of amniocentesis in pPROM improves perinatal outcome (Cotton et al 1984). Since microorganisms can exist in other reproductive tract compartments outside the amniotic fluid, amniocentesis at best provides only the minimum estimate of the incidence of subclinical intrauterine infection. Women with pPROM and advanced infections have short pPROM—delivery interval and severe oligohydramnios, both of which may preclude assessment by amniocentesis (Gonik et al 1985a, 1985b, Vintzileos et al 1985). On the other hand, intrauterine infection contained within the chorio-decidua but yet to reach the amniotic fluid may produce pPROM but yield a false-negative amniotic fluid culture. In one study where amniocentesis was performed at presentation after pPROM and repeated at the onset of spontaneous labour, 75% of patients with initial negative amniotic fluid cultures were positive when the procedure was repeated (Romero et al 1988). Even if the diagnosis of infection was promptly made by amniocentesis, we do not know whether fetal injury has already occurred. If such damage has not occurred, our interventions may not be sufficient to prevent it. Although an earlier meta-analysis of randomised controlled trials of antibiotic therapy in women with pPROM showed a prolongation of the latency period, reduced incidence of chorio-amnionitis, neonatal sepsis, pneumonia and intraventricular haemorrhage (Mercer & Arheart 1995), the 1999 Cochrane review showed no benefit from antibiotic use. At present in the UK, the routine use of antibiotics in the management of pPROM is not recommended. Furthermore, the antibiotic of choice, the optimal dose, duration of therapy and route of administration is unknown, and there is a risk of infection from resistant and subpathogenic organisms such as *Candida spp*.

BACTERIAL VAGINOSIS AND PREGNANCY OUTCOME

Bacterial vaginosis (BV) is a clinical syndrome of unknown aetiology characterised by an overgrowth of vaginal anaerobes such as *Gardnerella vaginalis*, *Bacteroides spp*. *Mycoplasma hominis* and *Mobiluncus spp* and variable degrees of depletion of protective lactobacilli. In an unselected population, the prevalence rate is 10–20% (Mead 1993). BV is the commonest cause of vaginal discharge in women of childbearing age, although 50% of sufferers are asymptomatic (Eschenbach et al 1988). The principle symptom of offensive fishy smelling vaginal discharge is often more apparent during menstruation or following unprotected intercourse. The vaginal pH is raised from the normal level of less than 4.5 to levels as high as 6 or 7. BV may be transient, intermittent or persistent but it tends to resolve spontaneously during pregnancy in 40–50% of cases (Hay et al 1994). It is currently not regarded as a sexually transmitted infection, and there is no benefit from treating male partners (Vejtorp et al 1988, Moi et al 1989).

The clinical diagnosis of BV is based on any three of Amsel's four composite criteria, comprising of the presence of characteristic discharge, raised vaginal pH, positive potassium hydroxide (whiff) test and the presence of clue cells on microscopy (Amsel et al 1983). Examination of a wet mount of vaginal fluid microscopically shows the presence of many small bacteria. These adhere to the epithelial cells giving them a fuzzy border, the clue cell. Gram staining of air-dried vaginal smears is a more reliable and reproducible method of diagnosis (Nugent et al 1991). Moreover, it detects the less florid but nevertheless abnormal intermediate flora. *Gardnerella vaginalis* is present in the vagina of 50–60% of healthy BV negative women (Sobel 1997) and its isolation from cultures of vaginal swabs is not diagnostic of BV. New rapid tests based on DNA probes for *G. vaginalis* genes (e.g. Affirm VPIII) and on the measurement of metabolic products of anaerobic bacteria such as proline aminopeptidase are being developed and evaluated (Thomason et al 1988, O'Dowd & Bourne 1994).

Many observational studies have confirmed that BV is associated with a 2–5-fold increase in the risk of mid trimester pregnancy loss and preterm delivery (Kurki et al 1992, Hay et al 1994a and b, McGregor et al 1994, Hillier et al 1995, Llahi-Camp et al 1996). BV is also associated with an increased risk of pPROM, chorio-amnionitis, amniotic fluid colonisation, low-birth-weight infants and postpartum endometritis (Silver et al 1989, Martius & Eschenbach 1990). The most common organisms cultured from the membranes, amniotic fluid and placentas of preterm births are BV related including *M. hominis* and fastidious anaerobic organisms (Hillier et al 1988).

Treatment

At present studies are evaluating the use of antibiotics to treat women in pregnancy with bacterial vaginosis. Studies of selected women at high risk of preterm birth have shown benefit from treatment with antibiotics (Morales et al 1994, Hauth et al 1995, McGregor et al 1995). However, these studies have been criticised either for their small sample sizes or design flaws. The role of screening and treatment is less clear in women without risk factors for preterm birth. Symptomatic women should of course be treated. The current recommendation by the Centres for Disease Control, Atlanta USA (1998) and the UK's Drug and Therapeutics Bulletin

(Anon 1998) is to screen for and treat BV in women at high risk of preterm delivery.

Two recent large randomised controlled trials of oral metronidazole for the treatment of BV in pregnancy did not show a reduction in the risk of preterm birth in low-risk pregnant women (McDonald et al 1997, Carey et al 2000). These studies, however, introduced therapy late in the second trimester of pregnancy using short courses of oral metronidazole. Screening late in pregnancy may miss cases where BV had resolved spontaneously, although such spontaneous resolution does not modify the risk of PTD (Gratacos et al 1998). Moreover, the efficacy of short courses of metronidazole for the treatment of BV in pregnancy is not clearly established. The question still remains whether screening for and treating BV earlier in pregnancy may yet be beneficial in the so-called low-risk pregnancy. The optimal time to introduce therapy is, however, unknown.

Antibiotic choice and route of administration

Women with BV may also have endometrial colonisation by BV organisms and subclinical endometritis (Korn et al 1995). Although topical clindamycin cream eradicates BV in pregnancy and reduces the activity of mucinase and sialidase in the vagina (McGregor et al 1994), it has not been shown to reduce the risk of PTD presumably because intravaginal medication may not eradicate BV organisms in the endometrial cavity (Joesoef et al 1995). If treatment is indicated in pregnancy the oral route is recommended. The standard treatment for bacterial vaginosis in the UK is oral metronidazole 400 mg twice a day for five days. Alternatively, oral clindamycin 300 mg twice a day for five days may be used. In our experience, recurrence of BV following successful treatment in pregnancy is unusual and re-screening is rarely warranted. Physicians have been wary of prescribing metronidazole during pregnancy because of reputed teratogenicity. Several metanalyses have reviewed pregnancies where it was prescribed and have shown no excess of birth defects (Anon 1998). The potential risks should be discussed with each individual woman and weighed against the benefits. Both oral and intravaginal clindamycin have been associated with pseudomembranous colitis, a potentially fatal condition. Women who develop diarrhoea following such treatment should cease treatment and seek medical advice. Given that the fetus and its immune system are involved in the infective process, antibiotic therapy alone may not be sufficient to reverse the effects of fetal infection and immune activation. The current practice of antenatal steroid administration to induce lung maturation in pregnancies at risk of PTD may favourably, albeit inadvertently, attenuate the inflammatory response.

INFECTION AND ADVERSE NEONATAL OUTCOME

Germinal matrix haemorrhage and intraventricular haemorrhage

Low gestational age is a major risk factor for intraventricular haemorrhage (IVH). However, infants with inflamed membranes and raised amniotic fluid IL-6 have a 3–4-fold increase in the risk of IVH compared to their peers without inflamed membranes (Morales 1987, Salafia et al 1995, Yoon et al 1995). The brain phagocytes, microglial cells, express IL-1β, IL-6 and TNF-α following stimulation by lipopolysaccharide (Hopkins & Rothwell 1995). The biologic effects of the pro-inflammatory cytokines released during intrauterine infection, can at least in part, explain the association between infection and intraventricular haemorrhage. TNF-α may produce generalised vasodilatation, increased vascular permeability, shock, and myocardial depression, all of which may lead to circulatory disturbances within the germinal matrix region of the developing fetal brain.

The germinal matrix zone is an unique but transient embryonic tissue of the fetal brain located immediately adjacent to the lateral ventricles. The motor nerves cells and their axons (white matter) in the matrix are perfused by a loose network of fragile and immature blood vessels supported by a single cell layer of endothelium with no muscularis or muscle coats. This deficiency perhaps reflects the fact that the germinal matrix is destined to involute at approximately 32–34 weeks' gestation. Furthermore, the zone is located at the vascular boundary of the cerebral circulation. This location as well as the fragile capillaries, predisposes the matrix zone to ischaemia and haemorrhage during fluctuations in cerebral blood flow secondary to sepsis or hypoxia. Since septic and hypoxic fetuses lack the auto-regulatory capacity to maintain a steady cerebral blood flow, dramatic alterations in the cerebral blood flow induced by TNF-α may lead to rupture within the tenuous germinal matrix vasculature. Bleeding into the matrix may subsequently rupture the single ependymal cell layer, which separates the matrix zone from the lateral ventricle and lead to IVH (Sarnat 1992).

Cytokines may further attenuate the already rather ineffective fetal blood–brain barrier, which protects the brain from blood borne proteins and toxins (Adinolfi 1985, Quagliarello et al 1991, Wright & Merchant 1994, Saija et al 1995). In humans, intrathecal TNF-α levels correlated with blood brain barrier damage (Sharief et al 1992). In severe cerebral malaria, brain haemorrhage correlates with TNF-α mediated cerebrovascular damage (Grou & Lou 1993). Cytokines mediate intravascular adhesion and transendothelial migration of leucocytes. Astrocytes treated with TNF-α express the message for adhesion molecules and may attract inflammatory leucocytes into the brain tissue, thereby increasing the damage (Hurwitz et al 1992, Merrill & Benvenista 1996). It is conceivable that the adhesion of leucocytes to the single endothelial cell vessels of the matrix zone may be followed by vascular damage and bleeding into the germinal matrix. Moreover, ventriculomegaly arising from IVH may compress adjacent periventricular capillaries causing ischaemia and further damage of fetal brain white matter.

Periventricular leukomalacia and cerebral palsy

Periventricular leukomalacia (PVL) or necrosis, is an acquired set of morphological abnormalities of the developing brain. It is defined on neurosonography as cystic, echolucent or hypoechoeic images in the cerebral white matter. PVL is the precursor lesion of cerebral palsy (CP) and predicts CP and other motor disabilities and neurodevelopmental disorders in 60–100% of affected preterm infants (Paneth et al 1994). The current consensus is that PVL is due to hypoxic-ischaemic injury or necrosis of the periventricular white matter resulting from impaired or increased perfusion of the germinal matrix zone during severe compromise of cardio-respiratory function. The cytokine TNF-α, released during host response to infection may induce circulatory collapse and in addition exert direct toxic effects on oligodendrocytes (Robbins et al 1987, Kahn & DeVellis 1994). Yoon et al has shown in two separate studies (1997, 2000) that infants at risk of developing PVL, and subsequently CP at three years of age, can be identified by prior antenatal exposure to high concentrations of pro-inflammatory cytokines. Studies in preterm infants have also demonstrated a correlation between positive amniotic fluid culture for microbes, raised amniotic fluid or umbilical cord blood concentrations of IL-1, IL-6, IL-8 and TNF-α and the development of PVL (Gomez et al 1995, Yoon et al 1996).

The long held belief that cerebral palsy is the result of antepartum and intrapartum hypoxic events is now relegated by recent epidemiologic, clinical and animal experimental evidence, which suggest a greater role for infection or inflammation in the pathogenesis of cerebral palsy (Bejar et al 1988, Murphy et al 1995, Grether & Nelson 1997, Yoon et al 1997), and it attributes a much more limited role to birth asphyxia (Nelson & Ellenburg 1986, Paneth 1986a,b). Even amongst very low-birth-weight preterm infants, those with chorio-amnionitis are at a greater risk of IVH and PVL (Dammann & Leviton 1997). Since IVH and PVL may be seen in stillborn babies and in infants delivered by elective caesarean section, and they may also appear late in the neonatal period, the role of central nervous system trauma in the etiology of these lesions is also in doubt.

Bronchopulmonary dysplasia

Bronchopulmonary dysplasia (BPD) is a form of chronic lung disease that affects approximately 20% of preterm babies who require mechanical ventilation. These infants are at increased risk of recurrent respiratory infections, failure to thrive, cardiovascular disease and neurodevelopmental delay. Pulmonary prematurity, barotrauma and supplemental oxygen are recognised major risk factors for BPD. Rojas et al (1995) observed that neonates who acquired nosocomial infections developed BPD more frequently than non-infected ones and proposed that infection caused pulmonary damage and predisposed to BPD. Subsequent studies have suggested a role for colonisation of the respiratory tract with *M. hominis* (Cassell et al 1991), *U. urealyticum* (Wang et al 1988), *C. trachomatis* (Numazaki et al 1986) and CMV (Sawyer et al 1987) in the risk of developing BPD. Postmortem examinations also show inflammatory changes more frequently in the lungs of infants who died from BPD than in those without BPD (Vapaavuori & Krohn 1971). Bronchopulmonary dysplasia starts with an initial influx of inflammatory mediators and neutrophils into the tracheo-bronchial effluent. This event appears to signal the development of the subacute and chronic fibroproliferative phase, which characterises BPD. The antigenic stimuli that initiate the inflammatory component of BPD and the repertoire of host cytokines that mediate the influx of neutrophils into the tracheo-bronchial tree are not yet fully understood. The likely candidates include the mycoplasmas. *M. hominis* and the *M. hominis* antigen are potent stimulators of the production of the chemotactic cytokine IL-8 by type II epithelial alveolar cells (Kruger & Baier 1997). A study of IL-8 and IL-6 levels in serial tracheal aspirates of preterm infants showed that high levels of these cytokines preceded the neutrophil influx seen in infants who develop BPD. This suggests that these cytokines either initiate the acute inflammatory cascade in the lungs or that they are early risk markers for BPD (Munshi et al 1997).

In at least a subset of infants that develop BPD, the inciting event may be antenatal exposure to infection and pro-inflammatory cytokines. Babies born to women with positive amniotic fluid cultures for microorganisms (Watts et al 1992), chorio-amnionitis (Watterburg et al 1996), and raised IL-1β level within 24 hours of birth were at increased risk of BPD. More recently, Yoon et al (1997) demonstrated significantly higher umbilical cord plasma IL-6 levels in preterm infants who developed BPD, compared with preterm babies who did not develop BPD.

SPECIFIC INFECTIONS THAT AFFECT THE FETUS

An expanded acronym STORCH (Table 22.1, replacing TORCH) may be applied to infections that may adversely affect the fetus or newborn.

Syphilis

Syphilis is a sexually transmitted infection caused by the spirochete *Treponema pallidum*. Acquisition of this organism

Table 22.1 STORCH—Specific infections that adversely effect the fetus, neonate or pregnant woman

S	Syphilis
T	Toxoplasmosis
O	Other
	Bacterial vaginosis
	Trichomonas vaginalis
	Group B streptococcus
	Escherichia coli
	Ureaplasma urealyticum
	Haemophilus influenzae
	Varicella
	Listeria monocytogenes
R	Rubella
C	Cytomegalovirus
H	Herpes
	HIV
	Hepatitis B
	Human papillomavirus
	Human parvovirus

occurs through sexual contact or across the placenta. It is common in many developing countries where up to 10% of pregnant women may have positive serological tests. In Western Europe and the United States the incidence has fallen progressively over the course of the second half of the twentieth century. An increase in incidence in the United States during the late 1980s was linked to drug misuse, as was a small epidemic in Bristol in the United Kingdom in 1998. Such outbreaks including the epidemic reported in Russia and Eastern Europe during the 1990s, reinforce the importance of continued vigilance and surveillance against this infection. The organism probably enters the host's body through inapparent breaks in the skin, which may occur during sexual intercourse.

Diagnosis

Primary syphilis presents as a painless genital ulcer three to six weeks after acquisition. In women the ulcer is most often on the cervix or in the vagina and it may therefore pass unnoticed. There is usually local lymphadenopathy. At this stage the infection is highly contagious. Secondary syphilis occurs six weeks to six months after infection, often just as the primary chancre is regressing. It usually presents as a symmetrical, non-pruritic, maculo-papular rash, which usually affects the palms of the hands and soles of the feet. It may vary from pale macules through to dense plaques resembling psoriasis. The rashes may be associated with a generalised lymphadenopathy and pyrexia, reflecting the systemic distribution of spirochetes. There may be lesions affecting the mucous membranes. In moist areas, the rashes may coalesce to form warty growths called *condylamata lata*, thought to arise because of host response to the presence of the treponemes and the deposition of immune complexes in the walls of vessels (Jorizzo et al 1986). The lesions of secondary syphilis actively shed spirochetes and caution must be exercised when handling patients with suspicious lesions. Other manifestations include alopecia, uveitis, and sensorineural deafness.

If no specific treatment is administered, the lesions regress after 2–4 weeks but may relapse during the following two years. At this stage the infection is called early latent, as it may be transmitted sexually during relapses, or transplacentally, giving rise to congenital syphilis. Subsequently, syphilis cannot be transmitted sexually and late latent infection ensues. About 20% of untreated patients will ultimately develop symptomatic cardiovascular tertiary syphilis including aortic aneurysm and insufficiency, probably due to vasculitis of the vasa vasorum, while 5–10% will develop neurosyphilis with meningo-vascular disease, or later, generalised paresis of the insane and tabes dorsalis.

Syphilis may infect the fetus at any time during gestation and it can be transmitted during any stage of maternal disease. The risk of fetal infection is proportional to maternal spirochetemia, which correlates with maternal disease stage. It is highest if primary or secondary maternal syphilis occurs during pregnancy when almost all fetuses will be infected, with 50% showing signs of congenital syphilis at birth. Early latent syphilis is associated with a 40% risk of congenital syphilis while the risk of transmission in later stages of disease decreases steadily to 10–15% of off-spring of women with late disease, usually after five years of maternal acquisition. The spectrum of congenital syphilis varies from a severe fetal infection causing intrauterine death, to a baby with symptomatic disease (early congenital syphilis).

Early congenital syphilis is described in babies born with symptomatic disease and children of less than two years of age. The immediate systemic distribution of the haematologically-acquired treponemes may affect any fetal organ system; this is the fetal equivalent of secondary syphilis in the adult. The syphilitic placenta is characteristically large, waxy and oedematous. The affected infants may be born with hepatitis, splenomegaly, lymphadenopathy, anaemia, maculopapular rash, mucous patches, condylomata lata, rhinorrhoea (snuffles), laryngitis with or without pneumonia, peri-osteitis, osteo-chondritis or active neurosyphilis. As in adult secondary syphilis, the skin lesions and mucous secretions from these infants are infectious. This pattern of presentation is, however, rare today because of prenatal screening and treatment. Late congenital syphilis is applied to children who subsequently develop the stigmata of congenital syphilis and in those over two years of age with Hutchingson's triad of interstitial keratitis, notched incisor teeth and sensorineural (eight nerve) deafness. Some infected children are asymptomatic.

Any woman presenting during pregnancy with genital ulcers, should be screened for syphilis and herpes. A dark ground microscope examination should be performed to look for *T. pallidum* and blood taken for serology. Two main classes of serological tests are employed for the diagnosis of syphilis. The non-treponemal antibody or flocculation tests (VDRL and RPR) are non-specific tests based on the detection of IgM and IgG to cardiolipin. Cardiolipin makes up 10% of the treponemal lipids but is also found in other mammalian tissues. The antibodies are produced in response to lipids released from damaged host's cells and from the cell surface of *T. pallidum*. Treponemal antibody tests (TPHA, TPI, FTA-absorbed) are group specific antibody tests based on the detection of the host's antibody produced against treponemal antigens. They confirm exposure to infection at some stage of life and remain positive for life, even after treatment. The three species of Treponema known to cause human disease are *T. pallidum* (syphilis), *T. pertenue* (yaws) and *T. carateum* (pinta). They are indistinguishable either by electron microscopy or (so for) by DNA analysis, but the diseases they produce are easily distinguishable clinically.

After treatment the VDRL titre falls progressively and will be non-reactive in most individuals after two years. Biological false-positive VDRL tests may occur in women with systemic lupus erythematosis or the antiphospholipid syndrome, usually at a titre of 1 : 8 or less. Therefore, if the VDRL is positive, but FTA and TPHA are negative an autoantibody screen should be performed and lupus antibody sought. Immigrants from tropical countries may have one of the tropical treponematoses, which are not sexually transmitted or transmissible to the fetus. Of these, yaws is still found in hot humid parts of sub-Saharan Africa and SouthEast Asia. Endemic non-venereal syphilis is found in the Sahel region of North Africa, the Middle East and the Gobi desert. Pinta is a milder disease, manifesting as patches of depigmentation and is found in isolated areas of South America. Even after treatment, individu-

Table 22.2 Screening for infection during pregnancy

Infection	Screening test	Action in antenatal clinic	Action for the neonate	Note
Universal in the UK, or in some parts of the UK				
Syphilis	Serum for VRDL/TPHA (ELISA)	Refer to specialist if reactive. If no history of prior treatment will need parenteral penicillin treatment for 12 days	Neonatal treatment might be indicated, especially if the mother was not treated with penicillin	Depending on the background prevalence, a positive screening test may not have a high positive predictive value
Rubella	Serum for rubella IgG	If negative avoid contacts and vaccinate in the puerperium		Perinatal rubella is preventable through vaccination in adolescence
Hepatitis B	Serum for surface antigen test	Check maternal liver function and refer to hepatitis clinic	Immunoglobulin and vaccination for the neonate	Universal precautions. Not an indication for routine elective caesarean section
HIV	Serum for HIV1 and HIV2 antibodies	Refer to specialist if reactive. Manage in multidisciplinary team Antenatal/perinatal antiretroviral treatment	Neonatal antiretroviral treatment Neonatal follow-up	Elective caesarean section Universal precautions
Asymptomatic bacteruria	MSU	Antibiotic treatment and retesting ± antibiotic prophylaxis		
May be indicated in some settings				
Group B streptococcus	High vaginal swab culture	None		According to local protocols women in preterm labour or with premature rupture of membranes may receive presumptive treatment
Herpes simplex	Serum antibodies to HSV2 Speculum examination in early labour for herpetiform ulcers	Women with known recurrent genital herpes may avoid an acute recurrence in labour if treated with prophylactic acylcovir		Offer caesarean section if herpetiform ulcers in labour
Toxoplasmosis	Serum IgG and IgM	Rising IgM titres suggest recent infection. Refer for specialist evaluation (cordocentesis)	Follow up	Routine in France but not in the UK as toxoplasmosis is too rare
Bacterial vaginosis	Vaginal pH or gram stain	Metronidazole or clindamycin in women at increased risk of preterm labour		Low risk intervention but high number of patient needed to treat to prevent one harmful outcome. Current recommendations are inconclusive
Chlamydia trachomatis	Urethral and cervical swabs First void urine for DNA detection		Tetracycline eye ointment prophylaxis in high prevalence populations	Women undergoing termination should either have presumptive treatment or a recent negative screening test
Gonorrhoea	Urethral and cervical swabs for culture		Tetracycline eye ointment prophylaxis in high prevalence populations Avoid breast feeding if possible	
Hepatitis C	Serum IgG			Universal precautions Not an indication for routine elective caesarean section
Malaria	Negative blood film does not exclude placental infection	Antenatal prophylaxis and possible insecticide treated bed nets in high prevalence populations		May present as maternal anaemia with negative blood film in hyperendemic area
Gastrointestinal parasites	Stool for ova and parasites	Screen immigrants from high prevalence countries		? presumptive treatment in high prevalence countries
Tuberculosis	Chest X-ray, sputum for AAFB	Screen immigrants from high prevalence countries		

als who have had these infections continue to have positive serological tests for syphilis. If syphilis cannot be excluded, they should be treated as though they have syphilis since a history of yaws does not exclude subsequent acquisition of syphilis.

Treatment

Penicillin is the treatment of choice for syphilis. For early syphilis (primary, secondary or early latent), procaine penicillin 1.2 MU daily, intramuscularly, for 12 days should be administered. Later stages of syphilis require 21 days of treatment. Particularly during early syphilis, a Jarisch–Herxheimer reaction may occur. This is mediated by the release of pro-inflammatory cytokines in response to dying organisms, and presents as a worsening of symptoms, and fever for 12–24 hours after starting treatment. It does not represent an allergic reaction and may be associated with uterine contractions and preterm labour. Women should be advised to return to hospital early if they feel uterine contractions. In anticipation of preterm labour, some clinicians admit women with primary or secondary syphilis to initiate treatment with intravenous penicillin.

Women who are allergic to penicillin represent a problem. Tetracycline, the second line treatment is contraindicated in pregnancy. Erythromycin is less reliable and indeed resistance has been reported. If it is to be used, it is best to administer it intravenously. The alternative is to perform penicillin desensitisation with assistance from a clinical allergist. It is essential that current and recent sex partners of women with syphilis are screened as well as her older children if the date of acquisition is unknown. Treatment in pregnancy should be instituted prior to 20 weeks to prevent the development of the stigmata of congenital syphilis (Wendel 1988). In one population studied in the USA, a third of the cases of syphilis seen in pregnant women were acquired during the course of the index pregnancy suggesting that rescreening may be an appropriate policy in some select populations (Goldmeier & Hay 1993).

Toxoplasmosis

Toxoplasmosis is caused by *Toxoplasma gondii*, an obligate intracellular protozoan parasite, which infects a wide variety of wild and domestic animals including household cats. It is usually acquired from eating uncooked meat or exposure to cysts deposited in soil contaminated with cat faeces. The prevalence varies widely according to eating habits. Thus, in France more than 70% of pregnant women have been infected and are immune before they fall pregnant, while in the UK only 10–20% of women are immune. An estimated one in 140 pregnant women in France and one in 400 in the UK acquire the infection during pregnancy. Primary infection, even during pregnancy, often passes unnoticed. It may cause a glandular fever like illness with atypical lymphocytes seen on a blood film. Occasionally it causes fulminating pneumonitis or fatal encephalomyelitis. Eye infections, presenting as choroido-retinitis can occur from either congenital or acquired infection. In AIDS, as immunity wanes, previously quiescent toxoplasma may recur, causing multiple brain abscesses. Approximately 10–25% of infections occurring

during the first trimester of pregnancy are transmitted to the fetus but these are likely to cause severe fetal damage. In the third trimester, 75–90% of infections are transmitted but the risk of fetal damage decreases from 65% in the first trimester to almost zero for those infected near delivery. Most congenitally infected infants are asymptomatic at birth but they may develop seqelae such as chorio-retinitis, strabismus, hydrocephalus or microcephaly, convulsions, developmental delay or deafness up until the child is several years old. Only 20% of newborns with congenital infection have sufficiently severe disease to display clinically apparent signs. Severely infected infants may have the classic tetrad of hydrocephalus or microcephaly, chorio-retinitis, convulsions and cerebral calcifications. Hydrocephalus results from subependymal proliferation of trophozoites with subsequent dissemination of toxoplasma in the ventricular system, which may lead to obstruction of the aqueduct of Sylvius or the foramen of Monro. In such cases, extensive neurological damage may occur and lead to neonatal death.

Diagnosis

At present only 10 or so severely affected babies are diagnosed per year in the UK. Routine screening in pregnancy is therefore not undertaken. A variety of serological tests are available to demonstrate past (IgG) and recent (IgM) infections. The Sabin–Feldman dye test is performed in reference laboratories. This test depends on the lysis of the trophozoite form of the organism by the patient's antibody in the presence of complement. It is highly specific but it requires living parasites and does not differentiate between IgG and IgM antibody subtypes. A high titre of antibody on the dye test (1–500 or higher) is suggestive but not diagnostic of current infection as titres may persist for several years. Enzyme linked immunosorbent assays are available and IgM antibody can also be measured. However, since specific IgG and IgM antibodies may persist in serum for many months, a single high IgM titre may not necessarily indicate a recent infection and a second high IgM titre is required to confirm the diagnosis of acute toxoplasmosis infection. The most definitive test is demonstration of the parasite in lymph node tissue or cerebrospinal fluid. It can be isolated by inoculation into mice. A presumptive clinical diagnosis can be made for congenital infection if the full clinical features are present and the infant has an elevated toxoplasma antibody titre. If the titre remains high for at least six months the diagnosis becomes definite. The presence of IgM antibody in cord blood is suggestive, but this can occur from a placental leak and repeat testing should be performed. A negative IgM test does not exclude congenital toxoplasmosis. Cordocentesis or amniocentesis may be used to diagnose prenatal infection. However, specific fetal antibodies are found in only 20% of affected fetuses, presumably because of the relative immaturity of the fetal immune system or possibly related to the suppressive effect of transplacentally acquired maternal IgG, which is present in all newborns of women with toxoplasmosis.

Treatment

Specific treatment is not necessary in mild or asymptomatic adult infection. Early treatment of acute toxoplasmosis may reduce the risk of congenital infection and pregnancy loss and also may modify the frequency of neonatal lesions (Krick & Remington 1978) A combination of sulphadiazine and pyrimethamine is used in symptomatic adults. Pyrimethamine, however, is potentially teratogenic and should not be used during the first trimester. Spiramycin, a macrolide antibiotic is less toxic and is devoid of teratogenic effects. A three-week course of 2–3 grams per day is administered during pregnancy. While this reduces the incidence of transplacental infection, it has not been shown definitively to reduce the incidence of clinical congenital disease. In France, where many more women acquire toxoplasma infection during pregnancy, women are screened antenatally, although the benefits of such a programme appear to be limited. Congenital toxoplasmosis should be treated with pyrimethamine and sulphonamide when diagnosed.

Prevention

Pregnant women should be informed of the mode of spread of toxoplasmosis from meat and cat faeces and should avoid eating rare steaks or hamburgers. They should exercise due care when handling raw meat, wash their hands with soap and water and avoid handling cats, particularly cat litter. Children's sandpits should be covered to prevent cats from defaecating in them. Infected kittens are far more infectious than infected adult cats. In high prevalence areas, women planning a pregnancy should ideally have serological tests to determine whether they are at risk of acquiring the infection during pregnancy. The patient with a positive specific IgG to *T. gondii* is protected against infection during pregnancy and her fetus is not at risk of congenital disease, provided she is not immunocompromised. A negative antibody status indicates susceptibility to acute infection and is an indication to institute preventive measures. Although *T. gondii* has been isolated from human breast milk (Langer 1963), there are no reports of transmission during breast feeding-feeding.

Cytomegalovirus

Cytomegalovirus (CMV) is a herpes virus and therefore has the ability to establish latency. It is the commonest cause of fetal and perinatal infection. In the UK, approximately 40% of pregnant women are susceptible at the beginning of their pregnancy. CMV is spread through the respiratory and genitourinary tract. Since the primary infection is frequently asymptomatic or produces only a mild non-specific glandular fever-like illness, the incidence of infection in pregnancy is reported as 0.5 to 1 percent, but is estimated to also be about 1% in seronegative women during pregnancy. Approximately 40% of these infections will be transmitted transplacentally to the fetus (Stagno et al 1982a). In healthy women, reactivation of latent CMV infection is unusual but it may occur in pregnancy, probably because of the relative depression of cell mediated immunity associated with pregnancy. There is no correlation between the rate of intrauterine infection (following acute maternal infection) and the gestational age of the pregnancy. Unlike toxoplasmosis and rubella, early intrauterine CMV infection does not seem to confer a greater risk of fetal damage (Preece et al 1983).

Over 90% of infected infants are asymptomatic with only 2–4% exhibiting sufficiently severe disease to be recognised clinically at birth (Stagno et al 1982a). Thus, of an estimated 1000 infected babies born per year in the UK, only about 100 are damaged by the virus. The principle features are microcephaly, blindness and deafness. Other manifestations include hepatosplenomegaly, jaundice, thrombocytopaenia and petechial haemorrhages, pneumonitis, chorio-retinitis, cerebral calcification and developmental delay. CMV is the commonest cause of mental retardation and childhood deafness related to puerpural infection (Simon & McCracken 1986) with another estimated 100 children born each year with sensorineural hearing loss as the only sign of congenital CMV infection.

Because the primary infection in the mother is usually asymptomatic the diagnosis is rarely made before birth. Congenital infection in the babies of women who acquire primary CMV infection in pregnancy is associated with more frequent and severe disease than infection in the off-spring of women with reactivated infection (Stagno et al 1982b). Following acute infection, the virus may be shed through all body secretions including blood, urine, saliva, tears and stools. In adults viral excretion may persist for weeks or months. In congenitally infected infants, viraemia (Lang & Noren 1968) and viriuria may persist for up to 5 months and 8 years respectively (MacDonald & Tobin 1978). The virus persists in the lymphocytes throughout life and can be transmitted by blood transfusion or transplantation. Infants who acquired CMV from the birth canal or later from the mother's mouth or milk may begin to excrete the CMV virus three to six weeks after birth (Stern 1975). Reactivation occurs intermittently with shedding in the genital, urinary or respiratory tract. In temperate countries infection is usually transmitted by close contact, kissing or sexual contact, with approximately 1–2% of the population being infected each year. In tropical countries, most infections take place in childhood and 60–70% of individuals are infected within six months of birth. The remaining individuals are mostly infected by the age of five and, therefore, there are few susceptible pregnant women. Previous maternal infection does not prevent congenital CMV infection nor protect against the occurrence of serious sequelae as was originally thought (Stern & Tucker 1975). The severity of serious complications may, however, be modified by prior exposure. Subsequent infection may be a result of recrudescence of previous infection or a primary infection by a new strain of CMV. Passively acquired maternal antibodies do not prevent the acquisition of primary CMV infection in the perinatal period. However, infants of CMV seronegative women are still at a greater risk of severe perinatal infections than infants born to seropositive mothers (Reynolds et al 1978, Fowler et al 1992).

Diagnosis

A definitive diagnosis of congenital CMV infection can be made by isolating the virus in cell culture from throat swabs, urine, blood or cerebrospinal fluid in the first three weeks of life. Since infants may secrete the virus for a prolonged period of time, isolation of the virus in the post-neonatal period does not confirm recent infection. Serological diagnosis is made by the demonstration of a rising titre of IgG antibody or specific CMV IgM antibody. Specific IgM antibodies, however, may persist for up to eight months hence a positive test result in early pregnancy could indicate CMV infection acquired prior to conception (Stagno et al 1985). Specific IgA antibodies may persist from a few months to a year. The congenital manifestations need to be differentiated from other congenital infections such as toxoplasmosis, rubella, herpes simplex and syphilis. The adult disease may be complicated by hepatitis or polyneuritis and occasionally it may present as genital ulceration mimicking herpes simplex.

Treatment

Specific antiviral agents such as ganciclovir are available for CMV. These agents are used in immunosuppressed individuals with AIDS or following transplantation. Trials of ganciclovir in infected infants have shown some benefit. Infants with congenital defects may require assistance with rehabilitation.

Rubella (German measles)

This togavirus that causes rubella, whose only known host is man, causes a self-limiting infection in adults or adolescents. Congenital infection, however, may produce devastating fetal and neonatal lesions. Rubella was differentiated from measles and scarlet fever by German investigators in the eighteenth century, hence the name association, but its effect in pregnancy remained unknown until 1941 when Gregg (1941) described the association between maternal rubella infection in pregnancy and congenital cataracts. In most countries between 70–90% of young adults are immune to rubella. In some parts of Asia only 50% are immune. In temperate climates, acquired disease is most common in the spring and early summer with local increases in incidence every 3–5 years.

The incubation period is 2–3 weeks and clinical manifestations include mild fever, sore throat, enlarged cervical glands and a rash that may be discreet or give a general pink flush to the trunk. Infection in children often passes unnoticed. Arthralgia is common in adults and the symptoms may persist for 3–7 days. Maternal viraemia occurs approximately seven days prior to the appearance of the typical rash. Fetal involvement may follow maternal viraemia and decidual infection. The placenta infected by rubella is small with poorly developed terminal villi and thrombotic vessels (Ornoy et al 1973). The virus induces a reduction in the rate of fetal cell growth and division and also interferes with blood supply. These events may manifest as early miscarriage, intrauterine or neonatal death, and neonatal or delayed disease (Ornoy et al 1973). Any symptoms suggestive of rubella during pregnancy should be investigated.

Congenital infection is summarised by the Gregg's triad of cardiovascular defects, eye defects and deafness. In addition, hepatitis, thrombocytopenia, bone involvement, microcephaly, behavioural changes and mental retardation have been reported. Miscarriages, stillbirths and preterm birth can occur. The diagnosis should be suspected in any small-for-gestational-age baby with congenital abnormalities. The congenital syndrome occurs most commonly following infection in early pregnancy when the incidence of congenital rubella syndrome may reach 70%. Many women elect to have a termination of pregnancy if the diagnosis is made at this stage of pregnancy. The anatomical changes are rare in late second trimester infections, however, hearing loss, psychomotor retardation and learning deficits may occur (Rowe 1973). There are no reports of congenital anomalies following third trimester infections but mental retardation and deafness may occur.

Three major categories of congenital rubella syndrome are recognised. In the *transient form*, the neonatal thrombocytopaenia, bone lesions, immunopathy, low birthweight and acute organ inflammation may regress or lead to death. In the *permanent category*, there is persistent inflammation with permanent sequelae including cataracts, retinopathy, congenital heart defects, deafness, microcephaly and mental retardation. The *delayed expression* of the effects of rubella infection is related to progressive internal vessel sclerosis leading to systemic or pulmonary hypertension and progressive central nervous system inflammation resulting in late onset chronic pan-encephalitis and hearing loss (Weil et al 1975). Hypothyroidism, caused by chronic lymphocytic thyroiditis, diabetes melitus, bile duct atresia and cirrhosis, may also occur.

Diagnosis

The virus can be isolated from over 90% of miscarried embryos of infected pregnancies and it appears that approximately half the cases are able to clear the infection as only 50% of proven maternal infections result in infants with persistent IgG or IgM antibodies. Up to 90% of neonates with congenital rubella syndrome continue to shed the virus. At age one, viral shedding occurs in only 10–15% and is rare after two years of age. Such prolonged persistence of the virus has been speculated to reflect a defective immune system. In clinical practice, the diagnosis is based on serological tests. At booking, maternal antibody levels are measured. If the antibody titre is low (< than 15 IU/ml) a booster vaccination should be given after delivery. A very high IgG antibody titre is suggestive of recent infection. Specific IgM is only detectable for 4–6 weeks in most cases. Non-immune women should be advised to stay away from known cases of rubella. If a woman is known to be immune, her fetus is not at risk. Susceptible pregnant women who develop a rash or are exposed should have serological testing, repeated after seven days of exposure and 2–4 weeks after the appearance of the rash. There is no specific treatment available. Congenital rubella can be diagnosed by detecting the virus and secretions from the throat, urine and faeces. It can also be found in cerebrospinal fluid, blood, eyes and ears. Excretion diminishes slowly and has ceased by the age of six months in 70% of cases. Presence of IgG antibody after six months of age is confirmatory and specific IgM may persist for 3–9 months.

Prevention

Since the introduction of the rubella vaccine in 1969 there has been a progressive and significant reduction in the incidence of congenital rubella to a current two cases per year for the whole of the UK. In the past, adolescent girls were vaccinated but in the last decade vaccination has been performed in infancy within the triple measles, mumps, rubella (MMR) vaccine. However, following the recent scares related to the measles vaccine, uptake has dropped below 90% in the UK meaning that a cohort of women susceptible to rubella will continue to present in pregnancy.

Varicella–zoster (chickenpox)

Varicella-zoster is another herpes virus. The disease, also known as chickenpox, is highly contagious and is predominantly seen in children. Less than 2% of varicella infections occur in individuals older than 20 years of age. In the UK, 90% of adults are immune to chickenpox. Shingles is a reactivation that can occur during pregnancy but it does not pose any threat to the fetus. Transmission occurs through droplet spread, with an incubation period of about two weeks. Patients are infectious from 24 hours prior to the appearance of the rash until all the lesions are crusted over, usually one week after eruption. Once the crusts resolve, viral particles can no longer be recovered from the skin lesions (Enders 1984). In children the illness is often mild and there may be only a handful of lesions. In adults there is usually a prodrome, with headache, general aches and pains and malaise. Clusters of vesicles emerge at different stages, usually most densely distributed centrally. If there is any doubt the diagnosis can be confirmed by electron microscopy and culture of vesicle fluid. Once the infection clears, latent infection of both sensory and motor nerve cells is established and can reactivate with dissemination of virus into a dermatome, causing the eruption recognised as shingles. This may be accompanied by damage to neurons, fibrosis, pain and post-herpetic neuralgia.

Pregnant women are more vulnerable to chickenpox and 10% of infected pregnant women develop pneumonitis, which can be fatal. Admission into the intensive care unit for monitoring of oxygen saturation and arterial blood gases is essential if pulmonary symptoms develop. In severe cases, intubation and ventilation may be required to maintain respiratory function. Smokers are more likely to develop this complication. Early intravenous administration of the viral DNA polymerase inhibitor, aciclovir, may ameliorate the severity. The evidence for the benefit of this intervention is not robust. Moreover, aciclovir is eliminated by glomerular filtration and tubal excretion of mostly unchanged drug. The dosage of aciclovir should, therefore, be adjusted according to creatinine clearance (Hankins et al 1987).

Varicella-zoster infection from 20 weeks up until four weeks prior to delivery typically does not affect the fetus. If infection occurs prior to 20 weeks of gestation there is a small risk, approximately 1%, of a congenital varicella syndrome. This consists of hypoplastic limbs, skin scarring and central nervous system anomalies such as mental retardation, cortical atrophy and microcephaly (Paryani & Arvin 1986). If a pregnant woman is exposed to chickenpox or shingles she should be tested for *Varicella zoster* antibody. If she is not immune, varicella-zoster immunoglobulin (VZIG) should be administered. The principal indication for this is the prevention of severe maternal complications. Presently, in the UK, supplies are limited, and so VZIG is only issued prior to 20 weeks or after 36 weeks, when labour is most likely to occur. In the acute phase of the infection, serological tests are negative. At present there is scanty evidence that VZIG prevents viraemia, neonatal varicella or congenital varicella syndrome. The possible role of antiviral agents has not yet been evaluated.

Since the incubation period of varicella-zoster is 8–21 days, disease in the newborn less than eight days of age, is likely to have been transmitted transplacentally (Brunell & Kotchmar 1981). Neonatal chickenpox can occur if the mother presents with symptoms or signs from two days before to five days after delivery, as the fetus has been exposed to the virus in the absence of maternal antibody. Neonatal varicella may be very severe although early reports of a mortality rate of up to 30% were an overestimate. Neonatal prognosis depends on the severity of maternal pneumonia and hypoxaemia. VZIG should be administered to the baby immediately if the mother develops chickenpox. If chickenpox develops during the first month of life intravenous aciclovir should be administered.

OTHER INFECTIONS ASSOCIATED WITH PREGNANCY LOSS AND PRETERM BIRTH

Parvovirus B19

Parvovirus B19 is a small single stranded DNA virus isolated in 1975 (Cossart et al 1975). Human infection causes acute aplastic crises with reduced red cell survival. In children it causes the viral exanthem—erythema infectiosum also known as *slapped cheek syndrome* or *fifth disease*. The latter term reflects the order in which it was discovered in relation to other viral exanthemas, measles being the first disease, scarlet fever second, rubella third and Duke's disease fourth. Parvovirus B19 may cause chronic anaemia in the immunosuppressed.

Approximately 30–60% of adults are seropositive for specific B19 IgG and are thus immune to infection. The virus is spread by respiratory secretions and hand to mouth contact. The incubation period is 4–20 days followed by viraemia. Subjects are, however, infectious 5–10 days after exposure, but before the onset of the rash. B19 infection is asymptomatic in 25% of adults and in over 50% of children who contract it. It may be associated with only mild symptoms of malaise or present with a macular rash. It can be associated with severe arthralgia. In non-immune pregnant women, the risk of infection depends on the degree of contact with infected persons. Without specific exposure, seroconversion still occurs in about 1% of pregnancies. Casual and brief exposure to children with B19 infection results in a 5% seroconversion rate, while prolonged exposures (e.g. teachers exposed during school epidemics) results in a 20% risk of infection. Illness within the household carries a 50% risk of infection in non-immune patients.

In approximately 15% of infections occurring during pregnancy the fetus becomes infected. B19 has a predilection for rapidly dividing cells, particularly erythroblasts. Thus, the major effect of infection is the destruction of red cell precursors leading to persistent and severe anaemia in utero and hydrops fetalis. This can resolve spontaneously or may require intrauterine blood transfusion. Fetal loss may occur but the virus is not considered to be teratogenic, and so far, there are no reported cases of B19 related malformations in human pregnancy. Congenital neonatal infection is also considered to be exceedingly rare.

Diagnosis

The diagnosis of parvovirus infection is confirmed by demonstrating virus specific IgM in maternal serum or demonstrating seroconversion with a previous specimen being negative. However, not all patients with B19 infections determined clinically will be B19 IgM positive. Specific antibodies should be sought in mothers who have the clinical features, or when hydrops fetalis develops. There is no specific treatment for parvovirus infection, but the baby should be monitored carefully with repeat ultrasound examinations. In utero transfusion may be necessary in cases of severe intrauterine anaemia and hydrops. The virus is not teratogenic.

Listeria monocytogenes

Listeria monocytogenes has been isolated from more than 50 species of domestic and wild animals including birds, fish, insects and crustaceans. It is found in sewage, water and mud. It can grow in refrigerated food including meat, eggs and dairy products, particularly soft cheeses. Asymptomatic carriage in man as well as animals is common with up to 29% of healthy people having detectable organism in the faeces (Lamont & Postlethwaite 1986). Such carriage is often transient. Cooking destroys it and, therefore, the risk of infection is greatest with uncooked food. Most infections are probably subclinical but pregnant women are more vulnerable to the infection. In the UK the incidence of congenital Listeria infection is approximately one in 37 000 births.

The organism has the ability to cross intact epithelial surfaces. Once it gains access into the body, *L. monocytogenes* functions as a facultative intracellular parasite growing within macrophages. T cell immunity is therefore important in the modulation of the disease (Mackaness & Hill 1969), and patients with AIDS are at a significantly increased risk from *L. monocytogenes* (Gellin & Broome 1989). In adults the anginose type of listeriosis may be confused with glandular fever. In the oculo-glandular form conjunctivitis and enlargement of the submandibular gland is found. Conjunctivitis may be associated also with meningo-encephalitis. Systemic infection, manifest in most organs, has occasionally been described including arthritis, peritonitis and chronic urethritis. A cutaneous form occurs in those exposed to infected animals, such as veterinary surgeons. In pregnancy, an episode of malaise, headache, fever, backache, conjunctivitis and diarrhoea associated with abdominal or loin pain may occur. Within three weeks of delivery there is often a further episode, which may be mild or subclinical. In 40% of cases fever is not marked at any time and the disease presents as a mild flu-like illness. In animals recurrent or persistent genital Listeria infection causes habitual abortion and it may do the same in man.

Listeria is transmitted through the transplacental or haematogeneous route. Newborn infection occurs in two forms. The early onset type from in utero infection manifests as septicaemia within two days of birth. This is associated with disseminated granulomas involving the liver, placenta and other solid organs. Usually the infant is born premature with signs of respiratory distress and there may be a rash. The late onset form of the disease presents predominantly as meningo-encephalitis after the fifth day and is not unlike late onset group B streptococcal disease. Approximately 30% of babies with early onset disease are born dead. In France, *L. monocytogenes* ranks third, after *E. coli* and group B streptococcus as a cause of neonatal sepsis. The organism has a predilection for infecting the central nervous system in the newborn (as in immunosuppressed adults). There may be only a low-grade fever and focal neurological signs may develop.

Diagnosis

Diagnosis requires a high index of suspicion. Specimens from affected sites including throat, liver, cerebrospinal fluid, vagina and placenta; urine, faeces or blood can be used for culture. Isolation is enhanced by cold passage at 4°C. Serological diagnosis is unsatisfactory, although finding a rising titre of Listeria specific IgM can be helpful.

Treatment

The organism is susceptible to penicillins, macrolides and tetracyclines. Ampicillin is the treatment of choice. Early and aggressive antibiotic treatment may allow continuation of pregnancy with a good outcome (Hume 1976, Fleming et al 1985, Cruikshank & Warenski 1989). Without recognition of the diagnosis the mortality for infantile listeriosis is as high as 90%. Early diagnosis and prompt treatment has reduced this figure to only 50%. The prognosis is worse in preterm babies.

Malaria

Malaria is prevalent throughout the tropics and is a major cause of mortality in both children and adults. Major polymorphisms such as thalassaemia and sickle cell trait provide a selection advantage in these areas because affected individuals are more resistant to severe manifestations of malaria. *Plasmodium falciparum* causes the most severe type of malaria that can present with hepatic and cerebral forms of infection. It is transmitted between human hosts by the female anopheles mosquito. Attempts to eradicate this intermediate host during the 1960s and 1970s with spraying of toxins such as DDT have now been abandoned. *P. falciparum* has been able to develop resistance to most antimicrobials, creating a need for new agents to be developed. The other strains of malaria seldom cause fatal disease but they cause considerable morbidity. They have not so far developed chloroquine resistance. Classically, infection caused by *P. ovale* and *P. vivax* produce a fever on alternate days (Tertian malaria) and *P. malarii* every third day (quartan malaria). The development of the parasite in the mosquito only occurs at warm temperatures. In the tropics, therefore, infection is rarely transmitted at altitudes above 2200 metres.

The principal feature of malaria is episodes of temperatures associated with rigors as the temperature rises followed by sweating as the temperature falls. There is headache, nausea and vomiting. With falciparum malaria the pyrexia may be continuous. The incubation period is approximately two weeks. In severe infections 20% or more of the red cells may be infected. Haemolysis occurs leading to anaemia. This may result in haemoglobinuria (blackwater fever), associated with acute renal failure. Hyponatraemia and disseminated intravascular coagulation may also occur. Cerebral malaria presents with disturbances in consciousness caused by obstruction of cerebral capillaries by infected red cells that have reduced deformability.

Pregnant women are at increased risk of severe manifestations of malaria, particularly hypoglycaemia. Infection may trigger a miscarriage or premature labour. In hyper-endemic areas it may present as severe anaemia, with a negative blood film. Recent trials evaluating the value of intermittent treatment in pregnancy have been reviewed (Yow et al 1980). Drugs given regularly and routinely were associated with fewer episodes of fever in the mother, fewer women with severe anaemia antenatally, and higher average birthweight in infants. Even non-falciparum malaria has been associated with intrauterine growth restriction. Congenital malaria has been described.

Diagnosis

The diagnosis should be suspected in anybody who has been to the tropics and presents with a febrile illness. A history of taking prophylaxis does not exclude the diagnosis, as no prophylaxis is 100% affective. A blood film should be requested and stained for malaria parasites. Repeated blood films should be taken during episodes of fever if the initial test is negative. As well as anaemia there may be thrombocytopenia and elevation of liver enzymes. Fever in the tropics or in those recently returned may be caused by many other infections including typhoid, food poisoning organisms, and viral infections such as dengue fever.

Treatment

Malaria is usually treated with quinine sulphate, initially administered intravenously. Individuals with falciparum malaria should be admitted to hospital and monitored closely as sudden deterioration requiring intensive care may occur. Non-falciparum malaria establishes chronic infection of the liver. If the individual is not returning to an endemic area acute treatment should be followed by a course of fansidar to eradicate such infection. Individuals living in endemic areas acquire immunity to malaria, but this is lost within a few months of moving away. Therefore, anyone travelling from the UK to an endemic area should consider taking prophylaxis. A combination of chloroquine and proguanil taken once weekly provides protection against non-falciparum malaria and falciparum in some areas. Malaria resistant to many antimicrobials is present in sub-Saharan Africa and South East Asia where even mefloquine resistance has been reported. The choice of prophylactic agent should, therefore, be made after consulting current recommendations giving details of resistant resistance patterns. Chloroquine is probably the least toxic prophylactic agent for pregnant women. Those travelling to areas of chloroquine resistance must balance the risk of malaria against the potential toxicity of prophylactic agents. It is safest to avoid travel to such areas when pregnant but, if the mother cannot be persuaded to delay travel, the potential risks and benefits of chemoprophylaxis must be discussed.

OTHER INFECTIONS AFFECTING THE FETUS

Group B streptococcus

Group B streptococcus (GBS) is a gut and genital tract commensal, which may be isolated from 15–30% of healthy women (Baker et al 1980, Christensen et al 1981). The fetal colonisation rate at birth from carrier mothers ranges between 40–75% in different studies (Christensen et al 1981, Baker & Kasper 1985). The attack rate, however, is only 2–3/1000 live births for early disease (less than one week of age) and 0.5/1000 live births for late onset disease (more than one week of age). Epidemiologically, the type III strain causes two-thirds of all invasive group B streptococcal disease in neonates and 90% of infections complicated by meningitis (Baker & Kasper 1985). Clinical virulence correlates with the type specific polysaccharide capsule and production of neuroaminidase (Shigeoka et al 1983). When the concentration of antibody to the type III polysaccharide is low, the likelihood of perinatal infection is increased (Baker et al 1981). Human sera containing high levels of antipolysaccharide IgG is known to be protective (Edwards et al 1980). A significant proportion of women whose infants had GBS septicaemia may be poor IgG responders to bacterial polysaccharide antigen and they may, therefore, remain susceptible to recurrent streptococcal disease in subsequent pregnancies (Christensen et al 1982). Since antibody testing is not available for routine practice, management protocols are based on detection of colonisation and antibiotic treatment (Boyer & Gotoff 1986, Lim et al 1986, Minkoff & Mead 1986, Morales et al 1986).

Prevention

The carriage of GBS is asymptomatic and can occur intermittently at any stage of pregnancy. GBS arrives in the vagina from the gut and it can, rarely, ascend into the uterine cavity by crossing intact fetal membranes to cause a severe and rapidly progressive neonatal infection. Neonatal death or upper maternal genital tract infection may follow, and it may progress to septicaemia and occasionally maternal death. In 30% of pregnant women with positive urine cultures, GBS may be one of the organisms isolated (Wood & Dillon 1981), suggesting that urine culture may be useful for GBS surveillance in pregnancy. Attempts have been made to screen for infection in early pregnancy and eradicate the organism with penicillin. However, recolonisation frequently occurs and this approach has not been shown to reduce the incidence of neonatal infection. In the USA, clinicians adopt either a screening, culture-based strategy or use the presence of clinical risk factors to identify women who require prophylactic antibiotic treatment in labour. With the screening based approach, low vaginal and rectal swabs are obtained at

369

35–37 weeks of gestation and transported to the lab for culture in a selective enriched broth medium. Combining vaginal and rectal swabs and the use of selective transport medium increases the rate of recovery of GBS by more than 25% and 50% respectively (Philipson et al 1995). The sensitivity of antenatal culture obtained between one and five weeks before delivery for the detection of GBS colonisation is 87% and the specificity 97% (Yancey et al 1996). GBS are universally sensitive to penicillin. The first dose should be administered ideally at least 4 hours prior to delivery. With this policy women who previously had GBS infected infant, preterm labour or GBS bacteriuria in the current pregnancy are also treated. In the risk based approach, intrapartum antibiotics are given in the presence of the following risk factors: ruptured membranes of greater than 18 hours duration, preterm delivery, intrapartum fever ≥38°C, a previously affected infant or GBS bacteriuria in the index pregnancy. Both strategies have produced dramatic reductions in the incidence of early onset GBS disease in the USA. The prevalence of GBS carriage is lower in the UK than in the USA and at present there are no good epidemiological data upon which to base a mass screening policy. This problem is, however, being addressed currently. It would be prudent for UK physicians to adopt one of the above preventive approaches, particularly in centres with a high incidence of GBS disease.

Herpes simplex virus

The herpes simplex virus is well adapted to its human host. Primary infection usually presents within seven days of exposure and may be accompanied by widespread lesions around the mouth and oro-pharynx in the case of oral herpes, around the vulva, vagina and cervix in women. If inoculation occurs on skin, a herpetic whitlow may result. In many populations more than 70–80% are exposed to oral herpes, herpes simplex virus type I (HSV1) during childhood. This gives some degree of cross protection against herpes simplex virus type II (HSV2), traditionally the causative agent of genital herpes, such that primary infection may be mild. With less exposure to infections in childhood in Western societies fewer young adults have been exposed to HSV1 and at present 50% of cases of genital herpes are now caused by this strain of virus. Primary infection may therefore follow oro-genital contact. Sero-prevalence studies suggest that 15–70% of the population have antibodies to HSV1, and approximately 20% to HSV2.

Primary genital herpes presents with soreness and irritation of the affected part. It may, however, pass completely unnoticed or manifest with a widespread eruption of vesicles followed by painful ulcers. Severe dysuria and peripheral nerve involvement may lead to urinary retention in women, requiring admission for analgesia and a temporary urinary catheterisation (urethral or even suprapubic). In pregnancy with reduced Th1 immunity recurrent herpes may be more severe than usual and mimic primary herpes. In primary herpes the lesions heal over the course of 2–3 weeks. Recurrences usually last 3–7 days and are more localised, similar to an oral cold sore. On examination vesicles and ulcers are seen. The cervix may be severely inflamed and haemorrhagic. More than half the men and women infected with genital herpes are unaware of its presence. HSV2 is more likely to cause symptomatic recurrences than HSV1. There is a wide individual variation in the frequency of recurrences. A few individuals have recurrences more often than six per year and some are incapacitated because of neurological symptoms such as pains going down the legs.

Diagnosis

The initial diagnosis is clinical, but it should always be confirmed by taking a swab from a vesicle or ulcer for culture or electron microscopy. Specific viral transport medium is essential. Serological tests which can distinguish between antibodies to HSV1 and HSV2 are now becoming available and they may be of benefit. Newer tests are also being developed, which may be helpful in certain situations. For instance, if a woman presents with an outbreak of herpes during pregnancy the virus can be typed. If she has antibody to that type of virus it is not a primary infection, as it takes several weeks for such antibodies to develop. Since the risk for the baby is far greater with primary herpes such information would be helpful for the obstetrician. Herpes simplex should be differentiated from other causes of genital ulcers such as syphilis, tropical genital ulcers and Behçet's syndrome, which classically presents with oral and genital ulceration and which may be accompanied by uveitis and central nervous system manifestations.

Treatment

In the non-pregnant woman primary herpes is treated with a five-day course of aciclovir 200 mg five times a day. This prevents further lesions from developing and allows current ulcers to heal. There is insufficient data to confirm that aciclovir is safe during pregnancy and the manufacturers (Glaxo-Wellcome) currently maintain a register. To date there is no excess of birth defects associated with its use but the potential benefits and risk must be discussed with individual mothers. Topical aciclovir cream has no place in the treatment of genital herpes.

Herpes is important in pregnancy because a devastating neonatal infection can occur with involvement of skin, liver and central nervous system. Neonatal mortality may reach 75%. This can be reduced to 40% if aciclovir is administered rapidly. This syndrome is more common in the USA than the UK: a rate of one in 33 000 live births in the UK compared with one in 5000 in the USA. The vast majority of these are associated with a primary herpes infection in the mother in the weeks prior to delivery. The baby then has no protective antibody and it is vulnerable to disseminated infection, or localised herpes encephalitis. If primary herpes presents around the time of delivery the case must be discussed with the paediatrician. Caesarean section will provide protection to the infant as long as the membranes have not ruptured for more than four hours. Genital swabs should be cultured from the mother and throat swabs from the baby. Intravenous aciclovir should be administered to the newborn. Women known to have recurrent herpes have also been offered caesarean section if a recurrence occurs at the time of delivery. The risk of infection to the baby from a maternal recurrence of herpes is very small indeed and many authorities no longer recommend caesarean section for this indication. The role of aciclovir administration for the last 2–4 weeks of pregnancy in women with recurrent herpes has not been fully evaluated because neonatal herpes in such cases is rare.

Infection during the first trimester may be associated with miscarriage. A congenital syndrome has also been described, although rare. It may be associated with micro-ophthalmia, choroidoretinitis and microcephaly. In adults, herpes simplex rarely causes serious manifestations such as encephalitis or recurrent aseptic meningitis. Many adults feel distressed on receiving a diagnosis of genital herpes as they have read that it is an incurable sexually transmitted disease. The diagnosis should be discussed sensitively and offers of further consultations, referral to a counselor (or health advisor in G-U medicine) should be made. Partners should be screened in a G-U clinic. Often the partner is unaware that he or she is carrying herpes infection, as by the time the index case has presented, the partner's infecting lesions will have healed.

Chlamydia trachomatis

Chlamydia trachomatis is an obligate intracellular parasite. Genital infection with serotypes D–K is the commonest bacterial sexually transmitted infection in developed countries. It is also very common in developing countries. In many tropical countries trachoma is endemic leading to blindness in the most severe cases. This is caused by serotypes A–C and transmission is thought to occur amongst household contacts. *C. trachomatis* is important in pregnancy because it causes neonatal eye infection (ophthalmia neonatorum) and neonatal pneumonitis.

Estimates of the prevalence of genital *C. trachomatis* infection vary between 2% and 10% of women in the UK. The organism is detected much more commonly in young sexually active women, particularly those under the age of 25. The spectrum of disease varies from chronic asymptomatic infection to cervicitis, endometritis, salpingitis (pelvic inflammatory disease) and intraperitoneal spread leading to perihepatitis (Fitz-Hugh Curtis syndrome). In men it causes non-gonococcal urethritis, which may present with urethral discharge and dysuria. Many male partners of women with *C. trachomatis*, however, are asymptomatic.

Pelvic inflammatory disease is uncommon during pregnancy and many pregnant women carrying *C. trachomatis* are only diagnosed after the newborn develops clinical disease. Where screening is undertaken, in communities with a high prevalence of *C. trachomatis*, asymptomatic infection will be detected. An infected cervix is friable, and bleeds easily on contact. This is associated with a purulent discharge from the cervical os, termed mucopurulent cervicitis. The changes induced by pregnancy may be similar so that the specificity of such findings is lower than in the non-pregnant woman.

Approximately 50% of babies born to women with chalmydial infection develop ophthalmia neonatorum. This usually presents about a week after birth with a red sticky eye, which may be bilateral. Chloramphenicol drops, which are commonly prescribed, will produce only partial resolution. A swab for *C. trachomatis* should be taken from the baby's eyes. The organism can also be sought in nasopharyngeal aspirates. The commonly used EIA tests for chlamydia infection are not sufficiently specific in this setting, culture, DNA detection based tests or direct immunofluorescence must be used.

Diagnosis

Diagnosis of chlamydial infection is made by detecting the organism. EIA tests are easily used to screen large numbers of samples but unfortunately the sensitivity is only about 60% or less. Tests that rely on amplification of DNA provide greater sensitivity and specificity and these will be used increasingly as routine. The organism can be detected with such tests in endocervical swabs, first pass urine samples, and even self-collected vaginal swabs.

Treatment

The treatment of choice for *C. trachomatis* in the non-pregnant woman is tetracycline, usually doxycycline. Tetracycline should be avoided in the second and third trimester of pregnancy because it binds to developing bones and teeth in the fetus causing brown staining of the teeth and dysplastic bones. Erythromycin 500 mg twice a day for two weeks is therefore prescribed. This causes nausea, and the pharmacokinetics are not reliable in pregnancy so a test of cure two weeks after completing treatment is obligatory. It is essential that male partners are screened and treated before sexual intercourse is resumed. Azithromycin as a single one-gram dose is licensed for the treatment of *C. trachomatis* and may be useful if the woman is unable to tolerate erythromycin. Although penicillins are not considered adequate treatment to eradicate *C. trachomatis*, co-amoxiclav is effective in preventing neonatal infection and may be used if macrolides are contraindicated. Definitive treatment with a tetracycline should be administered after completion of pregnancy and breast feeding. Newborn babies with ophthalmia neonatorum should be treated with tetracycline eye ointment. Because there is a risk of subsequent chalmydial pneumonitis, they should also be treated with a two-week course of erythromycin syrup.

Many women with *C. trachomatis* have subclinical endometritis, which may predispose to early pregnancy loss, chorio-amnionitis and preterm birth, and clinical post-partum endometritis. It has been associated with failure of implantation in women undergoing *in vitro* fertilisation (Witkin et al 1995). Such women and their partners should, therefore, be screened.

Chlamydia psittaci

This organism causes epidemic abortion in ewes. In humans it causes an atypical pneumonia. Exposure to lambing ewes, and their products of conception, can lead to infection of pregnant women. This results in intrauterine infection and abortion. It has occurred most commonly in vets and farm workers. All pregnant women should, however, be advised to avoid sheep during the lambing season.

Gonorrhoea

Neisseria gonorrhoea is a sexually transmissible agent causing cervicitis, urethritis, endometritis, salpingitis (PID) and perihepatitis in women. In men it causes urethritis and epididymitis. In both men and women it may lead to proctitis and pharyngitis. It is common worldwide although the incidence has decreased in developed countries since the Second World War. Infection in both sexes may be asymptomatic. Like chlamydia, gonorrhoea is commonest in young sexually active women, with the incidence declining over the age of 25. Its importance in obstetrics is because of a neonatal eye infection that if untreated can progress to blindness caused by corneal scarring. The introduction of silver nitrate drops as prophylaxis produced a dramatic decline in the incidence of this complication.

Diagnosis

The diagnosis is established by microscopy and culture. Gram stained microscopy of cervical, urethral and rectal swabs is performed, although the sensitivity of Gram stain is only 50% compared with culture, in women. The organism prefers a high carbon dioxide environment and it is cultured on selective media such as blood agar. Even with optimal conditions, a single set of cultures has a modest sensitivity of about 80–95% for detecting infection. If clinical suspicion is high, a second set of cultures should be taken. It is routine practice to perform two sets of cultures as a test of cure following treatment. DNA detection based tests are now available and these offer superior sensitivity compared with culture. At present, however, they do not allow the opportunity for antibiotic resistance testing, for which culture remains necessary.

Treatment

N. gonorrhoeae has demonstrated a great ability to acquire resistance to antibiotics. It readily exchanges plasmids with other bacterial species, and plasmid-mediated resistance to penicillin and tetracycline appear rapidly under selection pressure with such antibiotics. In many developing countries the price of antibiotics is prohibitive for most individuals, so that suboptimal doses are used. This encourages the development of resistant strains, which are then exported worldwide. Chromosomal mutation has also produced moderate levels of penicillin resistance and this is responsible for resistance to quinolones. Quinolones are contraindicated in pregnancy and, therefore, in a penicillin allergic woman or a woman with penicillin resistant infection a cephalosporin such as cefotaxime (2 g in a single i.m. dose) should be administered.

Newborns may present with ophthalmia neonatorum caused by gonorrhoeae a few days after birth. If N. gonorrhoeae is cultured, topical and systemic treatment should be administered according to antibiotic sensitivities. In a similar way to C. trachomatis, gonorrhoea is associated with chorioamnionitis and preterm birth.

HIV

The Human Immunodeficiency Virus (HIV) pandemic is spreading around the world and steady increases are reported in the numbers of infected women and children. Globally, the World Health Organization (WHO) estimates that in the year 2000, some 13 million women and 10 million children will have been infected with HIV worldwide (Chin 1991, Chin &

Lwanga 1991). The vast majority of the women will be in their reproductive years, live in developing countries and continue to have children. As at the end of December 1999, a total of 40 372 individuals with HIV infection have been reported in the UK HIV data set (AIDS and HIV infection 2000). Approximately 55% of diagnosed HIV positive individuals in the UK are women. This figure is set to rise as the promotion and uptake of antenatal testing increases following the Department of Health directive. In the UK, approximately 300 children are born to HIV infected women annually (Unlinked Anonymous Surveys Steering group 1997). As at the end of April 1999, follow-up data on 1470 babies born to HIV positive women in the UK showed that 578 (39%) of them were infected (AIDS and HIV infection 1999). Since the vast majority of HIV infected children acquired the infection by perinatal transmission (Quinn et al 1992), the prevention of vertical transmission is of paramount importance in reducing the prevalence of pediatric HIV.

Virology

The AIDS virus (HIV) is an RNA virus, characterised by the enzyme *reverse transcriptase*. It exists in two structurally similar forms, HIV-1 and HIV-2, sharing approximately 50% of their nucleotide sequence. HIV-1 is found mostly in North, Central and South America, Europe and Asia. HIV-2 is closely related to the Simian Immunodeficiency Virus (SIV) (about 75% DNA sequence identity between the two viruses) and is concentrated primarily in West Africa although pockets of cases have been reported in other parts of Africa, Europe, Asia and the USA. In man, the target host cells are particularly $CD4^+$ antigen-bearing T helper lymphocytes. The virus infects these key immune cells by attaching to the CD4 receptor and other cell membrane molecules and introducing its RNA into the cell. The viral enzyme *reverse transcriptase* uses this RNA as a template to effect a backward transcription of viral genome from RNA into DNA, which is then incorporated into the host's genome and subsequently, transcribed to produce viral RNA. The genetic material of the next generation of viral particles and the blue print required for their polyproteins is contained within this RNA. As the new viral particles mature, the enzyme *viral protease* cleaves the precursor proteins to generate viral enzymes and structural proteins. The mature viral particles bud from the host cell and can infect other cells.

The rapid and continuous replication of HIV impairs and eventually depletes the patient's $CD4^+$ T cell population. This progressive debilitation of the immune system and its network renders the patient susceptible to the opportunistic infections and neoplasia that characterise AIDS. During replication, mutations may occur in the DNA copies incorporated into the host's DNA because reverse transcription is inherently inaccurate. With each cycle of viral replication, which takes 48 hours, single point mutations arise, which may confer resistance to drugs.

Vertical transmission

Maternal to fetal or infant (vertical) transmission (VT) of HIV may occur during pregnancy, during childbirth or through breast feeding. Vertical transmission of HIV infection is reported in 15–20% of babies born to HIV positive women in European or American populations and in 25–35% in Africa and Asia (Peckham & Gibb 1995, Newell et al 1997). The risk of transmission is increased if the mother has more advanced HIV disease, as shown by a higher viral load (a measure of ongoing viral replication) or p-24 antigenaemia or a low CD4 T cell count (normal count 600–1500 cells/ml). Other risk factors include prolonged rupture of membranes and exposure to events that brings the fetus in contact with maternal blood such as vaginal or instrumental delivery, the use of a fetal scalp electrode, and episiotomy (Ryder et al 1989, Anon 1992, 1994, Peckham & Gibb 1995, Garcia et al 1999). Premature birth, low birthweight and breast feeding are also established risk factors associated with increased risk of vertical transmission. The exact mechanisms for perinatal transmission of HIV and the time during gestation that fetuses are at greatest risk are yet to be elucidated.

Viral DNA has been detected in fetal tissues as early as 12 weeks of gestation (Backe et al 1993). During pregnancy the HIV virus may reach the fetus by maternal–fetal transmission of infected lymphocytes as documented in children with severe combined immunodeficiency (Pollack et al 1982). At birth, HIV infection can be detected in 30–50% of infected children (Burgard et al 1992), suggesting that the remaining 50–70% of the infected infants without viral markers at birth may have been infected late in pregnancy, during delivery or postnatally, mainly through breast feeding. Although HIV placental infection (villitis) has not been reported, chorioamnionitis and placental infection by syphilis and malaria are known to enhance the likelihood of perinatal transmission (St Louis et al 1993, Bloland et al 1995). The observation that during vaginal delivery, the first-born twin is at greater risk of HIV infection compared with the second-born twin (Goedert et al 1991), provides evidence in support of intrapartum transmission of HIV and highlighted the possibility of preventing transmission by the use of elective caesarean section. Microtransfusions of maternal blood to the fetus occur during labour in some women, but its role in perinatal HIV transmission is unclear.

The risk of HIV infection in breast-fed infants born to women who acquired HIV postnatally is estimated at 29% (Dunn et al 1992). Children of postnatally infected mothers are at greater risk of infection compared with those of prenatally infected women because of the peak maternal viraemia that occurs in the former group as a result of primary infection, and the lack of transplacentally acquired antibodies. The additional risk of transmission through breast feeding in infants of prenatally infected women, over and above transmission in utero or during birth is estimated to be 14% (Dunn et al 1992). The duration of breast feeding is important and correlates with the risk of transmission. Nevertheless, in the rural settings of developing countries, the negative impact on overall infant morbidity and mortality of not breast feeding may outweigh the benefit of avoiding HIV transmission from breast milk. In a retrospective South African study, comparing exclusive breast feeding exclusive formula feeding and mixed breast and formula feeding, the rates of transmission were higher in the mixed feeding infants than in either the exclusive breast- or formula-feeding infants (Coutsoudis et al 1999).

Preventing vertical transmission

Recent advances in identifying the risk factors associated with perinatal HIV transmission have allowed interventions to be made to reduce mother–infant transmission. The finding that high maternal viral load correlates positively with perinatal transmission has driven the use of antiretroviral agents in pregnancy. However, there is paucity of data on the safety of these agents particularly in pregnancy. The benefits of non-pharmacological interventions such as elective caesarean section have been demonstrated in clinical studies, although the relevant trials were conducted before the introduction of combination regimens of the so-called Highly Active Anti-Retroviral Therapy (HAART). At present it is unknown whether elective caesarean section confers any additional benefit for infants of women on HAART with an undetectable viral load.

In a meta-analysis of 9 studies of transmission based on 1115 mother–infant pairs, viral loads $\geq 10\,000$ copies/ml were associated with 37% transmission rate, compared with 15% with viral loads of 1000–9999 copies/ml (Cao et al 1997). Zidovudine therapy was associated with a 50% reduction in transmission with viral loads of 10 000 copies/ml or more (Lancet, 1992). Another study reported 40% transmission with viral load >100 000 copies/ml and only 2% with viral loads of 1000 copies/ml. The rate of VT also correlates inversely with CD4+ lymphocyte count. Although current HAART reduces viraemia to <500 copies/ml with substantial reduction in the rates of VT anticipated, transmissions have occurred with undetectable viraemia (Mayaux et al 1997, Thea et al 1997) attributed to discrepancies between viral load in the genital tract secretions and in plasma (O'Shea et al 1998).

Antiretroviral therapy (ART)

The drugs used to treat HIV infection impair viral replication and so delay immunodeficiency and progression to AIDS. In the UK, three classes of antiretroviral agents are marketed for the suppression of HIV. The *Nucleoside Reverse Transcriptase Inhibitors* include agents such as zidovudine (AZT), lamivudine (3TC), didanosine (ddI), zalcitabine (ddC), and stavudine (d4T). These agents are activated within cells and they act by inhibiting reverse transcriptase and terminating the development of viral DNA chains. *The Non-Nucleoside Reverse Transcriptase Inhibitors* such as nevirapine and efavirenz also inhibit reverse transcriptase but only in HIV-1 and not in HIV-2. The *Protease Inhibitors* class prevent viral maturation and include nelfinavir, indinavir, ritonavir and saquinavir. Of all these agents, only zidovudine (AZT) is currently licensed for preventing mother–infant transmission of HIV.

Antiretroviral therapy in pregnancy aims to prevent VT and maintain maternal health without compromising the future treatment opportunities for the mother. In non-pregnant women with high CD4+ counts and low viral load, antiretroviral therapy is not indicated. In pregnancy ART is required to reduce the risk of VT but this has to be balanced against the risks of feto-maternal exposure with potential adverse effects and the emergence of resistant viral strains. The recommended optimal time to initiate therapy is late in the third trimester since less than 2% of mother to infant transmission is estimated to occur before the third trimester (Rouzioux et al 1995). This approach, however, leaves a gap for increased risk of VT in babies born prematurely who are already at increased risk of VT.

The role of single agent (mono-) therapy

The efficacy of zidovudine (AZT) monotherapy in reducing VT was demonstrated in a randomised double blind and placebo controlled trial ACTG 076 in 409 pregnant HIV positive women between 14 and 34 weeks of gestation with $CD4^+$ counts over 200 cells/mm³ (Connor et al 1994). The zidovudine regimen consisted of 100 mg orally five times per day antenatally; 2 mg/kg body weight intravenously for one hour in labour, followed by 1 mg/kg/hour until delivery and 2 mg/kg orally every six hours for six weeks for the neonate beginning at 8–12 hours after birth. The rate of vertical transmission was reduced by 67% in women treated with AZT (25.5% placebo v. 8.3% AZT). Apart from a mild self-limiting anaemia, no adverse effects were observed after a four-year follow-up. Initially, doubts existed as to whether AZT would be as effective in women with more advanced disease and different clinical characteristics and in women who had prior exposure to AZT who are potentially infected with zidovudine resistant virus strains. The relative or independent contributions of antepartum versus intrapartum and neonatal treatment were unknown, raising the question of whether a shorter duration of therapy could be just as effective. Furthermore, a shorter duration of therapy may reduce the toxic effects of AZT and the risk of development of zidovudine-resistant strains and make the intervention more practical and affordable in developing countries where perinatal transmission of HIV is a major public health problem. Further studies have since shown that AZT reduces the risk of VT regardless of low maternal $CD4^+$ cell counts (Boyer et al 1994, Mofenson et al 1999) and high viral load (Sperling et al 1996).

Nevirapine is the only other single drug (other than AZT) that has been shown in a randomised controlled trial to produce a significant reduction in vertical transmission. In the HIVNET 012 trial, 600 pregnant were randomised to receive AZT (600 mg orally at the onset of labour; 300 mg three-hourly until delivery and 4 mg/kg twice daily for one week for the newborn) or 200 mg nevirapine at the onset of labour and a single dose of 2 mg/kg of nevirapine for the neonate within three days of delivery (Guay et al 1999). At 14–16 weeks of age, 13.1% of the nevirapine group were HIV infected compared to 25.1% in the AZT group: a 47% reduction (Guay et al 1999). The question remains whether nevirapine adds any further benefit to the full AZT protocol. Nevertheless, nevirapine monotherapy is relatively cheap, easy to administer and has immense potential for use in developing countries (Marseille et al 1999).

Combination therapy

Triple therapy is recommended for pregnant women with advanced HIV disease, high viral load or low $CD4^+$ counts since the risk of mother to infant transmission correlates with these parameters (Taylor et al 1999). On the other hand, there is a paucity of safety data in human pregnancies with current ART agents, with the exception of zidovudine. With triple therapy, 49 babies are exposed for every protected baby (Taylor et al 1999). However, it is widely believed that the benefits of the marked reduction in viral load produced by triple therapy and the resultant reduction in transmission may outweigh the potential and unquantified risks of these ART agents for the newborn. For women with advanced HIV disease who are reluctant to expose their babies to combination ART, zidovudine monotherapy plus an elective caesarean section is recommended (Taylor et al 1999).

For women who present too late in pregnancy to allow formal virological/immunological assessment, the consensus guidelines recommend the zidovudine regimen with a possible addition of lamivudine and/or nevirapine (Taylor 1999). In women who conceive while on ART, treatment should be continued although a change to or the addition of zidovudine should be considered while it remains the main agent of proven efficacy and safety in human pregnancy. For mothers with zidovudine resistant virus, combination therapy with an alternative nucleoside ART should be considered.

OTHER VERTICALLY TRANSMISSIBLE VIRUS INFECTIONS

Human T cell leukaemia virus

Human T cell leukaemia virus (HTLV-1) is a retrovirus which establishes lifelong infection in infected individuals. The majority of such individuals remain asymptomatic but a small proportion may develop T cell leukaemia in adult life. It also causes tropical spastic paraparesis, which presents with demyelination of the spinal cord causing spastic weakness in the legs. Its prevalence is greatest in Japan, the Caribbean, the Indian Sub-continent and parts of Africa. It is transmitted sexually or through breast milk. If infection is identified the mother should be advised not to breast-feed. There is no specific treatment but barrier methods of contraception should be advised if the sexual partner is uninfected.

Hepatitis

Hepatitis A

This is an RNA virus, which is spread through the faecal–oral route. Approximately 50% of the UK population have antibodies from childhood infection but the prevalence is falling. The majority of individuals in developing countries acquire infection during childhood. It is usually a benign illness but occasionally fulminating hepatitis has been described in pregnant women. It has not been associated with congenital abnormalities. Individuals are most infectious before they develop jaundice. Some degree of protection may be provided through vaccination or administration of human immune globulin during the incubation period.

Hepatitis B

Hepatitis B is a more severe infection that may be followed by chronic carriage and disease ending in cirrhosis. It is transmitted sexually, through blood products, or vertically to the fetus from an infected mother. The majority of acute infections are not clinically recognised as only 20% of individuals develop jaundice. The earlier in life the infection occurs the more likely the person is to become a carrier. Of infants infected perinatally, 80% become carriers. Infection is particularly common in China and South East Asia but the virus is endemic in most tropical countries.

Pregnant women are screened for hepatitis B at booking. During acute infection hepatitis B surface antigen and e antigen are detectable in serum. Antihepatitis B core antibody appears after approximately six weeks and remains detectable thereafter as a marker of exposure. As the anti-e antibody develops, the e-antigen becomes undetectable. With clearance of the virus, the surface antigen also disappears and surface antibody becomes detectable. When the e-antigen is still present the individual is highly infectious. Only a small proportion of individuals who are surface antigen positive but e-antigen negative have replicating virus and are infectious. Therefore, to screen for chronic infection anti-core antibody is sought. If this is positive the other markers are tested to establish the degree of infectivity.

A proportion of individuals do not clear the acute infection and go on to develop chronic hepatitis. Treatment is available with interferon under the guidance of a liver specialist, and antiviral drugs with specific activity against hepatitis B are being introduced at present. Vertical transmission can be prevented by vaccination of babies born to mothers with hepatitis B. Hepatitis B immune globulin is given at birth additionally if the mother is eAg positive. Many countries with a higher prevalence of hepatitis B infection than the UK, and several European countries, have a policy of universal vaccination of all infants.

Hepatitis C

This is another RNA virus, which causes chronic hepatitis. Acute infection often passes asymptomatically but more than 50% of infected individuals have active hepatitis, which will progress to cirrhosis and possibly hepatocellular carcinoma. The prevalence varies widely across the world with the highest incidence in Egypt, possibly associated with the use of contaminated needles for mass treatment for schistosomiasis. In the UK infection is highly prevalent in those with a history of intravenous drug use. It may be transmitted sexually but transmission is not very efficient with only 1–2% of long-term partners becoming infected. Vertical transmission is uncommon and appears to correlate with Hepatitis C RNA viraemia (Giacchino et al 1998). The risk of transmission is, however, increased in those co-infected with HIV.

Hepatitis D

This is a defective virus that can only replicate in the presence of hepatitis B. Individuals who have this super infection are more likely to develop severe hepatitis.

Hepatitis E

This virus is spread through the oral–faecal route and causes acute hepatitis. It can, like hepatitis A, be fulminating in pregnant women, with up to 20% mortality. It is found mainly in tropical countries, where epidemics have occurred after natural disasters allow contamination of water with sewage. It is not thought to cause chronic hepatitis.

MATERNAL INFECTIONS

Trichomoniasis

Trichomonas vaginalis causes a severe vulvovaginitis in susceptible women. It is generally sexually transmitted although infection may persist asymptomatically for many months in women and in some men. In men it may cause urethritis but it is frequently asymptomatic. The incidence of trichomoniasis has fallen in the last decade in developed countries. It remains highly prevalent in many developing countries, where as many as 20–30% of pregnant women carry the infection (Klufio et al 1995, Mwakagile et al 1996). The women may present with a purulent vaginal discharge, which may be associated with severe inflammation causing soreness and itching with a tide mark extending on to the thighs. The diagnosis is made by detecting the organism on wet mount microscopy, with a sensitivity of approximately 50–60%. It can be cultured in specific medium such as Fineberg–Whittington. DNA detection based tests are showing that even culture is not 100% sensitive. The organism is detected much less frequently in men, but male partners should be screened for sexually transmitted diseases and treated with metronidazole.

Transient infection may be transmitted to newborn female infants who have stratified squamous epithelium in the vagina, similar to that of an adult because of the influence of high levels of maternal oestrogen in utero. They are, therefore, susceptible to infection and they may present with purulent vaginal discharge. As the influence of maternal oestrogen wanes over the first few weeks of life such infection usually resolves spontaneously and specific treatment is rarely necessary.

Trichomoniasis frequently coexists with disturbed vaginal flora that develops into bacterial vaginosis. The only established treatments for trichomoniasis are metronidazole or tinidazole that have hitherto been considered to carry a risk of teratogenecity. Recent reviews have concluded that there are extremely limited animal data to support such a claim, although there is some evidence of mutagenesis. Retrospective studies of women who have taken metronidazole during pregnancy have shown no excess of fetal abnormalities and it is, therefore, reasonable to treat symptomatic women with a five-day course of metronidazole 400 mg twice a day. It is sensible, however, to discuss the potential risks of any treatment with the mother so that she can make an informed decision. Clotrimazole has some activity against trichomoniasis and application of intravaginal clotrimazole pessaries may control symptoms until the end of the first trimester if a woman is particularly concerned about systemic treatment.

Vaginal candidiasis

Over three-quarters of women have at least one episode of vaginal candidiasis during their lifetime. A few women get frequent recurrences. The organism is carried in the gut, under the nails, in the vagina and on the skin. The yeast *Candida albicans* is implicated in more than 80% of cases. *Candida glabrata, C. krusei* and *C. tropicalis* account for most of the rest. Sexual acquisition is rarely important although the physical trauma of intercourse may be sufficient to trigger an attack in a predisposed individual. Candida is an opportunist, growing under favourable conditions. Symptomatic episodes are common in pregnancy. Its growth is favoured by the high levels of oestrogen, increased availability of sugars, and subtle alterations in immunity. The classical presentation is with itching and soreness of the vagina and vulva with a curdy white discharge that may smell yeasty but not unpleasant. Not all candida presents in the same way, in some cases there may be itching and redness with a thin watery discharge. The pH of vaginal fluid is normally between 3.5 and 4.5. The diagnosis can be confirmed by microscopy and culture of the vaginal fluid. Asymptomatic women from whom candida is grown in culture do not require treatment. Recurrent candida, or resistance to treatment is relatively uncommon. If this appears to be the case, it is important to consider other diagnoses particularly herpes simplex that causes localised ulceration and soreness, and dermatological conditions such as eczema and lichen sclerosus. In general it is better to use a topical rather than systemic treatment. This minimises the risk of systemic side effects, and exposure of the fetus. Vaginal creams and pessaries can be prescribed at a variety of doses and duration of treatment. For uncomplicated candida, a single dose treatment, such as clotrimazole 500 mg is adequate. If oral therapy has to be used, a single 150 mg tablet of fluconazole is usually effective, but its activity is limited to *Candida albicans* strains.

Postpartum endometritis

After delivery, the uterus and genital tract contain blood and products of conception, an environment highly conducive to the growth of microorganisms. The risk of infection is higher with preterm birth associated with chorio-amnionitis, emergency caesarean section and prolonged rupture of membranes. Postpartum endometritis may present with fever, purulent discharge and uterine tenderness, usually within a few days of delivery. Septicaemia and septic shock can occur if the early signs of infection are neglected. Cultures from the vagina, urine and blood should be obtained before antibiotic treatment is started. Postpartum endometritis is usually self-limiting but broad-spectrum antibiotics and occasionally uterine evacuation may be required. Fortunately, the classical puerperal fever associated with the group A streptococcus is now a rare event.

CONCLUSIONS

Two broad categories of perinatal infections have now emerged. On the one hand, the subclinical intrauterine infection associated with long-term fetal damage, irrespective of the gestational age at delivery. On the other hand, the established but increasingly rare and specific, mostly viral infections. Trials are underway evaluating the role of agents that dampen the fetal immune system, reducing the frequency and severity of chronic disabilities induced by prenatal exposure to infection and pro-inflammatory cytokines. It is anticipated that advances in antiviral therapy and the development of vaccines will ultimately lead to effective interventions in preventing pregnancy wastage and the neonatal stigmata associated with viral infections in pregnancy. The future of antenatal screening for these specific infections will be decided by their ever-falling prevalence rates and cost-benefit analyses. The control of HIV disease is a pressing problem worldwide, but more so in developing countries where inadequate resources, poverty, illiteracy and cultural attitudes especially towards breast feeding combine to perpetuate the spread of HIV.

KEY POINTS

- Subclinical intrauterine infection, the fetal inflammatory response syndrome and the actions of pro-inflammatory cytokines and inflammatory mediators may be the pathogenic processes responsible for a third of preterm births and a significant proportion of neurodevelopmental or motor disabilities and chronic lung disease.
- The risk of vertical transmission of HIV may be eliminated with the near total suppression of maternal viral load achieved by the newer HAART. This may obviate the need for prophylactic elective ceasarean section. However, the safety of these novel agents in pregnancy has first to be established.
- Screening for and treating bacterial vaginosis in pregnancy is beneficial in pregnant women at high risk of preterm delivery. The role of therapy in the general low-risk population has yet to be established.
- Clinicians should adopt either a screening, culture-based strategy or the risk-based approach for the detection of pregnant women colonised by group B streptococcus. Such women should receive prophylactic antibiotics in labour.

REFERENCES

Adinolfi M 1985 The development of the human blood-CSF-brain barrier. Dev Med Child Neurol 27:532–537

AIDS and HIV infection in the United Kingdom: monthly report 1999 Communicable Disease Report 9:277–280

AIDS and HIV infection in the United Kingdom: a monthly report 2000. Communicable Disease Report 10(4), 37–40.

Amsel R, Totten PA, Spiegel CA, Chen KC, Eschenbach D, Holmes KK 1983 Nonspecific vaginitis. Diagnostic criteria and microbial and epidemiologic associations. Am J Med 74:14–22

Anonymous 1994 Caesarean section and risk of vertical transmission of HIV-1 infection. The European Collaborative Study. Lancet 343:1464–1467

Anonymous 1998 Management of bacterial vaginosis. Drug Ther Bull 36:33–35

Backe E, Unger M, Jimenez E, Siegel G, Schafer A, Vogel M 1993 Fetal organs infected by HIV-1. AIDS 7:896–897

Baker CJ, Webb BJ, Kasper DL, Yow MD, Beachler CW 1980 The natural history of group B streptococcal colonization in the pregnant woman and her offspring. II. Determination of serum antibody to capsular polysaccharide from type III, group B Streptococcus. Am J Obstet Gynecol 137:39–42

Baker CJ, Edwards MS, Kasper DL 1981 Role of antibody to native type III polysaccharide of group B Streptococcus in infant infection. Pediatrics 68:544–549

Baker CJ, Kasper DL 1985 Group B streptococcal vaccines. Rev Infect Dis 7:458–467

Bang B 1962 Effect of lipopolysaccharides of Gram-negative bacilli in the rat litter in utero. Proc Soc Exp Biol Med 109

Bejar R, Curbelo V, Davis C, Gluck L 1981 Premature labor. II. Bacterial sources of phospholipase. Obstet Gynecol 57:479–482

Bejar R, Wozniak P, Allard M et al 1988 Antenatal origin of neurologic damage in newborn infants. I. Preterm infants. Am J Obstet Gynecol 159:357–363

Benedetti TJ, Valle R, Ledger WJ 1982 Antepartum pneumonia in pregnancy. Am J Obstet Gynecol 144:413–417

Benirschke K 1965 Routes and types of infection in the newborn. Am J Dis Child 99:714–721

Bennett PR, Rose MP, Myatt L, Elder MG 1987 Preterm labor: stimulation of arachidonic acid metabolism in human amnion cells by bacterial products. Am J Obstet Gynecol 156:649–655

Blanc W 1964 Pathways of fetal and early neonatal infection: viral placentitis, bacterial and fungal chorioamnionitis. J Pediatr 59:473

Bloland PB, Wirima JJ, Steketee RW, Chilima B, Hightower A, Breman JG 1995 Maternal HIV infection and infant mortality in Malawi: evidence for increased mortality due to placental malaria infection. AIDS 9:721–726

Boyer PJ, Dillon M, Navaie M et al 1994 Factors predictive of maternal-fetal transmission of HIV-1. Preliminary analysis of zidovudine given during pregnancy and/or delivery. JAMA 271:1925–1930

Boyer KM, Gotoff SP 1986 Prevention of early-onset neonatal group B streptococcal disease with selective intrapartum chemoprophylaxis. N Engl J Med 314:1665–1669

Brunell PA, Kotchmar GSJ 1981 Zoster in infancy: failure to maintain virus latency following intrauterine infection. J Pediatr 98:71–73

Bry K, Hallman M 1991 Synergistic stimulation of amnion cell prostaglandin E2 synthesis by interleukin-1, tumor necrosis factor and products from activated human granulocytes. Prostaglandins Leukot Essent Fatty Acids 44:241–245

Burgard M, Mayaux MJ, Blanche S et al 1992 The use of viral culture and p24 antigen testing to diagnose human immunodeficiency virus infection in neonates. The HIV Infection in Newborns French Collaborative Study Group [see comments]. N Engl J Med 327:1192–1197

Cao Y, Krogstad P, Korber BT et al 1997 Maternal HIV-1 viral load and vertical transmission of infection: the Ariel Project for the prevention of HIV transmission from mother to infant. Nat Med 3:549–552

Carey JC, Klebanoff MA, Hauth JC et al 2000 Metronidazole to prevent preterm delivery in pregnant women with asymptomatic bacterial vaginosis. N Engl J Med 342:534–540

Carroll SG, Papaioannou S, Ntumazah IL, Philpott-Howard J, Nicolaides KH 1996 Lower genital tract swabs in the prediction of intrauterine infection in preterm prelabour rupture of the membranes. Br J Obstet Gynecol 103:54–59

Cassell GH, Davis RO, Waites KB, et al 1983 Isolation of Mycoplasma hominis and Ureaplasma urealyticum from amniotic fluid at 16–20 weeks of gestation: potential effect on outcome of pregnancy. Sex Transm Dis 10:294–302

Cassell GH, Waites KB, Crouse DT 1991 Perinatal mycoplasmal infections. Clin Perinatol 18:241–262

Cassell GH, Waites KB, Watson HL, Crouse DT, Harasawa R 1993 Ureaplasma urealyticum intrauterine infection: role in prematurity and disease in newborns. Clin Microbiol Rev 6:69–87

Centers for Disease Control and Prevention. Recommendations and Reports. 1998 Guidelines for Treatment of Sexually Transmitted. January 23 1998, Vol. 47, # RR1. 1998

Chin J 1991 Global estimates of HIV infections and AIDS cases: 1991. AIDS 5 Suppl 2:S57–S61

Chin J, Lwanga SK 1991 Estimation and projection of adult AIDS cases: a simple epidemiological model. Bull World Health Organ 69:399–406

Christensen KK, Dahlander K, Esktrom A, Svenningsen N, Christensen P 1981 Colonization of newborns with group B streptococci: relation to maternal urogenital carriage. Scand J Infect Dis 13:23–27

Christensen KK, Christensen P, Lindberg A, Linden V 1982 Mothers of infants with neonatal group B streptococcal septicemia are poor responders to bacterial carbohydrate antigens. Int Arch Allergy Appl Immunol 67:7–12

Connor EM, Sperling RS, Gelber R et al 1994 Reduction of maternal-infant transmission of human immunodeficiency virus type 1 with zidovudine treatment. Pediatric AIDS Clinical Trials Group Protocol 076 Study Group. N Engl J Med 331:1173–1180

Cossart YE, Field AM, Cant B, Widdows D 1975 Parvovirus-like particles in human sera. Lancet 1:72–73

Cotton DB, Hill LM, Strassner HT, Platt LD, Ledger WJ 1984a Use of amniocentesis in preterm gestation with ruptured membranes. Obstet Gynecol 63:38–43

Cotton DB, Gonik B, Bottoms SF 1984b Conservative versus aggressive management of preterm rupture of membranes. A randomized trial of amniocentesis. Am J Perinatol 1:322–324

Coutsoudis A, Pillay K, Spooner E, Kuhn L, Coovadia HM 1999 Influence of infant-feeding patterns on early mother-to-child transmission of HIV-1 in Durban, South Africa: a prospective cohort study. South African Vitamin A Study Group. Lancet 354:471–476

Cruikshank DP, Warenski JC 1989 First-trimester maternal Listeria monocytogenes sepsis and chorioamnionitis with normal neonatal outcome. Obstet Gynecol 73:469–471

Cunningham FG, Morris GB, Mickal A 1973 Acute pyelonephritis of pregnancy: A clinical review. Obstet Gynecol 42:112–117

Dammann O, Leviton A 1997 Maternal intrauterine infection, cytokines, and brain damage in the preterm newborn. Pediatr Res 42:1–8

Dombroski RA, Woodard DS, Harper MJ, Gibbs RS 1990 A rabbit model for bacteria-induced preterm pregnancy loss. Am J Obstet Gynecol 163:1938–1943

Dunn DT, Newell ML, Ades AE, Peckham CS 1992 Risk of human immunodeficiency virus type 1 transmission through breastfeeding. Lancet 340:585–588

Edwards MS, Nicholson-Weller A, Baker CJ, Kasper DL 1980 The role of specific antibody in alternative complement pathway-mediated opsonophagocytosis of type III, group B Streptococcus. J Exp Med 151:1275–1287

Elder MG, Romero R, Lamonr RF eds. Preterm Labor. Gomez R, Romero R, Mazor M, Ghezzi F, David C, Yoon BH 1997 The role of infection in preterm labor and delivery. New York, Churchill Livingstone, pp 85–125.

Enders G 1984 Varicella-zoster virus infection in pregnancy. Prog Med Virol 29:166–196

Eschenbach DA, Hillier S, Critchlow C, Stevens C, DeRouen T, Holmes KK 1988 Diagnosis and clinical manifestations of bacterial vaginosis. Am J Obstet Gynecol 158:819–828

Fleming AD, Ehrlich DW, Miller NA, Monif GR 1985 Successful treatment of maternal septicemia due to Listeria monocytogenes at 26 weeks' gestation. Obstet Gynecol 66:52S–52 S

Fortunato SJ, Menon R, Lombardi SJ 1999 MMP/TIMP imbalance in amniotic fluid during PROM: an indirect support for endogenous pathway to membrane rupture. J Perinat Med 27:362–368

Fortunato SJ, Menon R, Lombardi SJ 2000 Amniochorion gelatinase-gelatinase inhibitor imbalance in vitro: a possible infectious pathway to rupture. Obstet Gynecol 95:240–244

Fowler KB, Stagno S, Pass RF, Britt WJ, Boll TJ, Alford CA 1992 The outcome of congenital cytomegalovirus infection in relation to maternal antibody status [see comments]. N Engl J Med 326:663–667

French JI, McGregor JA 1996 The pathobiology of premature rupture of membranes. Semin Perinatol 20:344–368

Garcia PM, Kalish LA, Pitt J et al 1999 Maternal levels of plasma human immunodeficiency virus type 1 RNA and the risk of perinatal transmission. Women and Infants Transmission Study Group. N Engl J Med 341:394–402

Garite TJ, Freeman RK, Linzey EM, Braly P 1979 The use of amniocentesis in patients with premature rupture of membranes. Obstet Gynecol 54:226–230

Gellin BG, Broome CV 1989 Listeriosis. JAMA 261:1313–1320

Giacchino R, Tasso L, Timitilli A et al 1998 Vertical transmission of hepatitis C virus infection: usefulness of viremia detection in HIV-seronegative hepatitis C virus-seropositive mothers. J Pediatr 132:167–169

Gilles HM, Lawson JB, Sibelas M, Voller A, Allan N, 1969, Malaria anaemia and pregnancy. Ann Trop Med Parasitol 63:245–263

Goedert JJ, Duliege AM, Amos CI, Felton S, Biggar RJ 1991 High risk of HIV-1 infection for first-born twins. The International Registry of HIV-exposed Twins. Lancet 338:1471–1475

Goldmeier D, Hay P 1993 A review and update on adult syphilis, with particular reference to its treatment [editorial]. Int J STD AIDS 4:70–82

Gomez R, Ghezza F, Romero R, Yoon BH, Mazor M, Berry SM 1998a Two thirds of human fetuses with microbial invasion of the amniotic cavity have a detectable systemic cytokine response before birth. Am J Obstet Gynecol 1997;176:(Suppl);S14. (Abstract)

Gomez R, Romero R, Ghezzi F, Yoon BH, Mazor M, Berry SM 1998b The fetal inflammatory response syndrome. Am J Obstet Gynecol 179:194–202

Gomez R, Ghezzi F, Romero R, Munoz H, Tolosa JE, Rojas I 1995 Premature labor and intra-amniotic infection. Clinical aspects and role of the cytokines in diagnosis and pathophysiology. Clin Perinatol 22:281–342

Gonik B, Cotton DB 1985a The use of amniocentesis in preterm premature rupture of membranes. Am J Perinatol 2:21–24

Gonik B, Bottoms SF, Cotton DB 1985b Amniotic fluid volume as a risk factor in preterm premature rupture of the membranes. Obstet Gynecol 65:456–459

Gratacos E, Figueras F, Barranco M et al 1998 Spontaneous recovery of bacterial vaginosis during pregnancy is not associated with an improved perinatal outcome. Acta Obstet Gynecol Scand 77:37–40

Grau GE, Lou J 1993 TNF in vascular pathology: the importance of platelet-endothelium interactions. Res Immunol 144:355–363

Gravett MG, Haluska GJ, Cook MJ, Novy MJ 1996 Fetal and maternal endocrine responses to experimental intrauterine infection in rhesus monkeys. Am J Obstet Gynecol 174:1725–1733

Gregg NM 1941 Congenital cataract following German measles in the mother. Trans Ophthal Soc Austr 3:35–46

Grether JK, Nelson KB 1997 Maternal infection and cerebral palsy in infants of normal birth weight. JAMA 278:207–211

Guay LA, Musoke P, Fleming T et al 1999 Intrapartum and neonatal single-dose nevirapine compared with zidovudine for prevention of mother-to-child transmission of HIV-1 in Kampala, Uganda: HIVNET 012 randomised trial. Lancet 354:795–802

Hankins GD, Gilstrap LC, Patterson AR 1987 Acyclovir treatment of varicella pneumonia in pregnancy. Crit Care Med 15:336–337

Hauth JC, Goldenberg RL, Andrews WW, DuBard MB, Copper RL 1995 Reduced incidence of preterm delivery with metronidazole and erythromycin in women with bacterial vaginosis. N Engl J Med 333:1732–1736

Hay PE, Morgan DJ, Ison CA et al 1994a A longitudinal study of bacterial vaginosis during pregnancy. Br J Obstet Gynaecol 101:1048–1053

Hay PE, Lamont RF, Taylor-Robinson D, Morgan DJ, Ison C, Pearson J 1994b Abnormal bacterial colonisation of the genital tract and subsequent preterm delivery and late miscarriage [see comments]. BMJ 308:295–298

Hillier SL, Martius J, Krohn M, Kiviat N, Holmes KK, Eschenbach DA 1988 A case-control study of chorioamnionic infection and histologic chorioamnionitis in prematurity. N Engl J Med 319:972–978

Hillier SL, Witkin SS, Krohn MA, Watts DH, Kiviat NB, Eschenbach DA 1993 The relationship of amniotic fluid cytokines and preterm delivery, amniotic fluid infection, histologic chorioamnionitis, and chorioamnion infection. Obstet Gynecol 81:941–948

Hillier SL, Nugent RP, Eschenbach DA et al 1995 Association between bacterial vaginosis and preterm delivery of a low-birth-weight infant. The Vaginal Infections and Prematurity Study Group [see comments]. N Engl J Med 333:1737–1742

Hopkins SJ, Rothwell NJ 1995 Cytokines and the nervous system. I: Expression and recognition. Trends Neurosci 18:83–88

Hume OS 1976 Maternal Listeria monocytogenes septicemia with sparing of the fetus. Obstet Gynecol 48:33S–33 S

Hurwitz AA, Lyman WD, Guida MP, Calderon TM, Berman JW 1992 Tumor necrosis factor alpha induces adhesion molecule expression on human fetal astrocytes. J Exp Med 176:1631–1636

Iams JD, Goldenberg RL, Meis PJ et al 1996 The length of the cervix and the risk of spontaneous premature delivery. National Institute of Child Health and Human Development Maternal Fetal Medicine Unit Network. N Engl J Med 334:567–572

Jauniaux E, Nessmann C, Imbert MC, Meuris S, Puissant F, Hustin J 1989 Morphological aspects of the placenta in HIV pregnancies [published erratum appears in Placenta May-Jun; 10(3):320]. Placenta 9:633–642

Joesoef MR, Hillier SL, Wiknjosastro G et al 1995 Intravaginal clindamycin treatment for bacterial vaginosis: effects on preterm delivery and low birth weight. Am J Obstet Gynecol 173:1527–1531

Jones SA, Challis JR 1990 Effects of corticotropin-releasing hormone and adrenocorticotropin on prostaglandin output by human placenta and fetal membranes. Gynecol Obstet Invest 29:165–168

Jones DA, Carlton DP, McIntyre TM, Zimmerman GA, Prescott SM 1993 Molecular cloning of human prostaglandin endoperoxide synthase type II and demonstration of expression in response to cytokines. J Biol Chem 268:9049–9054

Jorizzo JL, McNeely MC, Baughn RE, Solomon AR, Cavallo T, Smith EB 1986 Role of circulating immune complexes in human secondary syphilis. J Infect Dis 153:1014–1022

Kahn MA, De Vellis J 1994 Regulation of an oligodendrocyte progenitor cell line by the interleukin-6 family of cytokines. Glia 12:87–98

Klima G, Schmidt W 1988 [Immunohistochemical studies of the nature of connective tissue in fetal membranes]. Acta Histochem 84:195–203

Klufio CA, Amoa AB, Delamare O, Hombhanje M, Kariwiga G, Igo J 1995 Prevalence of vaginal infections with bacterial vaginosis, Trichomonas vaginalis and Candida albicans among pregnant women at the Port Moresby General Hospital Antenatal Clinic. P N G Med J 38:163–171

Korn AP, Bolan G, Padian N, Ohm-Smith M, Schachter J, Landers DV 1995 Plasma cell endometritis in women with symptomatic bacterial vaginosis. Obstet Gynecol 85:387–390

Krick JA, Remington JS 1978 Toxoplasmosis in the adult – an overview. N Engl J Med 298:550–553

Kruger T, Baier J 1997 Induction of neutrophil chemoattractant cytokines by Mycoplasma hominis in alveolar type II cells. Infect Immun 65:5131–5136

Kullander S 1977 Fever and parturition. An experimental study in rabbits. Acta Obstet Gynecol Scand Suppl 77–85

Kurki T, Sivonen A, Renkonen OV, Savia E, Ylikorkala O 1992 Bacterial vaginosis in early pregnancy and pregnancy outcome. Obstet Gynecol 80:173–177

Lamont RJ, Postlethwaite R 1986 Carriage of Listeria monocytogenes and related species in pregnant and non-pregnant women in Aberdeen, Scotland. J Infect 13:187–193

Lancet 1992 Risk factors for mother-to-child transmission of HIV-1. European Collaborative Study. Lancet 339:1007–1012

Lang DJ, Noren B 1968 Cytomegaloviremia following congenital infection. J Pediatr 73:812–819

Langer H 1963 Repeated congenital infection with Toxoplasma gondii. Obstet Gynecol 21:318–319

Lettieri L, Vintzileos AM, Rodis JF, Albini SM, Salafia CM 1993 Does idiopathic preterm labor resulting in preterm birth exist? Am J Obstet Gynecol 168:1480–1485

Lim DV, Morales WJ, Walsh AF, Kazanis D 1986 Reduction of morbidity and mortality rates for neonatal group B streptococcal disease through early diagnosis and chemoprophylaxis. J Clin Microbiol 23:489–492

Llahi-Camp JM, Rai R, Ison C, Regan L, Taylor-Robinson D 1996

Association of bacterial vaginosis with a history of second trimester miscarriage. Hum Reprod 11:1575–1578

Lopez B, Hansell DJ, Canete S, Keeling JW, Turnbull AC 1987 Prostaglandins, chorioamnionitis and preterm labour. Br J Obstet Gynaecol 94:1156–1158

MacDonald H, Tobin JO 1978 Congenital cytomegalovirus infection: a collaborative study on epidemiological, clinical and laboratory findings. Dev Med Child Neurol 20:471–482

MacDonald PC, Koga S, Casey ML 1991 Decidual activation in parturition: examination of amniotic fluid for mediators of the inflammatory response. Ann N Y Acad Sci 622:315–330

McDonald HM, O'Loughlin JA, Vigneswaran R et al 1997 Impact of metronidazole therapy on preterm birth in women with bacterial vaginosis flora (Gardnerella vaginalis): a randomised, placebo controlled trial. Br J Obstet Gynaecol 104:1391–1397

Mackaness GB, Hill WC 1969 The effect of anti-lymphocyte globulin on cell-mediated resistance to infection. J Exp Med 129:993–1012

Madinger NE, Greenspoon JS, Ellrodt AG 1989 Pneumonia during pregnancy: has modern technology improved maternal and fetal outcome? Am J Obstet Gynecol 161:657–662

Marseille E, Kahn JG, Mmiro F et al 1999 Cost effectiveness of single-dose nevirapine regimen for mothers and babies to decrease vertical HIV-1 transmission in sub-Saharan Africa. Lancet 354:803–809

Martius J, Eschenbach DA 1990 The role of bacterial vaginosis as a cause of amniotic fluid infection, chorioamnionitis and prematurity–a review. Arch Gynecol Obstet 247:1–13

Mayaux MJ, Dussaix E, Isopet J et al 1997 Maternal virus load during pregnancy and mother-to-child transmission of human immunodeficiency virus type 1: the French perinatal cohort studies. SEROGEST Cohort Group. J Infect Dis 175:172–175

McGregor JA, Lawellin D, Franco-Buff A, Todd JK, Makowski EL 1986 Protease production by microorganisms associated with reproductive tract infection. Am J Obstet Gynecol 154:109–114

McGregor JA, French JI, Lawellin D, Franco-Buff A, Smith C, Todd JK 1987 Bacterial protease-induced reduction of chorioamniotic membrane strength and elasticity. Obstet Gynecol 69:167–174

McGregor JA, French JI, Jones W et al 1994 Bacterial vaginosis is associated with prematurity and vaginal fluid mucinase and sialidase: results of a controlled trial of topical clindamycin cream. Am J Obstet Gynecol 170:1048–1059

McGregor JA, French JI, Parker R, et al 1995 Prevention of premature birth by screening and treatment for common genital tract infections: results of a prospective controlled evaluation [see comments]. Am J Obstet Gynecol 173:157–167

Mead PB, 1993 Epidemiology of bacterial vaginosis. Am J Obstet Gynecol 169:446–449

Mercer BM, Arheart KL 1995 Antimicrobial therapy in expectant management of preterm premature rupture of the membranes [see comments] [published erratum appears in Lancet 1996 Feb 10;347(8998):410]. Lancet 346:1271–1279

Mercer BM, Goldenberg RL, Das A et al 1996 The preterm prediction study: a clinical risk assessment system. Am J Obstet Gynecol 174:1885–1895

Merrill JE, Benveniste EN 1996 Cytokines in inflammatory brain lesions: helpful and harmful. Trends Neurosci 19:331–338

Minkoff H, Mead P 1986 An obstetric approach to the prevention of early-onset group B beta-hemolytic streptococcal sepsis. Am J Obstet Gynecol 154:973–977

Mofenson LM, Lambert JS, Stiehm ER et al 1999 Risk factors for perinatal transmission of human immunodeficiency virus type 1 in women treated with zidovudine. Pediatric AIDS Clinical Trials Group Study 185 Team. N Engl J Med 341:385–393

Moi H, Erkkola R, Jerye F et al 1989 Should male consorts of women with bacterial vaginosis be treated? Genitourin Med 65:263–268

Morales WJ, Lim DV, Walsh AF 1986 Prevention of neonatal group B streptococcal sepsis by the use of a rapid screening test and selective intrapartum chemoprophylaxis. Am J Obstet Gynecol 155:979–983

Morales WJ 1987 The effect of chorioamnionitis on the developmental outcome of preterm infants at one year. Obstet Gynecol 70:183–186

Morales WJ, Schorr S, Albritton J 1994 Effect of metronidazole in

patients with preterm birth in preceding pregnancy and bacterial vaginosis: a placebo-controlled, double-blind study. Am J Obstet Gynecol 171:345–347

Munshi UK, Niu JO, Siddiq MM, Parton LA 1997 Elevation of interleukin-8 and interleukin-6 precedes the influx of neutrophils in tracheal aspirates from preterm infants who develop bronchopulmonary dysplasia. Pediatr Pulmonol 24:331–336

Murphy DJ, Sellers S, MacKenzie IZ, Yudkin PL, Johnson AM 1995 Case-control study of antenatal and intrapartum risk factors for cerebral palsy in very preterm singleton babies. Lancet 346:1449–1454

Mwakagile D, Swai AB, Sandstrom E, Urassa E, Biberfeld G, Mhalu FS 1996 High frequency of sexually transmitted diseases among pregnant women in Dar es Salaam, Tanzania: need for intervention. East Afr Med J 73:675–678

Nelson KB, Ellenberg JH 1986 Antecedents of cerebral palsy. Multivariate analysis of risk. N Engl J Med 315:81–86

Newell ML, Gray G, Bryson YJ 1997 Prevention of mother-to-child transmission of HIV-1 infection. AIDS; 11 Suppl A:S165–S172

Nugent RP, Krohn MA, Hillier SL 1991 Reliability of diagnosing bacterial vaginosis is improved by a standardized method of gram stain interpretation. J Clin Microbiol 29:297–301

Numazaki K, Chiba S, Kogawa K, Umetsu M, Motoya H, Nakao T 1986 Chronic respiratory disease in premature infants caused by Chlamydia trachomatis. J Clin Pathol 39:84–88

O'Dowd TC, Bourne N 1994 Inventing a new diagnostic test for vaginal infection. BMJ 309:40–42

Offenbacher S, Katz V, Fertik G et al 1996 Periodontal infection as a possible risk factor for preterm low birth weight. J Periodontol 67:1103–1113

Ornoy A, Segal S, Nishmi M, Simcha A, Polishuk WZ 1973 Fetal and placental pathology in gestational rubella. Am J Obstet Gynecol 116:949–956

O'Shea S, Newell ML, Dunn DT et al 1998 Maternal viral load, CD4 cell count and vertical transmission of HIV-1. J Med Virol 54:113–117

Paneth N 1986a Etiologic factors in cerebral palsy. Pediatr Ann 15:191, 194–201.

Paneth N 1986b Birth and the origins of cerebral palsy [editorial]. N Engl J Med 315:124–126

Paneth N, Rudelli R, Kazam E, Monte W 1994 Brain damage in the preterm infant. London, MacKeith, pp 171–185.

Paryani SG, Arvin AM 1986 Intrauterine infection with varicella-zoster virus after maternal varicella. N Engl J Med 314:1542–1546

Peckham C, Gibb D 1995 Mother-to-child transmission of the human immunodeficiency virus. N Engl J Med 333:298–302

Philipson EH, Palermino DA, Robinson A 1995 Enhanced antenatal detection of group B streptococcus colonization. Obstet Gynecol 85:437–439

Pollack MS, Kirkpatrick D, Kapoor N, Dupont B, O'Reilly RJ 1982 Identification by HLA typing of intrauterine-derived maternal T cells in four patients with severe combined immunodeficiency. N Engl J Med 307:662–666

Preece PM, Blount JM, Glover J, Fletcher GM, Peckham CS, Griffiths PD 1983 The consequences of primary cytomegalovirus infection in pregnancy. Arch Dis Child 58:970–975

Quagliarello VJ, Wispelwey B, Long WJJ, Scheld WM 1991 Recombinant human interleukin-1 induces meningitis and blood-brain barrier injury in the rat. Characterization and comparison with tumor necrosis factor. J Clin Invest 87:1360–1366

Quinn TC, Ruff A, Halsey N 1990 Pediatric acquired immunodeficiency syndrome: special considerations for developing nations. Pediatr Infect Dis J 11:558–568

Rajabi M, Solomon S, Poole AR 1991 Hormonal regulation of interstitial collagenase in the uterine cervix of the pregnant guinea pig. Endocrinology 128:863–871

Reynolds DW, Stagno S, Reynolds R, Alford CAJ 1978 Perinatal cytomegalovirus infection: influence of placentally transferred maternal antibody. J Infect Dis 137:564–567

Rioux-Darrieulat F, Parant M, Chedid L 1978 Prevention of endotoxin-induced abortion by treatment of mice with antisera. J Infect Dis 137:7–13

Robbins DS, Shirazi Y, Drysdale BE, Lieberman A, Shin HS, Shin ML 1987 Production of cytotoxic factor for oligodendrocytes by stimulated astrocytes. J Immunol 139:2593–2597

Rojas MA, Gonzalez A, Bancalari E, Claure N, Poole C, Silva-Neto G 1995 Changing trends in the epidemiology and pathogenesis of neonatal chronic lung disease. J Pediatr 126:605–610

Romero R, Quintero R, Oyarzun E et al 1988 Intraamniotic infection and the onset of labor in preterm premature rupture of the membranes. Am J Obstet Gynecol 159:661–666

Romero R, Sirtori M, Oyarzun E et al 1989a Infection and labor. V. Prevalence, microbiology, and clinical significance of intraamniotic infection in women with preterm labor and intact membranes. Am J Obstet Gynecol 161:817–824

Romero R, Wu YK, Brody DT, Oyarzun E, Duff GW, Durum SK 1989b Human decidua: a source of interleukin-1. Obstet Gynecol 73:31–34

Romero R, Brody DT, Oyarzun E et al 1989c Infection and labor. III. Interleukin-1: a signal for the onset of parturition. Am J Obstet Gynecol 160:1117–1123

Romero R, Manogue KR, Mitchell MD et al 1989c Infection and labor. IV. Cachectin-tumor necrosis factor in the amniotic fluid of women with intraamniotic infection and preterm labor. Am J Obstet Gynecol 161:336–341

Romero R, Mazor M, Tartakovsky B 1991 Systemic administration of interleukin-1 induces preterm parturition in mice. Am J Obstet Gynecol 165:969–971

Romero R, Mazor M, Brandt F et al 1992 Interleukin-1 alpha and interleukin-1 beta in preterm and term human parturition. Am J Reprod Immunol 27:117–123

Romero R, Yoon BH, Mazor M et al 1993a A comparative study of the diagnostic performance of amniotic fluid glucose, white blood cell count, interleukin-6, and gram stain in the detection of microbial invasion in patients with preterm premature rupture of membranes. Am J Obstet Gynecol 169:839–851

Romero R, Yoon BH, Kenney JS, Gomez R, Allison AC, Sehgal PB 1993b Amniotic fluid interleukin-6 determinations are of diagnostic and prognostic value in preterm labor. Am J Reprod Immunol 30:167–183

Romero R, Yoon BH, Mazor M et al 1993c A comparative study of the diagnostic performance of amniotic fluid glucose, white blood cell count, interleukin-6, and gram stain in the detection of microbial invasion in patients with preterm premature rupture of membranes. Am J Obstet Gynecol 169:839–851

Rouzioux C, Costagliola D, Burgard M et al 1995 Estimated timing of mother-to-child human immunodeficiency virus type 1 (HIV-1) transmission by use of a Markov model. The HIV Infection in Newborns French Collaborative Study Group. Am J Epidemiol 142:1330–1337

Rowe RD 1973 Cardiovascular disease in the rubella syndrome. Cardiovasc Clin 5:61–80

Ryder RW, Nsa W, Hassig SE et al 1989 Perinatal transmission of the human immunodeficiency virus type 1 to infants of seropositive women in Zaire. N Engl J Med 320:1637–1642

Saija A, Princi P, Lanza M, Scalese M, Aramnejad E, De Sarro A 1995 Systemic cytokine administration can affect blood-brain barrier permeability in the rat. Life Sci 56:775–784

Salafia CM, Minior VK, Rosenkrantz TS et al 1995 Maternal, placental, and neonatal associations with early germinal matrix/intraventricular hemorrhage in infants born before 32 weeks' gestation. Am J Perinatol 12:429–436

Sangha RK, Walton JC, Ensor CM, Tai HH, Challis JR 1994 Immunohistochemical localization, messenger ribonucleic acid abundance, and activity of 15-hydroxyprostaglandin dehydrogenase in placenta and fetal membranes during term and preterm labor. J Clin Endocrinol Metab 78:982–989

Sarnat HB 1992 Role of human fetal ependyma. Pediatr Neurol 8:163–178

Sawyer MH, Edwards DK, Spector SA 1987 Cytomegalovirus infection and bronchopulmonary dysplasia in premature infants. Am J Dis Child 141:303–305

Schmidt W, Klima G 1989 [Experimental and histologic studies on fetal membrane tensility and membrane rupture]. Zentralbl Gynakol 111:129–141

Sebire NJ, Carroll SG, Newbold M, Nicolaides KH 1996 Preterm prelabour amniorrhexis: relation to histological chorioamnionitis. J Matern Fetal Med 5:227–231

Sharief MK, Ciardi M, Thompson EJ 1992 Blood-brain barrier damage in patients with bacterial meningitis: association with tumor necrosis factor-alpha but not interleukin-1 beta. J Infect Dis 166:350–358

Shigeoka AO, Rote NS, Santos JI, Hill HR 1983 Assessment of the virulence factors of group B streptococci: correlation with sialic acid content. J Infect Dis 147:857–863

Silver HM, Sperling RS, St, Gibbs RS 1989 Evidence relating bacterial vaginosis to intraamniotic infection. Am J Obstet Gynecol 161:808–812

Simon MW, McCracken GH 1986 Neonatal cytomegalovirus infection. J Ky Med Assoc 84:345–350

Skinner SJ, Campos GA, Liggins GC 1981 Collagen content of human amniotic membranes: effect of gestation length and premature rupture. Obstet Gynecol 57:487–489

Sobel JD 1997 Vaginitis. N Engl J Med 337:1896–1903

Sperling RS, Shapiro DE, Coombs RW et al 1996 Maternal viral load, zidovudine treatment, and the risk of transmission of human immunodeficiency virus type 1 from mother to infant. Pediatric AIDS Clinical Trials Group Protocol 076 Study Group. N Engl J Med 335:1621–1629

Stagno S, Pass RF, Dworsky ME et al 1982a Congenital cytomegalovirus infection: The relative importance of primary and recurrent maternal infection. N Engl J Med 306:945–949

Stagno S, Pass RF, Dworsky ME, et al 1982b Congenital cytomegalovirus infection: The relative importance of primary and recurrent maternal infection. N Engl J Med 306:945–949

Stagno S, Tinker MK, Elrod C, Fuccillo DA, Cloud G, O'Beirne AJ 1985 Immunoglobulin M antibodies detected by enzyme-linked immunosorbent assay and radioimmunoassay in the diagnosis of cytomegalovirus infections in pregnant women and newborn infants. J Clin Microbiol 21:930–935

Steinborn A, Gunes H, Roddiger S, Halberstadt E 1996 Elevated placental cytokine release, a process associated with preterm labor in the absence of intrauterine infection. Obstet Gynecol 88:534–539

Stern H, Tucker SM 1973 Prospective study of cytomegalovirus infection in pregnancy. Br Med J 2:268–270

Stern H 1975 Intrauterine and perinatal cytomegalovirus infections. J Antimicrob Chemother 5 Suppl A:81–85

St Louis ME, Kamenga M, Brown C et al 1993 Risk for perinatal HIV-1 transmission according to maternal immunologic, virologic, and placental factors. JAMA 269:2853–2859

Taniguchi T, Matsuzaki N, Kameda T et al 1991 The enhanced production of placental interleukin-1 during labor and intrauterine infection. Am J Obstet Gynecol 165:131–137

Taylor GP, Lyall EG, Mercey D et al 1999 British HIV Association guidelines for prescribing antiretroviral therapy in pregnancy (1998). Sex Transm Infect 75:90–97

Thea DM, Steketee RW, Pliner V et al 1997 The effect of maternal viral load on the risk of perinatal transmission of HIV-1. New York City Perinatal HIV Transmission Collaborative Study Group. AIDS 11:437–444

Thomason JL, Gelbart SM, Wilcoski LM, Peterson AK, Jilly BJ, Hamilton PR 1988 Proline aminopeptidase activity as a rapid diagnostic test to confirm bacterial vaginosis. Obstet Gynecol 71:607–611

Unlinked Anonymous Surveys Steering group 1997 Prevalence of HIV in England and Wales in 1997. Annual Report of the Unlinked Anonymous Prevalence Monitoring Programme. London: Department of Health

Vadillo-Ortega F, Gonzalez-Avila G, Villanueva-Diaz C, Banales JL, Selman-Lama M, Alvarado D 1991 Human amniotic fluid modulation of collagenase production in cultured fibroblasts. A model of fetal membrane rupture. Am J Obstet Gynecol 164:664–668

Vadillo-Ortega F, Hernandez A, Gonzalez-Avila G, Bermejo L, Iwata K, Strauss JF 1996 Increased matrix metalloproteinase activity and reduced tissue inhibitor of metalloproteinases-1 levels in amniotic fluids from pregnancies complicated by premature rupture of membranes. Am J Obstet Gynecol 174:1371–1376

Vane J 1994 Towards a better aspirin. Nature 367:215–216

van Meir CA, Matthews SG, Keirse MJ, Ramirez MM, Bocking A, Challis JR 1997 15-hydroxyprostaglandin dehydrogenase: implications in preterm labor with and without ascending infection. J Clin Endocrinol Metab 82:969–976

Vapaavuori EK, Krohn K 1971 Intensive care of small premature infants. II. Postmortem findings. Acta Paediatr Scand 60:49–58

Vejtorp M, Bollerup AC, Vejtorp L et al 1988 Bacterial vaginosis: a double-blind randomized trial of the effect of treatment of the sexual partner. Br J Obstet Gynaecol 95:920–926

Vince G, Shorter S, Starkey P et al 1992 Localization of tumour necrosis factor production in cells at the materno/fetal interface in human pregnancy. Clin Exp Immunol 88:174–180

Vintzileos AM, Campbell WA, Nochimson DJ, Weinbaum PJ 1985 Degree of oligohydramnios and pregnancy outcome in patients with premature rupture of the membranes. Obstet Gynecol 66:162–167

Wang EE, Frayha H, Watts J et al 1988 Role of Ureaplasma urealyticum and other pathogens in the development of chronic lung disease of prematurity. Pediatr Infect Dis J 7:547–551

Watterberg KL, Demers LM, Scott SM, Murphy S 1996 Chorioamnionitis and early lung inflammation in infants in whom bronchopulmonary dysplasia develops [see comments]. Pediatrics 97:210–215

Watts DH, Krohn MA, Hillier SL, Eschenbach DA 1992 The association of occult amniotic fluid infection with gestational age and neonatal outcome among women in preterm labor. Obstet Gynecol 79:351–357

Weil ML, Itabashi H, Cremer NE, Oshiro L, Lennette EH, Carnay L 1975 Chronic progressive panencephalitis due to rubella virus simulating subacute sclerosing panencephalitis. N Engl J Med 292:994–998

Wendel GD 1988 Gestational and congenital syphilis. Clin Perinatol 15:287–303

Wiqvist N, Lindblom B, Wikland M, Wilhelmsson L 1983 Prostaglandins and uterine contractility. Acta Obstet Gynecol Scand Suppl 113:23–29

Witkin SS, Kligman I, Grifo JA, Rosenwaks Z 1995 Chlamydia trachomatis detected by polymerase chain reaction in cervices of culture-negative women correlates with adverse in vitro fertilization outcome. J Infect Dis 171:1657–1659

Wood EG, Dillon HCJ 1981 A prospective study of group B streptococcal bacteriuria in pregnancy. Am J Obstet Gynecol 140:515–520

Wright JL, Merchant RE 1994 Blood-brain barrier changes following intracerebral injection of human recombinant tumor necrosis factor-alpha in the rat. J Neurooncol 20:17–25

Yancey MK, Schuchat A, Brown LK, Ventura VL, Markenson GR 1996 The accuracy of late antenatal screening cultures in predicting genital group B streptococcal colonization at delivery. Obstet Gynecol 88:811–815

Yoon BH, Romero R, Kim CJ et al 1995 Amniotic fluid interleukin-6: a sensitive test for antenatal diagnosis of acute inflammatory lesions of preterm placenta and prediction of perinatal morbidity. Am J Obstet Gynecol 172:960–970

Yoon BH, Romero R, Yang SH et al 1996 Interleukin-6 concentrations in umbilical cord plasma are elevated in neonates with white matter lesions associated with periventricular leukomalacia. Am J Obstet Gynecol 174:1433–1440

Yoon BH, Romero R, Yang SH et al 1996 Interleukin-6 concentrations in umbilical cord plasma are elevated in neonates with white matter lesions associated with periventricular leukomalacia. Am J Obstet Gynecol 174:1433–1440

Yoon BH, Jun JK, Romero R et al 1997 Amniotic fluid inflammatory cytokines (interleukin-6, interleukin-1beta, and tumor necrosis factor-alpha), neonatal brain white matter lesions, and cerebral palsy. Am J Obstet Gynecol 177:19–26

Yoon BH, Romero R, Jun JK et al 1997 Amniotic fluid cytokines (interleukin-6, tumor necrosis factor-alpha, interleukin-1 beta, and interleukin-8) and the risk for the development of bronchopulmonary dysplasia. Am J Obstet Gynecol 177:825–830

Yoon BH, Kim CJ, Romero R et al 1997 Experimentally induced intrauterine infection causes fetal brain white matter lesions in rabbits. Am J Obstet Gynecol 177:797–802

Yoon BH, Romero R, Park JS et al 2000 Fetal exposure to an intra-amniotic inflammation and the development of cerebral palsy at the age of three years. Am J Obstet Gynecol 182:675–681

Yow MD, Leeds LJ, Thompson PK, Mason EOJ, Clark DJ, Beachler CW 1980 The natural history of group B streptococcal colonization in the pregnant woman and her offspring. I. Colonization studies. Am J Obstet Gynecol 137:34–38

Zahl PA, Bjerknes C 1943 Induction of decidual-placental hemorrhage in mice by the endotoxins of certain Gram-negative bacteria. Proc Soc Exp Biol Med 54:329

Zakar T, Teixeira FJ, Hirst JJ, Guo F, MacLeod EA, Olson DM 1994 Regulation of prostaglandin endoperoxide H synthase by glucocorticoids and activators of protein kinase C in the human amnion. J Reprod Fertil 100:43–50

Zlatnik FJ, Gellhaus TM, Benda JA, Koontz FP, Burmeister LF 1990 Histologic chorioamnionitis, microbial infection, and prematurity. Obstet Gynecol 76:355–359

23

Urinary tract in pregnancy

John M. Davison, William Dunlop

The contribution of the author of the equivalent chapter in the second edition, on which this chapter draws extensively, is gratefully acknowledged.

INTRODUCTION

An understanding of the changes affecting the urinary tract during pregnancy is important for abnormalities must be assessed against gestational basal values, many of which are inappropriate for the non-pregnant state (Baylis & Davison 1998, Conrad & Lindheimer 1999). A brief account of the most significant alterations in renal physiology is presented before discussing urinary tract disorders which may complicate pregnancy.

PREGNANCY-INDUCED ALTERATIONS IN THE URINARY TRACT

In pregnancy there is marked dilatation of the urinary tract (Peake et al 1983). By the third trimester some 97% of women show evidence of stasis or hydronephrosis (Cietak & Newton 1985a). Dilatation is more pronounced on the right than the left at all stages of pregnancy (Fig. 23.1), perhaps because of the usual dextrorotation of the uterus. Nephrosonographic studies suggest that renal parenchymal volumes also increase during pregnancy (Cietak & Newton 1985b), probably the result of increases in intrarenal fluid predominantly. It appears that a 70% increment has occurred by the beginning of the third trimester but that there may be a slight reduction during the latter weeks of pregnancy (Cietak & Newton 1985b). Very occasionally these cause massive ureteral and renal pelvis dilatation (as well as

slight reduction in cortical width), but this is without ill-effect in the long term (Brown 1990). Rarely, the changes may be extreme and precipitate the overdistension syndrome and

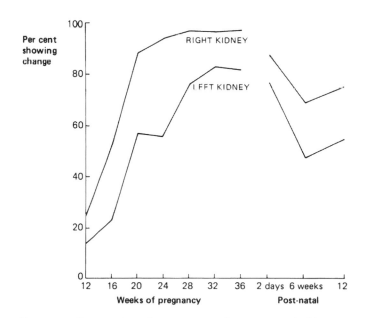

Fig. 23.1 Changes throughout pregnancy in percentage incidences for both kidneys of stasis and hydronephrosis with or without clubbing. Derived from the nephrosonographic data of Cietak & Newton (1985a).

hypertension (Satin et al 1993). Where there is a history of antivesicoureteric reflux surgery from childhood there may be increased risk of bilateral ureteric obstruction and possibly acute renal failure (Thorp et al 1999).

Renal haemodynamics

By the second trimester, renal blood flow (assessed indirectly as effective renal plasma flow) has increased, probably by as much as 70–80% (Roberts et al 1996). During the third trimester a significant reduction has been described, which cannot be attributed solely to the effects of maternal posture (Ezimokhai et al 1981). Since renal blood flow is one of the most important influences on the rate of filtration by the kidney, substantial increases in glomerular filtration rate (GFR) occur during pregnancy. The 50% increase is rather less than renal blood flow therefore filtration fraction, the proportion of renal plasma flow filtered at the glomerulus, decreases during early pregnancy (Baylis & Davison 1998).

In clinical practice, it is convenient to assess the glomerular filtration rate by means of the creatinine clearance, usually over a 24-hour period, in order to ensure reasonable accuracy. Serial investigations of groups of healthy women suggest that this has increased by 45% by the eighth week of pregnancy, from the LNMP or 6 weeks after conception. This increase is maintained throughout the second trimester, but a significant and consistent decrease in values equivalent to the non-pregnant occurs during the last weeks of pregnancy. Since the renal clearance of a substance bears a reciprocal relationship to its plasma concentrations, serum creatinine concentration falls during early pregnancy but it rises progressively during the third trimester. During pregnancy significant renal impairment may be present in women who have plasma concentrations of creatinine within the normal non-pregnant range, but on the other hand, increases in plasma creatinine concentrations (or decreases in creatinine clearance) during the third trimester of pregnancy may not imply pathological changes (Sturgiss et al 1994).

The augmented GFR of pregnancy is probably caused exclusively by increased renal blood flow, without coexistent glomerular hypertension and the evidence so far, albeit limited, argues against hyperfiltration as a result of increased intraglomerular pressure in normal human pregnancy (Roberts et al 1996). Studies of glomerular function and morphology in the rat have revealed no sustained increases in glomerular capillary blood pressure, no loss of nephrons, no persistent proteinuria and no morphological changes in animals that had completed five consecutive cycles of pregnancy, lactation: a long period in the lifespan of this species, compared with age-matched virgin controls (Davison & Baylis 1996).

Tubular function

Few constituents of the urine are excreted at the same rate as they are filtered at the glomerulus. Some substances, such as hippurate derivatives, are actively secreted into the urine but most are partially reabsorbed during passage through the nephron. In many cases of apparent tubular reabsorption a

degree of secretion by the kidney is also present, although it is difficult to determine the relative contributions of these two processes in human subjects (Baylis & Davison 1998).

Glucose is so avidly reabsorbed by the kidney that none is detectable by routine clinical testing in the urine of healthy non-pregnant individuals (Sturgiss et al 1994). However, during normal pregnancy, glucose excretion increases soon after conception. Excretion rates may be as much as 10 times those of non-pregnant women (20–100 mg/day) and there is marked variability both within and between days, the pattern bearing no demonstrable relationship to blood sugar concentrations. Some two-thirds of apparently healthy pregnant women will exhibit glycosuria to a degree conventionally considered clinically significant on repeated urinalysis. Conversely, not all women with impaired glucose tolerance during pregnancy are significantly glycosuric on routine testing. Glycosuria does not, therefore, provide reliable information about carbohydrate metabolism during pregnancy.

The extent to which glycosuria is provoked by pregnancy bears a significant relationship to the extent to which glucose is reabsorbed from the glomerular filtrate, not only during pregnancy but also in the same subjects in the non-pregnant state. It has been suggested that this phenomenon may be related to unsuspected renal tubular damage caused by previous urinary tract infections. Within a week of delivery, glucose excretion has returned to non-pregnant patterns. This is almost certainly a result of the reduction in GFR, for defects in glucose reabsorption can still be demonstrated by appropriate infusion protocols in women who have previously been severely glycosuric.

Changes in GFR are also partly responsible for the increased renal clearances of other urinary constituents and for reductions in their circulating concentrations. Of particular note in clinical practice are urea and uric acid, both of which decrease considerably during the first trimester of pregnancy (Conrad & Lindheimer 1999). However, during late pregnancy, the serum uric acid tends to increase. Part of this increase may reflect decreasing GFR, but there is also convincing evidence of altered renal handling. Renal reabsorption of uric acid decreases significantly during early pregnancy and rises gradually towards non-pregnant values thereafter (Dunlop & Davison 1977). The increased excretions of calcium (along with an inhibition of crystalluria) and protein are caused by alteration in tubular function as well as augmented renal haemodynamics (Sturgiss et al 1994). Increased total protein excretion should not be considered abnormal until it exceeds 400–500 mg in 24 hours, with the upper limit for albumin excretion being about 19 mg in 24 hours (Taylor & Davison 1998).

The distal renal tubule is actively concerned with volume homeostasis. Once again there is evidence of substantial change in this area of physiology during human pregnancy (Gallery & Lindheimer 1999). Total body water increases by between six and eight litres and there is a net retention of some 900 mmol of sodium. Although plasma osmolality is markedly reduced (by about 10 mosmol/l) from the early weeks of pregnancy, it is not associated with the water diuresis that would occur in the non-pregnant individual. While the process of osmoregulation is effective during pregnancy, there must be important changes in the osmotic thresholds that trigger control mechanisms, such as the sensation of thirst and the release of the antidiuretic hormone, arginine vasopressin (AVP). Other changes include a substantial increase in the metabolic clearance rate (MCR) of AVP, which rises fourfold after the first trimester, paralleling the appearance of, and marked increases in, circulating levels of a placental enzyme, vasopressinase (also called oxytocinase), which is a cystine aminopeptidase capable of inactivating large quantities of AVP *in vitro*. The MCR of 1-deamino-8-D-AVP (desmopressin acetate, dDAVP), an analogue of AVP that is resistant to enzyme degradation, is unchanged suggesting that the aminopeptidase enzymes are also active *in vivo* (Davison et al 1993, Lindheimer & Barron 1994). The osmoregulatory changes must be taken into account when managing women with known central diabetes insipidus (DI) and when diagnosing the rare syndrome of transient DI of pregnancy, which usually presents during the second trimester of pregnancy and remits postpartum.

These substantial alterations in physiological norms affect the interpretation of disordered renal function during pregnancy. A brief account of the changes of greatest clinical significance is provided in Table 23.1.

INFECTION OF THE URINARY TRACT

Definitions

The analysis of urine specimens during pregnancy is especially likely to be hampered by contamination at the time of collection with bacteria from urethra, vagina or perineum. This problem can be overcome by suprapubic aspiration of bladder urine, but this inconvenient procedure is distasteful to most patients and obstetricians. Another approach is to use the number of colony counts obtained upon culture of a fresh midstream urine specimen collected by a clean-catch technique involving anteroposterior swabbing of the vulva with water or a soap solution (not antiseptic) at least three times before starting micturition. True bacteriuria may then be defined as more than 100 000 bacteria *of the same species* per millilitre of urine, present in two consecutive specimens. Bacteriuria is frequently associated with discomfort on voiding, urgency and increased frequency of micturition, but these symptoms are common in pregnancy even in the absence of urinary tract infection. Conversely, asymptomatic (covert) bacteriuria, in which true bacteriuria is present without subjective evidence of urinary tract infection, may be of considerable clinical significance.

Bacteriuria originating from the upper urinary tract is more likely to recur and requires more rigorous surveillance and treatment. Numerous techniques have been used to investigate this problem without great success. The identification of antibody-coated bacteria in urine seemed promising but its precise value remains controversial (see Cunningham & Lucas 1994).

Pathogenesis

Bacteria originating in the large bowel probably colonise the urinary tract transperineally. By far the commonest infecting organism is *Escherichia coli*, responsible for 75–90% of bacteriuria during pregnancy. The pathogenic virulence of this organism, which is not the most plentiful in faeces, appears to derive from a number of factors, including resistance to vaginal acidity, rapid division in urine, adherence to cells and the production of chemicals which decrease ureteric peristalsis and inhibit phagocytosis (Stein & Fünfstuck 1999). Other organisms frequently responsible for urinary tract infection include *Klebsiella*, *Proteus*, coagulase-negative staphylococci and *Pseudomonas*. The interaction between host and infection is an exciting area of research and much is being discovered about the roles of uro-epithelial receptors, bacterial adhesions and induction of inflammatory responses (Lomberg et al 1992, Roche & Alexander 1992).

Asymptomatic bacteriuria

About 5% of young women are susceptible to bacteriuria. This is approximately the proportion found to be bacteriuric on routine screening during pregnancy (Stein & Fünfstuck 1999). Of those found to be non-bacteriuric on screening, only 1.5% develop bacteriuria later in pregnancy. Since the number of women in the initially uninfected group greatly exceeds the number with initial bacteriuria, however, this small percentage contributes substantially to the total population of pregnant women with urinary tract infection, accounting for some 30% of cases (Fig. 23.2).

Table 23.1 Physiological changes in common indices of renal function associated with human pregnancy: mean value (± 1 standard deviation)

Measurement	Units	Non-pregnant	Early pregnancy	Late pregnancy	Source
Effective renal plasma flow	ml/min	480 (72)	841 (144)	771 (175)	1
Glomerular filtration rate					
Inulin clearnace	ml/min	105 (24)	163 (19)	169 (22)	2
24-h creatinine clearance	ml/min	94 (8)	136 (11)	114 (10)	3, 4
Plasma					
Creatinine	μmol/l	77 (10)	60 (8)	64 (9)	5
Urea	mmol/l	4.3 (0.8)	3.0 (0.7)	2.8 (0.7)	5
Uric acid	μmol/l	246 (59)	189 (48)	269 (56)	6
Osmolality	mosmol/kg	288 (2.5)	278 (2.0)	280 (2.0)	7, 8

Sources: 1, Dunlop 1981; 2. Davison & Hytten 1974; 3. Davison & Noble 1981; 4. Davison et al 1980; 5. Lind, unpublished observations; 6. Lind et al 1984; 7. Davison et al 1981; 8. Davison et al 1988.

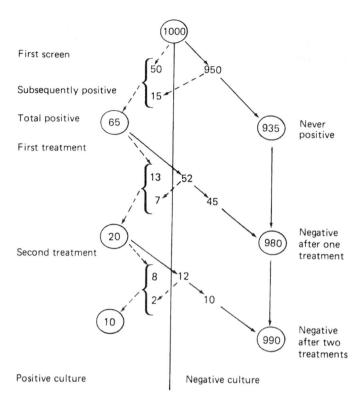

Fig. 23.2 Approximate outcome of screening and treatment for asymptomatic bacteriuria in 1000 women during pregnancy. Continuous arrows represent a change from positive to negative culture; interrupted arrows represent change towards positive culture. The 6.5% total positive rate comprises 5.0% positive on first culture and 1.5% subsequently positive. The first course of treatment produces a negative culture in 80% of bacteriuric women, but 15% of these develop recurrent bacteriuria. Second and subsequent courses of treatment produce negative cultures in only 40% of remaining bacteriuric women.

One antenatal study (Stenquist et al 1989), in which 99% of women took part in at least one screening, suggested that the rate of bacteriuria was highest between the 9th and 17th weeks of pregnancy. The 16th week was the optimal time for a single screen of bacteriuria calculated on the number of bacteria-free gestational weeks gained by treatment

Although asymptomatic bacteriuria has been implicated in several complications of pregnancy, including low birth-weight, fetal loss, pre-eclampsia and maternal anaemia, several of these apparent relationships may have resulted from inaccuracies in matching cases and controls and none is usually supported by subsequent studies (Martinell et al 1990). A meta-analysis of the better studies by Romero et al (1989) concludes that there was an association between untreated asymptomatic bacteriuria and low birthweight preterm delivery, and that therapy did reduce the incidence of low birth-weight babies. When evidence of previous parenchymal damage is present, however, there may be a greater propensity to hypertension (McGladerry et al 1992).

Not all untreated bacteriuric women develop symptoms of acute urinary tract infection during pregnancy and those found to have sterile urine when screened at antenatal booking will later contribute substantially to the pool of symptomatic women. Some, therefore, argued that screening programmes are not cost-effective (Campbell-Brown et al 1987). Chng & Hall (1982) found that as a predictor of symptomatic urinary infection, bacteriuria had a specificity of 89%, but a sensitivity of only 33%, and a false-positive rate of almost 90%. However, when their population was screened only by a single urine test an unusually high prevalence (11.8%) of bacteriuria was detected. Interestingly, they suggested that women with a history of previous urinary tract infection and current bacteriuria were 10 times more likely to develop symptoms during pregnancy than women without either feature. The overall cost effectiveness of screening for bacteriuria depends on its prevalence. In high-risk populations (prevalence >10%) it is likely to be valuable, whereas in low-risk populations (prevalence <5%) routine screening may well not be cost effective.

Most clinicians still treat asymptomatic bacteriuria. The agent chosen must not only be effective against the organism identified but also acceptable for use during pregnancy. Ampicillin and cephalosporins are commonly prescribed but short-acting sulphonamides may be equally effective. However, sulphonamides should be avoided during the last few weeks of pregnancy since they competitively inhibit the binding of bilirubin to albumin and they can increase the risk of neonatal hyperbilirubinaemia. Nitrofurantoin, which often causes nausea, may not be readily tolerated by pregnant women and it should also be avoided during late pregnancy because of the risk of haemolysis caused by deficiency of erythrocyte phosphate dehydrogenase in the newborn. The tetracyclines are not recommended during pregnancy because they predispose to dental staining in the child and (rarely) to acute fatty liver disease in the mother.

A two-week course of therapy is usually adequate and there is much controversy about short (especially single-dose) courses (Zinner 1992). Recurrent infection is common, however, affecting some 30% of bacteriuric women; after two courses of treatment about 15% will continue to have positive urinary cultures (Fig. 23.2). Recurrence may be caused either by relapse, when the same organism is found within six weeks of the initial infection, or to reinfection, when a different organism is detected. Treatment during pregnancy has little effect on the subsequent prevalence of bacteriuria, nor does persistent bacteriuria in women with normal urinary tracts contribute to chronic renal disease. Probably up to 20% of bacteriuric women have some abnormality of the urinary tract but in most this is minor and not clearly related to the disease. Postpartum intravenous urography is probably best reserved for bacteriuric women with a history of acute symptomatic infections before or during pregnancy, for those in whom bacteriuria is difficult to eradicate or for those in whom there is postpartum recurrence of disease (Schwartz et al 1999).

Symptomatic urinary tract infection

In the series of Chng & Hall (1982) 11.8% of bacteriuric women developed symptoms of urinary tract infection during pregnancy, whereas only 3.2% of women with sterile urine at initial screening did so. In the pregnant population as a whole, the incidence of symptoms was 4%. The upper urinary tract appears to be involved in a substantial proportion of cases: other workers estimate that acute pyelonephritis occurs in 1–2% of pregnancies, making it the most common renal complication of pregnancy (Cunningham & Lucas 1994, Schwartz et al 1999).

Acute pyelonephritis classically presents as a febrile illness associated with loin pain and vomiting, but there is considerable individual variation. The differential diagnosis includes other urinary tract pathology such as renal calculus or acute hydronephrosis (which can be recognised on ultrasound scanning or limited excretory urography), other causes of pyrexia such as respiratory tract infection, viraemia or toxoplasmosis (appropriate serological screening should be performed) and other causes of acute abdominal pain such as acute appendicitis, biliary colic, gastroenteritis, necrobiosis of a uterine fibroid or abruption of the placenta (Cunningham et al 1987). Acute pyelonephritis is associated with an increased incidence of premature labour and possibly also with intrauterine growth retardation or fetal death. The glomerular filtration rate may be reduced at the time of an acute episode during pregnancy in contradistinction to the usual lack of impairment of renal haemodynamics in non-pregnant patients.

Perhaps 20% of women with severe pyelonephritis develop complications in addition to renal dysfunction, including urinary obstruction, haematological dysfunction, perinephric cellulitis and abscess, septicaemic shock and pulmonary injury (Cunningham & Lucas 1994). Adult respiratory distress syndrome can be life-threatening (Cunningham et al 1987) and occurs in 8% of acute urinary infection patients if beta-mimetic tocolysis is given (Towers et al 1991). Prompt recognition and appropriate respiration support prevent severe hypoxaemia that may cause fetal death (Weinberger 1993).

Women with acute pyelonephritis are probably best managed in hospital. On admission, a midstream urine sample should be obtained, together with blood cultures in severely ill patients, but it will usually be necessary to begin antibiotic treatment before microbiological results are available. Recently it has been argued that urine and blood culture results are so rarely used to guide empirical therapy that the practice should be discontinued (MacMillan & Grimes 1991), thus saving much cost. The costs of urine culture and sensitivities are trivial, however, compared to the cost of hospitalization, which may be unnecessary for many patients with an uncomplicated infection (Wing et al 1999).

The chosen antibiotic must achieve high concentrations both in blood and in renal parenchyma. Ampicillin and the cephalosporins are widely favoured, but an aminoglycoside such as gentamicin may be of value in the acutely ill patient. The intravenous route of administration is preferred until pyrexia resolves, when oral therapy may be substituted. Antibiotic therapy should be continued for at least one month after an episode of acute pyelonephritis; thereafter, urine culture should be arranged at each antenatal visit.

Ultrasonic examination of the renal tract of pregnant women with pyelonephritis usually reveals significantly increased pelvicalyceal dilatation compared with normal physiological dilatation of pregnancy but as treatment does not necessarily produce a consistent decrease, the anomaly may antedate the acute infection (Twickler et al 1991).

Acute hydroureter and hydronephrosis

Rarely, pregnancy can precipitate the over-distension syndrome, with obstruction occurring at varying levels at or above the pelvic brim (Eckford et al 1991, Satin et al 1993). There is recurrent loin pain with increments in plasma creatinine but urinalysis reveals few or no red cells and repeat midstream urine specimens are negative. If positioning on the unaffected side, with appropriate antibiotics if needed, fails to resolve the situation, then urethral catheterization or ultrasound-guided percutaneous nephrostomy may be required (van Sonnenberg et al 1992).

CHRONIC RENAL DISEASE

There are conflicting views regarding pregnancy in women with renal disease (Jungers & Chauveau 1997). The majority view is that, with the exception of certain specific disease entities such as systemic lupus erythematosus, renal polyarteritis nodosa, scleroderma, perhaps IgA nephropathy, membranoproliferative glomerulonephritis and reflux nephropathy, the obstetric outcome is usually successful provided renal function is at most moderately compromised and hypertension is absent or minimal. If hypertension is present and it requires more than one drug for its control, the obstetric success becomes substantially less. In general, pregnancy does not have an adverse effect on the natural history of the renal disease (Davison & Baylis 1996, Williams 1997).

Renal dysfunction and its obstetric implications

It is inadvisable to assess renal function by plasma creatinine levels alone, as an individual may lose up to 50% of renal function, be symptom-free and still have a deceptively normal plasma creatinine level. Although a serum creatinine level of 75 µmol/l and a urea level of 4.5 mmol/l would be acceptable in non-pregnant subjects they are suspect in pregnant women (Table 23.1).

The ability to conceive and sustain a viable pregnancy is reduced more by the degree of functional impairment than by the nature of the underlying renal lesion. Fertility is diminished as renal function falls. When prepregnancy serum creatinine and urea levels exceed 275 µmol/l and 10 mmol/l respectively, normal pregnancy is rare. There are exceptions and successes have been documented in women with moderate to severe disease, including some treated by chronic dialysis (Okundaye et al 1998).

Prepregnancy counselling

Ideally, pregnancy is probably best restricted to women whose prepregnancy serum creatinine levels are 200 µmol/l or less and whose diastolic blood pressure is 90 mmHg or less. Whatever level is chosen, it should be recognised that degrees of impairment that do not cause symptoms or appear to disrupt homeostasis in non-pregnant individuals can certainly jeopardise pregnancy. The question has to be asked: 'Is pregnancy advisable?' (Table 23.2). In a woman with chronic renal disease who wishes to have a family, the sooner she conceives the better because in some, renal function will decline as they get older.

Effect of renal disease on pregnancy versus effect of pregnancy on renal disease

Clinicians do not always have the opportunity to counsel women with chronic renal disease before pregnancy. A patient with suspected or known renal disease often presents with pregnancy as a *fait accompli* and then the question is: 'Should pregnancy continue?' (Table 23.3). Also, think about the diagnosis of renal artery stenosis (Heybourne et al 1991). In view of the radically different obstetric and long-term outlooks in women with different degrees of renal insufficiency, it is important to consider the impact of pregnancy by categories of renal functional status prior to conception (Tables 23.4 and 23.5) (Cunningham et al 1990, Abe 1991, Imbascati & Ponticelli 1991, Jungers et al 1997, Bar et al 2000).

Table 23.2   Prepregnancy assessment: Is pregnancy advisable?

Factors to be considered
Type of chronic renal disease (see Table 23.6)
General health considerations
Diastolic blood pressure <90 mmHg
Renal function
Plasma creatinine <250 µmol/l
Plasma urea <10 mmol/l
Presence or absence of proteinuria
Review of all drug therapy

Table 23.3   Antenatal assessment: Should pregnancy continue?

Factors to be considered
Type of chronic renal disease (see Table 23.6)
General health considerations
Gestational age
Effect of pregnancy on blood pressure
Effect of pregnancy on renal function or plasma biochemistry
Review of all drug therapy
Past obstetric history

Table 23.4   Prepregnancy assessment: categories of renal functional status

Classification	Plasma creatinine (µmol/l)
Intact or mildly impaired renal function	≤125
Moderate renal insufficiency	≥125
Severe renal insufficiency	≥250

Table 23.5 Severity of renal disease and prospects for pregnancy[a]

Prospects	Category		
	Mild (%)	Moderate (%)	Severe (%)
Pregnancy Complications	26	47	86
Successful obstetric outcome[b]	96(85)	90(59)	25(71)
Long-term functional loss	<3(9)	25(80)	53(92)

[a]Estimates are based on data from 1973–1994 in 2370 women/3495 pregnancies and do not include collagen diseases. Numbers in parenthesis refer to prospects when complication(s) develop before 28 weeks' gestation.
[b]In recent years obstetric outcome has improved enormously for women with moderate and severe renal insufficiency. The infant survival rate was over 90% in 82 pregnancies in 67 women with moderate and severe disease from six tertiary referral centres, presumably reflecting the specialist obstetric and neonatal care at those centres (Jones & Hayslett 1996). Maternal complications were still inevitable (70%) and pregnancy-related loss of renal function occurred in almost 50%, of whom 10% progressed rapidly to end-stage failure. In another study (Jungers et al 1997) of 43 pregnancies in 30 women spanning 20 years, obstetric success was achieved in 82% (84% in 1985–1994, 55% in 1975–1984) but acceleration towards end-stage failure was evident in seven women (23%), all of whom had severe hypertension and heavy proteinuria prepregnancy.

Intact or mildly impaired renal function with minimal hypertension

Women with chronic renal disease but normal or only mildly decreased renal function at conception usually have a successful obstetric outcome and pregnancy does not adversely affect the course of their disease (Surian et al 1984, Hayslett 1985, Jungers et al 1997). Some authors suggest that this statement, although generally correct, should be tempered somewhat in lupus nephropathy, membranoproliferative glomerulonephritis and perhaps IgA and reflux nephropathies, which may be adversely affected by intercurrent pregnancy (Becker et al 1985, Nicklin 1991). When renal disease is detected or suspected for the first time during pregnancy (often because proteinuria or hypertension is first detected at the booking antenatal examination), it is usually surmised that renal function had been satisfactorily maintained until pregnancy brought an underlying mild lesion to clinical expression.

In most women with renal disease, the glomerular filtration rate increases during pregnancy, but the increases are usually less than those in normal pregnant women. Increased proteinuria is the most common effect of pregnancy in chronic renal disease, occurring in almost 50% of pregnancies (although rarely in women with chronic pyelonephritis), and it can be massive (often exceeding 3 g in 24 hours), frequently leading to nephrotic oedema. Between pregnancies and during long-term follow-up, hypertension, renal functional abnormalities and proteinuria are less common and less severe. When renal failure does supervene, it usually reflects the inexorable course of a particular renal disease (Jungers & Chauveau 1997).

Moderate and severe renal insufficiency

Prognosis has to be more guarded when renal function is moderately impaired before pregnancy (serum creatinine

125–250 µmol/l), but the number of cases reported is still small. Uncontrolled hypertension is a very important factor in the overall deterioration (Imbasciati et al 1984, Hou et al 1985, Imbasciati & Ponticelli 1991, Jungers et al 1997).

We generally recommend that pregnancy is best avoided in women who have lost 50% of their kidney function but some studies question this. Hou et al (1985) recorded a successful obstetrical outcome in 92% of the pregnancies in 22 women with serum creatinine levels of 190–300 µmol/l whose pregnancies were allowed to go beyond the second trimester. Many of these patients had high blood pressure and in 25% there was an accelerated decline in renal function. Therefore, although fetal survival is now improved in such women (Jones and Hayslett 1996) the maternal risks, especially complications of poorly controlled hypertension with acceleration towards end stage renal failure, might preclude encouraging such women to conceive or continue pregnancies which are already in progress (Table 23.5).

Most women with severe renal insufficiency (serum creatinine >250 µmol/l) are amenorrhoeic or anovulatory (Levy et al 1998). The likelihood of conceiving let alone having a normal pregnancy and delivery is, therefore, low but not impossible. Data on such patients are very limited but pregnancy can have an adverse effect on their disease (Jones & Hayslett 1996, Jungers et al 1997). In our opinion the risk of maternal complications (severe pre-eclampsia or bleeding) let alone renal failure are greater than the probability of a successful obstetric outcome. Nevertheless, some women elect to take these big risks (Stotland and Stotland 1997).

Antenatal assessment

Patients should be seen at two-week intervals until 32 weeks' gestation and weekly thereafter. Routine serial antenatal observations should be supplemented by:

- Assessment of 24-hour creatinine clearance and protein excretion
- Careful monitoring of blood pressure for early detection of hypertension and assessment of its severity
- Early detection of pregnancy-induced hypertension (pre-eclampsia)
- Assessment of fetal size, development and well-being
- Early detection of asymptomatic bacteriuria or urinary tract infection.

Renal function

If renal function deteriorates, reversible causes should be sought, such as urinary tract infection, subtle dehydration, or electrolyte imbalance, occasionally precipitated by inappropriate diuretic therapy. Near term, a 15–20% decrement in function, which affects serum creatine minimally, is permissible. Failure to detect a reversible cause of a significant decrement is a good reason to end the pregnancy by elective delivery. When proteinuria occurs and persists, but blood pressure is normal and renal function is preserved, the pregnancy can be allowed to continue.

Blood pressure

Most of the specific risks of hypertension appear to be mediated through superimposed pre-eclampsia, but excessive lowering of blood pressure may affect fetal growth (Von Dadelszen et al 2000). There is still controversy about the incidence of pre-eclampsia in those women with pre-existing renal disease. The diagnosis cannot be made with certainty on clinical grounds alone, because hypertension and proteinuria may be manifestations of the underlying renal disease (Gaber et al 1999). Treatment of hypertension is usually only undertaken at diastolic pressure >110 mmHg (see Chapter 24), but many would treat women with underlying renal disease more aggressively, believing this preserves function (Bakris 1996). Without doubt, perinatal outcome is poor in the presence of poorly controlled hypertension, nephrotic range proteinuria in early pregnancy or GFR ≤70 ml/minute prior to pregnancy or in the first trimester, whatever the type of renal disease (Abe 1996).

Fetal surveillance and timing of delivery

Serial assessment of fetal well-being is essential because renal disease can be associated with intrauterine growth restriction and, when complications do arise, the judicious moment for intervention is influenced by fetal status. Current management should minimise intrauterine fetal death as well as neonatal morbidity and mortality. Regardless of gestational age, most babies weighing 1500 g or more survive better in a special care nursery than in a hostile intrauterine environment. Delivery before 38 weeks may be necessary if:

- there are signs of impending intrauterine fetal death
- renal function deteriorates substantially
- uncontrollable hypertension supervenes
- eclampsia occurs.

Problems with particular renal diseases

Specific problems are associated with particular renal diseases (Table 23.6). The crux of the clinical situation is the balance between maternal prognosis and fetal prognosis—the effect of pregnancy on that disease and the effect of that disease on pregnancy. This balance is influenced by factors such as the degree of renal insufficiency and the presence or absence of hypertension, as well as the type of disease.

Acute and chronic glomerulonephritis

Acute glomerulonephritis is very rare as a complication of pregnancy and it can be mistaken for pre-eclampsia. The prognosis of chronic glomerulonephritis during pregnancy is hard to evaluate primarily because most reports are poorly documented, often failing to list the degree of functional impairment, the blood pressure prior to conception and the histological characteristics of the glomerulonephritis. One view is that most glomerular diseases are aggravated because of the hypercoagulable state that accompanies pregnancy, and patients are more prone to superimposed pre-eclampsia or hypertensive crises earlier in pregnancy (Epstein 1996).

Hereditary nephritis is an uncommon disorder, which may first manifest itself or exacerbate during pregnancy. It is

389

Table 23.6 Effects of pregnancy on established chronic renal disease

Renal disease	Effects
Chronic glomerulonephritis	Usually no adverse effect in the absence of hypertension. One view is that glomerulonephritis is adversely affected by the coagulation changes of pregnancy. Urinary tract infections may occur more frequently
IgA nephropathy	Risks of uncontrolled or sudden escalating hypertension and worsening of renal function
Pyelonephritis	Bacteriuria in pregnancy can lead to exacerbation. Multiple organ system derangements may ensue including adult RDS
Reflux nephropathy	Risks of sudden escalating hypertension and worsening of renal function
Urolithiasis	Infections can be more frequent, but ureteral dilatation and stasis do not seem to affect natural history
Polycystic disease (PKD)	Functional impairment and hypertension usually minimal in childbearing years
Diabetic nephropathy	Usually no adverse effect on the renal lesion, but there is increased frequency of infection, oedema, or pre-eclampsia
Systemic lupus erythematosus (SLE)	Controversial; prognosis most favourable if disease in remission >6 months prior to conception. Steroid dosage should be increased postpartum
Periarteritis nodosa	Fetal prognosis is dismal and maternal death often occurs
Scleroderma (SS)	If onset during pregnancy then can be rapid overall deterioration. Reactivation of quiescent scleroderma may occur postpartum
Previous urinary tract surgery	Might be associated with other malformations of the urogenital tract. Urinary tract infection common during pregnancy. Renal function may undergo reversible decrease. No significant obstructive problem but caesarean section often needed for abnormal presentation or to avoid disruption of the continence mechanism if artificial sphincter present
After nephrectomy, solitary kidney and pelvic kidney	Might be associated with other malformations of urogenital tract. Pregnancy well tolerated, dystocia rarely occurs with a pelvic kidney
Wegener's granulomatosis	Limited information. Proteinuria (± hypertension) is common from early in pregnancy. Immunosuppressives are safe but cytotoxic drugs are best avoided
Renal artery stenosis	May present as chronic hypertension or as recurrent isolated pre-eclampsia. If diagnosed then transluminal angioplasty can be undertaken in pregnancy if appropriate

a condition in which the patient has disordered platelet morphology and function. Pregnancy in women with this disorder has been successful from a renal viewpoint, but their pregnancies can be complicated by bleeding problems.

Pyelonephritis (tubulointerstitial disease)

The prognosis of pregnancy in women with chronic pyelonephritis seems similar to that of patients with glomerular disease in that its outcome is most favourable in normotensive patients with adequate renal function. Disease of an infectious nature has a propensity to exacerbate during pregnancy, and it may be minimised if the patient is well hydrated and rests frequently on her side, as ureteral obstruction by the enlarged uterus probably does not occur in this position. It has been suggested that patients with this condition are more prone to hypertensive complications during pregnancy, but in our experience they have a more benign antenatal course than women with glomerular disease.

Recurrent infection might be superimposed on vesicoureteric and intrarenal reflux and the resultant renal changes are termed reflux nephropathy. It is one of the most frequent diseases in women of childbearing age: a third of cases are clinically unmarked by pregnancy, up to 30% of women developing end-stage renal failure have reflux nephropathy and this is usually present before 40 years of age (Jungers & Chauveau 1997).

Polycystic renal disease

Polycystic renal disease may remain undetected during pregnancy, but careful questioning of pregnant women for a history of familial problems and the use of ultrasonography may lead to earlier detection. These patients do well when functional impairment is minimal and hypertension absent, which is often the case during childbearing years (Gabow 1993). They do, however, have an increased incidence of hypertension late in pregnancy, when their pregnancies are compared with those of sisters unaffected by this autosomal dominant disease.

There are other much rarer inherited renal disorders, some of which have an earlier onset than hereditary nephritis and polycystic renal disease. These include cystinosis, nephronophthisis, tuberous sclerosis and Von Hippel–Landau disease, in some of which antenatal diagnosis is technically possible (Davison & Baylis 1996, Grunfeld et al 1994).

Diabetic nephropathy

Because many patients have been diabetic since childhood, they probably already have microscopic changes in their kidneys. During pregnancy, diabetic women have an increased prevalence of bacteriuria and they may be more susceptible to symptomatic urinary tract infection. They also have an increased frequency of peripheral oedema and pre-eclampsia. Most women with diabetic nephropathy demonstrate the normal increments in renal function, and pregnancy does not accelerate deterioration of diabetic nephropathy (Coombs & Kitzmiller 1991, Hayslett & Reece 1994). It should be remembered, however, that prepregnancy diabetic nephropathy with plasma creatinine levels >125 μmol/l all too often progresses to renal failure during pregnancy.

Systemic lupus erythematosus

Systemic lupus erythematosus is a relatively common disease; its predilection to childbearing age makes the coincidence of systemic lupus erythematosus and pregnancy an important clinical problem (Grimes et al 1985). The profound disturbance of the immunological system in systemic lupus erythematosus, the complicated immunology of pregnancy, the multiple organ involvement and the complex clinical picture are just a few reasons for the vast literature. Suffice it to state here that there are differing opinions regarding the effects of pregnancy on lupus nephropathy. Transient improvements, no change, and a tendency to relapse have all been reported. Decisions regarding the status of the disease, as well as the assessment of the importance of having a baby to the patient and her partner, should be made on an individual basis. The majority of pregnancies succeed, especially when the maternal disease is in sustained, complete clinical remission for at least six months prior to conception. This applies even if the patient has severe pathological changes in her original renal biopsy and heavy proteinuria in the early stages of her disease. Continued signs of disease activity or increasing renal dysfunction reduce the likelihood of an uncomplicated pregnancy (Jungers et al 1982). From reviews of the literature it appears that as many as 19% experience decrements in GFR (progressive in 8%) and 42% have hypertension. The figures are worse if renal insufficiency (serum creatinine >125 μmol/l) antedates the pregnancy (Imbasciati & Ponticelli 1991, Nicklin 1991).

Lupus nephropathy may sometimes become manifest during pregnancy and when accompanied by hypertension and renal dysfunction in late pregnancy may be mistaken for pre-eclampsia. Some patients have a definite tendency to relapse, occasionally severely in the puerperium, and many advise steroids or an increase in steroid dosage at this time. The concept of the stormy puerperium is disputed, so others merely observe postpartum patients and do not institute or increase steroids unless signs of decreased renal function are noticed (Petri et al 1991).

Periarteritis nodosa

In contrast to lupus nephropathy, the outcome of pregnancy in women with renal involvement due to periarteritis nodosa is very poor, largely because of the associated hypertension, which is frequently of a malignant nature (Jungers & Chauveau, 1996). Although a few successful gestations have been reported, in most cases fetal prognosis is dismal and many pregnancies have ended with maternal deaths. This may merely reflect the nature of the disease itself, but it must, nevertheless, be taken into consideration when making a decision to go on with a pregnancy. Therapeutic termination of pregnancy (as an alternative form of management) may have less risk to the mother.

Scleroderma

This term includes a heterogeneous group of limited and systemic conditions causing hardening of the skin. Systemic sclerosis implies involvement of both skin and other sites, particularly certain internal organs. Renal involvement occurs in about 60% of patients, usually within 3–4 years of diagnosis. The combination of pregnancy and scleroderma is unusual because this infrequent disease occurs most often during the fourth and fifth decades and because patients with scleroderma tend to be relatively infertile. Whenever scleroderma has its onset during pregnancy, there is greater tendency for deterioration. Even after an uneventful and successful pregnancy, reactivation in the puerperium, with the use of converting enzyme inhibitors being necessary, can occur. Most maternal deaths have involved rapidly progressive scleroderma with pulmonary complications, infection, hypertension and heart failure.

Previous urinary tract surgery

Permanent urinary diversion is still used in the management of patients with congenital lower urinary tract defects; but since the introduction of self-catheterisation for neurogenic bladders, its use has declined in these patients. The most common complication of pregnancy is urinary infection, ranging from asymptomatic bacteriuria to severe pyelonephritis. Preterm labour occurs in 20% and there is some evidence that the use of prophylactic antibiotics throughout pregnancy reduces the incidence of this complication.

Renal function during pregnancy may decline, usually related to underlying infection or intermittent obstruction. With an ileal conduit, elevation and compression by the expanding uterus can cause outflow obstruction whereas with a ureterosigmoid anastomosis, ureteral obstruction may occur, with the changes usually reversing after delivery. A history of reflux surgery may lead to severe obstruction with renal failure and/or pre-eclampsia, reversible by stenting (Thorp et al 1999).

The mode of delivery is dictated by obstetric factors and not the presence of the urinary diversion. Abnormal presentation mainly accounts for a caesarean section rate of 25%, but of course minor genital tract abnormalities may contribute. Vaginal delivery is safe for women with an ileal conduit, augmentation cystoplasty or an ureterosigmoid anastomosis so long as one bears in mind that in the latter group, continence is dependent on an intact anal sphincter, which should be protected during vaginal delivery with an adequate mediolateral episiotomy.

Solitary kidney

Some patients have either a congenital absence of one kidney or marked unilateral hypoplasia. The majority, however, have lost a kidney because of pyelonephritis with abscess or hydronephrosis, unilateral tuberculosis, congenital abnormalities or tumour or following donor nephrectomy (Wrenshall et al 1996). In patients who had an infectious or structural renal problem, sequential prepregnancy investigation is needed for detection of any persistent infection.

There is no difference whether the right or left kidney remains as long as it is located in the normal anatomical position: if function is normal and stable, women with this problem seem to tolerate pregnancy well despite the superimposition of increases in glomerular filtration rate on the already hyperfiltering nephrons. Ectopic kidneys, usually pelvic, are more vulnerable to infection and are associated with decreased fetal salvage, probably because of an association with other malformations of the urogenital tract.

Urolithiasis

The prevalence of urolithiasis in pregnancy ranges from 0.3 to 0.35 per 1000 women (Maikranz et al 1994). Renal and ureteric calculi are one of the most common causes of non-uterine abdominal pain severe enough to necessitate hospital admission during pregnancy. When there are complications that need surgical intervention, pregnancy should not be a deterrent to intravenous urography, although there may be valid reluctance on the part of the clinician to consider radiological investigation. The absence of ureterics jets can be used when urolithiasis is suspected (Asrat et al 1998). It has been suggested that specific clinical criteria should be met before the undertaking of an intravenous urogram. For instance: microscopic haematuria, recurrent urinary tract symptoms, a sterile urine culture when pyelonephritis is suspected. The presence of two of these criteria points to a diagnosis of calculi in approximately 50% of gravidas, and an intravenous urogram is justifiable (Miller & Kakkis 1982).

Management should be conservative in the first instance, consisting primarily of adequate hydration, appropriate antibiotic therapy and pain relief with systemic analgesics (Maikranz et al 1994). The use of continuous segmental epidural block (T11 and L2) has been advocated, an approach that has long been used in non-pregnant patients with ureteric colic and which may even favourably influence spontaneous passage of the calculi. When the block is carefully confined to the relevant segments for pain relief, the patient micturates without difficulty, moves without assistance, and is at lower risk from thromboembolic problems than a drowsy patient immobilised in bed with pain, nausea and vomiting (Maikranz et al 1994).

An alternative approach involves placement of internal ureteral tubes or stents, between bladder and kidneys, under local anaesthesia, using cystoscopy or endoluminal ultrasound (Wolf et al 1992). The stent retains its position because it has a pig-tail or J-like curve at each end, and to prevent encrustation it can be changed every eight weeks. Also ultrasound-guided nephrostomy is a safe and effective method of relieving ureteric colic, or symptomatic obstructive hydronephrosis (van Sonnenberg et al 1992).

Wegener's granulomatosis

Despite the many potential dilemmas in these women there is a paucity of information on pregnancy. Proteinuria (with or without hypertension) is very common from early in pregnancy and the reports to date have described both complicated and uneventful pregnancies, including women taking azathioprine, alone or with cyclophosphamide (Harber et al 1999).

Nephrotic syndrome

The most common cause of nephrotic syndrome in late pregnancy is pre-eclampsia (Gaber et al 1999). This form has a poorer fetal prognosis than pre-eclampsia with less heavy proteinuria, but the maternal prognosis is similar. Other causes of nephrotic syndrome in pregnancy include proliferative or membranoproliferative glomerulonephritis, lipid nephrosis, lupus nephropathy, hereditary nephritis, diabetic nephropathy, renal vein thrombosis, amyloidosis and sec-

ondary syphilis. Some of these conditions do not respond to, and may even be seriously aggravated by, steroids, serving to emphasise the importance of establishing a tissue diagnosis before initiating steroid therapy.

The term nephrotic syndrome denotes the triad of heavy proteinuria, hypoalbuminaemia and generalised oedema, often associated with hyperlipidaemia. Since most of its manifestations derive from the excessive loss of protein in the urine, a more liberal definition is often used by nephrologists. This includes any renal disease characterised by proteinuria in excess of 3.5 g/24 h in the absence of depressed glomerular filtration rate. The prognosis of this syndrome is usually determined by the nature of the underlying glomerular problem.

If renal function is adequate and hypertension is absent, there should be few complications during pregnancy. Several of the physiological changes occurring during pregnancy may, however, simulate aggravation or exacerbation of the disease. For example, increments in renal haemodynamics as well as an increase in renal vein pressure may enhance protein excretion. Levels of serum albumin usually decrease by 5–10 g/l during normal pregnancy, and the further decreases that can occur in the nephrotic syndrome may enhance the tendency toward fluid retention. Despite oedema, diuretics should not be given, because these patients have a decreased intravascular volume and diuretics could compromise uteroplacental perfusion or aggravate the increased tendency to thrombotic episodes.

Questions that patients ask

Patient expectation is higher than ever. The questions commonly asked are usually quite simple. 'Is pregnancy advisable? Will the pregnancy be complicated? Will I have a live and healthy baby? Will I come to long-term harm?' (Table 23.5; Davison & Baylis 1996, Jungers & Chauveau 1997, Stotland & Stotland 1997, Williams 1997).

For any woman a balance must be struck between pregnancy outcome and the impact pregnancy has in the long term. Crucial determinants are the functional status of the kidneys at conception, the presence or absence of hypertension, and the nature of the renal lesion. If she wants to know if pregnancy will have a successful outcome, the answer is a qualified yes, provided her renal dysfunction is minimal. If dysfunction is moderate, there is still a fair chance that pregnancy will succeed, but the risks are much greater than in normal pregnancy. These statements have to be tempered somewhat in certain nephropathies, which appear to have a more problematical outcome during pregnancy. This is most true of collagen disorders affecting the kidney. Pregnancy outcome in the presence of focal glomerular sclerosis, reflux nephropathy, IgA nephropathy and mesangioproliferative glomerulonephritis is disputed.

Pregnancy does not adversely affect the natural history of the underlying renal lesion if kidney dysfunction is minimal and hypertension is absent at conception, again with the exception of certain collagen disorders. An important factor to be considered in long-term prognosis is the sclerotic effect that hyperfiltration might have in the residual (intact) glomeruli in kidneys of patients with moderate renal insufficiency, which could cause further progressive loss of renal function. Similarly, the compensatory changes in a woman with a single kidney are another form of hyperfiltration, which might over many years lessen the lifespan of that kidney. At the centre of this hypothesis is the implication that increases in glomerular pressure or glomerular plasma flow lead to sclerosis within the glomerulus (Brenner et al 1982), a concept that certainly cannot be ignored, since a pregnant woman with renal disease, like any healthy pregnant woman, experiences months of physiological hyperfiltration as part of the overall maternal adaptation to pregnancy. It seems unlikely, however, that there are any long-term sequelae in normal pregnancy (Baylis & Rennke 1985, Roberts et al 1996), and reassuring data are accruing from clinical practice and with research with animal models that has rigorously examined the mechanism controlling renal function in health and disease (Conrad & Lindheimer 1999).

RENAL TRANSPLANT PATIENTS

After transplantation, renal and endocrine functions return rapidly and normal sexual activity almost invariably ensues. About one in 50 women of childbearing age with a functioning renal transplant becomes pregnant. A total of 35% of all conceptions do not go beyond the initial trimester because of spontaneous miscarriage or therapeutic termination. Over 95% of pregnancies that do continue past the first trimester end successfully (Davison 1996). Over 10000 pregnancies are on record in women with a renal allograft, but of course many pregnancies, successful and unsuccessful, go unreported.

There are reports of transplants performed with the surgeons unaware that the recipient was in the second trimester of pregnancy (Sola et al 1988). The fact that mother, baby and kidneys came to no harm does not negate the importance of contraception counselling for all renal failure patients and the exclusion of pregnancy prior to transplantation.

Counselling and clinical considerations

The return of fertility and the possibility of conception in women of childbearing age who have transplants dictate appropriate counselling for all such patients (Levy et al 1998). Contraceptive advice should be routine. Couples who want a child should be encouraged to discuss all the implications, including the harsh realities of maternal prospects of survival. All involved must appreciate the possibility that the woman may not live to participate in the long-term care of her child (Table 23.7).

Prepregnancy guidelines
Individual centres formulate their own specific guidelines, but certain basic considerations cannot be ignored. Most advise that it is best to wait 18 months to two years posttransplant. This has turned out to be good advice because by then the patient will certainly have recovered from the major surgery

Table 23.7 Renal transplants and pregnancy: complications and outcome

Prospects	Incidence (%)
Pregnancy complications	49
Successful obstetric outcome	93 (70)
Long-term sequelae	12 (25)

These estimates are based on data reviewed in Davison (1994) for pregnancies which attained at least 28 weeks' gestation (1961–94). Figures in parentheses refer to prospects when pregnancy complications developed prior to 28 weeks' gestation.

and any sequelae, graft function will have stabilised and immunosuppression will be at maintenance levels. Consequently, potential teratogenic and suppressive effects and the risks of low birthweight or small-for-dates babies will be minimal.

A suitable set of guidelines for the advisability of pregnancy after renal transplant is given here, bearing in mind that these criteria are only relative indications:

- Good general health for about two years since transplantation
- Stature compatible with good obstetric outcome
- No proteinuria
- No significant hypertension or well controlled hypertension (the high incidence of hypertension in women with cyclosporin is a problem in this regard)
- No evidence of graft rejection
- No evidence of pelvicalyceal distension on a recent intravenous urogram
- Stable renal function plasma creatinine of 200 μmol/l or less
- Drug therapy reduced to maintenance levels: prednisone, 15 mg/day or less and azathioprine, 2 mg/kg bodyweight/day or less and cyclosporin A 5 mg/kg bodyweight/day or less.

Antenatal assessment

Pregnant renal transplant patients must be considered at high risk (Table 23.8). Antenatal care should be hospital-based and supplemented with attention to renal function surveillance, blood pressure control, bone disease, anaemia, detection of any infection (however trivial) and assessment of fetal well-being (see Davison 1996).

Table 23.8 Pregnancy in renal allograft recipients: antenatal watchpoints

Serial surveillance of renal function
Hypertension or pre-eclampsia
Graft rejection
Maternal infection
Fetal surveillance: intrauterine growth retardation
Premature rupture of membranes
Preterm labour
Decision of timing and method of delivery
Effects of drugs on fetus and neonate

Graft rejection and immunosuppressive therapy

Serious rejection episodes occur in 5% of pregnant renal allograft recipients where pregnancy is beyond the second trimester (Davison & Milne 1997). This incidence of rejection is no greater than that expected for non-pregnant allograft recipients, but it might be considered high because it is generally assumed that the privileged immunological state of pregnancy benefits the transplant. Furthermore, there are reports of reduction or cessation of immunosuppressive therapy during pregnancy without rejection episodes.

Whether pregnancy influences the course of subclinical chronic rejection, a problem present in most recipients, is unknown. No factors consistently predict which patients will develop rejection during pregnancy. There may also be a non-immune contribution to chronic graft failure because of the damaging effect of hyperfiltration through remnant nephrons, perhaps even exacerbated during pregnancy (Feehally et al 1986).

Difficulties can arise in distinguishing rejection from acute pyelonephritis, recurrent glomerulopathy, possibly severe pre-eclampsia and even cyclosporin A nephrotoxicity. Renal biopsy, which can be undertaken safely during pregnancy, might be necessary for definitive diagnosis. Ultrasonography alone may be very helpful because alterations in the echogenicity of the renal parenchyma and the presence of an indistinct corticomedullary boundary are indications of rejection.

Immunosuppressive therapy is usually maintained at prepregnancy levels, but adjustments may be needed if maternal leucocyte or platelet counts decrease. Azathioprine liver toxicity has been noted occasionally during pregnancy and responds to dose reduction (Armenti et al 1998, Ghandour et al 1998).

Cyclosporin A is supposedly more effective than conventional immunosuppression and its use throughout pregnancy is well established. Theoretically, some of the maternal physiological adaptations of pregnancy could be blunted by cyclosporin A: for example, its depressive effects on extracellular volume and renal haemodynamics may reduce a woman's ability to cope with the challenge of pregnancy to renal function and impair the placental circulation. More information is emerging (see Davison 1996) and overall the pregnancy success rates are comparable with those using routine immunosuppression. Reports from the recently established US National Transplantation Pregnancy Register are particularly enlightening (Armenti et al 1995, 1998) with birthweights reduced and intrauterine growth restriction, which is probably more related to hypertension or renal dysfunction than to cyclosporin A.

It will be interesting to monitor the impact of a new oral cyclosporin preparation, Neoral®, which has an improved drug biovailability in non-pregnant renal transplant patients where its use has enabled easier maintenance of blood drug concentrations in the therapeutic range. Data are slowly accruing for Tacrolimus (FK506, Prograf®) in renal recipients but good outcomes in liver recipients have been reported. There is a paucity of pregnancy data for mycophenolate mofetil (MMF, CellCept®), antithymocytic globulin (ATG, Atgam®) and orthoclione (OKT3®) although the latter has been used with steroids to treat acute rejection in pregnancy (Armenti et al 1998).

Renal function

The better the renal function before pregnancy the more satisfactory the obstetrical outcome, although one study indicates that increments in glomerular filtration rate in pregnancy are highest in women with the lowest initial GFR. In patients with satisfactory renal function before pregnancy, there may be a decline in GFR as well as the appearance of significant proteinuria during the third trimester (Toma et al 1999). These are usually transient and normal function returns postpartum. Permanent impairment of renal function is seen occasionally, especially where compromised prior to conception.

Hypertension

Hypertension, particularly before 28 weeks' gestation, is associated with adverse perinatal outcome (Sturgiss & Davison 1991). This may be due to the covert cardiovascular changes that accompany or are aggravated by chronic hypertension.

There is a 30% incidence of pre-eclampsia but, since the diagnosis is usually made by clinical criteria, it may be incorrect. In the absence of a renal biopsy, it may be difficult to distinguish pre-eclampsia from rejection and even recurrent glomerulopathy. Blood uric acid levels and 24-hour urinary protein excretion are often well above the norms for pregnancy in normotensive pregnant transplant patients. Increased values do not necessarily signify pre-eclampsia or herald its onset. Furthermore, although many of the hypertensive syndromes occurring in pregnant transplant recipients are quite severe, there is only one report of a patient in whom the condition progressed rapidly to eclampsia (Williams & Jelen 1979) with a subsequent pregnancy being normotensive and uneventful (Williams & Johnstone 1982).

Diabetes mellitus

The results of renal transplantations have been progressively improving in those patients whose end-stage renal failure was caused by juvenile onset diabetes mellitus (Remuzzi et al 1994). Inevitably pregnancies are now occurring in such women and the problems experienced are at least double those in other pregnant renal allograft recipients, perhaps related to the widespread, often covert, cardiovascular changes that accompany severe diabetes.

When women have received a pancreas as well as a kidney allograft the outlook may be considerably better (Calne et al 1988, Tyden et al 1989). For the future, the consensus is that simultaneous kidney and pancreas transplants are the treatment of choice for women with diabetic nephropathy (Light 1993), and inevitably these women will be potential mothers.

Timing and method of delivery

The factors previously discussed in relation to chronic renal disease also apply here. Timing depends on balancing fetal intrauterine jeopardy against neonatal morbidity and mortality, bearing in mind the mother's well-being at all times.

The transplanted kidney very rarely produces mechanical dystocia during labour and it does not sustain mechanical injury during vaginal delivery. Caesarean section is usually necessary only for purely obstetrical reasons. Regardless of the route of delivery, steroids must be augmented. Prophylactic antibiotics should be used for any surgical procedure, however trivial, for example, episiotomy.

Neonatal problems

There are hazards for the newborn (Table 23.9). Preterm delivery occurs in 50% and intrauterine growth restriction in at least 20% (range 8–40%), lower birthweights are seen in infants born to recipients less than two years posttransplant (Cunningham et al 1983, Ahlswede et al 1992) and cyclosporin A in some series has been associated with severe birthweight depression (Pickrell et al 1988, Haugen et al 1991, Armenti et al 1998, but see previous discussion).

Although there are no frequent or predominant congenital anomalies associated with chronic nephropathy (Raine et al 1992), one or more complications occur in about 40% of babies including respiratory distress syndrome, adrenocortical insufficiency, thrombocytopenia, leukopenia, cytomegalovirus and other infection, as well as development of hepatitis B surface antigen (HB Ag) carrier state.

Infectious hepatitis

These patients may have been exposed to multiple transfusions when on haemodialysis, and some may carry hepatitis B virus. These issues are discussed in detail elsewhere (see Chapter 22).

Breast-feeding

As there are substantial benefits to breast-feeding and since the baby has already been exposed to immunosuppressive drugs and their metabolites throughout pregnancy and their concentrations in mothers' milk are minimal, it could be argued that breast-feeding should be allowed. However, until these many uncertainties are resolved, breast-feeding should probably not be encouraged. Nonetheless, some mothers choose to breastfeed regardless!

Table 23.9 Neonatal problems in offspring of renal allograft recipients

Preterm delivery/small for gestational age
Respiratory distress syndrome
Depressed haematopoiesis
Lymphoid/thymic hypoplasia
Adrenocortical insufficiency
Septicaemia
Cytomegalovirus infection
Hepatitis B surface antigen carrier state
Congenital abnormalities
Immunological problems
Reduced lymphocyte phytohaemagglutin-reactivity
Reduced T-lymphocyte
Reduced immunoglobulin levels
Chromosome aberrations in lymphocytes

Long-term assessment

Azathioprine can cause transient gaps and breaks in the chromosomes of leucocytes. These defects may take almost two years to disappear spontaneously but in tissues not yet studied these anomalies may not be as temporary. The sequelae could be eventual development of malignancies in affected offspring or abnormalities in the reproductive performance in the next generation. There are some disturbing animal observations. For instance, fertility problems affect the female offspring of mice that have received low doses of 6-mercaptopurine, the major metabolite of azathioprine (equivalent to 3 mg/kg, Reimers & Sluss 1978). These offspring subsequently prove sterile, or if they conceive, have smaller litters and more dead fetuses than do unexposed dams. Thus, exposure in utero may not affect otherwise normal females until they embark on their reproductive careers.

Maternal follow-up after pregnancy

General outlook

The long-term impact, in terms of general well-being and renal prognosis, is difficult to quantify. The consensus is that it is safest to wait two years after transplantation before becoming pregnant. Pregnancy does occasionally and sometimes unpredictably cause irreversible declines in renal function. Recent studies, however, based on a comparison of groups of renal cadaver transplant recipients who did and did not become pregnant, concluded that pregnancy had no effect on graft function or survival (Rizzoni et al 1992, Sturgiss & Davison 1995, Armenti et al 1998). One exception, however, was a study from Finland which concludes that pregnancy does carry an increased risk of long-term reduced renal function and shorter graft survival and, furthermore, success in one posttransplant pregnancy does not guarantee success in repeated pregnancies (Salmela et al 1993). In this study, strangely, there were no graft losses in the controls and a low (36%) preterm delivery rate compared to the rest of the literature, possibly indicating longer pregnancies which theoretically might contribute to the long-term problems if time was bought at the expense of persistent hypertension and slowly dwindling renal function, which occurs even in late pregnancy in healthy women. More long-term studies are needed to assess this area, especially with the advent of new immunosupressive drugs and the emergence of national registries will help (Armenti et al 1995, Davison & Redman 1997).

Contraception

Oral contraceptives can produce subtle changes in the immune system, but this does not necessarily contraindicate their use. Low-dose oestrogen–progestogen preparations can be prescribed, although some authorities avoid them because of the possibility of causing or aggravating hypertension or further increasing the incidence of thromboembolism. If oral contraceptives are prescribed, careful and frequent surveillance is needed.

An intrauterine contraceptive device (IUCD) may aggravate menstrual problems, which in turn, may obfuscate signs and symptoms of abnormalities of early pregnancy, such as threatened miscarriage or ectopic pregnancy. The increased risk of pelvic infection associated with the IUCD makes this method worrisome in an immunosuppressed patient. In any case, the efficacy of these devices may be reduced by immunosuppressive and anti-inflammatory agents, possibly because of modification of the leucocyte response. Nevertheless, many patients request this method. Careful counselling and follow-up are essential.

Gynaecological problems

Long-term immunosuppression increases the risk of developing malignancy a hundred-fold (Newstead 1998). This is probably because of loss of immune resistance, chronic immunosuppression allowing tumour proliferation or prolonged antigenic stimulation of the reticuloendothelial system. The genital tract is an important site for cancer (Halpert et al 1986). Reports of cervical change range from cellular atypia to invasive squamous cell carcinoma. Carcinoma of the vulva has also been noted in young patients. Regular pelvic examinations and cervical cytology are essential in these women. Lastly, unusual malignancies have been reported including reactivation of latent choriocarcinoma (Lelievre et al 1978) and metastases from occult choriocarcinoma in a cadaver kidney (Manifold et al 1983).

PREGNANCY IN WOMEN ON LONG-TERM DIALYSIS

Reduced libido and relative infertility are common in women on haemodialysis and peritoneal dialysis but they can still conceive and must, therefore, use contraception if they wish to avoid pregnancy (Davison & Baylis 1996, Jungers & Chauveau 1997, Okundaye et al 1998). Although conception is not common (an incidence of one in 200 patients has been quoted), its true frequency is unknown because most pregnancies in dialysed patients probably end in early spontaneous miscarriage while there is also a high therapeutic termination rate in this group of patients.

Some women do achieve delivery of a viable infant, but most authorities do not advise attempts at pregnancy or its continuation, if present, when the woman has severe renal insufficiency. These women are prone to volume overload, severe exacerbations of their hypertension and superimposed pre-eclampsia and polyhydramnios. They also have a high fetal wastage at all stages in pregnancy. Even when therapeutic terminations are excluded the live birth outcome at very best is 40–50%. Fetal growth restriction and prematurity are common. However, as the debate continues more and more women are opting to take the chance of continuing with pregnancy (Hou & Firanek 1998).

Women frequently present in advanced pregnancy because pregnancy was not suspected earlier. Irregular menstruation is common in dialysis patients and missed periods are usually ignored. Urine pregnancy tests are unreliable (even if there is any urine available). Ultrasound is needed to confirm and to date the pregnancy.

There appear to be no specific advantages to any particular dialysis modality but, whatever the route, the dialysis strategy involves a 50% increase in hours and frequency and the following aims:

- Maintain serum urea <20 mmol/l (some would argue <15 mmol) as intrauterine death is more likely if levels are much in excess of 20 mmol/l. Success has occasionally been achieved despite levels of 25 mmol/l for many weeks.
- Avoid hypotension during dialysis, which can be damaging to the fetus. In late pregnancy the uterus and the supine posture may aggravate this by descreasing venous return.
- Ensure rigid control of blood pressure.
- Avoid rapid fluctuations in intravascular volume, by limiting interdialysis weight gain to about 1 kg until late pregnancy.
- Scrutinise carefully for preterm labour, as dialysis and uterine contractions are associated.
- Watch calcium levels closely to avoid hypercalcaemia.

Dialysis patients are usually anaemic, which is invariably aggravated further in pregnancy (Bagon et al 1998). Blood transfusion may be needed, especially before delivery. Caution is necessary because transfusion may exacerbate hypertension and impair the ability to control circulatory overload, even with extra dialysis. Treatment of anaemia with low-dose synthetic erthropoietin (rHuEpo) can be used in pregnancy without ill-effect and the need to increase the dose in an otherwise stable patient may be an indication that she is pregnant.

OBSTETRIC ACUTE RENAL FAILURE

Acute renal failure is a clinical syndrome characterised by sudden and marked decrease in GFR, increasing serum creatinine and urea and usually decreased urine output to <400 ml in 24 hours (Davison & Baylis 1996). Thus acute renal failure only describes the functional state of the renal tract without defining the pathology. For the most part, obstetric acute renal failure, whether during or after pregnancy, occurs in women with previously healthy kidneys. Such patients require multidisciplinary evaluation and treatment, the principles of which resemble those for the non-pregnant but there are also specific diagnostic and management points to bear in mind in pregnancy (Jungers & Chauveau 1997; Tables 23.10, 23.11 and 23.12).

Pregnancy complications that can be associated with acute renal failure

Septic abortion

There are many reasons why acute renal failure is associated with septic miscarriage. Dehydration and hypotension can lead to considerable renal ischaemia. Soap and lysol, common abortifacients, may have specific nephrotoxic effects. The marked haemolysis (with severe anaemia) caused by some bacteria and chemical abortifacients is, however, sufficient to provoke the renal shutdown. Most pregnancy sepsis is caused by gram-negative bacteria, and clostridia are

Table 23.10   Causes of acute renal failure in pregnancy

Urinary tract obstruction	Damage to ureters: during ceasarean section and repair of cervical/vaginal lacerations Pelvic haematoma Broad ligament haematoma
Volume contraction/hypotension	Antepartum haemorrhage (placenta previa) Postpartum haemorrhage: from uterus or extensive soft-tissue trauma Abortion Hyperemesis gravidarum Adrenocortical failure; usually failure to augment steroids to cover delivery in patient on long-term therapy
Volume contraction/hypotension and coagulopathy	Antepartum haemorrhage (abruptio placentae) Pre-eclampsia/eclampsia Amniotic fluid embolism Incompatible blood transfusion Drug reaction(s) Acute fatty liver of pregnancy (AFLP) Haemolytic uraemic syndrome (HUS)
Volume contraction/hypotension, coagulopathy and infection	Septic abortion Chorioamnionitis Pyelonephritis Puerperal sepsis

Table 23.11   Differential diagnosis of oliguria

	Prerenal failure (vasomotor nephropathy)	Acute tubular necrosis
History	Vomiting, diarrhoea, other causes of dehydration	Dehydration, ischaemic insult, nephrotoxin ingestion but no specific history in 50% of cases
Physical examination	Decreased blood pressure, increased pulse rate, poor skin turgor	May have signs of dehydration, but physical examination often normal
Urinalysis	Concentrated urine; few formed elements on sediment, but many hyaline cases	Isothenuria; sediment contains renal tubular cells and pigmented casts, but may be normal
Urinary sodium	<20 mEq/l; most <10 mEq/l	≥25, usually >60 mEq/l
Urine–plasma (U/P) ratios	High	Low
Osmolality	Often ≥1.5	<1.1
Urea	≥20	≤3
Creatinine	>40	<1 5
Fractional sodium excretion (U/P$_{Na}$/U/P$_{creatinine}$)	<1%	>1%
Renal failure index (U/P$_{Na}$/U/P$_{creatinine}$)	<1 <1	>1 >1

responsible for only 0.5% of cases in which patients develop shock. It is the latter bacterium that is responsible for one of the most devastating syndromes complication pregnancy.

Pyelonephritis

In the absence of complicating features such as obstruction, calculi, papillary necrosis and analgesic nephropathy, it is extremely rare for acute pyelonephritis to cause acute renal failure in non-pregnant subjects, but this association appears to be more frequent in pregnant women (Cunningham & Lucas 1994). It is known that acute pyelonephritis in pregnancy is accompanied by decrements in GFR, in contrast to

non-pregnant patients. It is has been suggested that the vasculature in pregnancy may be more sensitive to the vasoactive effect of bacterial endotoxins and cytokines.

Pre-eclampsia/eclampsia and HELLP Syndrome

The characteristic renal lesion is glomerular endotheliosis where the glomeruli are enlarged and ischaemic because of swelling of the intracapillary cells, with significant decreases in GFR (Gaber & Lindheimer 1999). Oliguria is not uncommon in these patients and may represent a normal response to short lived prerenal causes with reduced intravascular volume, poor fluid intake, vasospasm or decreased arterial pres-

Table 23.12 Conditions with haematologic and hepatic involvement linked to acute renal failure

	Pre-eclampsia	AFLP[a]	TTP[b]	HUS[c]	Viral or Drug-Induced Hepatitis
Symptoms					
Onset	>20 wk	>28 wk	Anytime	Anytime	Anytime
Nausea/vomiting	– or +	+++	+	+ to +++	+++
Abdominal pain	+ to +++	++	+	–	+/++
Signs					
Hypertension	+ to +++	–/+	+	+ to +++	–
Fever	–	–/+	+	–/+	–/+
Abnormal mental status	– to +++	– to +++	– to +++	–/+	–/+
Liver function tests					
Bilirubin	NL[d] to 5 × ↑	SL to 30 × ↑	↑ indirect	↑ indirect	5–40 × ↑
ALT (SGPT)	SL[e] to 100 × ↑	SL to 20 × ↑	NL to SL ↑	NL to SL ↑	SL to >100 × ↑
Glucose	NL	NL or ↓	NL	NL	NL or ↓
Ammonia	NL	↑	NL	NL	NL or ↑
Haematology					
White blood cell count	NL to ↑	↑↑	NL or ↑	NL or ↑	NL or ↑
Schistocytes	+/++	+/++	+++	+++	–
Normoblasts	–	+/++	+++	+++	–
Platelets	30 K to NL	20–150 K	5–100 K	5–100 K	NL
Prothrombin time	NL or SL ↑	NL to ↑↑↑	NL	NL	NL to ↑↑↑
Fibrinogen	NL or SL ↓	NL or ↓	NL	NL or SL ↓	↑, NL or ↓
Fibrin degradation products	NL or SL ↑	NL or ↑	NL	NL or SL ↑	NL
Antithrombin III	↓	↓	NL	NL	↓
Renal					
Creatinine	NL to 5 × ↑	NL to 10 × ↑	NL to 5 × ↑	Rapid & marked ↑	NL
Proteinuria	1+ to 4+	1+ to 4+	0 to 4+	0 to 4+	NL
Uric acid	↑	↑	NL or ↑	↑	NL

[a] AFLP, acute fatty liver of pregnancy
[b] TTP, thrombotic thrombocytopenic purpura
[c] HUS, haemolytic uremia syndrome
[d] NL, normal
[e] SL, slight

sure following antihypertensive treatment all predisposing to decreased urinary output. Of greater concern is prerenal failure presenting as oliguria after acute blood loss from abruptio placentae or postpartum haemorrhage, which is particularly dangerous if DIC supervenes.

Acute renal failure is usually due to acute tubular necrosis, but acute cortical necrosis may also occur. It is possible that acute tubular necrosis is the obligatory outcome of glomerular cell swelling and loss of anionic charge along with complete obliteration of the capillary lumen. If the ARF is related solely to pre-eclampsia without chronic hypertension, renal disease or both, before pregnancy, then long-term renal function is normal in about 80% of cases. Underlying chronic problems reduce this to 20%, with the rest needing long-term dialysis.

HELLP syndrome (*Haemolysis*, *Elevated Liver* enzymes and *Low Platelets*) was originally thought to be a rare complication of severe pre-eclampsia but as more attention has been paid to liver and haematological functions in gravidas it is now diagnosed more often. It is not clear, however, whether acute renal failure is a specific component of the HELLP syndrome itself or a complication of a particularly severe multisystem condition and it may even occur without the haemolysis, as ELLP syndrome (Sibai & Ramadan 1993; see Table 23.12).

Chronic renal disease

In women with moderate and severe renal disease, gestational complications are inevitable and pregnancy-related loss of renal function occurs in almost 50% of women, of whom 10% progress rapidly to end-stage renal failure shortly after delivery but also occasionally in late pregnancy, when dialysis may be implemented to prolong gestation (Jones & Hayslett 1996, Jungers et al 1997).

Acute renal failure specific to pregnancy

Acute fatty liver of pregnancy

Acute fatty liver of pregnancy, also called *obstetric pseudoacute yellow atrophy*, is a rare complication of late pregnancy or early postpartum period, occurring in approximately one in 13 000 deliveries (Pertuisit & Grunfeld 1994). It is characterised by jaundice, severe hepatic dysfunction, including coma and varying degrees of renal failure (Table 23.12).

The acute renal failure appears to be caused by haemodynamic factors, as in the hepatorenal syndrome, but some cases have been associated with DIC. Some believe that tetracyclines may precipitate this condition, but this antibiotic is no longer used in obstetric practice. In addition, reversible urea-cycle enzyme deficiencies (orthinine transcarbamylase and carbamyl phosphate synthetase) resembling those seen in Reye's syndrome have been described.

The clinician may be misled by a previously well patient who just feels unwell with vague abdominal pain, nausea and vomiting and perhaps a fever who then rapidly develops severe jaundice and hepatic encephalopathy. Common misdiagnoses are non-specific gastrointestinal disturbance, septicaemia or pre-eclampsia with liver involvement. It has been estimated that acute fatty liver of pregnancy and pre-eclampsia coexist approximately 20% of the time.

Treatment consists of supportive therapy for hepatic and renal failure and termination of the pregnancy although the efficacy of this for maternal survival has not been proven. The mortality rate is high, with death resulting primarily from hepatic rather than renal failure. The more recent literature, however, suggests that the prognosis for this condition has improved and more survivors are being recorded (Jungers & Chauveau 1997).

Haemolytic uremic syndrome

Haemolytic uremic syndrome also called *idiopathic postpartum renal failure, postpartum malignant nephrosclerosis* and *irreversible postpartum renal failure*, is rare and frequently fatal. It is characterised by the onset of renal failure 3–10 weeks postpartum, usually after an uneventful pregnancy and delivery. The patient develops marked azotemia and severe hypertension, frequently associated with microangiopathic haemolytic anemia and platelet aggregation with formation of microthrombi in the terminal portions of the renal vasculature. It should be remembered that renal failure, microangiopathic haemolytic anaemia, and thrombocytopenia may also be associated in gravidas with severe pre-eclampsia, HELLP syndrome, acute fatty liver of pregnancy and thrombotic thrombocytopenia purpura. Discrimination between these antenatal disorders may be difficult (see Table 23.12).

Many patients succumb despite treatment with dialysis, plasmaphoresis, exchange transfusion, immunosuppression, heparin, streptokinase, dipyridamole, aspirin or corticosteroids, alone or in combination. Others have survived but they required long-term dialysis or transplantation with a chance of recurrence of the haemolytic uraemic syndrome lesion in the graft.

Cortical necrosis of pregnancy

The incidence has decreased over the years to below one in 80 000. Although cortical necrosis may involve the entire renal cortex, resulting in irreversible renal failure, it is the patchy variety that occurs more often in pregnancy. It is more prevalent in multigravidas >30 years and may be associated with overwhelming septicaemia, placental abruption, unrecognised long-standing intrauterine death and occasionally pre-eclampsia with most presenting in the third trimester or the puerperium (Table 23.11).

There is an initial episode of severe oliguria, which lasts much longer than in uncomplicated acute tubular necrosis followed by a variable return of function and stable period of moderate renal insufficiency. Years later, for reasons still obscure, renal function may decrease again, often leading to end-stage renal failure.

Management of obstetric acute renal failure

Treatment of acute renal failure resembles that in nonpregnant populations and aims at retarding the appearance of uraemic symptomatology, acid-base and electrolyte disturbances and volume problems (i.e. overhydration when the patient is oliguric and dehydration during the polyuric phase). There must also be an awareness of the propensity of patients with acute renal failure to develop infection, a complication that can be serious in pregnant women. Many cases will respond to judicious conservative management, but if such an approach is unsuccessful dialysis will be necessary.

Dialysis in patients with acute renal failure can be prescribed prophylactically, that is, prior to the appearance of electrolyte and acidemia, or uraemic symptoms. Such prophylactic dialysis, although controversial, may be helpful in women with an immature fetus and in whom temporisation is desired.

When possible with acute renal failure, early delivery (as dictated by fetal maturity) should be undertaken. Blood losses should be replaced quickly to the point of overtransfusing slightly, because in the pregnant patient uterine bleeding may be concealed and so underestimated. It should also be remembered that the baby can be subject to rapid dehydration, because of increased levels of urea and other solutes within the fetal circulation precipitating an osmotic diuresis.

CONCLUSIONS

Women with renal disorders contemplating pregnancy, or in early pregnancy, ask four questions:

1. Is pregnancy advisable?
2. Will the pregnancy be complicated?
3. Will I have a live, healthy baby?
4. Will I be harmed in the longer term?

The following answers are relevant.

Chronic renal disease

Provided kidney dysfunction is minimal and hypertension is absent before pregnancy, then pregnancy is not contraindicated, and a successful and healthy obstetric outcome is usually the rule. Pregnancy does not adversely affect the course of the renal disease. This statement must be tempered somewhat as certain nephropathies, such as lupus nephropathy and perhaps mesangiocapillary glomerulonephritis, appear more sensitive to intercurrent pregnancy. It also does not apply to women who have scleroderma and periarteritis nodosa.

It must be emphasised that the degree of renal dysfunction or hypertension prior to pregnancy influences the incidence of both maternal and fetal complications. The main dangers are that women with moderate, and certainly those with severe dysfunction, will experience serious deterioration in renal function and accelerated progression of the underlying disease during pregnancy and post-delivery.

Dialysis

These patients are usually infertile, but contraception should not be neglected. On balance, pregnancy is probably contraindicated, since it is invariably complicated and poses major risks to the mother, with an uncertain and low chance of success. Even when therapeutic terminations are excluded, the live birth outcome is at best 40–50%.

Renal transplantation

Bearing in mind the criteria used in chronic renal disease—prepregnancy renal status or hypertension—certain generalisations can be made. If, according to a suitable set of guidelines, prepregnancy assessment is satisfactory, then pregnancy can be advised. Despite an overall five fold increase in the rate of complications, the chances of success are about 95%. If complications (usually hypertension, renal deterioration, and rejection) occur before 28 weeks, then successful obstetric outcome is reduced by 20%. More information is needed about the intrauterine effects and neonatal aftermath of immunosuppression which, at maintenance levels, is apparently harmless. From data available, it seems that pregnancy does not compromise long-term renal outlook.

Acute renal problems

In otherwise healthy women, these can be managed as in the non-pregnant population, bearing in mind fetal well-being, the judicious moment for intervention in the maternal interest and timely delivery of the baby.

KEY POINTS

- Assess and counsel the patient before pregnancy.
- Understand renal physiology and anatomy in normal pregnancy—the key to managing renal problems.
- Acute renal problems, in otherwise healthy women, can be managed as in the non-pregnant pregnant population, but remember the fetus.
- Chronic renal disorders are not a contraindication to pregnancy, provided kidney dysfunction is minimal and hypertension is absent (or well controlled), with there being no long-term maternal harm.
- All cases must be considered individually.

REFERENCES

Abe S 1991 An overview of pregnancy in women with underlying renal disease. Am J Kidney Dis 17:112–115

Abe S 1996 Pregnancy in glomerulonephritic patients with decreased renal function. Hypertension in Pregnancy 15:305–312

Ahlswede KM, Armenti VT, Mokritz MJ 1992 Premature births in female transplant recipients: degree and effect of immunosuppressive regimen. Surgical Forum 43:524–525

Armenti VT, Ahlswede KM, Ahlswede BA et al 1992 The National Transplant Registry: an analysis of 325 pregnancies in female kidney recipients. Journal of American Society of Nephrology 3:851P

Armenti VT, Ahlswede BA, Moritz MJ et al 1993 National Transplantation Registry: analysis of pregnancy outcomes of female kidney recipients with relation to time interval from transplantation to conception. Transplantation Proceedings 25:1036–1037

Armenti V, Ahlswede KM, Ahlswede B et al 1994 National Transplantation Pregnancy Register—outcome of 154 pregnancies in cyclosporine-treated female transplant recipients. Transpl 57:502–506

Armenti VT, Moritz MJ, Davison JM 1998 Medical management of the pregnant transplant recipient. Adv Renal Rep Ther 5:14–23

Armenti VT, Ahlswede KM, Ahlswede BA et al 1995 Variables affecting birthweight and graft survival in 197 pregnancies in cyclosporine-treated female kidney transplant recipients. Transpl 59:476–479

Armenti VT, Moritz MJ, Davison JM 1998 Drug Safety Issues in Pregnancy following Transplantation and Immunosuppression. Drug Safety Concepts Sep (3):219–232

Asrat T, Roossin MC, Miller EI 1998 Ultrasonographic detection of ureteral jets in normal pregnancy. Am J Obstet Gynecol 178(6):1184–1198

Bagon JA, Vernaeve H, De Muylder X, et al 1998 Pregnancy and Dialysis. Am J Kidney Dis 31: 756–765

Bailey RR 1992 Vesicoureteric reflux and reflux nephropathy. In: Cameron JS, Davison AM, Grunfeld JP, Kerr D, Ritz E (eds). Oxford textbook of clinical nephrology. Oxford University Press, Oxford, pp 1983–2001

Bakris GL 1996 Is the level of arterial pressure reduction important for preservation of renal function? Nephrol Dial Transplant 11:2383–2397

Bar J, Ben-Rafael Z, Padoa A et al 2000 Prediction of pregnancy outcome in subgroups of women with renal disease. Clin Nephrol 53:437–444

Barret RJ, Peters WA 1983 Pregnancy following urinary diversion. Obstetrics and Gynaecology 62:582–586

Baylis C, Rennke HG 1985 Renal hemodynamics and glomerular morphology in repetitively pregnant aging rats. Kidney Int 28:140–145

Baylis C, Davison JM 1998 The urinary system. In: Chamberlain G, Broughton-Pipkin F (eds). Clinical Physiology in Obstetrics. Blackwell, Oxford pp 263–307

Becker GJ, Fairley KF, Whitworth JA 1985 Pregnancy exacerbates glomerular disease. Am J Kidney Dis 6:266–272

Brenner BM, Meyer TW, Hostetter TH 1982 Dietary protein intake and the progressive nature of kidney disease: the role of hemodynamically mediated glomerular injury in the pathogenesis of progressive glomerular sclerosis in aging, renal ablation and intrinsic renal disease. N Engl J Med 307:652–659

Brown MA 1990 Urinary tract dilatation in pregnancy. Am J Obstet Gynecol 164:641–643

Brown MA, Gallery EAM 1994 Volume homeostasis in normal pregnancy and pre-eclampsia: physiology and clinical implications. Clin Obstet Gynecol 8:287–310

Burleson RL, Sunderji SG, Aubry RH et al 1983 Renal allo-transplantation during pregnancy. Transplantation 36:334–335

Calne RY, Brons EGM, Williams PF 1988 Successful pregnancy after paratopic segmental pancreas and kidney transplantation. Br Med J 296:1709

Campbell-Brown M, McFadyen IR, Seal DV, Stephenson ML 1987 Is screening for bacteriuria in pregnancy worthwhile? Br Med J 294:1579–1582

Chng PK, Hall MH 1982 Antenatal prediction of urinary tract infection in pregnancy. Br J Obstet Gynaecol 89:8–11

Cietak KA, Newton JR 1985a Serial qualitative maternal nephrosonography in pregnancy. Br J Radiol 58:399–404

Cietak KA, Newton JR 1985b Serial quantitative maternal nephrosonography in pregnancy. Br J Radiol 58:405–413

Conrad KP, Lindheimer MD 1999 Renal and cardiovascular alterations. In: Lindhiemer MD, Roberts JM, Cunningham FG (eds). Chesley's Hypertensive Disorders in Pregnancy (2E). Appleton and Lange, Connecticut, pp 263–326

Coombs GA, Kitzmiller JL 1991 Diabetic nephropathy and pregnancy. Clin Obstet Gynecol 13:505–515

Cunningham FG, Lucas MJ 1994 Urinary tract infections complicating pregnancy. Clin Obstet Gynecol 8:353–373

Cunningham GF, Lucas MJ, Hankins GDV 1987 Pulmonary injury complicating antepartum pyelonephritis. Am J Obstet Gynecol 156:797–807

Cunningham GF, Cox SM, Harstad TW et al 1990 Chronic renal disease and pregnancy outcome. Am J Obstet Gynecol 163:453–459

Cunningham RJ, Buszta C, Braun WE et al 1983 Pregnancy in renal allograft recipients and longterm follow-up of their offspring. Transpl Proc 15:1067–1070

Dadelszen von P, Ornstein MP, Bull SB et al 2000 Fall in mean arterial pressure and fetal growth restriction in pregnancy hypertension: a meta-analysis. Lancet 355:87–92

Davison JM 1988 The effect of pregnancy on longterm renal function in women with chronic renal disease and single kidneys. Clin Exp Hypertension B8:222A

Davison JM 1994 Pregnancy in renal allograft recipients: problems, prognosis and practicalities. Clin Obstet Gynecol 8:501–525

Davison JM, Baylis C 1996 Renal disease. In: de Swiet M (ed). Medical disorders in obstetric practice, 3rd edn. Blackwell Scientific Publications, Oxford, pp 226–305

Davison JM, Shiells EA, Philips PR et al 1993 Metabolic clearance of vasopressin and an analogue resistant to vasopressinase in human pregnancy. Am J Physiol 264:F348–353

Davison JM, Milne JEC 1997 Renal Disease in Pregnancy. In: Advances in Perinatal Medicine. Cockburn F (ed) Parthenon Group 152–157

Davison JM, Redman CWG 1997 Pregnancy post-transplant: the establishment of a UK Registry. Br J Obstet Gynaecol 104:1106–1107

Dunlop W, Davison JM 1977 The effect of normal pregnancy upon the renal handling of uric acid. Br J Obstet Gynaecol 84:13–21

Eckford SD, Gigngnell JC 1991 Ureteric obstruction in pregnancy—diagnosis and management. Br J Obstet Gynecol 98:1337–1340

Epstein FH 1996 Pregnancy and renal disease. N Engl J Med 335:277–278

Ezimokhai M, Davison JM, Philips PR et al 1981 Non-postural serial changes in renal function during the third trimester of normal human pregnancy. Br J Obstet Gynaecol 88:465–471

Feehally J, Bennett SE, Harris KPG et al 1986 Is chronic renal transplant rejection a non-immunological phenomenon? Lancet ii:486–488

First MR, Combs CA, Weiskittel P et al 1995 Lack of effect of pregnancy on renal allograft survival or function. Transpl 59:472–476

Gaber LW, Lindheimer MD 1999 Pathology of the kidney, liver and brain. In: Lindheimer MD, Roberts JM, Cunningham FG (eds) Chesley's Hypertensive Disorders in Pregnancy (2E). Appleton and Lange, Connecticut, pp 231–262

Gabow PA 1993 Autosomal dominant polycystic kidney disease. N Engl J Med 329:332–342

Gallery EDM, Lindhemicr MD 1999 Alterations in Vomue homestasis. In: Lindheimer MD, Roberts JM, Cunningham FG (eds). Chesley's Hypertensive Disorders in Pregnancy (2E.) Appleton and Lange, Connecticut, pp 263–326

Grimes DA, Le Bolt SA, Grimes KR et al 1985 Systemic lupus erythematosus and reproductive function: a case control study. Am J Obstet Gynecol 153:179–186

Grunfeld J-P, Choukroun G, Knebelman B 1997 Genetic diagnosis and counselling in inherited renal disease. In: Suki WN, Massry SG (eds) Therapy of renal diseases and related disorders (3 edn) Kluwer Academic Pub, pp 685–694

Halpert R, Fruchter RG, Sedlis A et al 1986 Human papillomavirus and lower genital neoplasia in renal transplant patients. Obstet Gynecol 68:251–258

Harber MA, Tso A, Taheri S et al 1999 Wegener's granulomatosis in pregnancy—the therapeutic dilemma. Nephrol Dial Transplant 14:1789–1791

Haugen G, Fauchald P, Sodal G 1991 Pregnancy outcome in renal allograft recipients: influence of cyclosporin A. Eur J Obstet Gynecol Reprod Biol 29:25–29

Hayslett JP 1985 Pregnancy does not exacerbate primary glomerular disease. Am J Kidney Dis 6:273–277

Hayslett JP, Reece EA 1994 Managing diabetic patients with

nephropathy and other vascular complications. Clin Obstet Gynecol 8:405–424

Heybourne KD, Schultz MF, Goodlin RC et al 1991 Renal artery stenosis during pregnancy: a review. Obstet Gynecol Survey 46:509–514

Hou SH, Grossman SD, Madias NE 1985 Pregnancy in women with renal disease and moderate renal insufficiency. Am J Med 78:185–194

Hou SH, Firanek C 1998 Management of the pregnant dialysis patient. Adv Renal Rep Ther 5:24–30

Imbasciati E, Ponticelli C 1991 Pregnancy and renal disease: predictors for fetal and maternal outcome. Am J Nephrol 11:353–362

Imbasciati E, Pardi G, Bozetti P et al 1984 Pregnancy in women with chronic renal failure. Proceedings of the 4th World Congress of the International Society for the Study of Hypertension in Pregnancy: 78

Jones DC, Hayslett JP 1996 Outcome of pregnancy in women with moderate or severe renal insufficiency. N Engl J Med 335:226–232

Jungers P, Dougados M, Pelissies C et al 1982 Lupus nephropathy and pregnancy. Arch Internal Med 142:771–776

Jungers P, Chauveau D 1997 Pregnancy in renal disease. Kid Intl 52:871–885

Jungers P, Houillier P 1995 Influence of pregnancy on the course of primary chronic glomerulonephritis. Lancet 346:1–22

Jungers P, Chauveau D, Choukronn G et al 1997 Pregnancy in women with impaired renal function. Clin Nephrol 47:281–288

Kincaid-Smith P, Whitworth JA, Fairley KF 1980 Mesangial IgA nephropathy in pregnancy. Clin Exp Hypertension 2:821–838

Lcikin JB, Arof HM, Pearlman LM 1986 Acute lupus pneumonitis in the postpartum period: a case history and review of the literature. Obstet Gynecol 68:298–318

Lelievre R, Ribet M, Gosselin B et al 1978 Chorio-carcinoma après transplantation. J Urol Nephrol 84:345–346

Levy DP, Giatris I and Jungers P 1998 Pregnancy and end-stage renal disease—past experience and new insights. Nephrol Dial Transplant 13: Editorial comments

Lewis GJ, Lamont CAR, Lee HA et al 1983 Successful pregnancy in a renal transplant recipient taking cyclosporin A. Br Med J 286:603

Light JA 1993 Experience with 50 kidney/pancreas transplants at the Washington Hospital Center. Dialysis and Transplantation 22:522–532

Lind T, Godfrey KA, Otum H et al 1984 Changes in serum uric acid concentrations during normal pregnancy. Br J Obstet Gynaecol 91:128–132

Lindheimer MD, Katz AI 1987 Gestation in women with kidney disease: prognosis and management. Clinical Obstetrics and Gynaecology 1:921–967

Lindheimer MD, Barron WM 1994 Water metabolism and vasopressin secretion during pregnancy. Clin Obstet Gynecol 8:311–331

Lomberg H, Jodal U, Leffler H et al 1992 Blood group non-secretors have an increased inflammatory response to urinary tract infection. Scand J Infectious Dis 24:77

Manifold IH, Champion AE, Goepel JR et al 1983 Pregnancy complicated by gestational trophoblastic disease in a renal transplant recipient. Br J Med 287:1025–1026

McFadyen IR, Eknyn SJ, Gardner NHN et al 1973 Bacteriuria of pregnancy. J Obstet Gynaecol Br Commonwealth 80:385–405

McGladdery SL, Aparicio S, Verrier-Jones K 1992 Outcome of pregnancy in an Oxford–Cardiff cohort of women with previous bacteriuria. Quart J Med 303:533–539

MacMillan MC, Grimes DA 1991 The limited usefulness of urine and blood cultures in treating pyelonephritis in pregnancy. Obstet Gynecol 78:745

Maikranz P, Lindheimer MD, Coe FC 1994 Nephrolithiasis and gestation. Clin Obstet Gynecol 8:375–386

Martinell J, Jodall U, Lipiu-Janson G 1990 Pregnancies in women with and without renal seaming after urinary infections in childhood. Br Med J 300:840–844

Miller DR, Kakkis J 1982 Prognosis, management and outcome of obstructive renal disease in pregnancy. J Rep Med 27:199–201

Newstead CG 1998 Assessment of risk of cancer after renal transplantation. Lancet 351:610–611

Nicklin JL 1991 Systemic lupus erythematosus and pregnancy at the Royal Women's Hospital, Brisbane 1979–1989. Austral N Zeal J Obstet Gynecol 31:128–133

Okundaye IB, Abrinko P, Hou SH 1998 Registry in pregnancy in dialysis patients. Am J Kid Dis 31:766–773

Peake SL, Roxburgh HB, Langlois S 1983 Ultrasonic assessment or hydronephrosis of pregnancy. Radiol 128:167–170

Pertuiset N, Grunfeld J-P 1994 Acute renal failure in pregnancy. Clinical Obstetrics and Gynaecology 8:333–351

Petri M, Howard D, Repke J 1991 Frequency of lupus flare in pregnancy: the Hopkins Lupus Pregnancy Center experience. Arthritis Rheumatism 34:1538–1545

Pickrell MD, Sawers R, Michael J 1988 Pregnancy after renal transplantation: severe intrauterine growth retardation during treatment with cyclosporin A. Br Med J 296:825

Powers RD 1991 New directions in the diagnosis and therapy of urinary tract infection. Am J Obstet Gynecol 164:1387–1389

Raine AEG, Margreiter R, Brunner FP et al 1992 Report on management of renal failure in Europe XXII, 1991. Nephrol Dial Transpl 7(suppl 2):7–35

Reimers TJ, Sluss PM 1978 6-Mercaptopurine treatment of pregnant mice: effects on second and third generations. Science 201:65–67

Remuzzi G, Ruggenenti P, Mauer SM 1994 Pancreas and kidney/pancreas transplants: experimental medicines or real impairment? Lancet 343:27–31

Rizzoni G, Ehrich JHH, Broyer M et al 1992 Successful pregnancies in women on renal replacement therapy: report from the EDTA Registry. Nephrol Dial Transpl 7:1–9

Roberts M, Lindheimer MD, Davison JM 1996 Altered glomerular permselectivity to neutral dextrans and heterporous membrane modelling in human pregnancy. Am J Physiol 270:F338–F343

Roche RJ, Moxon ER 1992 The molecular study of bacterial virulence: a view of current approaches illustrated by the study of adhesion in uropathogenic E. coli. Pediat Nephrol 6:587–596

Romero R, Oyazun E, Mazar M et al 1989 Meta-analysis of the relationship between asymptomatic bacteriuria and preterm delivery/low birthweight. Obstet Gynecol 73:576–582

Romero JC, Lahera V, Salom MG et al 1992 Role of endothelium dependent relaxing factor nitric oxide on renal function. Journal of American Society of Nephrology 2:1371–1387

Salmela K, Kyllonen LEJ, Holmberg C et al 1993 Impaired renal function after pregnancy in renal transplant recipients. Transpl 56:1372–1375

Satin AJ, Seikin GL, Cunningham FG 1993 Reversible hypertension in pregnancy caused by obstructive uropathy. Obstet Gynecol 81:823–825

Schwartz MA, Wang CC, Eckert L et al 1999 Risk factors for urinary tract infection in the postpartum period. Am J Obstet Gynaecol 181:547–553

Sola R, Ballarin J, Castrol et al 1988 Renal transplantation during pregnancy. Transpl Proc 20:270

Sibai BM, Kamadan MK 1993 Acute renal failure in pregnancies complicated by hemolysis, elevated liver enzymes and low platelets. Am J Obstet Gynecol 168:1682–1687

Stein G, Fünfstück R 1999 Asymptomatic bacteriuria—what to do. Nephrol Dial Transpl 14:1618–1621

Stenquist K, Dahlin-Nilsson I, Lidin-Janson G 1989 Bacteriuria in pregnancy. Frequency and risk of acquisition. Am J Epidemiol 129:372–379

Stotland NL, Stotland NE 1997 A Guest Editorial: The Mother and the Burning Building. Obstet Gynecol Surv 53(1)

Sturgiss SN, Davison JM 1991 Perinatal outcome in renal allograft recipients: prognostic significance of hypertension and renal function before and during pregnancy. Obstet Gynecol 78:573–577

Sturgiss SN, Davison JM 1995 Effect of pregnancy on longterm function of renal allografts. Am J Kid Dis An update (in press)

Sturgiss SN, Dunlop W, Davison JM 1994 Renal haemodynamics and tubular function in human pregnancy. Clin Obstet Gynecol 8:209–234

Surian M, Imbasciati E, Cosci P et al 1984 Glomerular disease and pregnancy: a study of 123 pregnancies in patients with primary and secondary glomerular diseases. Nephron 36:101–105

Taylor AA, Davison JM 1997 Albumin excretion in normal pregnancy. Am J Obstet Gynaecol 177:1559–1560

Thorp JA, Davis BE and Klingele C 1999 Severe early onset preeclampsia secondary to bilateral ureteral obstruction reversed by stenting. Obstet Gynecol 94:806–887

Toma H, Tanabe K, Tokumoto T et al 1999 Pregnancy in women receiving renal dialysis or transplantation in Japan: a nationwide survey. Nephrol Dial Transpl 14:1511–1516

Towers CV, Kaminskas CM, Garite TJ et al 1991 Pulmonary injury with antepartum pyelonephritis: can patients at risk be identified? Am J Obstet Gynecol 164:974

Twickler D, Little BB, Satin AJ et al 1991 Renal pelvicalyceal dilation in antepartum pyelonephritis: ultrasonographic findings. Am J Obstet Gynecol 165:1115–1119

Tyden G, Brattstrom C, Bjorkman U et al 1989 Pregnancy after combined pancreas-kidney transplantation. Diabetes 38(suppl 1):43–45

Van Sonnenberg E, Casola G, Talner LB et al 1992 Symptomatic renal obstruction or urosepsis during pregnancy: treatment by sonographically guided percutaneous nephrostomy. Am J Roentgenol 158:91–94

Weinberger SE 1993 Recent advances in pulmonary medicine (Part II). N Engl J Med 328:1462–1470

Whetam JCG, Cardelle C, Harding M 1983 Effect of pregnancy on graft function and graft survival in renal cadaver transplant patients. American Journal of Obstetrics and Gynecology 145:193–197

Williams DJ 1997 Renal Disease in pregnancy. Curr Obstet Gynaecol 7:156–162

Williams PF, Jelen J 1979 Eclampsia in a patient who had had a renal transplant. Br Med J 2:972

Williams PF, Johnstone M 1982 Normal pregnancy in renal transplant recipient with a history of eclampsia and intrauterine death. Br Med J 285:1535

Wing DA, Hendershott CM, Debuque L et al 1999 Outpatient treatment of acute pyelonephritis in pregnancy after 24 weeks. Vol. 94, No. 5 Part 1

Wolf MC, Hollander JB, Salisz JA 1992 A new technique of ureteral stent placement during pregnancy using endoluminal ultrasound. Surgical Gynecol Obstet 175:575–576

Wrenshall LE, McHugh L, Felton P et al 1996 Pregnancy after donor nephrectomy. Transplantation 62:1934–1936

Zinner SH 1992 Management of urinary tract infections in pregnancy: a review with comments on single dose therapy. Infection 4:S280–S285

Section 4
NORMAL LABOUR

24

The labouring mother

Sandy Oliver, Ann Oakley

The contribution of the author of the equivalent chapter in the second edition, on which this chapter draws extensively, is gratefully acknowledged.

In modern industrial societies the last 100 years have seen enormous changes in the reproductive roles of women and the management of childbirth. Average family size has decreased substantially, the average age at first childbirth has increased, and marriage has become less fashionable, with a consequent large rise in the proportion of one-parent families (Ditch et al 1998). Accompanying these changes has been an increased social emphasis on gender equality (Dex & Sewell 1995). It has become the norm for mothers to have paid employment at the workplace as well as looking after the home.

Although there have been substantial changes in the nature of women's activities, the roles of men and women at home and at work remain highly segregated (Scott 1994). Over half of employed women, but less than a fifth of employed men, work in sectors characterised by low pay (Department of Employment 1995). Within homes, women take the primary responsibility for the health-maintaining labour of housework, providing food, physical and emotional care.

Poverty and social exclusion are on the increase in the UK. The Acheson Report (1998) on inequalities in health described a pattern of increasing poverty and class differences in health outcomes among mothers and children. Widening income inequalities have their impact in disproportionate and specific ways on women with children (Graham 1998). Two-thirds of poor adults are women. State benefits fall short of the level necessary to maintain health (Middleton et al 1997), and this is particularly a problem among lone mothers (Leather 1996). In 1976, 8% of the UK population lived in households with incomes below the EC poverty line; by 1991 this was 24% (Goodman & Webb 1994). While under 10% of children in the UK lived in poverty in the late 1970s, this figure is now close to one-third of children (McGlone et al 1998).

These demographic and resource issues form the backdrop against which women's experiences of obstetric care need to be seen. As far as childbirth is concerned, the greatest change that has occurred over the last century is that reproduction has become a medical specialty and its control has been removed from the community and from women being now vested with medical and midwifery professionals instead. One consequence of this transformation is that the point of view of mothers themselves may be forgotten, and women may lack any formal input into processes of decision-making about their maternity care. In the UK, women strikingly lack influence in a system, the NHS, where they form the majority of users (Doyal 1998) as well as 75% of workers.

The exercise of articulating and making visible women's perspectives is considerably aided by two important twentieth-century social movements—feminism and the consumer movement in health care.

MOTHERS AND THE MEDICALISATION OF CHILDBIRTH

In the nineteenth century doctors played a minor role in the care of pregnant women. The predominant view was that pregnancy was not in itself a pathological condition but a natural physiological state (Johnstone 1913). Most women never saw a doctor in pregnancy, and most had their babies with the help of midwives (Donnison 1977, Versluysen 1981). This practice of women caring for women in childbirth was part of a long tradition of women's community health care (Oakley 1976). Healing the sick and caring for dependants was part of women's domestic role. Women's domestic knowledge embraced the recognition and use of painkillers, digestive aids, anti-inflammatory agents, ergot, belladonna and digitalis (Clark 1968, Chamberlain 1981).

The story of the male medical takeover of childbirth is well known (Carter & Duriez 1986). At its centre is the apocryphal story of the Chamberlen family who, in the seventeenth century, negotiated their way into upper-class homes with a magic box containing forceps and locked the door in order to guard their technological secret. Without effective antiseptics forceps would have carried a high risk of infection (Gélis 1991). The aspiring male midwives of the eighteenth and nineteenth centuries were not popular with labouring women or with doctors. Women were afraid of instruments and unhappy about permitting male access to their bodies during birth.

Midwifery was stereotyped as women's work (Hunt & Symonds 1991) and so those men who wanted to enter it had to contend with the dismissive attitudes of the medical profession, who regarded midwifery as something doctors ought not to get themselves embroiled in. An important factor in the development of the early lying-in hospitals in the eighteenth century was gaining control over client preferences by hospitalising them. One of the explicit aims behind the founding of the early maternity institutions was that medical men ought to be able to gain more experience of normal deliveries. The lying-in hospitals provided hospitalised delivery for poor women.

It is very hard to know how labouring women felt about the care available to them during these years of fundamental changes in the management of childbirth. The physician-accoucheur of the Westminster General Dispensary, Augustus Bozzi Granville, expressed the opinion, in 1819, that 'however distressed the poor mother may be, she will always prefer her own habitation, and the unbought, soothing cares of her own family, during her time of trial, to the spacious ward, and the precise attention of a hired matron and strange nurses' (Granville 1819). He also noted 'a decided aversion amongst lying-in women, against the inter-

ference of the Accoucheur, and the use of the most harmless instruments'. At this time the mother's risk of dying in childbirth was probably around 1 in 200. Puerperal fever accounted for about 40% of these deaths (Farr 1885). Infant mortality was around 150 per 1000 live births throughout the nineteenth century. Death of mother and child was therefore a real risk.

If hospitals were needed by the obstetrical specialists to build up their knowledge and control of clients, by the late nineteenth century they also held a particular attraction for women because they offered the possibility of pain relief in labour. Midwives delivering babies at home had no analgesia to offer mothers until R.J. Minnitt at Liverpool Maternity Hospital designed a portable apparatus for delivering gas and air in 1932. This may have been partly responsible for the move among middle-class mothers to have babies in hospital in the early decades of the twentieth century, a move which was associated with the unusual epidemiological picture of higher social class temporarily being associated with higher maternal mortality (Registrar-General 1930).

Place of delivery was first documented by the British Registrar-General in 1927, when 15% of all live births occurred in institutions; he thought the main reason for hospital birth was lack of home facilities. By 1954 the figure for institutional deliveries was 64% and, in that year, whatever mothers thought, the British Medical Journal (1954) was still able to declare that 'the proper place for the confinement is the patient's own home'. By 1960 the proportion of babies delivered in institutions had risen by only 1% since 1954 and this, not coincidentally, was the year in which one of Britain's most energetic consumer pressure groups in the maternity care field was born: the Association for Improvements in Maternity Services (AIMS), originally named the Society for the Prevention of Cruelty to Pregnant Women. These organisations are part of a widespread resistance to the medicalisation of childbirth (Haire 1972, Arms 1975, Houd & Oakley 1986, Wagner 1994, Moorhead 1996).

CONSUMERS' REVOLT?

The rise of groups such as AIMS, the National Childbirth Trust (NCT), the Maternity Alliance and a host of others has given prominence to the maternal (and paternal) point of view. Collectively they have provided a voice for what is incorrectly dubbed the consumer's perspective (Stacey 1976). Although many women belong to these organisations, many do not; membership is likely to be weighted towards the informed middle classes, which means that these pressure groups cannot be assumed to speak for all women. Having said that, it is of course necessary to query the assumption that all women share a single viewpoint on any specific issue, such as analgesia or position in labour, or more generally as to the overall management of childbirth. There is no reason to assume this. Women having babies do not form a homogeneous group (Riley 1977). In the same way not all obstetricians are in agreement about how to treat women in childbirth—there is a wide range of attitudes and great variation in clinical practice.

The consumers' revolt in childbirth has everywhere emphasised the same key themes: the right to information, the right to choose, respect for social and psychological aspects of childbearing and for the integrity, privacy and individuality of childbearing women and their families, and pregnancy and birth as normal physiological events. Over the last 15 years there has also been increasing stress on the need for obstetric procedures to be properly evaluated for effectiveness and safety before they enter routine practice.

Three other factors have contributed to the assertiveness of consumer organisations in maternity care. One is the women's movement, which has entailed an emphasis on appropriate health care for women. The second is medical sociology, which, as an academic-based discipline, has sought (among many other enterprises) to highlight the social dimension within medicine (Stacey & Homans 1978). The third is the development of the Cochrane Collaboration, an international movement committed to assembling and updating evidence about the effectiveness of health care interventions (Chalmers et al 1997). As a result of these developments, there are now systematic data which can be marshalled to answer questions about what women want in obstetric care, and which clinical and social interventions are effective, appropriate and safe.

The exercise of researching women's views is not simply a matter of health care professionals asking captive audiences in antenatal or postnatal clinics lists of pre-coded questions—an exercise which is likely to result in misleading responses (see, for example, Impey 1999) and certainly does not provide them with the opportunity to reflect on the meaning and health care implications of these experiences. Rather, our understanding of mothers' views is deepened by a diversity of approaches. Most research on women's experiences of maternity care has focussed on white women. We know much less about the attitudes and experiences of women from ethnic minorities (Katbamna 2000). Black and ethnic minority women are more likely than white women to be socially disadvantaged (Douglas 1998), and racial discrimination is an institutionalised feature of the maternity care system (Phoenix 1990). The increasing numbers of young, unmarried mothers (Department of Health 1997) mean that their views also deserve attention.

The rest of this chapter will explore some of what is known about the views of mothers about specific topics in the maternity care debate today, and how these relate to evidence of the effects of care. The following will be considered: place of birth; delivery personnel; so-called natural childbirth; analgesia; obstetric interventions, including induction of labour, instrumental delivery, monitoring in labour and caesarean section; and the relationship between evidence and processes of decision-making in maternity care.

PLACE OF BIRTH

In the late 1950s about one-third of deliveries in England took place at home. The proportion fell rapidly in the 1960s and 1970s to about 1% throughout the 1980s, and rose again slowly to nearly 2% in the mid 1990s (Department of Health 1997). Where do women want to have their babies? The proportion of women who would like to have their baby at home is generally higher than the proportion booked to do so (Macintyre 1977). The preference for home delivery appears to rise with parity and also with the experience of home delivery (Cartwright 1979, Chamberlain 1997) even when that experience was forced by a strike of hospital ancillary staff (Goldthorpe & Richman 1974).

Cartwright's survey (1979) suggests that birth at home may be more attractive to women because labour was significantly shorter at home, fewer women were left alone during labour and significantly fewer had episiotomies. Of the mothers at home, 57% held their babies as long as they wanted, compared with 29% in hospital. Table 24.1 shows reactions to pain relief. Again, the home birth group seem to do better, perhaps because it is easier for women to receive individualised care at home. This is reflected in the findings relating to communication between mothers and their attendants. Mothers in home and hospital groups were equally likely to have had worries during their labour and to have discussed these worries with someone, but those at home were more likely to say that the person they talked to was helpful (89% compared with 59% of the hospital group). Overall, 44% of the home group as against 34% of the hospital group said that labour and delivery had been pleasurable experiences (O'Brien 1978).

The overriding issue for mothers and their carers is safety, both physical and psychological. There is a vast body of evidence demonstrating that stress is bad for successful reproduction and that psychological stress has physiological manifestations in childbearing women (Oakley 1982). The supposedly superior physical safety of hospital delivery is constantly emphasised, but the message that emerges clearly from women's accounts of having a baby at home is the greater psychological safety of home birth (Kitzinger 1979). In part this is because the chances of maternal psychological stress are generally lower at home, where the mother's attendants are visitors in her home; she is not staying temporarily in the institution *they* run. This means that many of the procedures and routines that a mother is forced to accept by social pressures in hospital are avoided in the home. At home, social relationships are not influenced by the demands of a large bureaucratic structure dominated by an ethos of technical efficiency; instead they result from the needs and wishes of the individuals concerned. This is a point of overwhelming importance (Richards 1979).

As well as emphasising the enhanced psychological safety of home birth, consumer groups in the childbirth field have of course also tangled with the epidemiologists and statisticians

Table 24.1 Reactions to pain relief (from O'Brien 1978)

	Hospital birth (%) n=1730	Home birth (%) n=60
First given pain relief at right time	69	82
Given enough pain relief	72	87
On balance, felt glad about what they had	74	87

on the question of comparative perinatal mortality rates at home and in hospital. In doing so, they have made the point that many parents wish to be informed about the relative risks of different places of birth and are intelligent enough to understand the basic statistical arguments.

The Health Select Committee on Maternity Services (1992), which took evidence from women, health professionals and researchers, found 'no clear, overwhelming evidence' that hospital birth is safest and recommended that women be supported in home birth if they so choose.

In the absence of trials, the best available evidence about the safety of home birth is drawn from observational studies comparing planned home births with planned hospital births, using an intention-to-treat analysis for groups of women matched as well as possible, with lack of comparability being controlled for in statistical analysis. A meta-analysis of such studies (Olsen & Jewell 1999) has shown that in the home birth group there were fewer medical interventions: induction of labour, augmentation, episiotomy, operative vaginal birth and caesarean section. Furthermore there was a lower frequency of low Apgar scores and severe lacerations in the home birth group. In a study of women's experience in Essex, however, despite a government policy that now favours choice, only 13% of women said they were offered the possibility of giving birth at home; a third of those who gave birth at home had not been offered the possibility, but had actively sought and obtained a home birth (Gready et al 1995).

WHO SHOULD DELIVER?

Many complaints in the 1950s and 1960s highlighted the loneliness of labouring mothers in hospitals where staff were too busy or not sufficiently sensitive to stay with them; women's first preference, therefore, may be for *someone* to be with them.

A second commonly stated preference is for the birth attendant to be someone already known to the mother. When the mother delivers in hospital this is not very likely to happen: the London study already referred to found that 75% of the women had not previously seen the person who delivered their baby. As one of the women said 'It was *horrific* that the midwife and the pupil midwife who were there I'd never seen in my life before and I've never seen them again since. And yet they were *the* people in about the most vital and powerful experience of my life so far' (Oakley 1981). In historical and cross-cultural terms this is an unusual situation (Mead & Newton 1967). While it may be reassuring to feel that the person helping the mother to deliver the baby is technically expert, the positive impact of a familiar deliverer is likely to be considerable.

In the Essex study (Gready et al 1995), women who had previously met either a doctor or a midwife involved with their labour were significantly more likely to feel that health professionals always explained enough about what was happening in labour, that they always told them enough about why things were necessary, and that they always took enough notice of their views and wishes. They were also more likely to feel that they were fully involved in all the decisions about their care and they were significantly more likely to be happy with how involved they were with the decision-making.

A review of randomised controlled trials concludes that being cared for by a small team of midwives throughout pregnancy, labour and the postnatal period is favoured by women and has clinical benefits (Hodnett 1999a). All indicators of maternal satisfaction favoured this form of care. In addition, continuity of care by midwives was associated with an increased likelihood of labouring and giving birth without using any analgesia or anaesthesia, with a decreased likelihood of neonatal resuscitation, and, in one trial, with an increased likelihood of no medical intervention whatsoever (defined as spontaneous onset of labour, no augmentation, no analgesia or anaesthesia, spontaneous vaginal delivery, and no episiotomy).

On these grounds, those women who want a normal labour and delivery should prefer care by midwives; however, nothing is simple in the maternity care field, and a preference for doctors is often expressed. This is congruent with the professional claim that obstetricians are the people who know best how to secure healthy babies—in itself part of the medicalisation of life we are all socialised to accept (McKeown 1979).

An alternative approach is for women to be supported, in addition to a midwife who may be busy, by women who are experienced, either because they have given birth themselves or have had training as nurses, midwives, doulas, or childbirth educators. A systematic review of randomised controlled trials (Hodnett 1999b) found that women preferred continuous support and that such support reduced the likelihood of medication for pain relief, operative vaginal delivery, caesarean delivery, and a 5-minute Apgar score of less than 7; women were also more likely to be fully breast-feeding 4–6 weeks later. Hodnett concluded that, given the clear benefits and absence of known risks associated with intrapartum support, every effort should be made to ensure that all labouring women receive continuous support with the provision of comfort and encouragement.

NATURAL CHILDBIRTH OR HIGH-TECHNOLOGY DELIVERY?

Although natural childbirth is often associated with pain, and high technology with safety, these issues become interrelated in a complex way. The interaction between the unnatural and the medicalised arises from pregnancy and birth becoming the province of hospitals and doctors, as are other forms of illness. This is clearly appropriate for those mothers and fetuses who develop problems, but many consumer groups contend that it is not appropriate care for most mothers and fetuses, because it enhances the risk of complications. This was the substance of one of the early books in the present alternative childbirth movement, Suzanne Arms' *Immaculate Deception* (1975). Arms argues that women have been deceived by obstetricians into believing in an unobtainable ideal—the no-risk birth. They have been co-opted by the obstetrical establishment into accepting a hospitalised and interventionist management of childbirth in which a structure purported to minimise the risks of childbearing actually inflates these risks by incurring iatrogenic complications.

Anthropologists, however, point out that few human societies provide for childbirth as a purely natural or simply biological event. Childbirth everywhere is circumscribed by rules, rituals and prescriptions dictating how labouring women, their families and helpers should behave (Ford 1945). The stereotype of primitive childbirth as an unattended birth behind a bush describes an event 'as rare and remarkable as an American birth taking place in a taxi cab' (Mead & Newton 1967). Most importantly, the lack of modern medical facilities and therapies does not necessarily entail an attitude of non-interference; for example, herbs may be used to accelerate labour, abdominal stimulation, including external version, may be used, and manual removal of the placenta is by no means unknown (Oakley 1982).

In modern obstetric practice, the question is often asked 'do women really want natural childbirth?' The issue causes heated reactions on both sides. Some obstetricians condemn women's viewpoints as cranky, whimsical and dangerous, and women object that obstetricians are trying to frighten them into submission. It may be objected (by obstetricians) that they should not have to contend with something called *The Good Birth Guide*; neurosurgeons, after all, do not have to grapple with 'The Good Neurosurgery Guide'.

One explanation of these patterns is the fact that, by and large, women and obstetricians do have different perspectives on childbirth (Wagner 1994). A pooled analysis of data from two research projects in York and London showed that obstetricians and mothers differ in their view of the nature, context, control and criteria of success of childbirth. These differences are responsible for at least some of the conflicts that develop (Graham & Oakley 1981).

Women do not of course hold a single view about the pain of labour: their expectations and experiences vary and, indeed, an individual may hold one view when considering birth in the abstract and another in hindsight. Women may experience labour as they expected or they may find it more or less painful (Ounstead & Simons 1979, Macintyre 1981, Morgan et al 1982). Similarly, women have varying views on obstetric intervention. It is not only the prospect of interventions and their view in hindsight that may attract different opinions, women's attitudes may also be coloured by the circumstances in which they experienced interventions and whether they were employed to ease the labour or for the safety of mother or baby.

In Cartwright's study of induction (1979), the main reason women gave for not wanting labour induced was that they wanted the baby to come naturally. A study of British Asian women in Warwickshire found that 48% of mothers expressed a desire that nature should determine the timing and mode of birth. This desire was voiced most strongly by women who had experienced an unwelcome level of medical intervention in a previous birth. The chief reasons given for preferring a natural birth were firstly that women who had had induced labours with epidural analgesia and perhaps an instrumental delivery tended to feel they had not really given birth and, secondly, they were concerned that elective delivery led to a disturbed mother–child relationship (Homans 1980). In London, in the mid 1970s, 96% of a sample of women interviewed before delivery said that they would prefer a labour and delivery without medical intervention because such a birth would be more natural. In particular, 73% said that they would not like to have an induction, but 21% of these women did experience an induction (Oakley 1981).

It is commonly said that the desire for natural childbirth is limited to middle-class women, and it may also be objected that some women actively campaign for medical interventions. This follows from the point made earlier, that not all women want the same kind of birth experience. The matter of social class is complex. In a study in New England, Nelson (1983) found that there were two client models of childbirth, both of which were in competition with the medical model. Table 24.2 shows some dimensions of the two client models identified in this study. Significant differences exist between the two groups with respect to medication, artificial rupture of membranes (ARM) and fetal monitoring, but not for the other procedures shown in the table. Nelson summed up the differences thus:

> The working class women . . . favoured intervention because they thought it could bring the product easily, quickly and safely. The middle class women favoured a process which entailed safety (as they defined it) and personal participation, but excluded medical intervention in a natural process (Nelson 1983).

As Nelson points out, the preferences of working-class women in such settings may reflect inhibition, because they felt they were not able to control the birth process. In addition, middle-class women may have access to more information about childbirth. Account must also be taken of the fact that the social and economic position of the two groups is different. Working-class women have children at a younger age and have more accidental pregnancies and more limited material resources for childbearing. The pursuit of natural childbirth requires time, money and assertiveness, and will not occur at all unless it is seen to be a priority. It is clear that some women do not regard it as a priority.

Table 24.2 Planning for childbirth—choices about procedures by social class (from Nelson 1983)

	Percentage of women who wanted each procedure[a]	
	Working class (%)	Middle class (%)
Shave	20	20
Enema	42	46
Labour medication	57	11
Delivery medication	58	17
ARM[b]	59	4
Episiotomy	64	62
Fetal monitoring	90	55
Hold baby at birth	92	97

[a]Calculated on number in each group who expressed a choice. Total number of subjects in study = 322.
[b]Artificial rupture of membranes.

PAIN AND PAIN RELIEF

There is surprisingly little research that directly assesses the views of labouring women about pain. In 1982, 1000 women delivering at Queen Charlotte's Maternity Hospital were asked to grade the pain they felt in labour on a linear analogue scale (Morgan et al 1982). Those who had felt the most pain were mothers who had not received any analgesia and those who felt the least were those who had been given an epidural. One in three mothers experienced more pain than they had expected: this proportion was the same in all analgesic groups (Morgan et al 1982). Other surveys provide similar information; unfortunately, there has been no standard way of eliciting the information, so it is difficult to make direct comparisons between different studies. Cartwright (1979) included pain relief in her study of induction (Table 24.3). About one in four women said that they had not been given the right amount of pain relief. It is important to note that a drug or procedure given to alleviate pain may have other physical effects for the mother: Cartwright found that the proportion of women who felt nauseous or who vomited during labour was considerably higher in the epidural group than in any other.

Other surveys demonstrate regional and subcultural differences in attitudes to pain and pain relief. Analysis of data from the National Birthday Trust Fund survey of pain relief in labour (Social Science Research Unit 1992, unpublished report) found significant differences between ethnic groups. Asian women were more likely to describe the pain experienced as unbearable, and also more likely than other women to feel they had not been free to choose their method of pain relief. Comparison of mothers' and health professionals' perceptions of the same labours showed that health professionals were more likely than mothers to judge pain relief as effective; in other words, the professionals tended to underestimate the women's pain. Again, these differences were sharper for ethnic minority women.

It is known that individual pain thresholds vary. Although some health professionals and others may tend to see patterned differences between social groups in terms of attitudes to pain, for the British population at least, the notion that people in lower social classes have a high perception of pain and a greater prevalence of neuroticism has been shown to be false (Larson & Mercer 1984).

Satisfaction with childbirth, including feelings about the amount of pain experienced and relieved, evolves over time. It is necessary to know not only how mothers feel immediately or soon after delivery, but also what they make of the experience months or years later. The Queen Charlotte's study showed that the proportion of mothers dissatisfied with the experience of childbirth one year later was lowest in the group who had no analgesia. A recent American study examining mothers' recollections of their birth experiences with a 14–21-year period of follow-up found a striking consistency of recall over time. The significance attached to negative effects seemed to intensify over time, however, whereas the positive aspects tended to be recalled in a similar way over time (Shearer 1981).

There are methods other than medical for relieving labour pain. Fear, as described by Grantly Dick-Read (1942) and others, can lead to pain, thus the alleviation of fear by information and relaxation may directly affect pain. Contrary to some claims, however, there is no evidence that childbirth preparation classes on their own have an appreciable effect (Enkin 1982), although there is some evidence that they reduce the need for analgesia. Flynn et al (1978) found that ambulation in labour reduced the need for analgesia and had other effects, including higher Apgar scores and a reduced need for augmentation of labour with oxytocic drugs.

OBSTETRIC INTERVENTION

Consumer criticism of obstetrics was provoked by concern in the mid 1970s about rising induction rates (Gillie & Gillie 1974) and continues regarding rising caesarean section rates (Maternity Alliance 1983). In England, in 1994–1995, 21% of labours were induced and 15% of deliveries were by caesarean section (Department of Health 1997). The issues involved with these procedures relate both to what may be seen as the prevention of natural childbirth, and to the unwarranted promotion of medical and technological control, unwarranted in the sense that high rates of induction and caesarean section may entail more hazards than benefits for mothers and babies.

Macintyre (1981) asked the women in her Scottish study how they felt about the prospect of intervention during labour or delivery; her findings are shown in Table 24.4. Negative feelings were expressed by a third of the women; a very small proportion said they had positive feelings about the prospect.

Actively managed labour

The earliest step in managing labour is induction. Women comparing induced labour with a previous spontaneous

Table 24.3 Pain relief and induced and spontaneous labours (from Cartwright 1979)

	Induced labours (%)	Labours starting spontaneously (%)	All labours (%)
Pain relief			
None	11	21	19
Epidural/spinal anaesthesia	9	4	5
Other injection	72	62	64
Inhalant analgesia	4	6	5
Other	4	6	5
Amount of pain relief			
Enough	70	73	72
Would have liked more	7	7	7
Too much	9	7	8
Mixed views/other	14	13	13
Number of labours	522	1599	2134

Table 24.4 Women's feelings at 34 weeks' gestation about intervention during labour or delivery (from Macintyre 1981)

Feelings	% Women (n = 45)
Positive feelings about intervention	2
Accepting or indifferent	58
Negative feelings	36
Not asked	4
Total	100

labour reported the induced labour to be worse because of its greater pain and discomfort (Kitzinger 1975, Cartwright 1979). Similarly, women have found induced labour more painful than they expected (Stewart 1979), more women finding it so than those experiencing spontaneous labour (Lewis et al 1975).

Women whose labours are induced receive more pain relief (Kitzinger 1975, Stewart 1979, Yudkin et al 1979, Department of Health 1997). The increased use of analgesic drugs with induction is likely to have negative effects on the baby (Richards 1977, 1979) and induced labours tend to be shorter than those that begin spontaneously (Cartwright 1979). Shortening the length of labour, even spontaneous labour, sometimes appears to be a carrot held out by obstetricians to women to persuade them of the advantages of induced labour specifically, and the active management of labour in general. According to the active management of labour policy, as advocated and practised by O'Driscoll, it is important to assure women that their babies will be born within a definite time period 'because the prospect of prolonged labour is often a cause of serious concern' (O'Driscoll & Meagher 1980). In fact no one appears to have asked women which of the two alternatives they would prefer: a shorter more painful labour or a longer, possibly less painful one.

Surveys have shown that induced labours are far more frequently accompanied by fetal heart rate monitoring than spontaneous labours (Cartwright 1979, Yudkin et al 1979), and a causal link has been shown between oxytocin and internal electronic fetal monitoring (Tan & Hannah 1999a). The procedures involved in attaching scalp electrodes to the fetus are experienced by some women as painful (Oakley 1981) and monitors held in place externally by belts restrict movement, but these procedures were widely introduced while maternal reactions to continuous fetal heart rate monitoring generally received scant investigation. Of more than 500 articles on this topic published between 1970 and 1980, only two considered maternal attitudes. The following range of reactions was reported in one of these. The monitor was seen as:

- a protector, sometimes with quasi-magical powers
- an extension of the woman's own body
- an aid to communication
- an extension of the baby
- a distraction
- an aid to recognising the onset of contractions
- a mechanical monster

- a competitor for the husband's the midwife's, or the doctor's attention
- a facilitator of husband participation in labour
- a source of anxiety (Lumley & Astbury 1980).

A more recent randomised controlled trial of electronic fetal heart rate monitoring compared mothers' views of this technique with their views about intermittent auscultation. The electronically monitored women experienced more restriction of movement and were not more reassured by this method of monitoring than women exposed to the traditional alternative (Garcia et al 1985a).

Oxytocin-induced labours are associated with more epidurals (Tan & Hannah 1999a), although it is not entirely clear why. Are epidurals administered more often in these cases because women request them, because medical staff expect an induced labour to be more painful and advise the mother accordingly, or because it is more convenient to organise an epidural at the same time as the other procedures required for an induction? The greater use of epidurals in induced labour may be the consequence of a more general attitude to intervention among obstetricians, so that those who favour induction are also likely to favour epidurals. Obstetricians regard epidurals as increasing their job satisfaction and that of midwives, though most midwives in fact hold the view that this is not so (Cartwright 1979).

The more common use of epidural analgesia in induced as opposed to spontaneous labours in part explains the higher rate of instrumental delivery associated with induced labours (Cartwright 1979, Yudkin et al 1979, Department of Health 1997). Cartwright found differences in the incidence of instrumental delivery according to whether or not the husband was present (a higher rate characterised the husband-present group), and she suggests that 'possibly husbands agitate for something to be done—or possibly forceps are occasionally used as a reason for asking the husband to leave?'. Yudkin et al (1979) present the interpretation as being that the high rate of forceps deliveries among the induced women reflects not so much the inability of these women to deliver spontaneously, but rather the close attention of the supervising obstetrician; having started a woman's labour electively and closely followed it through to full dilation with fetal monitoring the obstetrician may well feel that he can ensure a successful delivery by intervening in the second stage as well.

Kirke (1975), in one of the very few studies of consumer attitudes carried out by doctors, reports that 'almost three quarters of those who had forceps deliveries said they either did not mind or were pleased about it, and one quarter were disappointed because they had wanted a natural birth'. It is difficult to know how to regard those who were pleased at having a forceps delivery. Would they have been very pleased if they had been offered a caesarean section instead? Similar questions apply to a survey by Impey (1999). A randomised controlled trial designed to compare the consequences for mothers and babies of the vacuum extractor versus forceps found that women allocated to vacuum extraction reported less pain at delivery but had more worries about their babies (Garcia et al 1985b).

There is some evidence that as is the case with fetal monitoring (Starkman 1976), instrumental delivery is more positively evaluated by the mother when it is seen as a solution to a real obstetric problem rather than as a routine procedure (Oakley 1981). The same probably holds for episiotomy, a procedure which has become more common in recent years and which appears to be considerably more painful and problematic for mothers than was originally recognised (Kitzinger 1981, Carroli et al 1999).

In a leading article on induction in labour in 1976, the British Medical Journal attempted to disentangle the main points emerging from the media debate on induction. The article took the view that since induction was only practised by clinicians 'in good faith for the good of the mother and the baby' its misrepresentation in the media must be 'disquieting evidence that doctors were not adequately communicating their intentions to their patients'.

Lack of information and inadequate discussion are certainly major themes in the studies of women's attitudes to induction that have been performed. The most detailed data are provided by Cartwright (1979). Only 57% of women whose labours were induced had discussed induction during pregnancy. Two out of five said they would have liked more information about it. Whereas middle-class women were more likely to have discussed induction beforehand, working-class women were more likely to feel deprived of adequate information about pregnancy and birth in general.

Given that the variation between different practitioners and institutions in induction rates is a matter of relatively public knowledge, and that hazards of the procedure are fairly openly discussed, it is hardly surprising that many women feel that induction of labour is not a purely clinical matter to be left to obstetricians, but one in which they themselves should be able to exercise choice (Friedson 1975). Indeed, 81% of the women in Cartwright's study indicated that in circumstances in which a doctor was uncertain about what clinical course to adopt in their case they would like the situation explained to them so that they could choose what should be done. This is surely a very important point: four-fifths of mothers would prefer to be involved in the decision-making process, but only a third of those whose labours were induced felt they had had any kind of choice. The desire of many women to take part in decisions about induction does not necessarily mean that they are opposed to induction.

Ounsted & Simons (1979) somewhat provocatively write: 'in addition to those women who insist on natural childbirth at all costs, there appears to be another group who may exert pressure on their obstetricians to induce labour in the absence of clear-cut medical reasons'. Although 6% of Cartwright's sample had tried to arrange not to have an induction, 2% recorded an attempt to have one. Adequate discussion of induction beforehand and good emotional support from medical staff during labour and delivery contribute to relatively comfortable experiences of induction (Kitzinger 1975, Cartwright 1979). Attitudes and reactions to childbirth are, in this sense, a function of many different variables, including women's prior experiences of birth and obstetric care, their confidence (or lack of it) in their body's ability to labour spontaneously, and the degree of unpredictability their social cir-

cumstances are able to support concerning the time of birth. Tables 24.5 and 24.6 from Cartwright's study show the same pattern as Table 24.7: the proportions of women who would prefer the same pattern of care for their next baby as they had for the last one are highest for the natural alternative in each case, i.e. no induction, no epidural, home birth.

Despite the worse pain and the attendant harms of medical pain relief and electronic fetal monitoring, there are circumstances in which women choose induction of labour. Systematic reviews of randomised controlled trials have confirmed that induction of labour by rupture of membranes at or near term has increased the use of anaesthesia or analgesia; oxytocin, but not prostaglandins, increased the use of electronic fetal monitoring. Prostaglandins, but not oxytocin, increased the rate of caesarean section (Tan & Hannah 1999a,b). Simultaneous benefits were decreases in the risks of maternal infection, neonatal infection and admission to neonatal intensive care. In these circumstances, in the trials which systematically collected information on women's views, women were more likely to view their care positively if labour was induced. The authors are unusual in advocating evidence-informed patient choice: that women with prelabour rupture of membranes at or near term should be informed of the benefits and risks of having their labour

Table 24.5 Preferences for induction in the next labour (from Cartwright 1979)

	Labour last time	
	Induced (%)	Not induced (%)
Prefer same as last time	17	93
Prefer not to have same as last time	78	5
Other comments	5	2
Number of mothers (= 100%)	552	1593

Table 24.6 Preferences for epidural analgesia in the next labour (from Cartwright 1979)

	Analgesia in the last labour	
	Epidural (%)	No epidural (%)
Prefer same as last time	63	82
Prefer not to have same as last time	34	13
Other comments	3	5
Number of mothers (= 100%)	110	2053

Table 24.7 Preferences for place of birth in the next pregnancy (from Cartwright 1979)

	Place of birth in the last pregnancy	
	Home birth (%)	Hospital birth (%)
Prefer same as last time	91	83
Prefer not to have same as last time	9	15
Other comment	–	2
Number of mothers (= 100%)	97	2083

induced and should be encouraged to choose the treatment option they would prefer.

Caesarean section

More research has been done in the USA than in the UK on the social and psychological costs of a caesarean section. It is interesting to note that a Consensus Development Task Force set up in 1979 by the National Institutes of Health to examine caesarean childbirth numbered a sociologist and a psychologist among its members; one of its assignments was to consider the 'psychological effects of Caesarean delivery on the mother, infant and family' (Shearer 1981).

It is significant that the operation of caesarean section is referred to in a different way from other forms of abdominal surgery; it is not called an operation, or surgery, but a section. Accompanying this difference in terminology, while it is accepted among surgeons that depression is a common consequence of major surgery, especially when carried out as an emergency procedure, the same assumption is not made about a caesarean section, but many of the psychological consequences of surgery in general also apply to caesarean section. These include a temporary response of emotional relief and elation at having survived the operation, worry about the mutilating effects of the operation on the body and its attractiveness to others, and a long-drawn-out period of physical and psychological discomfort (Janis 1958). It is worth noting that the care of the newborn involves activities that are likely to be forbidden to any patient on a surgical ward for some days (if not weeks) after abdominal surgery. It is presumably factors of this kind that account for the association between an admission to a psychiatric hospital in the first 90 days after childbirth and a caesarean delivery (Kendell et al 1981).

One British study (Trowell 1978) compared 16 mothers who had emergency caesarean sections under general anaesthetic with a control group of women who had spontaneously vaginally delivered. All were having first babies; the babies weighed over 2.49 kg (5.5 lb) and were not admitted to a special care unit. No section was performed for pressing obstetric reasons. At one month, observations showed that mothers who had had a caesarean section looked more but smiled less at their babies, and the caesarean babies were rated as being more tense. Striking differences emerged from the questioning of the mothers. Those who had had a caesarean section more often remembered birth as a bad experience, expressed doubts about their capacity to care for the baby and were depressed or anxious. As the author comments:

> These women had expected a normal vaginal delivery and had prepared themselves for this. They tended to feel a failure as a woman, unable to have a normal delivery and angry with the baby for not 'coming out', and there was some anger towards the hospital, although at the same time, an acknowledgement of the crisis that had occurred and a belief that the hospital had saved their and their baby's lives. Perhaps because of these feelings the Caesarean mothers were more anxious and apprehensive about parenthood and its responsibilities (Trowell 1978).

These sorts of attitudes were still present at one year, the mothers who had had a caesarean section being more likely to describe motherhood in negative terms, more likely to delay responding to their child's crying, and reporting that they first felt their child responded to them as a person at a later age. The group of mothers who had had a caesarean section expressed more anger in their handling of their children by shouting, smacking and losing their tempers. There were indications that the babies born by caesarean section had slower motor development (age of sitting unaided), and some interaction measures from the observations showed continuing differences between the groups. The groups in this study are small and, as the author herself emphasises, it was intended to be a pilot study.

Another study comparing perceptions of childbirth among socially similar groups of women having caesarean and vaginal deliveries found a generalised loss of self-esteem among the former (Marut & Mercer 1979).

The profound effects that can follow a caesarean section are recognised among women, and one of the more striking developments in recent years has been the growth of self-health groups offering support to mothers. The very existence of these groups is, of course, a clear indication of the psychological and social needs for support on the part of women who have undergone these procedures. As with induction, there are situations in which some women prefer an elective delivery by caesarean section to a vaginal one. Section rates are very high among private patients (Richards 1979); this may in part reflect a movement of women who want caesarean sections into the private sector, where they may be more likely to get them on demand.

EVIDENCE AND SHARED DECISION-MAKING

The broad spectrum of preferences amongst women having babies reflects variation in their health and social conditions. In order to respect the wishes of the labouring mother, those caring for her must find out how she approaches birth and her own role in it. The policy of patient partnership and the growing clinical approach of evidence-based health care have merged into the concept of evidence-informed patient choice. The extent to which this pertains in clinical encounters depends on attitudes towards patient choice, the nature of the evidence, personal preferences and the availability of interventions. Evidence-informed patient choice rests on the principle that patients should be able to take decisions themselves or share them with their clinician, as they wish, and that these decisions should also be informed by evidence of the effects of care.

As clinicians debate the relative merits of research evidence and personal experience for clinical practice, patients vary in their dependence on evidence, experience or personal values for their decisions about health care. For instance, ultrasound in early pregnancy (Neilson 1999) may be welcomed by some women for its effect on reducing the number of induced labours in hospitals where policies favour induction of post-term pregnancy; it may be avoided by others concerned about rare inaccuracies or adverse events; most often, however, it is welcomed by women for its positive impact on the social and emotional experience of normal pregnancy. Meanwhile, ultrasonographers themselves reject the research evidence about the effects of ultrasonography as outdated (Oliver et al 1996).

There are similar inconsistencies in decisions about who should provide care during pregnancy and childbirth. Women may be denied continuity of carer in pregnancy and childbirth or constant caregiver support in labour despite evidence of clinical benefit (Hodnett 1999a,b). Thus, evidence for decision-making may be considered open to interpretation or disregarded in favour of other influences such as expectations, emotional well-being, cost, and whether or not patients share those decisions.

In addition to questioning the weight that evidence may carry in decision-making, compared with these other influences, one may question the nature of the evidence and the claims that are made for a scientific basis of health services. The remainder of this chapter provides, from a lay perspective, a careful analysis and discussion of much of the evidence underpinning maternity care. Although science has been portrayed as trained and organised common sense (Huxley 1887), once laid out in a systematic fashion, reviews of obstetric interventions appear to generate knowledge more accurately described as trained and organised obstetricians' sense; this is different from the reviews of midwifery interventions, which appear to generate knowledge more accurately described as trained and organised midwives' sense. The analysis below illustrates the inherent subjectivity of scientific evidence and reveals how the organised nature of scientific knowledge makes it more open to critique, even from a lay perspective.

Evidence-based health care currently emphasises the value of randomised controlled trials and systematic reviews in decisions about treatment. Trials are designed to distinguish between (a) differences in outcome that are moderate but still worthwhile, and (b) differences in outcome that are too small to be of any material importance (Collins et al 1997). This argument has been used to support large-scale streamlined clinical trials, but *moderate*, *worthwhile*, and *of any material importance* are all subjective terms. When applied to outcomes of care they are qualitative as well as quantitative; it is not only the size of an effect but its nature that determines how highly we value it.

Within the medical model of childbirth, there is an overwhelming emphasis on mortality and its avoidance, and on physical morbidity. Within the social model of childbirth on the one hand, more holistic criteria of success are stressed; the mother's experience of birth is part of this, as is her emotional condition during the early years and months of motherhood, her relationship with the baby, the baby's long-term development and the whole nexus of relationships—the nuclear family, the extended family, the household—into which the baby is born.

Fortunately, in the Western world, childbirth is sufficiently safe for mortality to have limited use in studies that test efforts to improve care. This has not, however, led to wholesale application of more holistic criteria for success. Instead, surrogate outcomes have been applied in trials,

which are most often also obstetric interventions in their own right.

When systematic reviews relevant to women experiencing normal pregnancy or childbirth are analysed in terms of the interventions assessed in trials and the outcomes employed, their inherent subjectivity is readily apparent. Tables 24.8 and 24.9 show how frequently data appear in Cochrane reviews for various outcomes (1999). To be listed, data must have been collected in at least one included primary study and subsequently incorporated into a systematic review.

Of the 40 reviews relevant to normal pregnancy and childbirth, 28 include outcome data for obstetric intervention; 14 include outcome data for women's views of the intervention or outcome; nine include social, emotional and functional outcome data such as relationship with carers, anxiety and fatigue; and only four include outcome data for the mother–infant relationship (including breast-feeding). Outcome data about the babies' health appear in 28 reviews, although this is primarily for mortality (21 reviews), and physical measures at birth or subsequent medical treatment. In only four reviews are data available about the long-term health of babies. Only four reviews contain outcome data about women's views and social, emotional or functional outcomes. Three of these are primarily interventions that are central to the principles of radical midwifery: offering a com-

Table 24.8 Frequency of outcome data appearing in 40 reviews of interventions for healthy pregnancy and labour in *The Cochrane Library* 1999

Outcome measures	Number of reviews
Babies' health	28
Caesarean section	22
Induction of labour	14
Analgesia/anaesthesia	11
Instrumental delivery	10
Monitoring in labour	1
Any of the above obstetric interventions	28
Women's views	14
Social, emotional, functional outcomes	9
Long-term outcomes	9

Table 24.9 Frequency of outcome data about babies appearing in 40 reviews of interventions for healthy pregnancy and labour in *The Cochrane Library* 1999

Outcome measures	Number of reviews
Any measure of babies' health	28
Mortality	21
Birthweight	15
Apgar score	13
Admission to special/intensive neonatal nursery	12
Small for gestational dates	7
Infant infection	5
Birth asphyxia	2
Physical measures at or above 1 year	4
Psychosocial measures at or above 1 year	4

fortable birth place, encouragement and support (Homans 1980, Phoenix 1990, Hodnett 1999c).

Thus it is clear that maternity care has been assessed primarily in terms of obstetricians' interventions and little effort has been invested in assessing care from the perspective of women and their long-term experience of mothering. Consequently, not only do clinicians determine care, they also determine the evidence to support their decisions about care. For instance, a subjective clinical decision in the course of a trial to accelerate labour, or apply electronic fetal monitoring, simultaneously shapes the evidence on which such decisions will be made in future. Such subjectivity would not matter if it reduced only the precision of assessing health, but as these are the very foci of controversy, there is concern that the clinicians' subjective views are given undue weight in the design of randomised controlled trials.

This leads to the disquieting possibility that trials in maternity care may tell us less about the effect of care on the health of mothers and babies than they do about the impact of intervention on subsequent clinician behaviour. For instance, the authors of a systematic review of iron supplementation in pregnancy conclude that although blood iron is raised, no conclusions can be drawn in terms of any effects, beneficial or harmful, on outcomes for mother and baby, although routine iron supplementation may reduce the use of postpartum blood transfusion (Mahomed 1999). No mention is made of the risk of constipation despite this being of concern to pregnant women.

In childbirth, when spontaneous labour is accelerated by amniotomy, is the effect good for the mothers' experience because fewer women experience unbearable labour pain, or does the advantage lie in restraining clinicians from injecting women with oxytocics? (Fraser et al 1999).

Conversely, if the tendency of clinicians to intervene can be checked once, women should experience less subsequent intervention too. This appeared to be the case in a single-centre trial when clinicians adopted strict criteria for diagnosing the onset of labour; women were less likely to receive intrapartum oxytocics and analgesia, and mothers reported higher levels of control during labour and birth (Lauzon & Hodnett 1999).

The scale of intervention cascades (Wagner 1994) is unknown when national statistics ignore electronic fetal monitoring; it is not recorded in Maternity Hospital Episode Statistics in England despite its frequent use, even in hospitals without the facilities for measuring fetal scalp pH. Also notably absent from both these national statistics and reviews in *The Cochrane Library* is the use of drugs for accelerating spontaneous labour, another intervention whose benefits are debatable.

A HEALTHY BABY OR A GOOD EXPERIENCE?

If the consumer movement in maternity care has succeeded in saying anything loudly and clearly then it is surely this: that a healthy baby and a good experience are, for the majority of mothers, not different goals, but the same one. This message is brought out most sharply in the literature on mother–infant bonding which has stressed the fact that childbirth does not end with the delivery of the baby; a relationship, begun prenatally, has to be forged between the mother and the newborn and in the forging of this relationship obstetric procedures either may or may not help. Table 24.10 shows the association between some such procedures and breast-feeding as one indicator of the mothers' and babies' relationships with one another. Mothers who have caesarean deliveries and any type of analgesia or anaesthesia in labour and whose babies go into special care are more likely than other mothers to have stopped breast-feeding within two weeks of delivery. Of course these factors are interrelated but the statistical analysis showed that any factor causing a delay of more than four hours between delivery and the first breast-feed was likely to jeopardise the success of breast-feeding (Martin & Monk 1982).

Viewed more positively, a meta-analysis of randomised controlled trials showed that the continuous presence of a caregiver offering support during labour not only makes this a better experience for women by reducing the need for obstetric intervention and medical pain relief, but it benefits their health in the short and long term, their baby's health and their mothering relationship (Hodnett 1999b).

It is obvious that what obstetricians do may have long-term effects, especially when the link between early feeding and adult health is considered (Faulkner 1980). When childbirth is not successful and a perinatal death occurs, then the behaviour of obstetricians and paediatricians is not necessarily less important. Seeing and touching the dead baby are often important, and it is rare for those parents who have done so to regret it, while fantasies about the dead child's appearance may be a real obstacle to grieving

Table 24.10 Proportion of mothers who had stopped breast-feeding within 2 weeks by type of delivery, analgesia or anaesthesia and baby's postpartum care (from Martin & Monk 1982)

	Proportion (%) of mothers who had stopped breast-feeding within 2 weeks in England and Wales (n = 2499)
Delivery type	
Normal	19
Forceps/vacuum	19
Caesarean section	28
All mothers	19
Analgesia/anaesthesia	
Nothing	11
Gas and air	20
Injection (excluding epidural)	20
Epidural	22
General anaesthetic	28
All mothers	19
Baby's care	
No special care	18
Special care	23
All babies	19

for those who are not given this opportunity (Stringham et al 1982).

Examining medical evidence in terms of the concerns of childbearing women, or more directly, having those women examine the evidence themselves, underlines the unsettling truth that the more we know, the more we find we do not know. In the absence of evidence, or despite it, women may choose early ultrasound for social reasons, decline amniocentesis on moral grounds, or discard prescriptions for iron for fear of constipation. Women may even make opposing choices for identical reasons: peace of mind may be gained by continuous antenatal care of a known midwife for one woman, or consultant obstetric care for another; anxieties about childbirth may be allayed by the close proximity of high technology in hospital, or by the surroundings of the mother's own home; an atmosphere of panic during the third stage of labour may be avoided by an injection of Syntometrine in fear of haemorrhage, or by natural delivery of the placenta in its own time.

While women may be informed of relevant evidence, such as it is, their decisions must necessarily be largely based on uncertainty or faith. Women may decline or regret some obstetric interventions, or be unconvinced by the evidence underpinning maternity care, but still appreciate the information, support and opportunities for discussion offered by midwives and obstetricians.

CONCLUSION

This chapter has described how current maternity care and its evidence base is set within the context of falling mortality rates, increasing medicalisation of pregnancy and childbirth, greater variation amongst childbearing women in terms of their ethnicity, work commitments and family structures, increasing material deprivation among women and children, and a growing consumer movement. How these factors interrelate has implications for care during pregnancy and childbirth, how that care is evaluated and how decisions are made about care for individual women and their babies.

The welcome fall in mortality allows the longer-term view of health to influence decisions about care, but these decisions lack a firm evidence base because research evaluating care retains a predominantly short-term view. Issues central to consumer debates are those very issues in which there is little clear evidence about effects on the long-term health of women and their babies: place of birth, delivery personnel, analgesia and obstetric intervention.

The consumer movement and social medicine has not only highlighted a lack of congruence between clinicians' and women's priorities about maternity care and its evaluation, but also a huge variation in personal preferences amongst women themselves. Choice, for and by women, is invoked. Despite wide policy support for such choice, the medicalisation of childbirth, particularly the structures of health services and power relations within them, seriously constrains the availability of women's choice and the extent to which this choice is informed or evidence-based.

KEY POINTS

- Women perceive their experiences and care during pregnancy and childbirth differently from that expressed in routine statistics and evidence about the effects of that care.
- The wide variation in women's health, preferences for care, and social circumstances challenges how they should be cared for and how decisions about that care should be made.
- A critique of trials and systematic reviews of women's expressed views and their long-term family responsibilities draws attention to the inherent subjectivity of the current evidence base.

Women are diminished when:

- Clinicians make assumptions about women's experiences and preferences, for instance about pain and length of labour.
- Despite policies that explicitly support choice, in practice women's choice is curtailed.
- Evidence-based approaches favour professional knowledge over women's knowledge.
- Evidence is generated largely without the knowledge and insights of women.
- The long-term responsibilities women carry for their babies' health are not given the same attention in intervention research as the short-term responsibilities that clinicians carry.

Evidence is grounded in subjectivity when:

- Clinicians alone determine the choice of outcomes.
- Measurement of outcomes is largely a record of clinical intervention.
- Controversial topics are ignored by routine statistics, trials and systematic reviews.
- Research addresses the uncertainties of obstetricians, but not the uncertainties of women.
- Trials are short term or inadequate.
- The value of trials is seen more in their ability to distinguish small quantitative differences than to assess holistically the effects of intervention on health.

A vision for more holistic health care includes:

- Valuing and investing in clinicians' interpersonal skills as well as their technical skills.
- Recognising the inherent subjectivity of much current research evidence.
- Being explicit about the gaps in evidence.
- Necessarily and frankly making decisions about care in the dark.
- Including women in debates for setting priorities for research and services.

REFERENCES

Acheson Report 1998 Independent inquiry into inequalities in health. HMSO, London

Arms S 1975 Immaculate deception. Bantam Books, New York

British Medical Journal 1954 Editorial. BMJ 24:54

British Medical Journal 1976 Editorial. BMJ 1:729

Carroli G, Belizan J, Stamp G 1999 Episiotomy for vaginal birth (Cochrane Review). In: The Cochrane Library, Issue 4. Update Software, Oxford

Carter T, Duriez T 1986 With child: birth through the ages. Mainstream Publishing, Worcester

Cartwright A 1979 The dignity of labour. Tavistock, London

Chalmers I, Sackett D, Silagy C 1997 The Cochrane Collaboration. In: Maynard A, Chalmers I (eds) Non-random reflections in health services research. BMJ Publishing Group, London, pp 231–249

Chamberlain G, Wraight A, Crowley P 1997 Home births: the report of the 1994 confidential enquiry by the National Birthday Trust Fund. Parthenon Publishing, Carnforth, Lancs

Chamberlain M 1981 Old wives' tales. London, Virago

Clark A 1968 The working life of women in the seventeenth century. Frank Cass, London

Collins R, Peto R, Gray R, Parish S 1997 Large-scale randomised evidence: trials and overviews. In: Maynard A, Chalmers I (eds) Non-random reflections in health services research. BMJ Publishing Group, London, pp 197–230

Department of Employment 1995 New earnings survey. HMSO, London

Department of Health 1997 Government Statistical Service NHS maternity statistics, England: 1989–90 to 1994–95. Statistical Bulletin 1997. Department of Health, London

Dex S, Sewell R 1995 Equal opportunities policies and women's labour market status in industrialised countries. In: Humphries J, Rubery J, (eds) The economics of equal opportunities. Equal Opportunities Commission, Manchester

Dick-Read G 1942 Childbirth without fear. Heinemann, London

Ditch J, Barnes H, Bradshaw J (eds) 1998 Developments in family policies in 1996. The University of York and the European Commission, York

Donnison J 1977 Midwives and medical men. Heinemann, London

Douglas J 1998 Meeting the health needs of women from black and minority ethnic communities. In: Doyal L (ed) Women and health services: an agenda for change. Open University Press, Buckingham

Doyal L 1998 Introduction: women and health services. In: Doyal L (ed) Women and health services: an agenda for change. Open University Press, Buckingham

Enkin M 1982 Antenatal classes. In: Enkin M, Chalmers I (eds) Effectiveness and satisfaction in antenatal care. Spastics International Medical Publications, London

Farr W 1885 Vital statistics. Edward Stanford, London

Faulkner F 1980 Prevention in childhood of health problems in adult life. WHO, Geneva

Flynn AM, Kelly J, Hollins G, Lynch PF 1978 Ambulation in labour. BMJ 2:591–593

Ford CS 1945 A comparative study of human reproduction. Yale University Publications in Anthropology no 32, New York

Fraser WD, Krauss I, Brisson-Carrol G, Thornton J, Breart G 1999 Amniotomy for shortening spontaneous labour (Cochrane Review). In: The Cochrane Library, Issue 4. Update Software, Oxford

Friedson E 1975 Dilemmas in the doctor-patient relationship. In: Cox C, Mead A (eds) A sociology of medical practice. Collier-Macmillan, London

Garcia J, Corry M, MacDonald D, Elbourne D, Grant A 1985a Mothers' views of continuous electronic fetal heart rate monitoring and intermittent auscultation in a randomized controlled trial. Birth 12:79–85

Garcia J, Anderson J, Vacca A, Elbourne D, Grant A, Chalmers I 1985b Views of women and their medical and midwifery attendants about instrumental delivery using vacuum extraction and forceps. J Psychosom Obstet Gynaecol 4:1–9

Gélis J 1991 History of childbirth. Polity Press, Cambridge

Gillie L, Gillie O 1974 The childbirth revolution and the vital first hours. Sunday Times 13th October, 20th October

Goldthorpe WO, Richman J 1974 Maternal attitudes to unintended home confinement. Practitioner 212:845

Goodman A, Webb S 1994 For richer, for poorer: the changing distribution of income in the UK, 1961–91. Institute of Fiscal Studies, London

Graham H 1998 Health at risk: poverty and national health strategies. In: Doyal L (ed) Women and health services: an agenda for change. Open University Press, Buckingham

Graham H, Oakley A 1981 Competing ideologies of reproduction: medical and maternal perspective on pregnancy. In: Roberts H (ed) Women, health and reproduction. Routledge & Kegan Paul, London

Granville AB 1819 A report of the practice of the midwifery at the Westminster General Dispensary during 1818. Burgess and Hill, London

Gready M, Newburn M, Dodds R, Gauge S 1995 Birth choices— women's expectations and experiences. National Childbirth Trust, London

Haire D 1972 The cultural warping of childbirth. International Childbirth Education Association, Minneapolis

Health Committee 1992 Second Report, session 1991–2, volume 1. London, HMSO

Hodnett ED 1999a Continuity of caregivers for care during pregnancy and childbirth (Cochrane Review). In: The Cochrane Library, Issue 4. Update Software, Oxford

Hodnett ED 1999b Caregiver support for women during childbirth (Cochrane Review). In: The Cochrane Library, Issue 4. Update Software, Oxford

Hodnett ED 1999c Home-like versus conventional institutional settings for birth (Cochrane Review). In: The Cochrane Library, Issue 4. Update Software, Oxford

Homans H 1980 Pregnant in Britain: a sociological approach to Asian and British women's experiences. PhD thesis, University of Warwick

Houd S, Oakley A 1986 Alternative perinatal services. In: Phaff JML (ed) Perinatal health services in Europe: searching for better childbirth. Croom Helm, London

Hunt S, Symonds A 1991 The social meaning of midwifery. Macmillan, London

Huxley TH 1887 Introductory science primer. D. Appleton and Company, New York

Impey L 1999 Maternal attitudes to amniotomy and labor duruction: a survey in early pregnancy. Birth 26:211–217

Janis I 1958 Psychological stress: psychoanalytic and behavioural studies of surgical patients. John Wiley, New York

Johnstone RW 1913 A textbook of midwifery. Adam & Charles Black, London

Kathamna S 2000 Race and childbirth. Open University Press, Buckingham

Kendell RE, Rennie D, Clarke JA, Dean C 1981 The social and obstetric correlates of psychiatric admissions in the puerperum. Psychol Med 11:341–350

Kirke P 1975 The consumer's view of the management of labour. In: Beard R, Brudenell M, Dunn P, Fairweather D (eds) The management of labour. Proceedings of the third study group of the RCOG. RCOG, London

Kitzinger S 1975 Some mothers' experiences of induced labour. National Childbirth Trust, London

Kitzinger S 1979 Birth at home. Oxford University Press, Oxford

Kitzinger S (ed) 1981 Episiotomy. National Childbirth Trust, London

Larson AG, Mercer D 1984 The who and why of pain: analysing social class. BMJ 288:883–886

Lauzon L, Hodnett E 1999 Caregivers' use of strict criteria for diagnosing active labour in term pregnancy (Cochrane Review). In: The Cochrane Library, Issue 4. Update Software, Oxford

Leather S 1996 The making of modern malnutrition: an overview of food poverty in the UK. Caroline Walker Trust, London

Lewis BV, Rana S, Crook E 1975 Patient response to induction. Lancet i:1197

Lumley J, Astbury J 1980 Birth rites. Sphere Books, Melbourne

McGlone F, Millar J 1998 United Kingdom. In: Ditch J, Barnes H,

Bradshaw J (eds) Developments in family policies in 1996. The University of York and the European Commission, York

Macintyre S 1977 The management of childbirth: a review of sociological research issues. Soc Sci Med 11:477–484

Macintyre S 1981 Expectations and experiences of first pregnancy. Report on a prospective interview study of married primigravidae in Aberdeen. Occasional paper no 5. University of Aberdeen, Aberdeen

McKeown T 1979 The role of medicine. Basil Blackwell, Oxford

Mahomed K 1999 Iron supplementation in pregnancy (Cochrane Review). In: The Cochrane Library, Issue 4. Update Software, Oxford

Martin J, Monk J 1982 Infant feeding 1980. OPCS Social Survey Division, HMSO, London

Marut JS, Mercer RT 1979 The Caesarean birth experience. Nurs Res 28:260–266

Maternity Alliance 1983 One birth in nine—trends in Caesarean sections since 1978. Maternity Alliance, London

Mead M, Newton N 1967 Cultural patterning of perinatal behaviour. In: Richardson SA, Guttmacher AF (eds) Childbearing—its social and psychological aspects. Williams and Wilkins, Baltimore

Middleton S, Ashworth K, Braithwaite I 1997 Small fortunes: spending on children, childhood poverty and parental sacrifice. Joseph Rowntree Foundation, York

Moorhead J 1996 New generations: Forty years of birth in Britain. NCT Publishing, Cambridge

Morgan B, Bulpitt C, Clifton P, Lewis PJ 1982 Effectiveness of pain relief in labour: survey of 1000 mothers. BMJ 285:689–690

Neilson JP 1999 Ultrasound for fetal assessment in early pregnancy (Cochrane Review). In: The Cochrane Library, Issue 4. Update Software, Oxford

Nelson MK 1983 Working class women, middle class women and models of childbirth. Social Problems 30:285–296

Oakley A 1976 Wisewoman and medicine man: changes in the management of childbirth. In: Mitchell J, Oakley A (eds) The rights and wrongs of women. Penguin, Harmondsworth

Oakley A 1981 From here to maternity. Penguin, Harmondsworth

Oakley A 1982 Obstetric practice: cross-cultural comparisons. In: Stratton P (ed) Psychobiology of the human newborn. Wiley, New York

O'Brien M 1978 Home and hospital: a comparison of the experiences of mothers having home and hospital confinements. J Royal Coll Gen Pract 28:460–466

O'Driscoll K, Meagher D 1980 Active management of labour. WB Saunders, London

Oliver S, Rajan H, Turner H et al 1996 Informed choice for users of health services: views on ultrasonography leaflets of women in early pregnancy, midwives and ultrasonographers. BMJ 313:1251–1255

Olsen O, Jewell MD 1999 Home versus hospital for birth (Cochrane Review). In: The Cochrane Library, Issue 4. Update Software, Oxford

Ounstead M, Simons C 1979 Maternal attitudes to their obstetric care. Early Hum Dev 3:201–204

Phoenix A 1990 Black women and the maternity services. In: Garcia J, Kilpatrick R, Richards M (eds) The politics of maternity care. Clarendon Press, Oxford

Registrar-General 1930 Decennial supplement on occupational mortality. HMSO, London

Richards MPM 1977 The induction and acceleration of labour: some benefits and complications. Early Hum Dev 1:3–17

Richards MPM 1979 Perinatal morbidity and mortality in private obstetric practice. Journal of Maternal and Child Health September:341–345

Riley EDM 1977 What do women want? The question of choice in the conduct of labour. In: Chard T, Richards MPM (eds) Benefits and hazards of the new obstetrics. Spastics International Medical Publications, London

Scott AM 1994 Gender segregation and social change. OUP, Oxford

Shearer E 1981 National Institutes of Health consensus development task force on Caesarean childbirth. The process and the result. Birth and the Family Journal 8:25–30

Stacey M 1976 The health service consumer: a sociological misconception. In: Stacey M (ed) The sociology of the National Health Service. Monograph no 22. University of Keele, Staffordshire

Stacey M, Homans H 1978 The sociology of health and illness: its present state, future prospects and potential for health research. Sociology 12:281–307

Starkman M 1976 Psychological responses to the use of fetal monitor during labour. Psychosom Med 38:269–277

Stewart P 1979 Patients' attitudes to induction and labour. BMJ 2:749–752

Stringham JG, Riley JH, Ross A 1982 Silent birth: mourning a stillborn baby. Social Work July:322–327

Tan BP, Hannah ME 1999a Oxytocin for prelabour rupture of membranes at or near term (Cochrane Review). In: The Cochrane Library, Issue 4. Update Software, Oxford

Tan BP, Hannah ME 1999b Prostaglandins for prelabour rupture of membranes at or near term (Cochrane Review). In: The Cochrane Library, Issue 4. Update Software, Oxford

The Cochrane Library, Issue 4, 1999. Update Software, Oxford

Trowell J 1978 The effects of obstetric procedures on the mother/child relationship. A pilot study of emergency Caesarean section. Unpublished paper. Department for Children and Parents, Tavistock Clinic, London

Versluysen JC 1981 Midwives, medical men and 'poor women labouring of child'—lying-in hospitals in eighteenth century London. In: Roberts H (ed) Women, health and reproduction. Routledge & Kegan Paul, London

Wagner M 1994 Pursuing the birth machine. ACE Graphics, Camperdown, Australia

Yudkin P, Frumar AM, Anderson ABM, Turnbull AC, Yudkin P 1979 A retrospective study of the induction of labour. Br J Obstet Gynaecol 86:257–263

25

Endocrine control of labour

Mark Johnson, Phillip Bennett

INTRODUCTION

During pregnancy the uterus increases in size primarily by hyperplasia and hypertrophy and secondarily by simply stretching to accommodate the fetus, placenta and amniotic fluid. Propregnancy factors operate to inhibit myometrial contractility until near to term, when prolabour factors begin to operate. The latter have two effects: the cervix is remodelled to allow it to efface and dilate and the uterus is stimulated to begin coordinated contractions. It is suggested that labour is the result of the activation of a 'cassette of contraction-associated proteins' which act to convert the myometrium from a state of quiescence to a state of contractility (Lye 1994). These proteins include gap junction proteins, oxytocin and prostaglandin receptors, enzymes for the synthesis of prostaglandins and cytokines, and also components of cell signalling mechanisms which affect the way the uterus responds to receptor activation. It is likely that the factors that activate these proteins also have effects in the fetal membranes, resulting in the production of prostaglandins and cytokines, and in the uterus, leading to cervical remodelling.

PARTURITIONAL PHASES OF PREGNANCY

Pregnancy can be divided into four parturitional phases (0–3; Fig. 25.1). The first (phase 0, quiescence), during the first and second trimesters, is dominated by propregnancy factors and characterised by myometrial growth and quiescence. The factors involved include progesterone, nitric oxide, relaxin, corticotrophin-releasing hormone (CRH) and parathyroid hormone-related peptide (PTH-RP), prostacyclin, human placental lactogen, calcitonin gene-related peptide (CGRP),

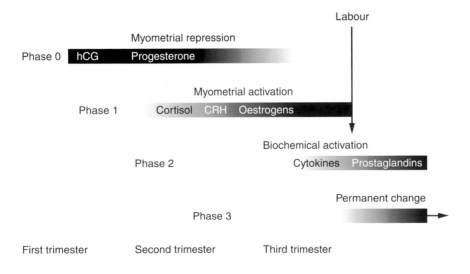

Fig. 25.1   The parturitional phases of pregnancy.

adrenomedullin and vasoactive intestinal polypeptide (VIP). During the second (phase 1, activation), which occurs in the early and mid third trimester, preparation for labour is made by the upregulation of relevant myometrial, cervical and fetal membrane proteins. This is probably an oestrogen-mediated process involving increased expression of gap junctions, contraction-related receptors and ion channels. Despite these changes, myometrial quiescence is maintained. The third (phase 2, stimulation) is labour itself. This occurs when the brake on myometrial contractility caused by propregnancy factors is released and prostaglandins, oxytocin and possibly CRH augment the underlying spontaneous contractility of the uterus. The fourth (phase 3, involution) occurs after labour and is primarily oxytocin mediated.

Phase 0: propregnancy factors

Progesterone

Progesterone, as its name suggests, is the principal propregnancy factor. In the human, progesterone is derived from the corpus luteum until approximately 7–8 weeks' gestation; thereafter the placenta is the dominant source. Progesterone has a negative effect on the expression and function of many of the contraction-associated proteins. It decreases uterine sensitivity to oxytocin through a non-genomic effect on the oxytocin receptor (Grazzini et al 1998). Progesterone is probably the most important factor in the enlargement of the uterus without increasing contractility. In many species, a withdrawal of progesterone immediately precedes the onset of labour. In some, the fall in progesterone is associated with an increase in oestrogen and in others with an increase in relaxin. The fall in progesterone and the increase in oestrogen probably act together to promote the expression and function of the 'contraction-associated proteins' while the fall in progesterone and increase in relaxin stimulate the process of cervical remodelling.

Progesterone withdrawal prior to labour is not thought to occur in the human or other primates; however, the progesterone antagonist (mifepristone, RU486) increases myometrial contractility (Haluska et al 1987), upregulates cervical IL-8 expression (Critchley et al 1996) and has been used successfully to induce labour (Elliot et al 1998). It is possible that in the human there is no actual or functional withdrawal of progesterone prior to labour, rather its propregnancy action is simply overwhelmed by prolabour factors. There are several alternatives to this view:

1. It is possible that there is a reduction in free, active progesterone rather than the total level (McGarrigle & Lachelin 1984).
2. Progesterone withdrawal may be a local event seen only within the fetal membranes (Mitchell & Wong 1993).
3. Functional progesterone withdrawal occurs because of a switch from expression of the B form to the A form of the progesterone receptor within the uterus near to term (Li & Lu 1995).
4. Functional progesterone withdrawal may occur as a result of competition between progesterone and increased concentrations of cortisol for the progesterone receptor (Karalis et al 1996).

Nitric oxide

Nitric oxide (NO) is a highly reactive free radical with diverse biological activities. During pregnancy, NO is suggested to promote myometrial quiescence and as such is considered a propregnancy factor (Buhimschi et al 1995). It is synthesised from L-arginine by nitric oxide synthase (NOS) that exists in at least three isoforms: type I, a constitutive, calcium-dependent neuronal form (nNOS); type II, an inducible, calcium-independent form (iNOS); and type III, a constitutive, calcium-dependent endothelial form (e/cNOS). NO donors have an inhibitory effect on pregnant human uterine contractility (Kumar et al 1965, Peng et al 1989). Although exogenous NO relaxes the uterus however, there is considerable doubt about the role of endogenous NO and the generation of NO within human myometrium (Bartlett et al 1999).

NO relaxes smooth muscle via activation of guanylate cyclase. A myometrial NO-cGMP relaxation pathway is present during pregnancy in animals and humans, but the cGMP response to NO is thought to decline before term (Yallampalli et al 1994, Buhimschi et al 1995). Uterine NOS activity has been reported to fall with the onset of labour in the rat and rabbit (Natuzzi et al 1993, Sladek et al 1993). In the human, e/cNOS is expressed in the non-pregnant uterus and both e/cNOS and iNOS in early pregnant human uterus (Telfer et al 1995). The expression of iNOS (assessed by immunostaining and Western analysis) has been found to fall significantly at term and again with the onset of labour (Bansal et al 1997); however, others using the same methods have failed to replicate these data (Bartlett et al 1999). Using reverse transcriptase polymerase chain reaction (RT-PCR) there was no correlation between gestational age and the expression of any of the NOS isoforms in human fetal membranes, placenta or myometrium, and no change with the onset of labour (Dennes et al 1999). Some have found that spontaneous myometrial contractions in vitro are unaltered by the administration of either L-arginine, the substrate for NOS, or L-NAME, a NOS inhibitor, suggesting that NO was unlikely to be involved in the maintenance of uterine quiescence (Jones & Poston 1997).

In contrast, others have reported that in vitro spontaneous myometrial contractions are reduced both by nitric oxide itself and by NO donor molecules (Ekerhovd et al 1999, Longo et al 1999), and in vivo glyceryl trinitrate (GTN, an NO donor) is as effective as ritodrine in prolonging pregnancy in women with preterm labour (Lees et al 1999). Topical GTN has been suggested to ripen the cervix, suggesting that NO, in the human at least, may also have a role as a prolabour factor in the cervix as well as a propregnancy role in the myometrium (Thomson et al 1997).

Relaxin

Animal data suggest that relaxin plays an important role in parturition, both as a propregnancy factor by promoting myometrial quiescence and as a prolabour factor by stimulating cervical remodelling; however, a major role for relaxin during human labour has yet to be found. Relaxin infusions in the rat have variable effects depending on their temporal relation to the time of onset of labour. Labour starting during a relaxin infusion is longer and associated with lower levels of oxytocin than control labours, but labour occurring after the cessation of the infusion is faster and associated with higher levels of oxytocin (Jones & Summerlee 1986). During lactation, relaxin infusion prevents the pulsatile release of oxytocin (essential to evoke a rise in intramammary pressure) (O'Byrne et al 1986), but increases the baseline release of oxytocin (Way & Leng 1992). In the human, the relationship between relaxin and oxytocin is not known. Oxytocin infusions during the menstrual cycle (Johnson et al unpublished observation) or during pregnancy at term (Hochman et al 1978) have no effect on circulating relaxin levels. Although relaxin levels appear to increase during breast feeding, no relationship between relaxin and oxytocin is seen either at this time or during labour (Johnson et al unpublished observation).

The administration of PGE_2 for the induction of second-trimester abortion results in an increase in circulating levels of relaxin (Seki et al 1987). In contrast, at term, the administration of $PGF_{2\alpha}$ has no effect on circulating relaxin levels (Hochman et al 1978). The addition of relaxin to cultures of fetal membranes obtained before the onset of labour inhibited prostaglandin release; however, the addition of relaxin to similar cultures of membranes obtained during labour increased prostaglandin release if the membranes were intact (López Bernal et al 1987). These data suggest that the response of relaxin to prostaglandins and the response of prostaglandin synthesis to relaxin is dependent on the stage of gestation. Relaxin, immunoreactivity observed in the fetal membranes prior to the onset of labour disappears after labour has begun (Bryant-Greenwood et al 1987). Porcine relaxin consistently inhibits spontaneous and induced myometrial contractions *in vitro* and *in vivo* in animal studies (Porter et al 1979, Goldsmith et al 1989). In the human, *in vitro* data conflict. Extracts of human corpora lutea and porcine relaxin have been demonstrated to inhibit both stimulated and spontaneous contractions of human myometrium *in vitro* (Szlachter et al 1980), but human relaxin (H2) has no effect (Petersen et al 1991). There are no data relating the *in vivo* administration of relaxin, whether porcine or human, to myometrial contractility. The relaxin receptor has been identified on human myometrial cells and in fetal membranes (Garibay-Tupas et al 1995, Osheroff & King 1995), but the post-receptor effects remain unclear.

Relaxin may exert its effects through several potential post-receptor mechanisms; these include cAMP generation, the opening of membrane potassium channels and the reduction in intracellular calcium levels. Relaxin has been shown to generate cAMP in several situations, but the time course of cAMP generation appears to follow that of mechanical relaxation of the uterus (Sanborn et al 1980, Kemp & Niall 1984). Indeed, *in vivo*, despite producing similar myometrial relaxation as β_2 agonists, cAMP levels increased relatively little (Downing et al 1992). Relaxin does inhibit MLKC activity, suggesting that some of its action is mediated through cAMP, however, other mechanisms must be responsible for its acute myometrial effects. Relaxin may open potassium channels and hyperpolarise the plasma membrane, but the evidence for this is conflicting (Downing & Hollingsworth 1993). Relaxin has been shown to increase calcium efflux and

antagonise oxytocin-induced increases in intracellular calcium and IP3 levels in animal studies (Ginsburg et al 1988, Anwer et al 1989).

In rats and pigs, removal of the activity of relaxin, either by ovariectomy or the administration of neutralising antibodies, results in labour, which is prolonged and attended by a high fetal mortality rate (Downing & Sherwood 1985). These findings are associated with reduced cervical elasticity (Downing & Sherwood 1985). This suggests that relaxin is important for normal cervical ripening. In the human, such studies have not been performed, but an analogous situation exists. Women with premature ovarian failure can only become pregnant after ovum donation. Such women do not have functional ovarian tissue and, consequently, there is no relaxin in their circulation (Johnson et al 1991). In cases where labour is allowed to start spontaneously cervical dilatation occurs successfully, although it may be slower than normal (Eddie et al 1990). This suggests that, in the human, relaxin is not essential for cervical dilatation. Moreover, the failure of recombinant human relaxin to induce labour or alter the structure of non-pregnant cervical samples *in vitro* has raised further questions about the role of endogenous relaxin in human labour (Brennand et al 1997). Overall, it seems that relaxin can cause myometrial relaxation, but the exact mechanisms involved are uncertain and the physiological importance of this inhibition, certainly in the human, is unproved.

Catecholamines

Catecholamines can act on the cell membrane or directly to alter myometrial contractility or cell metabolism. Catecholamine receptor expression is modulated by sex steroids. Progesterone stimulates β-receptor expression and oestrogen α-receptor expression (Bottari et al 1983). Cell membrane α-receptor excitation results in increased chloride conductance, which depolarises the membrane, and prolongation of the plateau part of the action potential by increased calcium conductance. The β_2 effect results from membrane stabilisation through increased potassium conductance and increased cAMP production (Bulbring & Tomita 1987). This is the basis of the use of β-mimetics in the management of preterm labour; however, the myometrium becomes refractory to prolonged treatment with β-mimetics because of reduced receptor expression, uncoupling of the β-receptor and increase in Gi activity (Dayes & Lye 1990, Lecrivain et al 1998).

Parathyroid hormone-related peptide (PTHrP) and calcitonin gene-related peptide (CGrP)

Both PTHrP and CGrP have been suggested to relax the myometrium. PTHrP is better known for its role in controlling transplacental transfer of calcium and controlling fetal calcium homeostasis. Many animal studies across several species suggest that PTHrP reduces uterine contractility (Shew et al 1991, Pitera et al 1998, Wu et al 1998). The data in the human are rather circumstantial to date, with increasing amniotic fluid levels of PTHrP reported to term; levels then decline with either rupture of membranes or the onset of labour (Ferguson et al 1992, Mitchell et al 1996). CGrP, in contrast, was first detected in the nerves supplying the uterus and reported to relax the non-pregnant uterus (Samuelson et al 1985). Later studies found that this effect was greater in the pregnant uterus but that it reduced with the onset of labour (Chan et al 1997). CGrP receptor expression is enhanced by progesterone and its excitation results in cGMP generation (Dong et al 1999, Yallampalli et al 1999).

Phases 1 and 2: prolabour factors

The placental clock

There is a substantial body of animal data to suggest that the fetus controls the time of onset of labour independent of whether pregnancy is maintained by the placenta, as in the sheep, or by the corpus luteum, as in the rat, pig and goat. The original observation that fetal hypophysectomy prevented the onset of labour in the sheep identified the crucial role played by the fetal adrenal in this animal (Liggins et al 1967). These data were supported by the ability of fetal infusions of ACTH, cortisol or dexamethasone to induce labour and bring about the endocrine changes found in spontaneous labour in the sheep (Liggins 1969). Finally, the progressive increase in cortisol output from the fetal adrenals in the last 20–25 days of gestation confirms the role of the fetal adrenal in the onset of labour in the sheep (Challis & Brooks 1989).

Fetal cortisol increases the expression of the P450 17α-hydroxylase and aromatase genes increasing the conversion of C21 to C19 steroids and the conversion of androgens to oestrogens (Tangalakis et al 1989). As progesterone is not a good substrate for placental 17α-hydroxylase, it is the delta-5 pathway of pregnenolone to 17-hydroxy-pregnenolone that is enhanced, resulting in increased levels of dihydro-epiandrosterone that is then aromatised to oestrogen (Mason et al 1989). The overall effect is to decrease placental progesterone output and increase oestrogen output. These changes are reflected in the decrease in progesterone and increase in oestrogen maternal serum concentrations. Similar changes can be induced by the administration of exogenous cortisol or by inhibitors of the 3β-hydroxysteroid dehydrogenase which converts pregnenolone to progesterone (Jenkin & Thorburn 1985, Mason et al 1989) (Figs 25.2, 25.3).

The mechanism that has been described in the sheep does not apply directly to the human although there are similarities that suggest a common evolutionary pathway. Both McLean and Challis have suggested that the time of onset of labour is determined by placental release of corticotrophin-releasing hormone (CRH; Jones et al 1989, McLean et al 1995). In the human, circulating maternal CRH levels begin to rise about 90 days before the onset of labour (Jones et al 1989, McLean et al 1995). CRH circulates principally in an inactive form, bound to CRH-binding protein (CRH-BP) derived from the maternal liver. CRH-BP is synthesised in the maternal liver and is negatively regulated by CRH, so that as circulating CRH levels increase so those of CRH-BP decrease. Typically, CRH concentrations exceed those of CRH-BP from about 37 weeks in the average pregnancy. Importantly, the regulation of hypothalamic CRH and placental CRH differs in that cortisol inhibits hypothalamic CRH release but enhances placental CRH release (Fig. 25.4).

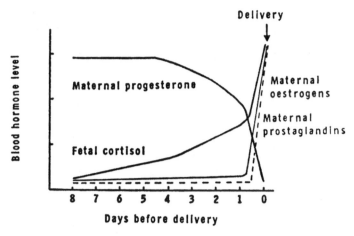

Fig. 25.2 Diagrammatic representation of the hormonal changes in the fetal and maternal circulation associated with parturition in the sheep. (After Flint et al 1975.)

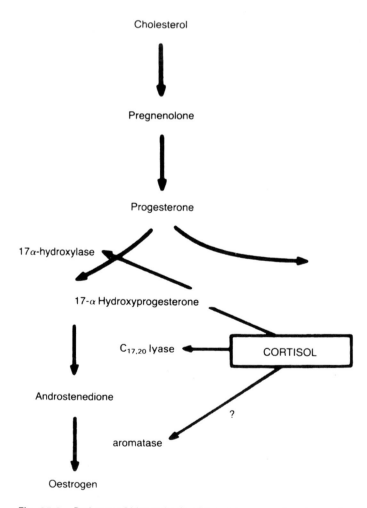

Fig. 25.3 Pathway of biosynthesis of progesterone and oestrogen in sheep placenta, indicating the possible sites of action of fetal cortisol on 17α-hydroxylase, $C_{17,20}$-lyase and aromatase. (From Liggins et al 1977.)

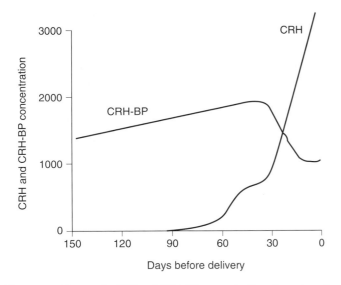

Fig. 25.4 Changes in CRH and CRH–BP concentrations in maternal circulation throughout pregnancy. (Adapted from McLean et al 1995.)

Both myometrium and fetal membranes express CRH receptors, linked to G-protein adenyl cyclase second messenger systems (Chen et al 1993, Grammatopoulos et al 1995, Liaw et al 1996, Rodriguez-Linares et al 1998). The increase in cellular cAMP levels would be expected to inhibit myometrial contractility through a reduction in myosin light chain kinase activity. Towards term, CRH-cAMP generation is reduced (Grammatopoulos et al 1996); this may contribute to the observation that CRH directly stimulates myometrial contractility at this time (Challis et al 1995). In addition, CRH upregulates expression of cyclo-oxygenase type 2 (COX-2) resulting in increased prostaglandin synthesis in both fetal membranes and myometrium (Jones and Challis 1990, Petraglia et al 1995, Alvi et al 1999). Overall, these data suggest that CRH promotes myometrial quiescence until late pregnancy, after which it stimulates myometrial contractility.

Oestrogens

Although maternal oestrogen concentrations do not rise acutely before human labour as they do in the sheep, there is a gradual rise in both oestriol and oestradiol concentrations during the third trimester, reaching a plateau at about 38 weeks (Buster et al 1979). In primates, increased oestrogen synthesis prior to labour is suggested to be mediated by increased androgen production by the fetal adrenal (Mecenas et al 1996). In some species, increased fetal adrenal activity is involved in the onset of labour. It has been suggested that in the human increased maternal oestriol levels may be a marker of preterm labour in some cases (Goodwin 1999). Modest increases in primate maternal plasma oestrogens may reflect more dramatic changes in concentration locally within the uterus. Oestradiol increases both oxytocin receptor expression and oxytocin synthesis within the uterus (Fuchs et al 1983). It does not, however, directly stimulate prostaglandin synthesis in prelabour amnion or in chorion (Gibb 1998) but it does increase prostaglandin synthesis in

amnion collected following labour (Olson et al 1983). The latter may, however, be secondary to stimulation of oxytocin synthesis and the increased oxytocin receptor density in amnion following labour (Challis et al 1995). Increased fetal dihydro-epiandrostenedione synthesis may occur in response to the increased placental CRH production via increased placental and fetal ACTH (Challis et al 1995). It appears, therefore, that CRH and oestrogens may be linked in the mechanism of the placental clock.

Oxytocin

The demonstration that extracts of the posterior pituitary stimulated uterine contraction, and the isolation of oxytocin as the active component, made it seem likely that oxytocin is important in the onset and progression of labour in the human. However, the failure to demonstrate an increase in the circulating levels of oxytocin with the onset of labour (Vasicka et al 1977), even in the presence of oxytocinase inhibitors (Yusoff Dawood et al 1978, Thornton et al 1992), raised doubts as to its importance in the human. These doubts were to some extent allayed by the observation of increased myometrial sensitivity to oxytocin with advancing gestation (Takahashi et al 1980), resulting from an increase in the myometrial expression of the oxytocin receptor (Fuchs et al 1984). This suggested that changes in plasma levels were not a necessary prerequisite for oxytocin to have a significant role in the onset of labour. Moreover, the demonstration of decidual oxytocin synthesis with the onset of labour suggests that oxytocin released from the decidua may act in a paracrine manner to stimulate myometrial contractility (Miller et al 1993). Changes in the local oestrogen : progesterone ratio may be important in the regulation of the synthesis of oxytocin (Richard & Zingg 1990) and the expression of the oxytocin receptor (Maggi et al 1992). Coincident with increases in myometrial receptor expression, decidual and fetal membrane oxytocin receptor mRNA expression is also increased during labour (Takemura et al 1994). Oxytocin binding to these tissues results in prostaglandin synthesis and release (Fuchs et al 1981, Moore et al 1988). That oxytocin antagonists stop preterm labour suggests that oxytocin may have an important role in labour (Akerlund et al 1986, Goodwin et al 1994).

OTR regulation occurs by transcriptional control (i.e. gene activity producing mRNA rather than changes in mRNA stability or modification of the protein). The promoter region of the OTR gene has been cloned. Deletion experiments show that approximately 1000 base pairs upstream of the coding region are needed for expression. It has long been thought that the OTR is upregulated by oestrogen and downregulated by progesterone (Maggi et al 1992). The OTR promoter does not, however, contain any full consensus oestrogen or progesterone response elements (ERE, PRE; Ivell & Walther 1999). Furthermore, in the tammar wallaby, which has a double uterine system but only becomes pregnant in one uterus, OTR expression only increases in the pregnant uterus at term and remains unchanged on the non-pregnant side (Parry et al 1997). Similarly, in the rat, if one uterine horn is tied to prevent implantation, oxytocin receptor and gap junction proteins are only expressed in the horn containing pregnancies (Ou et al 1998). These data suggest that OTR is modulated by local rather than by circulating factors.

Isolated myometrial strips contract spontaneously in the absence of oxytocin or other agonists (e.g. prostaglandins). These contractions can be inhibited using an oxytocin receptor antagonist (atosiban). This suggest the possibility that either myometrium releases oxytocin or other OTR ligands or that the receptor does not need oxytocin to initiate contractions (constitutive activity).

Prostaglandins

Labour is associated with increased prostaglandin synthesis by both the myometrium and fetal membranes (Turnbull 1977, Skinner & Challis 1985). Prostaglandin synthesis is particularly increased in the amnion, which is also a major site of arachidonic acid storage. Prostaglandins from the amnion must cross the chorion to reach their target tissues—the decidua, cervix and myometrium. Paradoxically, the chorion is rich in prostaglandin dehydrogenases (PGDH) and this might prevent or at least reduce prostaglandin transfer. Many individual cells have been shown to lack PGDH, however, and so prostaglandin transfer may be relatively unrestricted (Nackla et al 1986, Bennett et al 1990a, Challis et al 1991). Although these findings have been disputed (Roseblade et al 1990), prostaglandins injected into the amniotic cavity are able to induce labour, clearly demonstrating that at least some is able to cross to the chorion and stimulate myometrial contractility. The decidua is an alternative source of prostaglandins. Indeed, the increase in decidual prostaglandin synthesis with labour is of a similar magnitude to that seen in the amnion (Skinner & Challis 1985). Prostaglandins promote cervical ripening and stimulate uterine contractions directly and indirectly by upregulation of oxytocin receptors (Dyal & Crankshaw 1988, Garfield & Hertzberg 1990).

Prostaglandins are formed from the precursor arachidonic acid that is a substrate for at least three enzyme pathways (Fig. 25.5). Prior to labour, endogenous arachidonic acid metabolism in amnion is principally via the lipoxygenase enzyme pathways. With labour, there is a general increase in arachidonic acid metabolism and particularly in the cyclo-oxygenase (COX) pathway, which produces prostaglandins (Saeed & Mitchell 1983, Bennett et al 1993). The roles of the lipoxygenase metabolites of arachidonic acid within the uterus are unknown, although 5-HETE may play a role in prelabour (Braxton Hicks) contractions (Bennett et al 1987, Walsh 1989). The switch from lipoxygenase to cyclo-oxygenase (COX) metabolism is achieved by upregulation of COX expression (Fig. 25.6). There are two COX genes, the constitutively expressed COX-1 (2.8 kb) and the inducible COX-2 (usually greater than 4.0 kb; Hla et al 1986, DeWitt & Smith 1988, O'Banion et al 1991, Hla & Neilson 1992). COX-2 expression is induced by mitogens and inhibited by glucocorticoids (O'Banion et al 1991). The difference in transcript size between COX-1 and COX-2 is caused by a long 5′ untranslated region in the type 2 mRNA. Thus, although not identical, the COX-1 and COX-2 proteins are of similar size and show a high degree of homology. The two genes are on different chromosomes but have a similar intron and exon

arrangement. The COX-1 gene spans over 22 kb of genomic DNA while the COX-2 gene spans only 8 kb. The long 3′ untranslated portion of COX-2 contains multiple copies of the Shaw–Kamen sequence (AUUUA) which is typical of early response genes with rapid mRNA degradation.

COX-1 and COX-2 mRNA are present in the fetal membranes (Slater et al 1995) and, at term, COX-2 mRNA expression in the amnion is some 100-fold higher than COX-1. COX-1 expression does not change throughout pregnancy. In contrast, COX-2 expression in the fetal membranes increases throughout the third trimester and doubles with the onset of labour (Hirst et al 1993, Slater et al 1994, 1995). In the myometrium there is expression of COX-1 and COX-2 at similar levels but only COX-2 expression increases near to term and with the onset of labour (Slater et al 1999). At term, all fetal membrane PG synthesis is via COX-2 (Sawdy et al 2000).

Fetal membrane COX-2 expression is thought to be regulated by maternal CRH as in vitro CRH increases expression of COX-2 and prostaglandin synthesis in fetal membranes and the changes in fetal membrane COX-2 expression closely mirror the concentration of free CRH in the maternal circulation (Alvi et al 1999). It has also been suggested that platelet-activating factor (PAF) produced by the fetal lungs increases prostaglandin synthesis in amnion near to term (Hoffman et al 1990, Moya et al 1993). These prostaglandins may then cross to the decidua, cervix and myometrium to initiate labour. IL-1β also increases prostaglandin synthesis in the fetal membranes and myometrium by a combination of increased phospholipase activity, secondary to phosphorylation of PLA$_2$, and upregulation of COX-2 expression (Romero et al 1989, Skannal et al 1997). It is possible that increased COX-2 expression during pregnancy is induced by CRH, but that the increases closer to the onset of labour are induced by other factors such as IL-1β or PAF.

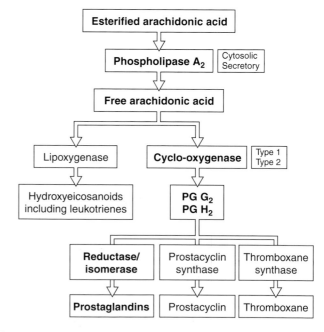

Fig. 25.5 Pathways for the metabolism of arachidonic acid.

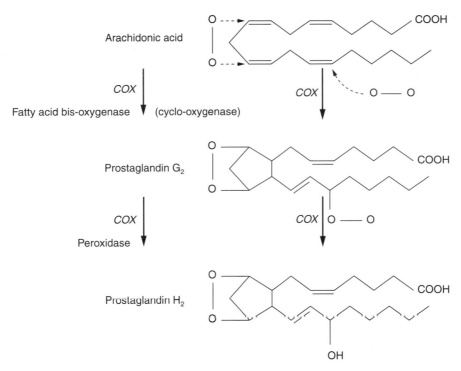

Fig. 25.6 The actions of the prostaglandin endoperoxide synthase, or cyclo-oxygenase enzymes.

The PAF and IL-1 receptors are expressed in fetal membranes, decidua and myometrium (Allport et al unpublished). PAF and IL-1β act to upregulate COX-2 expression through the transcription factor, nuclear factor κ-B (NFκB). The promoter region of COX-2 contains NFκB binding sites, as does those of IL-1β and IL-8. Activation of NFκB may precipitate a positive feedback loop of increased inflammatory and neutrophil attractant cytokines, leading to both a biochemical and cellular inflammatory reaction within the uterus. Generally, NFκB is considered to be a transcription factor associated with inflammation which functions as a homo- or heterodimer of the Rel family of proteins. The most biologically active combination is a heterodimer of the NFκB proteins p50 and p65, known as the classic NFκB. NFκB dimers normally exist in the cell cytoplasm bound by an inhibitor kappa B (IκB) protein. NFκB is activated through cell surface receptors, for example the receptor for the inflammatory cytokine IL-1β. Receptor activation leads to phosphorylation and degradation of IκB which then allows NFκB dimers to translocate to the nucleus and bind to the promoter (Kalkhoven et al 1996). A mutually negative interaction between NFκB and progesterone receptor has been described in which increasing the concentration of NFκB represses progesterone receptor function, and vice versa (Kalkhoven et al 1996). NFκB may play a role in the biochemical events associated with labour acting both to upregulate inflammatory/prolabour mediators, in particular COX-2, and to suppress progesterone receptor function.

Prostaglandin dehydrogenase

Fetal membrane COX-2 expression begins during the second trimester and increases towards term such that much of the COX-2 upregulation precedes labour. It is likely that this increase in prostaglandin synthetic capacity is balanced by the activity of prostaglandin dehydrogenase (PGDH) within the chorion. There is now good evidence that fetal membrane PGDH activity is upregulated by progesterone and downregulated by cortisol acting at the level of transcription (van Meir et al 1997, Patel et al 1999). The expression of PGDH falls with the onset of labour (Sangha et al 1994). The same group reported that a subgroup of patients presenting in idiopathic preterm labour had reduced chorionic PGDH expression, both at the mRNA and protein levels. PGDH activity is reported to be reduced in the chorion near to the cervix in normal labour and generally in the chorion in association with chorio-amnionitis (van Meir et al 1996). It is possible that chorionic PGDH expression is oppositely regulated by the same factors that regulate the prolabour gene cassette, and in particular COX-2, IL-1β and IL-8.

Endothelin

Although better known as a vascular peptide, endothelin does stimulate myometrial contractility itself and enhances the effects of oxytocin *in vitro* (Kaya et al 1998). Its levels increase in plasma and amniotic fluid in the third trimester, and endothelin receptor expression increases with the onset of labour (Yallampalli & Garfield 1994). The contractile effects of endothelin are mediated through the A-type receptor, excitation of which increases phosphoinositide generation (Dokhac et al 1995).

Inflammation and the onset of labour

Labour has been compared to an inflammatory reaction in both myometrium and cervix. There is a neutrophil and macrophage infiltration of upper and lower segments of the uterus with the onset of spontaneous labour, in part mediated through the increased expression of E-selectin or of IL-8 (Barclay et al 1993, Thomson et al 1999). Furthermore, there is a strong association between both term and preterm labour and increased production of the inflammatory cytokine interleukin-1β within the uterus (Romero et al 1990). IL-1β concentrations have been shown to be elevated in amniotic fluid in term labour and just prior to labour in patients with chorio-amnionitis (Romero et al 1992). Expression of IL-1β at the mRNA level is higher in fetal membranes after labour than before (Ammala et al 1997). The interaction between cytokines and COX-2 has been discussed above and, overall, cytokines can be divided into those that promote (IL-1α and β, IL-2, IL-6, IL-8, TNF-α) and those that inhibit (IL-4, IL-10) the onset of labour. The data regarding TGF-β are conflicting. It is reported to block IL-1α and TNF-α induced preterm delivery in the rabbit and to reduce IL-1 stimulated PGE_2 production by the placenta and TNF-α production by fetal membranes, but also to promote IL-8 activity and enhance myometrial contractility (Bry & Hallman 1993, Shimonovitz et al 1995, Arici et al 1996, Awad et al 1997, Fortunato et al 1997).

The cervix

The stroma of the cervix is made up of a network of collagen fibres, predominantly type I, proteoglycans and glycosaminoglycans. The latter include sulphated keratan, dermatan, chondroitins and hyaluronic acid. In addition, there is some smooth muscle in the human cervix, concentrated predominantly in the region of the internal os (Rorie & Newton 1967). Towards term, the cervix hypertrophies, becoming more vascular, oedematous and inflamed with a neutrophil polymorphonuclear leucocytosis (Junqueira et al 1980). Fibroblasts proliferate and synthesise glycosaminoglycans in response to prostaglandins, which they may also synthesise themselves (Liggins 1978). Collagen fibres are embedded in proteoglycan. Large-diameter fibres are associated with dermatan sulphate and chondroitin sulphate, while the finer, more loosely dispersed fibres are associated with hyaluronate. Relative increases in hyaluronidate enhance the susceptibility to collagenolytic digestion, and such changes have been described in the term human cervix (Kitamura et al 1980). The absolute amount and type of collagen present determines the physical properties of the cervix. Proteinases, which degrade collagen, are found to be increased in the term cervix. They include collagenase, PZ peptidase and acid proteinases (Ito et al 1977, 1979), and may be responsible for the reported changes in collagen content. Circulating levels of collagenase have also been related to cervical ripening, higher levels of collagenase being associated with improved cervical scores (Granstrom et al 1992).

At term, the application of prostaglandin E_2 topically to the cervix induces softening (Tromans et al 1981). The infusion of the oestrogen precursor, dehydro-epiandrosterone, increases the cervical concentration of oestrogens within 4 hours and results in high collagenase activity on subsequent culture *in vitro* (Mochizuki & Tojo 1980). The physiological importance of the action of oestrogen on the uterine cervix is still disputed, however, and the role of other hormones in its action is unclear. Prostaglandins increase cervical ripening at term by altering the glycosaminoglycan content of the cervix, inhibiting collagen synthesis and enhancing collagenase synthesis by macrophages (Murota et al 1977, Wahl et al 1979). Of cervices removed from spontaneous labours and those induced by oxytocin or PGE_2, PGE_2-treated cervices showed the greatest elasticity (Conrad & Ueland 1976). During the menstrual cycle in rhesus monkeys, relaxin was found to exaggerate the soft flaccid state of the cervix induced by the combination of progesterone and oestrogen (Hisaw & Hisaw 1964).

Much of the change in the cervix at term results from increased collagenase activity. Fibroblasts present in the cervix are capable of synthesising collagenase but there is also an accumulation of neutrophils which release collagenase into the cervix around the time of parturition. Cervical ripening therefore resembles an inflammatory reaction. It is thought that neutrophils are attracted into the cervix at term by the combination of increased prostaglandin synthesis and the neutrophil attractant peptide interleukin-8 (IL-8), whose expression may be mediated by the transcription factor NFκB (Kelly et al 1992, Calder 1994, Maradny et al 1995, Osmers et al 1995a,b, El Maradny et al 1996).

Infection

It is thought that, in most cases, infection ascends from the vagina, although it may also be transplacental or introduced during invasive procedures. It is probable that many cases of early preterm labour thought to be associated with cervical incompetence occur because vaginal pathogens enter the lower pole of the uterus through a modestly open cervix, where they set up an inflammatory reaction.

It seems logical that bacterial infection would initiate preterm labour by causing an inflammatory reaction within the uterus and effectively switching on parturitional phase 3 at an earlier stage. The mechanisms by which bacteria initiate infections are probably multifactorial. Bacteria do not directly synthesise prostaglandins (Bennett & Elder 1992), but they do release phospholipases which may liberate arachidonic acid from intracellular lipid pools, thereby increasing synthesis of prostaglandins (Lamont et al 1985, 1990). It has been demonstrated that bacteria release a substance which increases prostaglandin synthesis in amnion cells. This effect is probably mediated by phospholipase release (Bennett et al 1990b).

Another important mechanism by which bacteria might activate inflammatory mediators within the uterus is by the action of endotoxin. Endotoxin, or lipopolysaccharide, is a component of the cell wall of Gram-negative bacteria which has been shown to stimulate prostaglandin in a variety of tissues. Romero et al found that early spontaneous labour with preterm premature rupture of membranes was more likely when endotoxin was detected (Romero et al 1987). Endotoxin stimulates synthesis of inflammatory cytokines including IL-1β, IL-6 and tumour necrosis factor (TNF) in amnion cells and in intact fetal membranes (Romero et al 1988). Endotoxins also inhibit release of PAF acylhydrolase, the enzyme which inactivates PAF, from decidual macrophages (Narahara & Johnston 1993).

Phase 3: post labour

The involution of the uterus is primarily mediated by oxytocin released in response to breast feeding. After the first pregnancy, the cervix and myometrium appear to undergo irreversible change, such that in subsequent pregnancy the speed and length of labour is significantly different. Labour is more rapid and of shorter duration in multiparous women. This is probably a reflection not only of anatomical changes, but also of changes in the sensitivity of gestation-associated tissues to prolabour factors.

A UNIFIED HYPOTHESIS OF THE ONSET OF LABOUR IN HUMANS

The extent to which each of these factors associated with the control of the length of human pregnancy and the onset of labour are linked is currently far from understood. The current hypothesis is that during the first parturitional phase the uterus is under strong progesterone repression. During the second phase, rising oestrogen and CRH concentrations activate proteins such as cell surface receptors and gap junctions which will be needed for labour itself. CRH also increases the expression of IL-1β and of COX-2. Labour arises because a relatively rapid increase in synthesis of inflammatory mediators and the consequent influx of inflammatory cells cause cervical ripening and stimulate uterine contractions. These inflammatory factors are all positively regulated by inflammation-associated transcription factors such as NFκB. It is probable that the transition from parturitional phase 2 to phase 3 occurs once a certain threshold of CRH, or of IL-1β stimulated by CRH, is reached but the fetus may also signal its maturity through release of PAF from the lungs which adds to the IL-1β-induced activation of the inflammatory factors. Once phase 3 is entered, there are multiple positive feedback mechanisms which accelerate the processes of labour, which only stops once delivery is complete.

KEY POINTS

- In some mammals, the simple changes in the balance between oestrogens (*prolabour*) and progesterone (*propregnancy*) initiate labour.
- This is not the case in humans. Progesterone is not reduced but probably overwhelmed by the *prolabour* factors, many of which are produced by the fetus.
- Fetal oestrogen levels and prostaglandin production from the membranes, together with maternal oxytocin production, are important *prolabour factors*.
- The interaction of these positive and inhibitory actions is not fully worked out in the human but an hypothesis is presented.

REFERENCES

Akerlund M, Hauksson A, Lundin S, Melin P, Trojanar J 1986 Vasotocin analogues which competitively inhibit vasopressin stimulated contractions in healthy women. Br J Obstet Gynaecol 93:22–24

Alvi SA, Rajasingam D, Brown NL, Elder MG, Bennett PR, Sullivan MH 1999 The production of interleukin-1beta from human fetal membranes is not obligatory for increased prostaglandin output. Immunology 97:249–256

Ammala M, Nyman T, Salmi A, Rutanen EM 1997 The interleukin-1 system in gestational tissues at term: effect of labour. Placenta 18:717–723

Anwer K, Hovington JA, Sanborn BM 1989 Antagonism of contractants and relaxants at the level of intracellular calcium and phosphoinositide turnover in the rat uterus. Endocrinology 124:2995–3002

Arici A, MacDonald PC, Casey ML 1996 Modulation of the levels of interleukin-8 messenger ribonucleic acid and interleukin-8 protein synthesis in human endometrial stromal cells by transforming growth factor-beta 1. J Clin Endocrinol Metab 81:3004–3009

Awad SS, Lamb HK, Morgan JM, Dunlop W, Gillespie JI 1997 Differential expression of ryanodine receptor RyR2 mRNA in the non-pregnant and pregnant human myometrium. Biochem J 322:777–783

Bansal RK, Goldsmith PC, He Y, Zaloudek CJ, Ecker JL, Riemer RK 1997 A decline in myometrial nitric oxide synthase expression is associated with labor and delivery. J Clin Invest 99:2502–2508

Barclay CG, Brennand JE, Kelly RW, Calder AA 1993 Interleukin-8 production by the human cervix. Am J Obstet Gynecol 169:625–632

Bartlett SR, Bennett PR, Campa JS et al 1999 Expression of nitric oxide synthase isoforms in pregnant human myometrium. J Physiol 521:705–716

Bennett PR, Elder MG 1992 The mechanisms of preterm labor: common genital tract pathogens do not metabolize arachidonic acid to prostaglandins or to other eicosanoids. Am J Obstet Gynecol 166:1541–1545

Bennett PR, Elder MG, Myatt L 1987 The effects of lipoxygenase metabolites of arachidonic acid on human myometrial contractility. Prostaglandins 33:837–844

Bennett PR, Chamberlain GVP, Patel L, Elder MC, Myatt L 1990a Mechanisms of parturition: the transfer of prostaglandin E2 and 5-HETE across fetal membranes. Am J Obstet Gynecol 162:683–687

Bennett PR, Elder MG, Myatt L 1990b Secretion of phospholipases by bacterial pathogens may initiate preterm labor [letter]. Am J Obstet Gynecol 163:241–242

Bennett PR, Slater D, Sullivan M, Elder MG, Moore GE 1993 Changes in amniotic fluid arachidonic acid metabolism associated with increased cyclo-oxygenase gene expression. Br J Obstet Gynaecol 100:1037–1042

Bottari SP, Vokaer A, Kaivez E, Lescrainier JP, Vauquelin GP 1983 Differential regulation of alpha-adrenergic receptor subclasses by gonadal steroids in human myometrium. J Clin Endocrinol Metab 57:937–941

Brennand JE, Calder AA, Leitch CR, Greer IA, Chou MM, MacKenzie IZ 1997 Recombinant human relaxin as a cervical ripening agent. Br J Obstet Gynaecol 104:775–780

Bry K, Hallman M 1993 Transforming growth factor-beta 2 prevents preterm delivery induced by interleukin-1 alpha and tumor necrosis factor-alpha in the rabbit. Am J Obstet Gynecol 168:1318–1322

Bryant-Greenwood GD, Rees MC, Turnbull AC 1987 Immunohistochemical localisation of relaxin, prolactin and prostaglandin synthase in human amnion, chorion and decidua. J Endocrinol 114:491–496

Buhimschi I, Yallampalli C, Dong YL, Garfield RE 1995 Involvement of a nitric oxide-cyclic guanosine monophosphate pathway in control of human uterine contractility during pregnancy. Am J Obstet Gynecol 172:1577–1584

Bulbring E, Tomita T 1987 Catecholamine action on smooth muscle. Pharmacol Rev 39:49–96

Buster JE, Chang RJ, Preston DL et al 1979 Interrelationships of circulating maternal steroid concentrations in third trimester pregnancies. I. C21 steroids: progesterone, 16 alpha-hydroxyprogesterone, 17 alpha-hydroxyprogesterone, 20 alpha-dihydroprogesterone, delta 5-pregnenolone, delta 5-pregnenolone sulfate, and 17-hydroxy delta 5-pregnenolone. J Clin Endocrinol Metab 48:133–138

Calder AA 1994 Prostaglandins and biological control of cervical function. Aust NZJ Obstet Gynaecol 34:347–351

Calder AA, Greer IA 1992 Prostaglandins and the cervix. Baillieres Clin Obstet Gynaecol 6:771–786

Challis JR, Brooks AN 1989 Maturation and activation of hypothalamic-pituitary adrenal function in fetal sheep. Endocrine Rev 10:182–204

Challis JRG, Riley SC, Yang K 1991 Endocrinology of labour. Fetal Med Rev 3:47–66

Challis JR, Matthews SG, Van Meir C, Ramirez MM 1995 Current topic: the placental corticotrophin-releasing hormone–adrenocorticotrophin axis. Placenta 16:481–502

Chan KK, Robinson G, Pipkin FB 1997 Differential sensitivity of human nonpregnant and pregnant myometrium to calcitonin gene-related peptide. J Soc Gynecol Invest 4:15–21

Chen R, Lewis K, Perrin MH, Vale WW 1993 Expression cloning of a human corticotropin releasing factor receptor. Proc Nat Acad Sci USA 90:8967–8989

Conrad JT, Ueland K 1976 Reduction in the stretch modulus of human cervical tissue by prostaglandin E2. Am J Obstet Gynecol 126:218–223

Critchley HO, Kelly RW, Lea RG, Drudy TA, Jones RL, Baird DT 1996 Sex steroid regulation of leukocyte traffic in human decidua. Hum Reprod 11:2257–2262

Dayes BA, Lye SJ 1990 Characterization of myometrial desensitization to beta-adrenergic agonists. Can J Physiol Pharmacol 68:1377–1384

Dennes WJ, Slater DM, Poston L, Bennett PR 1999 Myometrial nitric oxide synthase messenger ribonucleic acid expression does not change throughout gestation or with the onset of labor. Am J Obstet Gynecol 180:387–392

DeWitt DL, Smith WL 1988 Primary structure of prostaglandin G/H synthase from sheep vesicular gland determined from the complimentary DNA sequence. Proc Nat Acad Sci USA 85:1412–1417

Dokhac L, LeStunff H, Naze S, Harbon S 1995 ETA receptors mediate activation of phospholipases C and D in rat myometrium. J Cardiovasc Pharmacol 26 (suppl 3):S307–S309

Dong YL, Fang L, Kondapaka S, Gangula PR, Wimalawansa SJ, Yallampalli C 1999 Involvement of calcitonin gene-related peptide in the modulation of human myometrial contractility during pregnancy. J Clin Invest 104:559–565

Downing SJ, Sherwood OD 1985 The physiological role of relaxin in the pregnant rat. 1. The influence of relaxin on parturition. Endocrinology 116:1200–1205

Downing SJ, Hollingsworth M 1993 Action of relaxin on uterine contractions—a review. J Reprod Fertil 99:275–282

Downing SJ, McIlwrath A, Hollingsworth M 1992 Cyclic adenosine 3′5′-monophosphate and the relaxant action of relaxin in the rat uterus in vivo. J Reprod Fertil 96:857–863

Dyal R, Crankshaw DJ 1988 The effects of some synthetic prostanoids on the contractility of the human lower uterine segment in vitro. Am J Obstet Gynecol 158:281–285

Eddie LW, Cameron IT, Leeton JF, Healy DL, Renou P 1990 Ovarian relaxin is not essential for dilatation of the cervix. Lancet 2:243

Ekerhovd E, Weidegard B, Brannstrom M, Norstrom A 1999 Nitric oxide-mediated effects on myometrial contractility at term during prelabor and labor. Obstet Gynecol 93:987–994

Elliott CL, Brennand JE, Calder AA 1998 The effects of mifepristone on cervical ripening and labor induction in primigravidae. Obstet Gynecol 92:804–809

El Maradny E, Kanayama N, Halim A, Maehara K, Sumimoto K, Terao T 1996 Biochemical changes in the cervical tissue of rabbit induced by interleukin-8, interleukin-1beta, dehydroepiandrosterone sulphate and prostaglandin E2: a comparative study. Hum Reprod 11:1099–1104

Ferguson JE II, Gorman JV, Bruns DE, Weir EC, Burtis WJ, Martin TJ, Bruns ME 1992 Abundant expression of parathyroid hormone-related protein in human amnion and its association with labor. Proc Nat Acad Sci USA 89:8384–8388

Flint APF, Anderson ABM, Steele PA, Turnbull AC 1975 The mechanism by which fetal cortisol controls the onset of parturition in the sheep. Biochem Soc Trans 3:1189–1194

Fortunato SJ, Menon R, Lombardi SJ 1997 Interleukin-10 and transforming growth factor-beta inhibit amniochorion tumor necrosis factor-alpha production by contrasting mechanisms of action: therapeutic implications in prematurity. Am J Obstet Gynecol 177:803–809

Fuchs AR, Husslein P, Fuchs F 1981 Oxytocin and the initiation of human parturition II. Stimulation of prostaglandin production in human decidual cells by oxytocin. Am J Obstet Gynecol 141:694–698

Fuchs AR, Periyasamy S, Alexandrova M, Soloff MS 1983 Correlation between oxytocin receptor concentration and responsiveness to oxytocin in pregnant rat myometrium: effects of ovarian steroids. Endocrinology 113:742–749

Fuchs AR, Fuchs F, Husslein P, Soloff MS 1984 Oxytocin receptors in pregnant human uterus. Am J Obstet Gynecol 150:734–741

Garfield RE, Hertzberg EL 1990 Cell-to-cell coupling in the myometrium: Emil Bozler's prediction. Prog Clin Biol Res 327:673–681

Garibay-Tupas JL, Maaskant RA, Greenwood FC, Bryant-Greenwood GD 1995 Characteristics of the binding of 32P-labelled human relaxins to the human fetal membranes. J Endocrinol 145:441–448

Gibb W 1998 The role of prostaglandins in human parturition. Ann Med 30:235–241

Ginsburg FW, Rosenberg CR, Schwartz M, Colon JM, Goldsmith LT 1988 The effect of relaxin on calcium fluxes in the rat uterus. Am J Obstet Gynecol 159:1395–1401

Goldsmith LT, Skurnick JH, Wojtczuk AS, Linden M, Kuhar MJ, Weiss G 1989 The antagonistic effect of oxytocin and relaxin on rat uterine segment contractility. Am J Obstet Gynecol 161:1644–1649

Goodwin TM 1999 A role for estriol in human labor, term and preterm. Am J Obstet Gynecol 180:S208–S213

Goodwin TM, Paul R, Silver H 1994 The effect of the oxytocin anatagonist atosiban on preterm uterine activity in the human. Am J Obstet Gynecol 170:474–478

Grammatopoulos D, Thompson S, Hillhouse EW 1995 The human myometrium expresses multiple isoforms of the corticotropin-releasing hormone receptor. J Clin Endocrinol Metab 80:2388–2393

Grammatopoulos D, Stirrat GM, Williams SA, Hillhouse EW 1996 The biological activity of the corticotropin-releasing hormone receptor–adenylate cyclase complex in human myometrium is reduced at the end of pregnancy. J Clin Endocrinol Metab 81:745–751

Granstrom LM, Ekman GE, Malmstrom A, Ulmsten U, Woessner JF Jr 1992 Serum collagenase levels in relation to the state of the human cervix during pregnancy and labor. Am J Obstet Gynecol 167:1284–1288

Grazzini E, Guillon G, Mouillac B, Zingg HH 1998 Inhibition of oxytocin receptor function by direct progesterone binding. Nature 392:509–512

Haluska GJ, Stanczyk FZ, Cook MJ, Novy MJ 1987 Temporal changes in uterine activity and prostaglandin response to RU486 in rhesus macaques in late gestation. Am J Obstet Gynecol 157:1487–1495

Hirst JJ, Teixeira FJ, Zakar T, Olson DM 1995 Prostaglandin endoperoxide-H synthase-1 and -2 messenger ribonucleic acid levels in human amnion with spontaneous labor onset. J Clin Endocrinol Metab 80:517–523

Hisaw FL, Hisaw FL 1964 Effect of relaxin on the uterus of monkeys (macaca mulatta) with observations on the cervix and symphysis pubis. Am J Obstet Gynecol 89:141–151

Hla T, Farrell M, Kumar A, Bailey JM 1986 Isolation of the cDNA for human prostaglandin H synthase. Prostaglandins 32:829–845

Hla T, Neilson K 1992 Human cyclooxygenase-2 cDNA. Proc Nat Acad Sc USA 89:7384–7388

Hirst JJ, Haluska GJ, Cook MJ, Novy MJ 1993 Plasma oxytocin and nocturnal uterine activity: maternal, but not fetal concentrations increase progressively during late pregnancy and delivery in rhesus monkey. Am J Obstet Gynecol 169:414–422

Hochman J, Weiss G, Steinetz BG, O'Byrne EM 1978 Serum relaxin concentrations in prostaglandin- and oxytocin-induced labor in women. Am J Obstet Gynecol 130:473–474

Hoffman DR, Romero R, Johnston JM 1990 Detection of platelet activating factor in amniotic fluid of complicated pregnancies. Am J Obstet Gynecol 162:525–531

Ito A, Nageneo K, Mori Y, Hirakawa S, Hayashi M 1977 PZ-peptidase activity in human uterine cervix during pregnancy at term. Clin Chim Acta 78:267–270

Ito A, Mori Y, Hirakawa S 1979 Purification and characterisation of an acid proteinase from human uterine cervix. Chem Pharm Bull (Tokyo) 27:969–973

Ivell R, Walther N 1999 The role of sex steroids in the oxytocin hormone system. Mol Cell Endocrinol 151:95–101

Jenkin G, Thorburn GD 1985 Inhibition of progesterone secretion by a 3 beta-hydroxysteroid dehydrogenase inhibitor in late pregnant sheep. Can J Physiol Pharmacol 63:136–142

Johnson MR, Abdalla H, Allman ACJ, Wren ME, Kirkland A, Lightman SL 1991 Relaxin levels in ovum donation pregnancies. Fertil Steril 56:59–61

Jones GD, Poston L 1997 The role of endogenous nitric oxide synthesis in contractility of term or preterm human myometrium. Br J Obstet Gynaecol 104:241–245

Jones SA, Challis JR 1990 Effects of corticotropin-releasing hormone and adrenocorticotropin on prostaglandin output by human placenta and fetal membranes. Gynecol Obstet Invest 29:165–168

Jones SA, Summerlee AJS 1986 Relaxin acts centrally to inhibit oxytocin release during parturition: an effect that is reversed by naloxone. J Endocrinol 111:99–102

Jones SA, Brooks AN, Challis JR 1989 Steroids modulate corticotropin-releasing hormone production in human fetal membranes and placenta. J Clin Endocrinol Metab 68:825–830

Junqueira LC, Zugaib M, Montes GS, Toledo OM, Krisztan RM, Shigihara KM 1980 Morphologic and histochemical evidence for the occurrence of collagenolysis and for the role of neutrophilic polymorphonuclear leukocytes during cervical dilation. Am J Obstet Gynecol 138:273–281

Kalkhoven E, Wissink S, van der Saag PT, van der Burg B 1996 Negative interaction between the RelA(p65) subunit of NF-kappaB and the progesterone receptor. J Biol Chem 271:6217–6224

Karalis K, Goodwin G, Majzoub JA 1996 Cortisol blockade of progesterone: A possible molecular mechanism involved in the initiation of human labour. Nat Med 2:556–560

Kaya T, Cetin A, Cetin M, Sarioglu Y 1998 Effect of endothelin-1 on spontaneous contractions and effects of nimodipine and isradipine on endothelin-1-induced contractions in myometrial strips isolated from normal pregnant and preeclamptic women. Acta Obstet Gynecol Scand 77:961–966

Kelly RW, Leask R, Calder AA 1992 Choriodecidual production of interleukin-8 and mechanism of parturition. Lancet 339:776–777

Kemp BE, Niall HD 1984 Relaxin. Vitam Horm 41:79–115

Kitamura K, Ito A, Mori Y 1980 The existing forms of collagenase in the human uterine cervix. J Biochem (Tokyo) 87:753–760

Kumar D, Zourlas PA et al 1965 In vivo effect of amyl nitrite on human pregnant uterine contractility. Am J Obstet Gynecol 91:1066–1068

Lamont RF, Rose M, Elder MG 1985 Effect of bacterial products on prostaglandin E production by amnion cells. Lancet 2:1331–1333

Lamont RF, Anthony F, Myatt L, Booth L, Furr PM, Taylor-Robinson D 1990 Production of prostaglandin E2 by human amnion in vitro in response to addition of media conditioned by microorganisms associated with chorioamnionitis and preterm labor. Am J Obstet Gynecol 162:819–825

Lecrivain JL, Cohen-Tannoudji J, Robin MT, Coudouel N, Legrand C, Maltier JP 1998 Molecular mechanisms of adenylyl cyclase desensitization in pregnant rat myometrium following in vivo administration of the beta-adrenergic agonist, isoproterenol. Biol Reprod 59:45–52

Lees CC, Lojacono A, Thompson et al 1999 Glyceryl trinitrate and ritodrine in tocolysis: an international multicenter randomized study. GTN Preterm Labour Investigation Group. Obstet Gynecol 94:403–408

Li J, Lu H 1995 The studies of the estrogen and progesterone receptor levels in the placenta, fetal membrane, uteroplacental bed and myometrium in patients with prolonged pregnancy. Chung Hua Fu Chan Ko Tsa Chih 30:536–538

Liaw CW, Lovenberg TW, Barry G, Oltersdorf T, Grigoriadis DE, de Souza EB 1996 Cloning and characterisation of the human corticotrophin releasing hormone 2 receptor cDNA. Endocrinology 137:72–77

Liggins GC 1969 Premature delivery of foetal lambs infused with glucocorticoids. J Endocrinol 45:515–523

Liggins GC 1978 Ripening of the cervix. Semin Perinatol 2:261–271

Liggins GC, Kennedy PC, Holm LW 1967 Failure of initiation of parturition after electrocoagulation of the pituitary of the fetal lamb. Am J Obstet Gynecol 98:1080–1086

Liggins GC, Fairclough RJ, Grieves SA, Forster CS, Knox BS 1977 Parturition in the sheep. In: Knight J, O'Connor M (eds) The fetus and birth. Elsevier/Excerpta Medica/North Holland, Amsterdam, pp 5–25

Longo M, Jain V, Vedernikov YP, Saade GR, Goodrum L, Facchinetti F, Garfield RE 1999 Effect of nitric oxide and carbon monoxide on uterine contractility during human and rat pregnancy. Am J Obstet Gynecol 181:981–988

López Bernal A, Bryant-Greenwood GD, Hansell DJ, Hicks BR, Greenwood FC, Turnbull AC 1987 Effect of relaxin on prostaglandin E production by human amnion: changes in relation to the onset of labour. Br J Obstet Gynaecol 94:1045–1051

Lye S 1994 The initiation and inhibition of labour—toward a molecular understanding. Semin Reprod Endocrinol 12:284–294

McGarrigle HH, Lachelin GC 1984 Increasing saliva (free) oestriol to progesterone ratio in late pregnancy: a role for oestriol in initiating spontaneous labour in man? BMJ 289:457–459

McLean M, Bisits A, Davies J, Woods R, Lowry P, Smith R 1995 A placental clock controlling the length of human pregnancy. Nat Med 1:460–436

Maggi M, Magini A, Fiscella A et al 1992 Sex steroid modulation of neurohypophysial hormone receptors in human nonpregnant myometrium. J Clin Endocrinol Metab 74:385–392

Maradny EE, Kanayama N, Halim A, Maehara K, Sumimoto K, Terao T 1995 Effects of neutrophil chemotactic factors on cervical ripening. Clin Exp Obstet Gynecol 22:76–85

Mason JI, France JT, Magness RR, Murry BA, Rosenfeld CR 1989 Ovine placental steroid 17 alpha-hydroxylase/C-17,20-lyase, aromatase and sulphatase in dexamethasone-induced and natural parturition. J Endocrinol 122:351–359

Mecenas CA, Giussani DA, Owiny JR et al 1996 Production of premature delivery in pregnant rhesus monkeys by androstenedione infusion. Nat Med 2:443–448

Miller FD, Chibbar R, Mitchell BF 1993 Synthesis of oxytocin in amnion, chorion and decidua: a potential paracrine role for oxytocin in the onset of human parturition. Regul Pept 45:247–251

Mitchell BF, Wong S 1993 Changes in 17 beta,20 alpha-hydroxysteroid dehydrogenase activity supporting an increase in the estrogen/progesterone ratio of human fetal membranes at parturition. Am J Obstet Gynecol 168:1377–1385

Mitchell MD, Hunter C, Dudley DJ, Varner MW 1996 Significant decrease in parathyroid hormone-related protein concentrations in amniotic fluid with labour at term but not preterm. Reprod Fertil Dev 8:231–234

Mochizuki M, Tojo S 1980 Hormonal aspects of cervical compliance. In: Natftolin F, Stubblefield PG (eds) Dilatation of the cervix. Raven Press, New York, pp 267–290

Moore JJ, Moore RM, Vander Kooy D 1988 Protein kinase C activation is required for oxytocin induced prostaglandin production in human amnion cells. J Endocrinol 72:1073–1080

Moya FR, Hoffman DR, Zhao B, Johnston JM 1993 Platelet-activating factor in surfactant preparations. Lancet 341:858–860

Murota S, Abe M, Otsuka K 1977 Stimulative effect of prostaglandins on the production of hexosamine-containing substances by cultured fibroblasts (3) induction of hyaluronic acid synthetase by prostaglandin F2α. Prostaglandins 14:983–991

Nackla S, Skinner K, Mitchell BF, Challis JRG 1986 Changes in prostaglandin transfer across human fetal membranes following spontaneous labour. Am J Obstet Gynecol 155:1337–1341

Narahara H, Johnston JM 1993 Effects of endotoxins and cytokines on the secretion of platelet-activating factor-acetylhydrolase by human decidual macrophages. Am J Obstet Gynecol 169:531–537

Natuzzi ES, Ursell PC, Harrison M, Buscher C, Riemer RK 1993 Nitric oxide synthase activity in the pregnant uterus decreases at parturition. Biochem Biophys Res Commun 194:1–8

O'Banion MK, Sadowski HB, Winn W, Young DA 1991 A serum and glucocorticoid regulated 4 kb mRNA encodes a cyclo-oxygenase related protein. J Biol Chem 266:23261–23266

O'Byrne KT, Eltringham L, Clarke G, Summerlee AJS 1986 Effects of porcine relaxin on oxytocin release from the neurohypophysis in the anaesthetised lactating rat. J Endocrinol 109:393–397

Olson DM, Skinner K, Challis JR 1983 Estradiol-17 beta and 2-hydroxyestradiol-17 beta-induced differential production of prostaglandins by cells dispersed from human intrauterine tissues at parturition. Prostaglandins 25:639–651

Osheroff PL, King KL 1995 Binding and cross-linking of 32P-labeled human relaxin to human uterine cells and primary rat atrial cardiomyocytes. Endocrinology 136:4377–4381

Osmers RG, Adelmann-Grill BC, Rath W, Stuhlsatz HW, Tschesche H, Kuhn W 1995a Biochemical events in cervical ripening dilatation during pregnancy and parturition. J Obstet Gynaecol 21:185–194

Osmers RG, Blaser J, Kuhn W, Tschesche H 1995b Interleukin-8 synthesis and the onset of labor. Obstet Gynecol 86:223–229

Ou CW, Chen ZQ, Qi S, Lye SJ 1998 Increased expression of the rat myometrial oxytocin receptor messenger ribonucleic acid during labor requires both mechanical and hormonal signals. Biol Reprod 59:1055–1061

Parry LJ, Bathgate RA, Shaw G, Renfree MB, Ivell R 1997 Evidence for a local fetal influence on myometrial oxytocin receptors during pregnancy in the tammar wallaby (Macropus eugenii). Biol Reprod 56:200–207

Patel FA, Clifton VL, Chwalisz K, Challis JR 1999 Steroid regulation of prostaglandin dehydrogenase activity and expression in human term placenta and chorio-decidua in relation to labor. J Clin Endocrinol Metab 84:291–299

Peng AT, Gorman RS, Shulman SM, DeMarchis E, Nyunt K, Blancato LS 1989 Intravenous nitroglycerin for uterine relaxation in the postpartum patient with retained placenta. Anesthesiology 71:172–173

Petersen LK, Svane D, Uldbjerg N, Forman A 1991 Effects of human relaxin on isolated rat and human myometrium and uteroplacental arteries. Obstet Gynecol 78:757–762

Petraglia F, Benedetto C, Florio P, D'Ambrogio G, Genazzani AD, Marozio L, Vale W 1995 Effect of corticotropin-releasing factor-binding protein on prostaglandin release from cultured maternal decidua and on contractile activity of human myometrium in vitro. J Clin Endocrinol Metab 80:3073–3076

Pitera AE, Smith GC, Wentworth RA, Nathanielsz PW 1998 Parathyroid hormone-related peptide (1 to 34) inhibits in vitro oxytocin-stimulated activity of pregnant baboon myometrium. Am J Obstet Gynecol 179:492–496

Porter DG, Downing SJ, Bradshaw JMC 1979. Relaxin inhibits spontaneous and prostaglandin-induced myometrial activity in anaesthetized rats. J Endocrinol 83:183–192

Rajasingam D, Bennett PR, Alvi SA, Elder MG, Sullivan MH 1998 Stimulation of prostaglandin production from intact human fetal membranes by bacteria and bacterial products. Placenta 19:301–306

Richard S, Zingg HH 1990 The human oxytocin gene promoter is regulated by estrogens. J Biol Chem 265:6098–6103

Rodriguez-Linares B, Phaneuf S, Lopez Bernal A, Linton EA 1998 Levels of corticotrophin-releasing hormone receptor subtype 1 mRNA in pregnancy and during labour in human myometrium measured by quantitative competitive PCR. J Mol Endocrinol 21:201–208

Romero R, Kadar N, Hobbins JC, Duff GW 1987 Infection and labor: the detection of endotoxin in amniotic fluid. Am J Obstet Gynecol 157:815–819

Romero R, Hobbins JC, Mitchell MD 1988 Endotoxin stimulates

prostaglandin E2 production by human amnion. Obstet Gynecol 71:227–228

Romero R, Durum S, Dinarello CA, Oyarzun E, Hobbins JC, Mitchell MD 1989 Interleukin-1 stimulates prostaglandin biosynthesis by human amnion. Prostaglandins 37:13–22

Romero R, Parvizi ST, Oyarzun E, Mazor M, Wu YK, Avila C, Athanassiadis AP, Mitchell MD 1990 Amniotic fluid interleukin-1 in spontaneous labor at term. J Reprod Med 35:235–238

Romero R, Mazor M, Brandt F, Sepulveda W, Avila C, Cotton DB, Dinarello CA 1992 Interleukin-1 alpha and interleukin-1 beta in preterm and term human parturition. Am J Reprod Immunol 27:117–123

Rorie DK, Newton M 1967 Histologic and chemical studies of the human cervix and uterus. Am J Obstet Gynecol 99:466–469

Roseblade CK, Sullivan MF, Khan F, Lumb MR, Elder MG 1990 Limited transfer of prostaglandin E2 across fetal membranes before and after labour. Acta Obstet Gynecol Scand 69:399–403

Saeed SA, Mitchell MD 1983 Conversion of arachidonic acid to lipoxygenase products by human fetal tissues. Biochem Med 30:322–327

Samuelson UE, Dalsgaard CJ, Lundberg JM, Hokfelt T 1985 Calcitonin gene-related peptide inhibits spontaneous contractions in human uterus and fallopian tube. Neuroscience Lett 62:225–230

Sanborn BM, Kuo HS, Weisbrodt NW, Sherwood OD 1980 The interaction of relaxin with the rat uterus. I. Effect on cyclic nucleotide levels and spontaneous contractile activity. Endocrinology 106:1210–1215

Sangha RK, Walton JC, Ensor CM, Tai HH, Challis JR 1994 Immunohistochemical localization, messenger ribonucleic acid abundance, and activity of 15-hydroxyprostaglandin dehydrogenase in placenta and fetal membranes during term and preterm labor. J Clin Endocrinol Metab 78:982–989

Sawdy RJ, Slater DM, Dennes WJ, Sullivan MH, Bennett PR 2000 The roles of the cyclo-oxygenases types one and two in prostaglandin synthesis in human fetal membranes at term. Placenta 21:54–57

Seki K, Uesato T, Kato K 1987 Serum relaxin concentrations in women following the administration of 16,16-dimethyl-trans-Δ2-prostaglandin-1 methyl ester during early pregnancy. Prostaglandins 33:739–742

Shew RL, Yee JA, Kliewer DB, Keflemariam YJ, McNeill DL 1991 Parathyroid hormone-related protein inhibits stimulated uterine contraction in vitro. J Bone Mineral Res 6:955–959

Shimonovitz S, Yagel S, Anteby E, Finci-Yeheskel Z, Adashi EY, Mayer M, Hurwitz A 1995 Interleukin-1 stimulates prostaglandin E production by human trophoblast cells from first and third trimesters. J Clin Endocrinol Metab 80:1641–1646

Skannal DG, Eis AL, Brockman D, Siddiqi TA, Myatt L 1997 Immunohistochemical localization of phospholipase A2 isoforms in human myometrium during pregnancy and parturition. Am J Obstet Gynecol 176:878–882

Skinner KA, Challis JR 1985 Changes in the synthesis and metabolism of prostaglandins by human fetal membranes and decidua at labor. Am J Obstet Gynecol 151:519–523

Sladek SM, Regenstein AC, Lykins D, Roberts JM 1993 Nitric oxide synthase activity in pregnant rabbit uterus decreases on the last day of pregnancy Am J Obstet Gynecol 169:1285–1291

Slater D, Berger L, Newton R, Moore GE, Bennett PR 1994 The relative abundance of type 1 to type 2 cyclo-oxygenase mRNA in human amnion at term. Biochem Biophys Res Commun 198:304–308

Slater DM, Berger LC, Newton R, Moore GE, Bennett PR 1995 Expression of cyclooxygenase types 1 and 2 in human fetal membranes at term. Am J Obstet Gynecol 172:77–82

Slater DM, Dennes WJ, Campa JS, Poston L, Bennett PR 1999 Expression of cyclo-oxygenase types-1 and -2 in human myometrium throughout pregnancy. Mol Hum Reprod 5:880–884

Szlachter N, O'Byrne E, Goldsmith L, Steinetz BG, Weiss G 1980 Myometrial inhibiting activity of relaxin-containing extracts of human corpora lutea of pregnancy. Am J Obstet Gynecol 136:584–586

Takahashi K, Diamond F, Bieniarz J, Yen H, Burd L 1980 Uterine contractility and oxytocin sensitivity in preterm, term and postterm pregnancy. Am J Obstet Gynecol 136:774–779

Takemura M, Kimura T, Nomura S et al 1994 Expression and localisation of human oxytocin receptor mRNA and its protein in chorion and decidua during parturition. J Clin Invest 93:2319–2323

Tangalakis K, Coghlan JP, Connell J et al 1989 Tissue distribution and levels of gene expression of three steroid hydroxylases in ovine fetal adrenal glands. Acta Endocrinol 120:225–232

Telfer JF, Lyall F, Norman JE, Cameron IT 1995 Identification of nitric oxide synthase in human uterus. Hum Reprod 10:19–23

Thomson AJ, Lunan CB, Cameron AD, Cameron IT, Greer IA, Norman JE 1997 Nitric oxide donors induce ripening of the human uterine cervix: a randomised controlled trial. Br J Obstet Gynaecol 104:1054–1057

Thomson AJ, Telfer JF, Young A et al 1999 Leukocytes infiltrate the myometrium during human parturition: further evidence that labour is an inflammatory process. Hum Reprod 14:229–236

Thornton S, Davison JM, Baylis PH 1992 Plasma oxytocin during the first and second stages of spontaneous human labour. *Acta Endocrinol (Copenh)* 126:425–429

Tromans PM, Beazely JM, Shronda PI 1981 Comparative study of oestradiol and prostaglandin E2 for ripening the unfavourable cervix before induction of labour. BMJ 88:679–681

Turnbull A 1977 The fetus and birth. Elsevier, London

Van Meir CA, Sangha RK, Walton JC, Matthews SG, Keirse MJ, Challis JR 1996 Immunoreactive 15-hydroxyprostaglandin dehydrogenase (PGDH) is reduced in fetal membranes from patients at preterm delivery in the presence of infection. Placenta 17:291–297

van Meir CA, Matthews SG, Keirse MJ, Ramirez MM, Bocking A, Challis JR 1997 15-hydroxyprostaglandin dehydrogenase:

implications in preterm labor with and without ascending infection. J Clin Endocrinol Metab 82:969–976

Vasicka A, Kumarsan P, Han GS, Kumaresan M 1977 Plasma oxytocin in initiation of labor. Am J Obstet Gynecol 130:263–273

Wahl LM, Olsen CE, Wahl SM, Sandberg AL, Mergenhagen SE 1979 Prostaglandin regulated macrophage collagenase. In: Horton JE (ed) Proceedings of mechanisms of localised bone loss. Special supplement to calcified tissue. Information Retrieval, New York, pp 181–190

Walsh SW 1989 5-Hydroxyeicosatetraenioc acid, leukotriene C4 and prostaglandin F2a in amniotic fluid before and during term and preterm labor. Am J Obstet Gynecol 161:1352

Way SA, Leng G 1992 Relaxin increases the firing rate of supraoptic neurones and increases oxytocin secretion in the rat. J Endocrinol 132:149–158

Wu WX, Bruns ME, Bruns D, Seaner R, Nathanielsz PW, Ferguson JE II 1998 Parathyroid hormone-related protein mRNA in sheep endometrium and myometrium during late gestation and labor. J Soc Gynecol Invest 5:127–131

Yallampalli C, Garfield RE 1994 Uterine contractile responses to endothelin-1 and endothelin receptors are elevated during labor. Biol Reprod 51:640–645

Yallampalli C, Izumi H, Byam-Smith M, Garfield RE 1994 An L-arginine-nitric oxide-cyclic guanosine monophosphate system exists in the uterus and inhibits contractility during pregnancy. Am J Obstet Gynecol 170.175–185

Yallampalli C, Gangula PR, Kondapaka S, Fang L, Wimalawansa S 1999 Regulation of calcitonin gene-related peptide receptors in the rat uterus during pregnancy and labor and by progesterone. Biol Reprod 61:1023–1030

Yusoff Dawood M, Raghavan KS, Pociask C, Fuchs F 1978 Oxytocin in human pregnancy and parturition. Obstet Gynecol 51:138–143

26

The mechanisms and management of normal labour

Philip J Steer

The contribution of the author of the equivalent chapter in the second edition, on which this chapter draws extensively, is gratefully acknowledged.

THE ONSET OF LABOUR

For evolutionary reasons, considered in Chapter 33, human childbirth is difficult. The human female pelvis is an uneasy compromise between the need for efficient walking and successful childbirth. The latter requires a wider pelvis than is ideal for running, which means that while women's performance in the marathon is gradually approaching that of men, they will always be slower at sprinting. The characteristic wiggle that many women exhibit while walking has even been proposed as a secondary sexual characteristic indicating fitness for reproduction.

Meanwhile, the fetus has its birthweight limited by maternal mechanisms, which include relatively short gestational length (Steer 1998a) and fetal growth restriction (Steer 1998b). The human fetus is born relatively immature, with a tendency to hypoglycaemia, hypothermia and respiratory distress due to immaturity of the lungs. There are a variety of mechanisms for the onset of labour, including spontaneous rupture of the membranes (SROM), silent dilatation of the cervix, and the onset of regular uterine contractions, which are often poorly synchronised. Preterm labour, with its associated high levels of neonatal mortality and morbidity, remains stubbornly high: 7% or more even in developed countries, and much higher in the developing world.

Even in otherwise healthy pregnancies, labour commences with SROM without contractions in 10–20% of labours. This is associated with an increased incidence of septic morbidity. While large prospective studies have shown that prompt induction of labour when women present at term with SROM results in a reduced level of maternal sepsis, increased maternal satisfaction (Hannah et al 1996), and less cost (Gafni et al 1997) than expectant management, the demand from women and midwives for so-called natural childbirth means that, in many cases, expectant management is still adopted. To conserve resources, women are even being encouraged to return home to await the spontaneous onset of labour. A recent study has confirmed that such a policy increases the subsequent need for maternal antibiotic therapy, subsequent delivery by caesarean section, and neonatal sepsis (Hannah et al 2000). In general therefore, there is much to commend a policy of induction of labour 6–12 hours after SROM, with either intravenous syntocinon or vaginal prostaglandin if the cervix is unripe (Tan & Hannah 2000). A recent prospective study of over 5000 women in six countries confirmed that women treated expectantly were more likely to feel negative about their subsequent labour, presumably because of its perceived protracted duration and increased need for intervention with antibiotics. Use of prostaglandins is associated with less need for analgesia and continuous fetal heart rate monitoring, but a higher incidence of chorioamnionitis (Tan & Hannah 2000), presumably because of a longer induction delivery interval. Known group B streptococcus carriers should always be induced promptly, and treated with intravenous penicillin (Hager 2000) or with erythromycin or clindamycin if allergic to penicillin.

Silent dilatation of the cervix can occur in a few women, especially those of a high parity, and this can result in babies being born before arrival (BBA). This carries a significant morbidity from trauma (the baby falling on the floor), hypothermia and inadequate resuscitation. Women at risk of this problem should be advised about coming into hospital promptly as soon as there is any sign of labour. Pre-emptive admission and even induction of labour by artificial rupture of membranes should be considered; oxytocics should be avoided as they can cause precipitate labour. Mothers should be advised that if the baby is born outside hospital and there is no qualified birth attendant, they should (a) make sure the baby does not fall on the floor, (b) keep it warm by wrapping it in a towel or clothing and (c) not interfere with the umbilical cord but allow spontaneous delivery of the placenta.

Keeping the baby warm by the mother cuddling it against her abdomen is a simple but effective manoeuvre.

Onset of contractions before the cervix is fully ripe is common, and a difficult clinical problem. It results in a prolonged latent phase of labour (Fig. 26.1), which can be up to 36 hours or more in some women. Not only is this demoralising for the woman, but it can lead to progressive fetal hypoxia, so careful fetal monitoring is necessary once uterine activity is established, even without progressive cervical dilatation. Some authorities have claimed that labour without cervical dilatation does not exist, but regular contractions reduce maternal placental bed blood flow and hence fetal oxygenation, whether or not labour is progressing. There is no clear advantage to augmenting labour in the latent phase, so the choice is usually between providing good analgesia, even if necessary with an epidural—after all, it can be removed again if progressive labour fails to become established and contractions cease — and fetal monitoring, or accelerating labour by artificial rupture of membranes and oxytocics if uterine activity subsequently proves to be poor. The latter approach can lead to failed induction, so the issues must be talked over fully with the woman and when possible, her partner, for a woman's recall of such discussions is often poor after a long labour; any decisions must be carefully recorded in the notes. Some women prefer to await nature's resolution of the problem, while others prefer to get on with it. Given that there is no clear clinical advantage to either policy, her preference should be the deciding factor.

THE MECHANISM OF LABOUR

Humans have a large brain and, therefore, a large head. The head is egg-shaped in cross-section, for aerodynamic reasons and to facilitate binocular vision (Fig. 26.2). Its largest transverse diameter is anteroposterior. In contrast, the shoulders are widest from side to side. It follows that the mother's pelvis, which is adapted to be as narrow as possible while still allowing birth, must have diameters that reflect this fetal asymmetry. The presence of the mother's legs either side of the pelvic outlet inevitably means that its side-to-side diameter is limited; its greatest diameter is anteroposterior (Fig. 26.3). The inlet must have its widest diameter from side to side therefore (Fig. 26.4), despite the disadvantage this confers to maternal ambulation, to allow the passage of the shoulders when the

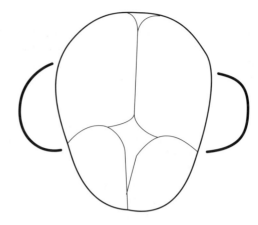

Fig. 26.2 Plan view of the human fetus, illustrating that the widest diameter of the fetal head is anteroposterior, whereas the shoulders are widest from side to side.

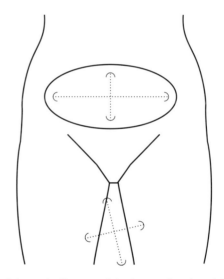

Fig. 26.3 Schematic diagram of the human female pelvis and legs, illustrating that the widest diameter of the pelvic inlet is from side to side, whereas the available space at the outlet is restricted laterally by the presence of the legs.

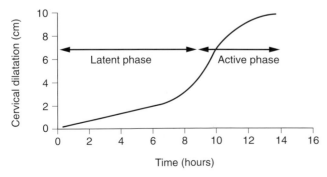

Fig. 26.1 The phases of labour.

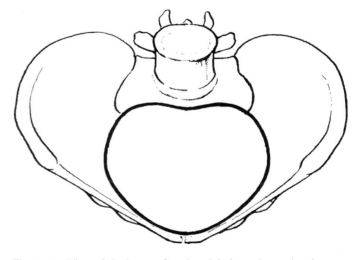

Fig. 26.4 View of the human female pelvis from above, showing pelvic inlet in heavy line.

head rotates into the occipito anterior position in order to emerge from the outlet. The inlet is heart shaped, with the fetal head engaging in the transverse or occipito-anterior (most commonly on the left side because of the presence of the maternal sigmoid colon posteriorly; Fig. 26.5).

Because the fetal head at term is at the limits of size that can pass through the maternal pelvis, moulding is necessary in many labours before the head can fit (Ch. 33). This means that in many pregnancies, engagement of the head does not occur until the onset of regular uterine contractions (Fig. 26.6). This is in fact the norm in most first pregnancies, and in most pregnancies in African women, because of the angle of the pelvic brim being almost parallel with the spine in this ethnic group (Fig. 26.7 shows the angle in White European women). Engagement occurs when there are contractions strong enough to push the fetus down into the pelvis, the fetus can move and flex into the right position, and sufficient

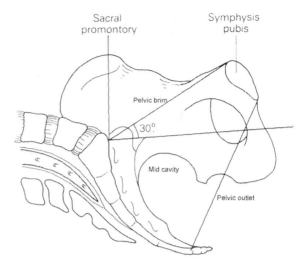

Fig. 26.7 Diagram of the human female pelvis, showing that the plane of the inlet is only 30° from being parallel with the spine.

moulding has occurred. The tight fit in the pelvis, and the moulding usually required, are shown in Figure 26.8. A summary of this mechanism is shown in Figure 26.9.

DURATION OF THE FIRST AND SECOND STAGES OF LABOUR

Because it is often difficult to define the onset of the first stage of labour, the measurement of its duration presents problems. It clearly ends with the delivery of the baby, but where does it begin? Is it when the mother first feels regular painful contractions? Most mothers think so, which is why in so many cases she will tell you that her labour lasted almost two days, when the obstetric record says eight hours. However, probably the only secure obstetric definition is progressive dilatation of the cervix, which means at least two vaginal assessments. The definition can, therefore, only be made securely at the time of the second assessment, although it

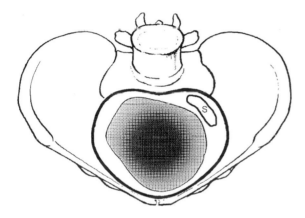

Fig. 26.5 View of the human female pelvis from above, showing the fetal head in a favourable position for engaging. S is the sigmoid colon; its presence favours engagement as occipito lateral or left occipito lateral, rather than right occipito lateral.

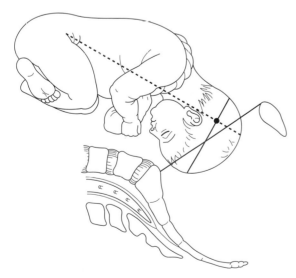

Fig. 26.6 Illustration of the fetal head entering the pelvis , but not yet engaged. The transection of the long axis of the fetus with the suboccipitobregmatic diameter indicates the level of the widest part of the fetal head, the biparietal diameter.

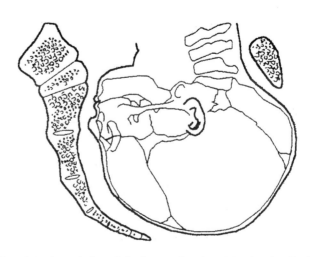

Fig. 26.8 Lateral view of the human female pelvis, showing the fetal head deeply engaged, with the vertex emerging at the introitus.

433

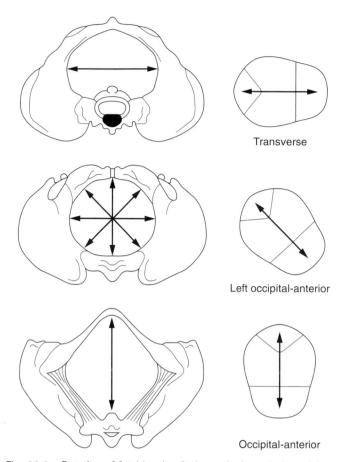

Fig. 26.9 Rotation of fetal head as it descends through the pelvis. The maximum diameter of the head matches that of the pelvis at each level (maximum diameter are indicated by an arrow).

Transverse

Left occipital-anterior

Occipital-anterior

regard the woman as being in labour. It is important to appreciate these uncertainties, as otherwise conflict can arise between the birth attendant and the woman herself as to whether she is in labour. A woman who has been unable to sleep for two days because of painful contractions does not appreciate being told she is not in labour, even if she does not meet the strict obstetric criteria.

The next problem in giving summary measures is that the durations of both the first and second stages of labour are not distributed in a Gaussian manner. Figures 26.10 and 26.11 give the distributions of the durations of first and second stages of labour for first and second labours from the St Mary's Maternity Information System database over 400 000 women in North West Thames (data analysed for 1988–1998 inclusive, singletons only). For first labours (n = 173 776), the mean duration of the first stage was 8.5 hours, the median (50% above and below) 8 hours, and the mode (most common value) only 6 hours. This decreases to 5.1 hours, 4 hours

may retrospectively be projected back to the first examination. The purpose of having such a stringent definition is to avoid inadvertent induction of labour. However, if at the first assessment the cervix is at least 4 cm dilated, with regular contractions, or there are regular contractions with ruptured

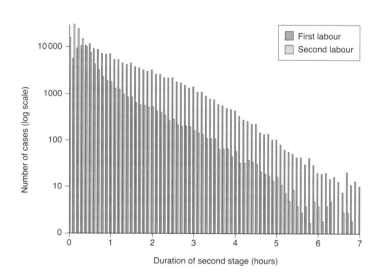

Fig. 26.11 Effect of partiy on the second stage of labour.

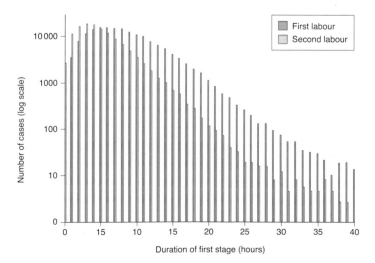

Fig. 26.10 Effect of parity on the duration of the first stage of labour.

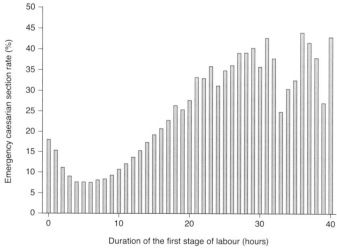

Fig. 26.12 Caesarean section rate in first labours, by duration of labour.

and 3 hours respectively for second labours (n = 156 757). Consequently, there is no simple answer to the question 'How long is my labour likely to be?' The same holds true for the second stage of labour, for which the summary measures were (first labours) 1.3, 0.9 and 0.5 hours and (second labours) 0.4, 0.2 and 0.1 hours. The log scale used emphasises clearly the long tail of the distribution of duration.

Is there a duration of labour that is normal? There is no clear discontinuity in the duration of labour that would enable one to define such a labour statistically. What is the likelihood of caesarean section? Is there a duration at which the likelihood is so high that there is no point in continuing the labour? Figure 26.12 shows that the lowest likelihood of caesarean section is at 4–6 hours. The likelihood in the first few hours is higher, because that is when babies that cannot tolerate labour (e.g. growth restricted fetuses) are often recognised and delivered. However, there is no subsequent time, even up to 40 hours or beyond, when the likelihood of caesarean section exceeds 50%. Therefore, the odds are always in favour of continuing if the mother wishes to try for a vaginal birth, so long as maternal and fetal condition are satisfactory.

But perhaps fetal condition deteriorates, and there is a point at which it is unwise to continue, because the baby is likely to be compromised. Figure 26.13 shows that a seriously low five minute Apgar score (three or less) is most likely in the first hour of labour. By five hours, the incidence of such a low score falls to less than one in 400, and remains at this low level for the next 11 hours. It is not until after more than 24 hours that the level exceeds one in 300, and even in the 405 births from labours lasting from 32 to 40 hours, there was only one baby with a five minute Apgar score of three or less. Therefore, there is no clear point at which one can say it is unwise for labour to continue, even from the point of view of the baby.

It seems likely, therefore, that the increasing caesarean section rate seen in all developed countries reflects maternal choice and socioeconomic factors, such as convenience, avoiding pelvic floor damage, higher income for obstetricians, rather than medical imperatives (Belizan et al 1999, Eftekhar & Steer 2000, Murray 2000, Roberts et al 2000).

MONITORING NORMAL LABOUR

Probably the major development in the last 50 years for monitoring normal labour has been the development of the partogram (Philpott 1972, Studd 1973). A typical example is shown in Figure 26.14. This allows all the important variables that need monitoring in labour to be summarised on a single sheet, so that it can all be viewed at once and one variable can readily be correlated with another.

The issue of fetal monitoring is covered comprehensively in Chapter 27. In relation to normal labour, there is no evidence that electronic fetal monitoring needs (EFM) to be used routinely. Intermittent auscultation appears to be sufficient and safe unless there are risk factors (Thacker et al 1995, Vintzileos et al 1995a, 1995b, Thacker & Stroup 2000). The most recent Cochrane review suggests that 'the only clinically significant benefit from the use of routine continuous EFM is a reduction in neonatal seizures. In view of the increase in caesarean and operative vaginal deliveries associated with the use of electronic fetal monitoring, the long-term benefit of this reduction must be evaluated in the decision reached jointly by the pregnant woman and her clinician to use continuous EFM or intermittent auscultation during labour'. A detailed guideline on electronic fetal monitoring has been prepared and released in April 2001 under the auspices of the Royal College of Obstetricians and Gynaecologists and the National Institute for Clinical Excellence (NICE).

SUPPORT FOR THE MOTHER

One to one midwifery support in normal labour is an ideal espoused by both the Royal College of Obstetricians and Gynaecologists and the Royal College of Midwives. Because such support is one of the few interventions to be supported by randomised clinical trials (Hodnett 2000), it behoves all obstetricians to help in the achievement of this goal. Amongst other things, such support can minimise the need for analgesia. Nevertheless, many women now request regional block for pain relief, and the use of such techniques increases year on year. This has led to a controversy as to whether the use of epidural anaesthesia per se leads to an increase in the operative delivery rate. (Chestnut 1994a, Chestnut et al 1994b, Morton et al 1994, Thorp et al 1994, Ramin et al 1995, Hemminki & Gissler 1996, Chestnut 1997a, 1997b, Alexander et al 1998, Halpern et al 1998). The general consensus from controlled studies is that, with the possible exception of blocks commenced in the latent phase of labour, epidurals do not necessarily lead to increases in the incidence of either instrumental delivery or caesarean section. However, observational studies commonly show such an association, and it may be that epidurals are used by women who are less motivated to either bear pain or to achieve a spontaneous delivery by making maximal bearing down efforts. It certainly makes sense that if a woman is tired and fed up with labour, she will ask for a regional block, and she will subsequently be less than keen to

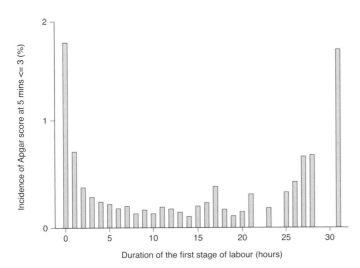

Fig. 26.13 Incidence of low five minute Apgar scores in first labours, by duration of labour.

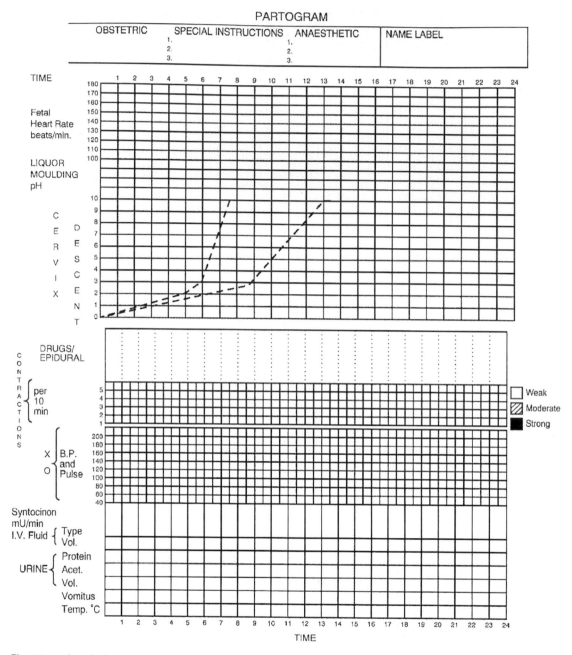

Fig. 26.14 A typical partogram.

exhaust herself further by making a huge effort to bear down. If this is true, then the real issue is whether assisted delivery by ventouse for failure of maternal effort carries any greater risk than spontaneous birth, given that (a) the baby is not stuck and (b) spontaneous birth may well take longer. Such a randomised study has yet to be performed.

THE IMPORTANCE OF CHOICE

One of the great surprises of the changes in the UK following the widespread approval of Changing Childbirth (Cumberlege et al 1993), which advocated a much greater role for maternal choice, is that women increasingly chose intervention rather than what is called natural childbirth. This is not what the activists had expected. At the Chelsea and Westminster Hospital in 1999, 59 women chose to have a caesarean section purely to avoid what was anticipated to be a normal labour (Eftekhar & Steer 2000). They had many reasons, but a predominant one was fear of damage to the maternal pelvis, with subsequent incontinence (Snooks et al 1986, Viktrup et al 1992, Sorensen et al 1993, Sultan et al 1994, Ryhammer et al 1995, Arrowsmith et al 1996, Fornell et al 1996, Lavin & Smith 1996, Walsh et al 1996, MacArthur et al 1997). Further studies are needed to determine whether elective caesarean section will in fact prevent such complications, or whether pregnancy itself is the culprit.

In the meantime, we need to be sensitive to the wishes of the mothers whose labours we supervise, while retaining a critical approach to new fashions, including that for routine elective caesarean section. It may be that the safety of the procedure is now so good that even a straightforward vaginal birth is not much safer, and that we are, therefore, within the realms of acceptable choice. On the other hand, the risks of repeat caesarean section, including placenta praevia and accreta, with the potential for maternal mortality cannot be ignored (Beckley et al 1991, Baker & D'Alton 1994, Chew & Biswas 1998, Zaideh et al 1998). There is much about the management of normal labour that we still need to know.

KEY POINTS

- The onset of labour is difficult to define and problems can arise when the various mechanisms (cervical ripening, rupture of the membranes and onset of regular contractions) are not properly synchronised.
- Rotational birth is necessary in the human because of the tight fit of the large fetal head through a maternal pelvis that is also fabricated for walking and running, and the widest diameter of the shoulders being at 90° to the widest diameter of the head.
- Partograms should be used as an aid to monitoring all pregnancies. Electronic fetal monitoring is optional unless there are risk factors.
- Women and their partners should be given as much choice in their management as possible, within safe limits.

REFERENCES

Alexander JM, Lucas MJ, Ramin SM, McIntire DD, Leveno KJ 1998 The course of labor with and without epidural analgesia. Am J Obstet Gynecol 178:516–520

Arrowsmith S, Hamlin EC, Wall LL 1996 Obstructed labor injury complex: obstetric fistula formation and the multifaceted morbidity of maternal birth trauma in the developing world. Obstet Gynecol Survey 51:568–574

Baker ER, D'Alton ME 1994 Cesarean section birth and cesarean hysterectomy. Clin Obstet Gynecol 37:806–815

Beckley S, Gee H, Newton JR 1991 Scar rupture in labour after previous lower uterine segment caesarean section: the role of uterine activity measurement. Br J Obstet Gynaecol 98:265–269

Belizan JM, Althabe F, Barros FC, Alexander S 1999 Rates and implications of caesarean sections in Latin America: ecological study. Br Med J 319:1397–1400

Chestnut DH 1994a Does epidural analgesia increase the incidence of cesarean section? Am J Obstet Gynecol 171:1398–1399

Chestnut DH, McGrath JM, Vincent RD Jr et al 1994b Does early administration of epidural analgesia affect obstetric outcome in nulliparous women who are in spontaneous labor? Anesthesiol 80:1201–1208

Chestnut DH 1997a Does epidural analgesia during labor affect the incidence of cesarean delivery? Reg Anesth 22:495–499

Chestnut DH 1997b Epidural analgesia and the incidence of cesarean section: time for another close look. Anesthesiol 87:472–476

Chew S, Biswas A 1998 Caesarean and postpartum hysterectomy. Singapore Med J 39:9–13

Cumberlege J et al 1993 Changing Childbirth. Part I: Report of the Expert Maternity Group. HMSO, London.

Efekhar K, Steer P 2000 Caesarean section controversy. Women choose caesarean section. Br Med J 320:1073

Fornell EK, Berg G, Hallbook O, Matthiesen LS, Sjodahl R 1996 Clinical consequences of anal sphincter rupture during vaginal delivery. J Am Coll Surg 183:553–558

Gafni A, Goeree R, Myhr TL et al 1997 Induction of labour versus expectant management for prelabour rupture of the membranes at term: an economic evaluation. TERMPROM Study Group. Term Prelabour Rupture of the Membranes. CMAJ 157:1519–1525

Hager WD, Schuchat A, Gibbs R, Sweet R, Mead P, Larsen JW 2000 Prevention of perinatal group B streptococcal infection: current controversies. Obstet Gynecol 96:141–145

Halpern SH, Leighton BL, Ohlsson A, Barrett JF, Rice A 1998 Effect of epidural vs parenteral opioid analgesia on the progress of labor: a meta-analysis. JAMA 280:2105–2110

Hannah ME, Ohlsson A, Farine D et al 1996 Induction of labor compared with expectant management for prelabor rupture of the membranes at term. TERMPROM Study Group. N Engl J Med 334:1005–1010

Hannah ME, Hodnett ED, Willan A, Foster GA, Di Cecco R, Helewa M 2000 Prelabor rupture of the membranes at term: expectant management at home or in hospital? The TermPROM Study Group. Obstet Gynecol 96:533–538

Hemminki E, Gissler M 1996 Epidural analgesia as a risk factor for operative delivery. Int J Gynaecol Obstet 53:125–132

Hodnett, ED 2000 Caregiver support for women during childbirth. The Cochrane Library, Issue 4. Update Software, Oxford: Electronic Citation.

Lavin J, Smith AR 1996 Pelvic floor damage. Modern Midwife 6:14–16

MacArthur C, Bick DE, Keighley MR 1997 Faecal incontinence after childbirth. Br J Obstet Gynaecol 104:46–50

Morton SC, Williams MS, Keeler EB, Gambone JC, Kahn KL 1994 Effect of epidural analgesia for labor on the cesarean delivery rate. Obstet Gynecol 83:1045–1052

Murray SF 2000 Relation between private health insurance and high rates of caesarean section in Chile: qualitative and quantitative study. Br Med J 321:1501–1505

Philpott RH 1972 Graphic records in labour. Br Med J iv:163–165

Ramin SM, Gambling DR, Lucas MJ, Sharma SK, Sidawi JE, Leveno KJ 1995 Randomized trial of epidural versus intravenous analgesia during labor. Obstet Gynecol 86:783–789

Roberts CL, Tracy S, Peat B 2000 Rates for obstetric intervention among private and public patients in Australia: population based descriptive study. Br Med J 321:137–141

Ryhammer AM, Bek KM, Laurberg S 1995 Multiple vaginal deliveries increase the risk of permanent incontinence of flatus urine in normal premenopausal women. Dis Colon Rectum 38:1206–1209

Snooks SJ, Swash M, Henry MM, Setchell M 1986 Risk factors in childbirth causing damage to the pelvic floor innervation. Intl J Colorectal Dis 1:20–24

Sorensen M, Tetzschner T, Rasmussen OO, Bjarnesen J, Christiansen J 1993 Sphincter rupture in childbirth. Br J Surg 80:392–394

Steer P 1998a Caesarean section: an evolving procedure? Br J Obstet Gynaecol 105:1052–1055

Steer P 1998b Fetal Growth. Br J Obstet Gynaecol 105:1133–1135

Studd JWW 1973 Partograms and nomograms in the management of primigravid labour. Br Med J iv:451–455

Sultan AH, Kamm MA, Hudson CN, Bartram CI 1994 Third degree obstetric anal sphincter tears: risk factors and outcome of primary repair. Br Med J 308:887–891

Tan BP, Hannah ME 2000 Prostaglandins versus oxytocin for prelabour rupture of membranes at or near term. Cochrane Database Syst Rev: CD000158

Thacker SB, Stroup DF, Peterson HB 1995 Efficacy and safety of intrapartum electronic fetal monitoring: an update. Obstet Gynecol 86:613–620

Thacker SB, Stroup DF 2000 Continuous electronic heart rate monitoring for fetal assessment during labor. Cochrane Database Syst Rev:CD000063

Thorp JA, Meyer BA, Cohen GR, Yeast JD, Hu D 1994 Epidural analgesia in labor and cesarean delivery for dystocia. Obstet Gynecol Survey 49:362–369

Viktrup L, Lose G, Rolff M, Barfoed K 1992 The symptom of stress incontinence caused by pregnancy or delivery in primiparas. Obstet Gynecol 79:945–949

Vintzileos AM, Nochimson DJ, Antsaklis A, Varvarigos I, Guzman ER, Knuppel RA 1995a Comparison of intrapartum electronic fetal heart rate monitoring versus intermittent auscultation in detecting fetal acidemia at birth. Am J Obstet Gynecol 173:1021–1024

Vintzileos AM, Nochimson DJ, Guzman ER et al 1995b Intrapartum electronic fetal heart rate monitoring versus intermittent auscultation: a meta-analysis. Obstet Gynecol 85:149–155

Walsh CJ, Mooney EF, Upton GJ, Motson RW 1996 Incidence of third-degree perineal tears in labour and outcome after primary repair. Br J Surg 83:218–221

Zaideh SM, Abu-Heija AT, El-Jallad MF 1998 Placenta praevia and accreta: analysis of a two-year experience. Gynecol Obstet Invest 46:96–98

27

Fetal monitoring in labour

Martin J. Whittle, William L. Martin

Material in this chapter contains contributions from the first and second editions and we are grateful to the previous author for the work done.

INTRODUCTION

In essence, the aim of the management of labour is to ensure the delivery of a healthy baby in good condition with the minimum of intervention. The value of fetal monitoring remains a much-debated topic and there is little evidence that continuous fetal heart rate monitoring has resulted in improvements in perinatal outcome. Conversely, it does appear to be associated with increased intervention rates (Neilson 1995). When continuous electronic fetal monitoring (EFM) is compared with intermittent auscultation, there is apparently little benefit in low-risk women, except when labour is prolonged or augmented, when EFM is associated with a reduction in neonatal seizure rate in the EFM group (MacDonald et al 1985).

One reason for the apparent ineffectiveness of EFM may be that the interpretation of the cardiotocogram (CTG, continuous recording of the fetal heart rate and uterine contractions) is generally performed badly, as suggested in the Confidential Enquiry into Stillbirths and Deaths in Infancy (CESDI) Report, 1997. This report highlighted the fact that in nearly 80% of intrapartum deaths an alternative course of action 'would reasonably be expected to or may have' resulted in a different outcome. The main reason for this failure appears to have been that attendants (obstetricians and midwives) did not recognise abnormalities in the CTG.

Birth asphyxia has become a common source of litigation,

resulting in costs amounting to around £60 million per annum in the UK, and although there is evidence that some of the neurological damage occurs before labour, in many cases settlements involve the clear misinterpretation of the CTG.

This chapter will discuss fetal monitoring during labour, including the pathophysiology of fetal heart rate changes. The use of the CTG and fetal blood sampling (FBS) with reference to the indications, interpretation and appropriate action required will be discussed, and finally the newer methods currently under evaluation will be mentioned.

Fetal physiology

Both neurogenic and humoral factors are involved in an appropriate fetal response to a hypoxic challenge or a mechanical stress.

Baseline fetal heart rate and variability

The baseline fetal heart rate (FHR) and variability are the result of the interaction between the sympathetic and parasympathetic nervous systems. Brainstem function, which is partly responsible for the autonomic nervous system activity, is further modulated by higher centres so that cerebral depression as a result of opiate-like drugs or hypoxia leads to a reduction in FHR variability. Baseline FHR falls gradually during pregnancy, probably as a result of increasing influence of the parasympathetic nervous system, but during normal labour there should be little overall change in the baseline rate.

In labour there is both increased corticosteroid and catecholamine production in the fetus, especially when there is hypoxia. The elevated catecholamine production produces fetal tachycardia, thus a rising baseline heart rate during labour may be an early feature of developing hypoxia.

Fetal oxygenation in labour

Fetal oxygenation is influenced by a number of interacting factors:

Uterine artery blood flow. During a uterine contraction the blood flow in the intramural vessels eventually becomes arrested such that replenishment of blood in the placental bed ceases. With relaxation of the uterus there is a reactive hyperaemia (Lees et al 1971), and providing uterine contractions are not excessively frequent (three in 10 minutes), the system has time to recover between contractions so that fetal oxygenation is maintained. If contractions are too frequent, the lack of recovery time between contractions will eventually result in the development of fetal hypoxia. Other factors which interfere with blood flow to the placental bed are hypotension (iatrogenic from posture or conduction anaesthesia) and certain pathological conditions such as diseases of the spiral arteries that feed the placental bed.

Placental gas transfer. There is normally a large oxygen pressure gradient across the placenta from the maternal side (Po_2 of 100–120 mmHg [13.3–16 KPa]) to the fetal side (Po_2 of 20–30 mmHg [2.7–4 KPa]). In a normal labour the fetus consumes 5 ml o_2/kg/min, the placenta twice that, and this demand changes little throughout the labour. In addition the fetus is well adapted to the low oxygen tension environment. Fetal haemoglobin (HbF) has a greater avidity for oxygen and carries more at low Po_2; the Bohr and Haldane effects ensure that there is maximal release of oxygen at the periphery.

Fetal blood supply. Blood coming from the placenta via the umbilical vein passes almost unhindered via the ductus venosus across the right atrium through the foramen ovale to the left atrium for pumping by the left ventricle into the aortic arch and neck and head vessels (Fig. 27.1). The

aortic arch and carotid bodies which contain the chemoreceptors are well positioned to sense any alteration in oxygen content of blood coming from the placenta via the umbilical vein and the fetus will show cardiovascular responses under these circumstances.

Fetal cardiac output. The fetal ventricles function in parallel, in contrast to the situation in the adult, with the left and right ventricles contributing respectively 55% and 45% of the fetal cardiac output (230 ml/kg/min). Seventy per cent of the overall cardiac output enters the descending aorta, 50% being directed towards the umbilical arteries and 10% to the fetal lungs (Wladimiroff & Moghie 1981).

The placental circulation can be regarded as a low-pressure, high-capacity system in which flow rate is pressure dependent. The system is responsive only to humoral factors because the umbilical vessels are not innervated. The fetal peripheral circulation will respond quickly to hypoxic stress through a mechanism of peripheral vasoconstriction, which helps to redistribute blood to vital areas such as the brain and heart. The increase in peripheral resistance also helps to maintain umbilical blood flow. However prolonged vasoconstriction causes pulmonary, gut and renal ischaemia, which may have adverse effects once the baby is delivered, especially in the preterm infant (respectively respiratory distress syndrome, ischaemic necrotising enteritis and renal insufficiency) ultimately anaerobic metabolism supervenes and acidosis develops.

Acid–base physiology

General

Acid–base balance is regulated partly by extra- and intracellular buffer systems, and partly by renal and respiratory compensation mechanisms. Extracellular buffering provides an immediate response to pH change, the carbonic acid–bicarbonate system being the most important. The intracellular response is slower, utilising haemoglobin and intracellular proteins to remove hydrogen ions. To maintain pH, volatile and fixed acids must be removed. Of the volatile acids, carbonic acid is the most important and is excreted via the lungs as carbon dioxide. The fixed acids are lactic acid, ketoacids, and phosphoric and sulphuric acids, and these must be buffered by bicarbonate from the extracellular fluid.

Maternal

Respiratory compensation provides a rapid response to an acid load in the form of expired carbon dioxide, which maintains a normal partial pressure of carbon dioxide ($Paco_2$). In the case of a respiratory acidosis, HCO_3 crosses the blood–brain barrier (BBB) by active mechanisms, thus several hours are required fully to activate the respiratory compensation mechanisms. In the case of metabolic acidosis, hydrogen ions cross the BBB freely, leading to a more immediate response. Renal compensation mechanisms excrete hydrogen ions to adjust pH but require hours to days to be fully effective.

Fetus

In the fetus the placenta is the organ of gas transfer. Rapid diffusion of CO_2 returns the pH to normal when acidosis

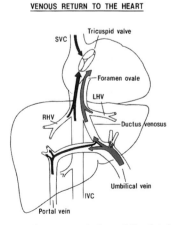

VENOUS RETURN TO THE HEART

Fig. 27.1 Diagrammatic representation of the fetal circulation.

develops, provided the uteroplacental unit is healthy. Intracellular and extracellular buffering systems are utilised but the renal compensation mechanisms are immature and relatively ineffectual. In practice, the 'renal' functions are carried out by the placenta.

Metabolic acidosis. Low pH, low CO_2, low HCO_3 very low base deficit. As the fetus becomes hypoxaemic, aerobic respiration cannot be supported and anaerobic respiration begins. The resulting lactic acid is initially buffered by the mechanisms discussed but ultimately there is a decrease in pH and HCO_3 as these mechanisms are overwhelmed. If the oxygen supply recovers, the process is reversed with the lactate being excreted by placental passage to the mother, and more slowly via the fetal kidneys. Lactate can also be used by the fetus as a substrate for energy production, provided it is well oxygenated.

Respiratory acidosis. Low pH, high pCO_2, raised HCO_3, moderately decreased base deficit. This may be seen after repeated episodes of cord compression, which lead to a rise in P_{CO_2} and a fall in pH. The result is an increase in fetal breathing movements (which has no effect on pH) and increased retention of bicarbonate by the fetal kidneys, which has a limited effect on restoring the pH towards normal. In general, such babies are found to have a mild respiratory acidosis at delivery (Westgate 1993).

Fetal monitoring

The aim of intrapartum monitoring is to identify developing hypoxia in the fetus with a view to intervening to deliver the baby before the development of permanent cerebral damage. It is estimated that only about 10% of cases of cerebral palsy have arisen from *intrapartum* misadventure (Nelson 1988, Yudkin et al 1995). The ideal method of monitoring would be non-invasive, acceptable to the mother and have a high sensitivity and specificity. Unfortunately, such a system does not yet exist and the following is a presentation of the currently available methods followed by a review of research into establishing other methods for intrapartum monitoring.

The preferred method of monitoring the fetus in labour has remained a controversial issue for many years. The first description of the fetal heart sounds was by Mayor in 1818, an observation confirmed by Kergaradec in 1821. The latter observed that a slowing of the fetal heart rate was often associated with a poor outcome. Evory Kennedy in Dublin in 1843 enhanced these observations by adding meconium staining of the amniotic fluid as a further feature of fetal distress. The definition of fetal distress—alterations in fetal heart rate and meconium-stained amniotic fluid—has been in existence, therefore, for many years.

The use of the fetal heart rate alone as a marker of fetal distress clearly has its limitations but intelligent use of the information derived from the continuous fetal heart rate and contractions trace and judicious use of fetal blood sampling to establish the fetal acid–base status does produce a system that can reasonably prevent the fetal compromise arising from oxygen deprivation. Unfortunately there is a tendency to overdiagnose fetal distress and this has led to

an increased incidence of operative delivery for this indication.

The relatively poor results from the use of fetal heart rate monitoring arise from three main factors:

1. The technique is somewhat crude and the physiology uncertain.
2. The training of staff, both midwives and obstetricians, in the use of the technique is almost uniformly poor (Confidential Enquiry into Stillbirths and Deaths in Infancy 2000).
3. The fear of litigious consequences if the baby is born in poor condition or subsequently develops mental or physical handicap, may lead to the defensive use of caesarean section when fetal distress is suspected.

Not all babies require continuous heart rate monitoring in labour and the results of the Dublin study tend to suggest this (MacDonald et al 1985), however it is not always possible to extrapolate from one centre's experience. In the Dublin study, there was a policy of one midwife to one mother throughout labour and there was a short and well-defined chain of command. Under these circumstances it is easy to ensure that regular ausculation will be both undertaken and recorded, and in the low-risk case with clear amniotic fluid this should suffice. While it can be argued that there are few advantages to any fetal heart rate monitoring in low-risk women in spontaneous labour, the Dublin study did suggest that, even in this group, if labour was prolonged or required augmentation, continuous electronic fetal monitoring identified more babies with milder acidosis than did traditional auscultation alone; convulsions following delivery were also more common in the latter group. In the more usual circumstances that exist in labour wards elsewhere in which staff are often heavily pressed, continuous fetal heart rate monitoring ensures that, whatever else is happening, the fetus is under constant supervision. There is certainly a need to monitor all fetuses for which a risk factor is present, when the labour is being induced or augmented, and probably when an epidural anaesthetic is in place.

DETECTION OF THE FETAL HEART RATE

Intermittent fetal heart rate monitoring

Intermittent heart rate monitoring is the traditional method, the rate being determined either from the heart sounds heard through a Pinard stethoscope or using a simple Doppler heart detector. The number of beats is usually counted over a minute and the heart rate calculated. This procedure is performed about 30–45 seconds after a uterine contraction and usually every 15 minutes in the first stage of labour and every 5 minutes in the second stage. The aim is to detect the ominous late decelerations associated with fetal hypoxia and as a technique it seems adequate when there are no complications. However, fetal status using this method is determined using just small samples of the overall heart rate, which provides only crude information about the fetus and gives no indication of impending or developing problems.

Continuous fetal heart rate monitoring

The benefit of continuous monitoring is that it offers sequential information concerning the fetal condition. One of the mistakes that the novice of fetal monitoring often makes is failing to assess the whole trace, merely concentrating on the 20 minutes or so placed in front of him.

Electronic detection of the fetal heart demands that the automatic counter is presented with a clear signal. When the fetal ECG is derived from a scalp clip (Fig. 27.2) it is the R wave that forms the counting source. The signal is usually electronically cleaned and provides accurate information, the rate being determined from the R–R interval. The continuous fetal heart rate trace reflects both short- and long-term variability in the baseline rate (see below).

Ultrasound using the Doppler principle can also be used as a continuous fetal heart rate detector. Various filtering techniques allow a reproduction close to that of the fetal ECG but spurious variability can produce interpretation difficulties so caution is needed. Further, there is group averaging of the Doppler signals so that the assessment of beat-to-beat variation is unreliable (Fig. 27.3). It is probably better to refer to ultrasound-derived data (i.e. all of the antenatal and some of the intrapartum results) on fetal heart rate variation as baseline variability.

Phonocardiography is rarely if ever used in the UK, although it is more frequent in Europe and especially Germany. The advantage of the technique is that the heart sounds are reasonably discernible from the background noise so that the method allows the fetal heart rate variability to be established with some reliability.

Indications for electronic fetal monitoring

Continuous fetal heart rate monitoring should be considered whenever risk factors exist. There are five circumstances under which continuous monitoring may be particularly valuable:

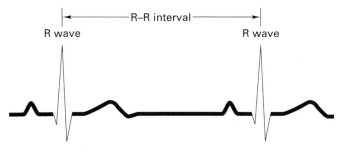

Computation of heart rate

Heart rate is inversely related to the duration of the R–R interval i.e., the longer the R–R interval, the slower the rate and vice versa

Hence, heart rate (beats per min) $= \dfrac{1}{\text{R–R interval (s)}} \times 60$

e.g., for an R–R interval of 0.5 s. heart rate (beats per min) $= \dfrac{1}{0.5} \times 60 = 120$

Fig. 27.2 Fetal ECG complex and the R–R interval.

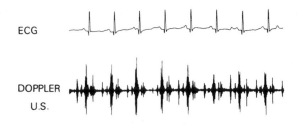

Fig. 27.3 Comparison between fetal ECG and ultrasound signals.

1. preterm labour
2. post-term pregnancy
3. meconium staining of the amniotic fluid
4. fetal growth retardation/small for dates/maternal disease
5. breech presentation.

The use of an admission test has been proposed as a method of ascertaining fetal status before, or early in, labour. Abnormalities in the baseline rate or the presence of decelerations indicate either that the baby would be unable to withstand labour (Arulkumaran & Ingemarsson 1990) or is at risk of adverse condition at delivery (see p. 446). Others (Fairlie et al 1989) have used Doppler waveform studies of the umbilical artery as an assessment of fetal condition; again, abnormal results are frequently associated with the development of fetal distress during labour (see p. 447).

In the absence of risk factors, a compromise which most women find acceptable is the strategy of running short traces intermittently, perhaps of 20–30 minutes duration every 2 hours, backed up by regular auscultation.

Fetal heart rate patterns

The fetal heart rate trace is analysed in terms of its baseline rate, baseline variability and periodic changes. The classification of fetal heart rate patterns developed by Hon (Hon & Quillighan 1967) is the only one now acceptable, and terms such as type 1 and type 2 decelerations should be discarded. The FIGO classification is complex, and the one shown in Table 27.1 is suggested.

Baseline fetal heart rate (Fig. 27.4)

The overall baseline rate used to be regarded as lying between 120 and 160 beats per minute (bpm); with the fetus at or close to term, a range between 110 and 150 bpm is now considered more acceptable (FIGO 1987). This rate probably represents a balance between the sympathetic and parasympathetic components of the autonomic nervous system. The variability of the baseline rate is derived from the continually changing beat-to-beat rate inherent in both fetus and adults. Loss of variability can occur as a natural phenomenon associated with normal rest–activity cycles but it can also indicate cerebral depression arising from hypoxia or narcotic drugs.

Changes in the baseline rate over time can be important indicators of developing hypoxia, the rate rising probably in response to increasing sympathetic drive.

Table 27.1 Classification (after Hon) of fetal heart rate deceleration patterns

1. Early decelerations (head compression)
   Occur with contractions
   Uniform onset and recovery
   Amplitude rarely greater than 40 bpm
   Probably benign
2. Variable decelerations (cord compression)
   Variable relationship to contractions
   'Ragged' waveform
   Variable amplitude
   Potentially dangerous to the fetus
3. Late decelerations (uteroplacental insufficiency)
   Occur late in relationship to the contractions
   Uniform onset and recovery
   Initially may be of low amplitude
   Indicate fetal hypoxia (50%)

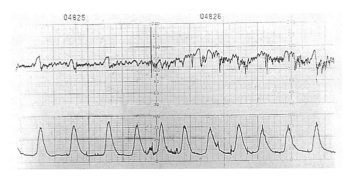

Fig. 27.4 Normal fetal heart rate pattern showing stable baseline rate with accelerations. Paper speed 1 cm/min.

Periodic changes (Fig. 27.5)

Early decelerations. These are relatively uncommon decelerations that are probably the result of fetal head compression and are vagally stimulated. They are subtle; the amplitude of the deceleration falls no lower than by 40 bpm and the waveform coincides with contractions. It is thought that they do not have any particular significance as far as the fetal condition is concerned and may arise from increased fetal intracranial pressure during a uterine contraction.

Variable decelerations. These are common and can be found at some time or another in almost all traces. They have not only erratic shapes and appearances but also a variable relationship to contractions, so that on occasion they can be late in timing. It is thought that they arise from compression of the umbilical cord, their inconsistent appearances resulting from differential compression of artery and vein. The former causes fetal blood pressure to rise and, via the baroreceptors, heart rate to fall. The latter reduces blood flow returning to the heart and lowers blood pressure, resulting in a compensatory acceleration in heart rate. Continued hypoxia stimulates chemoreceptors in the aorta, causing vasoconstriction and a rise in blood pressure. This redistributes flow and ensures oxygenation of the vital centres while maintaining vascular return to the umbilical vessels. Shallow or even deep but brief decelerations have little consequence for the fetus; persistent variable decelerations will eventually cause hypoxia.

Turning the woman on her side can often relieve the pattern. Oxytocin should certainly be discontinued if the decelerations persist. The use of amnioinfusion to relieve compression has been found effective in some circumstances (Owen et al 1990).

Complete cord compression will result in the development of profound respiratory and metabolic acidosis; cerebral damage will occur within 10–20 minutes (Smith 1987). These sudden problems are difficult to predict, and hypoxic damage may arise not only from the low oxygen levels in the fetal blood but also, probably, from major haemodynamic changes in the fetal cerebral vasculature. Unfortunately, events may occur so quickly that any action to deliver the baby may still result in death or damage. Conversely, the majority of babies can withstand, perhaps, up to five minutes of severe cord compression without significant damage, although a fairly profound respiratory acidosis may result.

Late decelerations. These are less common and represent the fetal response to hypoxia. Why the fetus responds in this way, in contrast to adults who develop tachycardia first, is uncertain. The initial responses are the results of the effect of hypoxaemia on the fetal chemoreceptors in the aortic arch which, when activated, cause fetal blood pressure to rise and, as a baroreceptor response, the fetal heart rate to fall. Thus in the initial stages the changes are entirely reflex-driven and physiological: blood flow to the brain, heart and adrenals is

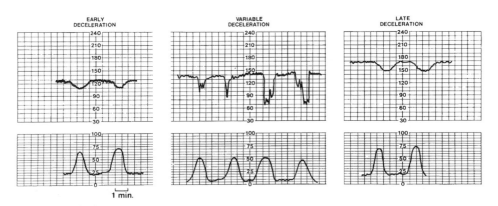

Fig. 27.5 Periodic deceleration patterns (schematic).

443

maintained or increased at the expense of carcass, kidney and gut. If hypoxia deepens, the fetal response changes such that fetal blood pressure falls rather than rises and the fetal heart rate pattern shows deep meandering decelerations, probably as a direct result of an hypoxic myocardium. If the hypoxia continues, catecholamine release is stimulated with unpredictable influences on the FHR. It is clearly the aim of fetal monitoring in labour to intervene before the development of these agonal patterns. The commonest causes of late decelerations are the development of maternal hypotension and excessive uterine activity. These are correctable factors and, if the FHR recovers, labour may be allowed to continue.

It is important to emphasise that only about 50% of fetuses showing late decelerations will be acidotic (Beard et al 1971). This is often held to be evidence that the technique of fetal heart rate monitoring is worthless but in actual fact the observation reflects the underlying physiology, a fetus not usually developing acidosis until lengthy hypoxia has eroded its buffering systems. In the presence of accelerations or a normal baseline variation (an indicator of an intact autonomic nervous system) acidosis is unlikely.

FETAL ACID–BASE MEASUREMENT

Whenever fetal heart rate monitoring is being employed it is vital that fetal acid–base status can be established from a scalp blood sample. This facility was only available in 50% of units in the UK in 1990; this figure is probably much higher now at around 80% (Wheble et al 1989). It should ideally be possible to measure pH, P_{CO_2}, and base deficit so that the nature (respiratory or metabolic) of the acidosis can be established. The limitations in interpreting fetal heart rate traces mean that the diagnosis of fetal distress should be confirmed in all possible cases by fetal blood pH prior to caesarean section for this indication. Using cord blood samples, Westgate (1993) established the normal range for pH, P_{CO_2}, and base deficit (BD) in 1716 subjects at delivery (Table 27.2). The normal range for arterial pH (representing the fetal situation) was 7.04–7.38 (median 7.26), for venous pH (representing the placental/maternal situation) the figures were 7.16–7.47 (median 7.35). The base deficit used was of the whole extracellular fluid (ecf) as this is more representative of buffering capacity in the fetus in which more buffering occurs outside the blood compartment compared with the situation in the adult where most buffering occurs in the blood compartment. The normal ranges for BD were −2.8 to 9.4 (median 2.3) and −1.4 to 8.8 (median 2.9).

These figures are in keeping with a recent consensus document from the International Cerebral Palsy Task Force (MacLennan 1999). The task force was set up to review the available literature on the development of cerebral palsy and try to identify objective indicators to determine whether an individual case of cerebral palsy was likely to have arisen due to intrapartum hypoxia. Current literature suggests that in 10% or so of cases of cerebral palsy is the origin in the perinatal period (Nelson 1988, Yudkin et al 1995). The consensus opinion with regard to defining metabolic acidaemia was that pathological acidaemia was present at a pH <7.00, BD >12 mmol/l. Below this level there is a significant risk of neurological deficit. Using paired cord samples (venous and arterial) a difference of P_{CO_2} of 25 mmHg (3.3 KPa) indicates acute rather than chronic (prelabour) acidosis.

Technique of fetal blood sampling

Fetal blood sampling is complementary to fetal heart rate assessment. When delivery is not imminent in the presence of a very abnormal CTG, FBS may not be appropriate and delivery preferable. Conversely, if progress is good and vaginal delivery imminent, FBS may prevent unnecessary intervention. There are no rules regarding the appropriate number of FBS; this will depend on the overall clinical picture. A patient whose labour is arrested at 3 cm dilatation who has already had two FBS probably needs to be delivered for indications other than suboptimal CTG alone. Similarly, no firm guidelines exist regarding the lower limit of gestation at which FBS should be used but less than 34 weeks would be reasonable. The indications and contraindications for FBS are listed in Table 27.3.

The FBS should be performed with the patient in the left lateral position to prevent supine hypotension. Epidural analgesia is not a requirement. Although sampling can be performed at 1–2 cm dilatation, it is seldom warranted as an abnormal heart rate at that degree of cervical dilatation probably indicates that delivery is required.

The necessary equipment is shown in Figure 27.6. The patient's right leg is held by an assistant and the perineum cleaned. A vaginal examination to check dilatation and posi-

Table 27.3 Indications and contraindications for fetal blood sampling

Indications
Persistent variable decelerations >45 minutes
Late decelerations >30 minutes
Meconium-stained liquor with a non-reassuring FHR trace
Monitoring in labour when the fetus is known to have heart block

Contraindications
Obvious indication for delivery (e.g. inadequate progress, breech presentation + abnormal CTG)
Face presentation
Maternal infection including HIV
Chorioamnionitis
Prematurity <34 weeks
Fetal condition, e.g. suspected haemophilia

Table 27.2 Cord blood gases—normal range (2.5th to 97.5th centiles) (from Westgate 1993)

	Artery	Vein
Ph	7.26 (7.04–7.38)	7.35 (7.16–7.47)
P_{CO_2} mmHg [KPa]	55 (37–81)	40 (27–59)
	[7.3 (4.9–10.8)]	[5.3 (3.6–7.9)]
Bdecf	2.3 (−2.8–9.4)	2.9 (−1.4–8.8)
Bdblood	3.7 (−1.7–12.4)	2.9 (−1.5–9.6)

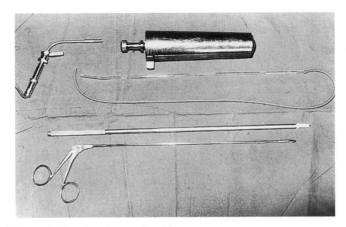

Fig. 27.6   Fetal scalp sampling kit.

tion of the cervix should be performed. The largest amnioscope available should be used. It is gently inserted, in the direction of the sacral hollow. Once the fetal head is reached, the amnioscope should be directed anteriorly. This has the effect of catching the anterior lip of the cervix, and once the obturator is removed, the fetal head should be seen. If cervix is obscuring the view, the amnioscope can be manipulated to lie behind the anterior cervical lip. Directing the amnioscope anteriorly fixes the fetal head against the symphysis pubis and often is enough to prevent liquor affecting the sampling and to prevent a poorly applied head from moving when the scalp is incised.

The head is cleaned and silicon grease applied in a circular motion which has the dual effect of making the blood come as a discrete bleb, making collection of blood easier, and to stick any hair onto the scalp, making sampling easier. An assistant sprays ethyl chloride onto the scalp; this causes a reactive hyperaemia, improving sample collection and making the capillary sample more representative of the oxygenated side of the fetal circulation. A guarded blade is pushed into the scalp for 2 mm at the most; this is nearly always accompanied by a 'pop'. The blade is then rotated through 90° and removed. This technique usually produces a bleb of blood that can then be collected in a capillary tube. The tube should be touched on the surface of the bleb, not on the scalp, for successful collection. If the sample does not draw up the tube, gently tapping the tip of the capillary tube on the scalp can start the capillary action. If the scalp is bleeding a lot, pressure should be applied with a dental roll while waiting for the assistant to return with the pH result.

The finding of falling scalp blood pH levels in labour indicates that a problem is impending and that action to deliver the baby will be necessary. The interpretation of the fetal scalp sample is usually based upon the values given in Table 27.4 with a pH value of ≤7.2 for scalp blood indicating significant acidosis. The values may be adjusted in the light of more recent evidence (Table 27.2; Westgate 1993, MacLennan 1999), however the figures in Table 27.2 are for cord gases at delivery, and a higher threshold for diagnosing acidosis is appropriate for fetal scalp samples as this allows a margin of safety.

Table 27.4   Interpretation of fetal blood sampling

	pH	Base deficit (mmol/l)	Action
Normal	>7.25	<6	Repeat if CTG abnormality continues
Preacidosis	>7.20–≤7.24	>6–≤10	Repeat 30–60 minutes depending on abnormality
Acidosis	<7.20	>10	Delivery

MANAGEMENT OF MONITORING IN LABOUR

The fetal heart rate changes are often taken out of the context of the woman's labour but they must be regarded as only a part of the decision-making process. Thus, if labour is progressing rapidly but the deterioration in the fetal heart rate patterns is gradual, then it is quite likely that a safe vaginal delivery is going to be possible. Conversely, deterioration in the face of slow progress in labour will almost certainly result in the need for operative delivery, often by caesarean section. Likewise the presence of abnormal fetal heart rate patterns in the face of minimal uterine activity is unlikely to result in a successful vaginal delivery. The presence of other risk factors, such as suspected growth restriction or prematurity, will also influence how the information from the fetal heart rate traces is used.

The main requirement for the fetus during labour is the maintenance of an adequate supply of oxygen. Figure 27.7 shows the components responsible, namely the uterine blood flow, the placenta and the umbilical circulation.

The *uterine blood flow* is influenced by a number of factors including uterine contractions and the maternal blood pres-

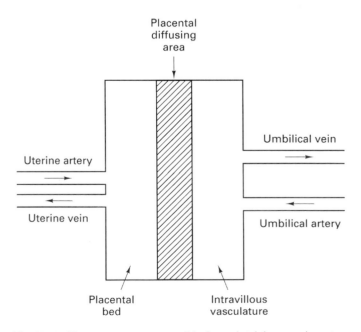

Fig. 27.7   The components responsible for maintaining an adequate oxygen supply to the fetus in labour.

sure which can be lowered by supine posture or conduction anaesthesia. The effects of reduced uterine blood flow on the fetal heart rate pattern often develop fairly slowly and in the early stages produce only subtle changes. Further deterioration is not, in itself, an indication for an immediate caesarean section but rather demands a search for the underlying cause, which can often be iatrogenic. Thus a reduction in the oxytocin infusion rate to lessen the uterine activity, or the repositioning of the woman to relieve hypotension will usually improve matters. Evaluation of the fetal condition by FBS will indicate the current acid–base status and allow more rational decision making (Recommendations arising from the 26th RCOG study group 1993).

The *placenta*, which get the blame for much that goes amiss in obstetrics, are only rarely implicated in the development of fetal heart rate abnormalities; as long as the placenta is still appropriately attached, it will continue to function well as a gas-exchange organ. Abruption does, of course, produce dramatic changes in the fetal heart rate but is a relatively rare event.

Compression of the *umbilical cord* causes rapid and sometimes dramatic fetal heart rate changes, in contrast to events in the uterine circulation. Most often these events are temporary and usually resolve spontaneously, but alteration of the woman's position and the more recently described use of amnioinfusion may also help. The assessment of the fetal acid–base status in the presence of variable decelerations can be unrewarding since rapid changes in pH can arise from the respiratory acidosis which develops during cord compression. Severe cord compression will occasionally produce profound effects, which sometimes result in death and damage before intervention is possible.

The importance of devising a clear management plan for these differing clinical circumstances cannot be overemphasised. Serious problems arise in the management of labour usually because of prevarication and lack of forward thinking (Confidential Enquiry into Stillbirths and Deaths in Infancy 1995). Explicit action plans are required so that all members of the team, and the woman herself, are aware of what is likely to happen. The obstetrician must learn to anticipate what information he might need to make his decision. It takes time and experience to develop these skills but they are vital if appropriate management of labour is to be achieved.

Second stage

The fetal acid–base status can change quite rapidly in the second stage but usually only when the mother is actively bearing down. This is a result of respiratory acidosis from rising carbon dioxide levels rather than oxygen lack producing a metabolic acidosis. Fetal heart rate patterns are difficult to interpret at this time but should not be ignored, especially if abnormal traces have occurred in the first stage.

ALTERNATIVE METHODS OF FETAL MONITORING

One of the weaknesses of continuous fetal heart rate monitoring is that it does not provide much quantitative informa-

tion about the fetal condition. Thus, in some circumstances, relatively minor heart rate changes may be found in a profoundly hypoxic baby while severe abnormalities may occur when the baby is only mildly affected. There has been a search for other techniques that may provide a more precise measure of the baby's condition.

Admission test

An admission test is performed for 20 minutes when the woman is admitted to the labour ward. Thereafter intermittent auscultation is performed for 1 minute after a contraction, every 15 minutes. The presence of a normal baseline, acceptable variability and two accelerations is considered normal, and thereafter intermittent auscultation may be carried out as the chance of the fetus developing hypoxia is small (Ingemarsson et al 1986). A suspicious trace is one without accelerations and either decreased variability, tachycardia or bradycardia or decelerations. A trace is deemed ominous in the presence of two or more abnormalities. In one study the incidence of fetal distress (defined as the need for operative delivery or normal delivery with an Apgar of <7 at 5 minutes) was 1.4% for those with reactive traces, 10.4% for suspicious traces and 40% for ominous traces (Ingemarsson et al 1986). In the cases in the reactive group that developed problems, fetal distress was diagnosed generally more than five hours after admission.

The combination of the assessment of amniotic fluid volume in early labour with intact membranes, and an admission CTG has the ability to identify those babies at risk of fetal distress. When the amniotic fluid index (AFI) (maximum pool depth in each of the quadrants combined) was more than 5 cm the outcome was better, even with a suspicious admission trace. In the presence of an AFI of less than 5 cm and despite a normal admission CTG, there were more operative deliveries, more admissions to the neonatal unit, and lower Apgar scores (Chua et al 1993).

Fetal stimulation tests

The fetal acoustic stimulation test

The acoustic stimulation test utilises an artificial larynx to stimulate the baby; the response is observed on the CTG. A prolonged acceleration for 3 minutes, two accelerations or acceleration for more than 1 minute is regarded as normal. The presence of an acceleration followed by a deceleration, or no response at all is regarded as abnormal. Fetal distress, using the same criteria as above, was seen in 1.7% of babies that exhibited a normal response to acoustic stimulation and a normal admission CTG. In 14% of those with an abnormal response to acoustic stimulation but a normal admission CTG there was fetal distress. Fetal distress also occurred in 6.1% of babies with an abnormal admission CTG but normal acoustic stimulation, and 56% of babies if both were abnormal (Ingemarsson et al 1986). Several studies have confirmed these findings and indicate that acoustic stimulation has a place as a screening test for fetal distress in labour.

In a recent report, Chauhan et al (1999) showed that of 271 fetuses subjected to acoustic stimulation in early labour, those with a non-reactive response were at increased risk of caesarean delivery for fetal distress (relative risk [RR] 4) and neonatal acidosis (pH ≤ 7.0; RR 5). This was a small study, however, and the confidence intervals were large, so further investigation is required.

Scalp stimulation test

A painful stimulus to the fetal scalp (e.g. fetal blood sample or pinching with a forceps) that results in an acceleration is unlikely to be associated with an acidotic pH on scalp sampling (Clarke et al 1984). If there is no response, half will have pH <7.20. The drawback with this method is the need to perform frequent vaginal examinations to carry out the test.

Fetal ECG

More detailed analysis of the ECG complex itself may prove advantageous although it would also require use of the continuous fetal heart rate trace and the use of a scalp electrode. Use of the various components of the fetal ECG has centred on the PR interval and the ST segment. The PR interval represents the conduction time for the atrioventricular node down the bundle of His. Under normal circumstances an increase in heart rate leads to a shortening of the PR interval and a decrease to a lengthening. In animal experiments, it was shown that the fetal response to hypoxaemia was a bradycardia and paradoxical shortening of the PR interval. One study in humans used the PR interval of the fetal ECG to monitor fetal condition. This led to a decrease in the number of FBS required with no increase in adverse outcome (van Wijngaarden et al 1996). A more recent randomised study, however, has suggested no significant advantages in the use of PR-interval analysis plus CTG compared with CTG alone (Strachan et al 2000).

Most interest has centred round the use of the ST segment. Animal work indicates that anaerobic respiration is associated with ST elevation in a normally grown fetus. In growth-restricted animals, ST depression and T wave inversion occur in response to hypoxia. This may be because the reserves in such fetuses for anaerobic metabolism are reduced and there is a direct effect of hypoxaemia leading to myocardial ischaemia and thus ST depression. Preliminary data using the ST segment changes of the ECG waveform do seem to provide a guide to the significance of certain fetal heart rate patterns and in a randomised study were found to reduce caesarean section rates for fetal distress (Westgate et al 1992).

Lactate measurement

The apparent paradox of a baby born with a low pH and a good Apgar score results from respiratory acidosis. In one study, 14% of babies born with acidaemia, as defined by umbilical cord pH, had Apgar scores >7 at 5 minutes. Of those with Apgar scores <7 only 19% were acidaemic (Sykes et al 1983). The rationale for lactate measurement is that the most significant abnormality of acid–base balance for the fetus is a metabolic acidosis. The end product of anaerobic respiration, as previously mentioned, is lactic acid resulting in a metabolic acidosis. Thus detection of lactic acid should correlate better with fetal outcome than pH alone. The technique used is identical to that already discussed for FBS, however lactate detectors are currently available that utilise very small amounts of fetal blood (5 μl) compared with conventional pH analysis (minimum of 35 μl). Based on current studies a lactate level >3.08 mmol/l is abnormal, 2.9–3.07 mmol/l is suspicious and ≤2.8 is normal (Nordstrom et al 1995). Studies to determine the utility of the technique continue but preliminary work found that the outcome in two groups, one where conventional FBS was used and the other where lactate level was used, was no different in terms of operative delivery or fetal outcome. However, as smaller samples are required for lactate measurement, a sufficient sample was more often obtained initially so fewer attempts at blood sampling were needed (Westgren et al 1998).

Computer assistance

Attempts have been made over many years to produce a computerised system that will interpret the CTG. These have been met with limited success although a reliable antenatal computerised CTG is in operation in clinical practice (Dawes et al 1991). Systems to interpret intrapartum CTGs have been developed but they have tended to assess the CTG in isolation whereas a clinician should consider the clinical situation as a whole. Keith et al (1995) performed a study to compare a computer system with 17 experts in assessing 50 complete intrapartum CTGs, including clinical data, relevant clinical information and FBS results. The system compared favourably with the experts and overall was found to perform more consistently. Of interest, however, was the finding that the experts made consistent and appropriate recommendations in the majority of cases, which probably indicates the result of appropriate training and experience gained over years of practice. The potential advantage of a computer program is that it can utilise years of experience immediately. As yet these systems are still being developed and evaluated and have not entered clinical practice. Given the findings of CESDI (1995) with regard to misinterpretation of traces and failure of action in the face of evidence of fetal compromise, such systems could be of considerable potential benefit.

Doppler for intrapartum monitoring

The use of Doppler velocimetry for intrapartum monitoring has been widely studied. Studies have shown that decelerations in labour correspond to a raised pulsatility index (PI; Fairlie et al 1989). Chua et al (1993) found that in cases where the admission CTG was suspicious but Doppler studies were normal, there were fewer operative deliveries, higher Apgar scores and fewer admissions to the neonatal unit than controls. In several studies the positive predictive value of, variously, the PI and S/D ratio, was poorly predictive of outcome but was probably as good as conventional CTG analysis (Feinkind et al 1989, Malcus et al 1991). In a recent systematic review and meta-analysis, the use of intrapartum umbilical artery Doppler velocimetry was a poor predictor of outcome as defined by the above criteria plus identification of the growth-restricted fetus (Farrell et al 1999). In view of this, Doppler study for the prediction of labour outcome has found little clinical use.

Doppler studies of the middle cerebral artery (MCA) have been performed in labour. There was no difference in PI of the MCA or internal carotid artery during or between contractions (Maesel et al 1994) and the velocity waveforms were similar to those obtained antenatally.

RESEARCH TECHNIQUES

The poor correlation that seems to exist between intrapartum evidence of hypoxia and eventual outcome has led to a search for other techniques with which to establish fetal compromise.

Pulse oximetry

Pulse oximetry allows measurements of oxygenation to be carried out. It is based on the premise that light transmission by blood varies with the change in blood volume in a tissue with each pulse. Two wavelengths of light are emitted by a source, one in the red range and one in the infrared. The differential absorption of the pulsatile component of the tissue at each wavelength compared with the non-pulsatile is calculated and compared with a standard curve to give oxygen concentration.

The sensor is placed against the fetal cheek; various methods have been employed to ensure that contact is maintained. Studies indicate that results may be obtained from 2 cm dilatation in between 45% and 60% of cases (Dildy et al 1993). Although results vary between studies, a SaO_2 of more than 30% is indicative of fetal well-being as this is the level below which anaerobic respiration begins (Nijland et al 1995). More recently this cut-off has been validated further (Kuhnert et al 1998) by the demonstration that SaO_2 of less than 30% for longer than 10 minutes correlated well with low scalp pH.

Near infrared spectroscopy

The technique of near infrared spectroscopy (NIRS) relies on the lucent nature of the fetal brain to light in the NIR range. There are three light-absorbing compounds in the fetal brain, oxy- and deoxyhaemoglobin and oxidised cytochrome oxidase. Thus emitted NIR light is altered when any of these components alter. It is possible to calculate changes in cerebral blood flow using this technique. The probe is similar to that for pulse oximetry and is placed on the fetal scalp away from the ears or face. Light at four wavelengths passes into the fetus via one channel and is collected through another.

Although NIRS is only a research tool at present, a few studies have been performed. As with oximetry, recordings can be made from 2 cm dilatation in up to 65% of labours. In normal labour the cerebral blood volume falls with uterine activity (Wyatt et al 1990). This probably reflects a head compression effect. If the interval between contractions is short (less than 2 minutes) then a fall in cerebral oxygen content was found and the level at which there was no change in oxygenation correlated with a contraction frequency of four in 10 minutes (Peebles et al 1994). There was a good correlation between fall in oxyhaemoglobin, which occurred after the onset of contraction, and late decelerations on CTG. The mean cerebral oxygen saturation ($SmcO_2$) is a parameter that can be obtained at the start of each labour. It is calculated over several contractions and reflects actual cerebral oxygen content. The normal range is 33–53%. There is a strong positive correlation between $SmcO_2$ and pH and a strong negative correlation with base deficit (Aldrich et al 1994).

There is a poor correlation between both acid–base status and hypoxaemia at birth and the development of neurological handicap, prevention of which is the whole aim of fetal monitoring. A concern with oximetry and NIRS is that the neurological damage may have already occurred by the time the fetus demonstrates central deoxygenation as a result of underperfusion. More detailed and prolonged research in these areas is clearly required.

CONCLUSIONS

Fetal monitoring in labour is currently performed using either intermittent auscultation or continuous electronic fetal monitoring in combination with fetal blood sampling. Many alternative methods have been investigated and others are under development, some of which have been discussed in this chapter, but as yet there is nothing new available. Although its place in low-risk labours may be questioned, the CTG is a very sensitive tool for identifying the fetus at risk of acidosis. It has a high false-positive rate, however, and therefore must be used in conjunction with FBS to achieve an acceptable intervention rate. Understanding the CTG is an integral part of modern obstetric care in the developed world, but after 25 years there is still a lack of consensus with regard to its interpretation; this is surprising as the definitions for interpretation have changed little in that time.

That CTG interpretation forms a major part of intrapartum obstetric care is demonstrated by the findings of a CESDI report (1995) which showed that amongst nearly 1300 intrapartum deaths in 1995 there was substandard care with regard to failure to recognise abnormalities and failure to take appropriate action in a majority of cases. This led to a recommendation from a recent Working Party report from the Royal College of Obstetricians and Gynaecologists, *Towards Safer Childbirth* (1999), for continuing education of staff with regard to CTG interpretation within obstetric departments. The 7th annual CESDI report (1998–1999) indicated that although multidisciplinary training in the use of CTG was available in over 75% of units, confirmed attendance was 88% for midwives but only about 50% for medical staff. The midwives most likely to attend were not necessarily those most likely to be responsible for women in labour, probably because of the difficulty of releasing critical staff for training. In addition, many midwives had to fund themselves to attend courses.

It is clear that considerable work needs to be done to improve matters but it is vital that change occurs so that the interpretation of CTG and communication of its results can become standardized and comprehensible to all concerned.

KEY POINTS

- The aim of fetal monitoring (FM) in labour is to identify hypoxia, so allowing intervention before the development of permanent cerebral damage.
- The value of FM as currently performed remains a much debated topic; there is little evidence that it improves perinatal outcome.
- Clinical interpretation of cardiotocography is generally performed badly with attendants failing to notice subtle changes; fetal blood sampling is underused.
- Much of the hypoxic cerebral damage occurs before labour.
- Adequate fetal tissue oxygenation depends on afferent uterine artery flow, adequate placental gas exchange, fetal blood flow and fetal cardiac output.
- The findings of FM in labour are detailed, their correct interpretation is outlined, and well-grounded action to be taken is described.

REFERENCES

Aldrich CJ, D'Antona D, Wyatt JS, Spencer JAD, Peebles DM, Reynolds EOR 1994 Fetal cerebral oxygenation measured by near infrared spectroscopy shortly before birth and acid–base status at birth. Obstet Gynecol 84:861–866

Arulkumaran S, Ingemarsson I 1990 Appropriate technology in intrapartum fetal surveillance. In: Studd J (ed) Progress in obstetrics and gynaecology, vol 8. Churchill Livingstone, Edinburgh, pp 127–140

Beard RW, Filshie GM, Knight CA, Roberts GM 1971 The significance of the changes in the continuous fetal heart rate in the first stage of labour. J Obstet Gynaecol Br Commonwealth 78:865–881

Chauhan SP, Hendrix NW, Devoe LD, Scardo JA 1999 Fetal acoustic stimulation in early labour and pathological fetal acidaemia: a preliminary report. J Matern Fetal Med 8: 208–212

Chua S, Arulkumaran S, Kurup A, Anandakumar C, Norshida S, Ratnam SS 1993 Search for the most predictive tests of fetal well-being in early labour. J Perinat Med 76: 606–612

Clarke SL, Gimovsky ML, Miller FC 1984 The scalp stimulation test: a clinical alternative to fetal scalp blood sampling. Am J Obstet Gynecol 148:274–277

Confidential Enquiry into Stillbirths and Deaths in Infancy (CESDI) 1997 4th Annual Report Concentrating on Intrapartum Related Deaths 1994–1995. Maternal and Child Health Research Consortium, Chiltern Court, Baker St, London

Confidential Enquiry into Stillbirths and Deaths in Infancy (CESDI) 2000 7th Annual Report 1998–1999. Maternal and Child Health Research Consortium, Chiltern Court, Baker St, London

Dawes GS, Moulden M, Redman CWG 1991 System 8000: computerized antenatal FHR analysis. J Perinat Med 19:47–51

Dildy GA, Clark SL, Loucks CA 1993 Preliminary experience with intrapartum fetal pulse oximetry in humans. Obstet Gynecol 81:630–635

Fairlie FM, Lang GD, Sheldon CD 1989 Umbilical artery velocity waveforms in labour. Br J Obstet Gynaecol 96:151–157

Farrell T, Chien PFW, Gordon A 1999 Intrapartum umbilical artery

Doppler velocimetry as a predictor of adverse perinatal outcome: a systematic review. Br J Obstet Gynaecol 106:783–792

Feinkind L, Abulafin O, Delke I, Feldman J, Minkoff A 1989 Screening with Doppler velocimetry in labour. Am J Obstet Gynecol 161:765–770

FIGO 1987 Int J Gynaecol Obstet 25:159–167

Hon EH, Quillighan EJ 1967 The classification of fetal heart rate. II. A revised working classification. Conn Med 31:779–784

Ingemarsson I, Arulkumaran S, Ingemarsson E, Tambyraja RL, Ratnam SS 1986 Admission test: a screening test for fetal distress in labour. Obstet Gynecol 69:800–806

Keith RDF, Beckley S, Garibaldi JM, Westgate JA, Ifeachor EC, Greene KR 1995 A multicentre comparative study of 17 experts and an intelligent computer system for managing labour using the cardiotocogram. Br J Obstet Gynaecol 102:688–700

Kuhnert M, Seelbach-Goebel B, Butterwegge M 1998 Predictive agreement between the fetal arterial oxygen saturation and fetal scalp pH: results of the German multicenter trial. Am J Obstet Gynecol 178:330–335

Lees MH, Hill JD, Ochsner AJ, Thomas CL, Novy MJ 1971 Maternal placental and myometrial blood flow of the rhesus monkey during uterine contractions. Am J Obstet Gynecol 110:68–81

MacDonald D, Grant A, Sheridan-Pereira M, Boylan P, Chalmers I 1985 The Dublin randomised controlled trial of intrapartum fetal monitoring. Am J Obstet Gynecol 152:524–539

MacLennan A 1999 A template for defining a causal relation between acute intrapartum events and cerebral palsy: international consensus statement. BMJ 319:1054–1059

Maesel A, Sladkevicius P, Valentin L, Marsal K 1994 Fetal cerebral blood flow velocity during labor and the early neonatal period. Ultrasound Obstet Gynecol 4:372–376

Malcus P, Gudmundsson J, Marsal K, Kwok HH, Vengadasalan D, Ratnam SS 1991 Umbilical artery Doppler velocimetry as a labour admission test. Obstet Gynecol 77: 10–16

Neilson JP 1995 EFM vs intermittent auscultation in labour [revised May 1994]. In: Keirse MJNC, Renfrew MJ, Neilson JP, Crowther C (eds) Pregnancy and childbirth module. In: The Cochrane Pregnancy and Childbirth Database [database on disc and CDROM]. The Cochrane Collaboration; Issue 2. Update Software, Oxford. BMJ Publishing Group, London

Nelson K 1988 What proportion of cerebral palsy is related to birth asphyxia? J Pediatr 112:572–574

Nijland R, Jongsma H, Nijhaus JG 1995 Arterial oxygen saturation in relation to metabolic acidosis in fetal lambs. Am J Obstet Gynecol 172:810–819

Nordstrom L, Ingemarsson I, Kublickas M, Persson B, Shimojo N, Westgren M 1995 Scalp blood lactate: a new test strip method for monitoring fetal well-being in labour. Br J Obstet Gynaecol 102:894–899

Owen J, Henson BV, Hauth C 1990 A prospective randomized study of saline solution amnioinfusion. Am J Obstet Gynecol 162:1146–1149

Peebles DM, Spencer JAD, Edwards AD, Wyatt JS, Reynolds EO, Cope M, Delpy DT 1994 Relation between frequency of uterine contractions and human fetal cerebral oxygen saturation studied during labour by near infrared spectroscopy. Br J Obstet Gynaecol 101:44–48

Recommendations arising from the 26th RCOG study group 1993 In: Spencer JAD (ed) Intrapartum fetal surveillance. RCOG Press, London, pp 387–393

Report of a Joint Working Party 1999 Towards safer childbirth. Minimum standards for the organisation of labour wards. RCOG Press, London

Smith NC 1987 Assessment of fetal acid-base status. In: Whittle MJ (ed) Clinical obstetrics and gynaecology, vol 1. Bailliere Tindall, London, pp 97–109

Strachan BK, Wijngaarden WJ, Sahota D, Chong A, James DK 2000 Cardiotocography only versus CTG and PR-interval analysis in intrapartum surveillance: a randomized multicentre trial. Lancet 355:456–459

Sykes GS, Molloy PM, Johnson P, Stirrat GM, Turnbull AC 1983 Fetal distress and the condition of the new born infants. BMJ 287:943–945

van Wijngaarden WJ, Sahota DS, James DK, Farrell T, Mires GJ, Wilcox M, Chang A 1996 Improved intrapartum surveillance with PR interval analysis of the fetal electrocardiogram: A randomized trial showing a reduction in fetal blood sampling. Am J Obstet Gynecol 1174:1295–1299

Westgate J 1993 The assessment of acid–base status at birth. MD Thesis, University of Plymouth, pp 114–143

Westgate J, Harris M, Curnow JSH, Greene KR 1992 Plymouth randomised trial of cardiotocogram only versus ST waveform analysis plus cardiotogram for intrapartum monitoring. Lancet 340:194–198

Westgren M, Kruger K, Ek S et al 1998 Lactate compared with pH analysis at fetal scalp blood sampling: a prospective randomised study. Br J Obstet Gynaecol 105:29–33

Wheble AM, Gillmer MDG, Spencer JAD, Sykes GS 1989 Changes in fetal monitoring practice in the UK: 1977–1984. Br J Obstet Gynaecol 96:1140–1147

Wladimiroff JW, McGhie JS 1981 M-mode ultrasonic assessment of cardiovascular geometry and function in the human fetus. Br J Obstet Gynaecol 88:870–875

Wyatt JS, Cope M, Delpy DT, Richardson CE, Edwards AD, Wray S, Reynolds EO 1990 Quantitation of cerebral blood volume in newborn human infants by near infrared spectroscopy. J Appl Physiol 68:1086–1091

Yudkin PL, Johnson A, Clover LM, Murphy KW 1995 Assessing the contribution of birth asphyxia to cerebral palsy in term singletons. Paediatr Perinatal Epidemiol 9:156–170

28

Obstetric analgesia and anaesthesia

Michael Harmer, Rachel Collis

INTRODUCTION

Labour is an intense and often unexpectedly painful experience, with as many as 30% of mothers finding it much more painful than expected (Morgan et al 1982). Although preparation and training in a variety of relaxation techniques may help some mothers, many request pharmacological methods of pain relief. Mothers, throughout history, have been given extracts of opium and hyoscine in an attempt to reduce suffering during prolonged difficult labours. Mothers now have the benefits of improved drug preparation and pharmacological knowledge, but regional analgesia, which has gained popularity since the early 1970s, remains the most reliable technique for the relief of pain in labour.

History

Early Chinese writings describe the use of opiates and soporifics during childbirth, while in the Middle Ages there was more dependence on self-administration of alcoholic drinks. However, in some groups the relief of childbirth pain was considered evil and led to the execution of those attempting to help the mother, a practice, fortunately, no longer in fashion. Dr James Young Simpson in 1847 gave the first recognised obstetric anaesthetic using ether, but perhaps it was not until John Snow in 1853 administered chloroform to Queen Victoria for the birth of Prince Leopold, that obstetric anaesthesia and analgesia gained respectability.

Of the agents still in current use, nitrous oxide was first used as an obstetric analgesic by Klikowitsch in 1881, but did not become widely available until the introduction of the Minnitt apparatus in 1934, which delivered a mixture of nitrous oxide in air. In 1961, the currently used 50 : 50 mixture of nitrous oxide and oxygen was described by Tunstall. While nitrous oxide has remained in use, other inhalational agents (trichloroethylene and methoxyflurane) administered in air via drawover vaporisers have come and gone.

The use of systemic analgesics in labour was not seen until 1902 when von Steinbuchel introduced the combination of morphine and scopolamine. In 1940, pethidine was first used and has remained the most commonly used systemic analgesic in obstetric practice in the UK to this day.

The earliest use of local anaesthetics in labour dates from 1910 when Stiasny applied cocaine to the vagina and vulva. Although spinal subarachnoid analgesia had first been performed in 1885, it was not until 1928 that Pitkin popularised its use in obstetric practice. Lumbar epidural analgesia was described by Dogliotti in the 1940s, but continuous lumbar epidural analgesia only became popular in the UK in the late 1960s.

The variety of techniques available for relieving labour pain should mean that every mother can find a method that will suit her. However, the actual technique used will vary according to local availability and other pressures; the provision of a full range of techniques may be hampered by lack of staff or funds.

NON-PHARMACOLOGICAL METHODS

Psychophysical methods

Psychoprophylaxis is often wrongly considered as a simple distraction technique, when in fact it is far more broad-based; the total package consists of antenatal preparation and education along with the development of various techniques of relaxation. In preparation for labour, the mother requires careful explanation of events that may happen, hopefully allaying her fear. This form of instruction has formed part of the basis of *natural childbirth* as first introduced by Dick-Read in the 1930s (Dick-Read 1944). Fumdamental to this philosophy is the belief that pain is the result of fear and misinterpretation of sensations associated with uterine contractions. If the mother learns how to relax fully and how to dissociate herself from the episode of contraction, labour can become an enjoyable experience. While some may scorn the aims of natural childbirth, it is prudent to remember that a relaxed and fully prepared mother is likely to be easier to manage should problems arise in labour.

While psychoprophylaxis may be of value in early labour, it is seldom satisfactory for the whole of labour. Studies on the efficacy of psychoprophylaxis are often difficult to compare with other approaches but one well-conducted study has been reported (Scott & Rose 1976). Two matched groups were compared; one had attended a full course of psychoprophylaxis classes based on the Lamaze method while the other had not. The results showed that the prepared group had a higher frequency of spontaneous vaginal delivery, which possibly related to the lower rate of epidural block employed in this group. In other aspects—length of labour, Apgar scores and incidence of fetal distress—there was no difference between the groups. In UK hospitals, where a wide range of pain relief methods is available, less than 5% of mothers use only psychophysical techniques.

Transcutaneous nerve stimulation

Transcutaneous nerve stimulation (TENS) involves the application of a variable electrical stimulus to the skin at the site of pain and is based upon the gate theory of pain control (Melzac & Wall 1965). Observational studies have shown there to be great or considerable relief of early labour pain in 20–24% of mothers with about 60% having slight relief (Robson 1979). It is said to be most helpful for backache. However, a controlled study of two parity groups comparing TENS and a placebo (Harrison et al 1986) showed that in terms of pain relief there was no difference between the groups. Nonetheless, mothers did find the apparatus reassuring and the study concludes that TENS may have a part to play in early or short labours.

SYSTEMIC OPIOID ANALGESIA

Systemic opioids, especially pethidine, are widely used for analgesia in labour. Since 1950, midwives in the United Kingdom have been allowed to give pethidine intramuscularly on their own initiative, without requiring it to be prescribed by a doctor. At the time, it was believed that it would have fewer side effects than morphine.

Pethidine's popularity seems not to have been based on its analgesic properties, but possibly more on its ease of administration, popularity with mothers, minimal cost and the midwife's autonomy over its use. The use of pethidine continues in many units, especially where there is not a full epidural service. In other units, especially where there is a high epidural up-take, the use of pethidine has diminished.

The pain of labour seems to be only partially amenable to systemic opioids (Rayburn et al 1989). Because of the episodic nature of labour pain the mother tends to receive little analgesia during contractions but may become oversedated at other times. This can lead to periods of respiratory depression and even hypoxia between contractions. Only about 25% of women feel that pethidine gave them good pain relief in labour (Morgan et al 1982).

Studies evaluating pethidine with other opioids have not been critical as to the analgesic usefulness of the drugs. In one study, despite 50 mg of intravenous pethidine 2–3 hourly, pain scores were reported as 6/10 in early labour and 9/10 in late labour (Rayburn et al 1989). These results are comparable with a more recent study that found no analgesic effect after the administration of either pethidine or morphine (Olofsson et al 1996). This study found that sedation increased successively after each dose, which may be why opioids are popular.

Patient-controlled intravenous administration of opioids has been investigated. It is theoretically possible to treat the pain of a contraction with an intravenous bolus of a drug, which will match the onset of pain and will have a diminishing effect between contractions. This should reduce the side-effects of sedation and respiratory depression. At present there are no opioids suitable for intravenous injection with an analgesic onset and elimination that can match the pattern of contractions. When patient controlled intravenous pethidine has been investigated there has been no consistent benefit in pain relief, but only a tendency to use less drug compared with intermittent intramuscular or intravenous groups. The evaluation of different opioids with various drug regimens is required.

Side-effects

In the doses commonly used for labour analgesia e.g. pethidine 50–150 mg/3–4 hourly, severe respiratory depression in the mother is uncommon. With these doses, however, there will be a significant delay in gastric emptying (Nimmo et al 1975). This places the mother at greater risk from acid aspiration syndrome, should she require emergency general anaesthesia. In some units, mothers who are given opioids are also given metoclopramide to reduce nausea and vomiting and increase gastric emptying and ranitidine to reduce gastric acidity.

Pethidine and the newborn

Pethidine along with the other opioids rapidly crosses the placenta into the baby. Babies who are becoming acidotic are particularly vulnerable from placental transfer (Gaylard et al 1990), as the drug becomes more ionised in the neonatal circulation and cannot pass back into the mother, as her blood levels diminish. The effect on the baby is greatest within 2–3 hours of maternal administration and after repeated doses. Intrauterine sedation may cause a reduction in baseline variability on the cardiotocograph (CTG), and make obstetric interpretation difficult. Babies tend to be born with lower Apgar scores, because of respiratory depression and are more likely to require treatment with naloxone. Babies who do not appear to have obvious respiratory depression at birth are more likely to be sleepy and are slower to establish feeding (Wiener et al 1979).

NITROUS OXIDE

Until 1983 when the Central Midwives Board withdrew approval for the use of trichloroethylene by unsupervised midwives, there were three agents available for use: nitrous oxide, trichloroethylene and methoxyflurane. Currently only nitrous oxide is available in the UK, the other inhalational agents having been withdrawn.

Nitrous oxide has been available throughout the last 100 years for analgesia in labour. Minnitt developed a device that mixed 50% nitrous oxide and air and was portable enough to be used by midwives during home delivery. The major drawback with this device was that the final mixture contained only 10% oxygen, which could be reduced further if the air inlet of the device became obstructed.

Nitrous oxide is analgesic in sub-anaesthetic concentrations and because of its low solubility in blood, rapidly achieves an analgesic concentration in the brain after five to six breaths (Waud & Waud 1970). The onset of analgesia can be matched with the onset of the contraction if used properly and the effects rapidly disappear between contractions. Intermittent use reduces the side-effects of nausea, sedation and disorientation.

Since 1960, nitrous oxide has been available as a 50:50 mixture with oxygen in a single cylinder (Entonox). A higher percentage of nitrous oxide is not beneficial as it does not improve analgesia but increases sedation, especially if taken between contractions (Cole et al 1970).

The effectiveness of Entonox as an analgesic is variable. In a survey, 46% of women found it satisfactory but 30% felt that they received no benefit from its use (Morgan et al 1982). In the only placebo-controlled study, Entonox was compared with compressed air over five contractions. There were no differences in pain scores between the groups nor did they differ from baseline recordings (Carstoniu et al 1994). The effectiveness of Entonox is probably very dependent on the way it is used with the maximum effect after 5–6 breaths being timed with the peak of a contraction.

Entonox has been studied with a background nasal infusion in an attempt to make it more effective. It was found that additional nasal Entonox was helpful. There was however more sedation and the overall additional effect was small (Arthurs & Rosen 1979). Entonox has also been supplemented with other inhalational anaesthetic agents. Isoflurane 0.2% has gained some popularity, with a high acceptability rate and a modest improvement in analgesia (Wee et al 1993). The concentration of these drugs has to be strictly controlled as anaesthesia can be rapidly induced if higher concentrations are used with 50% nitrous oxide.

Entonox is very popular in the UK because it is readily available, easy to use, the mother feels in control of its administration and it is an effective analgesic for some mothers.

Side-effects

Persistent hyperventilation, which can occur during use, can cause a respiratory alkalosis. The maternal oxygen dissociation curve is displaced to the left making oxygen less available to the baby. Hypoxia, because of reduced respiratory drive, may occur between contractions. The use of nitrous oxide for prolonged periods of time can cause exhaustion and the dry gases contribute to dehydration.

Nitrous oxide is also associated with abnormalities of vitamin B12 metabolism and the safety of chronic low-level exposure of health care workers has been questioned. There is no scientific evidence to support this but it would be especially relevant to midwives as nitrous oxide levels can be high in small under-ventilated delivery rooms.

Neonatal effect

The overall effect on the baby is small with intermittent use of nitrous oxide as a 50:50 mixture with oxygen. Although there is rapid placental transfer of the drug, elimination is also rapid.

Table 28.1 Non-regional techniques for labour analgesia

- The pain of labour seems only partly amenable to systemic opioids.
- Repeated doses sedate the mother and make the cardiotocograph difficult to interpret.
- Nitrous oxide is safe in a 50:50 mixture with oxygen.
- Prolonged use can cause maternal dehydration, exhaustion and respiratory alkalosis leading to placental vessel vasoconstriction and fetal acidosis.
- Transcutaneous nerve stimulation is safe but seems to give satisfactory pain-relief only in early labour.
- Other non-pharmacological methods such as phychoprophylaxis should not be dismissed as beneficial but studies have not yet been conclusive.

REGIONAL ANALGESIA

Central nerve blockade (epidural and spinal)

Spinal and epidural techniques for analgesia in labour have been available for the last 100 years, but have become popular in the last 30 years with the advent of 24-hour epidural services in many hospitals. The Mother's Hospital in Glasgow was the first to offer round-the-clock epidurals for any mother in 1965, and by 1997, 90% of units in the UK offered this service, with an average epidural rate of 24% (Burnstein et al 1999). The increasing availability and popularity of epidurals has caused controversy because of potential implications it has on obstetric care and because of common side-effects associated with the techniques.

The availability and use of analgesic techniques

While there are a number of analgesic techniques available to the mother, not all delivery units are able to offer the full range and as each mother is an individual, it is not surprising that there is wide variability in the type of analgesia used. The situation about availability and maternal usage was last comprehensively investigated in a national survey conducted by the National Birthday Trust (Chamberlain et al 1993). This survey was conducted over one week in 1990 and covers data from 15 900 mothers throughout the UK. In total, 293 obstetric units participated in the survey.

The availability of non-drug methods for pain relief is shown in Table 28.2. There was a high, possibly media-driven, availability of TENS. The relative unavailability of acupuncture or hypnosis probably reflects the time-consuming nature of these methods of analgesia.

The availability of drugs for pain relief is shown in Table 28.3. An epidural service was available in over 70% of units with approximately three-quarters of these providing a 24-hour service; in the other units availability was limited. Pethidine and Entonox were available in 97.6% and 99% of units, respectively.

Table 28.2 The availability of non-drug methods of pain relief (Chamberlain et al 1993)

Method	Units No.	%
TENS and relaxation	146	54.3
Relaxation	71	26.4
TENS alone	18	6.7
TENS, relaxation and hypnosis	12	4.5
TENS, relaxation and acupuncture	10	3.7
Acupuncture alone	3	1.1
All above	3	1.1
Acupuncture and relaxation	2	0.7
Hypnosis and relaxation	2	0.7
Acupuncture and hypnosis	1	0.4
Hypnosis alone	1	0.4

Table 28.3 The availability of drugs for pain relief

	Units No.	%
Entonox, pethidine and epidural	151	52.4
Entonox and pethidine	60	20.8
Entonox, pethidine, epidural and other	56	19.4
Entonox, pethidine and other	13	4.5
Entonox, epidural and other	3	1
Entonox only	2	0.7
Epidural only	1	0.3
Pethidine only	1	0.3
Other only	1	0.3

The actual main method of pain relief used by mothers in the survey, as recorded by the midwife, is presented in Table 28.4. The figures presented are not mutually exclusive as some mothers had significant use of more than one type of analgesia. The overall findings show that more than 50% of mothers had Entonox and about 40% received pethidine. Approximately 18% of mothers used an epidural in labour at this time although in an anaesthetic survey conducted in 1997, this rate had increased to 24%. Despite the high media profile of non-drug methods of pain relief, they were seldom used as the main method.

The effectiveness of the various methods of analgesia used was assessed by using the mothers' opinion as to whether a method was helpful to unhelpful. The benefit of the various methods is presented in Table 28.5. If one considers the ratio of helpful to unhelpful as a measure of the effectiveness of a method, it is clear that epidural analgesia is by far the most effective.

The conduct of spinal and epidural blockade

Nerve roots contain nerve fibres of different sizes. Some pain and sympathetic nerve impulses are carried in C fibres. They do not have an axonal covering and are readily penetrated by local anaesthetic solutions. Aδ fibres are intermediate in size and carry somatic pain associated with stretching of the perineum. Motor nerves are Aα and most difficult to block. The difference in nerve size has led to the concept of differential blockade. Correct local anaesthetic dosing can provide analgesia without anaesthesia. Anaesthesia is associated with dense motor blockade and unwanted paralysis. 'Motor loss is not infrequently a source of apprehension and complaint among our other-wise satisfied patient' (Crawford 1975).

Table 28.4 The frequency of main analgesic method used as recorded by the midwife

Method	Number	%
Entonox	5706	55.1
Pethidine	3916	37.8
Other narcotic analgesics	712	3.4
Relaxation	406	3.9
Epidural	1834	17.7
TENS	428	4.1
Massage	515	5.0
Other	24	0.2

Table 28.5 Methods of pain relief identified by the woman as helpful and unhelpful as a percentage of their use

Method	Helpful (%)	Unhelpful (%)
Relaxation	32	13
Massage	22	12
TENS	22	20
Pethidine	28	14
Entonox	43	13
Epidural	73	4

Absolute contraindications

Absolute contraindications to regional analgesia in labour are:

- the mother refuses permission for the epidural
- sepsis in the lumbosacral region involving the area through which the epidural needle will pass
- any condition that will lead to a maternal coagulopathy.

The fear in these last two situations is that the formation of an abscess or haematoma may cause spinal cord compression. Scott & Hibbard (1990), in a survey of over half a million obstetric epidurals, found only one case of an epidural abscess and one of an epidural haematoma. In both cases, surgical decompression was performed and there was a degree of neurological recovery.

Obstetric conditions that predispose to coagulopathy include moderate or severe pre-eclampsia, placental abruptions, prolonged retention of products of conception, recent spontaneous abortion and thrombocytopenia. If it is deemed necessary or desirable to use epidural analgesia in any mother in these groups, it is essential that coagulation studies should confirm normal clotting. Such tests must have been performed immediately (less than 30 minutes) before commencement of the procedure.

Full anticoagulation (but not low-dose heparin: Minihep) is an absolute contraindication to epidural analgesia. If it is necessary to give anticoagulants to a mother with an epidural *in situ*, a period of 30 minutes should pass after insertion of the catheter in order to ensure that any traumatised vessel has time to seal. After a dose of low molecular weight heparin (LMWH), a period of 12–24 hours must pass, depending on the dose, before insertion.

In any mother with coagulopathy, whether of pathological or therapeutic origin, it is also important that normal coagulation is present prior to the withdrawal of the catheter as damage can also be caused.

Relative contraindications

Progressive neurological disease has traditionally been considered a relative contraindication to regional analgesia in labour, on the grounds that such disease may be unpredictable, leading to relapse at any time. If a relapse coincides with the use of an epidural there could be a dispute over the possibility of damage having been caused by the epidural. It is advisable in any mother with such a disease to explain the situation at length (and document the explanation) prior to embarking upon epidural.

Epidural analgesia

A local anaesthetic solution given into the epidural space penetrates the neural covering of the nerve roots before entering the nerves, causing depolarisation and blockade. Pain during the first part of labour can easily be treated by bilateral blockade of the T10–12 nerve roots. As labour advances, pain arises from the pelvis, so the sacral nerve roots have also to be blocked. The nerve roots are thicker in the sacral region compared with thoracic and lumbar regions and local anaesthetics penetrate them slowly. This makes an epidural less useful in the later stages of labour (Chestnut et al 1990).

The major problem with epidural analgesia is that, unless a high concentration of local anaesthetic solution is used, the block can be slow in onset. If the local anaesthetic solution does not spread evenly in the epidural space, a patchy or unilateral block can result. Because of the plexus of veins in the epidural space, there can be a bloody tap on initial catheter placement and catheter migration into a blood vessel at any time during labour, leading to potential intravenous administration of local anaesthetic solutions. The proximity of the dura can result in accidental dural puncture on initial insertion of the Tuohy needle with a high incidence of post dural puncture headache, and catheter migration at any time during labour can cause dangerously high sensory and motor blockade (Crawford 1985).

Spinal analgesia

Spinal analgesia is more commonly associated with anaesthesia for caesarean section. Spinal anaesthesia has recently increased in popularity because of the introduction of pencil-point atraumatic spinal needles. In the past, a Quincke or cutting-tipped needle was the only type available. The problem was that the incidence of post dural puncture headache in obstetric patients was as high as 10% even with fine needles of a Quincke design (Tarkkila et al 1994). In contrast, the incidence of such headaches is less than 1% with 25G needles of the new design (Smith et al 1994).

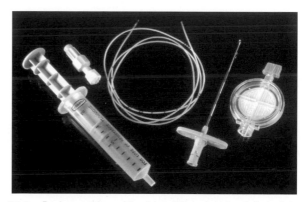

Fig. 28.1 Equipment for epidural insertion, showing left to right: loss of resistance syringe, catheter, Tuohy needle and filter.

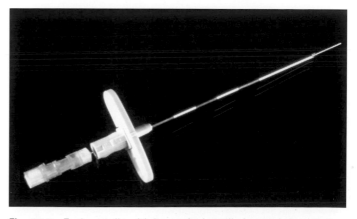

Fig. 28.2 Tuohy needle with long spinal needle inserted through it. Used for combined spinal–epidural technique.

Local anaesthetic solutions injected into the cerebrospinal fluid (CSF) have a quicker and more direct route into spinal nerves compared with injection into the epidural space, because of the absence of dural coverings. The dose of local anaesthetic can be reduced by a factor of five–ten times.

The advantage of spinal injection for labour pain relief is that a small dose of a local anaesthetic injected into the CSF will give almost instantaneous analgesia (Collis et al 1994). There is little risk of unilateral blockade and sacral analgesia is excellent. Intrathecal injection is an excellent technique for mothers requesting analgesia in late or rapidly progressing labour (Stacey et al 1993, Abouleish et al 1994) or where analgesia is required for instrumental vaginal delivery. The dose that is needed is so small that systemic toxicity is very unlikely. The major disadvantage is that as described, it is a single shot technique. Spinal analgesia will only last for one to two hours and as labour may continue for many more hours, it will become inadequate.

Spinal catheters. Spinal catheters can be positioned in the CSF to provide continuous spinal analgesia (Kestin et al 1992). The incidence of post dural puncture headache is the same as for the single shot technique, and depends entirely on the size of the hole made in the dura with the introducer needle. The finest catheter currently available in the UK is a 32G wire-supported microcatheter, which can be passed either through a 26G Quincke point, or a 24G Sprotte needle. However, this catheter has been associated in the USA with four cases of cauda-equina syndrome in surgical patients (Rigler et al 1991). Catheters smaller than 24G were subsequently withdrawn in the USA, although they are still available in the UK. A 24G catheter may be positioned using an 18G spinal needle but this is unacceptable for routine obstetric use because of the high incidence of post dural puncture headache.

Their usefulness will probably be limited to special circumstances such as analgesia for mothers who have had spinal surgery with internal splintage for severe kypho-scoliosis limiting access to the epidural space.

Combined spinal–epidural analgesia. Combined spinal–epidural (CSE) analgesia combines the benefit of rapid, reliable analgesia from a small dose of local anaesthetic intrathecally, and the flexibility to continue analgesia for as long as labour lasts with an epidural catheter (Rawal et al 1991).

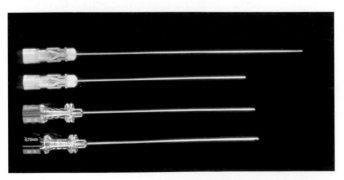

Fig. 28.3 Spinal needles commonly used. Bottom to top: 22G Sprotte, 24G Sprotte, 25G Whitacre, 27G 119 mm Whitacre for needle-through-needle combined spinal epidural.

There are several techniques for performing combined spinal–epidural analgesia.

- The single space needle-through-needle technique involves finding the epidural space with a Tuohy needle and, because of the narrow distance from the ligamentum flavum to the dura, deliberately puncturing the dura with a longer spinal needle. The initial injection is made into the CSF through the spinal needle. The spinal needle is withdrawn and an epidural catheter positioned in the epidural space. The technique can be performed with any spinal needle that is about 2 cm longer than the complete length of the Tuohy needle. The Tuohy needle supports the spinal needle and is therefore the perfect introducer for a very fine spinal needle, which in other circumstances can be technically difficult to use. The advantage is that by reducing the size of the spinal needle to 25G or 27G, the post dural puncture headache rate associated with the spinal injection can be as low as 0.03%. The disadvantage is that there is the additional expense of the long spinal needle. Also the technique has to be carefully taught, therefore it may not be universally available.

- A separate spinal injection can also be performed with a standard spinal needle and the epidural catheter inserted later in the usual way. The advantage of this double technique is that many anaesthetists are more familiar with the separate insertion of spinal and Tuohy needle. It may also reduce the risk of accidental dural puncture with the Tuohy needle if the mother is distressed and finding it difficult to lie still. The epidural catheter can then be more safely inserted, once the mother is comfortable from the initial spinal injection. The disadvantage is that the mother perceives the technique as two separate injections into her back.

Drugs

Local anaesthetics

Local anaesthetics act on nerve axons causing localised depolarisation, which prevents propagation of nerve impulses. Local anaesthetic solutions injected either into the epidural or subarachnoid space produce segmental blockade, depending on the spread of the local anaesthetic.

Local anaesthetics are used in labour analgesia and also anaesthesia for caesarean section. The major difference between the two uses is the concentration required. In labour, successful analgesia can be achieved with 0.125% bupivacaine or even less if mixed with an opioid (Chestnut et al 1990). For caesarean section, because the blockade of thoracic and sacral nerves must be more intense, bupivacaine 0.5% is required. The difference in bupivacaine requirement for labour and caesarean section is also seen with spinal injection. A dose of 2.5–5 mg bupivacaine will give good analgesia in labour but 10–15 mg bupivacaine is needed for caesarean section.

Lignocaine. Lignocaine is an amide-linked local anaesthetic, which was first synthesised in 1943. It has been widely used for all types of regional blockade but its use in obstetrics is limited. Although lignocaine has a rapid onset of action, its use during prolonged labour where repeated doses were required was problematic. When lignocaine was used for labour analgesia, successive top-ups were required at progressively shorter intervals and increased doses to maintain analgesia, a phenomenon known as tachyphylaxis. The mother became drowsy and enough lignocaine passed across the placenta to make the neonate floppy at birth.

Although lignocaine was almost abandoned after the introduction of bupivacaine, its use has increased more recently for topping-up an epidural that has been in use during labour, for caesarean section. It is reliable in producing a rapid dense block especially when adrenaline and bicarbonate are added (Fernando & Jones 1991). As a one-off top-up, it does not cause the side-effects, which were previously recognised.

Bupivacaine. Bupivacaine was introduced in 1963 and by the end of the 1960s had replaced lignocaine as the local anaesthetic of choice for epidural analgesia in labour. Bupivacaine was a great improvement because it does not cause tachyphylaxis and produces better motor–sensory separation. Bupivacaine is a mixture of the S and R stereoisomers of the drug and has been associated with cardiotoxicity. When it became available in the US, it was used in a concentration of 0.75%. There were a number of case reports of resistant ventricular fibrillation associated with inadvertent intravascular injection (Albright 1979). In the UK, where no more than 0.5% solutions are used, this has not been a documented problem with accidental intravascular injection. The pain of labour can be well treated with bupivacaine solutions of 0.125% (Bogod et al 1987). At these low concentrations cardiotoxicity is not a major risk, but a 0.5% solution has to be used for caesarean section, and toxicity may then occur.

Most of the cardiotoxicity is caused by the R (right-handed or dextro-rotatory) isomer of the drug, and experiments with the S (left-handed or levo-rotatory) isomer compared with racemic bupivacaine show it to be less toxic. This has led to the quest for single S-isomer local anaesthetics (Aberg 1972).

Ropivacaine. The S enantiomer of the N-alkyl piperidine series of local anaesthetics has recently become available. When compared with racemic bupivacaine in experimental animals, it caused fewer arrhythmias at the same dose (Pitkanen et al 1992). The therapeutic index of the S is greater and therefore safer. In practice, ropivacaine is less potent than bupivacaine (Capogna et al 1999) and the clear-cut reduction in toxicity of ropivacaine compared with racemic bupivacaine may not be so clear-cut if equipotent doses are used. The motor block may be shorter and less intense than bupivacaine and, therefore, this drug has gained some popularity for labour analgesia (Zaric et al 1996).

Levobupivacaine. Levobupivacaine is the S-isomer of bupivacaine. Levobupivacaine shows a similar reduction in cardiotoxicity to ropivacaine with far fewer fatal arrhythmias when given intravenously into experimental animals (Santos et al 1995). In contrast to ropivacaine however, the S-isomer does not seem to be less potent than the racemic mixture, which may make it a more useful drug (Lyons et al 1998). Large scale clinical surveillance will have to be undertaken

before levobupivacaine will be accepted into routine obstetric practice, because of the reliability of racemic bupivacaine.

Epidural and spinal opioids

These drugs have been increasingly accepted over the past 10 years in obstetric anaesthetic practice both for labour and caesarean section. They can be used alone during labour, especially intrathecally (Scott et al 1998, Leighton et al 1989), but more commonly as an adjunct to local anaesthetics (Collis et al 1995), where analgesia can be provided with marked local anaesthetic sparing. Opioids injected into the epidural or subarachnoid space readily pass into the substantia gelatinosa of the spinal cord, which contains opiate receptors. It is mainly at spinal cord level where opioids produce analgesia. The dose of an opioid can be reduced by a factor of 5–10 when injected into the CSF, compared with the epidural space (Camann et al 1992). When opioids are used in the epidural or subarachnoid space, the lower doses required confer advantages over systemic use. Opioids in the epidural space will be absorbed into the epidural veins, but the total dose is lower than that required systemically and the rate of intravascular absorption slower. Maternal blood levels are lower than after systemic administration, which reduces the placental transfer of the drugs. Opioid levels in the fetal circulation at delivery are low and behavioural scoring systems have failed to demonstrate any major adverse effects in the baby, of using epidural or subarachnoid opioids (Loftus et al 1995). This is in direct contrast to opioids given systemically to the mother, where high maternal peaks of these drugs facilitate rapid transfer of the drugs across the placenta into the fetus (Table 28.6).

Fentanyl. This is a short acting lipophilic drug that rapidly binds to opiate receptors in the spinal cord. With minimal spread in the CSF, the incidence of central side-effects of the drug is low. The incidence of serious side-effects, such as maternal respiratory depression, is very low, as is the incidence of nausea (Carrie et al 1981). It has been a popular drug in obstetric analgesia and can be given as a bolus or infusion. Fentanyl has a duration of action of between 4 and 6 hours when given epidurally, which makes it ideal for labour. By giving a bolus of fentanyl 50–100 μg and infusing it at a rate of 1–3 μg/hour with bupivacaine in the epidural space, the dose of bupivacaine can be reduced by 20–50%. Infusions of bupivacaine 0.0625% with fentanyl have been successfully used for labour analgesia (Chestnut et al 1990).

Table 28.6 A guide to doses of bupivacaine and opioides for labour analgesia

	Stat epidural dose	Infusion epidural dose	Stat intrathecal dose[a]
Bupivacaine	15–30 mg	0.0625–0.125%	2.5–10 mg
Fentanyl	50–100 μg	2–3 μg/ml	15–25 μg
Sufentanil	25–50 μg	1–2 μg/ml	5–15 μg
Pethidine	50–100 mg	–	10–20 mg
Diamorphine	2.5–5 mg	0.025 mg/ml	0.125–0.375 mg
Morphine	2.5–5 mg	–	0.1–0.25 mg

[a] Intrathecal drugs must be preservative free

Sufentanil. This is also a short-acting highly lipophilic drug, which has similar characteristics to fentanyl, and can be used intrathecally (Sia et al 1998) and mixed with a local anaesthetic in the epidural space (Vertommen et al 1994). It is more potent than fentanyl, especially when injected into the CSF. Doses of 5–10 µg have been used without local anaesthetics to produce rapid initiation of analgesia when injected into the CSF. Epidural sufentanil is approved in the USA for combined use with bupivacaine in obstetrics, but is not available in the UK. There is no substantial data that demonstrate a significant difference between it and an equipotent dose of fentanyl (Honet et al 1992).

Morphine. This has been used in the epidural and sub-arachnoid space for 15 years. It is not popular because it is much less lipophilic than fentanyl and it can cause late respiratory depression because of cephalic migration. Other side-effects such as nausea, drowsiness and pruritus are also more troublesome than with the more lipid soluble opioids. Analgesia is unreliable in labour if given in safe small doses of 100–200 µg intrathecally (Leighton et al 1989) but morphine has been used historically, in a much larger dose of 1.5 mg intrathecally (Scott et al 1980). Although this dose produced good analgesia during labour it is dangerous because of the high risk of maternal respiratory depression.

Because of its duration of action, morphine has gained popularity for analgesia after caesarean section. In a dose of 100 µg intrathecally (Palmer et al 1999) or 3–5 mg epidurally (Booker et al 1980, Asantila et al 1995), it is safe and effective, but respiratory monitoring is recommended for 12–24 hours after administration, which is impractical in some obstetric units.

Other adjuncts to local anaesthetics

Adrenaline (epinephrine). This is commonly added to local anaesthetics for epidural administration in doses of 25–100 µg. It increases the duration and intensity of blockade. The mechanism of action is likely to be vasoconstriction of epidural veins, thus reducing systemic absorption of local anaesthetics. Its other mechanism of action may be related to α_2-adrenergic agonism, which at spinal level may produce spinal analgesia. Adrenaline increases the likelihood of motor block (Lysak et al 1990) and is, therefore, of limited use in labour analgesia, but it can be useful during caesarean section.

Clonidine. Like adrenaline, clonidine produces spinal analgesia through α_2-adrenergic agonism. Clonidine intensifies and prolongs analgesia in a dose dependent fashion. It has been used in an infusion at 150 µg/h, where it increased the analgesia from 50 mg of bupivacaine by 100% (O'Meara & Gin 1993). Its major side-effects of sedation and hypotension are also dose related, and like adrenaline it intensifies motor blockade from local anaesthetics. For these reasons, its use for labour analgesia it probably limited.

Initiating analgesia in labour

Epidural space
The epidural space is the most common starting point for labour analgesia. Its major drawback is that the onset of analgesia may be delayed, patchy or unilateral. The rate of onset

Table 28.7 Drugs used in epidural or spinal anaesthesia and analgesia

- Local anaesthetics cause localised depolarisation of nerve fibres and segmental blockade.
- There is a 5–10-fold difference in the quantity of drug required between the epidural and subarachnoid space for local anaesthetics and opioids.
- Opioids reduce the quantity of local anaesthetic required for labour analgesia by 50%.
- The major benefit to the mother is a reduction in motor block.
- Opioids added to epidural or spinal bupivacaine for caesarean section improve the reliability of the technique.
- The long acting opioids morphine and diamorphine can provide safe and reliable analgesia after caesarean section.

and quality of analgesia can be improved by adding an opioid such as 25–100 µg of fentanyl (Janes & McCrory 1991), or increasing the initial dose of bupivacaine (Plaat et al 1996). The amount of bupivacaine required for rapid reliable analgesia is related to the stage and rate of labour (Capogna et al 1998). Better spread of local anaesthetic solutions can be achieved by increasing the volume in which the local anaesthetic is mixed. An example of this would be 20 ml of 0.125% bupivacaine rather than 10 ml of 0.25% bupivacaine. A good starting dose in early labour (less than 5 cm cervical dilatation) is 10–20 mg of bupivacaine mixed in 15 ml with normal saline and 20–100 µg of fentanyl. The dose of bupivacaine may have to be increased in advancing labour to 25–30 mg. If the larger doses are used, then the inevitable consequence is motor block in the legs. Once motor block is established, it rarely resolves until the epidural is discontinued. It is best practice to use the smallest initial dose possible and if analgesia is inadequate after 15–20 minutes, then to give an early top-up. After one dose of 25 mg of bupivacaine (10 ml of 0.25% bupivacaine), 30% of women will have motor block (Collis et al 1995), although this is still the most common starting dose in the epidural space for labour (Burnstein et al 1999).

The subarachnoid space
The major advantage of giving the first dose intrathecally is almost instantaneous analgesia, usually within 1 or 2 contractions even in rapidly advancing labour (Abouleish et al 1994). This analgesia, which is complete and gives especially good sacral analgesia, provides the mother with a great sense of relief. Doses of bupivacaine 2.5–5 mg (Stacey et al 1993) have been used to produce spinal analgesia successfully. Fentanyl 15–25 µg or sufentanil 5–10 µg is usually added to the smaller dose of bupivacaine for reliable analgesia. This analgesia typically lasts for 60–90 minutes. Although analgesia is profound, a differential block with little motor block is most evident when bupivacaine is used in this way.

The major disadvantages of a subarachnoid injection are:

- The incidence of post dural puncture headache.
- Anxiety about central nervous system infection.
- Spinal analgesia is most commonly a one shot technique and therefore analgesia from this route alone will be inadequate for most labouring women.

A CSE technique is therefore used if rapid onset of pain relief from a spinal injection is required, followed by epidural analgesia that can be continued until delivery. In a major comparison of epidural and CSE technique there were no excess of complication in the CSE group (Norris et al 1994).

The test dose

After an epidural catheter has been positioned in the epidural space, a test dose is given. As the epidural catheter placement is a blind technique it is necessary to test for accidental intravascular or intrathecal placement.

Intravascular injection of a test dose may cause subtoxic symptoms such as tingling around the mouth and ringing in the ears, caused by local anaesthetic toxicity, while adrenaline may cause a transitory tachycardia. Intravascular placement can usually be excluded, however, by careful aspiration of the epidural catheter.

An epidural catheter positioned in the epidural space initially may migrate into the subarachnoid space or into a blood vessel. The nurse or midwife, who is left to look after the epidural, must be constantly aware of the signs of misplacement. Those who are trained to give epidural top-ups must treat each administration into the epidural space as a test dose.

Continuing epidural analgesia in labour

Epidural analgesia can be administered as a bolus, continuous infusion or patient-controlled epidural analgesia (PCEA). It has rapidly become best practice to use dilute solutions of bupivacaine with fentanyl or sufentanil. Solutions as dilute as 0.0625% with fentanyl have been used successfully, although more commonly 0.08–0.1% bupivacaine solutions are used, as they are more reliable. A solution of 0.125% without an opioid can provide good analgesia (Bogod et al 1987).

Continuous infusion

After the initial analgesic dose, an infusion into the epidural space is usually started at 10–15 ml/h. This maintains the height of the block at about T10, and encourages spread to the sacral roots. An advantage of a continuous infusion is that compared to a bolus technique, there may be more consistent analgesia and smaller swings in sympathetic blockade and therefore less hypotension (Li et al 1985). From personal experience, it is also possible that there may be fewer episodes of moderate pain breakthrough. It has consistently been shown, however, that infusions use relatively more bupivacaine in early labour, while as labour advances, analgesia may become inadequate. The epidural then needs to be topped up using a bolus technique in addition to the infusion. The result is that an infusion compared to a bolus technique uses 50–100% more bupivacaine and is, therefore, associated with more motor block (Smedstad et al 1988).

Bolus top-ups

Bolus top-ups are usually described as a technique for labour analgesia that can be maintained by the midwife. Traditionally, the midwife gave 6–10 ml of 0.25% bupivacaine in divided doses, because of the risk of giving large amounts of bupivacaine through a misplaced catheter. As dilute bupivacaine/opioid mixtures have become commonplace, it is increasingly accepted as good practice for the pharmacy department to prepare these drugs. Accuracy and sterility can be maintained and trained midwives can use these drug mixtures safely.

Midwife controlled epidural boluses can result in a very high standard of analgesia. The midwife must be trained to respond to the mother's request for analgesia as soon as a sensation of discomfort returns, rather than wait for pain. With low concentration bupivacaine and opion mixtures, the time between discomfort and pain may only be a few minutes, and the onset of new analgesia slower than with the old high dose boluses. The major advance of this technique is analgesia can be tailored more specifically to the mother's analgesic requirement. A bolus technique may preserve the mother's mobility for longer (Collis et al 1999).

Patient-controlled epidural analgesia

Patient-controlled epidural analgesia allows the mother herself to give her own top-ups using a specially programmed pump. The important features in achieving good pain control is that the epidural catheter must be in the correct place with appropriate bilateral sensory blockade on initial dosing. There have been a number of regimens described, which vary from setting a small bolus of 2–4 ml with a 10–15 minute lockout to a larger bolus 6–10 ml with a 30 minute lockout (Gambling et al 1990, 1993). The first type is sometimes prescribed with an additional background infusion. The latter is very similar to the boluses a midwife could give, but allows the mother to give her own analgesia (Collis et al 1999, Paech et al 1995).

The safety feature of all these regimens is that a single dose given through a misplaced catheter will cause no harm. The opponents of this delivery system are concerned that the mother may give herself a top-up without her midwife knowing. She may develop hypotension without blood pressure recordings and treatment could be delayed.

Patient-controlled epidural analgesia has been made possible by the introduction of small portable infusion devices and many women have welcomed the additional control it gives. As with midwife-controlled boluses, there is a reduc-

Table 28.8 Techniques for regional anaesthesia and analgesia

- The most common starting place for labour analgesia is the epidural space.
- In advancing labour, analgesia is more reliable if started in the subarachnoid space using a technique called combined spinal and epidural analgesia.
- Analgesia can be maintained by delivering local anaesthetics and opioid mixtures into the epidural space by continuous infusion or top-ups. The mother can give her own top-ups using PCEA.
- A working epidural for analgesia in labour can be safely topped up for emergency caesarean section.
- Spinal anaesthesia is more reliable when anaesthesia is required *de novo*.

tion in bupivacaine usage and preservation of mobility. The mother must, however, be properly taught about the safety aspects of using the device and its limitations.

Why reduce motor blockade?

Although many women have been grateful for the introduction of an epidural service since the 1970s, it was recognised from the outset that the accompanying feeling of paralysis and helplessness was less welcome (Crawford 1975). Routine practice in the 1970s was epidural top-ups of 0.5% bupivacaine given in divided doses (Doughty 1975). It was slowly realised that 0.25% and then 0.125% bupivacaine was adequate for the treatment of most pain in labour (Vanderick et al 1974). The introduction of epidural opioids reduced the dose of bupivacaine that was required still further (Cohen et al 1987). This has dramatically reduced the degree of motor block from almost complete paralysis of hips, knees and ankles to a level of motor blockade where the mother has good knee and ankle movement, although commonly still has a degree of hip weakness (Russell & Reynolds 1996). The mother is able to move herself around the bed with little help, and her perception of the analgesia has improved with this reduction in motor blockade.

Walking in labour with an epidural

Walking in labour with regional analgesia was first described using a CSE technique (Collis et al 1994). It has since become apparent that if the starting dose of epidural analgesia is 10–15 mg of bupivacaine, it may also be possible to walk after epidural analgesia alone (Breen et al 1993, James et al 1998, Price et al 1998).

The introduction of the CSE in labour was originally studied because the spinal injection can provide reliable analgesia for advancing labour and emergency procedures. With the reduction in the initial bupivacaine dose from 5 to 2.5 mg and the addition of fentanyl or sufentanil, it was apparent that the initial dose given intrathecally could provide excellent analgesia with a low incidence of motor blockade.

The reduction in motor block made it obvious to the mothers that to stand and adopt other comfortable positions in labour was appropriate. The traditional approach to managing mothers with an epidural was that continuous fetal monitoring and haemodynamic instability would require the mother to remain in bed. The mother's wishes to stand and walk have challenged this view.

The only demonstrated benefit to date, of a mother being able to stand and walk with an epidural, is that she prefers it (Murphy et al 1991, Collis et al 1995b, 1999b). There is no evidence that it reduces the likelihood of instrumental delivery, for example. However, a mother's perception of a technique, with improved self-control and autonomy, must not be overlooked as a good reason for providing analgesia with the lowest possible incidence of motor block.

Measuring motor blockade

The safety aspect of the technique must be closely examined before allowing a mother to get out of bed with an epidural or CSE. The absolute lack of motor block is one of the most important aspects to examine. The traditional assessment of motor blockade with an epidural was with the Bromage scale. This assessment was made with the patient sitting in bed and examined motor power of the hips, knees and ankles, which are affected progressively with epidural blockade. The problem with this assessment is that the measurement of hip flexion is made after the mother has flexed her knee. She can then lift her heel off the bed because the greatest effect of gravity has been overcome and score Bromage 0, where in fact she does not have full motor power of her hips. The only way to test motor power is to do a straight leg raise while the mother is sitting in bed, and then a knee bend when the mother is standing. In this way, the full effect of gravity on muscle power is tested.

Proprioception

Proprioception is an important part of safe ambulation. Dorsal column function is one part of a triad of vestibular function and vision that allows the body to balance in the upright position, and allows a normal gait. If there is a reduction in dorsal column function it may make the mother more vulnerable to stumbling and falls. Studies have shown that there may be a marked reduction in dorsal column function with regional blockade, but there is an association with motor block (Parry et al 1998). Mothers who do not have motor block can balance normally and have a normal pregnant waddling gait. It would seem prudent, however, to allow walking only in a well-lit environment, on a flat surface and with an attendant.

Haemodynamic stability

Epidural and subarachnoid blockade is associated with hypotension and, therefore, intravenous preloading with a crystalloid solution is usual when initiating regional blockade in labour. The hypotension is caused by sympathetic blockade, which causes peripheral vasodilatation and venous pooling of blood. This in turn reduces venous return and cardiac output. The greatest potential fall in blood pressure usually occurs after the initial dose. With a reduction in the concentration of bupivacaine, when used with infusions or top-ups, the changes in sympathetic blockade are less and there has been a reduction in adverse episodes of hypotension.

Standing with an epidural or spinal may seem something of a cardiovascular challenge. It seems, however, that the mother adjusts physiologically, provided the development of sympathetic blockade is not too rapid and standing and walking does not cause a further drop in blood pressure. One of the dangers to the mother and fetus while in bed is aortacaval compression leading to supine hypotension. Aortacaval compression may not be fully corrected, even if the mother is placed in the full lateral position, and is only reduced (not abolished) in the supine position by lateral tilt. The mother with an epidural is at greater risk than normal of supine hypotension because the normal physiological counteraction of vasoconstriction in the lower limbs is abolished. It has been found that top-ups conducted with the mother standing have produced a smaller decrease in blood pressure compared to top-ups on her side in bed (Shennan et al 1995, al-Mufti et al 1997). This is almost certainly because of the absence of aorta-caval compression in the standing position, while muscle movement of the lower limbs will facilitate venous return.

CTG monitoring of the fetus has been routinely prescribed if the mother wishes to have an epidural. Hypotension in the mother leads rapidly to fetal heart rate abnormalities in the baby. Continuous CTG monitoring is usual in many situations where the uptake of epidural analgesia is the highest e.g. induction of labour and oxytocin augmentation, but with an epidural where motor and sympathetic block is minimal, the use of intermittent CTG monitoring may be appropriate in an otherwise normal labour. During a study where telemetry CTG monitoring was used, CTG abnormalities generally improved on walking and normal CTGs did not deteriorate.

Common side-effects of regional analgesia

Post dural puncture headache

Post dural puncture headache is a common problem in obstetric anaesthetic practice. Women of childbearing age are the most likely to complain of this typical headache after dural puncture. Dural puncture may be accidental during placement of an epidural catheter or deliberate during spinal injection. The incidence of headache is related to the size and type of needle that caused the hole.

After dural puncture with a 16 or 18G Tuohy needle, the incidence of headache is as high as 80% (Crawford 1972), the resulting headache can be severe, debilitating and difficult to treat. The incidence of headache following spinal injection with a Quincke (cutting tipped) needle, even of a 25G, may be 15–20% (Cesarini et al 1990). Spinal injection became more popular when a conical-tipped needle (Whitacre or Sprotte) was introduced, because the incidence of headache decreased dramatically. With a 24–25G needle; post dural puncture headache is seen in only 1% of cases or less (Shutt et al 1992). In a large audit of 27G Whitacre needles, used in a CSE technique, the post dural puncture headache rate was 0.3%. The headache associated with spinal needles is usually less severe and more readily treated than that following dural puncture with an epidural needle.

Diagnosis. The classical post dural puncture headache is fronto-occipital and radiates behind the eyes and into the neck. It is at its worst when upright especially sitting still and it tends to be relieved when lying down. It may also be associated with dizziness, tinnitus, hearing impairment, blurred or double vision and photophobia. It is caused by loss of CSF and the resulting traction on the meninges around the brain. Although it is usually thought of as a severe but benign headache, serious sequelae have been described such as cranial nerve palsy and subdural haematoma (Newrick & Read 1982). Without treatment it may resolve within two weeks but occasionally it may last for months or years.

Treatment. There is no evidence to show that post dural puncture headache is less common after dural puncture if the mother is prevented from bearing down in the second stage of labour. Bed rest after delivery is also not helpful as it does not prevent the headache but simply delays its onset.

Simple analgesics and hydration. This may be all that is required, especially if the headache is mild after a spinal injection.

Blood patch. This is the most effective treatment especially after accidental dural puncture with a Tuohy needle as the tear is large. Usually within 24–48 hours, a second epidural is sited under sterile conditions. 20 ml of the mother's blood is taken and slowly injected into the epidural space. This causes a plugging of the hole and the relief of symptoms can be instantaneous. The success rate of this treatment is about 80% after the first blood patch and can be repeated (Crawford 1980).

Drug therapy. Theophylline, ACTH and sumatriptan (Lhuissier et al 1996, Hutter 1997) have all been used in the treatment of post dural puncture headache. They seem to work most effectively when the headache is less severe but can reduce symptoms when the headache is severe if the mother does not want another epidural. The mechanisms of action are not clear, but as a one off treatment they seem to be safe for most women.

Backache

There has long been an association with epidural analgesia and new long term backache after delivery. In 1990, the British Medical Journal published the first of a retrospective series of studies looking at a large number of women that delivered in Birmingham over an eight-year period. It was thought from the first study that there was twice as much new backache (19% after epidural analgesia), than with other forms of analgesia (11%) (MacArthur et al 1990, Loughnan et al 1996). A detailed prospective study has since been conducted, which looked specifically at the rate of antenatal backache and its association with postnatal backache (Russell et al 1996). The conclusion from this study was that there is a stronger correlation of postnatal backache with pre-existing backache than epidural analgesia. It seems likely that an epidural is more likely to be blamed when antenatal backache has been forgotten. Close follow-up of these mothers has shown that most problems are related to poor posture and sacro-iliac strain (Breen et al 1994). The initial BMJ survey looked at a period of time when 0.5–0.25% bupivacaine was commonly used. The association between motor block and poor posture in labour, unprotected by the normal mechanisms of pain, was made. The recent studies, which have not shown an increase in new backache, have studied a period when more dilute bupivacaine was used. With the newer techniques, it is much easier to reduce the possibility of damaging poor posture in labour, and therefore the possibility of long-term problems. The ability to stand and walk with ultra low dose CSEs or epidurals may be the best protective mechanism against poor posture, because the mother retains the ability to change position regularly in labour.

ANAESTHESIA FOR CAESAREAN SECTION

There has been an increasing trend away from general anaesthesia for caesarean section to regional techniques; spinal, epidural or CSE. It was estimated almost 20 years ago that about 80% of caesareans could be done using a regional technique and in the UK (Davis 1982), general anaesthesia has come down to this level in many units. The clinical evidence to support this trend has been compelling, especially the reduction in deaths directly related to general anaesthesia and problems of airway management and aspiration. Although it has long been believed that general anaesthesia is more dangerous than a regional technique, deaths have usually been related to substandard care and, therefore, they should be avoidable. Avoidable deaths have also occurred following regional techniques. The safe practice of any anaesthetic relies upon understanding maternal physiology and how these changes influence anaesthetic practice.

General of regional anaesthesia

Requirement for general anaesthesia

There are a number of circumstances where, because of maternal request, maternal condition or obstetric urgency, a general anaesthetic is preferable.

Maternal request. This remains an important reason for performing a general anaesthetic. The reasons for wanting a general anaesthetic are varied, but they include the fear of backache, fear of the spinal or epidural needle, fear of hearing or seeing the operation and fear of being paralysed after the anaesthetic (Gajraj et al 1995).

Obstetric indications.

Extreme emergency e.g. placental abruption or cord prolapse where the fetus's life is threatened.

- In the severely distressed fetus, a high concentration of oxygen given to the mother may improve fetal oxygenation (Marx & Mateo 1971).
- General anaesthesia remains the most reliable technique for anaesthesia, and in most hands remains the quickest.
- In cases of placental abruption, a coagulopathy can develop rapidly and it may not be possible to measure and correct clotting abnormalities before insertion of a spinal or epidural needle.

Severe haemorrhage. General anaesthesia can provide better cardiovascular stability than a regional technique because sympathetic blockade is avoided. This is especially true if haemodynamic instability has already occurred.

Placenta praevia. In the elective setting, many obstetric anaesthetists will consider a regional technique for a posterior placenta praevia. Most choose a general anaesthetic for an anterior placenta praevia, especially where there has been a previous caesarean section with the possible complication of placenta accreta (Bonner et al 1995). Haemorrhage can be torrential and caesarean hysterectomy necessary. General anaesthesia may offer better haemodynamic stability and be more comfortable for the mother if the operation is prolonged.

Maternal indications.

Cardiac abnormalities. There are a small number of cardiac abnormalities where general anaesthesia has benefits over a regional technique. In severe pulmonary or aortic out-flow obstruction, sudden changes in afterload can cause cardiovascular decompensation. In cyanotic congenital heart disease, regional anaesthesia will also reduce the afterload and increase a right-to-left shunt, therefore, worsening central cyanosis.

Anatomical problems. There are a small number of mothers who have severe kyphoscoliosis (often with Harrington rod fixation), spina bifida or paraplegia. The technical problems that may be encountered with these mothers may make general anaesthesia necessary.

Low platelets. Are associated with pre-eclampsia; haemolytic anaemia, abnormal liver enzymes and low platelet syndrome (HELLP), and other rare complications associated with pregnancy such at thrombotic thrombocytopenic purpura (TTP). A platelet count above $80–100 \times 10^9/l$ is usually accepted as safe as long as coagulation is normal.

Coagulation problems. The mother may develop coagulation problems caused by sepsis, haemorrhage or pre-eclampsia. Under these situations, a clotting screen should be done before considering a regional technique. The mother may also be on anticoagulation therapy. Heparin and warfarin should ideally be stopped before delivery and coagulation tested.

Benefits of regional anaesthesia to the mother

The majority of women welcome the chance to be awake during the birth of their baby, especially if the mother's partner or close relative can accompany them. Mothers who are anxious or fearful about regional anaesthesia for caesarean section can often be persuaded to be awake for their operative delivery if the positive aspects are emphasised.

Safety. If regional anaesthesia is performed with great care and attention to maternal physiology, then it is probably fundamentally safer than general anaesthesia for caesarean section. The hazard of difficult airway associated with weight gain and oedema can be avoided, along with the problems of gastric regurgitation because of a physiological weakening of the gastro-oesophageal sphincter and an increase in gastric volume and acid production. The pregnant woman, however, is prone to supine hypotension, the effects of which can be greatly exaggerated during regional blockade. Poor management of this can result in severe hypotension, vomiting and unconsciousness, which in itself can increase the risk of acid aspiration. Although in the United Kingdom, maternal deaths associated with general anaesthesia have become increasingly rare, general anaesthesia still causes deaths.

Blood loss. There is an association with less bleeding at the time of caesarean delivery when a regional technique is used (Morgan et al 1984). The reason for an apparent reduction in blood loss with regional techniques may be the avoidance of volatile anaesthetic agents, which can cause uterine relaxation. However, reduced bleeding may be not only a result of the avoidance of volatile agents. During non-obstetric pelvic surgery where bleeding can be a major problem, operations carried out under epidural anaesthesia also result in less bleeding (Shir et al 1994).

Postoperative recovery. From casual observation, it is apparent that the mother who has had a regional technique recovers more rapidly from her caesarean section. This has been confirmed by an audit study (Morgan et al 1984). The mother is more likely to be mobile the following day, breastfeeding and caring for her baby, feeling hungry and thirsty. She develops fewer chest infections and is less likely to

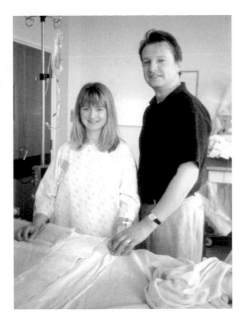

Fig. 28.4 Mother standing by bed with a mobile epidural (reproduced with permission).

develop postoperative pyrexia. She is less likely to feel depressed and tired both in the immediate postoperative period and after a week. She may also have an improved attitude towards the birth, making it easier to develop early bonding with her baby.

Postoperative pain. This is a major factor in the rate of recovery after any operation. Access to the intrathecal and epidural space makes it possible to use this route for administration of opioids. It has been shown, however, that after the same epidural opioids, mothers get better pain-relief if her epidural was topped up for her caesarean rather than receiving a general anaesthetic (Asantila et al 1995). Laboratory work suggests that there is a difference in transmission of pain impulses between the techniques in the central nervous system. Whatever the underlying mechanism, rapid pain-free recovery, which is characteristic after regional anaesthesia, is important after caesarean section.

Reducing the risk of pulmonary aspiration of gastric contents

The physiological changes that increase the risk of regurgitation and the risk of acid aspiration syndrome in a pregnant woman are:

- a reduction in lower oesophageal tone, a progesterone effect that occurs early in pregnancy
- a delay in gastric emptying with a tendency for higher gastric volume and a reduction in gastric pH, possibly a result of gastrin production from the placenta
- increase in reflux caused by an increase in intra-abdominal pressure from the enlarging uterus.

Heartburn is a very common symptom of pregnancy and is closely related to demonstrable gastric reflux (Hey et al 1977).

Feeding prior to caesarean section

Elective caesarean section. Fasting for an elective caesarean section is necessary. It was found that even with a light breakfast of tea and toast four hours prior to general anaesthesia, the volume of gastric contents was greater and the pH lower than in a control group who fasted for greater than six hours (Lewis & Crawford 1987). It would therefore seem prudent to insist on at least a six-hour fast before elective caesarean section.

Emergency caesarean section. Feeding in labour is much more controversial because of the often unpredictable necessity for caesarean section. Gastric emptying in labour may not be extended beyond the normal delay seen during pregnancy unless opioids or epidural analgesia are given (Carp et al 1992). It seems likely that prolonged labour associated with dehydration and ketosis will have a detrimental effect on the mother and fetus. Prolonged periods of fasting, especially withholding fluids, can be very unpleasant for the mother. Midwives and maternal pressure groups have demanded a more liberal approach to eating in labour. Many delivery units have an unselective policy, which allows mothers to eat and drink. In other units, either food or food and fluids are withheld depending on a number of criteria relating to the risk of obstetric intervention (Michael et al 1991). Mothers who have ingested food within the last 6–8 hours and have received an opioid or epidural will almost certainly have high volume, low pH stomach contents that are particulate in nature and very dangerous if aspirated.

Reducing gastric acidity

There is agreement that the volume, acidity and nature of aspirated material correlate with the severity of an aspiration syndrome. The published research that supports this is, however, largely based on animal experiments. The critical volume of aspiration is variably quoted, and may be between 0.4 ml/kg (25 ml) (Roberts & Shirley 1974) and 0.8 ml/kg (50 ml) (Raidoo et al 1990). It has been found that to produce an acid pneumonitis, the pH of the aspirate has to be less than 2.5. These figures are therefore used as a benchmark for the adequacy of therapeutic manoeuvres.

The prophylactic use of antacids

Magnesium trisilicate. This was the first antacid to be used in labour and caesarean delivery. In the 1980s its use was recommended. Although it was an effective drug at reducing gastric pH it was found to mix slowly with gastric contents and its particulate nature could cause a reaction in the lungs if aspirated (Gibbs et al 1979).

Sodium citrate. This is an unpalatable antacid with a short shelf life. When 30 ml of 0.3 molar sodium citrate is given 10–60 minutes before an elective caesarean section, it predictably raises the pH of gastric contents above 2.5 (Dewan et al 1985). After 60 minutes, the results are less predictable. Giving sodium citrate does not seem to increase the intragastric volume, in fact only 5% of mothers given 30 ml of sodium citrate were found to have a volume greater than 25 ml (Stuart et al 1996). These studies show that sodium citrate is a good antacid, which will reliably reduce the risk of acid pneumonitis at induction of anaesthesia. Problems of aspiration may occur, however, during emergence from anaesthesia, where the effect of sodium citrate is very much less predictable.

H₂ antagonists (cimetidine and ranitidine). These are both effective at reducing gastric pH and gastric volume (Rout et al 1993) especially when administered with metoclopramide. Ranitidine is now used in preference to cimetidine because cimetidine was associated with haemodynamic instability, when given parenterally. If an oral dose of ranitidine 150 mg is given more than 60 minutes before caesarean section then it is effective (Escolano et al 1996). This is the preferable route of administration for elective caesarean section and during labour where caesarean section is anticipated. Intravenous ranitidine is effective within half an hour of administration. In the event of an extreme emergency, it is still useful to give intravenous ranitidine because it will be effective by the time the mother emerges from anaesthesia.

Omeprazole. This is a H^+ ATPase proton pump inhibitor. It has been used since 1989 where a single oral dose of 80 mg was found to be effective at reducing intragastric volume and pH in the majority of mothers (Rocke et al 1994). It is well tolerated and seems to be free of fetal side effects. Intravenous omeprazole 40 mg is also effective at reducing pH and gastric volume if given at least 30 minutes before caesarean section. The draw back of omeprazole is that it is more expensive than ranitidine and does not seem to have any major advantages.

Metoclopramide. This is a dopaminergic antagonist, which can be used to accelerate gastric emptying and increase lower oesophageal tone. This is particularly useful if the mother complains of heartburn (Hey & Ostick 1978). Gastric emptying, which is delayed after the onset of labour and opioid administration, are both partially reversed by the use of metoclopramide (Murphy et al 1984). In conjunction with other drugs such as ranitidine or omeprazole, it is at its most useful. Its antiemetic effect conveys additional benefits and, as it has a low incidence of side-effects in the mother and fetus, its routine use can easily be justified.

General anaesthesia

Standards of care during induction of general anaesthesia

Preoxygenation. There is an increase in oxygen consumption at term by 20% compared with non-pregnant controls. In early labour, oxygen consumption increases by 40% and in the second stage may be as high as 100% greater than in the prepregnancy state. In the non-pregnant patient, careful pre-oxygenation will give at least three minutes of full saturation during apnoea. This is very much reduced, despite adequate denitrogination, in the labouring mother at term (Archer & Marx 1974).

Rapid sequence induction. During induction of anaesthesia, cricoid pressure must be applied. The backward pressure compresses the oesophagus onto the vertebral column, which is occluded while the airway remains patent because of the continuous ring of cartilage.

Failed intubation. It is important to remember that failure to intubate a mother' trachea will cause no harm as long as oxygenation is maintained and the airway remains clear. Unrecognised oesophageal intubation is a major hazard of a difficult intubation and has led to maternal deaths. End tidal CO_2 monitors are now mandatory equipment for the obstetric theatre, and will give early warning of tracheal intubation.

Failed intubation drill (Harmer 1997). When faced with a failed intubation the anaesthetist must quickly determine two things:

1. Is it possible to maintain oxygenation either through a laryngeal mask or facemask?
2. How urgent is the caesarean section?

The urgency of the caesarean section can be graded so that if oxygenation can be maintained, the need to continue surgery can be evaluated.

- Grade 1   The mother's life depends on completion of surgery e.g. massive haemorrhage or cardiac arrest
- Grade 2   Maternal pathology makes a regional technique unsuitable
- Grade 3   Sudden and severe fetal distress e.g. placental abruption or prolapsed cord
- Grade 4   Long-standing fetal distress showing signs of recovery between contractions
- Grade 5   Elective procedure

Grade 1: surgery should continue under almost any circumstances.

Grade 2: the safer option even if oxygenation is adequate is to wake the mother up and proceed with an awake fibre optic intubation if equipment and expertise allows.

Grade 3: if oxygenation can be maintained with good cricoid pressure then to save the life of the fetus, anaesthesia may continue, although this type of anaesthetic in the most skilled hands can be very difficult. If the mother's life is at risk because of continuing difficulties with airway management, the mother should be woken.

Grade 4 or 5: the safer option is to wake the mother and proceed with a regional technique.

There is some argument as to the best anaesthetic technique after these problems. A spinal anaesthetic will provide rapid anaesthesia especially when speed is a priority because of fetal distress. Haemodynamic stability can be more easily achieved with an epidural technique although a slow incremental epidural technique is advisable as a total spinal may occur. If expertise and equipment allow, an awake fibre optic intubation is probably the safest.

Induction and maintenance of anaesthesia

Induction–delivery interval. The time from induction of anaesthesia to delivery of the baby during general anaesthesia may affect the baby in two ways.

- Firstly, the baby may become progressively acidotic during anaesthesia. This effect is very much diminished if aorta-caval compression and hypotension is avoided. A high oxygen tension of 60–70% (Marx & Mateo 1971) will also improve the condition of the baby. The fetus will maintain good acid-base status for up to 30 minutes if maternal hypotension is avoideo (Crawford et al 1976).

- The second problem of prolonged induction to delivery interval is that the baby will progressively take up lipid soluble anaesthetic agents, while a gradient exists between the maternal and fetal circulation. During prolonged I–D intervals, the maternal-fetal transfer of thiopentone may continue for 40 minutes (Reynolds 1993), eventually reaching a higher level in the fetus than the mother. The inhalational agents have a more profound effect during a prolonged I–D time because the maternal levels are constant and a maternal-fetal gradient is maintained.

The influence of the uterine incision delivery interval (IDI) is controversial; if in excess of 180 seconds it is associated with low Apgar scores and fetal acidosis (Bader et al 1990). Excessive uterine manipulation may cause maldistribution of placental blood flow and enhance aorta-caval compression.

Maternal ventilation during general anaesthesia. *Oxygen:* During anaesthesia and caesarean delivery, a high inspired oxygen concentration is not only necessary because of the mother's increased metabolic requirements but also to improve the condition of the baby at birth.

Carbon dioxide: The anaesthetist controls the mother's partial pressure of CO_2. At term in the normal mother it is reduced to 4.1 kPa. This reduction allows elimination of CO_2 down a concentration gradient from fetus to mother. Once the mother is ventilated this level of $PaCO_2$ must be maintained for fetal well-being, but further reductions must be avoided. A $PaCO_2$ below 3.6 kPa is associated with fetal acidosis and increased time to sustained respiration after birth because of vasoconstriction in the umbilical vessels (Peng et al 1972).

Anaesthetic agents

Intravenous induction agents
There is a wide choice of intravenous induction agents that are commonly used for anaesthesia in the non-pregnant population. All can and have been used for induction of anaesthesia for caesarean section but thiopentone has remained the gold standard.

Thiopentone. Thiopentone can be safely used in a dose of 4 mg/kg. At this dose, the drug can be detected in the umbilical vein within seconds of induction, but the baby is protected from excessive sedation because of the fetal circulation through the liver. The advantage of thiopentone is that anaesthesia can be reliably produced in the mother because of its longer duration of action, while the baby is relatively unaffected (Hodgkinson et al 1978).

Propofol. Propofol has become a very popular induction agent for non-obstetric use. Propofol does not have a clear role during induction of anaesthesia for caesarean section (Capogna et al 1991).

Ketamine. Ketamine is indicated where massive obstetric haemorrhage has occurred. Its powerful sympathomimetic action can help to maintain cardiovascular stability and it may also be useful for anaesthesia during an asthma attack. Ketamine can be rapidly detected in the fetus, but in a dose of 1 mg/kg, the condition of the baby at birth compares favourably with thiopentone (Peltz & Sinclair 1973).

Etomidate. This may be a useful induction agent for caesarean section especially in the haemodynamically-compromised mother (Downing et al 1979). It causes less myocardial depression than thiopentone and less histamine release, making it useful for the asthmatic mother.

Neuromuscular blocking agents
Neuromuscular blocking drugs are used to facilitate intubation and maintain muscle relaxation during caesarean section. The fetus has minimal exposure, as the drugs do not cross the placenta in high enough concentration to cause paralysis.

Depolarising neuromuscular blocker
Succinyl choline (Suxamethonium). Succinyl choline remains the drug of choice in obstetric anaesthesia to achieve rapid intubating conditions within 90 seconds (Baraka et al 1986). It is used as part of a rapid sequence induction in a dose of 1–1.5 mg/kg. It is the only commonly available drug, which is metabolised rapidly with return of spontaneous respiration within 1–5 minutes. Succinyl choline must be avoided under the following conditions.

- 0.3% of the population have pseudocholinesterase deficiency. If a mother is known to have this condition, prolonged paralysis will occur requiring prolonged postoperative ventilation.
- Hyperkalaemia can result from the use of succinyl choline after burns or recent spinal cord transection.
- Hyperkalaemia may also occur if the mother has a severe demyelinating neurological condition.
- Severe rigidity and impossible intubation can occur if succinyl choline is used in a mother with a myotonia.
- Succinyl choline will also trigger malignant hyperthermia in a susceptible mother.

Non-depolarising neuromuscular blockers
Vecuronium, atracurium and rocuronium (Abouleish et al 1994) are widely used and have replaced pancuronium and D-tubocurarine because of their predictable, intermediate duration of action. After neuromuscular recovery from succinyl choline, they can be safely used to provide 20–30 minutes of muscle relaxation, which can then be easily reversed with glycopyrrolate or atropine and neostigmine, so the mother can rapidly regain control of her airway.

Magnesium sulphate
This has in recent years grown in popularity for both the control and treatment of pre-eclampsia and prevention of recurrent fitting in eclampsia. Mothers receiving these drugs are more likely to require surgical intervention where drug interaction between magnesium sulphate and the neuromuscular blocking drugs can be seen.

The fasciculations that are normally seen with succinyl choline may not occur but clinically succinyl choline works well in the presence of magnesium sulphate and the neuromuscular blockade is not prolonged (Stacey et al 1995).

The interaction of magnesium sulphate and the non-depolarising neuromuscular blocking drugs is more complicated. Here the block is enhanced by the interaction (Fuchs-Buder & Tassonyi 1996). Magnesium sulphate can also cause recurarisation (re-paralysis) in mothers previously exposed to neuromuscular blocking drugs. Mothers must be monitored closely for several hours after their anaesthetic for evidence of increasing muscle weakness. This is especially important where magnesium sulphate infusions are continued into the postoperative period.

Inhalational anaesthesia

Nitrous oxide. Nitrous oxide is an agent with limited lipid solubility that is used, mixed with oxygen, as a carrier gas for the other inhalational agents. Nitrous oxide passes into the fetus and will continue to increase in concentration for 15–20 minutes of maternal administration (Marx et al 1970). If more than 50% nitrous oxide is used with oxygen then it may contribute to depressed neonatal Apgar scores.

Nitrous oxide does not cause uterine muscle relaxation or interfere with oxytocin-induced uterine contraction and is therefore a useful carrier gas for the other inhalational agents so reducing their overall requirements.

The volatile anaesthetic agents. The halogenated anaesthetic agents halothane, enflurane and isoflurane have all been successfully used for caesarean section. All cause dose and time dependent neonatal depression. If any are used in a modest dose and the I–D interval is below 11 minutes, then there is no excess of neonatal depression (Warren et al 1983). All the volatile agents cause dose dependent uterine relaxation and potential haemorrhage as well as making the uterus less responsive to oxytocin.

Opioids. Opioids are not used as part of a standard rapid sequence induction. They are, however, recommended for anaesthesia if the mother is hypertensive. They are used to obtund the hypertension and tachycardia, which is associated with intubation using an induction agent alone. Once the baby is delivered it is very important that the mother is given an adequate dose of an opioid. This will provide balanced analgesia so the mother can wake reasonably pain free after her operation. Fentanyl 100–200 µg or morphine 10 mg are appropriate.

Postoperative analgesia

After general anaesthesia it is usual to have to rely on intramuscular or intravenous opioids. It is very important that mothers after caesarean section under general anaesthetic have regular access to opioids. This can either be by intramuscular morphine or pethidine up to one-hourly with appropriate sedation and respiratory monitoring or patient-controlled analgesia PCA morphine or pethidine (Harmer & Davies 1998).

Regional anaesthesia

The same high standard of care for the mother must apply to regional anaesthesia for caesarean section as much as general anaesthesia. This must include having a trained anaesthetic assistant, appropriate monitoring as set out by the Obstetric Anaesthetists Association and Association of Anaesthetists and full resuscitation drugs and equipment immediately available.

Table 28.9 General anaesthesia for caesarean section

- Anaesthesia for caesarean section should only be carried out in an operating theatre with adequate monitoring and a trained anaesthetic assistant.
- Mothers having, or at risk of having a caesarean section should have antacid prophylaxis with sodium citrate and an H2 antagonist such as ranitidine.
- Preoxygenation of the mother is essential as it increases the time that the anaesthetist has for intubation.
- A failed intubation drill should be known by everybody in the theatre.
- A prolonged induction to delivery time will progressively allow lipid-soluble drugs to accumulate in the fetus.

Regional anaesthesia and the baby

It is probably advantageous to the newborn to be vigorous at birth; this is characteristically seen after regional anaesthesia. The lack of drug effect means that the infant requires less intervention; can feed earlier and maternal–infant bonding may be encouraged. Caesarean delivery where there is a prediction of a long pre-delivery phase such as a repeat procedure makes a regional technique even more preferable to the baby.

Poor condition of the baby after a regional technique can be associated with the severe prolonged maternal hypotension, which can occur with poor regional technique (Corke et al 1982). Good anaesthetic technique is essential for the safety of the baby.

Aorta-caval compression

It is important to avoid aorta-caval compression during both regional and general anaesthesia, but the result of uncorrected compression is more serious after regional blockade (Clark et al 1976). Reducing aorto-caval compression is achieved by uterine displacement either in the lateral position, supine with tilt or manual lifting of the uterus.

Volume preloading

Crystalloid preloading. Crystalloids have been traditionally used as preloading fluid. The effectiveness of their use has been mainly studied in association with spinal blockade, where the incidence of hypotension is the highest at around 80%. The routine use of 1000 ml of a crystalloid solution does not reliably eliminate hypotension, with 40–60% of mothers still developing hypotension and requiring treatment with vasopressors (Rout et al 1993). Increasing the volume of the crystalloid infusion has little additional beneficial effect on the incidence of hypotension (Park et al 1996).

Colloid infusions. Colloid solutions have been studied, as the effects of crystalloids are known to be short lived and there is some evidence that they reduce the incidence of hypotension (Vercauteren et al 1996).

Vasopressors/ephedrine. Rout et al (1993) first questioned the routine preload. It seems that it is the avoidance of hypotension rather than use of ephedrine, which is important to the baby when assessed by Apgar, cord pH and NACS scores.

Phenylephrine. Although this drug is a pure α-agonist, and may have a direct vasoconstrictive effect on the placental vasculature, it can be used safely in bolus doses of 100 µg to safely control hypotension.

By avoiding large preloads, less time is required to initiate a spinal block, which may be important when rapid anaesthesia is required. Minimal preload will also avoid the risk of excessive fluid use, high CVP, pulmonary oedema and dilutional anaemia.

Block for caesarean section

There is continuing confusion as to the extent of the block required for caesarean section and how best to measure it prior to starting surgery. The extent of the block depends on the method by which it is tested, but a good block must be absence of cold sensation from T4 to S5, bilaterally with dense motor block of hip flexion and ankle dorsiflexion. Russell showed that if the block extended to T5 to light touch then the mother would have no pain during her operation (Russell 1995).

Differential zones of blockade

The measured spread of the block is determined by the method used for assessment. There are zones of differential blockade at the upper and lower edges of a regional block. During assessment of spinal and epidural blockade, testing for absence of cold sensation is two dermatomes higher than pinprick sensation, which in turn is at least two dermatomes higher than sensation to light touch (touching with a soft tissue) (Rocco et al 1985, Brull & Greene 1991).

Epidural blockade for caesarean section

Epidural blockade for elective caesarean section has become increasingly uncommon because spinal blockade is quicker and more reliable but it remains a safe option for topping-up an epidural already in use for labour analgesia.

Plain bupivacaine. Techniques using a test dose followed by 18 ml of 0.5% bupivacaine reduced time for establishing block to 30 minutes, but supplementation was still required in 30–50% of cases (Laishley & Morgan 1988).

Lignocaine. Lignocaine 2% used as a one-off bolus for caesarean section compared favourably with bupivacaine from the neonatal point of view, but was associated with a higher incidence of inadequate block than bupivacaine (Abboud et al 1983). The addition of adrenaline (1:200 000) and bicarbonate enhanced the effect of lignocaine (Norton et al 1988, Fernando & Jones 1991) and considerably improved the quality of the block with a reduction of intraoperative supplementation.

Spinal anaesthesia for caesarean section

Spinal anaesthesia is popular because of its relative simplicity, reliability and quicker onset time compared to epidural anaesthesia (Helbo-Hensen et al 1988). Adding opioids has further improved its reliability compared with epidural analgesia.

Combined spinal–epidural for caesarean section

The technique, which has already been described, can be used for elective and emergency caesarean section.

The advantages of the technique are:

- Ability to top-up an inadequate spinal block.
- Ability to top-up a spinal block during prolonged surgery.

- A smaller intrathecal dose can be used initially, which may increase haemodynamic stability, then anaesthetic infused via the epidural catheter used to extend the block slowly. This is especially useful if the mother has cardiovascular disease.
- The epidural catheter can be left *in situ* if required for postoperative analgesia.

Table 28.10 Regional anaesthesia for caesarean section

- Avoids the risk of failed intubation so is safer.
- The same standards of monitoring and availability of staff should be available as for general anaesthesia.
- Hypotension caused by sympathetic blockade can cause placental hypoperfusion and fetal acidosis.
- Aorto-caval compression compounds the problem and must be avoided by positioning the mother carefully on the operating table.
- Access to the epidural and subarachnoid space for opioids reduces intraoperative discomfort to the mother and can give safe long-lasting analgesia.

Local infiltration for caesarean delivery

If an emergency caesarean delivery is required and a general, epidural or subarachnoid anaesthetic cannot be performed, it is possible to perform this operation under local infiltration.

Drawbacks of local infiltration are as follows.

- A good field block may take some time to perform adequately.
- The patient must remain fully cooperative.
- Anaesthesia to the skin and immediate peritoneum can be performed relatively easily but traction of the internal organs will cause severe pain because there is no sacral or vagal nerve anaesthesia.
- The maximum dose of local anaesthetic such as lignocaine with adrenaline (epinephine) 1:200 000 is 7 mg/ml, which is approximately 500 mg for the average woman. This is only 25 ml of 2% lignocaine with adrenaline.

Performing local infiltration for caesarean section.

- A field block of the abdominal cutaneous nerves can be performed by subcutaneous injection towards the anterior edge of ribs 8–11 bilaterally.
- Additional infiltration over the incision site.
- After incision, infiltrate as you go into the retropubic space, rectus sheath and the peritoneum across the lower segment of the uterus (Beck 1942).

Intrathecal and epidural opioids

Intrathecal and epidural opioids can be added to the local anaesthetic solution to reduce intraoperative discomfort and give prolonged postoperative pain relief. See Table 28.6.

Diclofenac. Many studies have used intrathecal or epidural opioids in conjunction with rectal diclofenac 100 mg given at the end of surgery. Diclofenac has a marked morphine sparing effect and the suggested opioid doses are considerably less effective when given without a non-steroidal anti-inflammately drug (Luthman et al 1994). With diclofenac and a single dose of epidural diamorphine 3 mg, 92% of mothers said that their pain scores were mild or less and nobody required additional opioids other than oral co-dydramol.

Safety. The safety of using long-acting spinal opioids without high dependency facilities has been questioned. In obstetric patients, the incidence of respiratory depression with these doses of morphine or diamorphine is very low. As long as systemic opioids are avoided, one can use routine postoperative observations only.

CONCLUSION

The use of non-regional techniques is common but the analgesic effect is questionable. The psychological support that these methods provide, with improved relaxation and feeling of well-being, which maintain their popularity, has yet to be fully evaluated. Regional anaesthesia is popular, although up-take may have reached a plateau, because of the side-effects and continuing concerns that epidurals lead to obstetric intervention. In the past decade, obstetric anaesthesia has changed considerably with the replacement of bupivacaine for bupivacaine/opioid mixtures and the development of new techniques such as combined spinal-epidural analgesia, mobile epidurals and patient-controlled epidural analgesia. These changes in practice have been directed by research in the field, which in a large part have been stimulated by the increasing popularity of the British Obstetric Anaesthetists Association and the American equivalent The Society of Obstetric Anesthesiology and Perinatology.

KEY POINTS

- Non-regional techniques for labour analgesia have remained popular despite the lack of clear evidence of good analgesic effect.
- Epidural analgesia has moved away from the high dose bupivacaine to much lower dose bupivacaine/opioid mixtures.
- The remarkable reduction in weakness of the legs has introduced the concept of mobile epidurals.
- Recent introduction of the new techniques of combined spinal-epidural and patient-controlled epidural analgesia has further refined this.
- General anaesthesia now accounts for around 20% of anaesthetics for caesarean section.
- General anaesthesia is now safer with improved equipment and trained anaesthetic assistants, but dangers to the mother and baby still remain fundamental to the technique.
- Improved understanding of maternal physiology and pain pathways has improved the reliability of regional anaesthesia for caesarean section.
- Regional anaesthesia for caesarean section is the anaesthetic of choice because it is safer and reduces fetal and maternal morbidity. The mother in particular benefits from reduced bleeding, reduced postoperative pain, reduced chest complications and possibly reduced postoperative thrombosis.

REFERENCES

Abboud TK et al 1983 Epidural bupivacaine, chloroprocaine, or lidocaine for cesarean section—maternal and neonatal effects. Anesth Analg 62(10):914–919

Aberg G 1972 Toxicological and local anaesthetic effects of optically active isomers of two local anaesthetic compounds. Acta Pharmacol Toxicol 31(4):273–286

Abouleish E et al 1994 Rocuronium (Org 9426) for caesarean section [see comments]. Br J Anaesth 73(3):336–341

Abouleish A, Abouleish E, Camann W 1994 Combined spinal-epidural analgesia in advanced labour. Can J Anaesth 41(7):575–578

Albright GA 1979 Cardiac arrest following regional anesthesia with etidocaine or bupivacaine [editorial]. Anesthesiol 51(4):285–287

al-Mufti R et al 1997 Blood pressure and fetal heart rate changes with patient-controlled combined spinal epidural analgesia while ambulating in labour. Br J Obstet Gynaecol 104(5):554–558

Archer GW, Jr. Marx GF 1974 Arterial oxygen tension during apnoea in parturient women. British Journal of Anaesth 46(5):358–360

Arthurs GJ, Rosen M 1979 Self-administered intermittent nitrous oxide analgesia for labour. Enhancement of effect with continuous nasal inhalation of 50 per cent nitrous oxide (Entonox). Anaesthesia 34(4):301–309

Asantila R et al 1995 Epidural analgesia with 4 mg of morphine after caesarean section: Modulating effect of epidural block compared to general anaesthesia. Int J Obstet Anesth 4(2):89–92

Bader AM et al 1990 Maternal and fetal catecholamines and uterine incision-to-delivery interval during elective cesarean. Obstet Gynecol 75(4):600–603

Baraka A et al 1986 Pseudocholinesterase activity and atracurium v. suxamethonium block. Br J Anaesth 58 Suppl 1:91S–95S

Beck AC 1942 Detailed technique of a modified local anesthesia for Cesarean section. Am J Obstet Gynecol 44:558–569

Bogod DG, Rosen M, Rees GA 1987 Extradural infusion of 0.125% bupivacaine at 10 ml h-1 to women during labour. Br J Anaesth 59(3):325–330

Bonner SM, Haynes SR, Ryall D 1995 The anaesthetic management of Caesarean section for placenta praevia: a questionnaire survey [see comments]. Anaesthesia 50(11):992–994

Booker PD et al 1980 Obstetric pain relief using epidural morphine. Anaesthesia 35(4):377–379

Breen TW et al 1993 Epidural anesthesia for labor in an ambulatory patient. Anesth Analg 77(5):919–924

Breen TW et al 1994 Factors associated with back pain after childbirth. Anesthesiol 81(1):29–34

Brull SJ, Greene NM 1991 Zones of differential sensory block during extradural anaesthesia. Br J Anaesth 66(6):651–655

Burnstein R, Buckland R, Pickett JA 1999 A survey of epidural analgesia for labour in the United Kingdom. Anaesthesia 54(7):634–640

Camann WR et al 1992 A comparison of intrathecal, epidural, and intravenous sufentanil for labor analgesia. Anesthesiol 77(5):884–887

Capogna G, Calleno D, Sebastiani M 1991 Propofol and thiopentone for Caesarean section revisited. Maternal effect and neonatal outcome. Int J Obst Anesth 1:19–23

Capogna G et al 1998 Minimum local analgesic concentration of extradural bupivacaine increases with progression of labour. Br J Anaesth 80(1):11–13

Capogna G et al 1999 Relative potencies of bupivacaine and ropivacaine for analgesia in labour. Br J Anaesth 82(3):371–373

Carp H, Jayaram A, Stoll M 1992 Ultrasound examination of the stomach contents of parturients. Anesth Analg 74(5):683–687

Carrie LE, O'Sullivan GM, Seegobin R 1981 Epidural fentanyl in labour. Anaesthesia 36(10):965–969

Carstoniu J et al 1994 Nitrous oxide in early labor. Safety and analgesic efficacy assessed by a double-blind, placebo-controlled study. Anesthesiol 80(1):30–35

Cesarini M et al 1990 Sprotte needle for intrathecal anaesthesia for caesarean section: incidence of postdural puncture headache. Anaesthesia 45(8):656–658

Chamberlain G, Wraight A, Steer P 1993 Pain and its relief in childbirth. The results of a national survey conducted by The National Birthday Trust. London: Churchill Livingstone

Chestnut DH et al 1990 Continuous epidural infusion of 0.0625% bupivacaine-0.0002% fentanyl during the second stage of labor. Anesthesiol 72(4):613–618

Clark RB, Thompson DS, Thompson CH 1976 Prevention of spinal hypotension associated with Cesarean section. Anesthesiol 45(6):670–671

Cohen SE et al 1987 Epidural fentanyl/bupivacaine mixtures for obstetric analgesia. Anesthesiol 67(3):403–407

Cole PV et al 1970 Specifications and recommendations for nitrous oxide-oxygen apparatus to be used in obstetric analgesis. Anaesthesia 25(3):317–327

Collis RE et al 1994 Combined spinal epidural (CSE) analgesia: Technique, management, and outcome of 300 mothers. International Journal of Obstetric Anesth 3(2):75–81

Collis RE, Davies DWL, Aveling W 1995 Randomised comparison of combined spinal-epidural and standard epidural analgesia in labour. Lancet 345:1413–1416

Collis RE, Davies DW, Aveling W 1995b Randomised comparison of combined spinal-epidural and standard epidural analgesia in labour. Lancet 345(8962):1413–1416

Collis RE, Plaat FS, Morgan BM 1999 Comparison of midwife top-ups, continuous infusion and patient-controlled epidural analgesia for maintaining mobility after a low-dose combined spinal-epidural. Br J Anaesth 82(2):233–236

Collis RE, Harding SA, Morgan BM 1999b Effect of maternal ambulation on labour with low-dose combined spinal-epidural analgesia. Anaesthesia 54(6):535–539

Corke BC et al 1982 Spinal anaesthesia for Caesarean section. The influence of hypotension on neonatal outcome. Anaesthesia 37(6):658–662

Crawford JS 1972 Lumbar epidural block in labour: a clinical analysis. Br J Anaesth 44(1):66–74

Crawford JS 1975 Patient management during extradural anaesthesia for obstetrics. British Journal of Anaesth 47 suppl:273–275

Crawford JS et al 1976 A further study of general anaesthesia for Caesarean section. Br J Anaesth 48(7):661–667

Crawford JS 1980 Experiences with epidural blood patch. Anaesthesia 35(5):513–515

Crawford JS 1985 Some maternal complications of epidural analgesia for labour. Anaesthesia 40(12):1219–1225

Davis AG 1982 Anaesthesia for Caesarean section. The potential for regional block. Anaesthesia 37(7):748–753

Dewan DM et al 1985 Sodium citrate pretreatment in elective cesarean section patients. Anesth Analg 64(1):34–37

Dick-Read G 1944 Childbirth without fear. Heinemann, London

Doughty A 1975 Lumbar epidural analgesia—the pursuit of perfection. With special reference to midwife participation. Anaesthesia 30(6):741–751

Downing JW et al 1979 Etomidate for induction of anaesthesia at caesarean section: comparison with thiopentone. Br J Anaesth 51(2):135–140

Escolano F et al 1996 The efficacy and optimum time of administration of ranitidine in the prevention of the acid aspiration syndrome. Anaesthesia 51(2):182–184

Fernando R, Jones HM 1991 Comparison of plain and alkalinized local anaesthetic mixtures of lignocaine and bupivacaine for elective extradural caesarean section. Br J Anaesth 67(6):699–703

Fuchs-Buder T, Tassonyi E 1996 Magnesium sulphate enhances residual neuromuscular block induced by vecuronium. Br J Anaesth 76(4):565–566

Gajraj NM et al 1995 A survey of obstetric patients who refuse regional anaesthesia. Anaesthesia 50(8):740–741

Gambling DR et al 1990 Comparison of patient-controlled epidural analgesia and conventional intermittent 'top-up' injections during labor. Anesth Analg 70(3):256–261

Gambling DR et al 1993 Patient-controlled epidural analgesia in labour: varying bolus dose and lockout interval. Can J Anaesth 40(3):211–217

Gaylard DG, Carson RJ, Reynolds F 1990 Effect of umbilical perfusate pH and controlled maternal hypotension on placental drug transfer in the rabbit. Anesth Analgesia 71(1):42–48

Gibbs CP et al 1979 Antacid pulmonary aspiration in the dog. Anesthesiol 51(5):380–385

Harmer M 1997 Difficult and failed intubation in obstetrics. International Journal of Obstet Anesth 6(1):25–31

Harmer M, Davies KA 1998 The effect of education, assessment and a standardised prescription on postoperative pain management. The value of clinical audit in the establishment of acute pain services. Anaesthesia 53(5):424–430

Harrison RF et al 1986 Pain relief in labour using TENS. A TENS/TENS placebo controlled study in two parity groups. Br J Obstet Gynaecol 93:739

Helbo-Hansen S et al 1988 Subarachnoid versus epidural bupivacaine 0.5% for caesarean section. Acta Anaesthesiol Scand 32(6):473–476

Hey VM et al 1977 Gastro-oesophageal reflux in late pregnancy. Anaesthesia 32(4):372–377

Hey VM, Ostick DG 1978 Metoclopramide and the gastro-oesophageal sphincter. A study in pregnant women with heartburn. Anaesthesia 33(5):462–465

Hodgkinson R et al 1978 Neonatal neurobehavioral tests following cesarean section under general and spinal anesthesia. Am J Obstet Gynecol 132(6):670–674

Honet JE et al 1992 Comparison among intrathecal fentanyl, meperidine, and sufentanil for labor analgesia. Anesth Analg 75(5):734–739

Hutter CD 1997 Sumatriptan and postdural puncture headache [letter; comment]. Anaesthesia 52(11):1119

James KS et al 1998 Comparison of epidural bolus administration of 0.25% bupivacaine and 0.1% bupivacaine with 0.0002% fentanyl for analgesia during labour. Br J Anaesth 81(4):507–510

Janes EF, McCrory JW 1991 The loading dose in continuous infusion extradural analgesia in obstetrics. Br J Anaesth 67(3):323–325

Kestin IG et al 1992 Analgesia for labour and delivery using incremental diamorphine and bupivacaine via a 32-gauge intrathecal catheter [see comments]. British Journal of Anaesth 68(3):244–247

Laishley RS, Morgan BM 1988 A single dose epidural technique for Caesarean section. A comparison between 0.5% bupivacaine plain and 0.5% bupivacaine with adrenaline. Anaesthesia 43(2):100–103

Leighton BL et al 1989 Intrathecal narcotics for labor revisited: the combination of fentanyl and morphine intrathecally provides rapid onset of profound, prolonged analgesia. Anesth Analg 69(1):122–125

Lewis M, Crawford JS 1987 Can one risk fasting the obstetric patient for less than 4 hours? Br J Anaesth 59(3):312–314

Lhuissier C et al 1996 Sumatriptan: an alternative to epidural blood patch? [letter]. Anaesthesia 51(11):1078

Li DF, Rees GA, Rosen M 1985 Continuous extradural infusion of 0.0625% or 0.125% bupivacaine for pain relief in primigravid labour. Br J Anaesth 57(3):264–270

Loftus JR, Hill H, Cohen SE 1995 Placental transfer and neonatal effects of epidural sufentanil and fentanyl administered with bupivacaine during labor. Anesthesiol 83(2):300–308

Loughnan BA, Gordon H, Frank AO 1996 Long-term backache after childbirth. Study should have been randomised [letter; comment]. Br Med J 313(7059):755; discussion 755–756

Luthman J, Kay NH, White JB 1994 The morphine sparing effect of diclofenac sodium following caesarean section under spinal anaesthesia. Intl J Obstet Anesth 3(2):82–86

Lyons G et al 1998 Epidural pain relief in labour: Potencies of levobupivacaine and racemic bupivacaine. Br J Anaesth 81(6):899–901

Lysak SZ, Eisenach JC, Dobson CED 1990 Patient-controlled epidural analgesia during labor: a comparison of three solutions with a continuous infusion control [see comments]. Anesthesiol 72(1):44–49

MacArthur C et al 1990 Epidural anaesthesia and long term backache after childbirth. Br Med J 301(6742):9–12

Macfie AG et al 1991 Gastric emptying in pregnancy [see comments]. Br J Anaesth 67(1):54–57

Marx GF, Joshi CW, Orkin LR 1970 Placental transmission of nitrous oxide. Anesthesiol 32(5):429–432

Marx GF, Mateo CV 1971 Effects of different oxygen concentrations during general anaesthesia for elective caesarean section. Can Anaesthetists Soc J 18(6):587–593

Melzack R, Wall PD 1965 Pain mechanism: A new theory. Science 150:971

Michael S, Reilly CS, Caunt JA 1991 Policies for oral intake during labour. A survey of maternity units in England and Wales. Anaesthesia 46(12):1071–1073

Morgan BM et al 1982 Analgesia and satisfaction in childbirth (the Queen Charlotte's 1000 Mother Survey). Lancet 2(8302):808–810

Morgan BM et al 1984 Anaesthetic morbidity following caesarean section under epidural or general anaesthesia. Lancet 1(8372):328–330

Murphy DF et al 1984 Effect of metoclopramide on gastric emptying before elective and emergency caesarean section. Br J Anaesth 56(10):1113–1116

Murphy JD et al 1991 Bupivacaine versus bupivacaine plus fentanyl for epidural analgesia: effect on maternal satisfaction [see comments]. Br Med J 302(6776):564–567

Newrick P, Read D 1982 Subdural haematoma as a complication of spinal anaesthetic. Br Med J Clin Res Ed 285(6338):341–342

Nimmo WS, Wilson J, Prescott LF 1975 Narcotic analgesics and delayed gastric emptying during labour. Lancet 1(7912):890–893

Norris MC et al 1994 Complications of labor analgesia: epidural versus combined spinal epidural techniques [published erratum appears in Anesth Analg 1994 79(6):1217] [see comments]. Anesth Analg 79(3):529–537

Norton AC, Davis AG, Spicer RJ 1988 Lignocaine 2% with adrenaline for epidural caesarean section. A comparison with 0.5% bupivacaine [see comments]. Anaesthesia 43(10):844–849

Olofsson C et al 1996 Lack of analgesic effect of systemically administered morphine or pethidine on labour pain [see comments]. Br J Obstet Gynaecol 103(10):968–972

O'Meara ME, Gin T 1993 Comparison of 0.125% bupivacaine with 0.125% bupivacaine and clonidine as extradural analgesia in the first stage of labour. Br J Anaesth 71(5):651–656

Paech MJ et al 1995 Clinical experience with patient-controlled and staff-administered intermittent bolus epidural analgesia in labour. Anaesthesia Intensive Care 23(4):459–463

Palmer CM et al 1999 Dose-response relationship of intrathecal morphine for postcesarean analgesia. Anesthesiol 90(2):437–444

Park GE et al 1996 The effects of varying volumes of crystalloid administration before cesarean delivery on maternal hemodynamics and colloid osmotic pressure. Anesth Analg 83(2):299–303

Parry MG et al 1998 Dorsal column function after epidural and spinal blockade: implications for the safety of walking following low-dose regional analgesia for labour [see comments]. Anaesthesia 53(4):382–387

Peltz B, Sinclair DM 1973 Induction agents for Caesarean section. A comparison of thiopentone and ketamine. Anaesthesia 28(1):37–42

Peng AT, Blancato LS, Motoyama EK 1972 Effect of maternal hypocapnia v. eucapnia on the foetus during Caesarean section. Br J Anaesth 44(11):1173–1178

Pitkanen M et al 1992 Chronotropic and inotropic effects of ropivacaine, bupivacaine, and lidocaine in the spontaneously beating and electrically paced isolated, perfused rabbit heart. Regional Anesth 17(4):183–192

Plaat FS, Royston P, Morgan BM 1996 Comparison of 15 mg and 25 mg of bupivacaine both with 50 mug fentanyl as initial dose for epidural analgesia. Int J Obstet Anesth 5(4):240–243

Price C et al 1998 Regional analgesia in early active labour: combined spinal epidural vs. epidural. Anaesthesia 53(10):951–955

Raidoo DM et al 1990 Critical volume for pulmonary acid aspiration: reappraisal in a primate model. Br J Anaesth 65(2):248–250

Rawal N et al 1997 Combined spinal-epidural technique [see comments]. Regional Anesth 22(5):406–423

Rayburn WF et al 1989 Randomised comparison of meperidine and fentanyl during labour. Obstet Gynecol 74:604–606

Reynolds F 1993 Principles of placental drug transfer. In: Effects on the Baby of Maternal Analgesia and Anaesthesia. Saunders, London

Rigler ML et al 1991 Cauda equina syndrome after continuous spinal anesthesia [see comments]. Anesth Analg 72(3):275–281

Roberts RB, Shirley MA 1974 Reducing the risk of acid aspiration during cesarean section. Anesth Analg 53(6):859–868

Robson JE 1979 Transcutaneous nerve stimulation for pain relief in labour. Anaesthesia 34:357

Rocco AG et al 1985 Differential spread of blockade of touch, cold, and pinprick during spinal anesthesia. Anesth Analg 64(9):917–923

Rocke DA, Rout CC, Gouws E 1994 Intravenous administration of the proton pump inhibitor omeprazole reduces the risk of acid aspiration at emergency caesarean section [see comments]. Anesth Analg 78(6):1093–1098

Rout CC, Rocke DA, Gouws E 1993 Intravenous ranitidine reduces the risk of acid aspiration of gastric contents at emergency cesarean section. Anesth Analg 76(1):156–161

Rout CC et al 1993 A reevaluation of the role of crystalloid preload in the prevention of hypotension associated with spinal anesthesia for elective cesarean section. Anesthesiol 79(2):262–269

Russell IF 1995 Levels of anaesthesia and intraoperative pain at caesarean section under regional block. Int J Obstet Anesth 4(2):71–77

Russell R, Reynolds E 1996 Epidural infusion of low-dose bupivacaine and opioid in labour. Does reducing motor block increase the spontaneous delivery rate? Anaesthesia 51(3):266–273

Russell R, Dundas R, Reynolds F 1996 Long term backache after childbirth: prospective search for causative factors [see comments]. Br Med J 312(7043):1384–1388

Santos AC et al 1995 Comparative systemic toxicity of ropivacaine and bupivacaine in nonpregnant and pregnant ewes. Anesthesiol 82(3):734–740; discussion 27A

Scott DB, Rose NB 1976 Effect of psychoprophylaxis on labour and delivery in primipara. N Engl J Med 294:1205

Scott PV et al 1980 Intrathecal morphine as sole analgesic during labour. Br Med J 281(6236):351–355

Scott DB, Hibbard BM 1990 Serious non-fatal complications associated with extradural block in obstetric practice. Br J Anaesth 64(5):537–541

Shennan A et al 1995 Blood pressure changes during labour and whilst ambulating with combined spinal epidural analgesia. Br J Obstet Gynaecol 102(3):192–197

Shir Y, Raja SN, Frank SM 1994 The effect of epidural versus general anesthesia on postoperative pain and analgesic requirements in patients undergoing radical prostatectomy [see comments]. Anesthesiol 80(1):49–56

Shutt LE et al 1992 Spinal anaesthesia for caesarean section: comparison of 22-gauge and 25-gauge Whitacre needles with 26-gauge Quincke needles. Br J Anaesth 69(6):589–594

Sia AT et al 1998 Intrathecal sufentanil as the sole agent in combined spinal-epidural analgesia for the ambulatory parturient [see comments]. Can J Anaesth 45(7):620–625

Smedstad KG, Morison DH 1988 A comparative study of continuous and intermittent epidural analgesia for labour and delivery. Can J Anaesth 35(3 (Pt 1)):234–241

Smith EA et al 1994 A comparison of 25 G and 27 G Whitacre needles for caesarean section [see comments]. Anaesthesia 49(10):859–862

Stacey RG et al 1993 Single space combined spinal-extradural technique for analgesia in labour [see comments]. Br J Anaesth 71(4):499–502

Stacey MR et al 1995 Effects of magnesium sulphate on suxamethonium-induced complications during rapid-sequence induction of anaesthesia. Anaesthesia 50(11):933–936

Stuart JC et al 1996 Acid aspiration prophylaxis for emergency Caesarean section. Anaesthesia 51(5): 415–421

Tarkkila P, Huhtala J, Salminen U 1994 Difficulties in spinal needle use. Insertion characteristics and failure rates associated with 25-, 27- and 29-gauge Quincke-type spinal needles. Anaesthesia 49(8):723–725

Vanderick G et al 1974 Bupivacaine 0.125% in epidural block analgesia during childbirth: clinical evaluation. Br J Anaesth 46(11):838–841

Vercauteren MP et al 1996 Hydroxyethylstarch compared with

modified gelatin as volume preload before spinal anaesthesia for Caesarean section. Br J Anaesth 76(5):731–733

Vertommen JD, Lemmens E, Van Aken H 1994 Comparison of the addition of three different doses of sufentanil to 0.125% bupivacaine given epidurally during labour. Anaesthesia 49(8):678–681

Warren TM et al 1983 Comparison of the maternal and neonatal effects of halothane, enflurane, and isoflurane for cesarean delivery. Anesth Analg 62(5):516–520

Waud BE, Waud DR 1970 Calculated kinetics of distribution of nitrous oxide and methoxyflurane during intermittent administration in obstetrics. Anesthesiol 32(4):306–316

Wee MY, Hasan MA, Thomas TA 1993 Isoflurane in labour [see comments]. Anaesthesia 48(5):369–372

Wiener PC, Hogg MI, Rosen M 1979 Neonatal respiration, feeding and neurobehavioural state. Effects of intrapartum bupivacaine, pethidine and pethidine reversed by naloxone. Anaesthesia 34(10):996–1004

Zaric D et al 1996 The effect of continuous lumbar epidural infusion of ropivacaine (0.1%, 0.2%, and 0.3%) and 0.25% bupivacaine on sensory and motor block in volunteers: a double-blind study. Regional Anesth 21(1):14–25

29

The midwife's role in pregnancy and labour

Lesley Page

The contribution of the author of the equivalent chapter in the second edition, on which this chapter draws extensively, is gratefully acknowledged.

INTRODUCTION

The way women, their families and their babies are cared for around the time of birth is of profound and fundamental importance. The provision of an effective maternity service is one of the most important factors leading to a healthy and happy start to life and the family. For all the professions involved in providing maternity care, the aim is the same: to provide care that improves the physical health of mother and baby, and also to support psychological and family integrity. This includes the growth of secure bonds of love between the baby and parents, increased confidence and competence in parenting, and joy and celebration at the start of the new life. The professions of midwifery and obstetrics each play an important part in achieving this aim, and each makes a unique contribution. Working together to provide effective maternity services, while recognising the distinct contribution of each profession, is crucial to effective, efficient and appropriate perinatal care.

This chapter will focus on the role of the midwife in maternity services in the industrialised world. It is recognised that the particular problems of maternity care in the developing world are far greater. In general these are beyond the scope of this chapter; but the principles described, the humanisation of birth with effective and appropriate care are the same, and the avoidance of unnecessary interventions, are of relevance to the promotion of *safe motherhood* in any part of the world.

Midwives in different parts of the world practise in a variety of settings. In some countries midwifery has been subsumed into nursing and may be restricted in the main to care in the hospital. In other countries midwives may be community based. The degree to which midwives may practise autonomously varies tremendously. In some countries, for example Britain, every woman receives care from midwives. Most women in the National Health Service have their delivery by a midwife, unless they need an assisted or caesarean birth. All women receive some antenatal and all postnatal care in the community from midwives, and are cared for in hospital by midwives. In other countries nurses may be involved in some aspects of maternity provision.

In most parts of the industrialised world, even where midwifery holds a strong position, as in Holland, the practice of midwifery has been constrained over recent decades by a number of historical changes. These include the development and introduction of a large number of technical procedures, and the shift of the place of birth from home to hospital. The shift of the place of practice of midwifery from home to hospital has resulted in fragmented care, making a continuous personal relationship between individual midwives and women, which is the basis of effective midwifery, difficult if not impossible to achieve.

In general, midwives are entitled to practise autonomously where pregnancy and birth are normal and are responsible for seeking medical attention when there is a deviation from the norm or there is a medical complication. But what is the norm? The imposition of widespread antenatal and intrapartum screening, the routine introduction of active management of labour, and changing perceptions of risk have skewed and narrowed the perception of normal pregnancy and birth. The threshold for undertaking caesarean sections and assisted delivery is far lower than it was, and there is a powerful lobby from anaesthetists to encourage the uptake of epidural anaesthesia. Thus the norm is being skewed by these trends so that fewer women now have their care managed by midwives (English National Board for Nursing Midwifery and Health Visiting 1999). Key factors in the development of more effective midwifery practice will be rethinking the idea of the normal and developing ways of supporting physiological processes.

Where midwifery has been developed to enable midwives to practise fully, comparisons with medical or shared care have demonstrated that midwifery care is associated with a number of physical and psychological improvements in outcome.

Despite the restrictions experienced by midwives, women continue to value the special approach to pregnancy and birth that midwives bring, and are confident in their care (Page & Hutton 2000). A number of government reports, change of policy and legislation at national and local level, and published research measures all indicate that the tide is turning. Work is being undertaken in many parts of the world to educate midwives and organise midwifery practice in a way that allows midwives to play their full part in the maternity services. What can be described as a *New Midwifery* is being developed. This contains many of the traditional long-standing values of midwifery, while recognising that the clock cannot be turned back. Times have changed: the role of women has altered; families are different, societies and health services are increasingly complex, we live in a more global world and knowledge has proliferated. The challenge for the future will be to develop midwifery in a way that retains the characteristics that make it a crucial part of the provision of maternity services and so valuable to women and their families, while adapting to meet the needs of a rapidly changing society.

This chapter will draw on the characteristics of what has been called the *new midwifery*, and describe some of the most effective ways in which midwives and doctors work together; it will reframe the aims of midwifery to recognise the potential of a wider role for midwives. This is the potential to provide clinical care while also recognising the importance of pregnancy and birth as a transition to the new role and responsibility of parenthood, and the social significance and consequence of birth.

ENHANCING THE ROLE OF THE MIDWIFE

Changes in policy and practice

Awareness that midwifery could be used more efficiently and effectively has led to changes in the way midwives are organised in many parts of the world. The most radical changes have been seen in New Zealand and some Provinces of Canada where midwives have become primary Providers of health care, practising on a par with general practitioners, and reimbursed directly for services rather than being employees of hospitals or the maternity services. In Holland, midwives have always been independent practitioners, reimbursed by the health insurance companies. In some parts of the world, like Australia and the USA, change has concentrated on the creation of birth centres, homelike settings where care is usually provided by midwives who have a more autonomous role than they would in the general maternity services. In Britain, a number of changes in practice and policy have resulted in the development of different forms of working, which in many cases have resulted in midwives practising more autonomously. National policy documents on the maternity services have both reflected and brought about new thinking on the provision of maternity care and the role of midwives. Perhaps the most radical and well known of these policy documents, *Changing Childbirth* (1993), was adopted as new policy for the maternity services for England in 1994 and remains policy. Although the policy is specific for England, *Changing Childbirth* has had an influence on maternity care in many other parts of the world.

Changing Childbirth is based on three principles of good maternity care:

1. The woman must be the focus of maternity care. She should be able to feel that she is in control of what is happening to her and able to make decisions about her care, based on her needs, having discussed matters fully with the professionals involved.
2. Maternity services must be readily and easily accessible to all. They should be sensitive to the needs of the local population and based primarily in the community.
3. Women should be involved in the monitoring and planning of maternity services to ensure that they are responsive to the needs of a changing society. In addition, care should be effective and resources used efficiently.

Although this policy was general and to be applied to the whole of maternity provision, it was recognised that the development of midwifery within the maternity services was crucial to putting the policy into practice. The report has detailed aims and targets for achievement. These are summarised in 10 indicators of success; a number relate directly to midwifery and reinstatement of the role of the midwife.

1. All women should be entitled to carry their own casenotes.
2. Every woman should know one midwife who ensures continuity of her midwifery care – the named midwife.
3. At least 30% of women should have the midwife as the lead professional.
4. Every woman should know the lead professional who has a key role in the planning and provision of her care.
5. At least 75% of women should know the person who cares for them during their delivery.
6. Midwives should have direct access to some beds in all maternity units.
7. At least 30% of women delivered in a maternity unit should be admitted under the management of the midwife.
8. The total number of antenatal visits for women with uncomplicated pregnancies should have been reviewed in the light of the available evidence and the RCOG guidelines.

9. All front-line ambulances should have a paramedic able to support the midwife who needs to transfer a woman to hospital in an emergency.
10. All women should have access to information about the services available in their locality.

Much practical organisational change had started in advance of this change in policy, largely owing to the influence of the work of Flint in the *Know Your Midwife Project* (Flint & Poulengeris 1987). There were three approaches to change in midwifery practice:

1. to organise midwives to provide midwifery-led care, that is, take responsibility for the care of women with normal pregnancies
2. to provide greater continuity of care
3. to provide alternatives to hospital and home birth, namely birth centres or home-from-home schemes.

These developments occurred in a number of countries, including Britain, Australia, Iceland, America and Canada.

Home birth

Women should be free to decide where their baby is to be born, and whether or not they need to go to hospital for the birth. A number of women choose to have their babies at home. In general these are well-educated affluent women. The best current evidence indicates that this is no less safe than hospital birth for low-risk mothers and babies, where the service is backed up by a modern hospital system. There are a number of advantages to home birth. In general, the quality of personal support is better than can be achieved in the hospital system, and the rate of interventions is lower (Page 2000). Midwives have an important role in the provision of home birth services. This is an environment where midwives may come into their own, practising in a truly autonomous way. The approach and skills required for attendance at a home birth are quite different to those required in a hospital setting. The midwife needs to make good assessments and predict problems, and to be able to deal with all emergencies, until transfer is arranged. The provision of courses such as ALSO (Advanced Life Support in Obstetrics) has been invaluable to midwives attending out-of-hospital births.

Community-based care

Changing Childbirth emphasised the importance of shifting a large part of maternity care to the community. This may entail the provision of care in local surgeries or offices, where midwives or doctors practise, home-based antenatal visits, and community-based education for childbirth and parenting. In Britain, maternity services have always provided a strong community service in which community midwives make antenatal and postnatal visits to women at home and provide a service for the small number of women who have requested home birth. Some of the most successful developments of maternity care have been in the strengthening of local community-based services. The maternity service in Bath is one of the best examples of this approach. The most successful continuity of care schemes have been based on an integration of community and hospital care. In general, women report greater sensitivity from professionals, including midwives and doctors, practising in a community rather than a hospital setting.

Changes in the education of midwives

The preparation for entry to the register of midwives has changed radically in the UK and many other parts of the world. All preregistration programmes are at university level, the majority of these programmes awarding a degree. In addition, a number of programmes admit students of midwifery directly without the need to register as a nurse first. The clarification of midwifery as a profession distinct from nursing has been an important part of the development of midwifery autonomy. In addition to the higher level of preregistration midwifery education there are now a number of postgraduate programmes, educating midwives to the Masters and Doctoral level.

Relationship with medical colleagues

These changes to enhance the role of the midwife have often been supported or even implemented by medical colleagues. This does not mean they have been easy: inevitable overlapping of roles and confusion about the actual role, responsibility and accountability of midwives and doctors have created tensions. Finances enter into this for the funding of general practitioners for maternity services may be an important item in private practice. There is sometimes a mistaken belief that doctors need to take responsibility for the practice of midwives. This is not the case; the midwife is responsible and accountable for her own practice. It is important to clarify roles and responsibilities carefully and to identify differences.

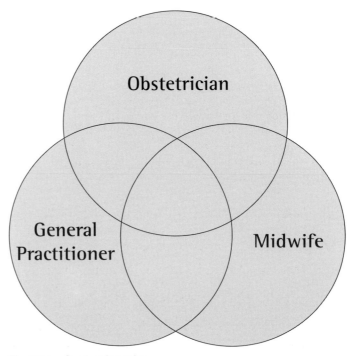

Fig. 29.1 Overlapping roles.

similarities and ways of working together in order to ensure that each profession is able to play a full and appropriate part in the provision of maternity services. So, in what ways do midwifery and medicine differ, and where are they similar?

In contrast to midwives, obstetricians specialise in care where there are complications of pregnancy and birth, and in surgical intervention. There is a growing field of specialism in fertility treatment and materno-fetal medicine. General practitioners provide maternity care as a part of their general practice, and for a number of GPs there is the potential for continuity in much of the life of the family. General practice obstetrics can be an important component of family practice. Increasingly, however, general practitioners only provide antenatal and postnatal care. The numbers of GPs providing the full range of maternity care are declining steadily.

Many of the problems of modern maternity services arise from failure to recognise the specialist skills and perspectives of medical care and to use it appropriately when it is really needed. A great deal of medical time seems to be spent in the oversight of healthy women in pregnancy, when this time could be better used elsewhere. For example, one area where substandard care is often identified is the provision of intrapartum care by junior medical staff in the delivery suite, where a senior experienced obstetrician is required (Department of Health et al 1996). When midwives identify problems they should be able to refer directly to an experienced obstetrician, rather than an obstetrician in training. Where the work of obstetricians has given them a substantial role in the care (and oversight of care) of women with normal pregnancies, the role of the midwife has often become that of acting as doctor's assistant. This is a very expensive use of a valuable resource. A number of studies over many years have described the frustration midwives have felt concerning constraints to their role.

Midwives are specialists in normal pregnancy and birth, and have the potential, when appropriately organised and empowered, to support physiological pregnancy and birth. This is not to suggest that midwives should work in isolation. On the contrary, collaboration and agreed processes and systems of referral are crucial to any health service. In reality there will always be some overlap in the roles of the three major care providers. The most important aspect of working out ways of practising together is to ensure that every woman has one named professional. This professional may be a midwife, obstetrician or general practitioner, who provides most of the hands-on care and is responsible for ensuring a personal, sensitive and high-quality service to individual women. This does not mean that the woman need only see one professional: for a number of women there will be times when consultation or referral will need to be made to another colleague, either from midwife to doctor or doctor to midwife. Clear processes and systems for consultation and referral between doctors and midwives are crucial.

THE SCOPE AND AIM OF MIDWIFERY PRACTICE

The *Midwife's Code of Practice* clearly states the duties, responsibilities and limits of the midwife. A midwife is a person who has been regularly admitted to a midwifery education programme duly recognised in the country in which it is located. She will have successfully completed the prescribed course of studies in midwifery and acquired the requisite qualifications to be registered and legally licensed to practise midwifery. She must be able to give the necessary supervision, care and advice to women during pregnancy, labour and the postpartum period, to conduct deliveries on her own responsibility and to care for the mother and the infant. This care includes preventative measures, the detection of abnormal conditions in mother and child, procurement of medical assistance and the execution of emergency measures in the absence of medical help. The midwife has an important task in health counselling and education, not only for the mothers but also within the family and the community. The work should involve antenatal education and preparation for parenthood and extends to certain areas of gynaecology, family planning and childcare. She may practise in hospitals, clinics, health units, domiciliary conditions or in any other service (UKCC 1998).

This international definition provides a clear outline of the scope of practice and is an important part of the framework for midwifery. However, it tells us little about the distinct nature of midwifery, the approach that makes it different to that of other professionals involved in maternity care. There are two characteristics of effective midwifery that make it unique. Firstly, midwives are specialists in the care of women with normal pregnancies and birth. Second, midwives have the potential to develop a personal relationship with women (the original meaning of midwife) through the whole of pregnancy, birth and the early weeks of life, that has been described in a number of ways, as a relationship of friendship, of partnership, or of skilled companionship.

The scope of midwifery is far wider than the physical health of mother and baby, although physical safety is, of course, basic to care. The aims of midwifery are threefold:

- to help the mother, and her family, make the transition to parenthood in the best way possible; that is, to emerge from childbirth physically and emotionally intact, with relationships within the family, particularly the attachment between baby and parents, as strong as possible, and to have the confidence, knowledge and commitment to care for the child until adulthood
- to support and protect physiological processes and healthy outcomes
- to provide comfort and alleviate distressing symptoms of pregnancy and birth and the postpartum period.

These aims are achieved in a number of ways and illustrated in Table 29.1. Each of these aims and how they may be achieved is described in detail in the remainder of the chapter.

Supporting an effective transition to parenthood

Pregnancy and birth are a time of personal transition when the mother and father undertake the most dramatic change of role and responsibility of their life. They take on the responsibility for caring for the infant who is totally depen-

Table 29.1 The aims of midwifery and how they are achieved

Aim	How the aim is achieved
Supporting the mother and her family in making an effective transition to the new role and responsibility of parenting	• Encouraging the mother to enlist support of family/friends/community • Providing a constant presence during labour and birth • Being *with woman*, rebuilding relationships between women and midwives • Developing new structures to allow continuity of carer • Using shared decision making (with women and their families) • Supporting attachment and bonding • Providing appropriate information/counselling/teaching • Promote breast-feeding
To support physiological processes while promoting healthy outcomes	• Use the principles of effective and appropriate care • Develop a risk prevention and assessment model • Be selective about the use of technology, medical interventions and screening
To help alleviate distressing symptoms and provide comfort, particularly during labour and birth and the postnatal period	• Attendance of a midwife the mother knows and trusts, particularly during labour and birth • Understand the basis of pregnancy symptoms and how to provide relief • Understand maternal ill health following birth and help prevent it whenever possible

dent at the start of life, and who will need love, guidance, care and provision for many years to come. The success of this transition is crucial to the health and well-being of the child, and indeed of future generations. To a great extent, the way this transition is made will be determined by past history and life circumstances, but the time around pregnancy and birth is a critical period that is also highly influential. Health professionals are in a position to support or destroy an effective transition. At one extreme, women may emerge from the experience of childbirth feeling more confident and competent (Simkin 1992); at the other, they may be left feeling depressed, distressed and unwell. Some women may even develop post-traumatic stress disorder, an extreme psychological distress reaction following exposure to a traumatic and threatening experience following birth (Lyons 1998). The concept of transition is particularly important to midwives, who have the potential to work in a close, continuous and sensitive relationship with women and their families. However, although health professionals are involved in care at a critical time, they are only part of the life of the family for a short duration. The support of family, friends and community is crucial.

Encouraging the mother to enlist support of family/friends/community

Social support is commonly conceived as having three dimensions: advice/information, tangible assistance and emotional support (presence, listening, reassurance, and affirmation) (Hodnett 1999a). Social support has a number of positive effects on both physical and emotional well-being. It is associated with enhanced physical health, and greater emotional well-being. Midwives may help to mobilise support, including practical help, for women in a number of ways. These might simply be by talking with the woman and her family of the need and importance of support. It may be by some minor social engineering, for example forming groups for education classes of women going through pregnancy at the same time

and in the same area. The provision of social support is more possible where the practice is arranged to provide community-based individual, continuous and sensitive care. Much of the work of enabling midwives to contribute to effective social support has taken place through the development of continuity of carer schemes.

Being with woman, *rebuilding the relationship*

The basis of effective midwifery lies in supporting the transition to parenthood through a positive and supportive relationship between the woman and her midwife. Historically the midwife was a part of the woman's community, understanding and to some extent sharing in similar daily lives. This may be more complex now when many communities are made up of a rich racial mix. Even now, when few midwives practice as part of the woman's community, women are likely to feel more comfortable in raising what may seem trivial questions or concerns with a sensitive midwife than with a doctor. Moreover midwives share intimately in aspects of the woman's pregnancy and birth.

The word midwife means *with woman* and has a number of implications, including the need to work in the best interests of the woman and her family, helping to achieve what is important to them as individuals.

Women entering the maternity services expect *care* from the professionals they meet. When women receive appropriate care, it has a powerful positive effect. The opposite, that has been described as uncaring, may have even more powerful negative effects. Care is a term we use constantly, yet it is a slippery concept and may be difficult to define. Studies of women's perspectives of the dimensions and attributes of caring are summarised in Table 29.2.

Women identify the need for kindness, connection, companionship and support. The direct words of women interviewed as part of the evaluation of One-to-One Midwifery Practice convey the power of a personal supportive relationship:

Table 29.2 Women's perspectives of the dimensions and attributes of caring: a fundamental framework for midwives (McCourt et al 2000)

Dimensions	Attributes
Attitude	A friendly presence, i.e. body language, tone of voice, use of language
Respect	For a woman's knowledge of herself; for a woman's need; that she has a right to receive care; that it is the woman's experience that is of most importance; that she is a woman and part of a family
Support	To enable and enhance the woman's experience, i.e. being with her when she needs the midwife psychologically and/or with her physical presence: to offer and provide the amount and type of help she needs rather than what the midwife wants to give
Reassurance	That a woman will know her carers; that she can easily access her carers; that physical and practical care will be provided to a high standard; that she will be treated honestly, by the type of words and language used with appropriate knowledge; by the midwife's presence and attitude
Interest	In her pregnancy; with listening and focusing upon her at that moment
Communication	In particular, the ability to communicate through the choice of words, tone of voice, presence, use of language, listening, interest and focus

'you had that person you knew you could turn to all the time'

and another woman said

'but my midwife, she was part of it, part of the birth, the baby'.

McCourt et al 2000, p 282

It is important for all midwives, whether or not they work in traditional fragmented structures, or in organisations that support the development of continuous relationships between midwives and mothers, to understand the importance of women receiving positive personal care. It is important too for such midwives to be aware of their own behaviour and communication skills and how women and families in their care perceive it. However, where midwives practise in fragmented systems of care it is far harder to provide this positive individual care, and women are far less likely to perceive their experience as caring. Sensitive care is of immense importance to women and they are more likely to perceive care as being sensitive when there is a continuous relationship with the caregiver.

Developing new structures to allow continuity of carer
Over the last two decades a number of changes have created greater continuity of care to enable personal relationships between women and their midwives and to support more sensitive care. The development of continuity of carer requires systems in which an individual midwife may act as the named or primary midwife for individual women, being responsible for and providing most of the hands-on care, while practising with a partner, or small number of partners, to allow time off. When well organised these schemes provide each woman with a midwife she knows and trusts. This is very important to women, and provides a very different experience of maternity to that of standard care.

The development of continuity of care schemes has been one of the major areas of debate amongst midwives over recent years. Once set up, these schemes are extremely effective, if appropriately organised. However, they require major shifts in both the structure and culture of the organisation. Following the publication of *Changing Childbirth*, nearly every maternity service in England had developed a pilot project to enable midwifery-led care, continuity of care, or both. Only a proportion of these innovations has been evaluated. In a structured review of 7 comparative studies of continuity of care schemes and midwifery-led care, Green et al (1998) found that these schemes were consistently associated with a lower use of epidurals and often of other forms of pain relief, and with less perineal trauma. There was no statistically significant difference between groups in rates of operative or assisted delivery. This may be because many of the developments have taken place in hospital settings; moreover, many developments were evaluated soon after their introduction. It is difficult to know to what extent the effects of these developments are restricted by the environment in which they are situated, or by the timing of the evaluation.

Two continuity of care schemes including 1815 women have been evaluated by randomised controlled trials. The comparison between continuity of care by midwives with non-continuity of care by a combination of physicians and midwives showed the following results; women were:

- less likely to experience antenatal admission to hospital
- more likely to attend antenatal education programmes
- less likely to have drugs for pain relief
- less likely to have a baby who required resuscitation
- less likely to have an episiotomy (more likely to have either a perineal or vaginal tear)
- more likely to be pleased with their antenatal, intrapartum and postnatal care
- less likely to experience clinic waiting times of more than 15 minutes
- less likely to feel not prepared for labour
- less likely to fail to enjoy labour
- less likely to perceive labour staff as unsupportive
- less likely to feel unable to discuss postnatal problems (Hodnett 1999b).

Two cohort studies of an innovative way of providing a high level of continuity of caregiver, One-to-One Midwifery, included 3000 women. The first cohort study took place soon after the inception of the scheme (Page et al 1999), the second when the innovation had become more routine and embedded in the service. The second cohort study of the One-to-One Midwifery Service showed an increase in differences in intervention rates between the first and second cohort.

Results in the second cohort indicated statistically significant differences in:

- assisted delivery or caesarean birth   OR   (95% CI) 0.60 (0.42,–0.85)
- episiotomy or perineal tear   OR   (95% CI) 0.43 (0.30,–0.64)
- epidural anaesthesia   OR   (95% CI) 0.37 (0.26,–0.53)
- labour duration minutes –98 minutes (mean difference not odds ratio) (–140,–56 minutes).

These results favoured the One-to-One group. Regression analysis was undertaken to adjust for potentially confounding variables and confirmed the differences between groups (Page et al 2001). This may indicate that an innovation needs time to become established; failure to show differences in rates of caesarean birth and assisted delivery in the first cohort, and other evaluations of innovation, may have occurred because the evaluation was premature. Other aspects of the evaluation showed this form of care to be highly cost effective and intensely satisfying to those midwives who choose to practise in this way.

An in-depth assessment of women's responses to care was undertaken as part of this study. Both qualitative and quantitative data indicate higher levels of satisfaction with birth, generally more positive responses to the experience and care, and higher scores of emotional well-being (McCourt & Page 1996, Page et al 2000).

What do such schemes need to be successful in providing good care for women while being satisfying to midwives? Midwives practising in continuity of care schemes are required to make an on-call commitment, but also need to balance professional and personal life, and to avoid unnecessary stress and burnout. The characteristics of systems that are effective for women and midwives are:

- occupational autonomy
- development of meaningful relationships with women
- social support.

Occupational autonomy allows the midwife to make decisions with women in her care, within her scope of practice. This also allows the midwife to organise her practice in a way that meets women's needs, while balancing her personal life and responsibilities. This is particularly important to a profession composed almost entirely of women. Midwives given occupational autonomy have the flexibility to arrange their work and on-call schedules in the best way to meet both professional and personal responsibilities. Such schemes can be self-managing and do not require the hierarchical and controlling management that has been a part of the traditional midwifery culture.

It should be obvious that the smaller number of midwives a woman has to get to know, the more likely she is to have good continuity of care. A named midwife working with a partner has been extremely successful in the One-to-One Midwifery Service that has been running for over 8 years. This service is very simply organised and covers two postal districts in London (W3 and W12). Women are either referred through the hospital system, or directly by a GP. Increasingly,

women self-refer. Each woman books with one named midwife who will provide most of her hands-on care. When the mother and baby are healthy the midwife will be the lead professional. If there are medical problems the midwife will work together with medical staff, while still providing all of the midwifery care. Each midwife works with a midwife partner who gets to know the woman, allowing the named midwife time off. The named midwife follows the woman through the system of care, providing a large proportion of the antenatal care in the woman's own home. The woman calls her midwife or the partner when she goes into labour. She may choose to deliver in one of two hospitals or at home; if booked for a hospital birth her early labour care may take place at home. The named midwife continues care into the postnatal period until at least day 10 and sometimes to day 28, when care is transferred to the health visitor. A high degree of continuity is achieved through the whole of the process.

Each midwife takes on a caseload of 40 births per year and has no other responsibilities. The amount of time spent is on average 37.5 hours a week. The working unit of the One-to-One service is a partnership. However, these partnerships work as a part of a group, who support each other, help balance the caseload, and undertake regular peer review of practice. The transition from working in a standard service, in which midwives are parts of teams providing only a fragment of the care for women, to professional autonomy can be a challenge for midwives. It often takes about 6 months to adapt to the new way of working. Midwifery and medical colleagues can do a great deal to support these developments and the midwives practising in them, by respecting professional autonomy, being supportive, having joint meetings and continuing education, and listening.

Using shared decision-making

The foundation of the *new midwifery* is what has often been described as a special relationship between women and their midwives. The purpose of this relationship is to provide support through the whole experience of pregnancy, to develop mutual trust between woman and midwife and to involve women in making decisions about their care. This means that talking about decisions need not happen in one visit but can go on over time. One of the most important principles of *Changing Childbirth* is the involvement of women in decisions about their care. These ideas have been summarised in the slogan of the 'three Cs' – continuity, choice and control.

It is important in such special relationships to avoid the development of undue dependency; indeed, the support is intended to increase the confidence and sense of personal autonomy in women. The concept of the skilled companion (Campbell, quoted in Page et al 2000) has been a useful metaphor for midwives. Pregnancy and birth are viewed as transitional and often transformative processes. This is a personal journey to a new life and role and responsibility. The midwife can be likened to the companion who supports the woman through this journey. There are four features to this companionship:

- a bodily presence that necessitates sensitivity
- the notion of helping another move forward on the journey with encouragement and hope

- *being with* rather than *doing to* in the sense of personal involvement, even with unpopular and difficult people
- the commitment is for the duration of the journey, recognising that both woman and midwife have their own lives to lead.

Recognition of the importance of personal autonomy for the woman and her partner in making decisions about their care and the care of their child, while taking into account evidence and expert advice, is the cornerstone of the relationship. In partnership, both midwife and woman are seen as having their own expertise: the collective knowledge and wisdom of the midwife and the specific self-knowledge and wisdom of the woman and her family (Guilliland, quoted in Page et al 2000).

Provide a constant presence during labour and birth

One of the most important outcomes of well-organised continuity of care schemes is to provide constant attendance at labour and birth. This constant presence of a trained midwife, nurse or doula and encouragement by comforting touch, words of praise and reassurance is associated with a number of improved outcomes for the mother and baby. A meta-analysis of 14 randomised controlled trials including more than 5000 women evaluated the effect of the continuous presence of a support person, which included reduction in:

- the likelihood of medication for pain relief
- operative vaginal delivery
- caesarean section
- 5-minute Apgar score less than 7
- the length of labour (slightly).

Six trials evaluated the effects of support on mother's views of their childbirth experience including:

- overall satisfaction
- failure to cope during labour
- finding labour to be worse than expected
- level of personal control during childbirth.

In each trial, results favoured the group who had received continuous support (Hodnett 1999a). It can be seen that this human support has a powerful positive effect on both physical and psychological outcomes.

Supporting attachment and bonding

Pregnancy and the birth of a baby mark the start of the most important love affair of human life, the love between the child and its parents.

> The midwife is a facilitator not only of the physical birth, but indeed also of the birth of the self, the family, and the potential for human love. The midwife, therefore, is in a unique position to play a critical role in the areas of both mental health promotion and the screening of parents and infants at risk of long-term social and emotional problems .... The human infant's attachment to the mother (or other primary caregiver) is seen as a prerequisite for survival and a test bed for all the other attachments that he or she will make in the future.
>
> Mills & Page 2000

All professionals have a part to play in early prevention, detection and intervention of mental health problems but midwives are perhaps the best placed to support parents and identify those who may need extra support, to promote a secure attachment. This is in part because of the amount of time they spend with parents in the perinatal period, and also because of the potential for a close relationship.

Attachment is defined as:

> The infant's development of an affectional bond, affective tie, or psychological bond to the primary caregiver, usually the mother during the last half of the first year of life. Infant attachment is thought to have a biological function to ensure infant survival, security and protection; it is considered a hypothetical construct of affection manifested by attachment behaviours which develop over time through a process of parent–child interaction.
>
> In contrast bonding usually refers to the affectional tie or bond of mother to infant believed to occur immediately after birth, perhaps to a sensitive or critical period.
>
> Klaus & Kennel 1976, quoted in Mills & Page 2000, p 293

Factors that affect the development of a secure attachment between the child and parents are complex and include:

- the parent's own experience from their parents
- the lifelong history of relationships
- the parents' own ability to love and support each other
- perinatal factors
- environmental stress
- the quality of support received by parents
- infant factors, health and temperament.

Relationship factors that occur long before the birth of the baby have the most profound impact, and the quality of the early parent–child relationship is the most consistent factor influencing the long-term mental, emotional and social health of the individual. However, the time around birth is a sensitive and critical period during which the potential of parents and baby to develop a secure attachment may be influenced.

The midwife may help to support the development of secure bonds of attachment in a number of ways that include the following:

- being aware of the importance of bonding and attachment and the theory underlying these concepts
- providing personal sensitive care if at all possible through a continuous relationship with the woman; this has the potential to provide a model of nurturing that may influence the sensitivity of care the mother shows her infant
- promoting physical closeness of mother and baby
- allowing undisturbed time together after birth
- helping the mother reflect on her experience of her own parents and her present life circumstances
- assessing the individual characteristics of the newborn, temperament and health, and explaining newborn behaviour to the parents
- advising on appropriate sources of support
- making referrals when necessary.

Providing appropriate information, counselling and teaching

It has been the tradition in Britain, over many years, for the midwife to provide or organise what is often known as parentcraft education. Effective midwifery requires an ability to promote health, help the woman and her family prepare for labour and birth, and develop essential skills and knowledge to prepare for caring for the baby. The provision of parentcraft classes is only a part of this process. Health promotion requires a political understanding of the components that contribute to health, a number of them outside the individual's control (for example environmental factors, material and social poverty). Midwives increasingly need a public health view of maternity care to understand the way in which individual health is affected by external circumstances. On an individual basis, the midwife has a huge potential to help in the education of the woman around the time of the birth of her babies. This may be accomplished in a number of ways, including:

- conducting all visits in a way that encourages the woman to ask questions
- building an approach to care that integrates the provision of information and discussion at all times
- assessing the learning needs of the woman and her family
- providing evidence-based information (for example MIDIRS leaflets), videos, stories or demonstrations in an appropriate form, recognising cultural differences in the way different women learn, and language barriers
- organising community learning and support groups
- using the principles of adult education in classes
- being prepared to raise issues and discuss them over time.

Midwives should recognise some of the problems inherent in education for childbirth. There is a huge tension when providing education in hospitals between a form of indoctrination – preparing the woman to accept the routines, unwritten rules, values and procedures of the institution – and at the other extreme the provision of external education that bears no relationship to the reality and limitations of care locally.

Promoting breast-feeding

The promotion of breast feeding is one of the most important things a midwife can do to enhance the long-term health and well-being of both baby and mother. In many developed countries breast feeding rates remain lower than those recommended by the World Health Organization (WHO) and the United Nations Children's Fund (UNICEF). There are a number of benefits to both baby and mother of breast feeding (see Ch. 40).

Midwives can promote breast-feeding in a number of ways. These include the provision of information, professional support and education within the mother's social circle, an early feed after birth, attention to the correct positioning of the baby, and providing consistent advice. Frequency and duration of breast-feeding should be unrestricted (Percival 2000).

Supporting physiological processes while promoting health

It is important to understand that much of the legislation that is the basis of the profession of midwifery was created to regulate and to limit the practice of midwives; for example, the Midwives Act of 1902 laid down the necessity of calling for medical aid in particular circumstances. Even now the emphasis is on midwives being able to recognise deviations from the norm, rather than emphasising their responsibility to recognise the normal and support it. The need to recognise deviations from the norm becomes very problematic in situations in which birth is recognised as normal only in retrospect, and risk assessment is likely to categorise the majority of women as high risk. It is particularly problematic when interventions are applied routinely and frequently to all women in a population, even those who do not need it. It means that most women have what is considered to be a complicated or high-risk pregnancy, and the scope of midwives to practise autonomously is limited.

This approach can be turned on its head to emphasise the importance of midwives in not only recognising the normal but also in taking the responsibility for preserving normal or physiological processes. It is important to make it clear from the outset that this is not allowing nature to take its course, but rather recognising when we can do no better than nature, while knowing when we must give nature a hand. We should only intervene in such a finely tuned and complex process as pregnancy and birth when we know that our intervention is likely to be of benefit. Much of the aim of midwifery is to protect and support normal or physiological pregnancy and birth.

Using the principles of effective and appropriate care

It is important for all professionals to understand that what we do in practice may not always benefit the women in our care. Midwives too must always be prepared to ask the questions:

- Is what I am planning likely to do more good than harm?
- Am I spending my time doing the right things?

The publication of the MIDIRS (Midwives Information in Research Service) digest, *Effective Care in Pregnancy and Childbirth* (1989), followed by the Cochrane Library, established clear standards for maternity care. New forms of care should be evaluated before being used widely in practice. The development of what has been called evidence-based medicine established the need to use good evidence as one source of information on which to make decisions. Recent policy documents, particularly *Changing Childbirth*, have emphasised the importance of making care sensitive to the personal needs of individuals, and of the importance of involving women in making decisions about their care. Effective practice requires an ability to use information about the preferences and values of the woman and her family, information arising from the best evidence available, and information arising from the clinical examination and history. This allows the weighing up of information, while taking into account the conclusions from population-based studies, that tell us more about populations than individuals, together with the individual health of a particular mother and baby, and their wishes. In midwifery, this is helped tremendously by a supportive and continuous relationship between the woman and her midwife.

Five steps of what is called evidence-based midwifery have been proposed to make this process more explicit.

1. getting to know the woman and her family
2. making a clinical assessment through the clinical examination and history
3. seeking and evaluating the evidence
4. talking it through
5. reflecting on outcomes and consequences (Page 2000).

Midwives nowadays are expected to use evidence to inform their practice. Huge problems may be created when protocols or guidelines are produced that do not reflect the best current evidence. The development of such guidelines requires collaboration and consensus in any institution in which doctors and midwives work together. At the minimum, guidelines should be referenced, and a rationale provided.

Developing a risk assessment model for midwifery

There is a simple explanation of the differences between midwifery and obstetrics. Obstetrics has developed the view that childbirth is only normal in retrospect. Midwifery views pregnancy and birth as a process that is a normal part of life, in which in most cases we can have confidence that the outcomes will be healthy. Although these two viewpoints are polemics that disguise great complexity they can both be held at the same time. Although, strictly speaking, the approaches of midwifery and of obstetrics as disciplines may differ, there are obstetricians who take a midwifery approach and midwives who take the obstetrical approach. However, much of modern maternity care is founded on routines and treatments that have been applied to women without discrimination, whatever their need (Chalmers et al 1989). The routine frequent use of ultrasound scanning, the use of routine electronic fetal monitoring, the imposition of the active management of labour and the widescale promotion of epidural anaesthesia are common in most parts of the industrialised world. The rate of assisted birth (forceps and vacuum extraction) is rising. Even in Britain, where intervention rates had been low in comparison with North America and Australia, the rise has recently been rapid (ENB 1999). There is little doubt that the culture of modern maternity care values intervention rather than a more passive wait-and-see approach, and values technology and medical intervention over human support. Midwives too are caught up in this wave, and continue to use interventions such as electronic fetal monitoring despite convincing evidence of lack of efficacy, especially for low-risk populations. It is difficult to assess to what extent these cultural norms reflect general changes in society or are shaped by professionals.

One of the important functions of modern midwifery will be to identify women and babies who are healthy, and to keep them that way, without unnecessary surgical or medical intervention. At the moment we are in a situation where childbirth has never been safer, yet it is still treated as a highly hazardous event. There will never be absolute safety in birth, but the treatment of all women as though they need interference reflects a desire to remove all risk. Strategies to identify groups of women who needed special care have largely failed.

Problems in risk assessment

The identification of women or groups of women who are at high risk was intended to direct specialist care and resources to those who needed them. Saxell reviewed the evidence and literature on risk in pregnancy. The review indicates poor predictive value of risk assessment. There are a number of problems, including a high level of false positives, difficulty in accumulating risk scores when the weighting is arbitrary, and the difficulty of using risk scores from populations in predicting risk of an adverse outcome in an individual. A culture of screening, testing and technology and risk assessment has shifted women's perceptions of pregnancy from a normal process to a risky process (Saxell 2000). It should be remembered that interventions hold their own risks; iatrogenesis (illness or injury caused by health care) is always a potential problem, so an attempt to reduce risk may create different risks. If midwives are to discriminate between women needing particular forms of support, or intervention, or place of birth, it is necessary to try to be more specific about risk as the probability of a particular adverse outcome in an individual and how it might be prevented. It is important to remember too that social and material deprivation, problems of substance abuse and addiction, are associated with higher rates of mortality and morbidity. Interventions to reduce risk therefore may not be medical but social. Saxell recommends interventions to reduce the root cause of risk: more money, educational programmes, better and safe housing, addiction treatment and counselling.

Like any intervention, risk assessment and prevention can create problems. It is important to remember that labelling a woman as being high risk may create anxiety that in itself may alter the outcome of the pregnancy, and at least spoil the enjoyment of it. It may also entail the use of valuable resources when they are not required; so, how can midwives approach risk assessment in a way that confirms where problems are not predicted, and identify who would benefit from the specialist care of midwives rather than obstetricians and who may give birth at home or use a low technology birth centre or hospital? How might they best reduce risk in pregnancy and birth for the women in their care?

As Saxell (2000) reminds us, for medicine risk is a statistical artefact, for the woman it is a subjective experience. The measurement of risk is 'weighted towards disaster and anxiety rather than peace of mind'. Labelling a woman as high risk is likely to create anxiety, and to become a self-fulfilling prophecy. The most reliable and specific assessment of risk is likely to be made by the professional who knows the woman and who can make an assessment of the probability of specific adverse outcomes. This should be based on an individual assessment of the condition of mother and baby, while taking into account good evidence on outcomes in populations. It is important also to recognise that psychological factors can be important (Page 2000, Saxell 2000). Assessment should be aimed at identifying those women who have positive indicators of good health and so can have midwifery-led care.

Saxell also recommends some very practical ways of avoiding risk in pregnancy and birth. These include:

- regular peer review of practice
- remaining up to date with emergency measures such as treatment of postpartum haemorrhage
- the provision of continuity of care
- discussing the pros and cons of particular forms of treatment during the pregnancy.

Finally, it is important to remember that there is no such thing as absence of risk. Moreover, different individuals will have different ideas of what constitutes an acceptable risk, and it is up to the individual woman to decide what is an acceptable risk (Saxell 2000).

Being selective and critical about the use of screening diagnostic tests, technology and medical interventions

Most modern maternity services now provide a whole battery of screening and diagnostic tests from early in pregnancy. In principle, women should opt in to these tests rather than needing to opt out of them. Midwives therefore need to provide women with information that they can understand about the advantages and disadvantages of such tests. This is no mean feat given their number and complexity. The provision and number of screening tests has increased dramatically in recent years and is likely to continue to rise, particularly with the development of genetic treatments. The detailed and pervasive screening of pregnancy has profound implications and consequences for individuals and society. Prenatal diagnosis and screening may lead to what has been described as 'the tentative pregnancy' (Katz Rothman 1994) – a tendency for women to put off or try to put off acceptance of the pregnancy and the baby until all is shown to be normal. Screening tests may reassure, but they can also cause unnecessary anxiety. In order to advise on such tests, help to interpret them to women, and reassure, midwives need to understand the difference between screening and diagnostic tests, concepts such as sensitivity and specificity, and positive predictive value. They need to understand how the value of such tests varies in accordance with the population in which it is used, for example populations with a low risk of the condition, or a high risk of the condition. This is particularly important to the interpretation of cardiotocographs, when the application in low-risk populations will lead to a large number of false-positive identification of fetal distress. They also need to understand that a number of factors, for example gestational age, may affect the interpretation of a number of prenatal screening tests.

If midwives are to promote physiological processes, to avoid unnecessary operative birth and make the experience positive they need to do a number of things (Table 29.3). These include:

- making an individual assessment of progress and health in labour and birth that includes all parameters of health
- using midwifery interventions appropriately (e.g. mobility and position in labour, massage)

- using intermittent auscultation to monitor the fetal heart in labour when pregnancy is normal
- helping women to avoid unnecessary epidural anaesthesia where possible by effective personal support, constant presence, words of encouragement and comforting touch, use of position, water and massage.

It is important, however, to recognise when intervention may be required. Progress of labour must be assessed and fetal and maternal health carefully evaluated. Up to 10% of all cases of cerebral palsy are caused by events during labour and birth, but everything possible should be done to avoid this. In some cases a timely intervention, such as performing an episiotomy, or using electronic fetal monitoring if, for example, second stage is extended, may prevent interventions such as operative or assisted birth.

Alleviating the distressing symptoms of pregnancy, labour, birth and the postnatal period

Understanding the basis of symptoms in pregnancy

Even when pregnancy is wanted, it is often accompanied by what were referred to as the discomforts of pregnancy. For many women the growth of another life inside her feels miraculous; for some it can be unwanted, a burden or a worry. For every woman the physical carrying of the baby and the dramatic physiological changes will bring about changes in body feel and image, and symptoms that can be inconvenient, distressing and very uncomfortable. It is important for the midwife to understand the physiological basis of these changes and how they might be relieved. In this way she can help the woman understand that changes are normal, how and why they occur, and to find some comfort.

The midwife is in a particularly good position to help in relation to the distressing symptoms of pregnancy shown in Table 29.4. Help and advice in these areas may include advice on life style and activities of daily living. Like anything else, though, such advice is an intervention. Women should be told whether or not the advice given is based on good evidence, or experience and the chances of it working.

Providing comfort and alleviation of symptoms, particularly during labour and birth

The role of the midwife is important at all stages of pregnancy, during and after birth. Yet labour and birth are critical and the most acute event. It is difficult therefore to avoid special attention to this climactic part of childbearing. In all history of various races, giving birth is the critical event. Where midwives play their full role they are able to manage labour and birth on their own responsibility without the involvement of a doctor, and their education should prepare them to assume this responsibility. This is one of the most psychologically challenging times of human life.

The birth of a child, especially a first child, represents a landmark event in the lives of all involved. For the mother particularly, childbirth has a profound physical, mental, emotional and social effect. No other event involves pain, emotional stress, vulnerability, possible physical injury or death, and permanent role change, and includes responsi-

Table 29.3 The midwifery matrix: avoiding unnecessary intervention in birth

Principle	Rationale	How?
Use individual assessment and support in labour, avoiding inappropriate use of the active management of labour	The important component of active management may be the constant presence of a caregiver (Thornton & Lilford 1994). Women progress at different rates and a standard target for dilatation does not allow for individual differences. Membranes should be left intact unless there is a reason to perform an artificial rupture. Amniotic fluid may play an important part in protecting the cord from compression during contractions	Stay with women in labour. Assessment of progress includes a number of parameters, including abdominal palpation, regular but not too frequent vaginal examinations assessing not only dilatation but application of presenting part, thickness of cervix, position and descent during contraction. Cervix may stretch during contraction with pressure from presenting part. Strength and duration of contractions should be palpated. Observation of the reaction of the mother to contractions is also an important indicator (Page & Tyson unpublished data 2000). Possibility of different pelvic shapes in women from different racial groups
Use mobility, and encourage the woman to move freely and change position to desire. Massage, water, birth pool (Beake 1999), etc. to help the woman cope with the pain of labour	Mobility and an upright posture make contractions less painful and more effective. MIDIRS leaflet (1996)	Demonstrate and encourage different positions. Rocking chair/leaning forward on back of bed, chair, birth ball, and partner. Moving and using pelvic rock during contraction. Help partner coach
Use intermittent auscultation unless there is a clear medical reason for electronic fetal monitoring (RCOG 1993) (e.g. thick meconium staining of the amniotic fluid Neilson 1993), IUGR, or medical complications such as pre-eclampsia, or if labour has been induced or stimulated with oxytocin	Electronic fetal monitoring associated with an increase in the operative and assisted delivery rate. No significant differences in rate of admission to neonatal intensive care nursery, perinatal death (Thacker & Stroup 1999)	Listen to the fetal heart every 15 minutes in first stage and after every contraction or at least every 10 minutes in second stage. Listen with a 'sonicaid' at the end and for a minute after every contraction. Accelerations in heart rate with fetal activity, palpation, after contraction, are reassuring. Assess amount of amniotic fluid as an important indicator of placental function (see Page 2000)
Help women cope with the pain of labour, avoid epidural anaesthesia where possible. Provide constant presence. Use entonox or TENS if necessary	The use of epidural anaesthesia is associated with an increase in the assisted delivery rate and the length of labour. Observational studies suggest there may be a greater incidence of backache following the use of an epidural (Howell 1999)	Stay with the woman, using words of praise and reassurance and using comforting touch where appropriate. However some women prefer not to be touched and request silence

Table 29.4 Symptoms of pregnancy

Sickness and nausea
Fatigue and sleeplessness
Feeling hot and sweaty
Physiological anaemia
Varicose veins and haemorrhoids
Breathlessness
Urinary frequency
Heartburn
Constipation
Cramps
Headache
Backache
Skin changes
Feelings of heaviness

bility for a dependent, helpless human being. Moreover, it generally all takes place within a single day. It is not surprising that women tend to remember their first birth experiences vividly and with deep emotion.

Simkin 1992, p 62

Labour and birth are by nature made up of extremes of pain, of physical hard work, of exhaustion, sometimes fear, and often joy. During such times there is an extreme sensitivity to the support, or lack of support, of others. All professionals at this time should treat any contact with the childbearing woman with the respect and sensitivity it deserves. Even brief contacts may be intensely supportive, or damaging, and may have long-term effects. The constant presence of the midwife, and her responsibility during this time, means that she has a particular role to play. This includes helping the woman to cope with the pain of labour, providing support and reassurance, developing a calm environment, and supporting physiological processes, while knowing when intervention is required. Helping women cope with the pain of labour is an important midwifery responsibility. Rather than seeing the pain of labour as pain that has to be removed at all costs, rather like a toothache, it should be recognised that, although extreme, it is pain with a positive end to it – the birth of the baby. Where women have constant attendance by a trained caregiver, words of praise and encouragement, and comforting touch, they are less likely to ask for pain relief, particularly an epidural, and are more likely to be satisfied with the experience. There is a place for pain relief in labour, but it must be emphasised that it has a number of adverse consequences and is best avoided if possible.

Midwives may help a great deal by promoting mobility and encouraging women to move as they wish during labour and birth. There are a number of props that may assist the woman, including swings, chairs, beanbags and other furniture. The birth room should be arranged to encourage movement, and it is best to avoid having the bed in the centre of the room. Water, in the form of showers, baths or birth pools, is a source of relief for the pain of labour. Massage may help, as may some forms of distraction.

Odent emphasised the importance of a darkened quiet space for the woman, so that she may draw into herself during labour, without distraction. LeBoyer emphasised the importance of gentle birth, the creation of a calm and quiet, darkened environment for the birth. In a number of places birth rooms have been decorated to make them more home-like and less clinical. This Laura Ashley treatment can be important so long as it does not distract from provision of sensitive personal care, and concentration on the provision of a calm quiet space in which there is little intrusion from strangers (Page 2000).

Recent research has highlighted the extent of ill health following birth. Maternal good health following birth is crucial not only to the mother, but also to the care of her family and her baby. Ill health following childbirth has a number of costs to individual, family and community. The first systematic review of ill health following birth, a study of 11 701 postpartum women, indicated a surprising amount of ill health. Just under half (47% of these women) reported at least one symptom within 3 months of the delivery of the child, which continued for more than 6 weeks and which had never been experienced before (McArthur et al 1991). There is currently much debate about ill health following birth and its causes and prevention. This is a topic of central importance to midwives. Much of the research is complex and difficult to interpret. An important area for future research and enquiry in midwifery will be related to duration of labour and the conduct of second stage. It seems that some of the ill health following birth, for example stress urinary and fecal incontinence, is associated with instrumental delivery, a large baby, or a difficult birth. There is much more to be learned about the possible effects of oxytocic augmentation in established labour, the effect of different types of bearing down efforts, and position for labour and birth, on genitourinary tract injury. Symptoms such as tiredness and headache following birth may well be amenable to midwifery advice and support on changes in life style to accommodate the intense demands of a newborn (Page 2000).

Space does not allow for adequate discussion of the proposal that women should be able to elect to give birth through caesarean section to avoid some of these problems, especially stress incontinence. The principle of demonstrating benefit should be observed in all maternity care, and current evidence does not support the belief that elective caesarean birth that is not medically indicated is better for mother or baby (Amu 1999).

CONCLUSION

Midwives have the potential to play an important and influential part in the provision of effective midwifery. Midwifery can provide an unique service that cannot be offered by any other professional group. Midwives are specialists in the care of healthy women with normal pregnancies. They also have an important part to play in accompanying women and their families in pregnancy and birth, supporting the transformation that a positive experience brings. In much of the modern maternity service the potential of midwifery is limited by inappropriate patterns of care, fragmented services and women with healthy pregnancies being looked after by medical and surgical specialists. Where organisational changes have been made, midwives are able to adjust and reach their full potential; however, midwifery has to a great extent been institutionalised in acute care hospitals, and change for and by midwives may not be easy. Despite this, development of the profession of midwifery is crucial. The pressure and practice of a strong midwifery profession will be an important way of ensuring that women enjoy pregnancy and birth as a natural part of life. It will be important in ensuring that the joy and excitement of birth is not clouded by uncalled-for anxiety and fear, that we do not face a future in which the majority of babies are brought into the world through an abdominal incision.

KEY POINTS

- The aim of all professionals in the maternity services is the same.
- All professionals should work together to ensure effective and appropriate care.
- Each professional group has a distinct and unique part to play in achieving the aim of care.
- Midwives are specialists in the care of healthy women with normal pregnancies.
- In addition to recognising that midwives should refer when medical attention is required there should be emphasis on midwives protecting normal or physiological processes.
- There should be agreed processes of referral and ease of referral between midwives and doctors.
- Midwives should be the lead professional for women with normal pregnancies.

REFERENCES

Amu O, Rajendran S, Bolajii II 1999 Maternal choice alone should not determine method of delivery. BMJ 317:463–465

Beake S 1999 Water birth: a literature review. MIDIRS Midwifery Digest 9(4):473–477

Chalmers I, Enkin M, Kierse MJNC 1989 Effective care in pregnancy and childbirth. Oxford University Press, Oxford

Department of Health 1993 Changing Childbirth. Part 1. Report of the Expert Maternity Group (Cumberlege report). HMSO, London

Department of Health, Welsh Office, Scottish Office Home and Health Department, Department of Health and Social Services, Northern Ireland 1996 Report on Confidential Enquiries into Maternal Deaths in the United Kingdom 1991–1993. HMSO, London

English National Board for Nursing Midwifery and Health Visiting 1999 Report on the Maternity Services. ENB, London

Flint C, Poulengeris P 1987 The Know your Midwife Project. Pub 49. Peckerman's Wood, London SE26 6RZ

Green JM, Curtis P, Price H, Renfrew MJ 1998 Continuing to care. The organization of midwifery services in the UK: a structured review of the evidence. Books for Midwives Press, Hale

Hodnett ED 1999a Caregiver support for women during childbirth (Cochrane Review). In: The Cochrane Library, Issue 4. Update Software, Oxford

Hodnett ED 1999b Continuity of caregivers for care during pregnancy and childbirth (Cochrane Review). In: The Cochrane Library, Issue 4. Update Software, Oxford

Howell CJ 1999 Epidural versus non epidural analgesia for pain relief in labour (Cochrane Review). In: The Cochrane Library, Issue 4. Update Software, Oxford

Katz Rothman B 1994 The tentative pregnancy: amniocentesis and the sexual politics of motherhood. Pandora, London

Lyons S 1998 Post-traumatic stress disorder following childbirth: causes, prevention and treatment. In: Clement S (ed) Psychological perspectives on pregnancy and childbirth. Churchill Livingstone, Edinburgh

McArthur C, Lewis M, Knox EG 1991 Health After Childbirth. HMSO, London

McCourt C, Page L 1996 Report on the evaluation of one-to-one midwifery. The Centre for Midwifery Practice, Thames Valley University, London

McCourt C, Hirst J, Page LA 2000 Dimensions and attributes of caring. In: Page LA (ed) The new midwifery: science and sensitivity in practice. Churchill Livingstone, Edinburgh

MIDIRS and the NHS Centre for Reviews and Dissemination Informed Choice for Professionals: positions in labour and delivery. 1996 MIDIRS, Bristol

Mills B, Page LA 2000 The growth of human love and commitment and implications for the midwife. In: Page LA (ed) The new midwifery: science and sensitivity in practice. Churchill Livingstone, Edinburgh

Neilson J 1993 Cardiotocography during labour: unsatisfactory technique but nothing better yet. BMJ 306:347–348

Page LA 2000 Putting science and sensitivity into practice. In: Page LA (ed) The new midwifery: science and sensitivity in practice. Churchill Livingstone, Edinburgh

Page LA, Hutton E 2000 Introduction: setting the scene. In: Page LA (ed) The new midwifery: science and sensitivity in practice. Churchill Livingstone, Edinburgh

Page L, McCourt C, Beake S, Hewison J, Vail A 1999 Clinical interventions and outcomes of One-to-One Midwifery Practice. J Public Health Med 21(4):243–248

Page L, Beake S, Vail A, McCourt C, Hewison J 2000 A comparative cohort study of clinical outcomes and maternal satisfaction with the One-to-One Midwifery Practice. Accepted for publication by the British Journal of Midwifery

Percival P 2000 Caring for the baby. In: Page LA (ed) The new midwifery: science and sensitivity in practice. Churchill Livingstone, Edinburgh

Royal College of Obstetricians and Gynaecologists 1993 Recommendations on intrapartum fetal surveillance in labour. In: Ward M, Spencer J (eds) Intrapartum fetal surveillance in labour. RCOG, London

Saxell L 1992 Risk: theoretical or actual. In: Page LA (ed) The new midwifery: science and sensitivity in practice. Churchill Livingstone, Edinburgh

Simkin P 1992 Just another day in a woman's life? Part 11: Nature and consistency of women's long term memories of their first birth experiences. Birth 19(2):64–81

Thacker SB, Stroup DF 1999 Continuous electronic heart rate monitoring versus intermittent auscultation for assessment during labour (Cochrane Review). In: The Cochrane Library, Issue 4. Update Software, Oxford

Thornton JG, Lilford RJ 1994 Active management of labour: current knowledge and research issues. BMJ 309:366–369

United Kingdom Central Council 1998 Midwives rules and code of practice. London: UKCC:25

30

The future of labour management

F. Goffinet, G. Bréart

INTRODUCTION

Before the middle of the twentieth century, management of childbirth was mostly a first aid procedure saving the mother and the baby from any damage induced by pregnancy or labour. It could be summarised as managed delivery of the second and third stages of labour. Antenatal care, although it started at the beginning of the century, did not have a great or universal effect until World War II. The wider spread of this led to the prevention of more labour problems and provided for a much better prepared woman and her fetus in labour. New means of monitoring appeared and management extended to include continuous monitoring of labour with both maternal partogram and fetal heart rate monitoring. Obstetric professionals and pregnant women became aware of the possibilities of ameliorating the pain of giving birth. Finally, after this period of relatively simple surveillance of labour, some experts suggested that policies should be established for taking care of labour, aiming to reduce the maternal and fetal risks associated with the events that surround childbirth. The maternal risks relate to dystocia, which leads to an elevated rate of prolonged labour, caesarean sections and instrumental deliveries. The fetal risks were fetal distress (asphyxia, meconium staining) and infection.

The principle of such management of labour was that, by monitoring the woman and the fetus from the first hours of labour (latent phase), the medical team could intervene early (and sometimes preventatively) to correct a situation that presented risks of dystocia or fetal distress. Several components are included in the management of labour policy. They include early admission to the maternity facility, early diagnosis of labour, individual support during the labour, the use of a partogram, artificial rupture of the membranes (ARM), oxytocin administration, effective anal-gesia and further continuous monitoring of mother and fetus. Thus, in the last 20 years, it was proposed that the management of labour ought to be an active management by the obstetrical professional team, taking over from the woman the control of labour and to some extent the timing of events.

MEDICALISATION OF LABOUR MANAGEMENT

Recent findings have not demonstrated any net health benefits from the active management of labour except for a reduction in the duration of labour. Some voices, of professionals as well as of women themselves, have been raised against this medicalisation of an act as natural as childbirth.

Medical intervention related to childbirth has increased steadily over recent decades. Consequently, in France, the caesarean rate has increased from 6.2% in 1972 to 10.8% in 1981 and 15.5% in 1995 (Blondel et al 1997). These data are in line with other Western European countries with the exception of Holland and Sweden. Other interventions are also used increasingly: oxytocin administration, ARM, epidural anaesthesia, continuous monitoring either by electronic fetal heart rate monitoring (EFM) or, more recently, by pulse fetal oxymetry. Other interventions increased at various times but they have more recently declined in frequency such as forceps and vacuum extractions. The increased rates of some interventions have continued in recent years, although perinatal results over the same period have been essentially stable, those of cerebral palsy in particular. Table 30.1 reviews the trends of disabilities in children, born from 1972 through 1981, at ages nine to 14 years, together with the parallel trends in the management of labour, such as rates of continuous fetal heart rate monitoring, prolonged labour and

Table 30.1 Trends in the frequency of perinatal death, motor and sensory disabilities in children aged 9–14 years) and parallel trends in perinatal care interventions in France

	1972 %	1976 %	1981 %
Interventions during labour			
Fetal heart rate recording	5.7	29.0	69.7
Prolonged labour	6.7	3.8	1.5
Caesarean section	6.2	8.5	10.9
Outcomes			
Perinatal mortality	2.1	1.6	1.2
Motor, mental or sensory disabilities	0.1	0.1	0.11

caesarean section (Breart & Rumeau-Rouquette 1996). Initially, active management of labour was associated with a low caesarean rate, in association with the increase in earlier interventions (Lopez-Zeno et al 1992), more recently, clinical trials and meta-analysis suggest that accelerated management and, in particular, early use of oxytocin and ARM do not yield this benefit (Frigoletto et al 1995, Cammu & Van Eekhout 1996, Fraser et al 1998). Moreover, no benefits to fetal health have been found (Fraser et al 1998).

Some obstetric professionals (both obstetricians and midwives) and the women having the babies have strongly protested against this hyper-medicalisation of all deliveries when there is no clear health justification. It may nonetheless be argued that this medicalisation which has progressively developed in recent decades has brought with it some health benefits, even though these are hard to demonstrate. Consequently, today, the level of safety in childbirth in developed nations seems high but even if this is so, is any further medicalisation necessary? One of the future issues in assessing how childbirth should be managed is the possible de-escalation of the number of interventions systematically applied. If not we risk an ever-increasing augmentation of medicalization with its negative consequences without any improvement in maternal or perinatal results. Along with this, the other fundamental points that need to be taken into account are the preferences and the degree of satisfaction of both the women and the professionals. In most areas of medicine, patient satisfaction has become an important element in management decisions. This should perhaps be even more true for decisions about childbirth, which in the eyes of many is considered to be a natural, normal event rather than a medical condition.

Benefits of medical intervention

Individual support, ARM, correctly paced oxytocin administration, effective analgesia and continuous monitoring of mother and fetus all have positive effects that are unlikely to be challenged in the future, although the indications for their use and the decision thresholds vary according to the obstetrician and the hospital's policy. One way of examining the existing data in relation to the benefits or otherwise of these various components of accelerated labour management is to review the meta-analysis in the Cochrane database.

Continuous support during labour from caregivers (nurses, midwives, doulas or lay people) appears to result in several benefits for mother and child and has no harmful effects (Hodnett 2000a). It reduces the likelihood of analgesia administration, operative vaginal delivery, caesarean delivery and the 5-minute Apgar score of less than seven in the newborn. Moreover, women in the group who received continuous support had more positive views of their childbirth experiences than women without such support. Furthermore, one trial has shown that early labour assessment performed by caregivers may have some positive outcomes for women in term pregnancies, by increasing the perceived level of the women's control during labour and childbirth (Lauzon & Hodnett 2000). However, the latter review includes only one trial. In the future, if obstetricians, midwives and the women themselves choose the least possible intervention, this one-to-one care should nonetheless be proposed systematically. It requires increased financial resources because the efficacy of such support appears to rest in the concept of one caregiver for each woman. This could be helped by the recruitment of experienced women to stay with the labouring mother throughout labour. Although a recent study did not find any important benefits (Langer et al 1998), the meta-analysis by Zhang et al of four randomised trials carried out among nullipara in the lower socioeconomic class showed that such psychosocial support shortened the duration of labour by 2.8 hours (95% CI 2.2–3.4) and also reduced oxytocin administration (Relative risk (RR) = 0.46, 95% Confidence interval (CI) 0.3–0.7), operative vaginal deliveries (RR = 0.46, 95% CI 0.4–0.7) and caesarean sections (RR = 0.54, 95% CI 0.4–0.7) (Zhang et al 1996). This psychosocial support is especially helpful when it comes from an untrained female supporter or doula and less helpful when it is supplied by the partner, family or friends. One study found that the women with this support had a more positive perception of their labour and their delivery (Langer et al 1998); in addition, a higher proportion of them chose to breast-feed their babies. The authors concluded that more than the psychosocial support itself, the attitude of the obstetric team affected the outcome of labour.

Some technical interventions have also been proven helpful. One example is amnioinfusion for meconium-stained fluid in labour. It is associated with improvements in perinatal outcome, particularly in settings where facilities for perinatal surveillance are limited (Hofmeyr 2000). Meconium aspiration syndrome was reduced by 76% in the amnioinfusion group (RR = 0.24, 95% CI 0.12–0.48).

In the Cochrane database, the available data do not support a conclusion that the other interventions used to accelerate labour are useful when considered individually. More studies, preferably randomised controlled, are needed. This leads us to consider which interventions should be systematically proposed to women in labour.

What intervention should be proposed to all women?

Most of these interventions, if evaluated individually, have not shown clear benefits when they are proposed to women at low risk. Some, such as ARM are even suspected of being more harmful than beneficial when used systematically (Goffinet et al 1997). Various policies use different decision thresholds, for example the type of partogram chosen where some recommend an action line four hours to the right of the alert line, others recommend a line displaced by only two or three hours. The decision thresholds among nullipara or multipara vary substantially according to report, regarding when to administer oxytocin or effectuate an ARM (O'Driscoll et al 1984, World Health Organization 1994). These differences make it difficult to interpret the results of systematic reviews (Fraser et al 1998).

We should also examine in this context some of the conclusions in the Cochrane database about components of management of labour that have not been shown to be valuable or for which some benefits may be counterbalanced by disadvantages. Systematic ARM, although it allows a significant reduction in the duration of labour, can lead to an increase in the number of caesarean sections for acute fetal distress (Fraser et al 2000). Restrictive episiotomy policies appear to have a number of benefits, amongst them a low requirement for medical intervention during labour (Carroli & Belizan 2000).

Because some pregnant women prefer and require little or no medical intervention during labour, homebirth rates are rising slightly (e.g. in UK: 0.9% in 1989; 2.1% in 1997) and many home-like birth centres have been established near conventional labour wards. Meta-analysis shows some benefits from home-like settings for childbirth such as lower rates of intervention. Also, they are associated with higher levels of patient satisfaction with care (Hodnett 2000b). This could of course be because of the concomitant increased support from caregivers. However, the authors conclude that both caregivers and the labouring woman in home-like settings must be alert for signs of complications such as uterine inertia or clinical signs of fetal distress. Similarly, in large randomised trials continuous EFM during labour is not associated with a reduction in perinatal mortality although there is a reduction in the rate of neonatal seizures. There is, however, an increase in the rate of operative deliveries (Thacker & Stroup 2000). The authors concluded that the pregnant woman and her clinician should jointly decide whether to use continuous EFM or intermittent fetal heart auscultation. This is one example of the increasing trend in relation to interventions for which no definitive benefits can be established and the choice should be left to the woman with the obstetrician or midwife providing her with full information about the consequences of this or that decision.

In meta-analyses of studies of the best position for the woman during the second stage of labour, either an upright or lateral position, compared with supine or lithotomy positions, was associated with several benefits (reduction of assisted deliveries and episiotomies) but also with the possibility of an increased risk of blood loss >500 ml (Gupta &

Nikodem 2000). The conclusion was that women should be encouraged to give birth in the position they find most comfortable. They should be allowed to make an informed choice about the position they might wish to assume for delivery of their babies.

If no benefit has been shown and if the women giving birth and their obstetricians and midwives are not satisfied with these systematic interventions, should these managements continue to be imposed? We must stress that in the control groups in the comparative trials, the rates of ARM, oxytocin, pain relief and perfusions have generally been elevated (Langer et al 1998). It is, therefore, possible that the failure to demonstrate that some interventions associated with accelerated management of labour have a useful effect may be explained by the lack of contrast in the intervention rates in many studies.

Are women satisfied with labour management?

Beyond some groups who succeed in making their voices heard but whose representativeness is uncertain, how satisfied are the women to whom acceleration is applied? Objective data concerning women's satisfaction about this are very sparse, because this outcome has rarely been measured in clinical trials. Reid (1994) reported that the patients allocated to early augmentation had higher satisfaction scores than those with delayed augmentation. In a randomised trial of an early labour assessment programme, McNiven et al (1998) found significant decreases in the duration of labour, the use of epidural analgesia for pain, and oxytocin use to augment labour in the early labour assessment group. More importantly these women evaluated their labour and birth experience more positively than did the women in the direct admission group. In another randomised controlled trial of three different partograms the women preferred active management of labour, ie: the two-hour ARM compared with three or four hours laid down in partograms between alert and action lines (Lavender et al 1998).

The debate around the interventions associated with active management have focussed on the caesarean section rates, but other considerations can be very important to individual women, who might, therefore, prefer acceleration for non-medical reasons. It has been demonstrated that ARM alone, used systematically, leads to a significant and substantial diminution in the duration of labour (Fraser et al 1998). In future, the satisfaction of women must become one of the principal outcomes of randomised trials of aspects of labour management.

The opinion of women is, therefore, counting more in the management of labour. For example, the diminution in the number of women who attempt a trial of labour after having had a previous caesarean section is essentially linked to the patients' choice (Leitch & Walker 1998). Questions about the pelvic risks (urinary incontinence or prolapse) associated with vaginal deliveries may have influenced women obstetricians, 30% of whom expressed a preference for an elective caesarean rather than a vaginal delivery in one study (Al-Mufti et al 1996). Similarly, such serious intrapartum complications as persistent neonatal brachial plexus injury or fetal death increased the subsequent caesarean section delivery rate of the obstetrician involved in these events (Turrentine & Ramirez 1999). McGurgan showed in a national confidential questionnaire performed in 1998–1999 that there is a high significant correlation ($p < 0.01$) between the expression of a personal preference for caesarean section for a range of scenarios and working in an obstetric unit with a caesarean section rate of >16% (McGurgan 1999). Professionals then will inform their patients but they will also influence them. Similarly, there is evidence that morbidity resulting from caesarean sections performed after a trial of labour is higher than that resulting from elective operations and even that an elective caesarean section does not protect the anal sphincter mechanism any better than vaginal delivery (McMahon et al 1996, Fynes et al 1998). When this information is available to the overall population of pregnant women, will many of them still request an elective caesarean section?

THE FUTURE OF LABOUR MANAGEMENT

If there is no demonstrated medical indication for some of the decisions that must be made about care in childbirth, the woman should receive clear explanations of the choices and choose the policy that she prefers. Further, it is essential that the obstetric team are comfortable with the medical management applied.

In the future, each team will probably have to set out a policy of its major systematic medical choices and philosophy. We can even imagine that hospitals and other maternity units might provide pregnant women with a written assessment of the results available in the literature of the various components of interventions. Such statements should be accompanied by data about the frequency in their unit of various interventions such as their rates of caesarean deliveries, operative vaginal deliveries, regional pain relief, ARM, oxytocin administration and long or slow labours. The women then can choose more freely where they wish to give birth if they live in an area with several delivery units.

Impey and Boylan (1999) foresee that informed choice will lead to three styles of intrapartum care. Some women will choose a birth-plan calling for minimal intervention, some will request elective caesarean sections. The rest will prefer a short labour with a high chance of a normal delivery. The birth-plans of these women will describe active management of labour.

CONCLUSIONS

Many of the interventions introduced into the modern delivery suite have been introduced simply because they were thought to be good ideas. Few have been subject to randomised controlled trials; when they have been, the results are unimpressive and often unhelpful to normal women in normal labours with normal babies. Extrapolation from the perceived needs of women with maternal or fetal problems in labour does not necessarily fulfil the needs of normal women.

REFERENCES

Al-Mufti R, McCarthy A, Fisk NM 1996 Obstetricians' personal choice and mode of delivery [letter] [see comments]. Lancet 347:544

Blondel B, Breart G, du Mazaubrun C et al 1997 The perinatal situation in France. Trends between 1981 and 1995]. J Gynecol Obstet Biol Reprod 26:770–780

Breart G, Rumeau-Rouquette C 1996 [Cerebral palsy and perinatal asphyxia in full term newborn infants]. Arch Pediatr 3:70–74

Cammu H, Van Eeckhout E 1996 A randomised controlled trial of early versus delayed use of amniotomy and oxytocin infusion in nulliparous labour [see comments]. Br J Obstet Gynaecol 103:313–318

Carroli G, Belizan J 2000 Episiotomy for vaginal birth (Cochrane review)

Dujardin B, De Schampheleire I, Sene H, Ndiaye F 1992 Value of the alert and action lines on the partogram [see comments]. Lancet 339:1336–1338

Fraser W, Vendittelli F, Krauss I, Breart G 1998 Effects of early augmentation of labour with amniotomy and oxytocin in nulliparous women: a meta-analysis. Br J Obstet Gynaecol 105:189–194

Fraser W, Turcot L, Krauss I, Brisson-Carrol G 2000 Amniotomy for shortening spontaneous labor (Cochrane review)

Frigoletto FD, Jr., Lieberman E, Lang JM et al 1995 A clinical trial of active management of labor [published erratum appears in N Engl J Med 1995; 333(17):1163] [see comments]. N Engl J Med 333:745–750

Fynes M, Donnelly VS, O'Connell PR, O'Herlihy C 1998 Cesarean delivery and anal sphincter injury. Obstet Gynecol 92:496–500

Goffinet F, Fraser W, Marcoux S, Breart G, Moutquin JM, Daris M 1997 Early amniotomy increases the frequency of fetal heart rate abnormalities. Amniotomy Study Group. Br J Obstet Gynaecol 104:548–553

Gupta J, Nikodem V 2000 Woman's position during second stage of labour (Cochrane review)

Hodnett E 2000a Caregiver support for women during childbirth (Cochrane review)

Hodnett E 2000b Home-like versus conventional institutional settings for birth (Cochrane review)

Hofmeyr G 2000 Amnioinfusion for meconium-stained liquor in labour (Cochrane review)

Impey L, Boylan P 1999 Active management of labour revisited. Br J Obstet Gynaecol 106:183–187

Langer A, Campero L, Garcia C, Reynoso S 1998 Effects of psychosocial support during labour and childbirth on breastfeeding, medical interventions, and mothers' wellbeing in a Mexican public hospital: a randomised clinical trial. Br J Obstet Gynaecol 105:1056–1063

Lauzon L, Hodnett E 2000 Caregivers' use of strict criteria for diagnosing active labour in term pregnancy (Cochrane review)

Lavender T, Alfirevic Z, Walkinshaw S 1998 Partogram action line study: a randomised trial. Br J Obstet Gynaecol 105:976–980

Leitch CR, Walker JJ 1998 The rise in caesarcan section rate: the same indications but a lower threshold. Br J Obstet Gynaecol 105:621–626

Lopez-Zeno JA, Peaceman AM, Adashek JA, Socol ML 1992 A controlled trial of a program for the active management of labor. N Engl J Med 326:450–454

McGurgan P 1999 Active management of labour revisited [letter; comment]. Br J Obstet Gynaecol 106:1002

McMahon MJ, Luther ER, Bowes WA, Jr, Olshan AF 1996 Comparison of a trial of labor with an elective second cesarean section [see comments]. N Engl J Med 335:689–695

McNiven PS, Williams JI, Hodnett E, Kaufman K, Hannah ME 1998 An early labor assessment program: a randomized, controlled trial. Birth 25:5–10

O'Driscoll K, Foley M, MacDonald D 1984 Active management of labor as an alternative to cesarean section for dystocia. Obstet Gynecol 63:485–490

Reid M 1994 What are consumer views of maternity care? In: Chamberlain G, Patel N (eds) The future of maternity services. RCOG Press, London

Thacker S, Stroup D 2000 Continuous electronic heart rate monitoring for fetal assessment during labor (Cochrane review)

Turrentine MA, Ramirez MM 1999 Adverse perinatal events and subsequent cesarean rate. Obstet Gynecol 94:185–188

World Health Organization partograph in management of labour. 1994 World Health Organization Maternal Health and Safe Motherhood Programme [see comments]. Lancet 343:1399–1404

Zhang J, Bernasko JW, Leybovich E, Fahs M, Hatch MC 1996 Continuous labor support from labor attendant for primiparous women: a meta-analysis. Obstet Gynecol 88:739–744

31

Preterm labour and delivery of the preterm infant

Stephen A. Walkinshaw

The contribution of the author of the equivalent chapter in the second edition, on which this chapter draws extensively, is gratefully acknowledged.

Prematurity and its consequences remain a major health problem. The mortality following preterm birth has fallen steadily over the last two decades (Cooke 1992); however, the long-term consequences, both respiratory and neurological, have not improved at the same rate in recent years.

DEFINITION

A preterm infant is defined as one who is born at less than 259 days (37 completed weeks) of pregnancy (WHO 1977). As menstrual dating may be inaccurate in up to 20% of women, gestation should be based on the best clinical estimate, including ultrasound. Extreme prematurity is usually defined as gestations less than 28 completed weeks. The lower limit of preterm birth varies, depending on national definitions of stillbirth. WHO has recommended that all births over 500 g should be registered to allow uniformity, as very few infants under this weight will survive. Underreporting of live births of very immature infants (Powell et al 1987), makes comparison of preterm birth rates between countries unreliable. Even within countries comparison can be difficult (UK CESDI reports).

Because of these difficulties, much epidemiological work has used birthweight as a standard. Low birthweight is defined as less than 2501 g, very low birthweight (VLBW) as less than 1501 g, and extremely low birthweight (ELBW) as less than 1000 g. However, such data are less helpful, given that outcome is much more closely aligned with gestational age than birthweight.

Preterm labour is defined as the occurrence of regular uterine activity which produces either cervical effacement or dilatation prior to 37 completed weeks of gestation (Anderson 1977). The term threatened preterm labour is often used to describe pregnancies complicated by episodes of clinically significant uterine activity but without cervical change.

INCIDENCE

In developed countries the incidence of preterm birth varies between 5 and 10% (Villar & Ezcurra 1994). Over long periods, some areas have shown a decline, such as in Aberdeen, from 9.3% in 1951–1955, to 6.8% in 1976–1980 (Hall 1985). Over shorter periods, rates in Haguenau in France have fallen from 8.2% in 1972 to 5.6% in 1981 (Papiernik et al 1985). Recently there has been concern in both the USA and Canada with evidence of a rise in the preterm birth rate (Goldenberg & Rouse 1998, Joseph et al 1998). This appears to be due to an increase in preterm multiple births, an increase in late preterm births in singleton pregnancies, possibly as a consequence of increasing obstetric intervention, and better registration of live births at the margins of viability.

In practical terms, preterm births at the mature end of the gestation range are less important although numerically high. Deliveries under 32 weeks account for between 1 and 1.5% of births (van den Berg & Oeschli 1984, Wariyar et al 1989), and deliveries under 28 weeks account for 0.22–1.5% of births (Hall et al 1997), with most areas having a rate of 0.5–0.7% of births. There may be a recent increase as a result of more complete reporting. These distinctions are important, as over two-thirds of deaths in preterm infants occur in infants born at less than 28 weeks.

The incidence of threatened preterm labour, because of problems of definition, is not available, but is likely to be higher than that of spontaneous preterm delivery. In one study, one-third of women with preterm uterine activity went home undelivered within 48 h (Kragt & Kierse 1990). In most trials of tocolysis, where preterm uterine activity is an entry criterion, more than 50% of pregnancies deliver after 37 weeks.

Preterm premature rupture of the membranes (preterm PROM) occurs in 1–2% of all pregnant women (Gibbs & Blanco 1982, Cox et al 1988) but is implicated in around half of women eventually delivering spontaneously preterm.

EPIDEMIOLOGY

Preterm labour and delivery are not homogeneous entities. Four major categories can be identified:

- elective preterm delivery such as for alloimmunisation or growth restriction
- complicated emergency delivery such as abruptio placentae
- preterm PROM
- uncomplicated spontaneous preterm delivery.

The last two account for around half of all preterm births, with elective delivery occurring in 16–18%, and complicated emergency delivery in one quarter (Halliday 1988, Wariyar et al 1989).

The classic epidemiological associations of preterm labour and preterm PROM are those of poverty and social disadvantage (Table 31.1).

Maternal characteristics

There is probably an increased risk of preterm delivery in women under 18–20 years of age and in women over 35 years of age in most populations (Lumley 1993, Meiss et al 1995, Martius et al 1998, Ancel et al 1999), although not all studies have shown this (Mercer et al 1996). Primiparity is associated with a higher rate of preterm delivery independent of maternal age (Bakketeig & Hoffman 1981). Being unmarried may be a strong risk factor in some North American populations (Wen et al 1990) and in European populations (Ancel et al 1999) but is only significantly associated with preterm birth in Australian women over the age of 25 years (Lumley 1993). The relationship is strongest in deliveries under 32 weeks (Ancel et al 1999).

Ethnicity has always been an issue in preterm labour and delivery. Much of the difference in the incidence of low birthweight between developed and developing areas is due to the excess of growth-restricted infants, with the rate of preterm births being similar. In North American studies however (Garn et al 1977, Wen et al 1990) there is a consistently increased risk for black women, independent of social class. This has been confirmed, particularly for primigravidae, in the large prospective study of Mercer and colleagues (Mercer et al 1996). The magnitude of the risk is greatest for extremely preterm deliveries (Schoendorf et al 1992).

Although maternal nutritional studies have not shown any clear relationship with preterm births, low maternal prepregnancy weight (less than 50 kg) and poor weight gain (less than 0.24 kg per week) are associated with an increased risk (Wen et al 1990, Barros et al 1992). In recent studies in North America, the UK and Europe, low weight or body mass index is consistently associated with an increased risk of spontaneous preterm birth (Meiss et al 1995, Mercer et al

Table 31.1 Associations with preterm labour

	Relative risk
Maternal characteristics not modifiable during pregnancy	
Age less than 18 years	1.5–3.4
Age more than 35 years	1.3–1.8
Unmarried (not cohabiting)	2.2
Unemployed	2.3
African origin, primigravida	1.9
Maternal characteristics potentially modifiable during pregnancy	
Low BMI (<20)	1.5–1.8
Cigarette smoking	1.3
Heavy work	2.1–3.3
Stress (perceived)	1.2–1.8
Substance abuse	2.5–6
Past reproductive history	
Two previous first trimester losses	2.9
Two previous therapeutic terminations of pregnancy	2.5
Second trimester loss	4.2
One previous preterm delivery	2–5
Two previous preterm deliveries	4–7.6
Pregnancy complications not amenable to intervention	
Multiple pregnancy	
Pre-existing maternal illness	
Fetal malformation	
Pre-eclampsia	
First- or second-trimester bleeding	1.6–2.0
Pregnancy complications amenable to intervention	
Asymptomatic bacteriuria	2–4
Bacterial vaginosis	1.4–1.8
Cervical incompetence	
Uterine anomalies	
Sexually transmissible disease	
Screening tests during pregnancy in unselected pregnancies	
Cervical length less than 1st centile	14
Cervical length less than 5th centile	9.5
Fetal fibronectin	7.5
Maternal plasma CRH in second trimester	3.5

1996, Ancel et al 1999). Maternal height does not appear to be a factor.

Cigarette smoking results in an excess of births under 34 weeks' gestation, the greatest risk being to those smoking more than 20 cigarettes per day (Meyer 1977). Although initially attributed to an excess of abruptio placentae, placenta praevia and preterm PROM, more recent epidemiological studies have shown a stronger relationship with spontaneous preterm birth (Kyrklund-Blomberg & Cnattingius 1998). A large population study from Sweden (Cnattingius et al 1999) suggested odds ratios of preterm birth of 1.3–1.6, and strongly suggested both a dosage effect and a more marked effect on the risk of very preterm birth. Shah & Bracken (2000) have systematically reviewed the relationship between smoking and preterm birth. They suggested a relative risk of 1.27, with consistency across studies. They too suggested a dose–response effect at mild to moderate smoking

values. As a consequence of these recent findings, it may be that smoking is a causal rather than an epidemiological factor in preterm birth. Such a link is plausible, with known effects of smoking on collagen synthesis and on some proinflammatory cytokines.

An increased risk as a consequence of alcohol consumption remains unproven. Cocaine use increases the rate of preterm delivery (relative risk 2.4), in part a consequence of a higher risk of abruptio placentae (Volpe 1992). Opiate use has persistently been implicated in preterm birth but it has been difficult to disentangle the effect of opiates from that of confounding social factors. More recent data (Boer et al 1993, Walkinshaw et al 1993), controlling for social circumstances, confirm an excess of preterm births in opiate users.

Regular moderate exercise may actually reduce the incidence of preterm delivery (Berkowitz et al 1982). Vigorous activity into the third trimester may increase the risk (Kulpa et al 1987). Scandinavian data (Henriksen et al 1995) emphasised the link with heavy work where a woman was standing or walking in excess of 5 hours per day at work. Despite myths, sexual activity is not implicated in preterm birth (Lumley & Astbury 1989).

The physical and psychological stress of work itself has been implicated in some studies (Mercer et al 1996) but not in all (Meiss et al 1995). The clearest evidence derives from French work (see Luke & Papiernik 1997 for detailed review) demonstrating an association between preterm birth and an index of occupational fatigue based on posture, machine work, physical effort, repetition and workplace environment (Mamelle et al 1984). Others have subsequently demonstrated similar, but less marked, associations for both heavy manual and highly stressful work (Klebanoff et al 1990, Launer et al 1990).

Psychological stress (Copper et al 1996) has been implicated. This group, using extensive psychometric testing on unselected women, demonstrated a clear link between the stress element of their score and preterm delivery. Furthermore, the greater the stress score, the higher the risk. Danish data (Hedegaard et al 1996) examining both life events and the stress generated by them, also showed that events perceived as highly stressful were associated with preterm birth. Stress as an underlying causal factor is plausible in two ways. Stress may lead to increases in corticotrophin releasing factor, which has been implicated in the initiation of labour. Stress may also lead to other behavioural changes, such as the use of drugs which carry risk.

A lack of antenatal care has been suggested as a primary risk factor, even allowing for differences in access and utilisation (Murray & Bernfield 1988), but others have challenged this assumption (Tyson et al 1990). Considering what occurs in antenatal clinics and parent education classes in the UK, it is difficult to identify which components of prenatal care before 34 weeks would be likely to have an impact on preterm delivery.

Past reproductive history

The risk of preterm birth following induced or spontaneous early miscarriage has been debated. Lumley (1993) has demonstrated relative risks of 1.7, 2.9 and 5.9 for preterm labour less than 28 weeks for one, two and three prior spontaneous miscarriages, although Holbrook et al (1989) suggested no increase in risk unless there are more than two preceding early losses. Second trimester loss has consistently been associated with preterm birth, and the association is more marked with early preterm birth (Ancel et al 1999).

There remains controversy over the risk imparted by induced abortion. Lumley's data (Lumley 1993) showed similar risks for induced as for spontaneous loss. Recent Danish population data (Zhou et al 1999) showed remarkably similar risk ratios.

The strongest predictor of preterm birth is previous preterm birth and this is consistent across studies (Wen et al 1990, Mercer et al 1996, Ancel et al 1999). The risk increases if there has been more than one previous preterm birth, and the more preterm the first birth, the less likely the subsequent pregnancy is to go to term (Hoffman & Bakketeig 1984). The magnitude of risk varies from between 2 and 5 with a single previous preterm birth (Wen et al 1990, Mercer et al 1996, Ancel et al 1999) to a relative risk of 4–7.6 (Mercer et al 1996, Ancel et al 1999) if there have been two or more previous preterm births. The relationship linking the degree of previous prematurity with subsequent preterm birth has been clarified by Mercer (Mercer et al 1999). The risk of preterm birth before 32 weeks was 1 in 10 if the previous preterm birth was before 28 weeks, 1 in 15 if between 28 and 34 weeks, and 1 in 28 if between 35 and 36 weeks' gestation.

Uterine abnormalities such as uterus didelphus, unicornus, or women with Asherman's syndrome or leiomyomas are less likely to deliver at term, but are rare causes of preterm birth.

Current pregnancy complications

Many pregnancy complications are associated with preterm birth, and many of these are included in complex risk scores for the prediction of preterm labour (Creasy et al 1980). Their precise relationship with prematurity is considered in their individual chapters.

Multiple gestation makes up the largest single group, accounting for just under 2% of all births, with almost half being born preterm. For similar reasons polyhydramnios frequently results in preterm delivery (Kirbinen & Jouppila 1978).

Any severe maternal medical condition may result in preterm birth, as often for maternal as for fetal reasons. Similarly, acute maternal illness, especially systemic infection, can precipitate labour. Together these groups contribute substantially to elective preterm delivery.

Bleeding in pregnancy carries a risk irrespective of timing (Turnbull 1977). Threatened first- or early second-trimester miscarriage doubles the risk of subsequent preterm labour (Meis et al 1995, Mercer et al 1996).

Pregnancies complicated by fetal malformation, in particular multiple anomalies, renal anomalies and anterior abdominal wall defects, deliver preterm more often than expected. Some preterm births in this group are iatrogenic, often without clear advantage to the fetus.

The association between asymptomatic bacteriuria and preterm labour remains unclear (Wang & Smaill 1989, Meiss et al 1995, Mercer et al 1996), with some studies supportive (Romero et al 1991). Randomised trials of antibiotics for this condition appear to demonstrate a reduction in preterm delivery (Smaill 2000).

The putative relationship between preterm delivery and assisted conception is interesting insofar as it raises interesting speculation on links between the aetiology of difficult reproduction and that of preterm labour. The relationship persists even after correcting for age and multiple pregnancy.

Genital tract infection or colonisation

The role for infection in preterm labour

The results of epidemiological, molecular, microbiological, animal and clinical studies suggest that infection and inflammation play a role in up to 50% of pregnancies ending in spontaneous preterm birth:

1. Clinical and histological chorio-amnionitis is more common in the placenta and membranes of preterm deliveries (Russell 1979, Hillier et al 1988). This relationship is maintained after adjustment for socioeconomic confounding variables.
2. Maternal and neonatal sepsis is more common after preterm delivery than term delivery.
3. Amniotic fluid cultures are more frequently positive in preterm labour (Romero et al 1988a), with an average rate of 13%, and this is higher where specialist microbiological and molecular techniques are used to detect fastidious organisms. Those with positive cultures are more likely to develop chorio-amnionitis, to be refractory to tocolytics and to rupture the membranes spontaneously compared with those with negative cultures. The incidence of positive cultures is higher in cases of preterm PROM (34%).
4. Amniotic fluid in preterm labour contains other biochemical evidence of inflammation, such as increased leucocyte counts, lower glucose levels, higher prostaglandin levels, and evidence of increased cytokine activity (interleukins (IL)-1, -6, -8, tumour necrosis factor (TNF), platelet-activating factor (PAF).
5. Studies demonstrate associations between specific microorganisms and preterm labour. These include *Neisseria gonorrhoea*, group B streptococci, *Chlamydia trachomatis* (Alger et al 1988), *Mycoplasma hominis* and *Ureoplasma ureolyticum* (Lamont et al 1987), *Gardnerella vaginalis*, *Bacteroides* species and *Haemophilus* species (McDonald et al 1991, Kurki et al 1992). Some of these associations have been challenged (Romero & Mazor 1988) and data, particularly from screening studies during early pregnancy, are conflicting. The most convincing study remains that of Macdonald and colleagues, who demonstrated significant independent risk of preterm delivery for two groups of organisms, namely those associated with bacterial vaginosis and a group of virulent enteropathogens. This risk is most marked in preterm deliveries under 34 weeks. Subsequently Hillier

(Hillier et al 1995), in a very large prospective study of unselected women, suggested that women with bacterial vaginosis had a relative risk of preterm delivery of 1.5. This was similar to the relative risk shown by McDonald, and is similar to that from the other large prospective study in the USA (Goldenberg et al 1996a) with relative risks of 1.8 and 1.7.

6. Randomised trials of antibiotic treatment of asymptomatic bacteriuria, preterm labour and preterm PROM show reductions in maternal and neonatal infectious morbidity.
7. Experimental evidence demonstrating interplay between bacterial products and initiation of prostaglandin synthesis.

Mechanisms for bacteria as a cause of preterm labour

The mechanism of preterm labour is likely to be triggered by a number of different pathways, although the final pathways activating prostaglandin synthesis and receptor changes may be similar. Pathological distension, such as that seen in multiple pregnancies or hydramnios, may stretch gap junctions, affect oxytocin receptors and alter IL-8 synthesis. The decidual haemorrhage of placental abruption or subchorionic haemorrhage may act either through similar inflammatory mechanisms, as occur in infection, or via direct effects of thrombin on the membranes. There is now discussion of a placental clock, perhaps mediated by corticotrophin-releasing factor (CRF) (Lockwood 1999), and premature signals may occur in this system. Factors which alter the maternal glucocorticoid axis, such as stress, may trigger CRF release. CRF increases directly prostanoid production in the choriodecidua. Therefore the pathways outlined in Figure 31.1 simply demonstrate the mechanisms by which bacteria might initiate preterm labour.

Microorganisms must first breach the cervical barrier before initiating changes in the membranes and structures in the lower uterine segment. Defence is initially maintained by the physical mucous cervical plug and the presence of secretory IgA in cervical fluid. Proteases are produced in abundance by many bacteria inhabiting the female genital tract (McGregor et al 1986). IgA-specific proteases are produced by both *N. gonorrhoea* and ureoplasmas (Plaut 1978, Kapatais-Zoumbos et al 1985). Mucinase and neuraminidase are also produced by many genital microorganisms (McGregor 1988) and may disrupt the mucin plug.

Once through the initial barrier, bacteria may initiate preterm labour via a number of routes. The key processes are the stimulation of the production of prostaglandins and the release of a number of immune mediators, such as PAF or 5-hydroxytryptamine (5-HT), which stimulate smooth muscle cells directly.

The prostaglandin pathways are accessed via several routes. Bacteria may directly metabolise arachidonic acid. Both phospholipase A_2 and C can be released from microorganisms (Bejar et al 1981, McGregor 1988) and these may be able to release arachidonic acid from appropriate stores in the amnion. However, the major route is via the effects of released bacterial toxins in initiation of the inflammatory process in the decidua and chorio-amnion. These endotoxins may directly stimulate prostaglandin synthesis in the amnion and chorion (Lamont et al 1985), or via the release from the chorion of cytokines such as IL-6 (Dudley et al 1992). The most dramatic effects of these endotoxins are on the decidua, and particularly on cells of bone marrow origin, such as monocytes and macrophages, which make up half of all decidual cells (Vince et al 1990). These cells are stimulated to produce large quantities of proinflammatory cytokines, particularly PAF, IL-1, TNF, colony-stimulating factors, IL-6 (Casey et al 1989, Romero et al 1990a), and chemokines such as IL-8 and macrophage inhibitory protein 1α (Gomez et al 1997). These in turn stimulate prostaglandin synthesis in both decidua and amnion (Romero et al 1989, Mitchell et al 1991, Gomez et al 1997).

Once activated, this complex cycle of cytokine stimulation becomes established, with mutual enhancement of the differing immune mediators which is difficult to reverse despite the simultaneous increase in inhibitory cytokines such as transforming growth factor (TGF β) and IL-10.

Other ecosanoids are produced, such as thromboxane and the leukotrienes. These may cause local circulatory disturbance, and the leukotrienes are potent chemotactic agents (Lopez Bernal et al 1990), thus fuelling the inflammatory process. Free radical damage occurs, and other mediating substances derived from decidual cells, and which can directly stimulate myometrial cells, are released. Other released cytokines, such as IL-2 and IL-4, have important roles in cell-mediated immune processes. It is easy to see that, once bacterial products have initiated this complex immunological, endocrinological and biochemical process, labour may be inevitable.

The final route by which microorganisms may initiate labour is by membrane disruption. Proteases are produced by both decidual cells and bacteria. Bacterial proteases are often very non-selective but some genital bacteria produce elastase and collagenase. Such enzymes could reduce the tensile strength of membranes (McGregor et al 1987) and there is good evidence that the proteases produced by some genital organisms have this capability (Sbarra et al 1987). Once the membranes are ruptured, labour is initiated by a combination of normal factors and by the processes outlined above. The potential pathways and interactions are outlined in Figure 31.1.

PREDICTION OF PRETERM DELIVERY

Much effort has been expended in attempts to identify groups of women at high risk of preterm delivery who might benefit from increased surveillance and the potential early use of therapy to abort threatened preterm labour. A number of different approaches have been used.

Risk factor scoring

Many scoring systems have been constructed, all based on epidemiological risk factors such as those outlined in Table 31.1. In all, past reproductive history plays the major role,

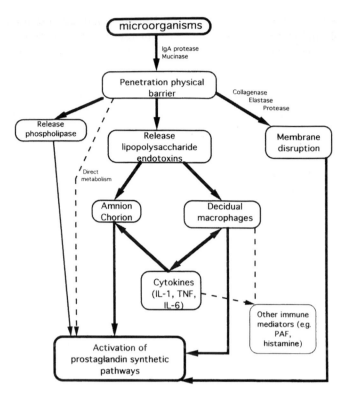

Fig. 31.1 Mechanisms by which infection could cause preterm labour.

with a history of previous preterm births, second-trimester miscarriages and cone biopsy all scoring highly (Creasy et al 1980, Holbrook et al 1989). Many other risk factors, such as abdominal surgical procedure in pregnancy, stilboestrol exposure and uterine malformation are rare and are poor predictors of the bulk of preterm delivery. Overall the performance of risk scoring, though easily applied, has been poor. Pooled results give a sensitivity of only 40% and a false-positive rate of almost 80% (see McLean et al 1993). The wealth of better epidemiological data published in the last 5 years may allow modification of clinical risk assessment which might be best utilised in nulliparous women to direct them towards other more sensitive screening tests as described below.

Clinical cervical assessment

It has been widely assumed that premature effacement or dilatation of the cervix is related to an increased risk of preterm delivery. The evidence to support this is poor. Positive predictive values of cervical changes range from 4 to 30% (Leveno et al 1986, Mortensen et al 1987), and sensitivities are less than 50%. Others have reported no additional advantage over risk factor scoring (Blondel et al 1990). The largest study is from France and considers length and dilatation of the cervix (see Papiernik 1993). Between 19 and 31 weeks' gestation in nulliparae, dilatation of the os was associated with an adjusted relative risk of 1.8–3.6, and a short cervix with an adjusted risk of 2.2–2.8.

Ultrasound cervical assessment

The relationship between the length of the cervix assessed by transvaginal ultrasound and preterm delivery was initially described in 1990 (Anderson et al 1990). Subsequent work has described normal values (Anderson 1991, Iams et al 1996, Heath et al 1998a) with the mean length in the second trimester lying between 34 and 40 mm. Consistently, 20–25 mm lies around the 5th centile and 10–13 mm at the 1st centile of most studies. Accuracy of the measurement, both inter- and intraobserver, is plus or minus 3–4 mm. Transabdominal ultrasound can be used for measurement, but it is felt that accuracy is compromised, and this is borne out in the range of normal mean values seen, from 32 to 53 mm.

The concept of the cervix has therefore changed from a static competent or incompetent organ to an organ with continuous properties, which can change dynamically with uterine contractions, gestation or position in the antenatal period.

Iams and colleagues (Iams et al 1996) screened a large unselected population. Women with a cervical length less than 20 mm had an 11% risk of delivering before 35 weeks. Values less than the 5th centile (22 mm) carried a relative risk of 9.5, and those less than the 1st centile a risk of 14. The overall sensitivity was 23% and predictive value 26% for delivery under 35 weeks.

Others have looked at women at high risk of preterm delivery (Berghella et al 1997, 1999) and described similar relative risks.

As a result of such studies, transvaginal evaluation of the cervix is one of the best predictive factors, particularly for nulliparous women, although the sensitivity remains low. Better results may be possible where other risk factors are identified. This work is already underway, particularly examining the interaction between cervical length, fetal fibronectin and previous preterm delivery (Iams et al 1998). The presence of a short cervix in a woman who has previously delivered an extremely preterm infant doubles her existing risk; conversely, a normal length almost returns the risk to background.

KEY POINTS: RISK FACTORS

- Assessment of risk of preterm delivery should be a formal part of each antenatal visit.
- Concentrate on identification of modifiable risk factors:
  - weight, smoking, drugs
  - life style, stress, working pattern
  - urinary and vaginal infection.
- Use key non-modifiable demographic, past reproductive history and current pregnancy risk factors to consider secondary screening by ultrasound or biochemistry.

Fetal fibronectin

Fetal fibronectin is an oncofetal protein that is expressed in the first half of pregnancy. It is thought to be an adhesion molecule involved in maintaining the integrity of the choriodecidual extracellular matrix. After 20 weeks it is not usually detectable until membrane rupture. It is hypothesised that preterm labour is preceded by progressive enzymatic or mechanical disruption of the extracellular matrix, allowing release of intact or degraded fetal fibronectin. There is also some evidence that inflammatory products may increase the production of fetal fibronectin.

Preliminary studies suggested that, in women presenting with preterm uterine activity, measurement of fetal fibronectin levels by means of a simple vaginal swab has an 82% sensitivity in the prediction of those going on to deliver preterm, with a positive predictive value of 83% (Lockwood et al 1991). Early antenatal studies indicated sensitivities of 70–80% in the prediction of preterm delivery although the false-positive rates remain high (Lockwood et al 1993, Nageotte et al 1994).

Subsequently there have been a number of studies in high- and low-risk pregnancies. In low-risk pregnancies a positive result at 24 weeks' gestation carries a 10% risk of delivery before 28 weeks, with a sensitivity of 63% and a relative risk of 59 (Goldenberg et al 1996b). This sensitivity falls to 25% when delivery at less than 32 weeks is the outcome. Faron and colleagues (Faron et al 1998) systematically reviewed the screening literature to 1997. From the data available to them, in low-risk women, the likelihood of delivery before 37 weeks with a positive fibronectin was 7.5, and most studies of low-risk subjects have been close to this value.

In high-risk women, sensitivities are improved, with the higher prior risk giving sensitivities of up to 80% (Leeson et al 1996). Other work has shown that a positive fetal fibronectin may particularly identify those preterm labours and deliveries most closely linked with infection (Goldenberg et al 1996a). Serial testing at 24 and 26 weeks may reduce the false-positive rate. One study (Goldenberg et al 1997) has shown a fivefold reduction in risk of delivery before 32 weeks if only one of the tests is positive; the risk is 5%, compared with 25% if both are positive. Fetal fibronectin may also be a better second line test in women with a past history of preterm birth (Iams et al 1998) than cervical length estimation. If both tests are used in this group, then if both are positive, two-thirds of women will deliver before 35 weeks, and if both are negative, the risk is similar to the background risk.

Other biochemical markers

Attempts to utilise progesterone, oestradiol and mediators of the inflammatory process have not shown any promise as screening tests. Plasma CRH, a peptide produced by the syncitiotrophoblast, is implicated in the initiation of labour, both term and preterm. Placental and fetal membrane production of prostaglandins E_2 and F_2 are regulated by CRH, and it potentiates the action of oxytocin. The bioavailability of CRH increases in the weeks leading up to the onset of labour. Recent studies (Leung et al 1999, McLean et al 1999), looking at CRH levels in mid-pregnancy in unselected women, have shown some promise, with likelihood ratios of 3.5 and sensitivities of 24–73%, depending on the level examined. For very high levels (McLean et al 1999) the subsequent risk of preterm delivery may be as high as 1 in 3.

Serum alpha-fetoprotein (AFP) has been suggested but sensitivity is poor (McLean et al 1999). Angionen, a marker of angiogenesis secondary to ischaemia or inflammation, is raised in second-trimester amniotic fluid in pregnancies going on to deliver early, but there is no clear cut-off value (Spong et al 1997). Preliminary data on human chorionic gonadotrophin (hCG) in cervical secretions in high-risk pregnancies (Bernstein et al 1998) shows promise, with predictive values in the range of those seen with fetal fibronectin.

Further data from the preterm prediction study of the Maternal-Fetal Medicine Network in the US has implicated plasma granulocyte-stimulating factor levels, with odds ratios of between 4 and 10 for delivery within a 4 week period after the test and predicted between one-third and one-half of deliveries in that period (Goldenberg et al 2000a). Similarly, this group (Goldenberg et al 2000b) analysed a number of factors in cervical secretions. Both cervical lactoferrin and sialidase values were related to preterm delivery but sensitivities were low.

Uterine activity monitoring

The development of non-invasive sensing devices and computer technology have made it possible to detect uterine activity in the home, with data being transmitted by telephone. Its use is based on measurement of contraction frequency, and the documented increase in this in the 24–48 h before delivery. Initial work suggested sensitivities of 57–80% (Katz et al 1986, Main et al 1988) in high-risk groups, with positive predictive values of 32–72%. Subsequent studies (Hill et al 1990, Knuppel et al 1990) have confirmed the possibility that this type of monitoring, with daily nursing support and intensive obstetric supervision, may reduce the incidence of preterm birth.

The relative efficacy of these predictive factors are included in Table 31.1. Risk assessment for preterm delivery should be a formal and defined part of each antenatal contact. Particular attention should be directed at life style issues where the risk could be altered, such as drugs or smoking. Where the risk cannot easily be changed, e.g. previous preterm delivery or young age, then consideration could be given to using a second-line screening test, such as fetal fibronectin or vaginal ultrasound, to determine higher risk subgroups. The next decade is likely to see the emergence of targeted clinics for women at risk of preterm delivery. Such clinics would allow better evaluation and education, directed therapy and the production of a patient group capable of quickly testing new interventions.

PREVENTION OF PRETERM LABOUR

Identification of women at risk by some sort of screening is important, but even 100% sensitivity would be ineffective if appropriate therapy is not available either to prevent preterm labour or to modify its outcome. Prevention would be the primary aim, but another approach would be early identification, which would allow time for administration of drugs that might modify neonatal outcome. Therapies that have had some success are outlined in Table 31.2.

Table 31.2 Possible interventions to reduce preterm delivery in antenatal period

Cervical cerclage where three or more spontaneous losses beyond first trimester

Treatment and confirmed eradication of bacteriuria

Treatment of sexually transmissible diseases

Smoking cessation programmes

Work pattern planning

Substance abuse programmes, e.g. methadone replacement and reduction

Targeted psychological counselling

Antibiotic treatment of bacterial vaginosis in women with previous preterm delivery

(Cervical cerclage for demonstrable short cervix on screening)

Educational strategies

Approaches that could have value include the teaching of groups of women to recognise early symptoms of preterm labour, with the premise that earlier presentation may modify outcome, or specific interventions aimed at individual risk factors such as work habits, smoking, drug abuse or stress.

The most widely quoted education programme study is that from France, where an entire population was subjected to an education programme that focused both on an appreciation that excess physical effort or heavy work may predispose to preterm uterine activity and on the ability to recognise early the features of early preterm labour. Although none of the work was carried out as a controlled trial, representative samples of the French population have been studied at intervals (see Papiernik 1993 for a review of this work). The preterm delivery rate declined from 7.9% in 1972 to 4.1% in 1988–1989. Delivery under 34 weeks' gestation declined from 3.3 to 1.3% over this period. Similar reductions in very preterm births were demonstrated in the more detailed study in Haguenau carried out as part of the assessment of this programme (Papiernik et al 1985), with a fall in deliveries under 32 weeks from 1.5 to 0.5% over 10 years. Some of this fall may be due to well-documented changes in the population over this period, including a reduction in parity, and reductions in births at both extremes of age.

Randomised trials of high-risk women have shown no reduction in preterm births by use of education programmes (Main et al 1985, Mueller-Huebach et al 1989, Goldenberg et al 1990). The largest trial (Collaborative Group on Preterm Birth Prevention 1993) did not show any reliable benefit from an education programme. A systematic review (Hueston et al 1995) showed no reduction in perinatal mortality, low birthweight or preterm delivery. They did find an increase in the diagnosis of preterm labour and concluded that such approaches appeared to increase intervention without clinical benefit.

Pregnancy is often used as a trigger for smoking cessation programmes, but in the UK few hospitals have a systematic approach to this. In the latest systematic review (Lumley et al 2000), smoking cessation interventions can reduce the number of women smoking by 50%, both where cessation is self-reported and where biochemically validated. In trials where pregnancy outcome is given, a 17% reduction (odds ratio 0.83) in preterm births was seen, although there were no differences in perinatal mortality.

The recognition that stress and stressful life events may increase the risk of preterm delivery allows possible psychological interventions. There is little specific work, but trials of social and psychological support in various settings have not shown a reduction in preterm births. However, where such support has been targeted at high-risk situations (Mamelle et al 1997), significant reductions in preterm delivery can be achieved, even in women with cervical changes.

Home uterine activity monitoring

Systematic reviews of early trials (Keirse 1993a, Colton et al 1995) suggested a modest benefit (odds ratio 0.67–076) in preterm births but trials were of variable quality and small. Since then, two large trials (Collaborative Home Uterine Monitoring Study Group 1995, Dyson et al 1998) and one trial in a very high-risk group (Brown et al 1999) with better quality, have shown no difference in preterm birth with the addition of home monitoring to the usual nurse support and education. In Dyson's trial there were increased interventions with more visits and more use of tocolytics, without benefit. At present, home uterine activity monitoring does not appear to have a place in preventative care.

Pharmacological intervention

Studies using fish oil supplementation show prolongation of pregnancy (Olsen et al 1992) but it is too soon to tell if preterm delivery will be affected by such therapy.

Treatment of asymptomatic bacteriuria with antibiotics appears to reduce the likelihood of delivery of an infant weighing less than 2500 g, odds ratio 0.6 (95% CI 0.45–0.80) (Smaill 2000). One of the trials involving specifically group B streptococci also demonstrated a reduction in preterm PROM (Thomsen et al 1987). Although the overall impact on preterm delivery within the population will be small, such therapy should be offered where screening for bacteriuria takes place.

Two interesting interventions have received less notice, namely the use of magnesium supplementation and the use of progesterone. Magnesium sulphate is a well-established tocolytic in established preterm labour and probably acts by interfering with the uptake, binding and distribution of intracellular calcium in smooth muscle (Altura et al 1987). Three trials with 1700 women (Kovacs et al 1988, Spatling & Spetling 1988, Sibai et al 1989) examined the effects of routine oral magnesium supplementation on preterm delivery. The odds ratio for premature delivery in the supplemented group was 0.67 (95% CI 0.47–0.94). Reduction of preterm births by one-third would be a major achievement for such simple and safe therapy and more large studies are required. Trials of 17α-hydroxyprogesterone caproate in the prevention of miscarriage have demonstrated an unexpected benefit in reduction in preterm birth, with an odds ratio of 0.5 (CI

0.3–0.85) (Prendeville 1993), which similarly demands further, more detailed study, although weekly intramuscular injections are required.

Antibiotics

The demonstration of a causal link between microbiological colonisation and preterm birth opens the way to prevention by antibiotic prophylaxis. Clearly where the organism involved is pathogenic, such as chlamydia or neisseria, then treatment will be indicated. More contentious is the possibility of screening for bacterial vaginosis and treating detected cases. McGregor (McGregor et al 1995) made a powerful case for this within a prospective screen and treat programme, which showed a 50% reduction in preterm births, particularly in the early preterm group, after treatment with oral clindamicin, compared with historical controls. However, randomised trials have been less convincing. In a systematic review of studies till mid-1998 (Brocklehurst et al 2000) involving 1500 women, no reduction in preterm births was seen. Local therapy appears to be no better (Vermeulen & Bruinse 1999), nor does therapy directed against group B streptococcus. A recent very large trial of 2000 women with bacterial vaginosis (Carey et al 2000) demonstrated no differences in preterm delivery before 37 or 32 weeks or in preterm PROM.

The only consistently positive finding has been that there does appear to be benefit to women with bacterial vaginosis who have had previous preterm deliveries (Vermeulen & Bruinse 1999; Brocklehurst et al 2000). It may be worth considering screening and treating such pregnancies.

Cervical cerclage

Elective cerclage may have a place in the prevention of preterm birth in very high-risk women (three or more previous preterm deliveries). Subanalysis of the large European trial (MRC/RCOG Working Party on Cervical Cerclage 1993) suggests reduction of the risk of delivery before 33 weeks in these women by about one-quarter by the use of cerclage. Overall there is a trend to a reduction in preterm birth in all women with previous second-trimester loss or preterm delivery.

The emergence of cervical length as a predictor for preterm delivery has led to attempts to target women with a short cervix for cervical cerclage. Early uncontrolled work (Heath et al 1998b) was encouraging but others did not find benefit (Guzman et al 1998). In a patient preference study no differences were found in the preterm delivery rate or in the days gained after diagnosis (Berghella et al 1999). Careful randomised studies will be needed. Preliminary data from these are not encouraging (Rust et al 2000) but studies are small.

MANAGEMENT OF PRETERM LABOUR

Diagnosis of preterm labour and preterm premature rupture of membranes

It is often difficult to distinguish between threatened preterm labour and real preterm labour. Many women present with uterine activity in the third trimester, with up to 10% of women with normal pregnancies progressing to term complaining of painful uterine activity preterm (Iams et al 1990a). Up to one-third of women subsequently presenting with preterm labour reported no prodromal symptoms (Iams et al 1990b). Given the risks of the possible therapeutic interventions and the anxiety produced in families, more accurate differentiation of true from false preterm labour would be valuable.

Clinical evaluation

Attempts have been made to define a group of symptoms likely to result in preterm delivery based on the placebo arms of randomised trials to prevent preterm labour (Ingemarrson 1976). These all include regular contractions (at intervals of less than 10 min for 30 min, or eight in 60 min) accompanied by either cervical effacement or change in dilatation and effacement. Changes in parameters assessed by digital vaginal examination are best quantified using the Bishop score. Where uterine activity follows vaginal bleeding then delivery is more likely (Macones et al 1999).

Preterm PROM can sometimes present a similar diagnostic dilemma. Here the differential diagnosis lies between PROM, watery vaginal discharge and urinary incontinence. A careful history may help, but commonly other tests are required after speculum examination to examine and sample the fluid present in the vagina. These include ferning of amniotic fluid on a glass slide, with an accuracy of 96% and a false-negative rate of 5–10% (Friedman & McElin 1969); or the use of the alkalinity of amniotic fluid to alter the colour of nitrazine paper, with a maximum accuracy of over 90%, but a false-positive rate of up to 15% and false-negative rate of 10%. Fetal fibronectin can be used where there is doubt; if negative, it is highly unlikely that the membranes are ruptured. A positive test may be more difficult to interpret given the link between positive fetal fibronectin and preterm delivery in women with intact membranes. Amniotic fluid volume assessment by ultrasound may aid clarification but has yet to be appropriately evaluated. The use of fetal fibronectin has made intra-amniotic instillation of dye obsolete.

Use of fetal fibronectin in women with preterm uterine activity

The original work on fibronectin was in women in suspected preterm labour (Lockwood et al 1991). Subsequent studies (Bartnicki et al 1996, Rizzo et al 1996, Peaceman et al 1997) have shown in excess of 50% likelihood of delivery within 7–14 days in women with preterm uterine activity and a positive fetal fibronectin. More importantly, the risk of delivery within 7 days in women without cervical change who have a negative test is only 1 in 200 (Peaceman et al 1997). Fetal fibronectin has been shown to be a better discriminator than clinical indices (Peacemen et al 1997, Rozenberg et al 1997). Such discrimination should allow better targeting of therapy and resources, and might reduce the need for in utero transfer. Results from clinical audits of its use have shown similar sensitivities and predictive values to research studies (Chuileannain et al 1998).

Cervical ultrasound in women with preterm uterine activity

A number of groups have looked at the utilisation of vaginal ultrasound measurement of the cervix as a predictor in women with preterm uterine activity. Although predictive values of around 50% have been demonstrated (Rizzo et al 1996, Rozenberg et al 1997), it is less efficient as a test than fetal fibronectin. In clinical terms much might depend on available expertise on the delivery suite.

Once a diagnosis of putative preterm labour is made, management is centred on a number of questions:

1. Why is the woman in preterm labour?
2. How is the fetus (and its parents)?
3. What therapy is indicated?
4. What monitoring should be used in labour?
5. How should the fetus be delivered?

KEY POINTS: DIAGNOSIS

- Clinical diagnosis should be much more rigorous than current standards.
- Maternity units should have an agreed definition of what constitutes suspected preterm labour likely to lead to delivery, and which would result:
  - in the use of steroids and tocolysis
  - in discussions with parents about survival and outcome
  - in fetal monitoring
  - in discussion about obstetric intervention.
- More widespread use of fetal fibronectin testing on delivery suite would improve diagnosis.
- More widespread use of amniocentesis in preterm PROM and in persistent uterine activity without cervical change would improve diagnostic accuracy.

Why is the woman in preterm labour?

This is essentially an aetiological work-up (Table 31.3). It will include a full history and clinical examination, fetal fibronectin testing, ultrasound examination with cervical length estimation and comment on funnelling if expertise is

Table 31.3 Investigation of suspected preterm labour

Full blood count, C-reactive protein
Kleihauer test
Plasma urea and electrolytes
Urine microscopy/culture
High vaginal/cervical swabs or aliquot of liquor for infection/colonisation
Fetal fibronectin (unless clear ruptured membranes)
Ultrasound examination: fetal position, size, liquor; cervical length if available skills
Amniocentesis: for Gram stain, glucose, white cell count; LDH or IL-6 if possible

available, and possibly amniocentesis. The key clinical diagnoses to be excluded are fetal death, multiple pregnancy, uterine malformation, cervical incompetence, maternal systemic disease, infection and placental abruption.

All investigative modalities need to be available 24 h a day, and individuals skilled in ultrasound and third-trimester amniocentesis must be similarly available. Maternal white blood cell counts and C-reactive protein (CRP) estimates may give an index of general infection, although results must be interpreted using normal pregnancy ranges. Particular care is needed if glucocorticoid therapy has already been initiated as the leucocyte count may be markedly elevated. CRP levels below 30 mg/l may be normal, although persistent values above 20 mg/l are highly suggestive of chorioamnionitis (Fisk 1988). Kleihauer testing may detect occult fetomaternal haemorrhage suggestive of concealed abruption. More recently it has been suggested that AFP is a more sensitive index of fetomaternal haemorrhage, although third-trimester normal ranges are less well described.

Urine microscopy is essential to exclude urinary tract infection as a cause of preterm labour, as appropriate antibiotics will be required before successful suppression of labour is achieved. Genital tract infection, especially group B streptococcal infection, should be tested for.

Ultrasound plays a key role in the assessment of preterm labour. Its diagnostic functions include the diagnosis of multiple pregnancy, confirmation and quantification of polyhydramnios, determination of fetal presentation, diagnosis of previously unsuspected malformation, and, in skilled hands, identification of subchorionic haemorrhage. Maternity units delivering preterm infants need to ensure the availability at all times of someone skilled enough to perform these complex assessments.

Role of amniocentesis in suspected preterm labour

Although popular in North America, amniocentesis is less practised on labour wards in the UK. With intact membranes, the incidence of positive culture is around 13% (Romero & Mazor 1988). In experienced hands it is not associated with significant risk of ruptured membranes (Dunlow & Duff 1990). There is good evidence that the presence of organisms in the amniotic cavity is associated with an increased risk of ruptured membranes and of failed tocolysis (Romero & Mazor 1988).

Culture results take too long to be useful in the immediate management of preterm labour. A number of rapid markers of inflammation and infection have been examined and correlated both with positive liquor culture and with rapid delivery. Gram staining is the gold standard of acute investigation (Romero et al 1988b) in terms of prediction of a positive amniotic fluid culture and of delivery within 36 h (Garry et al 1996). However, other simple tests such as white cell counts >50 cells/dl (Romero et al 1991), glucose levels less than 16 mg/dl (Romero et al 1990b) and leucocyte esterase activity (Egley et al 1988) also have good predictive values. More recently amniotic fluid complement levels (C3 more than 6 mg/dl) and lactic dehydrogenase (LDH) levels greater than 419 units/l have been shown to have high predictive value (Garry et al 1996, Elimian et al 1998). Of the more sophisticated tests, IL-6 assays (greater than 17 ng/ml) show the best predictive value (Yoon et al 1995), and simple kits are becoming available.

Such information is useful clinically in determining a subset of women who are likely to deliver, are likely to be refractory to tocolysis, are at higher risk of chorio-amnionitis, and are at risk of neonatal sepsis in order to maximise care. All of these tests are applicable to any labour ward, and should perhaps be more widely utilised.

How is the fetus?

The next question to be addressed before deciding on therapy is that of fetal well-being. This is approached using conventional cardiotocography and by ultrasound assessment.

Accurate knowledge of gestation is central to the management of preterm labour and it may be necessary to assess gestational age where this is uncertain. Given the social class and age-related associations of preterm labour, late presentation for antenatal care and concealed pregnancy are more common in these higher risk groups than in the general obstetric population. Gestational assessment is less accurate in the late second and early third trimester. Routine measurements of biparietal diameter (BPD), femur length, head circumference and abdominal circumference should be made. Where possible transcerebellar diameter or foot length should be assessed, as these measurements are less affected by deviations in fetal growth (Mercer et al 1987, Reece et al 1987) and are the most accurate measures of gestation at this stage.

Liquor volume should be assessed as this may help differentiate the growth-restricted from the preterm fetus. Maximum pool depth or amniotic fluid index may be used and it is better to utilise gestationally adjusted reference ranges (Nwosu et al 1993) rather than absolute values. Growth is difficult to assess in the absence of good data about gestational age, and is made more so by the view that growth restriction is more common in preterm then in term deliveries (Tamura & Sabbagha 1984). Weight can be estimated using a number of formulae but no single formula stands out (Robson et al 1993); however, those of Hadlock (Hadlock et al 1985) and Shepard (Shepard et al 1982) are most commonly used. More sophisticated methods of determining appropriateness of growth relative to maternal characteristics (Wilcox et al 1993) or relative to previous ultrasound measurements (Deter et al 1986) are possible but may not yet be applicable in the labour ward. Strenuous efforts to determine gestation and weight accurately are important at the lower limits of viability in order to prevent fetuses from being erroneously labelled previable.

While carrying out such assessments, some impression of fetal activity and general behaviour can be made. Fetal breathing activity is not as useful a test of well-being under these conditions as its absence has been proposed as a predictor of true preterm labour (Agustsson & Patel 1987).

Well-being is normally assessed by cardiotocography. This is evaluated using standard criteria modified for use in the preterm fetus. Both fetal heart rate reactivity and amplitude of accelerations are reduced prior to 32 weeks (Natale et al 1984). Isolated variable decelerations are common and not of pathological significance. Caution is required in defining fetal distress by cardiotocography alone in the preterm fetus, and recourse to other biophysical assessment and even fetal cord blood sampling may be necessary in the extremely preterm to decide on the best management.

Following these extensive investigations, clinicians are in a position to determine which therapies, including immediate delivery, are appropriate to optimise outcome.

Therapies to improve outcome: delaying delivery

Several drugs are now available to delay delivery in spontaneous preterm labour and where possible these should be utilised to allow other therapies that may improve outcome to be given. There are few complete contraindications to the inhibition of preterm labour (Table 31.4). Current drugs used are beta-mimetics, prostaglandin synthetase inhibitors, magnesium sulphate, calcium-channel blockers, oxytocin receptor antagonists, nitric oxide antagonists and antibiotics.

Table 31.4 Contraindications to suppression of preterm labour

Absolute contraindications
Fetal death
Fetal congenital anomaly incompatible with life
Clear clinical chorio-amnionitis
Fetal condition requiring immediate delivery
Maternal condition requiring immediate delivery
Relative contraindications
Significant vaginal bleeding
Pre-eclampsia
Fetal distress
Fetal growth restriction
PROM with evidence of intra-amniotic bacterial colonisation

Beta-adrenergic agonists (beta-mimetics)

Mechanism of action. The action of the commonly used drugs (ritodrine, salbutamol, terbutaline) is dependent on interaction with β_2-adrenergic receptor sites on myometrial cell membranes. Their activity depends on the alkyl substitutions on the ethylamine side-chain and the hydroxyl groups at the 3 and 5 positions of the benzene ring. The agonist–receptor complex activates adenylate cyclase, resulting in an increase in intracellular cyclic adenosine monophosphate (cAMP; Roberts 1984). In turn this activates a protein kinase which causes both phosphorylation of membrane proteins in the sarcoplasmic reticulum responsible for reducing intracellular calcium concentrations, and an inhibition of myosin light-chain kinase activity which prevents the actin–myosin interaction necessary for smooth muscle contraction.

Safety. Maternal side effects of beta-mimetics are well documented and are described in Table 31.5. The metabolic effects are a result of β_2-receptor stimulation, which promotes hepatic glycogenolysis and thus hyperglycaemia. The effect is transient, peaking at 3–6 h after treatment starts (Young et al 1983). Transient hypokalaemia almost always occurs as a consequence of a redistribution of potassium from extracellular to intracellular compartments. Total body potassium is

Table 31.5 Maternal side-effects of beta-agonists

Palpitations
Tremor
Restlessness
Agitation
Rash
Nausea and bloating
Elevated transaminases
Anaemia
Paralytic ileus
Glucose intolerance
Hypokalaemia
Myocardial ischaemia
Arrhythmia
Pulmonary oedema

not changed and there are no reports of adverse effects. No replacement therapy is indicated.

Most of the concern over the use of beta-agonists centres on the severe cardiovascular side effects. These have been well reviewed recently (Lamont 2000). The risk of pulmonary oedema is 0.3% of cases (Canadian Preterm Labour Investigators Group 1992). This does not usually occur within the first 24 h of therapy and its aetiology is multifactorial. There is a high output state with possible capillary endothelial leaks. Vasodilatation leads to systemic hypotension with compensatory rises in heart rate, stroke volume, cardiac output and eventually systolic blood pressure. Tachycardia may initially maintain the blood pressure but excessive rises in heart rate lead to decompensation with a marked fall in stroke volume. Heart failure with pulmonary oedema then occurs. Other factors may also act in this direction. Arrhythmias are described, and although usually benign, serious pathology may be unmasked by beta-mimetic therapy. Symptomatic myocardial ischaemia, usually localised to the subendocardial region, has been described (Benedetti 1983), although most women have the normal response to sustained tachycardia, namely depression of the ST segment and flattening or inversion of the T wave from relative hypoperfusion of the subendocardial region. The findings urge extreme caution where pre-existing cardiac disease is even suspected, and alternative therapies should be explored.

Many of the reported severe cases, including deaths, were associated with the intravenous infusion of very large volumes of crystalloid fluid. There is some evidence that the use of sodium chloride solution compared with dextrose solution is associated with an increased likelihood of fluid retention (Philipsen et al 1981). Whatever the cause, the injudicious use of beta-agonists can be lethal, and appropriate monitoring needs to be in place (see below).

Fetal side effects are confined in practical terms to a tachycardia and hypoglycaemia. No long-term effects have been noted.

Administration. All delivery suites should have clear guidelines for the management of women on beta-agonist therapy and in the UK these should be consistent with the RCOG recommendation. They should include guidance on the indications and contraindications for use, preliminary investigations, dosage schedules and frequency of increasing dose, instructions for maintenance of intravenous therapy, duration of therapy, maternal and fetal monitoring required with special attention to calculation of fluid balance, and indications for abandoning therapy or adding further drugs. The maximum duration of therapy should be stated clearly, as should the chain of command for re-initiating treatment. There should be clear objectives to the therapy.

Beta-agonists should only be used where there is good evidence of preterm labour (see above) (Fig. 31.2). Preliminary investigations will include a full cardiovascular history and examination, and measurement of plasma electrolytes and haematocrit. An electrocardiogram should be performed if there is any suspicion of a cardiac problem.

Beta-adrenergic agonists should be given as continuous intravenous infusions, diluted in 5% dextrose or half strength saline solution. They should be given as high concentration solutions to minimise the amount of fluid given; the use of syringe pumps is one way to achieve this. At the very least, calibrated infusion pumps are necessary, and the drug should be given as a separate infusion from other i.v. fluid administration. Administration schedules vary but the initial dose should be the minimum recommended. The dose should be increased every 10–20 min until uterine activity is less than one contraction in 15 min, or until maternal side effects ensue. The maternal heart rate should not be allowed to exceed 140 b.p.m. The dose should then be stabilised and the infusion maintained for 12–24 h. Gradual tapering of the dose should be commenced after a few hours, and there is increasing evidence that the dose required for maintenance of intravenous tocolysis is much less than previously thought. Some work remains to be carried out on dosage regimens and there may be practical advantages to giving a loading dose with a reduced sliding scale compared with standard incre-

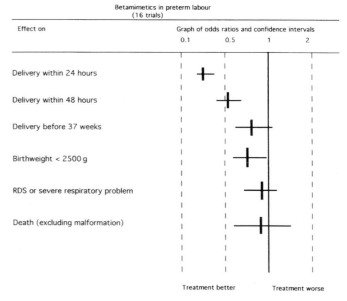

Fig. 31.2 Meta-analysis of effects of beta-agonists in preterm labour.

mental regimens (Holleboom et al 1996a). The major objectives of tocolytic therapy are to allow time for maternal and fetal transfer to a place with appropriate neonatal facilities or to buy time for therapies which may directly influence fetal outcome, such as corticosteroids. These objectives are usually achievable in 24–36 h, and continuation of intravenous treatment beyond this period should only occur in unusual circumstances, such as difficulties in finding appropriate neonatal care or where the fetus is thought previable and therapy appears effective. Other drugs (see below) can be used where effective tocolysis for 24 h seems unlikely or where there are contraindications to beta-agonists. Prior to their use, critical review of the suspected aetiology should be undertaken, and consideration should be given to exclusion of infection by direct examination of the amniotic fluid (via amniocentesis).

Detailed maternal monitoring is mandatory. It should include regular auscultation of the lung bases, half-hourly to hourly measurement of vital signs, 12-hourly plasma electrolyte measurement, strict input/output charting, and continuous pulse oximetry. In addition to standard midwifery observations, continuous cardiotocography is helpful, as much for information on the frequency of uterine activity as for fetal heart rate monitoring.

Following the tapering of intravenous treatment, some clinicians advocate the use of oral therapy (see below).

Prostaglandin synthetase inhibitors

Mechanism of action. Prostaglandins play a key role in both stimulating uterine activity and in facilitating cervical dilatation. Indomethacin (the only drug of this class to be studied to any extent) when given orally or rectally, has a peak action at around 2 h, and a half-life of 2.6–11.2 h (Duggan et al 1972). It acts by inhibiting cyclo-oxygenase, the enzyme which converts fatty acids into prostaglandin endoperoxides. Its action is reversible and enzyme activity resumes as drug levels fall. *In vitro*, spontaneous contractions of myometrial strips are abolished by the addition of indomethacin (Garrioch 1978). The drug passes freely to the fetus, with equivalent levels in the fetus at 5–6 h after the maternal dose, independent of gestational age (Moise et al 1990).

Safety. Maternal side effects are uncommon and usually minor (gastrointestinal disturbance, headache, vertigo, tinnitus). Postpartum haemorrhage has been reported. The classic contraindications and cautions relating to prostaglandin synthetase inhibitors should be recognised, namely history of duodenal ulceration, allergy to salicylates, known coagulation disorder, or known hepatic or renal dysfunction.

The main concerns regarding indomethacin, in contradistinction to ritodrine, are fetal (Table 31.6). Prostaglandins play a central role in maintaining ductal patency (Sideris et al 1983). Ductal constriction with concomitant tricuspid regurgitation in human fetuses exposed to indomethacin has been demonstrated, and the duct is sensitive from as early as 27 weeks' gestation (Moise 1993). However, the mean gestation at which ductal constriction occurs is 31 weeks, with, in some studies, 70% of fetuses exhibiting this side effect beyond

Table 31.6 Fetal side-effects of indomethacin

Constriction of ductus arteriosus
Persistent fetal circulation
Hydrops
Oligohydramnios
Bleeding disorders
Necrotising enterocolitis/perforation
Grade 3 and 4 intraventricular haemorrhage
Cerebral palsy

31 weeks. Fetal urinary output decreases after indomethacin therapy. The mechanism is unrelated to alterations in renal blood flow (Mari et al 1990) and is probably a combination of changes in the central and peripheral effects of antidiuretic hormone and arginine vasopressin, and changes in proximal tubular absorption. Indomethacin can lead to alterations in haemostasis. These drugs can cause platelet dysfunction, inactivating cyclo-oxygenase. The effects of indomethacin are transient as the binding to the enzyme is reversible. Experimentally there is decreased intestinal blood flow following fetal exposure to indomethacin (Meyers et al 1991) and there seems to be a specific risk to the terminal ileum. In the human fetus, ductal constriction with tricuspid regurgitation is associated with alterations in Doppler measures of cerebral blood flow velocity waveforms consistent with increased flow (Mari et al 1989).

Despite these effects, trials using short courses of indomethacin have not demonstrated major neonatal problems. Early detailed case–control studies suggested an increase in intraventricular haemorrhage, particularly severe haemorrhage leading to periventricular leucomalacia (Baerts et al 1990), but recent Australian and US studies have not found increased frequencies of grade 3 and 4 intracranial haemorrhage (Souter et al 1998, Vermillion & Newman 1999). Localised ileal perforation, often delayed and in otherwise well babies (Vanhaesebrouk et al 1988), and necrotising enterocolitis (Major et al 1991) appeared to be increased following the use of indomethacin tocolysis in early case–control studies but in the larger, better US study (Vermillion & Newman 1999) no difference in necrotising enterocolitis was seen. Other complications such as chronic lung disease and pulmonary hypertension were not increased in this study.

Nevertheless, caution is advised above 30 weeks' gestation, where there is existing oligohydramnios, where fetal coagulopathy is possible (e.g. allo-immunisation), and in the growth-restricted fetus already at risk of necrotising enterocolitis and severe intraventricular haemorrhage.

Administration. Before use, fetal size and liquor volume should be estimated using ultrasound, and maternal contraindications sought. The usual daily dose is between 150 and 300 mg, and the commonest regimen in preterm labour is 100 mg rectally followed by 25 mg orally every 6 h. It is rarely justified to continue therapy beyond 48 h. Liquor volume should be assessed every 12–24 h. If long-term use is considered, detailed ultrasonography may be valuable to detect alterations in ductal and cerebral blood flow.

Magnesium sulphate

Mechanism of action. *In vitro* studies demonstrate that magnesium can completely inhibit spontaneous contractility in gravid uterine muscle strips (Hall et al 1959). Its precise mode of action *in vivo* is not fully understood, but involves alterations in uptake, binding and distribution of calcium in smooth muscle cells (Altura et al 1987). Magnesium concentration is regulated by the kidney, with most of an extraneous load being excreted within 24 h. Calcium excretion is also increased, further reducing available intracellular calcium.

Safety. Until recently the major safety concerns for the use of magnesium related to maternal effects. Flushing and perspiration occur shortly after commencement of the loading infusion. Other side effects occur at higher infusion rates (2.5–4 g/h) and can be alleviated by a reduction in the rate of infusion or by injection of 1 g calcium gluconate. Serious side effects are uncommon. Chest pain may be due to myocardial ischaemia, and is usually associated with multiple therapy rather than magnesium alone. Pulmonary oedema occurs in 1% of cases (Elliot 1983), and again is more likely in complex cases involving dual therapy, prolonged therapy or medical complications. While deep tendon reflexes are still present, there is little risk of respiratory depression, and this clinical sign is a useful marker of toxicity.

Long-term therapy has been linked with radiographic abnormalities of the long bones (Holcolm et al 1991). Short-term side effects mimic those in the mother, with a reduction in fetal heart rate and variability, a decrease in fetal breathing, and hypotonia with poor respiratory effort at birth. Of major recent concern was the premature closure of a large trial of magnesium in preterm labour as a consequence of an unacceptably increased perinatal mortality rate and this increased death rate has been confirmed in a recent systematic review (Gyetvai et al 1999).

Administration. Women with muscle disorders or renal impairment should not receive magnesium tocolysis.

Magnesium sulphate is commonly given as an initial loading dose of 4–6 g over 30 min, followed by an infusion of 2–3 g/h for the first hour. Magnesium should be given in 5% dextrose. If uterine quiescence does not occur, then the rate can be increased by 0.5 g/h every 30 min until uterine activity ceases or side effects supervene. Once effective tocolysis is achieved, the rate is maintained at the lowest effective dose or at 2 g/h, whichever is the lowest, for 12 h. It is then tapered off at a rate of 0.5 g/h. In most regimens oral beta-agonists are started at this point. As with other tocolytics, failure to suppress uterine activity should trigger a more aggressive search for the cause of labour, and therapy should not be continued beyond 48 h, save in exceptional circumstances.

Careful attention to fluid balance and reflexes form the key elements to maternal monitoring. Where possible, serum magnesium levels should be evaluated, especially where rates of 6–8 g/h are thought necessary. Ineffective tocolysis at magnesium levels greater than 7 mg/dl should prompt reconsideration of infection or concealed abruption as the cause of preterm labour.

Nifedipine

Mechanism of action. Nifedipine is a type 2 calcium-channel blocker which inhibits inward calcium flow through cell membranes. *In vitro* it inhibits myometrial contractions in a number of settings, by reducing basal tone and the amplitude and frequency of contractions (Smith et al 2000). It is absorbed rapidly from the oral mucosa and from the gastrointestinal tract, with detectable levels within minutes of administration. Peak levels are achieved in pregnancy at around 40 min following administration and its elimination half-life is around 80 min (Ferguson et al 1989). The mechanism of uterine muscle relaxation is by reducing available calcium within myometrial cells.

Safety. Adverse effects include dizziness, flushing, headache and peripheral oedema, all a consequence of vasodilatation; these occur in one in six women, and can sometimes lead to discontinuance of therapy (Talbert & Bussey 1983). Severe side effects are extremely rare. In normotensive women there is a reduction in blood pressure but this is very small. Although the drug crosses the placenta and clearance from the fetus is delayed, fetal side effects are negligible. (Smith et al 2000) and the only major problem is that of fetal distress precipitated by acute hypotension.

Administration. There is no consensus on dosage or frequency for tocolysis with nifedipine. A starting dose of 20 mg seems common, with 10–20 mg 4–6-hourly thereafter. Blood pressure should be monitored carefully.

Oxytocin antagonists

Mechanism of action. Atosiban is a synthetic competitive inhibitor of oxytocin. Its binding to myometrial cell oxytocin receptors results in a dose-dependent inhibition of intracellular calcium release, a reduction in oxytocin-mediated prostaglandin release and a reduction in myometrial contractility. Given intravenously, plateau levels are reached in 1–2 h. It does cross the placenta in small quantities.

Safety. The commonest side effects are maternal nausea and vomiting. Arthralgia and chest pain have been described. At the moment there appear to be few significant fetal side effects.

Administration. Dosage regimens require a high-dose bolus with continuing infusion rates of around 300 µg/min. These produce a consistent and effective reduction of uterine activity in preterm labour over 28 weeks without observable fetal or maternal side effects (Andersen et al 1989, Goodwin et al 1994).

Other tocolytics

Evidence that nitroglycerine can reduce smooth muscle tone via GMP-mediated effects on calcium flux led to studies examining the use of glycenyl trinitrate (GTN) patches as therapy. Early uncontrolled data were encouraging, as was an early small trial (Smith et al 1999). However a larger trial (Lees et al 1999) with 250 women was unable to demonstrate any advantage over conventional tocolysis with ritodrine. Side effects were common, particularly headache.

There is ongoing work with newer oxytocin antagonists (Williams et al 1998) and preliminary work with COX-2 inhibitors (such as nimesulide), although hopes for fewer fetal side effects because of increased selectivity of action on uterine muscle have not so far been fulfilled.

Tocolytic efficacy

It is now clear that at present, in most cases, tocolysis can only offer short-term delay of labour. Although this brief delay does not of itself appear to be translated into improvements in mortality, most studies predate the widespread use of antenatal steroids and contained significant numbers of pregnancies beyond 34 weeks. It seems reasonable to assume that delays of 48 h, which allow the administration of steroids, will significantly reduce perinatal mortality and serious morbidity. However, an alternative argument is that delay in delivery, particularly where intrauterine infection or placental abruption is the trigger, may expose the fetus to a longer period of danger, and thus perinatal outcome is not improved. Delay in delivery also allows safer transfer to appropriate neonatal facilities.

More prolonged delays may be possible using indomethacin (Gyetvai et al 1999) or nifedipine (Oei et al 1999), and a few studies have suggested that prolonged betamimetic therapy is occasionally effective.

Placebo-controlled trials are available for beta-mimetics, indomethacin, magnesium sulphate and atosiban. Trials with nifedipine have been comparative, mainly with beta-mimetics. Recent systematic reviews (Gyetvai et al 1999, Oei et al 1999) allow some 'ranking' in terms of odds ratios for delay at 48 h and 1 week and these are shown in Table 31.7.

The reduction in deliveries within 48 h and 7 days with indomethacin is impressive. Observational and other studies suggest that indomethacin can often rescue failed beta-agonist tocolysis but that the reverse rarely occurs. However, although sepsis was reduced in the trials examined, perinatal mortality was not. In indomethacin trials steroid use was very low. Given the concerns, particularly at later gestational age, of fetal side effects, the failure of apparently effective indomethacin tocolysis to improve outcome is worrying and is probably the main reason for its use not being whole heartedly recommended.

Systematic examination of magnesium as a tocolytic has never been impressive, with poor methodology and poor description of outcomes. Its clear failure to delay delivery beyond 7 days, coupled with serious concerns that it may actually increase perinatal mortality, suggest that this drug has little role as a first-line tocolytic (Gyetvai et al 1999) (although despite this it is still very widely used in the USA, probably for historical reasons).

The value of nifedipine and atosiban lies in their low risk to both mother and fetus. Nifedipine has the added benefit of oral administration. The possibility that it may also delay delivery beyond 7 days is exciting. However, there are no large studies of nifedipine and only 680 women were included in the systematic review. In addition there are no placebo-controlled trials. It is therefore difficult to recommend its use in preference to more established therapy. Atosiban's advantage is that it is safe; its disadvantage is that it is expensive. It may be most useful as rescue therapy where side effects have occurred or where first-line therapy is contraindicated.

At present ritodrine is the mainstay of tocolytic therapy; however, in current practice, this may have to be challenged. Indomethacin is a better tocolytic, a single dose being effective in many women at term (Reiss et al 1976). Both atosiban and nifedipine may be therapeutically equivalent, but have a much more acceptable side effect profile for mother and fetus.

It is surprising that no new trials are planned, particularly as the use of fetal fibronectin, cervical ultrasound or amniocentesis in women presenting with preterm uterine activity would allow much better selection of pregnancies truly at risk of delivery. This may be due to the increasing expense of carrying out trials of any medication during pregnancy, because of the adverse medico-legal climate.

Antibiotics

The increasing evidence implicating infection as a major aetiological factor in preterm labour makes it logical to suppose that appropriate antibiotics might interrupt or modify the process. Antibiotic treatment of asymptomatic bacteriuria appears to prolong pregnancy (Smaill 2000). A number of studies have been performed using ampicillin or erythromycin in preterm labour with intact membranes and in preterm PROM, both with labour and without. The data from preterm labour with intact membranes is unconvincing to date, although numbers remain small. Systematic reviews (Egarter et al 1996a, 1996b, King & Flenady 2000) have demonstrated no reduction in preterm birth, no prolongation of pregnancy and no reduction in neonatal sepsis, although there have been significant reductions in maternal sepsis and necrotising enterocolitis. However surprisingly, both reviews have shown increased rates of perinatal death (odds ratio just over 3) in the antibiotic-treated group.

The large multicentre ORACLE trial finished recruitment in May 2000 and this should clarify whether antibiotics are of benefit in unselected women with preterm uterine activity and intact membranes. At present there are no grounds for antibiotic use in this group.

Maintenance of tocolysis

It seems logical that tocolysis should be maintained by oral therapy after successful initial parenteral therapy. Only two drugs have been studied to any extent, magnesium and beta-agonists. Only one trial (Ricci et al 1991) has evaluated magnesium against placebo, and no advantage in terms of prolongation of pregnancy or improved outcome was demonstrated. Although oral ritodrine and terbutaline are widely used, there are few trials comparing their effect with placebo.

Table 31.7 Relative efficacy of tocolytic drugs

Drug	Odds ratio delivery	
	Less than 48 h	Less than 7 days
Indomethacin	0.12	0.07
Nifedipine	0.48[a]	
Magnesium	0.52	1.54
Ritodrine	0.56	0.65
Atosiban	0.67	0.59

[a] Estimated from Gyetvai et al (1999) and Oei et al (1999).
Derived from data in Gyetvai et al (1999).

Two recent systematic reviews have examined the effectiveness of prolonged oral tocolysis (Meirowitz et al 1999, Sanchez-Ramos et al 1999), but there were no differences in rates of preterm delivery, recurrent preterm labour, incidence of serious neonatal complications of perinatal mortality. A gain of just over 4 days was found in the treatment group (Sanchez-Ramos et al 1999).

Others have tried systemic therapy with continuous subcutaneous infusion of terbutaline (Guinn et al 1998) but demonstrated only a day's prolongation of gestation.

One group have used aggressive oral therapy, arguing that to achieve adequate oral tocolysis, then therapeutic levels of ritodrine need to be maintained (Holleboom et al 1996b). To achieve this they gave 80 mg of slow release ritodrine three times daily. They did demonstrate clinically important differences in the need for repeat treatment and delivery under 35 weeks' gestation. This approach may be worth further study.

Therapies to improve outcome: improving fetal lung maturity

Corticosteroids

The use of corticosteroids in circumstances where preterm delivery is expected or imminent is of proven value, and is strongly recommended in all such circumstances unless there are specific contraindications.

Mechanism of action. Steroids exert their effect via enhanced production and release of pulmonary surfactant. Surfactant glycerophospholipid and protein synthesis is regulated by a number of factors, including corticosteroids. At the molecular level, glucocorticoids have a complex action on transcription and post-transcriptional modification of surfactant protein A. This protein is closely involved with surfactant proteins B and C in structural change of the lamellar bodies, and in rapid formation of phospholipid surface films. Secretion of phospholipids may be in part regulated by surfactant protein A. The interaction of stimulatory and inhibitory effects are dose-dependent and time-dependent, and effects may differ at differing stages in development (see Mendelson et al 1993). In contrast, surfactant protein B and C expression are stimulated in a dose-dependent manner, which may be an indirect effect, mediated through other messengers.

Glucocorticoids are also implicated in lung morphogenesis, and in phospholipid synthesis itself (Gonzales et al 1986). The dependence of much of the effect of steroids on receptor-mediated gene transcription explains much of the time effect seen with therapy.

Safety. Maternal concerns have centred around pulmonary oedema and infection. Cases of pulmonary oedema have been associated with concomitant tocolytic therapy, rather than therapy with corticosteroids alone. Other side effects of corticosteroids are well documented. Given the short duration of therapy, only gastrointestinal haemorrhage is a potential, serious risk and steroids may be contraindicated where this is an issue.

There are now sufficient data to dispel the fear that, with intact membranes, there is increased maternal infectious morbidity (Crowley 1993). Experimental studies support the lack of effect of these doses of corticosteroids on maternal resistance to infection (Cunningham & Evans 1991).

There also appears to be no increase in neonatal infection following corticosteroid administration. Other concerns around neonatal morbidity have focused on long-term effects, given the reduction in immediate morbidity and mortality demonstrated. Growth and psychomotor development have been studied in cohorts of infants from several of the trials. There is no evidence that these are impaired over 3, 6 or 10–12 years (MacArthur et al 1982, Collaborative Group on Antenatal Steroid Therapy 1984, Howie 1986, Smolders-de-Has et al 1990). Available evidence in fact suggests that steroids protect against neurological abnormality. The single potential long-term adverse outcome reported to date is that of a reduction in the number of boys reaching puberty (Smolder-de-Has et al 1990). Lung growth appears normal.

Administration. Twenty-four milligrams of betamethasone or dexamethasone, or 2 g of hydrocortisone should be administered in 24 hours as divided doses. The most popular regimens are 8 mg 12-hourly or 12 mg 12-hourly.

Contraindications to use include a history of gastrointestinal haemorrhage, overt chorio-amnionitis, and other contraindications to corticosteroid use. Caution is necessary in hypertensive pregnancies and in diabetic pregnancies. Infants of diabetic mothers are more likely to develop hyaline membrane disease and its use should be encouraged in these pregnancies. Diabetic control requires very close supervision to avoid ketoacidosis, and women may have to be managed on regimens akin to those utilised in labour.

For most women, use will be combined with that of tocolysis to delay delivery to allow optimal action of steroids. For others with pregnancy complications requiring elective early delivery, consideration should be given as to whether delivery can be postponed for 24–48 h to allow steroid administration. This will include pregnancies complicated by intrauterine growth restriction, hypertensive disease, allo-immunization and antepartum haemorrhage. Individual clinical judgement is required, but with foresight many of these deliveries can be predicted. Prophylactic steroids are probably not given often enough in such cases.

Efficacy. The efficacy of corticosteroids is not in doubt (Crowley et al 1990, Crowley 1993) and the key results are summarised in Figure 31.3. All groups benefit from therapy and the maximum benefit accrues if delivery occurs between 24 h and 7 days after treatment (odds ratio 0.31). Usage rates of corticosteroids before preterm delivery still vary enormously, but can and perhaps should approach 75–80% (Cooke et al 1993). Active dissemination programmes can lead to more rapid improvements in corticosteroid use (Leviton et al 1999).

Special care is required with prophylactic usage. Delivery should be delayed only until corticosteroid therapy is completed in both intrauterine growth restriction and hypertensive disease. Further delay may be the contributing factor in the increase in intrauterine deaths seen with hypertensive disease in the various trials.

More recently there has been controversy over the use of repeated doses of corticosteroids in high-risk groups. This approach gained popularity as a consequence of data in the

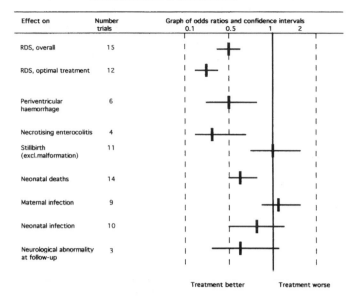

Fig. 31.3 Effects of antenatal corticosteroids.

trials showing that the beneficial effect of steroids was lost after 10 days, coupled with early experimental data showing that further exposure to steroids resulted in further surfactant release. Subsequent experimental work has, however, suggested that repeated exposure may affect lung, tissue and brain growth, although not all studies have shown this. Clinical studies have also been conflicting, and none have been able adequately to control all the relevant variables. The most persuasive clinical study suggesting harm was a secondary analysis of one of the thyroid-releasing hormone (TRH) trials (Banks et al 1999) where most variables are controlled. In one of the largest retrospective studies (Elimian et al 2000), not only was no harm demonstrated but there was a substantial reduction in respiratory distress syndrome with repeated doses of steroids.

At present attempts are being made to mount a large trial. It is hoped that better identification of women admitted in suspected preterm labour will reduce unnecessary use of courses of steroids and thus repeat courses. Attention should be given to the possible effect on single course use when considering any current change in clinical practice.

Antenatal administration of a single course of corticosteroids is the most effective perinatal intervention currently available to obstetricians. Attempts should be made to administer the drug to all eligible women.

Thyroid-releasing hormone

The finding that both T_4 and T_3 stimulate production of phosphatidylcholine in human lung explants (Gross et al 1980), with T_4 enhancing choline incorporation and the possibility that the effect on phospholipid production might be synergistic with that of steroids if given together (Gonzales et al 1986), led to exploration of the use of thyroid hormone during pregnancy to further improve outcome. As the placenta is relatively impermeable to thyroid hormone, clinical studies have utilised either intra-amniotic injection of thyroid hormone or intravenous injection of maternal thyroid-releasing hormone (TRH) in doses between 200 and 400 µg, 8–12 h apart, for 4–6 doses.

Early trials were encouraging, but the large ACTOBAT trial (Australian Collaborative Trial of Antenatal Thyrotrophin-releasing Hormone 1995) showed no added benefit. The trial was criticised for using a lower dose of TRH, and three other large trials were started in the USA, South America and Europe to evaluate the higher dose regimen. The reports of the first two studies (Ballard et al 1998, Collaborative Santiago Surfactant Group 1998) with over 1300 pregnancies showed no additional benefit, and subsequently the third trial was stopped (Alfirevic et al 1999). Later information on long-term follow-up from the ACTOBAT trial (Crowther et al 1997) has raised concerns about developmental milestones and, as a result of the accumulative data, TRH is not thought to be of value.

Therapies to improve outcome: prevention of intraventricular haemorrhage

Corticosteroids themselves have an effect in reducing rates of periventricular haemorrhage (Fig. 31.3). As most severe haemorrhage occurs shortly after birth, other strategies have been considered in an attempt to reduce this serious morbidity.

Antenatal vitamin K and phenobarbitone

Phenobarbitone can reduce mean arterial blood pressure peaks in preterm infants. Dramatic changes in blood pressure and cerebral blood flow have been implicated in the genesis of intraventricular haemorrhage. Vitamin K reduces haemorrhagic disease of the newborn, and maternal administration results in therapeutic cord levels. Both were therefore possible prophylactic therapies to reduce the incidence of periventricular haemorrhage.

Initial small trials in both were encouraging; however, the large trial of Thorpe and colleagues (Thorpe et al 1994), using both in a well-designed study, demonstrated only a small and not statistically significant reduction in both total intraventricular haemorrhage and in severe bleeding. More recently a very large trial of phenobarbitone with good follow-up did not demonstrate any differences in either grade 3 or 4 intracranial haemorrhage or periventricular leucomalacia (Shankaran et al 1997).

It would appear that neither treatment confers additional benefit and it may be that the increasing use of steroids and artificial surfactant has rendered these possible beneficial therapies obsolete.

Intrapartum monitoring of the preterm fetus

Once labour is established and it is decided to allow labour to progress, issues regarding intrapartum monitoring of the preterm fetus must be addressed. There are three issues: namely, who should be monitored, which form of monitoring should be used, and how should monitoring be interpreted?

There is strong evidence that metabolic acidaemia in the preterm fetus has a closer relationship with poor neurodevelopmental outcome than in the term fetus (Low et al 1981, Mires et al 1991, Gaudier et al 1992). Hypoxia and acidosis can affect lecithin production and surfactant formation. It is therefore vital that intrapartum asphyxia be avoided to improve outcome.

The issues around who should be monitored are contentious. Monitoring should be considered in any case where abnormalities of monitoring would result in action. This requires judgement on viability and ultimate prognosis, as well as the potential risks of operative intervention, including classical caesarean section, on the mother. Close collaboration with paediatric colleagues is essential, with reference to published and local survival and handicap figures.

At gestations of 26 weeks and above, all labours should be monitored, unless there is good evidence of severe growth restriction with an estimated weight less than 500 g.

For a normally grown fetus at 26 weeks, current intact survival rates are over 50%. Given increasing survival even at gestations below 26 weeks, many obstetricians now monitor all labours at or above 24 weeks' gestation. However, there is a significant handicap rate at these gestations (25% severe and 25% mild or moderate) and parents need to be involved in discussions. At gestations below 22 weeks there is little realistic chance of survival at present, and monitoring should rarely be considered. Survival rates at 23–24 weeks are improving, although handicap rates are high, and at present decisions should be on an individual basis. All these issues should be discussed with midwifery and neonatal paediatric colleagues initially, and then with the parents, before reaching a joint decision. Difficulties in interpreting monitoring at this gestation should form part of the discussion.

Issues around the method of monitoring to be used follow the same pattern as for term fetuses (Neilson & Grant 1993). There remains scanty evidence to support widespread use of continuous electronic fetal heart rate monitoring in normal labours. In the preterm fetus the issue has been addressed by Luthy and colleagues (Luthy et al 1987, Shy et al 1990) in a randomised trial. They did not demonstrate any benefit of electronic fetal heart rate monitoring either in immediate neonatal outcome (Apgar scores, acidaemia, intracranial haemorrhage) or in neurological development. For uncomplicated preterm labours, it may therefore be appropriate to monitor using structured intermittent auscultation.

If continuous electronic fetal heart rate monitoring is used to monitor the preterm fetus, then it must be appreciated that cardiovascular physiology in the preterm fetus differs from that at term (Natale et al 1984). It is not appropriate to interpret findings as for a term fetus. Variable decelerations are extremely common, 55–75% (Ingemarrson et al 1980, Zanini et al 1980), and there is a poor correlation with pH. Variable decelerations with a late component, and those with an overshoot, seem most associated with acidosis. Tachycardia and reduced baseline variability are commonly seen in acidaemia (Westgren et al 1982), although the relationship for reduced variability has been challenged (Mires et al 1993). Late decelerations are ominous (Westgren et al 1982, Mires et al 1993). Follow-up of preterm infants with ominous continuous electronic fetal heart rate monitoring

has shown a relationship with neurodevelopmental outcome, especially in the very preterm (Westgren et al 1986).

Interpretation of continuous electronic fetal heart rate monitoring is complex in the preterm, and such records need to be examined by appropriately trained medical staff who understand the complexities of the physiology of the preterm fetus. This should allow both better recognition of ominous records and prevention of unnecessary intervention based on term criteria.

Delivery of the preterm fetus

The preterm fetus should be delivered in a unit where appropriate neonatal care can be provided. Earlier evidence (Paneth et al 1987) that neonatal outcome is better in central units has been given support by recent comparisons of different-sized neonatal units (International Neonatal Network 1993), strongly suggesting better outcome, especially in the very preterm, in the largest units.

The ideal mode of delivery will vary, dependent on the indication for delivery. For complicated pregnancies where delivery is deliberately preterm on maternal or fetal grounds, there may be cogent reasons for recourse to caesarean section. For the majority of preterm births, however, there are few data to support liberal use of abdominal delivery. Mode of delivery correlates poorly with outcome (Kitchen et al 1985). Analysis of long-term neonatal outcome in inborn infants delivering in Liverpool over the last decade shows no relationship between mode of delivery and outcome. Barely 100 women have been recruited into randomised trials (Grant 1993) of elective versus selective caesarean section, and no conclusion can be drawn from this data.

For cephalic presentations with preterm labour or preterm PROM, vaginal delivery is the preferred option. Oxytocin may be used (as in preterm PROM) but with great caution. Both prolonged labour and precipitate labour are risk factors for intracranial haemorrhage. Analgesia should be adequate. There is no necessity for routine use of epidural analgesia, although there is some evidence that outcome is better than if opiate analgesia is used. There is no evidence that forceps delivery, applied routinely, confers any fetal advantage, and as it confers maternal detriment, its use should be abandoned. All texts suggest liberal use of generous episiotomy to prevent sudden decompression of the head of the preterm infant, although the evidence for such a policy is flimsy (Lobb & Cooke 1986).

Delivery of the preterm breech generates as much controversy as for term breech delivery. There are no adequate trials, and retrospective, prospective and cohort studies are plagued with selection bias (see Keirse 1989), making rational decision-making virtually impossible. At gestations under 26 weeks, there is unlikely to be a benefit from caesarean section. Above this, the majority of breech presentations between 26 and 32 weeks' gestation presenting in labour are delivered by caesarean section. A number of randomised trials have failed to recruit adequate numbers, and it seems unlikely that a definitive answer to the best mode of delivery will be found.

Caesarean section of the preterm uterus is not necessarily

an easy option, and should not be seen as a way of avoiding trauma. A poorly formed lower segment in the very preterm may make classical caesarean section, low vertical incision, J and T incisions, and trauma likely. Delivery of a fragile preterm infant through a small low transverse uterine scar in a thick lower segment is likely to be as traumatic as a well-conducted normal or vaginal breech delivery.

Summary

The key to successful management is a well-structured and comprehensive set of guidelines dealing with diagnosis, therapy and delivery, with early and close involvement of senior staff. Neonatal mortalities of 2 or less per 1000 are achievable with this closely linked and comprehensive perinatal approach.

KEY POINTS: MANAGEMENT

- There is almost no contraindication to antenatal corticosteroids.
- Short-term tocolysis should be employed unless clear contraindication.
- Choice of tocolysis is complex, but increasingly beta-mimetics seem the least preferred option.
- Indomethacin is the most effective tocolytic, but there remains concern over fetal safety.
- Mode of delivery should be vaginal unless there are other obstetric considerations which influence type of delivery.
- Continuous electronic fetal monitoring is recommended, but given the difficulties in interpretation, decisions on intervention should be taken at senior level.
- Families should have continuous support from an experienced midwife.
- Paediatric staff should be involved in discussion with parents as early as possible.
- All medical staff should have agreed outcome statistics, based on published, regional and local data.

PRETERM PREMATURE RUPTURE OF THE MEMBRANES

Many of the factors and management decisions discussed for preterm labour are relevant for preterm PROM, but some issues differ.

Aetiology and risk factors

Many of the risk factors described earlier apply equally to preterm PROM. In particular, previous preterm delivery (odds ratio 2.8), early pregnancy bleeding (odds ratio 2.4 for first-trimester bleeding, odds ratio 4.4 for second-trimester bleeding) and cigarette smoking (odds ratio 2.1) emerge as important variables in women subsequently presenting with preterm PROM (Harger et al 1990).

The mechanism by which bleeding in the first half of pregnancy predisposes to preterm PROM is unclear but could include ascending infection or disruption of nutritional support to part of the membranes. The data on smoking are controversial but consistent (Meyer & Tonascia 1977) and the mechanism may be mediated through damage to decidual blood vessels.

The aetiology may vary with gestation. The primary aetiological mechanism is again infection, as outlined in Figure 31.1. Where organisms have been sought from amniotic fluid, positive cultures have been found in about one-third (Carroll et al 1996). *Chlamydia trachomatis* has been implicated (Gravett et al 1986), as has group B streptococcus (Alger et al 1988). Interest is now focused on the role of apparently less-pathogenic organisms, such as those involved in bacterial vaginosis (Gravett et al 1986, McDonald et al 1991).

Organisms may stimulate membrane peroxidase systems, releasing free radicals, which may cause local tissue necrosis or cleave peptide collagen bonds. Local necrosis may also arise via the effect of the secretion of bacterial phospholipases on cytokine production, particularly thromboxane and the leukotrienes. Collagen types III and V may play a central role. In addition, there may be destabilisation of lysosomal membranes which could result in deactivation of IgA and IgG with reduced volume of mucus (Gomez et al 1997, Polzin & Brady 1998).

Management issues in preterm PROM

There are a number of complex issues to be dealt with in the management of preterm PROM, as outlined in Table 31.8. The argument between expectant versus interventional management is driven by fear of serious maternal morbidity and poor survival rates in early preterm PROM. Loss rates are clearly linked to gestation at delivery rather than infection (Newton et al 1987). For pregnancies where labour does not ensue rapidly after rupture of the membranes, the risk of infection has been overstated (Kappy et al 1979). In the absence of clear evidence of infection, most clinicians now advocate an expectant approach up to 36 weeks. One area where this may be challenged is where group B streptococcus is isolated. The effectiveness of intrapartum antibiotics may be reduced if expectant management is pursued (Newton et al 1987).

Maternal risks

Infection is the major risk, with chorio-amnionitis complicating up to 25% of cases. Serious maternal infection is rare, perhaps up to 2%, but should not be underestimated. Both maternal death and postpartum hysterectomy secondary to sepsis have been reported. In 60 consecutive cases of preterm

Table 31.8 Issues in preterm PROM

Viability
Maternal infection
Antibiotics
Tocolysis
Use of corticosteroids
Antenatal fetal monitoring
Home or hospital monitoring

PROM under 22 weeks managed in Liverpool, two women had sepsis severe enough to warrant treatment in an intensive care unit. Postnatal sepsis is also common, affecting 10% of cases. Placental abruption is also said to be more common after preterm PROM, although some studies have disputed this. Digital vaginal examination may contribute to infection (Lewis et al 1991), although the data are not strong.

Monitoring for developing sepsis relies on conventional clinical surveillance, and the presence of symptomatic infection is an absolute indication for delivery. C-reactive protein estimates seem the most reliable monitoring tool (Fisk 1988), although cut-off values need to be modified for pregnancy. Persistent levels above 20 mg/l or single estimates above 30–40 mg/l are highly suggestive of infection. In more detailed studies both CRP and white cell count were poor predictors of the presence of a positive amniotic fluid or fetal blood culture (Carroll et al 1996).

Preterm PROM at less than 24 weeks' gestation

The question of viability arises when preterm PROM occurs early. Survival is related both to the gestation at membrane rupture and to the gestation at delivery (Carroll et al 1995). The risk of chorio-amnionitis is high, and the risk of pulmonary hypoplasia can exceed 50% at very early gestations (Rotschild et al 1990). There is good evidence that the development of pulmonary hypoplasia is dependent on the gestation of membrane rupture rather than duration (Rotschild et al 1990). Prediction is difficult, but nomograms of chest circumference or lung length (Roberts & Mitchell 1990) may help. Where preterm PROM occurs at less than 26 weeks' gestation, 30–50% will gain 1 week of more gestation, with one-quarter gaining 4 weeks' gestation (Bartfield & Carlan 1998).

Where preterm PROM occurs at less than 24 weeks, then parents should be advised of the likely poor outcome, of the small risk of serious infection for themselves, and of how the pregnancy will be monitored. In the study of Taylor & Garite (1984) with a mean gestational age at preterm PROM of 23 weeks, only 10% of pregnancies produced a neurologically normal long-term survivor. More recent studies (Carroll et al 1995) have shown better survival, and our own prospective data where membrane rupture occurs before 22 weeks shows survival in 25%, with intact survival of 20%. Parents should have an option, particularly where membrane rupture occurs at less than 20 weeks, of terminating the pregnancy.

Antenatal corticosteroids are not indicated before 24 weeks in these cases. The role of antibiotics is considered below, but should probably be limited to treating specifically identified organisms such as beta-haemolytic streptococcus or chlamydia.

No therapy is currently available to replace or maintain successfully amniotic fluid in these circumstances, although some interesting approaches to plugging the cervix are under investigation (Quintero et al 1999). Spontaneous resealing of the membranes is described in around 4% of cases, and it is more likely in earlier gestations (Mercer et al 1992).

Preterm PROM between 24 and 34 weeks' gestation

Around 70–80% of these pregnancies will deliver within 1 week, half within 4 days (Bartfield & Carlan 1998). At this stage viability is possible with delivery but in the absence of infection or evidence of fetal distress, delaying delivery is the management choice. The role of amniocentesis is uncertain, although it may be valuable where there is equivocal evidence of infection, such as a mild pyrexia or elevated CRP. As discussed previously, Gram staining of the liquor is the best option (Carroll et al 1996).

The use of parenteral tocolysis in women with preterm PROM in established or suspected labour is controversial. There is little doubt that in the presence of ruptured membranes, tocolysis is less effective. Few randomized trials have specifically addressed the issue of prolongation of pregnancy in this group. The trials of Christensen (Christensen et al 1980) and Weiner (Weiner et al 1988) did suggest some short-term gains akin to those seen in overviews of tocolytic therapy, but no improvement in outcome. Steroids were not used in either trial. If considering tocolysis in these circumstances, then infection needs to be excluded, and this may be another group where amniocentesis may be helpful.

Evidence now favours the use of steroids in preterm PROM (Crowley 1993). In an analysis of 11 trials, there was a reduction in respiratory distress syndrome of the same order of magnitude as demonstrated for all infants (odds ratio 0.5, 95% CI 0.38–0.66) without any significant increase in neonatal infection. After much debate the American College of Obstetricians and Gynaecologists recommended its use in 1995. Its value has been confirmed in prospective studies (Elimian et al 1999). Recently a moderate-sized randomised trial in women with preterm PROM has confirmed the clinical benefits in terms of reduced perinatal mortality (Pattinson et al 1999). Maternal leucocyte counts will rise in response to steroid administration, and C-reactive protein estimates are helpful in determining if the rise is infectious in origin.

If labour does not occur, then fetal and maternal monitoring will be instituted. The non-stress test alone may be helpful, with high sensitivity for chorio-amnionitis and neonatal sepsis (Vintzileos et al 1986a), although the false-positive rate remains around 40%. Amniotic fluid volume itself has been proposed as a predictor (Gonick et al 1985, Vintzileos et al 1985), with maximum pools less than 1 cm being associated with increased infection rates. It is not as sensitive or specific as the non-stress test, but may be useful.

A number of biophysical parameters have been used to predict infection. Fetal breathing activity is reduced after preterm PROM (Roberts et al 1991a) and a number of groups have documented an association between reduced breathing and subsequent sepsis (Vintzileos et al 1986b, Goldstein et al 1988); however, although very sensitive, false-positive rates are 50%. Fetal movement, total fetal activity and fetal biophysical profile scoring show similar predictive abilities (Roberts et al 1991b), with sensitivities in excess of 90%, negative predictive values around 95% but with false-positive rates of 25–40%. The very detailed studies of Carroll and colleagues with both amniotic fluid and fetal blood parameters highlight the poor predictive value of all non-invasive surveillance (see Carroll et al 1995b). Given current information, the most appropriate monitoring appears to be frequent ultrasound assessment of fetal activity and breathing, with amniocentesis reserved for exclusion of false-positive non-invasive results. None of these strategies have been subjected to an appropriate trial.

Whether such intensive monitoring should be hospital based is also open to debate. The only trial of hospital versus home (Carlan 1993), although small, demonstrated no differences. Subsequent small observational studies have supported the view that home or outpatient monitoring may increase latency periods. It has been suggested that if all monitoring has been normal for 72 h, the woman lives close to the hospital, and has reliable transport and communication links, then outpatient monitoring should be considered (Bartfield & Carlan 1998).

Preterm PROM between 34 and 36 weeks' gestation

Technically such pregnancies are preterm PROM, although survival is expected. There are no good data to guide management, and individual hospitals have developed their own guidelines, often based on local audit. Given the evidence from the Term PROM trial (Hannah et al 1996) that conservative management is safe for up to 4 days, it seems illogical to prolong pregnancies above 34 weeks' gestation for longer than this. Active steps to promote delivery may be justified at 36 weeks.

Antibiotics

The use of antibiotics in preterm PROM is currently unresolved, although the multicentre ORACLE trial finished recruitment in 2000. Many groups advocate routine use of antibiotics, although regimens vary. A systematic review in 1996 (Egarter et al 1996a, 1996b) suggested a significant reduction in neonatal sepsis and intraventricular haemorrhage. A subsequent detailed review (Mercer & Lewis 1997) examined all aspects of antibiotic therapy in preterm PROM. There was a significant increase in pregnancies undelivered at 7 days, but the mean prolongation in days was small, and they estimated that only 15% of pregnancies would benefit from such intervention. They found a small but not significant reduction in postpartum endometritis. Significant reductions in neonatal sepsis and intraventricular haemorrhage were confirmed, although overall perinatal mortality was not reduced. The most recent Cochrane review (Kenyon & Boulvain 2000) confirms a significant reduction in delivery at 48 h and 7 days, chorio-amnionitis, postpartum maternal infection, neonatal sepsis, and need for ventilation at 28 days. Despite these advantages, no reduction in perinatal death can be demonstrated. The failure to improve outcome given these data is puzzling, but may be due to failure to utilise corticosteroids; ruptured membranes and the fear of infection are frequently cited as contraindications for their use. It may, however, reflect masking of infection with associated poor outcome balancing the gains of prolongation of gestation.

In summary, most women with preterm PROM will progress to preterm labour within 48 h, and their management is not different from those admitted in preterm labour. For the smaller group of women who do not labour, expec-

tant management with surveillance of both mother and fetus for evidence of sepsis is appropriate. Strategies for both are empirical, as no trials have been conducted. Intervention should occur only if there is evidence of clinical maternal infection or evidence of fetal infection, preferably based on invasive testing of amniotic fluid rather than on non-invasive ultrasound tests with high false-positive rates. For women with very early preterm PROM, full information on outcome should be available, and discussion of termination should be considered.

KEY POINTS: PRETERM PROM

- Outcome in early preterm PROM is related to gestation at membrane rupture and gestation at delivery.
- Where preterm PROM occurs at less than 24 weeks, termination of pregnancy is a controversial option.
- Most women will labour within 4–7 days
- Antenatal corticosteroids should be used unless clinical infection.
- Tocolysis can be used, but infection must be excluded, preferably by amniocentesis.
- There is increasing evidence that antibiotic therapy can delay delivery and reduce infective morbidity.
- Where delivery does not occur within 4 days:
  - fetal surveillance using ultrasound and/or cardiotocography has a high negative predictive value
  - all fetal monitoring tests have a poor positive predictive value
  - amniocentesis should be used more often as back up to non-invasive monitoring
  - the issue of inpatient versus outpatient surveillance is not resolved
  - there is no consensus on timing of elective delivery.
- Where preterm PROM occurs at 34–36 weeks' gestation, delivery should occur as for term PROM.

PARENTS

It is important to involve parents at every stage of the management of preterm labour and delivery. The woman will require skilled midwifery and medical support, not least because most parent education does not commence until the third trimester. For women in their first ongoing pregnancy (especially given the sociodemographic associations of preterm delivery), labour itself, and operative delivery especially, are ordeals suddenly thrust upon them. Family support is vital and there should be no restrictions placed on companionship in labour in these circumstances.

Careful attention should be focused on explaining what tests will be performed, what drugs will be used and their effects, how the baby will be monitored, and what the expectations might be. All involved in such care should be aware of local survival rates by weight and gestation, and early involvement of neonatal paediatric colleagues is to be encouraged. Where possible, the parents should visit the neonatal unit before delivery, and if elective preterm delivery is contemplated, the entire family should visit.

Postnatally, midwifery and medical staff need to be aware of the different potential reactions. Parents may react to the separation from their baby by infrequent visiting. There may be distress following a visit to the neonatal unit, with the baby attached to complex equipment and often not looking like a proper baby. The daunting difficulties in maintaining breast milk production under these circumstances should not be underestimated.

Neonatal intensive care units often have well-developed support systems for parents and other family members, but it is important that the obstetric and midwifery team remain involved and interested.

Follow-up is important, both from the point of view of continuing support for the family, but also to discuss the reasons for preterm delivery and to discuss the management of future pregnancies.

REFERENCES

Agustsson P, Patel N 1987 The predictive value of fetal breathing movements in the diagnosis of preterm labour. Br J Obstet Gynaecol 94:860–863

Alfirevic Z, Boer K, Brocklehurst P et al 1999 Two trials of antenatal thyrotrophin-releasing hormone for fetal maturation: stopping before the due date. Antenatal TRH trial and the thyroneth trial groups. Br J Obstet Gynaecol 106:898–906

Alger LS, Lovchik JC, Habel JR et al 1988 The association of Chlamydia trachomatis, Neisseria gonorrhoeae, and group B streptococci with preterm premature rupture of the membranes and pregnancy outcome. Am J Obstet Gynecol 159:397–404

Altura BM, Altura BT, Carella A et al 1987 Mg^{2+}–Ca^{2+} interacts in contractility of smooth muscle: magnesium versus organic calcium channel blockers on myogenic tone and agonist-induced responsiveness of blood vessels. Can J Physiol Pharmacol 65:729–745

Ancel PY, Saurel-Cubizolles MJ, Di Renzo GC, Papiernik E, Breart G 1999 Very and moderate preterm births: are the risk factors different? Br J Obstet Gynaecol 106:1162–1170

Andersen LF, Lyndrup J, Akerlund M, Melin P 1989 Oxytocin receptor blockade: a new principle in the treatment of preterm labour? Am J Perinatol 6:196–199

Anderson A 1977 Preterm labour: definition. In: Anderson A (ed) Proceedings of the fifth study group of the Royal College of Obstetricians and Gynaecologists. RCOG, London

Anderson HF 1991 Transvaginal and transabdominal ultrasonography of the uterine cervix during pregnancy. J Clin Ultrasound 19:77–81

Anderson HF, Nugent CE, Wanty SD, Hayashi RH 1990 Prediction for risk of preterm delivery by ultrasonographic measurement of cervical length. Am J Obstet Gynecol 163:859–867

Australian Collaborative Trial of Antenatal Thyrotrophin-releasing Hormone (ACTOBAT) for prevention of neonatal respiratory disease 1995 Lancet 345:877–882

Baerts W, Fetter WF, Hop WJ et al 1990 Cerebral lesions in preterm infants after tocolytic indomethacin. Dev Med Child Neurol 32:910–918

Bakketeig LS, Hoffman HJ 1981 Epidemiology of preterm birth: results from a longitudinal study of births in Norway. In: Elder MG, Hendricks CH (eds) Preterm labour. Butterworth, London, pp 17–46

Ballard RA, Ballard PL, Cnaan A et al 1998 Antenatal thyrotropin-releasing hormone to prevent lung disease in preterm infants. North American thyrotropin-releasing hormone study group. N Engl J Med 338:493–498

Banks CA, Cnaan A, Morgan MA et al 1999 North American thyrotrophin-releasing hormone study group. Multiple course of

antenatal corticosteroids and outcome of premature neonates. Am J Obstet Gynecol 181:709–717

Barros FC, Huttly SRA, Victoria CG et al 1992 Comparison of the causes and consequences of prematurity and intrauterine growth retardation: a longitudinal study in Southern Brazil. Pediatrics 90:238–244

Bartfield MC, Carlan SJ 1998 The home management of preterm premature ruptured membranes. Clin Obstet Gynecol 41:503–514

Bartnicki J, Casal D, Kreaden US, Saling E, Vetter K 1996 Fetal fibronectin in vaginal specimens predicts preterm delivery and very-low-birth-weight infants. Am J Obstet Gynecol 174:971–974

Bejar R, Curbelo V, Davis C, Gluck L 1981 Premature labour. Bacterial sources of phospholipase. Obstet Gynecol 57:479–482

Benedetti TJ 1983 Maternal complications of parenteral betasympathomimetic therapy for premature labour. Am J Obstet Gynecol 145:1–6

Berghella V, Tolosa JE, Kuhlman K, Weiner S, Bolognese RJ, Wapner RJ 1997 Cervical ultrasonography compared with manual examination as a predictor of preterm delivery. Am J Obstet Gynecol 177:723–730

Berghella V, Daly SF, Tolosa JE et al 1999 Prediction of preterm delivery with transvaginal ultrasonography of the cervix in patients with high risk pregnancies: does cerclage prevent prematurity. Am J Obstet Gynecol 181:809–815

Berkowitz GS, Kelsey JL, Holford TR et al 1982 Physical activity and the risk of spontaneous preterm labour. J Reprod Med 28:581–585

Bernstein PS, Stern R, Lin N et al 1998 Beta-human chorionic gonadotropin in cervicovaginal secretions as a predictor of preterm delivery. Am J Obstet Gynecol 179:870–873

Blondel B, Le Coutour X, Kaminski M et al 1990 Prediction of preterm delivery: is it substantially improved by routine vaginal examination? Am J Obstet Gynecol 162:1042–1048

Boer K, Samlal RAK, Smit BJ, Kreijenbroek ME, Hogerzeil HV 1993 Twenty years' drug policy in obstetric care in Amsterdam. In: Koppe JG, Eskes TKAB, van Geijn HP, Weisenhann PF, Ruys JH (eds) Care, concern and cure in perinatal medicine. Parthenon Press, Carnforth, Lancashire, pp 221–231

Brocklehurst P, Hannah M, McDonald H 2000 Interventions for treating bacterial vaginosis in pregnancy (Cochrane review) In: The Cochrane library, issue 1. Update Software, Oxford

Brown HL, Britton KA, Brizendine EJ et al 1999 A randomized comparison of home uterine activity monitoring in the outpatient management of women treated for preterm labor. Am J Obstet Gynecol 180:798–805

Canadian Preterm Labour Investigators Group 1992 Treatment of preterm labour with beta-adrenergic agonist ritodrine. N Engl J Med 327:308–312

Carey JC, Klebanoff MA, Hauth JC et al 2000 Metronidazole to prevent preterm delivery in pregnant women with asymptomatic bacterial vaginosis. National institute of child health and human development network of maternal–fetal medicine units. N Engl J Med 342:534–540

Carlan ST 1993 Home versus hospital monitoring for preterm premature rupture of the membranes. Obstet Gynecol 81:61–64

Carroll SG, Blott M, Nicolaides KH 1995a Preterm prelabor amniorrhexis: outcome of live births. Obstet Gynecol 86:18–25

Carroll SG, Papaioannou S, Davies ET, Nicolaides KH 1995b Maternal assessment in the prediction of intrauterine infection in preterm prelabor amniorrhexis. Fetal Diagn Ther 10:290–296

Carroll SG, Philpott-Howard J, Nicolaides KH 1996 Amniotic fluid gram stain and leukocyte count in the prediction of intrauterine infection in preterm prelabour amniorrhexis. Fetal Diagn Ther 11:1–5

Casey ML, Cox SM, Beutler B, Milewich L, McDonald PC 1989 Cachectin/tumour necrosis factor-alpha formation in human decidua. Potential role of cytokines in infection-induced preterm labour. J Clin Invest 83:430–436

Christensen KK, Ingemarsson I, Leideman T et al 1980 Effect of ritodrine on labour after premature rupture of the membranes. Obstet Gynecol 55:187–190

Chuileannian FN, Bell R, Brennecke S 1998 Cervicovaginal fetal fibronectin testing in threatened preterm labour: translating research findings into clinical practice. Aust NZ J Obstet Gynaecol 38:399–402

Cnattingius S, Granath F, Petersson G, Harlow BL 1999 The influence of gestational age and smoking habits on the risk of subsequent preterm deliveries. N Engl J Med 341:943–948

Collaborative Group on Antenatal Steroid Therapy 1984 Effects of antenatal dexamethasone administration in the infant: long-term follow up. J Pediatr 104:259–267

Collaborative Group on Preterm Birth Prevention 1993 Multicentre randomised, controlled trial of a preterm birth prevention program. Am J Obstet and Gynecol 169:352–366

Collaborative Home Uterine Monitoring Study (CHUMS) Group 1995 A multicenter randomized controlled trial of home uterine monitoring: active versus sham device. Am J Obstet Gynecol 173:1120–1127

Collaborative Santiago Surfactant Group 1998 Collaborative trial of prenatal thyrotropin-releasing hormone and corticosteroids for prevention of respiratory distress syndrome. Am J Obstet Gynecol 178:33–39

Colton T, Kayne HL, Zhang Y, Heeren T 1995 A metaanalysis of home uterine activity monitoring. Am J Obstet Gynecol 173:1499–1505

Cooke RWI 1992 Annual audit of neonatal morbidity in preterm infants. Arch Dis Child 67:1174–1176

Cooke RWI, Walkinshaw SA, Ryan S 1993 Steroids for babies. Lancet 341:569

Copper RL, Goldenberg RL, Das A et al 1996 The preterm prediction study: maternal stress is associated with spontaneous preterm birth at less than thirty-five weeks' gestation. National institute of child health and human development maternal–fetal medicine units network. Am J Obstet Gynecol 175:1286–1292

Cox S, Wilow MI, Leveno KJ 1988 The natural history of preterm rupture of the membranes: what to expect of expectant management. Obstet Gynecol 71:558

Creasy RK, Gummer BA, Liggins GC 1980 A system for predicting spontaneous preterm birth. Obstet Gynecol 55:692–695

Crowley P 1993 Corticosteroids after preterm prelabour rupture of the membranes. In: Enkin M, Keirse MJNC, Renfrew M, Neilson JP (eds) Pregnancy and childbirth module. Cochrane database of systematic reviews (review no. 04395 vol disk issue 2). Update Software, Oxford

Crowley PA 1995 Antenatal corticosteroid therapy: a meta-analysis of the randomized trials, 1972 to 1994. Am J Obstet Gynecol 173:322–335

Crowley P, Chalmers I, Keirse MJNC 1990 The effects of corticosteroid administration before preterm delivery: a review of the evidence from controlled trials. British Journal of Obstetrics and Gynaecology 97:11–25

Crowther CA, Hiller JE, Haslam RR, Robinson JS 1997 Australian collaborative trial of antenatal thyrotropin-releasing hormone: adverse effects at 12-month follow-up. ACTOBAT Study Group. Pediatrics 99:311–317

Cunningham DS, Evans EE 1991 The effects of betamethasone on maternal cellular resistance to infection. Am J Obstet Gynecol 165:610–615

Deter RL, Rossavik IK, Harrist RB, Hadlock FP 1986 Mathematical modelling of fetal growth: development of individual growth curve standards. Obstetrics and Gynecology 68:156–161

Dudley DJ, Trautman MS, Edwin SS et al 1992 Biosynthesis of interleukin-6 by cultured human chorion laeve cells: regulation by cytokines. J Clin Endocrinol Metab 75:1081–1086

Duggan DE, Hoggans AF, Kwan KC et al 1972 The metabolism of indomethacin in man. J Pharmacol Exp Ther 181:563–569

Dunlow SG, Duff P 1990 Microbiology of the lower genital tract and amniotic fluid in asymptomatic preterm patients with intact membranes and moderate to advanced degrees of cervical effacement and dilatation. Am J Perinatol 7: 235–238

Dyson DC, Danbe KH, Bamber JA et al 1998 Monitoring women at risk for preterm labor. N Engl J Med 338:15–19

Egarter C, Leitich H, Husslein P, Kaider A, Schemper M 1996 Adjunctive antibiotic treatment in preterm labor and neonatal morbidity: a meta-analysis. Obstet Gynecol 88:303–309

Egarter C, Leitich H, Karas H et al 1996 Antibiotic treatment in premature rupture of membranes and neonatal morbidity: a meta-analysis. Am J Obstet Gynecol 174:589–597

Egley CC, Katz VL, Herbert WNP 1988 Leukocyte esterase: a simple bedside test for the detection of bacterial colonisation of amniotic fluid. Am J Obstet Gynecol 159:120–122

Elimian A, Figuerosa R, Canterino J, Verma U, Aguero-Rosenfield M, Tejani N 1998 Amniotic fluid complement C3 as a marker of intra-amniotic infection. Obstet Gynecol 92:72–76

Elimian A, Verma U, Canterino J, Shah J, Visintainer P, Tejani N 1999 Effectiveness of antenatal steroids in obstetric subgroups. Obstet Gynecol 93:174–179

Elimian A, Verma U, Visintainer P, Tejani N 2000 Effectiveness of multidose antenatal steroids. Obstet Gynecol 95:34–36

Elliot JP 1983 Magnesium sulfate as a tocolytic agent. Am J Obstet Gynecol 147:277–284

Faron G, Boulvain M, Irion O, Bernard PM, Fraser WD 1998 Prediction of preterm delivery by fetal fibronectin: a meta-analysis. Obstet Gynecol 92:153–158

Ferguson JEI, Schutz T, Pershe R, Stevenson DK, Blaschke T 1989 Nifedipine pharmacokinetics during preterm labor tocolysis. Am J Obstet Gynecol 161:1485–1490

Fisk NM 1988 Modification to selective conservative management in preterm premature rupture of the membranes. Obstet Gynecol Surv 43:328–334

Friedman ML, McElin TW 1969 Diagnosis of fetal ruptured membranes: clinical study and review of the literature. Am J Obstet Gynecol 104:544–550

Garn SM, Shaw HA, McCabe KD 1977 Effects of socioeconomic status and race on weight defined and gestational prematurity in the United States. In: Reed DM, Stanley FJ (eds) The epidemiology of prematurity. Urban and Schwartzenburg, Baltimore, p 127

Garrioch DB 1978 The effect of indomethacin on spontaneous activity in the isolated human myometrium and on the response to oxytocin and prostaglandin. Br J Obstet Gynaecol 85:47–52

Garry D, Figueroa R, Aguero-Rosenfeld M, Martinez E, Visintainer P, Tejani N 1996 A comparison of rapid amniotic fluid markers in the prediction of microbial invasion of the uterine cavity and preterm delivery. Am J Obstet Gynecol 175:1336–1341

Gaudier FL, Goldenberg RL, Peralta M et al 1992 Prediction of long term neurologic handicap in very low birth weight infants. Am J Obstet Gynecol 166:419

Gibbs RS, Blanco JD 1982 Premature rupture of the membranes. Obstet Gynecol 60:671–679

Goldenberg RL, Rouse DJ 1998 Prevention of preterm birth. N Engl J Med 339: 313–320

Goldenberg RL, Davis RO, Cooper RL et al 1990 The Alabama preterm birth prevention project. Obstet Gynecol 75:933–939

Goldenberg RL, Thom E, Moawad AH, Johnson F, Roberts J, Caritis SN 1996a The preterm prediction study: fetal fibronectin, bacterial vaginosis, and peripartum infection. NICHD maternal fetal medicine units network. Obstet Gynecol 87:656–660

Goldenberg RL, Goldenberg RL, Mercer BM et al 1996b The preterm prediction study: fetal fibronectin testing and spontaneous preterm birth. NICHD maternal fetal medicine units network. Obstet Gynecol 87:643–648

Goldenberg RL, Mercer BM, Iams JD et al 1997 The preterm prediction study: patterns of cervicovaginal fetal fibronectin as predictors of spontaneous preterm delivery. National institute of child health and human development maternal–fetal medicine units network. Am J Obstet Gynecol 177:8–12

Goldenberg RL, Andrews WW, Guerrant RL et al 2000a The preterm prediction study: cervical lactoferrin concentration, other markers of lower genital tract infection, and preterm birth. National institute of child health and human development maternal–fetal medicine units network. Am J Obstet Gynecol. 182:631–635

Goldenberg RL, Andrews WW, Mercer BM et al 2000b The preterm prediction study: granulocyte colony-stimulating factor and spontaneous preterm birth. National institute of child health and human development maternal–fetal medicine units network. Am J Obstet Gynecol 182:625–630

Goldstein I, Romero R, Merrill S et al 1988 Fetal body and breathing movements as predictors of intra-amniotic infection in preterm premature rupture of the membranes. Am J Obstet Gynecol 159:363–368

Gomez R, Romero R, Mazor M, Ghezzi F, David C, Yoon BH 1997 The role of infection in preterm labor and delivery. In: Elder MG, Romero R, Lamont RF (eds) Preterm labor. Churchill Livingstone, Edinburgh, pp 85–126

Gonick B, Bottoms SF, Cotton DB 1985 Amniotic fluid volume as a risk factor in preterm premature rupture of the membranes. Obstet Gynecol 65:456–459

Gonzales LW, Ballard PL, Ertsey R et al 1986 Glucocorticoids and thyroid hormones stimulate biochemical and morphological differentiation of human fetal lung in organ culture. J Clin Endocrinol Metab 62:678–691

Goodwin TM, Paul R, Silver H et al 1994 The effect of the oxytocin antagonist atosiban on preterm uterine activity in the human. Am J Obstet Gynecol 170:474–478

Grant AM 1993 Elective vs selective Caesarean delivery of the small baby. In: Enkin M, Keirse MJNC, Renfrew M, Neilson JP (eds) Pregnancy and childbirth module. Cochrane database of systematic reviews (review no 06597 vol disk issue 2). Update Software, Oxford

Gravett MG, Nelson HP, DeRouen T et al 1986 Independent association of bacterial vaginosis and chlamydia trachomatis infection with adverse pregnancy outcome. JAMA 256:1988–1993

Gross I, Wilson CM, Ingelson LD et al 1980 Fetal lung in organ culture. III Comparison of dexamethasone, thyroxine, and methylxanthines. J Appl Physiol 48:872–877

Guinn DA, Goepfert AR, Owen J, Wenstrom KD, Hauth JC 1998 Terbutaline pump maintenance therapy for prevention of preterm delivery: a double-blind trial. Am J Obstet Gynecol 179:874–878

Guzman ER, Forster JK, Vintzileos AM, Ananth CV, Walters C, Gipson K 1998 Pregnancy outcomes in women treated with elective versus ultrasound-indicated cervical cerclage. Ultrasound Obstet Gynecol 12:323–327

Gyetvai K, Hannah ME, Hodnett ED, Ohlsson A 1999 Tocolytics for preterm labor: a systematic review. Obstet Gynecol 94:869–877

Hadlock FP, Harrist RB, Sharman RS et al 1985 Estimation of fetal weight with the use of head, body and femur measurements: a prospective study. Am J Obstet Gynecol 151:333–337

Hall DG, McGaughey HS, Corey EL et al 1959 The effects of magnesium therapy on the duration of labour. Am J Obstet Gynecol 78:27–32

Hall MH 1985 Incidence and distribution of preterm labour. In: Beard RW, Sharp F (eds) Preterm labour and its consequences. Proceedings of the thirteenth study group of the Royal College of Obstetricians and Gynaecologists. Royal College of Obstetricians and Gynaecologists, London, pp 5–13

Hall MH, Danelian P, Lamont RF 1997 The importance of preterm birth. In: Elder MG, Romero R, Lamont RF (eds) Preterm labour. Churchill Livingstone, Edinburgh, pp 1–28

Halliday HL 1988 Care of the preterm babies in the first hour. Care Crit Ill 4:7–12

Hannah ME, Ohlsson A, Farine D et al 1996 Induction of labor compared with expectant management for prelabor rupture of the membranes at term. TERMPROM study group. N Engl J Med 334:1005–1010

Harger JH, Hsing AW, Tuomala RE et al 1990 Risk factors for preterm premature rupture of the fetal membranes: a multicenter case–control study. Am J Obstet Gynecol 163:130–137

Heath VCF, Southall Tr, Souka AP, Elisseou A, Nicolaides KH 1998a Cervical length at 23 weeks of gestation: prediction of spontaneous preterm delivery. Ultrasound Obstet Gynecol 12:312–317

Heath VC, Souka AP, Erasmus I, Gibb DM, Nicolaides KH 1998b Cervical length at 23 weeks of gestation: the value of Shirodkar suture for the short cervix. Ultrasound Obstet Gynecol 12:318–322

Hedegaard M, Henriksen TB, Secher NJ, Hatch MC, Sabroe S 1996 Do stressful life events affect duration of gestation and risk of preterm delivery. Epidemiology 7:339–345

Henriksen TB, Hedegaard M, Secher NJ 1995 Standing and walking at work and birthweight. Acta Obstet Gynecol Scand 74:509–516

Hill WC, Fleming AD, Martin RW et al 1990 Home uterine activity monitoring is associated with a reduction in preterm birth. Obstet Gynecol 76:13s–18s

Hillier SL, Martius J, Krohn M, Kiviat N, Holmes KK, Eschenbach DA 1988 A case–control study of chorioamniotic infection and histologic chorioamnionitis in prematurity. N Engl J Med 319:972–978

Hillier SL, Nugent RP, Eschenbach DA et al 1995 Association between bacterial vaginosis and preterm delivery of a low birth weight infant. The vaginal infections and prematurity study group. N Engl J Med 333:1737–1742

Hoffman HJ, Bakketeig LS 1984 Risk factors associated with the occurrence of preterm birth. Clin Obstet Gynecol 27:539–552

Holbrook RH, Laros RK, Creasy RK 1989 Evaluation of a risk-scoring system for prediction of preterm labour. Am J Perinatol 6:62–68

Holcolm WL, Schackelford GD, Petrie RH 1991 Magnesium tocolysis and neonatal bone abnormalities. Obstet Gynecol 78:611–614

Holleboom CA, Merkus JM, van Elferen LW, Keirse MJ 1996a Randomised comparison between a loading and incremental dose model for ritodrine administration in preterm labour. Br J Obstet Gynaecol 103:695–701

Holleboom CA, Merkus JM, van Elferen LW, Keirse MJ 1996b Double-blind evaluation of ritodrine sustained release for oral maintenance of tocolysis after active preterm labour. Br J Obstet Gynaecol 103:702–705

Howie RN 1986 Pharmacological acceleration of lung maturation. In: Villee CA, Villee DB, Zuckerman J (eds) Respiratory distress syndrome. Academic Press, London, pp 385–396

Hueston WJ, Knox MA, Eilers G, Pauwels J, Lonsdorf D 1995 The effectiveness of preterm-birth prevention educational programs for high-risk women: a meta-analysis. Obstet Gynecol 186:705–712

Iams JD, Stilson R, Johnson FF, Williams RA, Rice R 1990a Symptoms that precede preterm labour and preterm premature rupture of the membranes. Am J Obstet Gynecol 162:486–490

Iams JD, Johnson FF, Hamer C 1990b Uterine activity and symptoms as predictors of preterm labour. Obstet Gynecol 6:42s–46s

Iams J, Goldenberg R, Meis P et al 1996 The length of the uterine cervix and the risk of spontaneous premature delivery. N Engl J Med 334:567–572

Iams JD, Goldenberg RL, Mercer BM et al 1998 The preterm prediction study: recurrence risk of spontaneous preterm birth. National institute of child health and human development maternal–fetal medicine units network. Am J Obstet Gynecol 178:1035–1040

Ingemarsson E, Ingemarsson I, Solum T et al 1980 A one-year study of routine fetal heart rate monitoring during the first stage of labour. Acta Obstet Gynaecol Scand 59:297–300

Ingemarsson I 1976 Effect of terbutaline on premature labour: a double blind placebo controlled study. Am J Obstet Gynecol 125:520–524

International Neonatal Network 1993 The CRIB (clinical risk index for babies) score: a tool for assessing initial neonatal risk and comparing performance of neonatal intensive care units. Lancet 342:193–198

Joseph KS, Kramer MS, Marcoux S et al 1998 Determinants of preterm birth rates in Canada from 1981 through 1983 and from 1992 through 1994. N Engl J Med 339:1434–1439

Kapatais-Zoumbos K, Chandler DKF, Barlie MF 1985 Survey of immunological A protease activity among selected species of ureoplasmas and mycoplasmas: specificity for host immunoglobulin. Infect Immun 47:704–709

Kappy KA, Cetrulo CL, Knuppel RA 1979 Premature rupture of the membranes: a conservative approach. Am J Obstet Gynecol 134:655–661

Katz M, Gill PJ, Newman RB 1986 Detection of preterm labour by ambulatory monitoring of uterine activity: a preliminary report. Obstet Gynecol 68: 773–778

Keirse MJNC 1989 Preterm delivery. In: Chalmers I, Enkin M, Keirse MJNC (eds) Effective care in pregnancy and childbirth, vol 1. Pregnancy. Oxford University Press, Oxford, pp 1270–1292

Keirse MJNC 1993a Home uterine activity monitoring for preventing preterm delivery. In: Enkin M, Keirse MJNC, Renfrew M, Neilson JP (eds) Pregnancy and childbirth module. Cochrane database of systematic reviews (review no 06656 vol disk issue 2). Update Software, Oxford

Kenyon S, Boulvain M 2000 Antibiotics for preterm rupture of membranes (Cochrane review). In: The Cochrane library, issue 1. Update Software, Oxford

King J, Flenady V 2000 Antibiotics for preterm labour with intact membranes (Cochrane review). In: The Cochrane library, issue 1. Update Software, Oxford

Kirbinen P, Joupilla P 1978 Polyhydramnios. A clinical study. Ann Chir Gynaecol Senniae 67:117–123

Kitchen W, Ford GW, Doyle LW et al 1985 Caesarean section or vaginal delivery at 24 to 28 weeks gestation: comparison of survival and neonatal and two-year morbidity. Obstet Gynaecol 66:149–157

Klebanoff MA, Shiono PH, Rhoads GG 1990 Outcomes of pregnancy in a national sample of resident physicians. N Engl J Med 323:1040–1045

Knuppel RA, Lake MF, Watson DL et al 1990 Preventing preterm birth in twin gestation: home uterine activity monitoring and perinatal nursing support. Obstet Gynecol 76:24s–27s

Kovacs L, Molnar BG, Huhn E, Bodis L 1988 Mg substitution in pregnancy: a prospective randomised double blind study. Geburtshilfe Frauenheilkd 48:595–600

Kragt H, Kierse MJNC 1990 How accurate is a woman's diagnosis of threatened preterm delivery? Br J Obstet Gynecol 97:317–323

Kulpa PJ, White BM, Visscher R 1987 Aerobic exercise in pregnancy. Am J Obstet Gynecol 156:1395–1403

Kurki T, Sivonen A, Renkonen OV, Savia E, Ylikorkala O 1992 Bacterial vaginosis in early pregnancy and pregnancy outcome. Obstet Gynecol 80:173–177

Kyrklund-Blomberg NB, Cnattingius S 1998 Preterm and smoking. Am J Obstet Gynecol 179:1051 1055

Lamont RF 2000 The pathophysiology of pulmonary oedema with the use of beta-agonists. Br J Obstet Gynaecol 107:439–444

Lamont RF, Rose M, Elder MG 1985 Effects of bacterial products on prostaglandin E2 production by amnion cells. Lancet ii:1131–1133

Lamont RF, Taylor-Robinson D, Wigglesworth JS, Furr PM, Evans RT, Elder MG 1987 The role of mycoplasmas, ureoplasmas, and chlamydiae in the genital tract of women presenting in spontaneously early preterm labour. J Med Microbiol 24:253–257

Launer LJ, Villar J, Kestler E et al 1990 The effect of maternal work on fetal growth and duration of pregnancy: a prospective study. Br J Obstet Gynaecol 97:62–70

Lees CC, Lojacono A, Thompson C et al 1999 Glyceryl trinitrate and ritodrine in tocolysis: an international multicenter randomized study. GTN preterm labour investigation group. Obstet Gynecol 94:403–408

Leeson SC, Maresh MJ, Martindale EA et al 1996 Detection of fetal fibronectin as a predictor of preterm delivery in high risk asymptomatic pregnancies. Br J Obstet Gynaecol 103:48–53

Leung TN, Chung TK, Madsen G, McLean M, Chang AM, Smith R 1999 Elevated mid-trimester maternal corticotrophin-releasing hormone levels in pregnancies that delivered before 34 weeks. Br J Obstet Gynaecol 106:1041–1046

Leveno KJ, Cox K, Roark ML 1986 Cervical dilatation and prematurity revisited. Obstet Gynecol 68:434–435

Leviton LC, Goldenberg RL, Baker CS et al 1999 Methods to encourage the use of antenatal corticosteroid therapy for fetal maturation: a randomized controlled trial. JAMA 281:46–52

Lewis DF, Major CA, Towers CV, Harding JA, Asrat T, Garite TJ 1991 Effects of digital vaginal exams on latency period in preterm premature rupture of the membranes. Am J Obstet Gynecol 164:381

Lobb MO, Cooke RWI 1986 The influence of episiotomy on the neonatal survival and incidence of periventricular haemorrhage in the very-low-birthweight infants. Eur J Obstet Gynaecol Reprod Biol 22:17–21

Lockwood CJ 1999 Stress-associated preterm delivery: the role of corticotropin-releasing hormone. Am J Obstet Gynecol 180:S264–266

Lockwood CJ, Senyei AE, Dische MR et al 1991 Fetal fibronectin in cervical and vaginal secretions as a predictor of preterm delivery. N Engl J Med 325:669–674

Lockwood CJ, Wein R, Lapinski R et al 1993 The presence of cervical and vaginal fetal fibronectin predicts preterm delivery in an inner-city obstetric population. Am J Obstet Gynecol 169:798–804

Lopez Bernal A, Hansell DJ, Khong TY, Keeling JW, Turnbull A 1990 Placental leukotriene B4 release in early pregnancy and in term and preterm labour. Early Hum Dev 23:93–99

Low JA, Karchmar J, Brockhoven L et al 1981 The probability of fetal metabolic acidosis during labour in a population at risk as determined by clinical factors. Am J Obstet Gynecol 141:941–951

Luke B, Papiernik E 1997 The effects of lifestyle on prematurity. In: Elder MG, Romero R, Lamont RF (eds) Preterm labor. Churchill Livingstone, Edinburgh, pp 127–152

Lumley J 1993 The epidemiology of preterm birth. Baillière's Clin Obstet Gynaecol 7:477–498

Lumley J, Astbury J 1989 Advice for pregnancy. In: Chalmers I, Enkin M, Keirse MJNC (eds) Effective care in pregnancy and childbirth, vol 1. Pregnancy. Oxford University Press, Oxford, pp 237–254

Lumley J, Oliver S, Waters E 2000 Interventions for promoting smoking cessation during pregnancy (Cochrane Review). In: The Cochrane library, issue 1. Update Software, Oxford

Luthy D, Shy K, van Belle G et al 1987 A randomised trial of electronic fetal heart rate monitoring in preterm labour. Obstet Gynecol 69:687–695

MacArthur BA, Howie RN, Denzoete JA, Elkins J 1982 School progress and cognitive development of 6-year old children whose mothers were treated antenatally with betamethasone. Pediatrics 70:99–105

McDonald HM, O'Loughlin JA, Jolley P, Vigneswaran R, McDonald PJ 1991 Vaginal infection and preterm labour. Br J Obstet Gynaecol 98:427–435

McGregor J 1988 Prevention of preterm birth: new initiatives based on microbial–host interactions. Obstet Gynecol Surv 43:1–14

McGregor JA, Lawellin D, Franco-Buff A et al 1986 Protease production by microorganisms associated with reproductive tract infection. Am J Obstet Gynecol 154:109–114

McGregor JA, French JI, Lawelin D et al 1987 In vitro study of bacterial protease-induced reduction of chorioamniotic membrane strength and elasticity. Obstet Gynecol 69:167–174

McGregor JA, French JI, Parker R et al 1995 Prevention of premature birth by screening and treatment for common genital tract infections: results of a prospective controlled evaluation. Am J Obstet Gynecol 173:157–167

McLean M, Walters WA, Smith R 1993 Prediction and early diagnosis of preterm labor: a critical review. Obstet Gynecol Sur 48:209–225

McLean M, Bisits A, Davies J et al 1999 Predicting risk of preterm delivery by second-trimester measurement of maternal plasma corticotropin-releasing hormone and alpha-fetoprotein concentrations. Am J Obstet Gynecol 181:207–215

Macones GA, Segel SY, Stamilio DM, Morgan MA 1999 Predicting delivery within 48 hours in women treated with parenteral tocolysis. Obstet Gynecol 93:432–436

Main DM, Gabbe S, Richardson R et al 1985 Can preterm deliveries be prevented? Am J Obstet Gynecol 151:892–898

Main DM, Katz M, Chiu G et al 1988 Intermittent weekly contraction monitoring to predict preterm labour in low risk women: a blinded study. Obstet Gynecol 72:757–761

Major CA, Lewis DF, Harding JA et al 1991 Does tocolysis with indomethacin increase the incidence of necrotising enterocolitis in the low birthweight neonate. Am J Obstet Gynecol 164:361

Mamelle N, Gabbe SG, Richardson D et al 1984 Prematurity and occupational activity during pregnancy. Am J Epidemiol 119:309–322

Mamelle N, Segueilla M, Munoz F, Berland M 1997 Prevention of preterm birth in patients with symptoms of preterm labour: the benefits of psychologic support. Am J Obstet Gynecol 177:947–952

Mari G, Moise KJ, Deter RL et al 1989 Doppler assessment of the middle cerebral artery during constriction of the fetal ductus arteriosus after indomethacin therapy. Am J Obstet Gynecol 161:1528–1531

Mari G, Moise KJ, Deter RL et al 1990 Doppler assessment of the renal blood flow velocity waveform during indomethacin therapy for preterm labour and polyhydramnios. Obstet Gynecol 75:199–201

Martius JA, Steck T, Oehler MK, Wulf KH 1998 Risk factors associated with preterm (< 37 + 0 weeks) and early preterm birth (<32 +0 weeks): univariate and multivariate analysis of 106 345 singleton births from the 1994 statewide perinatal survey of Bavaria. Eur J Obstet Gynecol Reprod Biol 80:183–189

Meirowitz NB, Ananth CV, Smulian JC, Vintzileos AM 1999 Value of maintenance therapy with oral tocolysis: a systematic review. J Matern Fetal Med 8:177–183

Meis PJ, Michielutte R, Peters TJ et al 1995a Factors associated with preterm birth in Cardiff, Wales. I. Univariable and multivariable analysis. Am J Obstet Gynecol 173:590–596

Meis PJ, Michielutte R, Peters TJ et al 1995b Factors associated with preterm birth in Cardiff, Wales. II. Indicated and spontaneous preterm birth. Am J Obstet Gynecol 173:597–602

Mendelson CR, Alcorn JL, Gao E 1993 The pulmonary surfactant protein genes and their regulation in fetal lung. Semin Perinatol 17:223–232

Mercer BM, Lewis R 1997 Antibiotic therapy for preterm labour and preterm premature rupture of the membranes. In: Elder M, Romero R, Lamont RF (eds) Preterm labour. Churchill Livingstone, Edinburgh, pp 299–317

Mercer BM, Sklar S, Shariatmader A et al 1987 Fetal foot length as a predictor of gestational age. Am J Obstet Gynecol 156:350–355

Mercer B, Moretti M, Rogers R, Sibai B 1992 Antibiotic prophylaxis in preterm premature rupture of the membranes: a prospective randomised double blind trial of 220 patients. Am J Obstet Gynecol 166:794–802

Mercer BM, Mercer BM, Goldenberg RL et al 1996 The preterm prediction study: a clinical risk assessment system. Am J Obstet Gynecol 174:1885–1893

Mercer BM, Goldenberg RL, Moawad AH et al 1999 The preterm prediction study: effect of gestational age and cause of preterm birth on subsequent obstetric outcome. National institute of child health and human development maternal–fetal medicine units network. Am J Obstet Gynecol 181:1216–1221

Meyer M 1977 Effects of maternal smoking and altitude on birth weight and gestation. In: Reed DM, Stanley FJ (eds) The epidemiology of prematurity. Urban and Schwarzenberg, Baltimore, pp 81–104

Meyer MB, Tonascia JA 1977 Maternal smoking, pregnancy complications and perinatal mortality. Am J Obstet Gynecol 128:494–502

Meyers RL, Gadalpan E, Cluman RI 1991 Patent ductus arteriosus, indomethacin and intestinal distention: effects on intestinal bloodflow and oxygen consumption. Paediatr Res 29:569–574

Mires GJ, Agustsson P, Forsyth JS, Patel N 1991 Cerebral pathology in the very low birth weight infant: predictive value of peripartum metabolic acidosis. Eur J Obstet Gynecol Reprod Med 42:181–185

Mires GJ, Owen P, Lee CP, Patel NB 1993 Electronic fetal heart rate monitoring in prematurity. In: Spencer JAD, Ward RHT (eds) Intrapartum fetal surveillance. RCOG, London, pp 95–109

Mitchell MD, Dudley DJ, Edwin SS, Lundin-Schiller S 1991 Interleukin-6 stimulates prostaglandin production by human amnion and decidual cells. Eur J Pharmacol 192:189–191

Moise KJ 1993 The effect of advancing gestational age on the frequency of fetal ductal constriction secondary to maternal indomethacin use. Am J Obstet Gynecol 168:1350–1353

Moise KJ, Ou C-N, Kirshon B et al 1990 Placental transfer of indomethacin in the human pregnancy. Am J Obstet Gynecol 162:549–554

Mortensen OA, Franklin J, Lofstrand T et al 1987 Prediction of preterm birth. Acta Obstet Gynaecol Scand 66:507–512

MRC/RCOG Working Party on Cervical Cerclage 1993 Final report of the MRC/RCOG multicentre randomised trial of cervical cerclage. Br J Obstet Gynaecol 100:516–523

Mueller-Heubach E, Reddick D, Barnett B et al 1989 Preterm birth prevention: evaluation of a prospective controlled randomised trial. Am J Obstet Gynecol 160:1172–1178

Murray JL, Bernfield M 1988 The differential effect of prenatal care on the incidence of low birth weight among blacks and whites in a prepaid health care plan. N Engl J Med 319:1385–1391

Nageotte MP, Casal D, Senyei AE 1994 Fetal fibronectin in patients at increased risk for premature birth. Am J Obstet Gynecol 170:20–25

Natale R, Nasello C, Turluik R 1984 The relationship between movement and accelerations in the fetal heart rate between 24 and 32 weeks gestation. Am J Obstet Gynecol 148:591–595

Neilson JP, Grant AM 1993 The randomised trials of intrapartum electronic fetal heart rate monitoring. In: Spencer JAD, Ward RHT (eds) Intrapartum fetal surveillance. RCOG, London, pp 77–93

Newton ER, Kennedy JL, Louis F et al 1987 Obstetric diagnosis and perinatal mortality. Am J Perinatol 4:300–308

Nwosu EC, Welch CR, Manasse P, Walkinshaw SA 1993 Longitudinal assessment of amniotic fluid index. Br J Obstet Gynaecol 100:816–819

Oei SG, Mol BW, de Kleine MJ, Brolmann HA 1999 Nifedipine versus ritodrine for suppression of preterm labour; a meta-analysis. Acta Obstet Gynaecol Scand 78:783–778

Olsen SF, Sorensen J, Secher NJ et al 1992 Randomised controlled trial of effect of fish-oil supplementation on pregnancy duration. Lancet 339:1003–1007

Paneth N, Kiely JL, Wallenstein S, Susser M 1987 The choice of place of delivery. Effect of hospital level on mortality in all singleton births in New York City. Am J Dis Child 141:60–64

Papiernik E 1993 Prevention of preterm labour and delivery. Baillière's Clin Obstet Gynaecol 7:499–522

Papiernik E, Bouyer J, Dreyfus J et al 1985 Prevention of preterm birth: a perinatal study in Haguenau, France. Pediatrics 76:154–158

Pattinson RC, Makin JD, Funk M et al 1999 The use of dexamethasone in women with preterm premature rupture of membranes: a multicentre, double-blind, placebo-controlled, randomised trial. Dexiprom study group. S Afr Med J 89:865–870

Peaceman AM, Andrews WW, Thorp JM et al 1997 Fetal fibronectin as a predictor of preterm birth in patients with symptoms: a multicenter trial. Am J Obstet Gynecol 177:13–18

Philipsen T, Erikson PS, Lyngaard F 1981 Pulmonary edema following ritodrine–saline infusion in preterm labour. Obstet Gynecol 58:304–308

Plaut AG 1978 Microbial IgA proteases. N Engl J Med 298:1459–1462

Polzin WJ, Brady K 1998 The etiology of premature rupture of the membranes. Clin Obstet Gynecol 41:810–816

Powell PG, Pharoah POD, Cooke RWI 1987 How accurate are the perinatal statistics in your region? Community Med 9:226–231

Prendeville WJ 1993 17 Alphahydroxyprogesterone caproate in pregnancy. In: Enkin M, Keirse MJNC, Renfrew M, Neilson JP (eds) Pregnancy and childbirth module. Cochrane database of systematic reviews (review no 04399 vol disk issue 2). Update Software, Oxford

Quintero RA, Morales WJ, Allen M, Bornick PW, Arroyo J, LeParc G 1999 Treatment of iatrogenic previable premature rupture of membranes with intra-amniotic injection of platelets and cryoprecipitate (amniopatch): preliminary experience. Am J Obstet Gynecol 181:744–749

Reece EA, Goldstein I, Pilu G, Hobbins J 1987 Fetal cerebellum growth unaffected by intrauterine growth retardation: a new parameter for prenatal diagnosis. Am J Obstet Gynecol 157:632–638

Reiss U, Atad J, Reuinstein I et al 1976 The effect of indomethacin in labour at term. Int J Obstet Gynaecol 143:369–374

Ricci JM, Hariharan S, Helfgott A, Reed K, O'Sullivan MJ 1991 Oral tocolysis with magnesium chloride: a randomised controlled prospective clinical trial. Am J Obstet Gynecol 165:603–610

Rizzo G, Capponi A, Arduini D, Lorido C, Romanini C 1996 The value of fetal fibronectin in cervical and vaginal secretions and of ultrasonographic examination of the uterine cervix in predicting premature delivery for patients with preterm labor and intact membranes. Am J Obstet Gynecol 175:1146–1151

Roberts AB, Mitchell JM 1990 Direct ultrasonographic measurement of fetal lung length in normal pregnancies and pregnancies complicated by prolonged rupture of the membranes. Am J Obstet Gynecol 163:1560–1566

Roberts AB, Goldstein I, Romero R, Hobbins J 1991a Fetal breathing movements after preterm premature rupture of the membranes. Am J Obstet Gynecol 164:821–825

Roberts AB, Goldstein I, Romero R, Hobbins JC 1991b Comparison of total fetal activity measurement with the biophysical profile in predicting intra-amniotic infection in preterm premature rupture of the membranes. Ultrasound Obstet and Gynecol 1:36–39

Robson SC, Gallivan S, Walkinshaw SA, Vaughan J, Rodeck CH 1993 Ultrasonic estimation of fetal weight: use of targeted formulas in small for gestational age fetuses. Obstet Gynecol 82:359–364

Romero R, Mazor M 1988 Infection and preterm labour. Clin Obstet Gynecol 31:553–584

Romero R, Mazor M, Wu YK et al 1988a Infection in the pathogenesis of preterm labour. Semin Perinatol 12:262–279

Romero R, Emamian M, Quintero R 1988b The value and limitations of the gram stain in the diagnosis of intraamniotic infection. Am J Obstet Gynecol 159:114–119

Romero R, Mazor M, Wu YK, Avila C, Oyarzun E, Mitchell MD 1989 Bacterial endotoxin and tumour necrosis factor stimulate prostaglandin production by human decidua. Prostaglandins, Leukot Essent Fatty Acids 37:183–186

Romero R, Avila C, Santhanam U, Seghal PB 1990a Amniotic fluid interleukin 6 in preterm labour. J Clin Invest 85:1392–1400

Romero R, Jimenez C, Lohda AK 1990b Amniotic fluid glucose concentrations: a rapid and simple method for the detection of intra amnionitis in preterm labour. Am J Obstet Gynecol 163:968–974

Romero R, Avila C, Brekue CA, Morotti R 1991 The role of systemic and intrauterine infection in preterm parturition. Ann NY Acad Sci 622:355–375

Rotschild A, Ling EW, Puterman ML, Farqhuarson D 1990 Neonatal outcome after prolonged preterm rupture of the membranes. Am J Obstet Gynecol 162:46–52

Rozenberg P, Goffinet F, Malagrida L et al 1997 Evaluating the risk of preterm delivery: a comparison of fetal fibronectin and transvaginal ultrasonographic measurement of cervical length. Am J Obstet Gynecol 176:196–199

Russell P 1979 Inflammatory lesions of the human placenta. I. Clinical significance of acute chorioamnionitis. Am J Diagn Gynecol Obstet 1:127–137

Rust O, Atlas R, Jones K, Benham B, Balducci J 2000 A randomized trial of cerclage vs no cerclage in patients with sonographically detected 2nd trimester premature dilation of the internal os. Am J Obstet Gynecol 182:S13

Sanchez-Ramos L, Kaunitz AM, Gaudier FL, Delke I. 1999 Efficacy of maintenance therapy after acute tocolysis: a meta-analysis. Am J Obstet Gynecol 181:484–490

Sbarra AJ, Thomas GB, Cetrulo CL et al 1987 Effect of bacterial growth on the bursting pressure of fetal membranes in vitro. Obstet Gynecol 70:107–110

Schoendorf KC, Hogue CJR, Rowley D et al 1992 Mortality among infants of black as compared to white college educated parents. N Engl J Med 326:1522–1526

Shah NR, Bracken MB 2000 A systematic review and meta-analysis of prospective studies on the association between maternal cigarette smoking and preterm delivery. Am J Obstet Gynecol 182:465–472

Shankaran S, Papile LA, Wright LL et al 1997 The effect of antenatal phenobarbital therapy on neonatal intracranial hemorrhage in preterm infants. N Engl J Med 337:466–471

Shepard MJ, Richards VA, Berkowitz RL et al 1982 An evaluation of two equations for predicting fetal weight by ultrasound. Am J Obstet Gynecol 142:47–54

Shy K, Luthy D, Bennett F et al 1990 Effects of electronic fetal heart rate monitoring as compared to periodic auscultation on neurologic development of premature infants. N Engl J Med 322:588–593

Sibai BM, Villar MA, Bray E 1989 Mg supplementation during pregnancy: a double blind randomised controlled clinical trial. Am J Obstet Gynecol 161:115–119

Sideris EB, Yokochi K, Van Helder T et al 1983 Effects of indomethacin and prostaglandins E2, 12 and D2 on the fetal circulation. Adv Prostaglandin, Thromboxane Leukot Res 12:477–486

Smaill F 2000 Antibiotics for asymptomatic bacteriuria in pregnancy (Cochrane review). In: The Cochrane library, issue 1. Update Software, Oxford

Smith GN, Walker MC, McGrath MJ 1999 Randomised, double-blind, placebo controlled pilot study assessing nitroglycerin as a tocolytic. Br J Obstet Gynaecol 1106:736–739

Smith P, Anthony J, Johanson R 2000 Nifedipine in pregnancy. Br J Obstet Gynaecol 107:299–307

Smolders-de-Has H, Neuvel J, Schmand B, Treffers PE, Koppe JG, Hoeks J 1990 Physical development and medical history of children who were treated antenatally with corticosteroids to prevent respiratory distress syndrome. Pediatrics 86:65–70

Souter D, Harding J, McCowan L, O'Donnell C, Mcleay E, Baxendale H 1998 Antenatal indomethacin: adverse fetal effects confirmed. Aust NZ J Obstet Gynaecol 38:11–16

Spatling L, Spatling G 1988 Mg supplementation in pregnancy: a double blind study. Br J Obstet Gynaecol 95:120–125

Spong CY, Ghidini A, Sherer DM, Pezzullo JC, Ossandon M, Eglinton GS 1997 Angiogenin: a marker for preterm delivery in midtrimester amniotic fluid. Am J Obstet Gynecol 176:415–418

Talbert RL, Bussey HI 1983 Update on calcium channel blocking agents. Clin Pharmacol 2:403–416

Tamura RK, Sabbagha RE 1984 Diminished growth in fetuses born preterm after spontaneous labour or rupture of the membranes. Am J Obstet Gynecol 148:1105–1110

Taylor J, Garite TJ 1984 Premature rupture of the membranes before fetal viability. Obstet Gynecol 64:615–620

Thomsen AC, Morup L, Brogaard Hansen K 1987 Antibiotic elimination of group B streptococci in urine in prevention of preterm labour. Lancet i: 591–593

Thorpe JA, Parriott J, Ferette-Smith D, Meyer BA, Cohen GR, Joynson J 1994 Antepartum vitamin K and phenobarbitol for preventing intraventricular haemorrhage in the premature newborn: a randomised double-blind, placebo controlled trial. Obstet Gynecol 83:70–76

Turnbull AC 1977 Aetiology of preterm labour. In: Anderson A (ed) Proceedings of the fifth study group of the Royal College of Obstetricians and Gynaecologists. RCOG, London, pp 56–70

Tyson J, Guzick D, Rosenfield CR et al 1990 Prenatal care evaluation and cohort analyses. Paediatrics 85:195–204

van den Berg BJ, Oechsli F 1984 Prematurity. In: Bracken MB (ed) Perinatal epidemiology. Oxford University Press, Oxford, pp 69–85

Vanhaesebrouk P, Thiery M, Leroy JG et al 1988 Oligohydramnios, renal insufficiency, and ileal perforation in preterm infants after in utero exposure to indomethacin. J Paediatr 113:738–743

Vermeulen GM, Bruinse HW 1999 Prophylactic administration of clindamycin 2% vaginal cream to reduce the incidence of spontaneous preterm birth in women with an increased recurrence risk: a randomised placebo-controlled double-blind trial. Br J Obstet Gynaecol 106:652–657

Vermillion ST, Newman RB 1999 Recent indomethacin tocolysis is not associated with neonatal complications in preterm infants. Am J Obstet Gynecol 181:1083–1086

Villar J, Ezcurra EJ 1994 Preterm delivery syndrome: the unmet need. New perspectives for the effective treatment of preterm labour: an international consensus. Res Clin Forums 16:9–38

Vince GS, Starkey PM, Jackson MC, Sargent IL, Redman CW 1990 Flow cytometric characterisation of cell populations in human pregnancy decidua and isolation of decidual macrophages. J Immunol Methods 132:181–189

Vintzileos AM, Campbell WA, Nochimson DJ, Weinbaum PJ 1985 Degree of oligohydramnios and pregnancy outcome in patients with premature rupture of the membranes. Obstet Gynecol 66:162–167

Vintzileos AM, Campbell WA, Nochimson DJ, Weinbaum PJ 1986a The use of the nonstress test in patients with premature preterm rupture of the membranes. Am J Obstet Gynecol 155:149–153

Vintzileos AM, Campbell WA, Nochimson DJ, Weinbaum PJ 1986b Fetal breathing as a predictor of infection in premature rupture of the membranes. Obstet Gynecol 67:813–817

Volpe JJ 1992 Effect of cocaine use on the fetus. N Engl J Med 327:399–407

Walkinshaw SA, Siney C, Kidd M, Manasse P, Morrison C 1993 Outcome of pregnancy in opiate dependent women within a methadone treatment programme. In: First international conference on practical obstetrics, Paris, p 156

Wang E, Smaill F 1989 Infection in pregnancy. In: Chalmers I, Enkin M, Keirse MJNC (eds) Effective care in pregnancy and childbirth. Oxford University Press, Oxford, pp 534–564

Wariyar U, Richmond S, Hey E 1989 Pregnancy outcome at 24 to 31 weeks gestation: mortality. Arch Dis Child 64:670–677

Weiner CP, Renk K, Klugman M 1988 The therapeutic efficacy and cost-effectiveness of aggressive tocolysis for premature labor associated with premature rupture of the membranes. Am J Obstet Gynecol 159:216–222

Wen SW, Goldberg RL, Cutter GR, Hoffman HJ, Cliver SP 1990 Intrauterine growth retardation and preterm delivery: perinatal risk factors in an indigent population. Am J Obstet Gynecol 162:213–218

Westgren M, Holmquist P, Svenningsen N, Ingemarsson I 1982 Intrapartum fetal monitoring in pre-term deliveries: prospective study. Obstet Gynecol 60: 99–106

Westgren M, Malcus P, Svenningen N 1986 Intrauterine asphyxia and long term outcome in pre term fetuses. Obstet Gynecol 67:512–516

WHO 1977 Manual of the international classification of diseases, injuries and causes of death, vol 1. World Health Organization, Geneva

Wilcox MA, Johnson IR, Maynard PV, Smith SJ, Chilvers CED 1993 The individualised birthweight ratio: a more logical outcome measure of pregnancy than birthweight alone. Br J Obstet Gynaecol 100:342–347

Williams PD, Bock MG, Evans BE, Freidinger RM, Pettibone DJ 1998 Progress in the development of oxytocin antagonists for use in preterm labor. Adv Exp Med Biol 449:473–479

Yoon BH, Romero R, Kim CJ et al 1995 Amniotic fluid interleukin-6: a sensitive test for antenatal diagnosis of acute inflammatory lesions of preterm placenta and prediction of perinatal morbidity. Am J Obstet Gynecol 172:960–970

Young DC, Toofanian A, Leveno KJ 1983 Potassium and glucose concentrations without treatment during ritodrine tocolysis. Am J Obstet Gynecol 145:105–106

Zanini B, Paul RH, Huey JR 1980 Intrapartum fetal heart rate: correlation with scalp pH in preterm fetuses. Am J Obstet Gynecol 136:43–47

Zhou W, Sorensen HT, Olsen J 1999 Induced abortion and subsequent pregnancy duration. Obstet Gynecol 94:948–953

32

Prolonged pregnancy

Patricia Crowley

The contribution of the author of the equivalent chapter in the second edition, on which this chapter draws extensively, is gratefully acknowledged.

DEFINITION

Post-term, post-dates, prolonged and postmature are all terms officially accepted by the World Health Organization (1994) to describe pregnancy that continues for 294 days or more following the first day of the last menstrual period (LMP), assuming valid dates and a regular 28-day cycle. The term 'postmature' has also been used to refer to a clinical syndrome with additional features ranging from dry cracked skin (stage 1 postmaturity) to meconium staining and birth asphyxia (stage 2 postmaturity), and respiratory distress, convulsions and fetal death (stage 3 postmaturity) (Clifford 1954). In this chapter I will refer mainly to pregnancies of 294 days and over, but will also touch on the management of pregnancies of 41 weeks and over as intervention is commonly practised at this time.

INCIDENCE OF POST-TERM PREGNANCY

It is impossible to state the true incidence of post-term pregnancy. Published rates for prolonged pregnancy vary from a rate of 14.9% for Norwegian women with registered menstrual dates (Bjerkdal & Bakketeig 1975) to 2.2% for women with singleton pregnancies without fetal abnormality whose dates were based on mid-trimester ultrasound (Gardosi et al 1997). The real incidence of prolonged pregnancy probably lies somewhere in between these two rates. A true estimate of the incidence of post-term pregnancy would require access to a population with meticulous documentation of obstetric data, accurate pregnancy dating and a complete absence of obstetric intervention. (Such an estimate would still only apply to

the population studied, and would not be generalisable across ethnic groups, for example.) Some of these criteria were met by the study by Bierman et al (1965) of 3000 pregnancies on the Hawaiian island of Kauai, where 14% of pregnancies were of 42 weeks or more. It would now be assumed, however, that this series exaggerated the incidence of post-term pregnancy by including women with invalid dates. In general, accurate dating using mid-trimester ultrasound and a low level of obstetric intervention are mutually exclusive features of published series of post-term pregnancy.

The varying rates of preterm delivery and of elective delivery prior to 42 weeks substantially alter the incidence of prolonged pregnancy. This is well illustrated by the change in incidence of prolonged pregnancy in Britain from 11.5% in 1958 (Butler & Bonham 1963) to 4.4% in 1970 (Chamberlain et al 1978), coinciding with a rise in the rate of induction of labour from 13% in 1958 to 26% in 1970. Fabre et al (1996), using data from the Spanish Perinatal Mortality Study, reported a reduction in the incidence of post-term births from 8.1% in 1980 to 5.0% in 1992. Recently, Roberts et al (1999) reported a reduction in prolonged pregnancy in New South Wales from 4.6% in 1990 to 2.8% in 1996. The decline in prolonged pregnancy was associated with increasing rates of induction at 41 weeks.

Ultrasound estimation of gestational age

In modern obstetric practice, the use of ultrasound during the first half of pregnancy to determine gestational age reduces the apparent incidence of post-term pregnancy. Ultrasound measurement of biparietal diameter and femur length in the second trimester of pregnancy is more accurate in predicting the date of the onset of spontaneous labour than menstrual dates, even when these are reliable (Mongelli et al 1996). The discrepancy between menstrual and ultrasound dates increases with the apparent gestational age at birth according to LMP, with 72% of pregnancies presumed to be post-term by menstrual dates being less than 42 weeks by ultrasound dates (Gardosi et al 1997). Gardosi & Geirsson (1998) argue that routine ultrasound is the method of choice for dating all pregnancies. However, Henriksen et al (1995) caution that basing pregnancy management on mid-trimester biometry in preference to menstrually derived dates may introduce a bias, inflating the incidence of preterm birth and reducing the incidence of post-term birth in female infants and in the infants of smokers, because of their smaller size. Tunon et al (1999) failed to detect any increased risk of adverse outcome in pregnancies that were post-term according to the last menstrual period estimate but not according to the ultrasound estimate. The most robust evidence in favour of routine use of ultrasound to establish gestational age comes from the systematic review by Neilson (1999) which shows that routine ultrasound in the first half of pregnancy significantly reduces the incidence of induction for post-term pregnancy (odds ratio for induction 0.61, 95% confidence interval (CI) 0.52–0.72) without any increase in adverse outcomes.

AETIOLOGY

The effects of anencephaly and of placental suphatase deficiency on the duration of pregnancy are interesting examples of extreme post-term pregnancy, but throw little light on the aetiology of the majority of cases of prolonged pregnancy. It is likely that the majority of pregnancies of greater than 42 weeks' duration represent the upper range of a normal distribution. Prolonged pregnancy tends to repeat itself. Analysis of data from the Norwegian Birth Registry showed that a woman delivering post-term in her first pregnancy had a relative risk of a second post-term pregnancy of 2.2, and a woman with two post-term pregnancies had a 3.2-fold relative risk of a third post-term pregnancy (Bakketeig & Bergsjo 1989). Swedish Medical Birth Registry data confirm these results and also indicate a tendency for daughters of mothers who deliver post-term to have prolonged pregnancies (Mogren et al 1999) but these factors account for only a small proportion of the overall population attributable risk for post-term pregnancy. Low vaginal levels of fetal fibronectin at 39 weeks are predictive of an increased likelihood of post-term pregnancy (Lockwood et al 1994). Prolonged pregnancy could result from variations in the corticotrophin releasing hormone (CRH) system during pregnancy such as an alteration in the number or expression of myometrial receptor subtypes, altered signal-transduction mechanisms, or an increase in the capacity of CRH-binding hormone protein to bind and inactivate CRH (Grammatopoulis & Hillhouse 1999). Research on the mechanisimg leading to preterm labour may lead to greater understanding of the aetiology of post-term pregnancy.

RISKS ASSOCIATED WITH POST-TERM PREGNANCY

Methodological issues

Just as obstetric intervention makes an accurate assessment of the incidence of post-term pregnancy impossible, any statistics relating to the risks of post-term pregnancy are influenced by interventions aimed at reducing these risks.

Traditionally, perinatal mortality rates of babies delivered at 42 weeks or more are compared with rates in babies delivered at 37–41 weeks. Yudkin et al (1987) argued that the convention of presenting gestation-specific stillbirth rates, using the number of births at a given gestation as the denominator, underestimates the true risk of intrauterine fetal death in late pregnancy. They proposed that the number of deaths in utero should be expressed per thousand babies still in utero for each 2-week period of pregnancy. With this method, the risk of unexplained stillbirth was least in preterm pregnancies, rising fourfold after 39 weeks to a maximum at 41 weeks. At this time, it was also four times higher than at 33 weeks, in contrast to the rate, which was 19 times lower.

Comparisons between perinatal mortality rates at and beyond 42 weeks and those at 37–41 weeks inclusive should also be viewed in the light of the differing risk profiles of the two groups. In modern obstetric practice, women with twins, pre-eclampsia, diabetes, advanced maternal age, previous perinatal death and recurrent antepartum haemorrhage are all likely to be delivered at 37–41 weeks. Women who reach 42 weeks are likely to represent a low-risk population.

Before the increased use of ultrasound to detect serious congenital malformations, babies with lethal malformations were more likely to be delivered post-term and accounted for up to 30% of perinatal deaths in post-term pregnancies (Naeye 1978). Early detection of lethal malformations with termination of pregnancy or elective delivery now reduces this potential source of bias in large cohort studies.

A further potential source of bias could arise in cases where intrauterine death occurs before 42 weeks' gestation and delivery occurs after 42 weeks' gestation. With the availability of effective methods of induction of labour, a long latent period between intrauterine death and delivery is now unusual and unlikely to contribute greatly to perinatal mortality statistics post-term.

Perinatal mortality

Tables 32.1 and 32.2 present a sample of some large published case series of comparisons between gestation-specific perinatal mortality rates. There is a consistent tendency for perinatal mortality rates to increase after 42 weeks. Table 32.2 shows how Hilder et al (1998) applied the concept developed by Yudkin et al (1987) of mortality risks per 1000 ongoing pregnancies to gestation-specific mortality risks. The risks of post-term pregnancy are magnified using this method.

Table 32.1 Perinatal mortality rates; term versus post-term pregnancies

Authors	Source	Outcome	37–41 weeks inclusive	42 weeks and more
Crowley 1989	62 804 hospital births 1979–86	Corrected perinatal mortality rate	4.5	6.7
O'Herlihy & Robson 1993	31 255 hospital births 1987–91	Corrected perinatal mortality rate	3.8	5.0
Campbell et al 1997	444 241 births Norway 1978–87	Relative risk of perinatal death	1	1.30 (95% CI 1.13–1.50)
Fabre et al 1996	547 923 births Spain 1980–92	Stillbirth rate	3.3	3.6
		Early neonatal mortality rate	1.7	2.8
		Perinatal mortality rate	4.9	6.4

Table 32.2 Gestation-specific perinatal mortality 37–43 weeks

Author	Source	Outcome	38–39	39–40	40–41	41–42	42–43	>43
Bakketeig & Bergsjo 1989	157 577 births Sweden 1977 & 1978	Perinatal mortality rate	7.2	3.1	2.3	2.4	3	4
Ingemarsson & Kallen 1997	914 702 births Sweden 1982–91	Stillbirth rate nulliparae	2.72	1.53	1.23	1.86	2.26	
		Neonatal mortality nulliparae	0.62	0.54	0.54	0.9	1.03	
		Stillbirth rate multiparae	2.1	1.42	1.35	1.4	1.51	
		Neonatal mortality multiparae	0.55	0.45	0.53	0.5	0.86	
Hilder et al 1998	171 527 births London 1989–91	Stillbirth rate per 1000 births	3.8	2.2	1.5	1.7	1.9	2.1
		Infant mortality rate per 1000 births	4.7	3.2	2.7	2	4.1	3.7
		Stillbirth rate per 1000 OP	0.56	0.57	0.86	1.27	1.55	2.12
		Infant mortality per 1000 OP	0.7	0.83	1.57	1.48	3.29	3.71

OP, Ongoing pregnancies

Timing of perinatal death

Increases in antepartum, intrapartum and early neonatal mortality associated with post-term pregnancies have been reported in various studies. Recently published data from the North East Thames Region show that infant mortality is also increased in this group (Hilder et al 1998). The series is not corrected for congenital malformations which could contribute to increased rates of neonatal and postneonatal death, however the authors were of the opinion that this did not explain the increase. A detailed analysis of the deaths in the Crowley (1989) study indicated a specific increase in intrapartum and neonatal asphyxial deaths. In an analysis of a large cohort of post-term births in Sweden, Ingemarsson and Kallen (1997) showed that the increased risk of stillbirth after 41 weeks' gestation applied only to primiparae (Table 32.2). Neonatal mortality was increased after 42 weeks for both primiparae and multiparae. Divon et al (1998), using a subset of the same Swedish data, showed a significant rise in the odds ratio for fetal death from 41 weeks' gestation onwards (odds ratios 1.5, 1.8, and 2.9 at 41, 42, and 43 weeks, respectively). In this study, odds ratios for neonatal mortality were not significantly dependent on gestational age.

Effect of birthweight

Birthweight less than two standard deviations below the mean for gestational age was associated with significantly higher odds ratios for both fetal and neonatal mortality rates at every gestational age examined (with odds ratios ranging from 7.1 to 10.0 for fetal death and from 3.4 to 9.4 for neonatal death) (Divon et al 1998). Campbell et al (1997) also identified babies who were small for gestational age as a particularly high-risk group for both stillbirth and neonatal death in post-term pregnancies. In their study of 65 796 post-term births in Norway, birthweight less than the 10th centile was associated with a 5.68 relative risk of perinatal death (95% CI 4.37–7.38) compared with birthweight between the 10th and 90th centiles. Clausson et al (1999) showed a similar relationship between small for gestational age babies and perinatal death in post-term pregnancies in a large Swedish study. Among post-term small for gestational age births, the odds ratios were 10.56 (95% CI 6.95–16.05) for stillbirth and 5.00 (95% CI 3.04–8.22) for infant death. When births with congenital malformations were excluded, the risk of infant death decreased considerably.

Earlier Swedish epidemiological work (Bakketeig & Bergsjo 1989) challenges the view that intrauterine growth retardation explains the increase in perinatal mortality after 42 weeks. These authors showed that perinatal mortality differences persist within birthweight groups. For example, among babies weighing 3625–3874 g the perinatal mortality rate increased from 0.9 to 1.3 to 3.4 to 4.4 as the gestational age increased from 40 to 41, 42 and 43 weeks or more, respectively. Campbell et al (1997) showed that birthweight above the 90th centile was protective against perinatal death in post-term pregnancies. Babies who were large for gestational age had a relative risk of 0.51 of perinatal death (95% CI 0.26–1.0) compared with babies between the 10th and 90th centiles.

Perinatal mortality in home births after 42 weeks

In a population-based study of 7002 planned home births in Australia (Bastian et al 1998), 50 perinatal deaths occurred, giving a perinatal mortality rate of 7.1 per 1000. The mortality rate among babies weighing more than 2500 was higher than the national average (relative risk 1.6, 95% CI 1.1–2.4). Seven of 44 (15.9%) perinatal deaths with a known gestational age occurred in post-term pregnancies. Six of these were the result of intrapartum asphyxia.

Neonatal encephalopathy

Babies delivered post-term are at increased risk of neonatal convulsions. In a case–control study of early neonatal seizures in Cardiff babies born during 1970 to 1979, 54 babies with convulsions were identified among 41 144 singleton babies delivered after 37 weeks. Twenty-six of the babies with convulsions were delivered after 41 weeks, giving an odds ratio of 2.7 (95% CI 1.6–4.8) (Minchom et al 1987). In a study of 89 babies with early neonatal seizures born over a 4-year period in Dublin, 27 were delivered after 42 weeks compared with 6 of 89 controls (odds ratio 4.73, 95% CI 2.22–10.05) (Curtis et al 1988).

Cerebral palsy

A proportion of babies with neonatal encephalopathy subsequently develop cerebral palsy. A history of neonatal encephalopathy is accepted as evidence of a predominantly intrapartum origin for cerebral palsy whereas its absence is thought to denote a cerebral insult earlier in the antenatal course. Gaffney et al (1994) examined the obstetric background of 141 children born after 37 weeks, without apparent congenital malformation, who went on to have cerebral palsy. Forty-one children with evidence of neonatal encephalopathy were compared with 100 who showed no evidence of neonatal encephalopathy. In this series, babies with neonatal encephalopathy were more likely to be delivered at 42 weeks or more (odds ratio 3.5, 95% CI 1–12.1). Babies of primiparae, born at 42 weeks or more, were particularly at risk (odds ratio 11.0, 95% CI 1.2–102.5).

Meconium-stained amniotic fluid

Meconium-stained amniotic fluid is rare before 34 weeks' gestation. The incidence of meconium-stained amniotic fluid increases as pregnancy advances, reaching approximately 30% at 40 weeks and 50% at 42 weeks (Meis et al 1978, Miller & Read 1981, Steer et al 1989). This common finding is not a specific indicator of fetal hypoxia, however there is good evidence that cord arterial pH is lower in babies who show fetal heart rate abnormalities with meconium-stained fluid than in cases of fetal heart rate abnormalities with clear liquor (Steer et al 1989). Meconium-stained amniotic fluid occurred in 9 of 11 intrapartum and neonatal deaths in Crowley's (1989) series of deaths in association with post-term pregnancy. Meconium aspiration syndrome is increased in post-term pregnancy (Grausz & Heimler 1983, O'Herlihy & Robson 1993, Clausson et al 1999).

Fetal distress

Fetal distress is an imprecise term and reports of gestation-specific incidences may be biased. The large Norwegian Birth Registry study (Campbell et al 1997) recorded a 1.68 (95% CI 1.62–1.72) relative risk of fetal distress, and this has also been reported elsewhere (Klapholz & Friedman 1977, Grausz & Heimler 1983). The increased risk of fetal distress in post-term versus term babies persisted after stratification for size for gestational age; however, the absolute risk increased as size for gestational age fell.

Other complications of labour

Dystocia, shoulder dystocia and obstetric trauma are all increased in post-term pregnancy (Campbell et al 1997). Here the risks increase with increasing fetal weight, but gestational age remains a risk factor independent of birthweight. In a case-matched study of 285 women with uncomplicated singleton post-term pregnancy and spontaneous onset of labour and 855 women with uncomplicated singleton term pregnancy, Luckas et al (1998) showed that caesarean section was significantly more common in women with post-term pregnancy (relative risk (RR) 1.90, 95% CI 1.29–2.85). The increase was equally distributed between caesarean sections performed for failure to progress in labour (RR 1.74, 95% CI 1.02–3.04) and fetal distress (RR 2.00, 95% CI 1.14–3.61). Again, the possibility of bias in management arising from the knowledge that a pregnancy is post-term cannot be excluded as a factor in the increase in caesarean section rates.

MANAGEMENT OF POST-TERM PREGNANCY

Assuming that the increased risks of adverse outcomes associated with post-term pregnancy are genuine effects and not epidemiological artefacts, obstetricians can respond in a number of ways. Options include induction at term to prevent pregnancies reaching 42 weeks, routine induction at 42 weeks (or shortly before), and selective induction at 42 weeks in cases identified by tests as being at risk of adverse outcome. Fortunately, the benefits and hazards of some of these strategies have been evaluated in randomised controlled trials. Randomised or quasi-random trials comparing elective induction at term versus expectant management and elective induction after 41 weeks versus monitoring of post-term pregnancies were identified using the search strategy described by the Cochrane Pregnancy and Childbirth Group (Crowley 1999) and formed the basis of a systematic review of management options in post-term pregnancy (Crowley 1999). The main outcomes of interest are those already identified in the analysis of post-term pregnancy risks, namely perinatal mortality, neonatal encephalopathy, meconium-stained amniotic fluid, and caesarean section. In addition, evidence was sought relating to the effect of the various management options on maternal satisfaction.

Induction at or before 40 weeks

Pre-emptive induction of labour, where women with uncomplicated pregnancies were routinely offered induction at or before 40 weeks, was practised in some obstetric units in some countries in the 1970s. Six randomised trials compare a policy of routine induction at 39 weeks (Cole et al 1975, Martin et al 1978), or 40 weeks (Tylleskar et al 1979, Breart et al 1982, Sande et al 1983, Egarter et al 1989) with either expectant management of an indefinite duration or expectant management until 42 weeks' gestation. These trials reveal no evidence of any major benefit or risk to routine induction at 40 weeks. Two perinatal deaths of normally formed babies occurred in the expectant arm of these trials and none in the induction arm. Obviously, this is not a significant difference. There was no effect on caesarean section (odds ratio 0.60, 95% CI 0.35–1.03), instrumental delivery or use of analgesia in labour. Not surprisingly, given the relationship between gestational age and meconium staining of the amniotic fluid in labour, induction around 40 weeks reduces the incidence of meconium staining in labour (odds ratio 0.50, 95% CI 0.31–0.86). Unfortunately, the authors of these trials did not address the important question of women's views of induction of labour at this stage of pregnancy. The authors of these trials missed a golden opportunity in failing to measure women's satisfaction with their care.

Induction after 41 weeks

Perinatal outcomes

Fourteen trials, involving 6284 women, were identified in which induction of labour after 41 weeks' gestation is compared with expectant management using a variety of tests to monitor the post-term pregnancy (Henry 1969, Katz et al 1983, Suikkari et al 1983, Cardozo et al 1986, Augensen et al 1987, Dyson et al 1987, Witter & Weitz 1987, Bergsjo et al 1989, Martin et al 1989, Heden et al 1991, Hannah et al 1992, Herabutya et al 1992, NICHD 1994, Roach & Rogers 1997). The trial conducted by Hannah et al (1992) is much larger than all other trials and contributes considerable weight to the meta-analysis. A systematic review of these trials indicates that induction of labour is associated with some benefits (Table 32.3). There is a reduced risk of perinatal death in normally formed babies (odds ratio 0.23, 95% CI 0.06–0.90). The incidence of meconium-stained amniotic fluid is reduced (odds ratio 0.73, 95% CI 0.65–0.83) but this does not affect the rate of meconium aspiration (odds ratio 0.82, 95% CI 0.49–1.37). There is no effect on fetal heart rate abnormalities during labour. Induction increases the rate of neonatal jaundice (odds ratio 3.39, 95% CI 1.42–8.09), although this finding is based on a small number of trials.

Maternal outcomes

The systematic review provides good evidence that induction of labour after 41 weeks' gestation does not increase the

Table 32.3 Perinatal deaths in trials of routine versus selective induction of labour in post-term pregnancy

Before 41 weeks					
Breart et al 1982	0/481	0/235		0.0	Not estimable
Cole et al 1975	0/118	0/119		0.0	Not estimable
Egarter et al 1989	0/188	1/168		10.0	0.12 (0.00,6.09)
Martin et al 1978	0/131	1/134		10.0	0.14 (0.00,6.98)
Sande et al 1983	0/76	0/90		0.0	Not estimable
Tylleskar et al 1979	0/57	0/55		0.0	Not estimable
Subtotal (95% CI)	0/1051	2/801		20.0	0.13 (0.01,2.07)
Chi-square 0.00 (df=1) Z=1.45					
After 41 weeks					
Augensen et al 1987	0/214	0/195		0.0	Not estimable
Bergsjo et al 1989	0/94	1/94		10.0	0.14 (0.00,6.82)
Cardozo et al 1986	0/195	1/207		10.0	0.14 (0.00,7.24)
Dyson et al 1987	0/152	1/150		10.0	0.13 (0.00,6.73)
Hannah et al 1992	0/1701	2/1706		20.0	0.14 (0.01,2.17)
Heden et al 1991	0/109	0/129		0.0	Not estimable
Henry 1969	0/55	2/57		19.9	0.14 (0.01,2.23)
Herabutya et al 1992	0/57	0/51		0.0	Not estimable
Katz et al 1983	1/78	0/78		10.0	7.39 (0.15,372.41)
Martin et al 1989	0/12	0/10		0.0	Not estimable
NICH 1994	0/235	0/175		0.0	Not estimable
Suikkari et al 1983	0/66	0/53		0.0	Not estimable
Witter & Weitz 1987	0/103	0/97		0.0	Not estimable
Subtotal (95% CI)	1/3071	7/3002		80.0	0.23 (0.06,0.90)
Chi-square 3.48 (df=5) Z=2.10					
Total (95% CI)	1/4122	9/3803		100.0	0.20 (0.06,0.70)
Chi-square 3.61 (df=7) Z=2.53					

caesarean section rate (Table 32.4). The typical odds ratio of 0.86 (CI 0.76–0.98) is actually compatible with a reduction in the risk of caesarean section. This result is weighted by the reduced risk of caesarean section in the Hannah et al (1992) trial where women in the induction arm had a lower rate of caesarean section (5.7%) for fetal distress than those allocated to expectant management (8.3%). The reduced rate of caesarean section associated with induction of labour appeared to contradict a traditionally held view among obstetricians that induction of labour increases the likelihood of delivery by caesarean section, and so a number of secondary analyses were carried out. These showed that induction of labour after 41 weeks of pregnancy does not increase the caesarean section rate, irrespective of parity, cervical ripeness, method of induction or ambient caesarean section rates.

Women's views of induction for post-term pregnancy

It is regrettable that randomised trials give little information on women's views of induction versus conservative management. Only one trial assessed maternal satisfaction with induction of labour (Cardozo et al 1986). These authors showed that satisfaction was related to the eventual outcome of labour and delivery, rather than to the mode of onset of labour. Women's views are likely to be influenced by the local culture, by the attitude of their caregivers, and by practical considerations such as the duration of paid maternity leave. Few obstetricians, midwives or childbirth educators are capable of giving women unbiased information about the risks of post-term pregnancy and the benefits and hazards of induction of labour. In a prospective questionnaire study of women's attitudes towards induction of labour for post-term

Table 32.4 Caesarean section in trials of routine versus selective induction of labour in post-term pregnancy

Before 41 weeks					
Breart et al 1982	10/481	16/235		42.6	0.26 (0.11,0.60)
Cole et al 1975	5/118	9/119		25.4	0.55 (0.19,1.62)
Egarter et al 1989	2/188	3/168		9.5	0.59 (0.10,3.48)
Martin et al 1978	4/106	1/124		9.4	4.01 (0.68,23.65)
Sande et al 1983	4/76	1/90		9.3	4.11 (0.69,24.38)
Tylleskar et al 1979	1/57	1/55		3.8	0.96 (0.06,15.62)
Subtotal (95% CI)	26/1026	31/791		100.0	0.60 (0.35,1.03)
Chi-square 12.92 (df=5) Z=1.86					
After 41 weeks					
Augensen et al 1987	14/214	20/195		3.3	0.61 (0.30,1.24)
Bergsjo et al 1989	27/94	39/94		4.6	0.57 (0.32,1.04)
Cardozo et al 1986	25/195	20/207		4.3	1.37 (0.74,2.55)
Dyson et al 1987	22/152	41/150		5.3	0.46 (0.26,0.80)
Hannah et al 1992	360/1701	418/1706		63.8	0.83 (0.71,0.97)
Heden et al 1991	10/109	9/129		1.9	1.35 (0.53,3.44)
Henry 1969	0/55	1/57		0.1	0.14 (0.00,7.07)
Herabutya et al 1992	27/57	24/51		2.9	1.01 (0.48,2.15)
Katz et al 1983	16/78	7/78		2.1	2.49 (1.03,6.02)
Martin et al 1989	3/12	1/10		0.4	2.62 (0.31,21.94)
NICH 1994	55/235	32/175		7.1	1.36 (0.84,2.19)
Witter & Weitz 1987	30/103	27/97		4.3	1.07 (0.58,1.97)
Subtotal (95% CI)	589/3005	639/2949		100.0	0.87 (0.77,0.99)
Chi-square 22.40 (df=11) Z=2.14					
In women with Bishop score of ≤ 6					
Dyson et al 1987	22/152	41/150		29.9	0.46 (0.26,0.80)
Herabutya et al 1992	27/57	24/51		16.2	1.01 (0.48,2.15)
Katz et al 1983	16/78	7/78		11.6	2.49 (1.03,6.02)
Martin et al 1989	3/12	1/10		2.0	2.62 (0.31,21.94)
NICH 1994	55/235	32/175		40.1	1.36 (0.84,2.19)
Subtotal (95% CI)	123/534	105/464		100.0	1.02 (0.75,1.38)
Chi-square 13.98 (df=4) Z=0.13					
In primigravidae					
Breart et al 1982	18/293	15/139		4.6	0.52 (0.24,1.11)
Cardozo et al 1986	13/18	95/107		1.3	0.25 (0.06,1.05)
Dyson et al 1987	21/106	38/110		7.5	0.48 (0.26,0.87)
Egarter et al 1989	1/99	3/88		0.7	0.32 (0.04,2.32)
Hannah et al 1992	329/1153	381/1155		85.6	0.81 (0.68,0.97)
Tylleskar et al 1979	1/20	1/18		0.3	0.90 (0.05,14.96)
Subtotal (95% CI)	383/1689	533/1617		100.0	0.75 (0.64,0.88)
Chi-square 6.84 (df=5) Z=3.48					

In multigravidae

			Weight	OR (95% CI)
Breart et al 1982	4/188	2/96	6.0	1.02 (0.19,5.63)
Cardozo et al 1986	12/100	2/100	14.9	4.61 (1.56,13.63)
Dyson et al 1987	1/46	3/40	4.4	0.31 (0.04,2.26)
Egarter et al 1989	1/81	0/77	1.1	7.03 (0.14,354.91)
Hannah et al 1992	31/548	37/551	72.5	0.83 (0.51,1.36)
Tylleskar et al 1979	1/89	0/80	1.1	6.68 (0.13,338.47)
Subtotal (95% CI)	50/1052	44/944	100.0	1.09 (0.72,1.66)

Chi-square 11.20 (df=5) Z=0.41

In women induced with prostaglandin

			Weight	OR (95% CI)
Cardozo et al 1986	25/195	20/207	5.1	1.37 (0.74,2.55)
Dyson et al 1987	22/152	41/150	6.4	0.46 (0.26,0.80)
Egarter et al 1989	2/188	3/168	0.6	0.59 (0.10,3.48)
Hannah et al 1992	360/1701	418/1706	77.1	0.83 (0.71,0.97)
Herabutya et al 1992	27/57	24/51	3.5	1.01 (0.48,2.15)
NICH 1994	39/174	32/175	7.3	1.29 (0.77,2.17)
Subtotal (95% CI)	475/2467	538/2457	100.0	0.85 (0.74,0.98)

Chi-square 9.94 (df=5) Z=2.29

In women induced with oxytocin

			Weight	OR (95% CI)
Augensen et al 1987	14/214	20/195	13.2	0.61 (0.30,1.24)
Bergsjo et al 1989	27/94	39/94	18.2	0.57 (0.32,1.04)
Breart et al 1982	10/481	16/235	9.4	0.26 (0.11,0.60)
Cole et al 1975	5/118	9/119	5.6	0.55 (0.19,1.62)
Heden et al 1991	10/109	9/129	7.4	1.35 (0.53,3.44)
Henry 1969	0/55	1/57	0.4	0.14 (0.00,7.07)
Katz et al 1983	16/78	7/78	8.4	2.49 (1.03,6.02)
Martin et al 1978	4/106	1/124	2.1	4.01 (0.68,23.65)
NICH 1994	16/91	32/175	15.1	0.95 (0.49,1.84)
Sande et al 1983	4/76	1/90	2.1	4.11 (0.69,24.38)
Tylleskar et al 1979	1/57	1/55	0.8	0.96 (0.06,15.62)
Witter & Weitz 1987	30/103	27/97	17.3	1.07 (0.58,1.97)
Subtotal (95% CI)	137/1582	163/1446	100.0	0.84 (0.65,1.08)

Chi-square 24.93 (df=11) Z=1.34

In trials where caesarean section rate was <10%

			Weight	OR (95% CI)
Augensen et al 1987	14/214	20/195	39.2	0.61 (0.30,1.24)
Cole et al 1975	5/118	9/119	16.6	0.55 (0.19,1.62)
Egarter et al 1989	2/188	3/168	6.2	0.59 (0.10,3.48)
Heden et al 1991	10/109	9/129	21.9	1.35 (0.53,3.44)
Henry 1969	0/55	1/57	1.3	0.14 (0.00,7.07)
Martin et al 1978	4/106	1/124	6.1	4.01 (0.68,23.65)
Sande et al 1983	4/76	1/90	6.1	4.11 (0.69,24.38)
Tylleskar et al 1979	1/57	1/55	2.5	0.96 (0.06,15.62)
Subtotal (95% CI)	40/923	45/937	100.0	0.89 (0.58,1.39)

Chi-square 9.23 (df=7) Z=0.49

In trials where caesarean section rate was >10%

			Weight	OR (95% CI)
Bergsjo et al 1989	27/94	39/94	4.8	0.57 (0.32,1.04)
Cardozo et al 1986	25/195	20/207	4.5	1.37 (0.74,2.55)
Dyson et al 1987	22/152	41/150	5.6	0.46 (0.26,0.80)
Hannah et al 1992	360/1701	418/1706	67.3	0.83 (0.71,0.97)
Herabutya et al 1992	27/57	24/51	3.0	1.01 (0.48,2.15)
Katz et al 1983	16/78	7/78	2.2	2.49 (1.03,6.02)
Martin et al 1969	3/12	1/10	0.4	2.62 (0.31,21.94)
NICH 1994	55/235	32/175	7.5	1.36 (0.84,2.19)
Witter & Weitz 1987	30/103	27/97	4.6	1.07 (0.58,1.97)
Subtotal (95% CI)	565/2627	609/2568	100.0	0.87 (0.77,1.00)

Chi-square 19.79 (df=8) Z=1.99

pregnancy, Roberts & Young (1991) found that, despite a stated obstetric preference for conservative management, only 45% of women at 37 weeks' gestation were agreeable to conservative management if undelivered by 41 weeks. Of those actually undelivered by 41 weeks' gestation only 31% still desired conservative management. This significant decrease was unaffected by parity or certainty of gestational age. In a subsequent study, Roberts et al (1994) offered women a choice between induction and conservative management at 42 weeks. Forty-five per cent of women opted for conservative management. In both studies, therefore, the majority of women opted for induction of labour.

Tests of fetal well-being in prolonged pregnancy

Women who opt for conservative management of post-term pregnancy are generally advised to participate in some form of fetal assessment while awaiting spontaneous onset of labour. A non-reassuring test usually provokes delivery. In the earlier randomised controlled trials, women allocated to conservative management were monitored with amnioscopy or urinary oestriol measurement. The protocol in recently published trials usually offered cardiotocography and either ultrasound assessment of amniotic fluid volume or a biophysical profile score. This is typical of current clinical practice. The intervals between tests varied between 3 and 7 days. No currently used method of monitoring post-term pregnancy is backed up by good evidence of effectiveness. There is observational evidence to suggest that post-term pregnancies at high risk of adverse outcome can be identified by these tests but little evidence to prove that their use improves outcome.

Ultrasound assessment of amniotic fluid

Ultrasound monitoring of amniotic fluid volume was first described in 1980 when a subjective classification of normal, reduced or absent amniotic fluid was described based on the presence or absence of echo-free space between the fetal limbs and the fetal trunk or the uterine wall (Crowley 1980). In order to test the value of the classification, 150 patients with pregnancies of 42 weeks or greater duration underwent ultrasound examination in the 48 hours prior to delivery. The patients classified as having reduced or absent amniotic fluid had a statistically significant excess incidence of meconium-stained liquor, fetal acidosis, birth asphyxia and meconium aspiration. Manning et al (1981) described a semi-quantitative method based on the largest vertical pool of amniotic fluid and used a 1 cm pool depth as the cut-off for intervention in a population of babies with suspected growth retardation. This was subsequently modified to 2 cm to improve detection of the growth-retarded infant (Chamberlain et al 1984). Crowley et al (1980) found an increase in adverse outcomes in post-term pregnancies where the maximum pool depth was less than 3 cm. Fischer et al (1993) found that a maximum vertical pool of less than 2.7 cm was the best predictor of abnormal perinatal outcome.

Phelan et al (1987) described the 'amniotic fluid index' which is the sum of the maximum pool depth in four quadrants. Fischer et al (1993) found that maximum pool depth performed better than amniotic index in predicting adverse

outcomes in post-term pregnancies. Alfirevic et al (1997) randomly allocated women with post-term pregnancy to monitoring using either maximum pool depth or amniotic index. Both groups underwent computerised fetal heart rate monitoring every three days in addition to amniotic fluid measurements. The threshold for intervention was a maximum pool depth of less than 1.8 cm or an amniotic fluid index of less than 7.3 cm. These figures had been identified as the 3rd centiles for the local population. The number of women found to have an abnormal amniotic fluid index was significantly higher than the number found to have an abnormal maximum pool depth, and more women underwent induction of labour in the amniotic fluid index arm of the trial. There were no perinatal deaths and no statistically significant differences in perinatal outcome between the two groups.

Biophysical profile

One randomised controlled trial (Alfirevic & Walkinshaw 1995) compares monitoring of prolonged pregnancy using a modified biophysical profile score (consisting of computerised cardiotocography, amniotic fluid index and the rest of the components of the conventional biophysical profile) with simple monitoring using cardiotocography and measurement of amniotic fluid depth. The more complex method of monitoring post-term pregnancy is more likely to yield an abnormal result, but does not improve pregnancy outcome as evidenced by umbilical cord pH. This is the only one of four trials (Manning et al 1984, Platt et al 1985, Nageotte et al 1994, Alfirevic & Walkinshaw 1995) comparing biophysical profile scoring with other forms of monitoring to deal exclusively with post-term pregnancy. A systematic review (Alfirevic & Neilson 1999) of these trials yields insufficient data to show that biophysical profile measurement is better than any other method of antenatal monitoring. Observational studies indicate that low biophysical scores identify babies at higher risk of adverse outcome (Manning et al 1985). Evidence of ability to predict adverse outcome must not be interpreted as proof of the ability to prevent these outcomes. An observational study of biophysical profile scoring in the management of prolonged pregnancy showed that the 32/293 women who had abnormal biophysical profiles had significantly higher rates of neonatal morbidity, caesarean section for fetal distress and meconium aspiration than the women with reassuring biophysical profiles (Johnson et al 1986).

Cardiotocography

Antenatal cardiotocography has been widely used for more than 20 years to monitor pregnancies at moderate to high risk. Observational studies have reported very low rates of perinatal loss in high-risk pregnancies monitored in this way (Keegan & Paul 1980, Mendenhall et al 1980). Four randomised controlled trials comparing cardiotocography (CTG) with other methods of antepartum fetal monitoring (Brown et al 1982, Flynn et al 1982, Kidd et al 1985, Lumley et al 1993) were the subject of a systematic review (Pattison & McCowan 1999). Women with post-term pregnancy were included in these trials. On the basis of the information presented in this review, the antenatal CTG has no significant effect on perinatal outcome or interventions such as early elective delivery. Miyazaki and Miyazaki (1981) reported a series of 125 women with post-term pregnancies where a reactive CTG was recorded within one week of delivery. Ten adverse outcomes were reported from this group: four antepartum deaths, one neonatal death, one case of neonatal encephalopathy and four cases of fetal distress on admission in early labour. The poor performance of antenatal cardiotocography in this series and in the randomised trials may relate to errors in interpretation or excessive intervals between tests (a normal cardiotocogram provides only short-term reassurance about fetal well-being, probably 24 hours at most and often less). Numerical analysis using computerised calculations of the baseline rate and variability may reduce the potential for human error (Dawes et al 1991).

Fetal movement counting

Fetal movement counting is another test used commonly in the supervision of post-term pregnancies that is not backed up by firm evidence of efficacy. Two randomised trials have addressed the question of whether clinical actions taken on the basis of fetal movement improve fetal outcome (Neldam 1980, Grant et al 1989). The larger of these trials involved over 68 000 women. These trials collectively provide evidence that routine formal fetal movement counting does not reduce the incidence of intrauterine fetal death in late pregnancy. Routine counting results in more frequent reports of diminished fetal activity, with a greater use of other techniques of fetal assessment, more frequent admission to hospital and an increased rate of elective delivery. It may be that fetal movement counting in post-term pregnancy will perform more effectively than it does in low-risk pregnancies. Women will be required to pay extra attention to fetal movements for less than one week in the majority of cases and will usually be attending at intervals of three days for other tests.

Perinatal deaths in the randomised trials

The eight perinatal deaths that occurred among women in the randomised trials of induction versus conservative management provide a small amount of additional anecdotal evidence concerning the sensitivity of the tests used to monitor expectantly managed post-term pregnancies. Seven of the deaths occurred in those allocated to expectant management. Two deaths in the Hannah et al (1992) trial occurred despite adherence to the monitoring protocol of daily movement counting and three times weekly cardiotocography and ultrasound assessment of amniotic fluid volume. These babies were both relatively small, weighing 2600 g and 3175 g. In the Dyson et al (1987) trial, a neonatal death from meconium aspiration occurred in a 43-week baby delivered for acute fetal bradycardia during spontaneous labour. Fetal heart rate monitoring and ultrasound assessment of amniotic fluid had been reassuring 48 hours before the spontaneous onset of labour. One of the deaths in the Henry (1969) trial was attributed to gestational diabetes. The second occurred due to fetal meconium aspiration in a woman who refused induction following detection of meconium at amnioscopy. The deaths in the Bergsjo et al (1989) and the Cardozo et al (1986) trials, due to pneumonia and abruptio placentae

respectively, are unlikely to be related to the method of fetal monitoring used. One normal baby in the induction arm of these trials (Katz et al 1983) died from asphyxia following emergency caesarean section in labour for meconium-stained amniotic fluid and prolonged bradycardia.

CONCLUSIONS

Effective management of post-term pregnancy begins at booking. Where resources allow it, routine early pregnancy ultrasound should be provided for all consenting women and the expected date of delivery should be based on the ultrasound measurements (Gardosi & Geirsson 1998, Neilson 1999). At 41 weeks' gestation, based on this early ultrasound examination, women should be offered an assessment by a consultant obstetrician. Prior to this consultation, women should have access to a brief patient information document summarising the key points of current evidence in relation to post-term pregnancy management.

Assessment by the consultant obstetrician should begin with a careful review of the dates and supporting ultrasound evidence with documentation of any risk factors such as a caesarean section scar, gestational diabetes or hypertensive disease. An ultrasound assessment of amniotic fluid and fetal abdominal circumference should be performed with an emphasis on diagnosing intrauterine growth restriction. Elective delivery should be advised in any case of intrauterine growth restriction in view of the particularly high perinatal mortality in this group of post-term babies (Campbell et al 1997). A vaginal examination to assess the state of the cervix will inform discussions with the woman about management options and facilitate selection of the most appropriate method of induction of labour.

Women should be informed that pregnancy after 41 weeks is associated with a small increased risk of perinatal mortality and that induction of labour may reduce that risk (Crowley 1999). However, up to 500 women may need to undergo induction of labour to prevent one perinatal death. Irrespective of the findings on vaginal examination, women should be informed of the evidence that induction of labour does not increase the likelihood of delivery by caesarean section. Any woman who requests induction of labour after 41 weeks' gestation should have this carried out. Those who wish to wait should be monitored with daily cardiotocography, and ultrasound monitoring of amniotic fluid maximum pool depth at intervals of three days. Computerised cardiotocography should be used if available. Its use may reduce the risk of errors in interpretation of this test. Delivery should be offered in cases where the amniotic fluid maximum vertical pool is less than 2.7 cm. Care should be taken to ensure that this is a cord-free pool. Women with accurate dates opting for conservative management at 42 weeks' gestation should be informed of the high statistical probability of spontaneous labour within a few days. However, they should also be aware that delivery following an abnormal ultrasound assessment or cardiotocogram may be by caesarean section and may be associated with some fetal morbidity.

Current evidence suggests that cervical ripening with PGE_2 gel should be performed in women with unfavourable cervical findings. In view of the high incidence of meconium stained amnotic fluid in post-term pregnancies, early amniotomy is indicated. Electronic fetal heart rate monitoring should be considered in all cases of post-term pregnancy, especially where there is meconium-stained fluid and oligohydramnios. There is growing evidence from randomised trials that amnioinfusion in cases of heavy meconium staining of amniotic fluid during labour will reduce the incidence of meconium aspiration syndrome (Hofmeyr et al 1998, Mahomed et al 1998).

KEY POINTS

- A pregnancy that continues for 294 days or more is considered prolonged (synonyms: post-term, post-dates and postmature).
- The majority of prolonged pregnancies represent the upper end of the range of normal distribution; they tend to repeat in subsequent pregnancies.
- Perinatal mortality is increased in prolonged pregnancy despite the fact that prolonged pregnancies may represent an otherwise low-risk population as many pregnancies with problems will have ended before 41 weeks.
- Evidence from randomised trials indicate that induction of labour is assiciated with a reduced risk of perinatal death with no effect on the risk of caesarean section.

REFERENCES

Alfirevic Z, Neilson JP 1999 Biophysical profile for fetal assessment in high risk pregnancies (Cochrane Review). In: The Cochrane Library, Issue 1, 1999. Update Software, Oxford

Alfirevic Z, Walkinshaw SA 1995 A randomised controlled trial of simple compared with complex antenatal fetal monitoring after 42 weeks of gestation. Br J Obstet Gynaecol 102:638–643

Alfirevic Z, Luckas M, Walkinshaw SA, McFarlane M, Curran R 1997 A randomised comparison between amniotic fluid index and maximum pool depth in the monitoring of post-term pregnancy. Br J Obstet Gynaecol 104:207–211

Augensen K, Bergsjo P, Eikeland T, Ashvik K, Carlsen J 1987 Randomized comparison of early versus late induction of labour in post-term pregnancy. BMJ 294:1192–1195

Bakketeig L, Bergsjo P 1989 Post-term pregnancy: magnitude of the problem. In: Chalmers I, Enkin M, Keirse MJNC (eds) Effective care in pregnancy and childbirth. Oxford University Press, Oxford, pp 765–775

Bastian H, Keirse MJ, Lancaster PA 1998 Perinatal death associated with planned home birth in Australia: a population based study. BMJ 317:384–388

Bergsjo P, Gui-dan H, Su-qin Y, Zhi-zeng G, Bakketeig LS 1989 Comparison of induced vs non-induced labor in post-term pregnancy. Acta Obstet Gynecol Scand 68:683–687

Bierman T, Siegel E, French F, Simonian K 1965 Analysis of the outcome of all pregnancies in a community. Am J Obstet Gynecol 91:37–45

Bjerkdal T, Bakketeig LS 1975 Medical registration of births in Norway during the 5-year period 1967–71. Time trends and differences between counties and municipalities. Institute of Hygiene and Social Medicine, University of Bergen, Bergen, Norway, p 71

Breart G, Goujard J, Maillard F, Chavigny C, Rumeau-Rouquette C, Sureau C 1982 Comparison of two obstetrical policies with regard to artificial induction of labour at term. A randomised trial. J Obstet

Biol Reprod (Paris) 11:107–112

Brown VA, Sawers RS, Parsons RJ, Duncan SLB, Cooke JD 1982 The value of antenatal cardiotocography in the management of high risk pregnancy: A randomised controlled trial. Br J Obstet Gynaecol 89:716–722

Butler NR, Bonham DG 1963 Perinatal mortality. Churchill Livingstone, Edinburgh

Campbell MK, Ostbye T, Irgens LM 1997 Post-term birth: risk factors and outcomes in a 10-year cohort of Norwegian births. Obstet Gynecol 89:543–548

Cardozo L, Fysh J, Pearce JM 1986 Prolonged pregnancy: the management debate. BMJ 293:1059–1063

Chamberlain PF, Manning FA, Morrison I, Harman CR, Lange IR 1984 Ultrasound evaluation of amniotic fluid volume. 1. The relationship of marginal and decreased amniotic fluid volumes to perinatal outcome. Am J Obstet Gynecol 150:245–249

Chamberlain R, Chamberlain G, Howlett B, Masters K 1978 British births 1970, vol 2. Obstetric care. Heinemann Medical, London

Clausson B, Cnattingius S, Axelsson O 1999 Outcomes of post-term births: the role of fetal growth restriction and malformations. Obstet Gynecol 94:758–762

Clifford SH 1954 Postmaturity with placental dysfunction. Clinical syndrome and pathological findings. J Pediatr 44:1–13

Cole RA, Howie PW, MacNaughton MC 1975 Elective induction of labour. A randomised prospective trial. Lancet 1:767–770

Crowley P 1980 Non quantitative estimation of amniotic fluid volume in suspected prolonged pregnancy. J Perinat Med 8:249–251

Crowley P 1989 Post-term pregnancy: induction or surveillance? In: Chalmers I, Enkin M, Keirse MJNC (eds) Effective care in pregnancy and childbirth. Oxford University Press, Oxford, 1989, pp 776–791

Crowley P 1999 Interventions for preventing or improving the outcome of delivery at or beyond term (Cochrane Review). In: The Cochrane Library, Issue 1, 1999. Update Software, Oxford

Crowley P, O'Herlihy C, Boylan P 1980 The value of ultrasound measurement of amniotic fluid volume in the management of prolonged pregnancies. Br J Obstet Gynaecol 91:444–448

Curtis P, Matthews T, Crowley P et al The Dublin Collaborative Seizure Study 1988: Do early neonatal seizures indicate quality of perinatal care? Arch Dis Child 63:1065–1068

Dawes GS, Moullden M, Redman CWG 1991 System 8000: Computerised antenatal FHR analysis. J Perinant Med 19:47–51

Divon MY, Haglund B, Nisell H, Otterblad PO, Westgren M 1998 Fetal and neonatal mortality in the postterm pregnancy: the impact of gestational age and fetal growth restriction. Am J Obstet Gynecol 178:726–731

Dyson D, Miller PD, Armstrong MA 1987 Management of prolonged pregnancy: induction of labour versus antepartum testing. Am J Obstet Gynecol 156:928–934

Egarter CH, Kofler E, Fitz R, Husselein P 1989 Is induction of labour indicated in prolonged pregnancy? Results of a prospective randomised trial. Gynecol Obstet Invest 27:6–9

Fabre E, Gonzalez de Aguero R, de Agustin JL, Tajada M, Repolles S, Sanz A 1996 Perinatal mortality in term and post-term births. J Perinat Med 24:163–169

Fischer RL, McDonnell M, Bianculli RN, Perry RL, Hediger ML, Scholl TO 1993 Amniotic fluid volume estimation in the postdate pregnancy: A comparison of techniques. Obstet Gynecol 81:698–704

Flynn A, Kelly J, Mansfield H, Needham P, O'Conor M, Viegas O 1982 A randomized controlled trial of non-stress antepartum cardiotocography. Br J Obstet Gynaecol 89:427–433

Gaffney G, Flavell V, Johnson A, Squier M, Sellers S 1994 Cerebral palsy and neonatal encephalopathy. Arch Dis Child 70:F195–200

Gardosi J, Geirsson R 1998 Routine ultrasound is the method of choice for dating pregnancy. Br J Obstet Gynaecol 105:933–936

Gardosi J, Vanner T, Francis A 1997 Gestational age and induction of labour for prolonged pregnancy. Br J Obstet Gynaecol 104:792–797

Grammatopoulis D, Hillhouse E 1999 Role of corticotropin releasing hormone in onset of labour. Lancet 354:1546–1549

Grant A, Elbourne D, Valentin L, Alexander S 1989 Routine formal fetal movement counting and risk of antepartum late death in normally formed singletons. Lancet 8659:345–349

Grausz JP, Heimler R 1983 Asphyxia and gestational age. Obstet Gynecol 62:175–179

Hannah ME, Hannah WJ, Hellman J, Hewson S, Milner R, Willan A 1992 Canadian Multicenter Post-Term Pregnancy Trial Group. Induction of labour as compared with serial antenatal monitoring in post-term pregnancy. A randomized controlled trial. N Engl J Med 326:1587–1592

Heden L, Ingemarsson I, Ahlstrom H, Solum T 1991 Induction of labor vs conservative management in prolonged pregnancy: controlled study. Int J Feto-maternal Med 4:148–152

Henriksen TB, Wilcox AT, Hedegaard M, Secher NJ 1995 Bias in studies of preterm and postterm delivery due to ultrasound assessment of gestational age. Epidemiology 6:533–537

Henry GR 1969 A controlled trial of surgical induction of labour and amnioscopy in the management of prolonged pregnancy. J Obstet Gynaecol Br Commonwealth 76:795–798

Herabutya Y, Prasertsawat PO, Tongyai T, Isarangura N, Ayudthya N 1992 Prolonged pregnancy: the management dilemma. Int J Gynaecol Obstet 37:253–258

Hilder L, Costeloe K, Thilaganathan B 1998 Prolonged pregnancy: evaluating gestation-specific risks of fetal and infant mortality. Br J Obstet Gynaecol 105:169–173

Hofmeyr GJ, Gulmezoglu AM, Buchmann E et al 1998 The Collaborative Randomised Amnioinfusion for Meconium Project (CRAMP): 1. South Africa. Br J Obstet Gynaecol 105:304–308

Ingemarsson I, Kallen K 1997 Stillbirths and rate of neonatal deaths in 76,761 postterm pregnancies in Sweden, 1982–1991: a register study. Acta Obstet Gynecol Scand 76:658–662

Johnson JM, Harman CR, Lange IR, Manning F 1986 Biophysical scoring in the management of the postterm pregnancy: An analysis of 307 patients. Am J Obstet Gynecol 154:269–273

Katz Z, Yemini M, Lancet M, Mogilner BM, Ben-Hur H, Caspi B 1983 Non-aggressive management of post-date pregnancies. Eur J Obstet Gynecol Reprod Biol 15:71–79

Keegan KA, Paul RH 1980 Antepartum fetal heart rate testing. IV. The non-stress test as the primary approach. Am J Obstet Gynecol 136:75–80

Kidd L, Patel N, Smith R 1985 Non-stress antenatal cardiotocography—a prospective randomized clinical trial. Br J Obstet Gynaecol 92:1156–1159

Klapholz H, Friedman EA 1977 The incidence of intrapartum fetal distress with advancing gestational age. Am J Obstet Gynecol 127:405–407

Lockwood CJ, Moscarelli RD, Wein R, Lynch L, Lapinski RH, Ghidini A 1994 Low concentrations of vaginal fetal fibronectin as a predictor of deliveries occurring after 41 weeks. Am J Obstet Gynecol 171:1–4

Luckas M, Buckett W, Alfirevic Z 1998 Comparison of outcomes in uncomplicated term and post-term pregnancy following spontaneous labor. J Perinat Med 26:475–479

Lumley J, Lester A, Anderson I, Renou P, Wood C 1993 A randomised trial of weekly cardiotocography in high risk obstetric patients. Br J Obstet Gynaecol 90:1018–1026

Mahomed K, Mulambo T, Woelk G, Hofineyr GJ, Gulmezoglu AM 1998 Collaborative Randomised Amnioinfusion for Meconium Project (CRAMP): 2. Zimbabwe. Br J Obstet Gynaecol 105:309–313

Manning FA, Hill LM, Platt LD 1981 Qualitative amniotic fluid volume determination by ultrasound: Antepartum detection of intrauterine growth retardation. Am J Obstet Gynecol 151:304–308

Manning FA, Lange IR, Morrison I, Harman CR 1984 Fetal biophysical profile score and the nonstress test: a comparative trial. Obstet Gynecol 64:326–331

Manning FA, Morrison I, Lange IR, Harman CR, Chamberlain PF 1985 Fetal assessment based upon fetal biophysical profile scoring: experience in 12,620 referred high-risk pregnancies. I Perinatal mortality by frequency and etiology. Am J Obstet Gynecol 151:343–350

Martin DH, Thompson W, Pinkerton JHM, Watson JD 1978 A randomised controlled trial of selective planned delivery. Br J Obstet Gynaecol 85:109–113

Martin JN, Sessums JK, Howard P, Martin RW, Morrison JC 1989 Alternative approaches to the management of gravidas with prolonged post-term postdate pregnancies. J Miss State Med Assoc 30:105–111

Meis P, Hall M, Marshall J, Hobel CJ 1978 Meconium passage: A new classification for risk assessment during labor. Am J Obstet Gynecol 131:509–520

Mendenhall HW, O'Leary J, Phillips KO 1980 The nonstress test: the value of a single acceleration in evaluating the fetus at risk. Am J Obstet Gynecol 136:87–91

Miller FC, Read JA 1981 Intrapartum assessment of the postdate fetus. Am J Obstet Gynecol 141:516–520

Minchom P, Niswander K, Chalmers I et al 1987 Antecedents and outcome of very early neonatal seizures in infants born at or after term. Br J Obstet Gynaecol 94:431–439

Miyazaki FS, Miyazaki BA 1981 False reactive nonstress tests in postterm pregnancies. Am J Obstet Gynecol 140:269–276

Mogren I, Stenlund H, Hogberg U 1999 Recurrence of prolonged pregnancy. Int J Epidemiol 28:253–257

Mongelli M, Wilcox M, Gardosi J 1996 Estimating the date of confinement: ultrasonographic biometry versus certain menstrual dates. Am J Obstet Gynecol 174:278–281

Naeye R 1978 Causes of perinatal mortality excess in prolonged gestation. Am J Epidemiol 108:429–433

Nageotte MP, Towers CV, Asrat T, Freeman RK 1994 Perinatal outcome with the modified biophysical profile. Am J Obstet Gynecol 170:1672–1676

National Institute of Child Health and Human Development Network of Maternal-Fetal Medicine Units 1994 A clinical trial of induction of labor versus expectant management in postterm pregnancy. Am J Obstet Gynecol 170:716–723

Neilson JP 1999 Ultrasound for fetal assessment in early pregnancy (Cochrane Review). In: The Cochrane Library, Issue 1, 1999. Update Software, Oxford

Neldam S 1980 Fetal movement as an indication of fetal wellbeing. Lancet 1:1222–1224

O'Herlihy C, Robson M 1993 The intrapartum risks of prolonged pregnancy and meconium aspiration. In: Spencer JAD, Ward RHT (eds) Intrapartum fetal surveillance. RCOG Press, London, pp 111–125

Pattison N, McCowan L 1999 Cardiotocography for antepartum fetal assessment (Cochrane Review). In: The Cochrane Library, Issue 1, 1999. Update Software, Oxford

Phelan JP, Smith CV, Broussard P, Small M 1987 Amniotic fluid volume assessment with the four quadrant technique at 36–42 weeks' gestation. J Reprod Med 32:540–542

Platt LD, Walla CA, Paul RH, Trujillo ME, Loesser CV, Jacobs ND, Broussard PM 1985 A prospective trial of the fetal biophysical profile vs the nonstress test in the management of high-risk pregnancies. Am J Obstet Gynecol 153:624–633

Roach VJ, Rogers MS 1997 Pregnancy outcome beyond 41 weeks gestation. Int J Gynaecol Obstet 59:19–24

Roberts CL, Taylor Henderson-Smart D 1999 Trends in births at and beyond term: evidence of a change? Br J Obstet Gynaecol 106:937–942

Roberts L, Cook E, Beardsworth SA, Trew G 1994 Prolonged pregnancy: two years experience of offering women conservative management. J Royal Army Medical Corps 140:32–36

Roberts LJ, Young KR 1991 The management of prolonged pregnancy, an analysis of women's attitudes before and after term. Br J Obstet Gynaecol 98:1102–1106

Sande HA, Tuveng J, Fonstelien T 1983 A prospective randomized study of induction of labor. Int J Gynaecol Obstet 21:333–336

Steer P, Eigbe F, Lissauer T, Beard R 1989 Inter-relationships among abnormal cordiotocograms in labor, meconium staining of the amniotic fluid, arterial cord blood pH and Apgar scores. Obstet Gynecol 74:715–721

Suikkari AM, Jalkanen M, Heiskala H, Koskela O 1983 Prolonged pregnancy: induction or observation. Acta Obstet Gynecol Scand Suppl 116:58

Tunon K, Eik-Nes SH, Grottum P 1999 Fetal outcome in pregnancies defined as post-term according to the last menstrual period estimate, but not according to the ultrasound estimate. Ultrasound Obstet Gynecol 14:12–16

Tylleskar J, Finnstrom O, Leijon I, Hedenskog S, Ryden G 1979 Spontaneous labor and elective induction—a prospective randomized study. Effects on mother and fetus. Acta Obstet Gynecol Scand 58:513–518

Witter FR, Weitz CM 1987 A randomised trial of induction at 42 weeks of gestation vs expectant management for postdates pregnancies. Am J Perinatol 4:206–211

World Health Organization 1994 International Classification of Disease. ICD-9CM, 76b.2

Yudkin PL, Wood L, Redman CW 1987 Risk of unexplained stillbirth at different gestational ages. Lancet 8543:1192–1194

33

Cephalopelvic disproportion and abnormal uterine action

Philip J. Steer

The contribution of the author of the equivalent chapter in the second edition, on which this chapter draws extensively, is gratefully acknowledged.

INTRODUCTION

One of the most common questions women ask is why human labour is often difficult and complicated. It is a natural process, and therefore, if the woman is healthy and she has taken all reasonable steps to prepare herself for labour, it is reasonable to expect that birth should be straightforward. Why is this often not the case? The answer may lie in an evolutionary conflict between the need to run and the need to think.

The reasons our ancestors began to walk upright some four million years age can never be known for certain. However, they probably relate to a change in the climate of Africa, where our Australopithecine ancestors lived. Drier seasons meant that dense rainforest gave way to open grasslands. Originally tree dwellers, our ancestors had increasingly to move across open Veldt to move from one area of cover to another. Erect locomotion has a number of advantages—an expanded field of vision (especially in tall grass) and 40% less body area exposed to direct rays of the noon sun are arguably the most important (the need for temperature control also lead to loss of body hair and an increase in sweat gland density). An erect person is also more exposed to cooling breezes, as anyone who has been tempted to sunbathe horizontally on a beach and then had to stand up to cool off can testify.

The Australopithecines, who formed a variety of species from the lightly built *Australopithecus Afarensis* to the heavily built *Australopithecus robustus*, flourished from about four million years ago until about two million years ago. They were probably scavengers and had brains only about the size of a modern chim-

panzee (Johanson et al 1990)—about 450–550 ml. However, their skeleton from the waist down (including the pelvis) was very similar in shape to that of modern homo sapiens, although much smaller—the Australopithecines were only just over a metre tall. Apes give birth comparatively easily because they have large pelvises and their babies' heads at birth are comparatively small compared with the human (Fig. 33.1).

Because there is plenty of room, the fetal head of the apes can go straight through the mother's pelvis during labour, and it emerges with the face anterior so that the mother can readily resuscitate her own baby by clearing its pharynx. When the Australopithecines adapted to the upright posture, an important part of the process was a narrowing of the pelvis so that the forces generated during walking could be transmitted efficiently from the femurs, through the pelvis, to the spine. So long as the fetal head remained small, this could be accommodated, although it did require that the baby be born with the head in the occipito transverse position (Fig. 33.2).

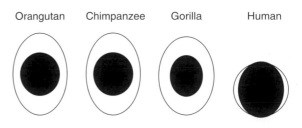

Fig. 33.1   Orangutan, Chimpanzee, Gorilla and Human—relationship of the fetal head to the maternal pelvis.

Chimpanzee   A.L. 288-1   Human

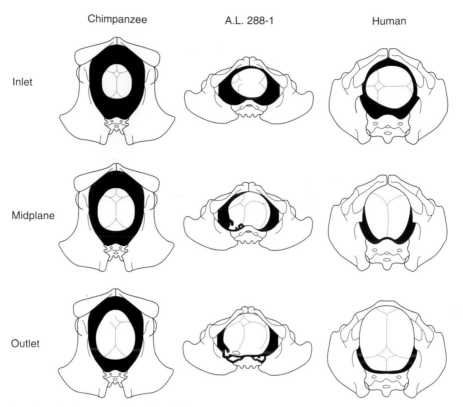

Inlet

Midplane

Outlet

Fig. 33.2 Fetal head passing through the maternal pelvis—Chimpanzee, Australopithecus Afarensis skeleton number A.L. 288-1 (known as 'Lucy') and Human.
Reproduced with permission from: K. Rosenberg and W. Trevethan. Bipedalism and human birth: the obstetrical dilemma revisited. Evolutionary Anthropology 4:161–168, 1996.

The next development was the appearance of *Homo habilis* two million years ago and then *Homo erectus* about 1.5 million years ago. This species was probably a more effective team player, because of the development of a larger brain (500–900 ml), and possibly as a result, spread widely across Africa and even into Asia. The process of brain enlargement continued rapidly, so that in old *Homo sapiens*, *Homo neanderthalis*, and modern man, reaches 1000–2000 ml. This meant babies being born with larger heads, resulting in the relative disproportion seen in Figure 33.1. For the fetus to negotiate the pelvis successfully, rotational birth had to develop (Fig. 33.2).

Mothers can to a large extent regulate the growth of their fetuses so that they are born at a size that will allow birth (Steer 1998a), but babies that are too small (preterm or growth restricted) have problems such as respiratory distress, hypoglycaemia and hypothermia, and they have high perinatal mortality rates. The baby benefits from being big, despite the damage that this can do to the mother's pelvis during birth (Steer 1998b). Thus, the scene is set for a conflict between the interests of the fetus and the mother, the conflict between the advantages of thinking—large brain—and running fast—small pelvis. This conflict has led to many late pregnancy problems, not only difficult birth, but possibly also pre-eclampsia (Haig 1993).

To allow the relatively large fetal head at term to negotiate the mother's pelvis effectively, a number of factors must be operating.

1. The uterus must contract efficiently. Human uterine contractions are much stronger than those of most other mammals, and the uterine muscle is therefore much thicker.
2. The fetal head must mould effectively. The ability of the skull bones to overlap reduces the biparietal diameter substantially, although excessive moulding can damage the brain beneath.
3. The fetal head must move in the correct way through the pelvis. Engagement in the transverse and midcavity flexion of the head with rotation to occipito anterior is the most favourable mechanism, as it minimises the presenting diameters at each level of the pelvis.
4. The diameters of the pelvis must be maximised. This is facilitated by relaxin-induced elasticity of the cartilaginous joints, especially the symphesis pubis (symphesis dysfunction caused by a loose joint, which is painful during locomotion, is a common problem in late pregnancy). Maternal squatting can also increase the pelvic diameter by up to a centimetre.
5. The cervix must give way easily; ripening in later pregnancy is an essential prerequisite for successful labour.

Abnormal uterine action

Uterine action in labour is variously considered to be abnormal if it falls into one of the following categories:

1. *Hypotonic:* too little.
2. *Hypertonic:* too much.
3. *Incoordinate:* abnormal in pattern.
4. *Inefficient:* not associated with progressive cervical dilatation.

Incoordinate contractions (irregular in shape and timing) are probably of no significance unless they are also hypotonic (Seitchik & Chatkoff 1977).

MEASUREMENT OF UTERINE ACTIVITY

The three terms used to describe the main components of a uterine contraction are basal tonus, active pressure (peak pressure above basal tonus) and frequency (Fig. 33.3). True quantification of uterine activity can only be performed by measuring intrauterine pressure with an intrauterine catheter; manual palpation has been shown to be inaccurate at assessing the true active pressure (Arrabal & Nagey 1996). Studies using intrauterine catheters have shown that the best predictor of likely cervical dilatation rates is a combination of the frequency of contractions and the peak active pressure of contractions (maximum intrauterine pressure during a contraction minus baseline tone) (Steer et al 1984). Peak active pressure is more closely related to cervical dilatation rate than the frequency of contractions (Steer et al 1984), whereas the frequency is more strongly associated with fetal oxygenation (Peebles et al 1994).

The reported range of normal baseline tonus varies from 0.8 to 2.6 kPa (5–20 mmHg) depending on the measuring technique used (external pressure transducer connected to a fluid-filled intrauterine catheter or internal catheter-tipped pressure transducer) and the position of the transducer relative to the upper level of amniotic fluid within the uterus (see Ch. 29). Values greater than 3 kPa are likely to represent hypertonus and will compromise maternal blood flow into the placental bed resulting in fetal hypoxia.

A widely used combined measure of overall uterine activity is the Montevideo Unit (MU) (Caldeyro-Barcia et al 1957). This is defined as the mean active pressure of contractions per ten minutes multiplied by the mean frequency. It is most simply calculated by adding up the peak active pressure of each contraction for a ten-minute period (Fig. 33.3). Another widely used measure is the area under the contraction curve above baseline tone, usually called the uterine activity integral (UAI). The SI units for UAI are kiloPascalseconds. 125 MU is approximately equivalent to 1000 kPas/15 min.

NORMAL LEVEL OF UTERINE ACTIVITY IN LABOUR

Uterine action cannot be categorised as hypotonic or hypertonic without knowledge of the normal levels of uterine action. Unfortunately, there is no precise agreement about what constitutes normal. The population mean level of uterine activity depends on the population studied. The selection for study of women progressing rapidly in labour (often described arbitrarily as normal) is likely to result in a higher mean level of observed uterine activity than if a total unselected population sample is studied. This is because the rate of cervical dilatation in labour is proportional to the level of uterine action (Steer et al 1984), and so women selected as having normal (i.e. rapid) rates of cervical dilatation will inevitably have higher levels of uterine activity than the average for the population. The rate of cervical dilatation is also inversely proportional to the resistance to progress, a hypothetical concept which involves pelvic and fetal size, presentation, and consistency of the soft tissues and cervix (Rossavik 1978). For any particular level of uterine activity, the higher the resistance, the slower is the rate of cervical dilatation. Therefore, if women are short and have large babies so that their resistance to progress is high, for a particular level of uterine activity they will have a lower rate of

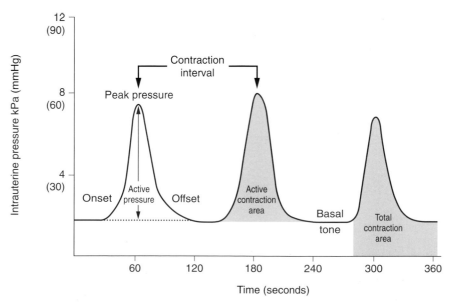

Fig. 33.3 Terminology of uterine contractions.

cervical dilatation than women with less resistance, for example, grand multiparae (Al-Shawaf et al 1987). Therefore, to enable true comparison of results, researchers should quote values of uterine action in relation to groups specified in terms of parity, height, birthweight and rate of cervical dilatation. Most reported studies lack this type of information and, consequently, they are difficult to compare with each other. However, despite their lack of precise comparability, a number of important conclusions can be drawn from the reported data (Fig. 33.4).

Firstly, uterine action increases by about 50% as labour progresses. Secondly, mean uterine activity levels fall somewhere between 1000 and 1500 kPas/15 min or 125–190 MU. Most studies give a similar distribution around the mean value such that the 10th percentile is about 700 kPas/15 min and the 90th percentile is about 1800 kPas/15 min. This translates to between three and five contractions of the average peak active pressure of 40 mmHg per ten minutes. By analogy with other distributions (such as birthweight) where the 10th and 90th percentiles are used as the boundaries of normality, it seems reasonable to designate levels <700 kPas/15 min as hypotonic and >1800 kPas/15 min as hypertonic. This is equivalent to less than 90 MU (e.g. three contractions of 30 mmHg per ten minutes) or more than 225 MU (e.g. five contractions of 45 mmHg per ten minutes).

HYPOTONIC UTERINE ACTIVITY

Most cases of slow progress in labour are associated with hypotonic uterine activity and they are, therefore, likely to respond to oxytocics (Steer et al 1985). This suggests that in most cases there is not an inherent defect in the ability of the uterus to contract but that uterine contractility is at an early stage of its evolution. Such a conclusion is supported by the report of Hemminki et al (1985) who showed that 83% of

women progressing slowly in labour subsequently developed normal levels of uterine activity when managed expectantly (ambulation was encouraged) rather than being given oxytocics. A similar evolution of activity was seen in women progressing slowly in labour and nursed in the lateral recumbent position with epidural anaesthetic rather than being ambulant (Bidgood & Steer 1987).

However, in a few cases, hypotonic uterine activity fails to respond to oxytocics. In some cases, this appears to be because of a deficiency in oxytocin receptors (Fuchs et al 1984, Phaneuf et al 2000). In others it may be because of inhibition by high levels of endogenous adrenaline. Bourne & Burn (1927) noted that 'the effect of emotion appears to be to delay the uterine contractions in labour'. They investigated the effects of injections of adrenaline into labouring patients and demonstrated that the intravenous injection of five minims of adrenaline produced complete cessation of uterine contractions for 12 minutes, following which contractions began again. This foreshadowed the use of sympathomimetics for the treatment of preterm labour.

Mitrani et al (1975) hypothesised that since adrenaline exerts its suppressive effect on uterine activity via the uterine muscle beta-receptors, a beta-blocker such as propranolol could be used to treat hypotonic uterine activity. They treated 10 primigravidae in dysfunctional labour with intravenous propranolol at the rate of 1 mg/min for four minutes. The authors observed a marked increase in uterine activity in all cases; in two cases there was tachysystole with hypertonus sufficient to produce fetal bradycardia.

The active management of labour has been examined in many prospective studies, and the only component that has been shown in meta-analyses to be effective in reducing intervention rates and improving outcome is the presence of a supportive birth partner, or Doula (Hodnett 2000). It may be that such support works by reducing stress and thus bringing about a reduction of beta adrenergic activity.

In relation to the pharmacological augmentation of slow labour, oxytocin remains the only widely used uterine stimulant, although prostaglandins are widely used following prelabour rupture of the membranes. Studies of small doses of misoprostol for the augmentation of labour in the presence of inadequate uterine activity are currently being planned. Induction and augmentation of labour are discussed fully in Chapter 35.

HYPERTONIC UTERINE ACTIVITY

Spontaneous uterine hypercontractility without placental abruption is rare, probably occurring in not more than one in 3000–4000 pregnancies. Most cases of hypoxia in spontaneous labour are a result of intrauterine growth restriction, with consequent inability of the fetus to withstand the normal stress of labour, rather than excessive uterine activity. Nonetheless, cases of excessive uterine activity without obvious causes are sometimes seen. There is no evidence that an unusually high active pressure of contractions (i.e. above 12 kPa) is associated with any clinical problem. However, an increase in the frequency or duration of contractions, or a

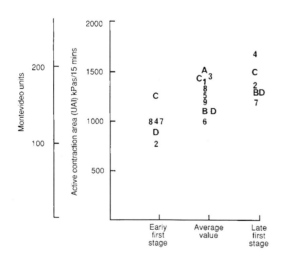

Fig. 33.4 Normal levels of uterine activity in spontaneous labour. 1, Zambrana et al (1960); 2, Poseiro & Noriega-Guerra (1961); 3, Cibils & Hendricks (1965); 4, El Sahwi et al (1967); 5, Krapohl et al (1970); 6, Mendez-Bauer et al (1975); 7, Pontonnier et al (1975); 8, Lindmark & Nilsson (1977); 9, Flynn et al (1978); A, Cowan et al (1982); B, Steer et al (1984); C, Gibb et al (1984); D, Arulkumaran et al (1984).

rise in baseline tone, may all lead to problems with fetal oxygen supply by interfering with blood supply to the maternal intervillous space of the placenta.

Excessive duration of contractions

Figure 33.5 illustrates a case of spontaneous labour where the duration of contractions averaged 120 seconds. Frequency and baseline tone were normal. Figure 33.5a shows small decelerations synchronous with contractions, which became larger two hours later (Fig. 33.5b). After a further two hours (Fig. 33.5c) the decelerations became prolonged and a fetal blood sample showed a pH of 7.15. Delivery was effected by caesarean section as the cervix was still only 6 cm dilated. Frequency and basal tonus remained normal throughout.

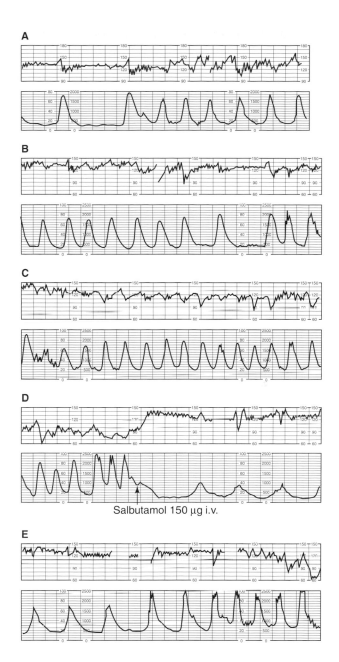

Fig. 33.6 (a)–(e) An example of spontaneous uterine hypercontractility—excessive frequency of contractions.

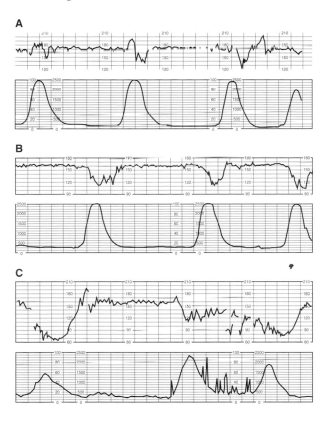

Fig. 33.5 (a)–(c) An example of spontaneous uterine hypercontractility—prolonged duration of contractions.

Excessive frequency of contractions

Figure 33.6 illustrates a case of spontaneous labour where contraction frequency became excessive without obvious cause (the traces illustrated form a continuous sequence). Contraction frequency was normal initially (Fig. 33.6a) but as contractions increased to six every 10 minutes, early fetal heart rate (FHR) decelerations appeared (Fig. 33.6b). As the frequency increased to seven every 10 minutes, the decelerations became larger (Fig. 33.6c). Eventually, intrauterine pressure failed to return to a normal tonus between contractions and a persistent fetal bradycardia developed (Fig. 33.6d). A slow intravenous infusion of salbutamol (150 μg)

was given with immediate reduction in the frequency and active pressure of contractions, and recovery of the FHR. The contractions then continued to be normal until the second stage (Fig. 33.6e), when some mild hypertonus recurred. However, a healthy infant was born after only 15 minutes in the second stage. A recent (2000) Cochrane review of three prospective randomised trials concluded that 'Betamimetic therapy appears to be able to reduce the number of fetal heart rate abnormalities and perhaps reduce uterine activity'; however the evidence is still insufficient to recommend tocolysis as a routine treatment strategy except as short term therapy in an emergency, or while preparing for delivery by caesarean section (Kulier & Hofmeyr 2000).

Hypertonic uterine action with placental abruption

Placental abruption occurs in about one in 100 pregnancies, and is severe enough to kill the fetus in one in every eight cases. Death may occur because of extensive placental separation but, in many cases, the excessive uterine activity produced by the massive release of prostaglandins from the disrupted decidua is also a major factor. Odendaal (1976) has drawn attention to the high mean frequency of contractions seen in association with abruption. Mean contraction frequency recorded in 37 studied cases was 7.9 in 10 minutes, with some occurring as often as 16 in 10 minutes. The importance of excessive contraction frequency as a sign in the diagnosis of abruption has been emphasised by Saunderson & Steer (1978). They pointed out that the high frequency of contractions seen with abruption means that associated late decelerations can be misinterpreted as increased baseline variability, or a reduced baseline rate with accelerations. Such a case is shown in Figure 33.7. The contractions were recorded with an external tocodynamometer, so true baseline tone is not shown. In the initial half of the tracing, without careful synchronisation of the FHR changes with the contractions it would be easy to interpret it as showing a baseline FHR of 125 beats/min with frequent accelerations. In the latter half of the tracing, however, the reduced baseline variability and the increasing amplitude of the late decelerations make the correct diagnosis more obvious. Figure 33.8 shows a similar case with intrauterine pressure recording. The initial baseline tone is set rather high, at 25 mmHg; however, the subsequent rise of baseline tone by 25 mmHg to 50 mmHg, the abnormal contraction pattern, and the excessive frequency of contractions are all typical of abruption. The FHR pattern is grossly abnormal, with loss of variability and late decelerations. The baby was delivered by emergency caesarean section with a cord artery pH of 6.98; however, it made a good long-term recovery.

Hyperstimulation with oxytocics

One of the commonest causes of uterine hyperactivity in modern clinical practice is the use of oxytocics. Bourne & Burn warned against the careless use of oxytocin in 1927 (Bourne & Burn 1927) and Liston & Campbell echoed their warnings in 1974. The use of oxytocin at infusion rates up to 40 mU/min is associated with a uterine hyperstimulation rate of 30–40% (Caldeyro-Barcia et al 1957, Bidgood & Steer 1982, Seitchik & Castillo 1982, Mercer et al 1991). The more physiological school of augmentation advocates measuring uterine activity by direct measurement of the pressure achieved during contractions and only giving oxytocin if there is a demonstrable deficiency in the strength of the contractions (Bidgood & Steer 1982). Oxytocin dose rate is titrated upwards until a target value of uterine activity is reached (usually 1500–1700 kPas/15 min, or 150–200 Montevideo Units). The usual infusion rate of oxytocin required to induce this level of uterine activity at term is 2–8 mU/min, with a mean of 4 mU/min (Caldeyro-Barcia et al 1957, Steer et al 1985, Blakemore et al 1990). The American College of Obstetricians and Gynecologists has recommended that oxytocin infusion to induce or augment labour should commence at an initial dose of 0.5–1 mU/min, increasing by 1–2 mU/min every 30–60 minutes. Retrospective studies have confirmed that there is no evident advantage to using higher dosage regimens (Foster et al 1988, Wein 1989). The active management of labour school, however, start at higher doses (7 mU/min) and recommend increases up to 40 mU/min in most cases (O'Driscoll et al 1984). There is no conclusive evidence that either of these

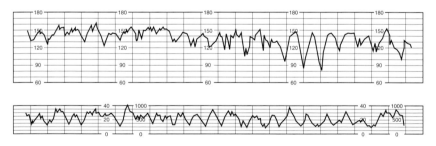

Fig. 33.7 Uterine hypercontractility associated with placental abruption, recorded with an external tocodynamometer.

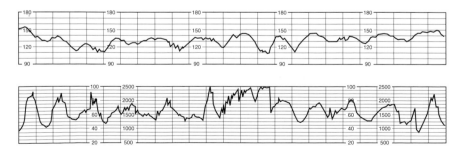

Fig. 33.8 Uterine hypercontractility associated with placental abruption, recorded with a catheter-tip pressure transducer.

two approaches, either physiological or active, is superior one from the other. However, the data sheet for Syntocinon (the synthetic oxytocin used in clinical practice) lists absolute contraindications to its use in labour as including 'hypertonic uterine inertia' (i.e. failure of the cervix to dilate despite a high level of uterine contraction), 'mechanical obstruction to delivery' (which is often only suspected when the cervix fails to dilate) and 'fetal distress'. Therefore, caution should always be exercised when giving oxytocin in the absence of intrauterine pressure measurement, and it should be withheld or stopped if the FHR becomes in any way abnormal. Failure to observe these precautions is a major source of litigation in both the USA and UK and it is almost always indefensible. An obvious example of oxytocin-induced hypertonus is shown in Figure 33.9. Figure 33.10 illustrates a case where oxytocin was administered because of slow cervical dilatation despite apparently normal uterine activity as assessed by external tocograph. The abnormal uterine activity that occurred almost immediately syntocinon was started is obvious. There was an associated temporary increase in fetal heart rate variability indicating mild hypoxia, followed by a brief fetal tachycardia, indicating increased fetal adrenergic activity in response to the fetal stress.

Prostaglandin administration is also associated with abnormal uterine action. Figure 33.11 shows the excessively frequent and incoordinate contractions that occurred following the vaginal administration of a 2.5 mg prostaglandin E_2 pessary used to induce labour. Large late decelerations indicated the resulting fetal hypoxia and emergency delivery by caesarean section was necessary.

INEFFICIENT UTERINE ACTIVITY

By definition, any level or type of uterine activity that does not produce progressive cervical dilatation is inefficient. Some workers prefer this term to expressions such as hypotonic, incoordinate, and hypertonic. However, the cervix may fail to dilate despite apparently normal contractions, because of cephalopelvic disproportion or cervical dystocia. Some authorities recommend the use of oxytocics in this situation, despite the risk of uterine hyperstimulation, but this is a controversial issue and more properly considered in Chapter 35.

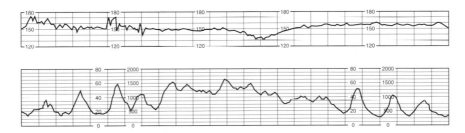

Fig. 33.9 Uterine hypercontractility associated with oxytocin infusion—acute hyperstimulation.

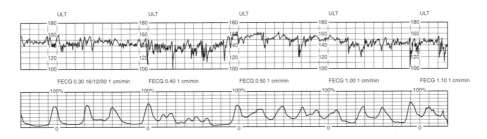

Fig. 33.10 Cardiotocograph tracing recorded using external transducers (1 cm per minute). Initial normal uterine activity is converted to a hyperstimulation pattern by the administration of intravenous syntocinon. Following the initial hyperstimulation there is a temporary increase in fetal heart rate variability indicating mild hypoxia, followed by a brief tachycardia indicating fetal adrenergic stimulation.

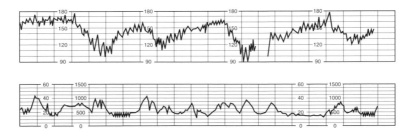

Fig. 33.11 Uterine hypercontractility associated with vaginal prostaglandin administration.

The role of the cervix in slow labour

Gough et al (1990) have suggested that a major factor in inefficient uterine action is a low force generated between the fetal presenting part (usually the head) and the lower segment or cervix. They studied 31 women in slow labour, and they found that once uterine activity levels had been normalised by appropriate oxytocin infusion, women who eventually needed caesarean section for inadequate cervical dilatation rates had poor forces (mean, 16.5 g wt; range, 6–31) between the presenting part and the cervix compared with those who achieved a vaginal delivery (mean, 45 g wt; range, 22–100). This was despite similar levels of uterine activity in both groups. Their observations were subsequently confirmed by Allman and co-workers (Allman et al 1996a, 1996b). These findings can be explained by the hypothesis that cervical dilatation is an active process that requires the application of an effective stretching force. If this force is inadequate to overcome the stretch threshold, then progressive dilatation will not take place. It can be imagined that poor forces will be applied to the cervix, even when the contractions of the uterine body are strong, if there is malpresentation, malposition or inadequate moulding of the fetal presenting part. The association of abnormal head to cervix forces with malposition has since been confirmed by Pitman et al (Antonucci et al 1997, Pitman et al 1997). It therefore appears that however strong the uterine contractions, if they cannot deliver an adequate force to the cervix, it will fail to dilate.

Margono et al (1993) have suggested that another factor which might prevent cervical dilatation is inadequate fundal dominance, a concept introduced by Caldeyro et al (1950) and elaborated by Jeffcoate (1963). This concept suggests that, in order to be effective, uterine contractions should commence at the cornua of the uterus (the designated pacemaker sites) and sweep downwards over the uterus. If the lower segment contracts at the same time, or before the upper segment, the effect may be to prevent descent of the head, and thus reduce the effective dilating force. Margono et al (1993) studied 22 women in labour, 15 of whom had active phase arrest of labour, by inserting two intrauterine catheters, one into the lower segment area and the other up to the fundus. They showed that in the 16 women who delivered vaginally, the upper segment pressures were always higher than those in the lower segment. In the six who were delivered by caesarean section, the pressures were higher in the lower segment. Olah et al (1994) have demonstrated that in the latent phase of labour almost 50% of women in labour exhibit contractions of the cervix, and have since suggested that if this persists into the active phase, such women are at increased risk of caesarean section. In such cases, the use of oxytocin is likely to be ineffective, and may even be counterproductive.

POSTURE IN LABOUR AND ABNORMAL UTERINE ACTION

Most obstetricians now appreciate that the supine position can cause the uterus to compress the inferior vena cava, thus causing supine hypotension and sometimes fetal hypoxia (Aldrich et al 1995, Carbonne et al 1996). Fewer however appreciate that the supine position can also cause abnormal uterine activity. This phenomenon was first noted by Williams in 1952 (Williams 1952). In the case he reported, uterine activity with the parturient in the sitting position was normal, with a contraction frequency of three in 10 minutes and an active pressure of 5.3 kPa (40 mmHg). When the woman was allowed to lie supine, the contraction frequency rose to 6.4 in 10 minutes and the active pressure fell to 2.1 kPa (16 mmHg). A similar example recorded by the author is shown in Figure 33.12. The change in pattern is abrupt and dramatic. In this case the FHR pattern continued to be normal, but in some cases the increase in contraction frequency is associated with changes indicating hypoxia. Caldeyro-Barcia et al (1960) reported positional changes in uterine activity could be observed in 94% of women in spontaneous labour, and in 76% of those in oxytocin-induced labour.

The mechanism by which the supine position can produce abnormal uterine action in this way is completely unknown. Some workers (Mendez-Bauer et al 1975, Flynn et al 1978) have suggested that the erect posture improves the pattern of uterine activity and that it is associated with more rapid progress in labour; however, subsequent work has shown that uterine activity is similar in pattern and efficiency in the recumbent lateral position, provided the supine position (flat on the back) is avoided (Williams et al 1980). In fact, if the effect of gravity in the upright position had a significant

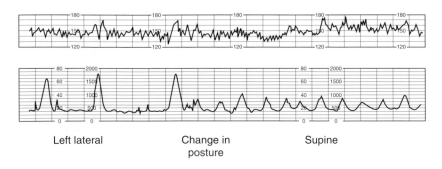

Left lateral   Change in posture   Supine

Fig. 33.12 Effect of posture on uterine activity.
Reproduced with permission from: K. Rosenberg and W. Trevethan. Bipedalism and human birth: the obstetrical dilemma revisited. Evolutionary Anthropology 4:161–168, 1996.

prompting effect on labour, as proponents of active childbirth have suggested, then labouring in water (where the effects of gravity are completely nullified) would lead to slow progress. In fact, no such effect is observed (Schorn et al 1993). Studies of posture in the second stage of labour have led to a similar conclusion: that so long as the mother avoids the supine position, she should be encouraged to take up any position she finds comfortable, secure in the knowledge that it is unlikely to affect her progress (de Jong et al 1997, Bonfim-Hyppolito 1998, Gupta & Nikodem 2000).

THE MANAGEMENT OF ABNORMAL UTERINE ACTION

The key to appropriate management is the recognition of the category of abnormality. It is particularly important to recognise promptly hypertonic uterine activity, as it is potentially harmful to the fetus. In addition, the diagnosis of uterine hyperactivity may be the first clue to a diagnosis of placental abruption.

Placental abruption

Abruptio placentae is not only likely to have serious implications for the fetus because of interference with placental gaseous exchange, but it can also have major consequences for the mother (particularly blood loss leading to shock, and coagulopathy (Chs 14 & 20). In severe cases, with lower abdominal pain and vaginal bleeding or the signs of shock (pallor, sweating, tachycardia and hypotension) the diagnosis may be obvious, but in the early stages of abruption the possibility is all too easily overlooked. For example, the lower abdominal pain and uterine irritability may be misattributed to a urinary tract infection.

In any pregnant woman, the occurrence of spontaneous uterine contractions with a frequency exceeding one every two minutes should lead one to consider the diagnosis of placental abruption.

In addition, the mother may give a history of continuous lower abdominal pain, or backache, which persists between contractions. She may give a history of bleeding per vaginam; this may be quite slight and it is sometimes only elicited on direct questioning. Examination is likely to show uterine tenderness, which is often localised but in severe cases will spread to include the entire uterus.

Cardiotocography has an important place in the early diagnosis of abruption, because it facilitates recognition of tachysystolia (excessively frequent contractions). In addition, the interference with placental perfusion which occurs in abruption often causes fetal hypoxia, resulting in abnormal fetal heart rate patterns. In their early stages, these abnormalities (such as loss of variability and shallow late decelerations) are not readily detectable using the Pinard stethoscope. Because of their subtlety it is important that the cardiotocography should be performed carefully, with particular attention to the placement of the external tocodynamometer (contraction transducer). Ideally the mother should be in the semi-Fowler position, sitting up at about 60° to the horizon-

tal, supported by pillows, with the tocodynamometer sited firmly in the midline about 12 cm below the fundus of the uterus. If the mother is lying on her side, then the tocodynamometer should be placed in a similar position but displaced about 10 cm towards the upper side. Only tachysystolia is demonstrable using an external contractions transducer, since neither baseline tone nor amplitude of contractions can be measured in absolute terms using commercially available tocodynamometers. The demonstration of raised baseline tone requires the insertion of an intrauterine catheter. Ideally this should have a catheter-tipped pressure transducer, for the maximum error in measurement of baseline tone using this type of catheter is about 2 kPa (15 mmHg) because of variations in hydrostatic pressure at different points within the uterus. In contrast, if a fluid-filled catheter with external pressure transducer is used, unless the transducer is placed carefully at the same level as the uterus, very large offsets in measured baseline tone can occur, making the assessment of true baseline tone unreliable.

Once the diagnosis of abruption has been made, management depends on whether the fetus remains in good condition and upon the state of the cervix. If the mother's condition is satisfactory and if the FHR remains normal then conservative management can proceed with continuing and continuous monitoring of maternal condition, uterine activity and FHR.

If the fetus is sufficiently mature and the cervix is favourable, an induction of labour by artificial rupture of the membranes is probably advisable in case there is a further and larger abruption later on. If the FHR pattern is abnormal or if there is any concern over the mother's condition, immediate delivery is the only safe treatment. Caesarean section will often be the method of choice, particularly if the cervix is unfavourable or if the FHR abnormality is severe.

Attempts to suppress uterine activity with tocolytics such as ritodrine or salbutamol should never be made in the presence of placental abruption for raised intrauterine tone limits the inflow of blood into the uterus and if the tone is reduced, it may precipitate further catastrophic intrauterine bleeding. In addition, if the mother is developing tachycardia and hypotension, these will be exacerbated by tocolytics. This is in contrast to the situation with antepartum haemorrhage caused by placenta praevia, where the bleeding is not restricted by raised intrauterine tone but instead is often provoked by uterine contractions. In this situation tocolytics can be used relatively safely and often result in the cessation of bleeding. However, the same caveats about the use of tocolytics in placenta praevia apply with respect to maternal condition: they should not be used if tachycardia and hypotension suggest haemodynamically significant blood loss.

Uncomplicated tachysystolia

If abruption can be ruled out as a cause of excessive uterine contractions, then tocolytics can be used with advantage to reduce the level of uterine action to within normal limits. They are particularly useful as an emergency measure if hypercontractility is secondary to an oxytocic such as prostaglandin E_2 whose action cannot easily be terminated.

Oxytocin has a short half-life in the blood; if hyperstimulation occurs with oxytocin use, it is usually sufficient to discontinue the infusion. The effect will wear off within 5–10 minutes.

Inadequate uterine activity

This is usually diagnosed initially because of a slow rate of cervical dilatation. The rate of dilatation below which progress is designated slow varies from one obstetric unit to another but in the UK usually lies between 1 cm an hour and 1 cm every two hours. About 75% of slow labours are caused by inadequate levels of uterine activity (Steer et al 1985), and most of these will respond effectively to intravenous oxytocin infusion at a rate between 2 and 8 mU/min (techniques for augmentation of labour are covered fully in Ch. 35). Ideally such infusion should be monitored by intrauterine pressure measurement, particularly in women of high parity, in those with a uterine scar and in those where the fetus is known to be at particular risk (e.g. small-for-gestational-age). If intrauterine pressure monitoring is not available, then contraction frequency should not be stimulated beyond one contraction every two minutes, and the rate of infusion should be reduced by half as soon as there is any sign of abnormality of the FHR pattern, and reduced further if the abnormality persists.

Incoordinate uterine action

There is no need to treat incoordinate uterine action so long as the FHR and the rate of cervical dilatation remain normal. As previously mentioned, the role of oxytocin in the management of incoordinate activity, where both overall levels of activity and rates of cervical dilatation are low, remains controversial. The author's experience is that the cervical dilatation rate increases in parallel with any increase in uterine activity, even if that uterine activity appears incoordinate. It, therefore, seems appropriate to use oxytocin infusion in the first instance, and in many cases improvement in the level of uterine activity and the rate of cervical dilatation will occur. Prostaglandins are not recommended as they have an inherent tendency to produce incoordinate uterine contractions and they may make the situation worse. If, however, there is a poor response to oxytocin, further measures may be tried. It must be emphasised that at present there are no firm scientific data to support the use of these measures.

Firstly, the posture of the woman should be adjusted; while the supine position should always be avoided any other position in which uterine activity improves should be maintained. If this is not effective then adequate analgesia must be ensured. This will usually be a regional block such as an epidural anaesthetic. This can sometimes produce an improvement in uterine activity and also provides analgesia, which is important in prolonged labour; if the mother is comfortable and fetal condition is satisfactory, it may be possible to wait long enough so that even a slow rate of cervical dilatation will result in a vaginal delivery. Care should be taken to continue observing the FHR pattern and uterine contractions as the anaesthetic is administered, particularly if an oxytocin infusion is being given; if the uterus suddenly becomes more sensitive and there is hypertonus, fetal hypoxia may result. If there is also hypotension from the epidural (despite preloading the circulation with fluid) the effect on the fetus can be catastrophic. If there is still no improvement in the overall level of uterine activity, then sedation with 150 mg pethidine may be tried as a last resort. At the present time there is insufficient evidence on which to recommend the use of beta-blockers such as propranolol.

FETAL HEAD MOULDING

Head moulding refers to the changes in the fetal cranial bone relationships that occur in response to the compression forces applied during labour. In normal term labour with vertex presentation, the suboccipito-bregmatic diameter shortens and the mentovertical diameter lengthens (Carlan et al 1991). This is accomplished partially through the unbending or straightening of the parietal bones as well as the better known mechanism of overlapping sutures. First born babies have to achieve significantly higher degrees of moulding of the head than those born to parous women (Sorbe & Dahlgren 1983). Oxytocin stimulation during labour as well as instrumental delivery results in greater fetal head moulding (Sorbe & Dahlgren 1983). All these findings suggest that poor fetal head moulding is a significant factor contributing to the need for operative delivery. However, there is currently no known way to facilitate head moulding.

ASSESSMENT OF THE FETAL HEAD/MATERNAL PELVIS RELATIONSHIP

It would seem to be obvious that a fetal head which is too large, or a maternal pelvis which is too small, would lead to the need for delivery by caesarean section. Maternal X-ray pelvimetry was used for many years in the belief that a mother with a small pelvis (for example, a true conjugate less than 10 cm if the presentation was cephalic and 11 cm if breech) should be delivered by caesarean section. However, this belief overlooked the fact that small mothers have small babies, and during the 1990s it has become apparent that routine X-ray pelvimetry is not useful. For example, a study from Glasgow showed that routine X-ray pelvimetry following caesarean section for dystocia was not predictive of the success or otherwise of a subsequent trial of labour (Krishnamurthy et al 1991). A subsequent trial of antepartum X-ray pelvimetry, allowing the assessment of fetal head size as well as maternal pelvic size, also failed to show any benefit (Thubisi et al 1993). Despite this, a survey in 1995 showed that 97% of maternity units in the UK continued to use X-ray pelvimetry (Morrison et al 1995). Subsequent studies (Van Loon et al 1997, Ferguson et al 1998) have shown that even modern techniques such as digital radiography, fetal head size assessment using ultrasound, and magnetic resonance imaging have little predictive value. A review in the Cochrane Collaboration has concluded that there is no evidence to support the use of pelvimetry with cephalic presentations. This is probably not because the measurements made are completely inaccurate, but because they cannot predict the efficiency of uterine action, the position and presentation of the head and its moulding, the compliance of the cervix, and the changes in the dimensions of the maternal pelvis, which will occur in a subsequent labour. As many of these papers say, the only true pelvimeter is labour. Impey & O'Herlihy (1998) were able to define only 83 cases of unequivocal cephalopelvic disproportion from over 42 000 births. Of these, they were able to study subsequent labours in 40. Twenty-seven (68%) of these delivered vaginally, seven with larger babies than at the first birth.

The role of pelvimetry for breech presentation is also doubtful. Even studies using magnetic resonance imaging have failed to show any advantage for the fetus (Van Loon et al 1997), and following the recent multicentre trial showing a two thirds reduction in perinatal mortality, neonatal mortality, or serious neonatal morbidity when babies presenting by the breech are delivered by elective caesarean section rather than being allowed a trial of vaginal birth (Hannah et al 2000), it seems likely that all future trials of vaginal birth will only occur at the mother's specific request.

KEY POINTS

- The success of labour depends not only on the size of the maternal pelvis and the size of the fetal head, but the presentation and position of the fetus, the degree of fetal head moulding, the efficiency of the uterine contractions and the compliance of the cervix and soft tissues.
- It is the Peak Pressure of contractions that Produces Progress, but the Frequency that aFFects the Fetus.
- Progress in labour is best predicted by measuring intrauterine pressure and measuring active contraction area (Uterine activity integral, UAI; kPas/15 min) or Montevideo Units (MU, total peak pressure of contractions per ten minutes).
- Manual estimation of uterine activity is inaccurate and unreliable.
- Slow progress in labour is most commonly caused by hypotonic uterine activity *but*
- Use of syntocinon when the uterine action is already normal often causes uterine hyperstimulation and fetal hypoxia.
- Maternal supine position should be avoided in labour or delivery; the left lateral or supported squat are preferable. If the lithotomy position is necessary, lateral tilt is advisable.
- Spontaneous uterine hypercontractility (tachysystole, hypertonus) is usually caused by placental abruption.
- Small frequent contractions seen on the cardiotocograph in association with late decelerations is characteristic of significant placental abruption.

REFERENCES

Aldrich CJ, D'Antona D, Spencer JA, Wyatt JS, Peebles DM, Delpy DT et al 1995 The effect of maternal posture on fetal cerebral oxygenation during labour. Br J Obstet Gynaecol 102:14–19

Allman AC, Genevier ES, Johnson MR, Steer PJ 1996a Head-to-cervix force: an important physiological variable in labour. 2. Peak active force, peak active pressure and mode of delivery. Br J Obstet Gynaecol 103:769–775

Allman ACJ, Genevier ESG, Johnson MR, Steer PJ 1996b Head-to-cervix force: an important physiological variable in labour. 1. The temporal relationship between head-to-cervix force and intrauterine pressure during labour. Br J Obstet Gynaecol 103:763–768

Al-Shawaf T, Al-Moghvaby S, Akiel A 1987 Normal levels of uterine activity in primigravidae and women of high parity in spontaneous labour. J Obstet Gynaecol 8:18–23

Antonucci MC, Pitman MC, Eid T, Steer PJ, Genevier ES 1997 Simultaneous monitoring of head-to-cervix forces, intrauterine pressure and cervical dilatation during labour. Med Eng Phys 19:317–326

Arrabal PP, Nagey DA 1996 Is manual palpation of uterine contractions accurate? Am J Obstet Gynecol 174:217–219

Bidgood KA, Steer PJ 1982 A randomized control study of oxytocin augmentation of labour. 2. Uterine activity. Br J Obstet Gynaecol 94:518–522

Bidgood KA, Steer PJ 1987 A randomized control study of oxytocin augmentation of labour. 1. Obstetric outcome. Br J Obstet Gynaecol 94:512–517

Blakemore KJ, Nai-Geng Q, Petrie R, Paine L 1990 A prospective comparison of hourly and quarter hourly oxytocin dose increase intervals for the induction of labor at term. Obstet Gynecol 75:757–761

Bomfim-Hyppolito S 1998 Influence of the position of the mother at delivery over some maternal and neonatal outcomes. Int J Gynaecol Obstet 63 Suppl 1 S67–S73

Bourne A, Burn JH 1927 The dosage and action of Pituitary extract and the ergot alkaloids on the uterus in labour, with a note on the action of adrenalin. J Obstet Gynaecol Br Emp 34:249–272

Caldeyro R, Alvarez H, Reynolds SRM 1950 A better understanding of uterine contractility through simultaneous recording with an internal and a seven channel external method. Surg Gynecol Obstet 91:641–650

Caldeyro-Barcia R, Sica-Blanco Y, Poseiro JJ, Gonzalez-Panniza V, Mendez-Bauer C, Fielitz C et al 1957 A quantitative study of the action of synthetic oxytocin on the pregnant human uterus. J Pharmacol 121:18–31

Caldeyro-Barcia R, Pose SV, Sica-Blanco Y, Mendez-Bauer C, Fielitz C, Gonzalez-Panniza V 1960 Effect of position changes on the intensity and frequency of uterine contractions during labor. Am J Obstet Gynecol 80:284–290

Carbonne B, Benachi A, Leveque ML, Cabrol D, Papiernik E 1996 Maternal position during labor: effects on fetal oxygen saturation measured by pulse oximetry. Obstet Gynecol 88:797–800

Carlan SJ, Wyble L, Lense J, Mastrogiannis DS, Parsons MT 1991 Fetal head molding. Diagnosis by ultrasound and a review of the literature. J Perinatol 11:105–111

de Jong PR, Johanson RB, Baxen P, Adrians VD, van der WS, Jones PW 1997 Randomised trial comparing the upright and supine positions for the second stage of labour. Br J Obstet Gynaecol 104:567–571

Ferguson JE, Newberry YG, DeAngelis GA, Finnerty JJ, Agarwal S, Turkheimer E 1998 The fetal-pelvic index has minimal utility in predicting fetal-pelvic disproportion. Am J Obstet Gynecol 179:1186–1192

Flynn AM, Kelly J, Hollins G, Lynch PF 1978 Ambulation in labour. Br Med J 2:591–593

Foster TC, Jacobson JD, Valenzuela G, Brindley BE, Sokol RJ 1988 Oxytocin augmentation of labor; a comparison of 15 and 30 minute dose increment intervals. Induction and augmentation of labor: basis and methods for current practice. Obstet Gynecol Surv 43:730–743

Fuchs AR, Fuchs F, Husslein P, Soloff MS 1984 Oxytocin receptors in the human uterus during pregnancy and parturition. Am J Obstet Gynecol 150:734–741

Gough GW, Randall NJ, Genevier ES, Sutherland IA, Steer PJ 1990 Head to cervix forces and their relationship to the outcome of labor. Obstet Gynecol 75:613–618

Gupta JK, Nikodem VC 2000 Woman's position during second stage of labour. Cochrane Database Syst Rev CD002006

Haig D 1993 Genetic conflicts in human pregnancy. Quarterly Rev Biol 68:495–532

Hannah ME, Hannah WJ, Hewson SA, Hodnett ED, Saigal S, Willan AR 2000 Planned caesarean section versus planned vaginal birth for breech presentation at term: a randomised multicentre trial. Term Breech Trial Collaborative Group. Lancet 356:1375–1383

Hemminki E, Lenck M, Saariksoki S, Henriksson L 1985 Ambulation versus oxytocin in protracted labour: a pilot study. Europ J Obstet Gynecol Reprod Biol 20:199–208

Hodnett ED 2000 Caregiver support for women during childbirth. The Cochrane Library, Issue 4. Update Software, Oxford

Impey L, O'Herlihy C 1998 First delivery after cesarean delivery for strictly defined cephalopelvic disproportion. Obstet Gynecol 92:799–803

Jeffcoate JNA 1963 Physiology and mechanism of labour. In: Claye A, Bourne A, (eds). British Obstetric and Gynaecological Practice William Heinemann, London pp 145–183

Johanson DC, Edey MA 1990 Lucy—the beginnings of humankind. Penguin books, London

Kulier R, Hofmeyr GJ 2000 Tocolytics for suspected intrapartum fetal distress (Cochrane Review). In: The Cochrane Library. Update Software, Oxford

Krishnamurthy S, Fairlie F, Cameron AD, Walker JJ, Mackenzie JR 1991 The role of postnatal x-ray pelvimetry after caesarean section in the management of subsequent delivery. Br J Obstet Gynaecol 98:716–718

Liston WA, Campbell AJ 1974 Dangers of oxytocin induced labour to fetuses. Br Med J iii:606–607

Margono F, Minkoff H, Chan E 1993 Intrauterine pressure wave characteristics of the upper and lower uterine segments in parturients with active-phase arrest. Obstet Gynecol 81:481–485

Mendez-Bauer C, Arroyo J, Garcia RC, Menendez A, Lavilla M, Izquierdo F et al 1975 Effects of standing position on spontaneous uterine contractility and other aspects of labor. J Perinat Med 3:89–100

Mercer B, Pilgrim P, Sibai B 1991 Labor induction with continuous low dose oxytocin infusion: a randomized trial. Obstet Gynecol 77:659–663

Mitrani A, Oettinger M, Abinader EG, Sharf M, Klein A 1975 Use of propranolol in dysfunctional labour. Br J Obstet Gynaecol 82:651–655

Morrison JJ, Sinnatamby R, Hackett GA, Tudor J 1995 Obstetric pelvimetry in the UK: an appraisal of current practice. Br J Obstet Gynaecol 102:748–750

Odendaal HJ 1976 The frequency of uterine contractions in abruptio placentae. South African Med J 50:2129–2131

O'Driscoll K, Foley M, MacDonald D. 1984 Active management of labour as an alternative to cesarean section for dystocia. Obstet Gynecol 63:485–490

Olah KS, Gee H, Brown JS 1994 The effect of cervical contractions on the generation of intrauterine pressure during the latent phase of labour. Br J Obstet Gynaecol 101:341–343

Peebles DM, Spencer JAD, Edwards AD, Wyatt JS, Reynolds EOR, Cope M et al 1994 Relation between frequency of uterine contractions and human fetal cerebral oxygen saturation studied during labour by near infrared spectroscopy. Br J Obstet Gynaecol 101:44–48

Phaneuf S, Rodriguez LB, Tambyraja RL, MacKenzie IZ, Lopez BA 2000 Loss of myometrial oxytocin receptors during oxytocin-induced and oxytocin-augmented labour. J Reprod Fertil 120:91–97

Pitman M, Antonucci M, Eid T, Genevier E, Johnson M, Steer P 1997 Head-to-cervix force: profiles beats peaks. J Obstet Gynaecol 17:S19

Rossavik IK 1978 Relation between total uterine impulse, method of delivery and one-minute Apgar score. Br J Obstet Gynaecol 85:847–851

Saunderson PR, Steer PJ 1978 The value of cardiotocography in abruptio placentae. Br J Obstet Gynaecol 85:796–779

Schorn MN, McAllister JL, Blanco JD 1993 Water immersion and the effect on labor. J Nurse Midwifery 38:336–342

Seitchik J, Castillo M 1982 Oxytocin augmentation of dysfunctional labor. Am J Obstet Gynecol 144:899–905

Seitchik J, Chatkoff ML 1977 Intrauterine pressure wave form characteristics of successful and failed first stage labor. Gynecol Invest 8:246–253

Sorbe B, Dahlgren S 1983 Some important factors in the molding of the fetal head during vaginal delivery—a photographic study. Int J Gynaecol Obstet 21:205–212

Steer PJ, Carter MC, Beard RW 1984 Normal levels of active contraction area in spontaneous labour. Br J Obstet Gynaecol 91:211–219

Steer PJ, Carter MC, Beard RW 1985 The effect of oxytocin infusion on uterine activity levels in slow labour. Br J Obstet Gynaecol 92:1120–1126

Steer P 1998a Fetal Growth. Br J Obstet Gynaecol 105:1133–1135

Steer P 1998b Caesarean section: An evolving procedure? Br J Obstet Gynaecol 105:1052–1055

Thubisi M, Ebrahim A, Moodley J, Shweni PM 1993 Vaginal delivery after previous caesarean section: is X-ray pelvimetry necessary? Br J Obstet Gynaecol 100:421–424

van Loon AJ, Mantingh A, Serlier EK, Kroon G, Mooyaart EL, Huisjes HJ 1997 Randomised controlled trial of magnetic-resonance pelvimetry in breech presentation at term. Lancet 350:1799–1804Wein P 1989 Efficacy of different starting doses of oxytocin for induction of labor. Obstet Gynecol 74:863–868

Williams EA 1952 Abnormal uterine action during labour. J Obstet Gynaecol Br Emp 59:635–641

Williams RM, Thom MH, Studd JW 1980 A study of the benefits and acceptability of ambulation in spontaneous labor. Br J Obstet Gynaecol 87:122–126

34

Abnormal fetal presentation and position

Justus Hofmeyr

Material in this chapter contains contributions from the first two editions. We are grateful to the previous authors for the work done.

In early pregnancy the fetus frequently changes position within the uterine cavity. It is remarkable that by term as many as 95% of fetuses have adoped the cephalic presentation. The association between various clinical factors and malpresentation suggests that adopting the cephalic presentation is an active process whereby an active, normally proportioned fetus in an average volume of amniotic fluid finds the position of best fit in the available intrauterine space (Stevenson 1951). This position is usually with the flexed legs accommodated in the broader fundal region and the head in the narrower lower segment of the uterus.

Many factors have been found to occur more frequently in women with a malpresentation. These may be grouped into factors related to intrauterine shape, fetal shape, fetal mobility and general factors:

Altered intrauterine shape:
- uterine anomalies, e.g. bicornuate, septate (Ben-Rafael et al 1991, Michalas 1991)
- space-occupying lesions, e.g. uterine myomata, ovarian tumours
- placenta praevia and cornual placenta (Stevenson 1950, Fianu & Vaclavinkova 1978)
- multiparity (lax abdominal wall, more rounded intrauterine space)
- polyhydramnios
- oligohydramnios.

Altered fetal shape:
- fetal anomaly, e.g. anencephaly, hydrocephaly
- extended fetal legs (Tompkins 1946)
- multiple pregnancy.

Altered fetal mobility:
- fetal compromise or decreased activity (Moessinger et al 1982)
- impaired fetal growth (Westgren et al 1985b)
- neurological impairment
- fetal death.
- Short umbilical cord (Soernes & Bakke 1986)

General:
- nulliparity (breech) (Westgren et al 1985b)
- prematurity
- previous breech presentation (Tompkins 1946)
- anticonvulsant therapy (Robertson 1984)
- contracted pelvis (Rannay 1973).

Neurological impairment is common following breech birth, being as high as 19.6% in one study, irrespective of the method of delivery (Danielian et al 1996). Impairment is thus often a cause rather than a result of breech birth. Failure to adopt the cephalic presentation may be seen as failure of the fetus to achieve its first developmental milestone. In some cases, however, abnormal presentation may be a chance occurrence or associated with factors unrelated to fetal well-being, such as cornual placental position (Fianu & Vaclavinkova 1978).

During the early stages of labour a favourable presentation and position is one in which the well flexed baby's head is entering the mother's pelvis with the occiput directed towards the side wall or some point between it and the symphysis pubis.

Human evolution and the upright posture have resulted in a forward curvature of the lower sacrum and a curved birth canal (Morgan 1972). Delivery of a child came to involve two processes: pushing it through a rigid bony canal, the entrance to which was wider from side to side while the exit was larger from front to back, and also negotiation of a right-angled bend halfway down the canal followed by traversing strong perineal muscles designed more for keeping things in than letting them out (Stewart 1984a; Fig. 34.1).

These changes were accompanied by an increase in the size of the human brain required to develop and utilise the skills needed by humans in order to remain the dominant animal (Moore 1970). These disadvantages are normally overcome by what are known as the mechanics of labour. The bigger parts of the baby, such as the head, shoulders and breech, enter the pelvis with their largest diameters running transversely. They rotate as they descend so that the same diameters leave the pelvis in an anterior–posterior direction.

As the spine is inserted into the back of the skull, pressure directed along it will make the head flex (Fig. 34.2). Thus, before labour commences or in its early stages the occipito-frontal diameter of the head is in the transverse diameter of the pelvis. As it descends it flexes so that the presenting diameter becomes the suboccipito-bregmatic, identical in length with the biparietal diameter at 9.5 cm. These form a circle to apply pressure equally all round the cervix, resulting in a reflex that stimulates fundal contractility and subsequently more downward pressure. When the head reaches the gutter formed by the levator muscles deep in the pelvis, the occiput, which is larger than the sinciput and lies lower in the pelvis, is funnelled forwards to present at the vulval opening. With further downward pressure it can emerge from the pelvis outlet, finally extending as it does so and returning to a neutral position in relation to the shoulders. Subsequent external rotation of the head is a reflection of the shoulders following the same spiral course through the pelvis.

Using these mechanics, most babies negotiate the pelvis safely. However, in a small number of cases the presentation is not cephalic or, if it is, the head rotates the wrong way in midpelvis or extends instead of flexing and these mechanisms

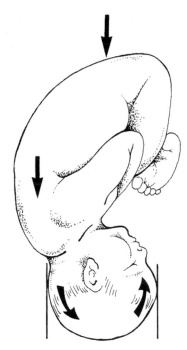

Fig. 34.2 Fundal pressure directed down fetal spine promotes flexion rather than extension of head.

cannot apply. Such problems form the basis of this chapter. In high-income countries the tendency is to manage them by caesarean section. This solution has been criticised because it is a major procedure for the mother (Yudkin & Redman 1986). Caesarean section is not always available in low-income countries.

DEFINITIONS

- The *attitude* of the fetus describes the relationship of the fetal head and limbs to the trunk. Usually this is one of flexion.
- The *lie* of the fetus is its relationship to the long axis of the uterus. This can be longitudinal, oblique or transverse.
- The *presentation* is that part of the fetus presenting in the lower pole of the uterus or at the pelvic brim.
- The *presenting part* is that part of the presentation that lies immediately inside the internal os of the cervix.
- The *position* defines the relationship of the presentation or the presenting part to the maternal pelvis.
- The *denominator* is that part of the presenting part that denotes the position. For a cephalic presentation with the vertex as the presenting part, the denominator is the occiput. With a face as the presenting part it is the chin and for a breech it is the sacrum.

OCCIPITO–POSTERIOR POSITIONS OF THE HEAD

Occipito-posterior position means that the occiput, the denominator for the position of the head, points posteriorly in

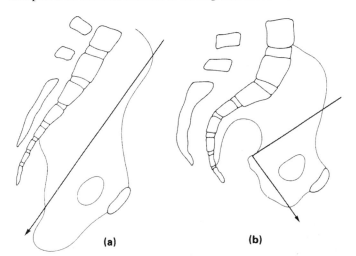

Fig. 34.1 (a) Gorilla pelvis showing straight birth canal. (b) Human pelvis showing birth canal with right-angle turn.

the pelvis, either directly at the sacrum (direct occipito-posterior) or to one side of it in the region of the sacroiliac joints (left or right occipito-posterior). This may be the case during the antenatal period or at any time in labour right up to delivery. The head rotates during labour, and discussion of these positions therefore has to include women in whom the occiput points sideways (occipito-lateral, occipito-transverse). It is accepted that 10–20% of cephalic presentations enter labour with the occiput directed posteriorly (Myerscough 1982). Some rotate to occipito-anterior so that, by the time of delivery, only 5% remain occipito-posterior or have arrested in the occipito-lateral position while turning towards the front.

Occipito-posterior position of the fetal head is one of the commonest causes of a high head at term, and can be recognised by the difficulty in locating the fetal back, the scaphoid concave area between the pubic symphysis and umbilicus and the prominence of the fetal limbs anteriorly. The fetal heart may also be more difficult to locate, as it can either be heard directly anteriorly or out in the flanks.

There are several possible causes for the abnormal position. Braxton Hicks contractions may not be strong enough to push the head into the brim and make it flex prior to the onset of labour (Fig. 34.3a). Conversely, the extended head presents an oblong-shaped outline to the lower segment so that the stimulus to fundal contractility may be irregular and incomplete (Fig. 34.3b). Hypertonus in the fetus can prevent the normal flexed attitude in utero.

The babies of women with either anthropoid or android pelves are more likely to be occipito-posterior. The anthropoid pelvic shape is very uncommon but is usually large; the baby presents directly occipito-posterior for the whole labour and delivers easily in that position. Viewed from above, the more commonly found android pelvis is triangular in shape with the apex at the symphysis pubis so that the larger part of the fetal head finds more room in the back of the pelvis and turns into the sacral curve as it descends (Stewart 1984b).

The fact that the baby's spine is juxtaposed to the mother's means that downward pressure along the spine is more likely to extend the head than flex it, thus increasing the diameters presented to the pelvic brim. Since the head is rarely directly occipito-posterior, the biparietal, its largest transverse diameter, fits poorly into the space between the sacral promontory and the pectineal line while the smaller bitemporal measurement has all the space available from the sacroiliac joint to the back of the symphysis pubis (Fig. 34.4). Uterine contractility is adversely affected because the cervix is not stimulated correctly by the oblong surface presented by the extended head (Fig. 34.3b). When the occiput eventually meets the pelvic floor it may fail to rotate to the front, partly because of the long way it has to travel, through three-eighths of a circle (135°), and partly because the posterior shoulder remains caught on the wrong side of the mother's sacral promontory. In many cases the head rotates through 45° and can go no further, ending up as deep transverse arrest. Some turn the same distance but posteriorly and become persistent occipito-posterior positions. Neither delivers or can be delivered as easily as a well-flexed head in the normal occipito-anterior position. Thus, progress of labour is

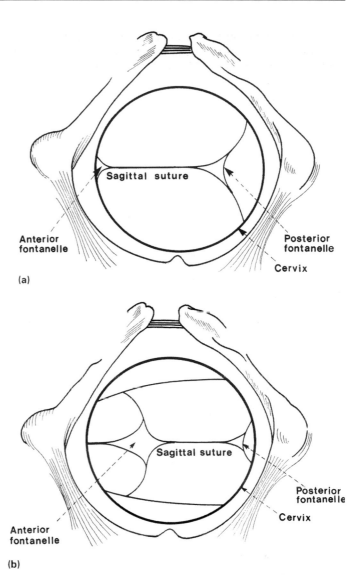

(a)

(b)

Fig. 34.3 (a) Flexed head presenting as a circle to the cervix. Biparietal diameter 9.5 cm; suboccipito-bregmatic diameter also 9.5 cm. (b) Deflexed head presenting a rectangular surface to the cervix. Biparietal diameter 9.5 cm; occipito-frontal diameter 11.5 cm.

marred by misapplication of the head to the cervix, the largest transverse diameter of the head trying to pass through the smallest diameter of the pelvic brim, and the tendency of the head to deflex and present increasingly greater diameters as it descends in the pelvis. In a small number of cases this extension continues so that first the baby's brow and then its face becomes the presenting part.

KEY POINTS

- Malpresentation is associated with poor application of the presenting part to the cervix, and poor progress of labour.
- Maternal posture to correct malpresentations requires further evaluation.

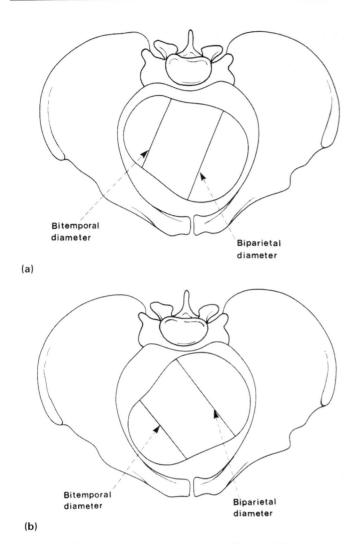

(a)

(b)

Fig. 34.4 (a) Left occipito-anterior position. Biparietal diameter (9.5 cm) lying between the sacroiliac joint and the summit of the symphysis pubis. Bitemporal diameter (8.5 cm) occupies the smaller sacrocotyloid dimension. (b) Left occipito-posterior position. Biparietal diameter squeezed into the sacrocotyloid while the bitemporal has excess space.

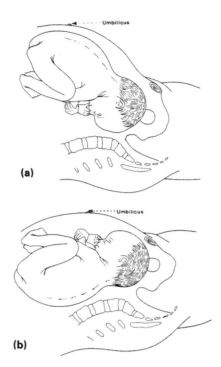

Fig. 34.5 Lateral view of abdomen near term. (a) Occipito-anterior position: maternal umbilicus at summit of abdominal swelling. (b) Occipito-posterior with umbilicus inferior to summit.

The resultant trend towards prolonged labour, possibly with operative delivery, increases morbidity for both mother and child. Phillips & Freeman (1974), in a retrospective review of 1082 cases born vaginally, reported an operative delivery rate of 66% with 22% requiring rotation. There was more puerperal pyrexia and so many episiotomies extended posteriorly that the authors recommended never using a midline technique. Friedman et al (1977) examined 656 children aged between 3 and 4 years and found that a history of prolonged labour and mid-forceps either together or independently had an adverse effect on subsequent intelligence.

The diagnosis of an occipito-posterior position can be suspected antenatally on abdominal palpation. With the baby lying on its back when the mother is examined, its flexed legs mean that the maximum protrusion of the maternal abdomen viewed from the side is well above the umbilicus with a sharp fall down to the xiphisternum and a gentle slope towards the symphysis pubis (Fig. 34.5). The head will feel smaller because the sinciput is anterior and the back may be difficult to palpate clearly.

Management of the occipito-posterior position

Maternal posture has been suggested as a method of correcting abnormal positions. Systematic review of the literature (Hofmeyr & Kulier 1999a) revealed one rather small trial (Andrews & Andrews 1983). Lateral or posterior position of the presenting part of the fetus was far less likely to persist following ten minutes in the hands and knees position than in a control position (sitting) (relative risk 0.25, 95% confidence interval 0.17–0.37). Further research is needed to determine whether this technique has any real clinical benefits.

Once labour is under way some cases of occipito-posterior position progress at a normal rate and either rotate to occipito-anterior spontaneously or deliver as face to pubis. These cause no problem apart from a tendency towards perineal damage during face to pubis delivery. Most cases come to light because of failure to progress in labour, and a vaginal examination reveals the abnormal position. It is essential that such examinations are thorough and produce as much information as possible. Abnormal positions often entail moulding and caput formation as labour progresses and it is easier to define the suture lines on the fetal skull in the early stages.

During vaginal examination, the degree of deflexion of the fetal head should also be noted. The bony pelvis should also be assessed, and the thickness and elasticity of the maternal soft tissues may be relevant to subsequent attempts at operative delivery. Application of the cervix to the presenting part is assessed, especially during a contraction. Observations about the colour of the amniotic fluid and whether the cord can be palpated are also important. Augmentation of labour may be required to maintain adequate progress. The fetus should preferably be continuously monitored. Labour with an occipito-posterior position may be particularly painful. Back pain is a common feature and epidural analgesia should be offered.

In some cases, the head will descend to the pelvic floor and deliver spontaneously either with the occiput anterior or in the direct occipito-posterior position. The latter may require a sufficiently large episiotomy to prevent excess tearing of the perineum. Provided progress is being made and the baby's condition remains good, patience and care will result in a spontaneous delivery for many women. However, if the head remains high a full reassessment of the case is essential. There is no point in doing X-ray pelvimetry as, even with a large pelvis, failure of the head to descend to a level where forceps or vacuum extraction can be safely applied will necessitate an abdominal delivery (Bottoms et al 1987).

For some women a change of position in the second stage of labour may be helpful. Squatting, semi-squatting, lying on the side or using a birth cushion or chair may enable the woman who feels the urge to push to do so more effectively than lying on her back, even when propped up with pillows. Failure of conservative measures to assist delivery will lead to operative vaginal delivery.

Operative vaginal delivery

Operative vaginal delivery must start with careful palpation of the abdomen. If any part of the head can be felt above the symphysis pubis its station in the pelvis is higher than may have appeared to be the case on vaginal examination, usually because of moulding or caput or both. While such a finding is not an absolute contraindication to vaginal delivery it acts as a warning not to persist if the first attempt is unsuccessful. If the success of vaginal delivery is in any doubt, it should be performed as a formal trial of vaginal delivery in the operating theatre, prepared for immediate caesarean section in the event of failure (Lowe 1987).

The woman is put into the lithotomy position and if then vaginal examination shows the head to be directly occipito-posterior and low in the pelvis, a direct application of a curved Neville Barnes-type forceps or vacuum extractor with a suitable episiotomy and gentle traction should deliver the baby. However, if the head fails to descend it will be necessary to rotate it to occipito-anterior. This will also be the case if the head is in the oblique occipito-posterior position or has arrested at mid-cavity in the deep transverse position. The anaesthesia used depends on the procedure undertaken: pudendal nerve block may be used, or if there is not an epidural in place, a single-shot spinal block may be inserted quickly, making certain that a wedge is placed under one of the woman's buttocks when she is returned to the lithotomy position.

Manual rotation of the head

For manual rotation from the left occipito-posterior or lateral position, the right hand is used, and for right-sided positions the left hand is used. The fetal head is grasped transversely between thumb and fingers, and rotated by a pronation movement of the forearm. The other hand may help by pulling the anterior shoulder abdominally in the same direction. The fingers of the abdominal hand are then inserted between the lateral aspect of the head and the vaginal wall to prevent the head rotating back while guiding the first blade of the forceps into position. In the case of rotation from the left occipito-posterior or lateral position, the right forceps blade is thus applied before the left, and the position of the handles needs to be reversed before locking.

Correct application means that the handles will close easily with the operator rechecking the suture lines before using any traction. Non-closure demands that the blades be removed and the vaginal assessment repeated.

Forceps rotation

The choice between forceps and vacuum delivery depends on several factors, including operator experience. Ten randomised trials comparing the two instruments in general (not specifically for rotational deliveries', have been reviewed (Johanson & Menon 1999a). Use of the vacuum extractor was associated with significantly less maternal trauma (odds ratio 0.41, 95% confidence interval 0.33–0.50) and with less general and regional anaesthesia. Fewer caesarean sections were carried out in the vacuum extractor group; however, the vacuum extractor was associated with an increase in neonatal cephalahaematomata and retinal haemorrhages. Serious neonatal injury was uncommon with either instrument.

Forceps have the advantage over manual rotation that the blades are thinner than human fingers so that the operator keeps the head low when applying them. In the direct or oblique occipito-posterior position the blades of a Kielland's type of instrument can be applied directly. Rotation is then performed with one hand while the sagittal suture is palpated frequently to ensure that it is turning with the forceps. Rotation may be helped by either pulling down or pushing up the head a centimetre or two, or by gentle posterior angulation of the handles. Since there is no pelvic curve the handles of the forceps must always be directed more posteriorly than with axis traction forceps. In the direct occipito-posterior position, rotation can be either clockwise or anticlockwise, usually towards the side on which the back has been palpated abdominally. With an obliquely posterior head the rotation is towards the side on which the occiput already lies. As soon as the occipito-anterior position is attained the same forces are used for delivery.

An alternative is the use of Barton's forceps (see Ch. 36). A sharp angle makes the posterior blade easier to apply than Kielland's forceps and rotation occurs spontaneously as traction is applied (Parry-Jones 1968).

Vacuum extractor

The vacuum extractor has the advantage that it occupies no space to the side of the baby's head. When properly applied, it actually flexes the baby's head, reducing the diameter presenting to the pelvic outlet from the occipito-frontal to the smaller suboccipito-bregmatic. In addition, with traction the head can rotate to whichever position enables it to be delivered most easily. Review of randomised trials has shown that, for rotational deliveries, the metal cup is more suitable than the soft cup (Johanson & Menon 1999b). Details are given in Chapter 36.

KEY POINT

- Vacuum extraction causes less maternal trauma than forceps delivery, but is associated with an increase in neonatal cephalahaematomata and retinal haemorrhages.

Two further points should be emphasised in connection with operative delivery for abnormal cephalic positions: episiotomy and failed forceps delivery.

Episiotomy

The fact that the head is extended in a face to pubis delivery means that the episiotomy may need to be larger than for an occipito-anterior position. With instrumental delivery there is a temptation to do the episiotomy before inserting either the forceps or the vacuum in order to make the application easier. This should be avoided: failure to effect the delivery and subsequent caesarean section means that the patient will have a wound on her abdomen and in her perineum. In addition, insertion or rotation of the forceps may extend the episiotomy. The operator should aim to reserve the incision until vaginal delivery is certain, by which stage even a midline incision may be adequate (although some have recommended never performing a midline episiotomy with a direct occipito-posterior delivery because of the risk of extension into a third-degree tear).

Episiotomy discomfort worries many puerperal women more than anything else (Reading et al 1982) and great care should be taken in its performance and repair. Midline incisions are easier to suture than mediolateral ones (Coats et al 1980). A subcuticular repair (Kettle & Johanson 1999a) with polyglycolic suture material (Kettle & Johanson 1999b) is better than other techniques although a recent randomised controlled trial has suggested that repairing the skin layer may be altogether unnecessary (Gordon et al 1998).

Failed forceps or vacuum delivery

No surgeon likes a procedure to fail but it is important to remember that a forceps delivery which requires a strong pull is occasionally followed by shoulder dystocia. Acker and his colleagues (1986) have shown that secondary arrest or a prolonged second stage with mid-cavity forceps is a warning sign for this complication. While in theory it can be overcome by a variety of manoeuvres, including replacement of the head and later caesarean section (Sandberg 1985), in practice fetal mortality and morbidity are high.

If rotation cannot be achieved, or if a large vacuum cup properly applied comes off, or if firm one-handed traction with forceps applied to a head in the direct occipito-anterior position fails to deliver the baby, caesarean section must be undertaken (Lowe 1987).

FACE AND BROW PRESENTATIONS

Face and brow presentations are similar in many respects and may be considered together. Both conditions result from hyperextension of the fetal neck, usually cases of occipito-posterior position which extend first into a brow and then into a face, sometimes before labour but usually as labour is progressing. Anencephaly or tumours of the fetal neck may rarely be associated. Cruikshank & Cruikshank (1981) quote an incidence of one in 500 for the face and one in 1500 for the brow as presenting parts. The chin is the denominator when the face is presenting but traditionally there is no such marker for a brow presentation; it is thought that the large occipito-mental diameter can never pass through a pelvis and therefore no mechanism is necessary. The diameters of the face are the normal biparietal (9.5 cm) and the submento-bregmatic, which is the same as the occipito-frontal of a deflexed vertex (11.5 cm). However, labour can be more difficult with an extended head because the facial bones do not mould as satisfactorily as the parietal bones; if the chin rotates posteriorly, then the large area of skull comprising the vertex and the occiput cannot follow the face out under the symphysis.

The principal complication for the mother is that of operative delivery, commonly caesarean section. For the baby there exists the danger of trauma due to excessive moulding of the presenting part. The excess oedema of eyelids, nose, lips and cheeks found when the face presents looks alarming but resolves quickly. Vaginal operative delivery must be done with care to avoid causing damage to these organs.

The diagnosis is suspected on palpation when the head will be high or will feel larger than normal on the same side as the fetal back with a sharp angulation between the fetal back and the occiput. Often an ultrasound scan or X-ray is done to exclude abnormality and shows extreme extension of the fetal neck. Most cases appear for the first time in labour, when vaginal examination demonstrates the root of the nose and the two orbital ridges of a brow presentation, or the nose, the mouth and the two orbital hollows of a face. Occasionally the mouth can be mistaken for the anal orifice.

Management of face and brow presentation

There is no point in attempting to correct the abnormality prior to the onset of labour, the advent of which it is to be hoped will lead to the head flexing and the vertex becoming the presenting part. If there is an overriding requirement to deliver the baby, elective caesarean section is usually a wiser choice than inducing labour with the high presenting part, even if the cervix is suitable.

When a brow presentation is encountered in early labour a limited period of observation is justified as conversion to a vertex or face presentation occasionally occurs. For a persistent brow presentation, a caesarean section is required.

A face presentation may be allowed to deliver spontaneously provided that the chin is already anterior or is rotating forwards. Should it be mento-posterior, it is usually high in the pelvis; although rotation forceps can be successfully applied, most operators will opt for caesarean section as the wiser choice.

Manipulations such as Thorn's manoeuvre—walking the fingers over the head—often will turn a brow into a vertex but the complication is so rare that few people are experienced. Provided the head is engaged, it is possible to treat a forward-facing brow as an exaggerated occipito-posterior position. It can be flexed with a vacuum cup placed as posteriorly as possible, or rotated to occipito-anterior with Kielland's forceps, then flexion will occur automatically.

Most normal-sized brow presentations are undeliverable as such, but rare exceptions to this rule do occur. The author has attended an easy spontaneous brow delivery of a baby weighing over 4000 g.

TRANSVERSE LIE

A transverse lie involves the long axis of the fetus lying at right angles to that of the uterus. The incidence is 2% early in the third trimester but only 0.3% at term. Spontaneous resolution occurs in 80–90% of cases before delivery. Most cases have no obvious aetiology and presumably result from laxity of the abdominal musculature in a multiparous woman. However, this must not be assumed until pelvic masses such as placenta praevia, fibroids and ovarian cysts have been excluded, along with fetal malformations, including twins. Rarely the cause is an abnormal uterus with the baby fixed in a transverse lie, its back pointing towards the lower segment. Antenatal diagnosis is usually easy, the two poles of the fetus being felt on either side of the abdomen. Ultrasound must be done to detect any abnormalities, including a low-lying placenta. Only when this has been done should a vaginal examination be performed.

Once labour starts, the diagnosis is made in the same manner but vaginal examination can confirm the lie by feeling a shoulder or the baby's ribs. The shoulder can feel like the breech, hence the importance of doing ultrasound scans in the delivery suite.

Management of transverse lie

Provided the gestational age has been confirmed, a persistently transverse or unstable lie should be managed conservatively until 37 weeks' gestation. At that stage external cephalic version, repeated when necessary, has been suggested, but the reversion rate is high. As the volume of amniotic fluid diminishes nearer term the uterus may close down on the fetus and hold it in a longitudinal lie. The mother must be given strict instructions to come into hospital if there is any sign of labour and many units will prefer to admit her two or three weeks before term for daily observation.

There are three methods of managing these cases after 37 weeks: conservative, stabilising induction, and elective caesarean section.

The conservative approach involves keeping the mother in hospital in the hope that the lie will straighten either before labour or when it starts. This approach is expensive and disruptive to the patient's family life; there is the risk of rupture of the membranes with cord prolapse.

Stabilising induction is done by first performing external cephalic version. This is easier to perform if the baby is facing

downwards (Fig. 34.6a) than if it is facing upwards (Fig. 34.6b). An oxytocin infusion is started while the longitudinal lie is maintained by gentle lateral pressure on the uterus. Once the head enters the pelvic brim the membranes are ruptured and the infusion continued. Edwards & Nicholson (1969) produced excellent results with this approach, but although it works well with patients of low parity, in the grand multipara the tendency is for the membranes to rupture spontaneously before the head enters the brim and the lie then becomes oblique or reverts to transverse as the amniotic fluid drains out.

Elective caesarean section is performed if stabilising induction cannot easily be achieved.

If the transverse lie is first diagnosed in labour, placenta praevia and fetal abnormality must be excluded by ultrasound, which can also sometimes demonstrate a cord in the lower segment (Lange et al 1985). Provided these complications are not present, external version to a longitudinal lie may be attempted between contractions, with the use of a beta-stimulant to relax the uterus if necessary. In a prospective uncontrolled study this was successful in 10 of 12 cases (Phelan et al 1985). If successful, amniotomy may be performed to stabilise the head in the pelvic brim. The bladder is kept empty with an indwelling catheter and a normal labour may be anticipated if the fetus remains longitudinal. Vaginal examination is done when the membranes rupture to exclude cord prolapse; this or failure of the fetus to stabilise demands immediate caesarean section. If the diagnosis is not suspected until after the membranes have ruptured the uterus will be wrapped tightly around the baby, making abdominal palpation more difficult. Careful vaginal examination will reveal an arm, a shoulder or some ribs, all of which can be mistaken for a breech presentation. Immediate caesarean section is essential to prevent ruptured uterus in all cases where the baby is alive. Even when it is dead, a section will be the safest procedure for the mother in most obstetricians' hands.

Internal version is contraindicated even with a live fetus and intact membranes, because while the cervix may appear fully dilated, once the procedure ruptures the membranes the

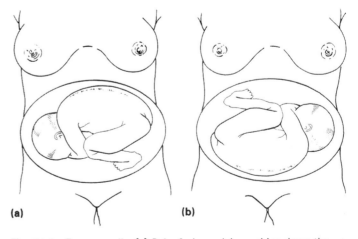

(a) **(b)**

Fig. 34.6 Transverse lie. **(a)** Baby facing pelvis: pushing down the head produces flexion and makes version easy. **(b)** Baby facing maternal diaphragm: pushing down the head extends the fetal spine and makes version difficult.

uterus will clamp down on the baby and the cervix will then be found to be only 6 or 7 cm dilated with subsequent entrapment of the aftercoming head.

Malpresentation of a second twin

Transverse lie in labour is most commonly found with a second twin. This differs from a singleton pregnancy in that the cervix has already been fully dilated. There are no data from randomised trials to guide the choice between caesarean section, external cephalic or podalic version, or internal podalic version. The author's policy is as follows. During the birth of the first twin, the most experienced attendant identifies (a portable ultrasound scanner is often helpful here) and guides the head of the second twin towards the pelvis. If this is unsuccessful, external cephalic version or, failing that, external podalic version is attempted, with tocolysis if necessary. The abdomen is steadied with a hand along each side of the uterus to maintain a longitudinal lie while oxytocin infusion is commenced, and once the presenting part descends, membranes are ruptured. External cephalic version for the second twin was successful in 11 of 12 transverse lies and 16 of 18 breech presentations (Tchabo & Tomai 1992), but in another study was associated with increased complications (Goeke et al 1989).

In the case of breech presentation, provided the fetal heart rate is satisfactory, expulsion with assistance to delivery of the aftercoming head is preferable to breech extraction. If transverse lie cannot be corrected, internal podalic version may be considered (Drew et al 1991) provided certain criteria are met. The second sac should be intact or only recently ruptured; the volume of amniotic fluid should be judged adequate; and the uterus should be soft or able to be relaxed with tocolysis. Helped by suitable analgesia and occasionally general anaesthesia a hand pushes up the membranes, grasps one or preferably both feet (identified by the heel) and pulls it down through the membranes, tearing them as it emerges. It is important not to release amniotic fluid before grasping the foot as the uterus clamps down on the baby and by the time the foot is located attempts to turn the baby can harm it and rupture the uterus. Once the breech enters the pelvis, if there is no evidence of fetal distress, oxytocin may be started and routine breech delivery conducted. In the event of fetal distress, breech extraction is performed. This often entails manoeuvres to deliver extended arms and head caused by the traction (see breech delivery).

KEY POINTS

- Non-longitudinal lie may be corrected by external cephalic version in early labour or prior to labour induction. If version is contraindicated or unsuccessful, caesarean section is needed.
- For malpresentation or abnormal lie of the second twin, the choice lies between external cephalic version, caesarean section, and if there is an experience operator, internal version and breech extraction.

COMPOUND PRESENTATION

A compound presentation is uncommon, and is diagnosed in labour by vaginal examination. In most cases there is a limb beside the fetal head. Provided the head is descending with contractions it usually pushes its way past the limb and labour continues normally. A high unstable presentation should be managed in the same way as a transverse lie, with repeated vaginal examinations to exclude cord prolapse and monitor alterations in the presentation.

BREECH PRESENTATION

The incidence of breech presentation varies with fetal maturity. Scheer & Nubar (1976) reported a 16% incidence at 32 weeks, falling to 7% at 38 weeks and 5% at 40 weeks. After 36 weeks the chance of spontaneous version is 25% (Westgren et al 1985b), and it may occur even after 40 weeks. Planned elective caesarean section for breech presentation should therefore be delayed as long as possible. The presentation should be checked immediately before surgery. Breech presentation should not be considered abnormal until late in pregnancy and causes no problems unless premature labour intervenes. Nearer term, a breech presentation may be caused by spatial factors or failure of the fetus to move into the cephalic presentation.

Faber-Nijolt and his colleagues (1983) considered that the mild neurological dysfunction found after breech birth was not always the result of the vaginal delivery while O'Connell & Keane (1985) have described several inherent differences in breech babies. Torgrim & Bakke (1986) reported that breech babies have shorter cords than cephalic-presenting babies, but whether this is a result of their lack of mobility or whether the short cord actually prevents them turning in utero is not clear.

The mechanism of breech labour involves the bitrochanteric diameter (9.25 cm) entering the pelvis in the transverse plane, rotating in mid-cavity and presenting at the pelvic outlet in the anterior–posterior diameter. The buttocks deliver in this position and then the whole body rotates to allow the shoulders to do exactly the same. Delivery of the anterior shoulder occurs as the head enters the pelvis in the transverse diameter, hopefully flexed as much as possible. Internal rotation then occurs so that the chin appears at the perineum, followed by the face, and then flexion allows the remainder of the skull to leave the pelvis. Thus there are no difficulties about the mechanics: the problem of a vaginal delivery is that the largest and least compressible part of the baby comes out last.

The irregular outline of the breech means that spontaneous rupture of the membranes may be followed by cord prolapse. Although the soft breech is less likely than the head to compress the cord, the cord may still go into spasm and cause acute fetal hypoxia. The ill-fitting breech can also be associated with slower labour, particularly in multiparous women. The much-feared complication at the end of labour is that of the bitrochanteric diameter being smaller than the biparietal, so that the breech and the lower limbs fit through a cervix or pelvis which is not sufficiently large for the after-coming head.

The small baby is unlikely to have bony problems but, as the head is relatively larger than in the mature baby, it may be caught in a partially dilated cervix and cause acute asphyxia. This can happen to the larger baby, especially if a foot pressing on the maternal rectum causes the mother to push before full dilatation.

In both premature and mature babies, the skull does not have sufficient time to mould when passing through the pelvis; Wigglesworth & Husemeyer (1977) have shown the danger of damage to the occipital bone (occipital diastasis) which increases the possibility of intracranial haemorrhage. Nevertheless, most premature breeches suffer more from the complications of immaturity than the actual mode of delivery, and good management in labour rarely allows a mature breech to get into trouble.

Diagnosis in the antenatal period should be made by abdominal palpation. Careful assessment of the fetal lie and presentation should be routine, particularly in late pregnancy. When the breech presents, the mother may report subcostal discomfort, or kicking felt in the lower abdomen. On palpation, the presenting part lacks the firmness of the fetal head and there is no recess between head and shoulders. The fetal head in the upper abdomen is confirmed by ballottement: it can be moved freely back and forth. Movement of the breech, which is accompanied by movement of the whole trunk, is characteristically more sluggish. Clinical diagnosis is not infallible. An experienced clinician examining 138 women detected only 3 of 8 breech presentations and falsely diagnosed 6 (Thorp et al 1991). About a third of all breech presentations are first detected during labour (Cally et al 1993). If the presentation persists, ultrasound examination is performed to exclude fetal abnormality and demonstrate the placental site as well as confirming the diagnosis.

Management of breech presentation has traditionally distinguished between multiparous and parous mothers; however, the maturity of the baby is of greater importance. Preterm breeches suffer from immaturity as well as from the mode of delivery and should therefore be considered separately from larger babies.

Management of the preterm breech in labour

The incidence of breech presentation in babies born before 37 weeks is approximately 15%. Some mothers arrive in hospital with ruptured membranes or a small antepartum haemorrhage but few contractions, and yet are found a few hours later with the cervix fully dilated and a bearing-down sensation, having had no obvious labour. Others labour, but at 6 or 7 cm push the small limbs and body through the cervix, which remains insufficiently stretched to allow passage of the aftercoming head.

On admission to the delivery suite the mother's records should be checked to see that fetal abnormality has been ruled out. Even if this is the case ultrasound must be employed to confirm it, to exclude a low-lying placenta, to make an estimate of fetal weight, and to assess fetal breathing, the presence of which suggests that labour is unlikely to proceed (Besinger et al 1987). Anderson (1981) reported that

in up to 80% of cases where the mother thinks she is in premature labour contractions cease spontaneously and the pregnancy continues. If labour contractions persist and the gestational age is below 32 weeks, steroids should be administered to enhance fetal lung maturity (Crowley 1999) and intravenous tocolytics administered in the hope of delaying labour for at least 24–48 hours.

The fetal heart rate must be monitored as in some cases the cord will be in the lower segment of the uterus. Should labour progress, the suitability for vaginal delivery must be assessed. To prevent the mother pushing before full dilatation an epidural block should be advised (Crawford 1985). This will also relax the pelvic floor, reducing pressure on the fetal head when it passes through as well as facilitating any vaginal manoeuvre that may become necessary. The actual delivery is the same as for a mature breech but there is some evidence that delivery in an intact sac is better for the baby than rupturing the membranes (Goldenberg & Nelson 1984). The infant must be handled particularly gently, with a paediatrician present for the birth.

Should the cervix clamp down on the head, rapid infusion of a tocolytic may relax it somewhat but this is not always immediately available so the head should be flexed with one hand abdominally and the middle finger of the vaginal hand in the baby's mouth. Turning the baby into the transverse diameter may make it easier to deliver through the cervix. If this is unsuccessful, scissors with the intracervical blade guarded by a finger are used to incise the cervix at 4 and 8 o'clock. The previously described manoeuvre should then deliver the head. The edges of the cervical incisions are grasped with sponge-holding forceps and are usually easy to suture as the cervix hangs down into the vagina.

Caesarean section for preterm breech

The current trend is to perform caesarean section for all preterm breech babies although evidence from randomised trials is inadequate to inform practice (Grant 1999).

Bodmer et al (1986) felt that, since head entrapment killed seven out of 55 premature breech babies born between 25 and 28 weeks' gestation, perhaps caesarean section should be undertaken for all babies weighing less than 1000 g. Karp and his colleagues (1979) had already tried to distinguish between the various types of presenting part and felt that small footling breeches should always be delivered by caesarean section, but that those with extended legs could be allowed a trial of labour.

At present it would seem reasonable to consider caesarean section for babies thought to weigh between 1000 and 1500 g, allowing the others to progress in labour and always remembering how difficult it can be to assess fully a premature breech baby in early labour.

Reporting from a hospital where the policy is to utilise abdominal delivery, Westgren et al (1985a) remarked that many cases advanced so quickly that it was not possible to estimate the baby's weight before delivery was imminent. Conceding that the study was retrospective, they had difficulty in showing that caesarean section produced a statistically better result but reported that 25% of the deaths in the vaginally delivered group resulted from head entrapment.

Management of the mature breech baby

If the malpresentation persists at 37 weeks, external cephalic version (ECV) should be considered. Prior to the mid-1970s, external cephalic version was usually attempted before term because it was believed that the procedure would seldom be successful at term. External cephalic version before term entered routine obstetric practice on the basis of the self-evident immediate effectiveness of the procedure as well as reassuring results from several non-randomised trials, and in spite of the negative results of the only randomised trial reported prior to 1980 (Brosset 1956). The popularity of ECV before term waned after the mid-1970s, partly because of reports of perinatal mortality associated with the procedure, and the increasing perception of caesarean section as a safer option than ECV or breech delivery. Review of randomised trials has confirmed the ineffectiveness of ECV before term (Hofmeyr 1999a), though reports of its use continue to appear (Kornman et al 1995).

Subsequent studies showed that with the use of tocolysis, ECV could be achieved in a substantial proportion of women with breech presentation at term. ECV at term differs in many fundamental ways from that performed before term. These include the fact that the fetus is mature and may be delivered more readily in the event of complications, and that spontaneous version without ECV attempt, or reversion after successful ECV, is less common at term. Six randomised trials of external cephalic version at term have been reviewed (Hofmeyr & Kulier 1999b). External cephalic version at term was associated with a significant reduction in non-cephalic births (relative risk 0.42, 95% confidence interval 0.35–0.50) and caesarean section (relative risk 0.52, 95% confidence interval 0.39–0.71). There was no significant effect on perinatal mortality (relative risk 0.44, 95% confidence interval 0.07–2.92). It was calculated that if external cephalic version were attempted in 2% of pregnant women in the United Kingdom, this would result in 15 000 attempts each year, 5100 fewer breech births and 2100 fewer caesarean sections (Hofmeyr 1991). The two randomised trials in black African women (Hofmeyr 1983, Mahomed et al 1991) showed higher success rates than the trials in mainly White European women. This may be because descent of the presenting part into the pelvis is more common in White Europeans making external cephalic version more difficult (Fortunato et al 1988, Hofmeyr et al 1986). Studies of the use of external cephalic version as part of routine hospital policy have reported immediate success rates of 35% (Thunedborg et al 1991), 49% (Hanss 1990), 51% (Laros et al 1995), 59% (Pluta et al 1981) and 60% (Marchick 1988). After the external cephalic version attempt, women who are rhesus-negative receive anti-D immunoglobulin.

Routine tocolysis appears to reduce the failure rate of external cephalic version at term inprimiparal but not in parous women. Other methods of facilitating the procedure which have not yet been adequately evaluated are the use of fetal acoustic stimulation in midline fetal spine positions, epidural analgesia and transabdominal amnioinfusion (Hofmeyr 1999b).

The factors thought to prevent spontaneous version are among those that make external cephalic version more difficult. These are nulliparity (Tan et al 1989), anterior placenta (Kirkinen & Ylostalo 1982), lateral or cornual placenta (Hofmeyr et al 1986), decreased liquor (Kirkinen & Ylostalo 1982, Fortunato et al 1988), low birthweight (Kirkinen & Ylostalo 1982), descent of the breech into the pelvis (Fortunato et al 1988), obesity (Fortunato et al 1988), posteriorly located fetal spine (Fortunato et al 1988), extended legs and firm abdominal muscles (Westgren et al 1985b). Others have found less success with non-frank breech presentation. Lau et al (1997) have investigated which factors are associated with an increased chance of successful external cephalic version. An active policy of version with tocolysis cannot yet be justified in women with a history of antepartum haemorrhage or hypertension.

The benefits of external cephalic version for the mother are clear. The risk of operative vaginal breech delivery, usually with forceps (Tatum et al 1985), or caesarean section is greatly reduced. The risks of the external cephalic version procedure are small, but include possible negative psychological effects in the event of failure (Van De Pavert et al 1990).

The risks and benefits for the fetus are less clearly defined. It is common for fetal heart rate tracings to be non-reactive for 20–40 minutes after the procedure, probably indicating a tendency for the fetus to enter a quiet sleep state during the procedure. Temporary bradycardia is less common (Hofmeyr & Sonnendecker 1983). Placental abruption has been reported following external cephalic version (DeRosa & Anderle 1991). Against the small procedure-related risk must be weighed the risk of persistent breech presentation, including cord prolapse and complications of breech birth. Even if elective caesarean section is planned, complications may result from precipitate breech labour and birth. Caesarean breech delivery is not without the risk of trauma to the baby (Tatum et al 1985), and caesarean section itself may carry increased neonatal risks such as pulmonary hypertension (Heritage & Cunningham 1987). Randomised trials reviewed to date have been too small to address the issue of perinatal mortality. Of 612 women entered into these trials, there have been no procedure-related fetal losses, and perinatal death has occurred in one of the external cephalic version group and three of the control group (Hofmeyr & Kulier 1999b).

Successful external cephalic version has been reported in 82% of 56 women with one or two previous caesarean sections (Flamm et al 1991) and in one other small trial (Schachter et al 1994), but larger trials are needed to establish its safety.

Two small trials of external cephalic version during labour have reported excellent success rates provided the membranes are intact (Fortunato et al 1988, Ferguson & Dyson 1991). Theoretical advantages during labour are that the maximum time for spontaneous version has been allowed, the fetal condition can be monitored continuously until delivery, in the event of failure caesarean section can be performed without delay if the features are not favourable for vaginal breech delivery, and anti-D serum need be given only to those Rh negative women whose babies are Rh positive. Electively delaying external cephalic version until labour has the disadvantages that the opportunity may be lost because of ruptured membranes or rapid labour. However, for women who present in labour with breech presentation, intact membranes and no contraindications, external cephalic version appears to be a good option.

The contraindications and technique for external cephalic version have been described elsewhere (Hofmeyr 1999b).

Elkins (1982) describes 71 women with confirmed breech presentation after the 37th week of gestation. All were instructed to adopt the knee–chest position for 15 minutes every 2 hours of waking time for 5 days. A total of 65 babies underwent spontaneous version and all had normal vaginal deliveries. Of the six who failed to turn, two had low-lying placentas, two had unusually short cords and one mother had a bicornuate uterus; all six underwent caesarean section. There were no perinatal deaths in either group and no evidence of side-effects or complications from the manoeuvre. The results of randomised trials of a modified knee–chest procedure have been inconclusive (Hofmeyr & Kulier 1999c).

Management of the persistent breech presentation

Failure of version means that a decision must be made whether a baby in breech presentation should be delivered by elective caesarean section or be allowed to go into labour. During the 1970s caesarean section was being used increasingly: in the US for breeches it rose from 11.6% in 1970 to 79.1% in 1985. Cheng & Hannah in 1993 pointed out that a percentage of mothers sectioned for breech experienced significant morbidity. In 1982, Green et al reported that a caesarean section rate increase from 22% to 94% produced no significant improvement for breech babies either in the short or long term.

The routine use of caesarean section for breech presentation has become widespread without evidence from randomised trials that the benefits of such a policy outweigh the risks (Hofmeyr 1989). The interpretation of studies that compare outcome after vaginal breech delivery and cephalic birth is confounded by the fact that breech presentation per se appears to be a marker for poor perinatal outcome. Thus poor outcomes following vaginal breech delivery may be the result of underlying conditions causing breech presentation rather than damage during delivery.

In a review of two randomised trials and seven cohort studies, the risk difference between trial of labour and planned caesarean section for any perinatal injury or death was 1.1% (Gifford et al 1995), findings similar to a previous review (Cheng & Hannah 1993). However, cohort studies are fundamentally flawed by the fact that factors that influence the choice of method of delivery may have more to do with the outcome for the baby than the method of delivery. In addition, the selection criteria for allowing a trial of labour in the studies included in these reviews may differ from those used today, and little attention was given to the skill and experience of the clinician at delivery. For these reasons, information from randomised trials is required to determine whether benefits (if any) of routine caesarean section for the infant are sufficient to justify subjecting mothers to the increased current and future risks of caesarean section. Caesarean section is associated with increased maternal morbidity (Department of Health 1989), subsequent reproductive function is compromised, and there may be negative emo-

tional effects (Garel et al 1990). Another problem associated with a policy of routine elective caesarean section for breech delivery is that with time vaginal breech delivery skills are lost. This may impair the outcome in unanticipated breech deliveries.

The recent Term Breech Trial has shown convincingly that planned vaginal breech birth is associated with more perinatal morbidity than planned caesarean section (Hannah et al 2000, Hofmeyr & Hannah 2001).

Criteria have been developed from clinical experience to minimise the risk of vaginal breech delivery. Ultrasound, after excluding abnormality and placenta praevia, should be used to estimate the fetal weight. If this is more than 3750 g, a caesarean section may be indicated. The fetal attitude is also important and, even with a small baby, extension of the head is an unfavourable finding. Westgren et al (1981), on the basis of an observational trial, advocated abdominal delivery if the fetal neck was extended in any way.

Vaginal delivery is usually restricted to frank and complete breech presentations. If the body and thighs at term together pass easily through the pelvis, there is unlikely to be disproportion. Footling or kneeling presentations are unfavourable as the body may pass through an inadequate pelvis or incompletely dilated cervix.

Breech labour should take place in an institution with resident staff skilled in breech delivery, and facilities for safe emergency caesarean section (Bingham & Lilford 1987).

Inducing labour prematurely in an attempt to achieve a smaller baby would have to be done so early in the pregnancy that the chances of successful induction would be much reduced. Induction for other reasons is not totally contraindicated but most obstetricians would regard two pregnancy complications as a reason for caesarean section.

Management of labour in the mature breech

Once labour commences, cervical dilatation and descent of the breech should be plotted on a partogram, as with a cephalic presentation. Vaginal examination is done to exclude cord prolapse and to confirm whether the breech is flexed or extended. Oxytocin infusion is permissible only to accelerate a dilatory labour in its early stages, not to try to deliver an over-sized breech through the pelvis. As with premature breeches, epidural anaesthesia both relieves pain and prevents the mother pushing involuntarily before full cervical dilatation. Failure of the cervix to dilate at a standard rate or of the breech to descend should be accepted as indicating that the baby is larger (or the pelvis smaller) than the prelabour assessment had implied, and caesarean section will be required. Descent is regarded as adequate when the breech reaches the level of the ischial spines when the cervix is 6 cm dilated, and the pelvic floor at full dilatation. There is no need to encourage maternal efforts immediately the cervix is fully dilated but, once she does start pushing, failure of the breech to descend should lead to caesarean section rather than breech extraction.

If labour progresses satisfactorily, preparation should be made for an assisted breech delivery. This involves a standard forceps trolley on which there is also a sterile razor and a scalpel with a no. 1 blade. The mother is in the lithotomy position with a wedge under one side of the buttocks. If she does not have epidural analgesia, it will be necessary to infiltrate the perineum and preferably do a pudendal block once the breech has descended on to it. Episiotomy is reserved until the fetal anus has appeared at the vulva. Once done, maternal effort should deliver the baby's buttocks and, with flexed legs, the lower limbs. With extended legs the operator will have to flex each knee joint separately, pushing it to the side of the baby so that the foot pops out. Only once the delivery has commenced may oxytocin be added to the intravenous infusion to maximise uterine contractions, particularly with epidural analgesia as the physiological second stage oxytocin surge is blocked.

The mother is encouraged to bear down until the trunk up to the scapula becomes visible. Cord pulsation is checked and a small loop pulled down to prevent traction on the cord. The mother is asked to push again and the shoulders should deliver one at a time, along with the arms folded over the chest.

Failure of the shoulders to deliver is dealt with by lifting up the baby's legs and trunk, which enables a finger to reach an elbow joint; flexing it, and delivering it across the chest. This is repeated for the other side. Gentle rotation of the fetal trunk at the same time will assist this manoeuvre. Rarely, the baby's abdomen is facing the operator: if so, the trunk is turned and, as the mother pushes, one shoulder will deliver under the symphysis with further rotation producing the other. With extended arms it is necessary to slide an index finger along the baby's scapula over the shoulder and down into the antecubital fossa to deliver the elbow between the body and the side of the vulva. These manoeuvres virtually always deliver the shoulders.

At this stage the baby's head may start to appear without any further effort on the operator's part. Should maternal effort not push down the head, more assistance is needed as the occiput must be low enough in the pelvis to hinge around the back of the symphysis and not be caught above it. Simply permitting the baby to hang may delay progress: the manoeuvre can cause extension rather than flexion of the head as the head swivels on an axis through the biparietal eminences (Fig. 34.7). Therefore, while the baby is hanging feet down, the operator must insert two fingers behind the symphysis pubis to push up an anterior lip of cervix which is often dragged down by the occiput and will slow its final descent (Fig. 34.8). This will also tend to flex the head, an action which can be further assisted by some suprapubic pressure and renewed maternal effort.

Once the hairline is visible the head is delivered. The baby's feet are grasped and, using as much traction as required to keep the body straight and take weight off its neck, they are swung outwards and upwards to be held by an assistant, using a towel to make certain they do not slip. The operator then applies a Neville–Barnes type or Piper's forceps and delivers the head slowly, sucking out the mouth as soon as it can be seen, and remembering that the final part of the head only appears as the face flexes on to the chest. Unlike a conventional forceps application, a breech delivery means that the smallest part of the baby's skull appears at the vulva first with the large parietal area at the back of the pelvis. Thus, if the forceps handle is straightened out too soon after

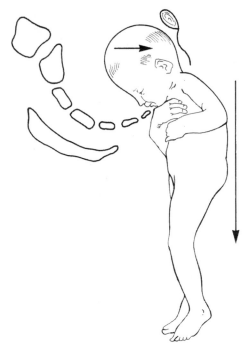

Fig. 34.7 Trunk of breech allowed to hang. Traction on fetal spine would extend, not flex the head. Contrast this with Figure 34.2.

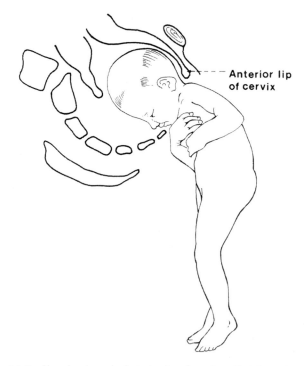

Fig. 34.8 Hanging breech. Anterior lip of cervix pulled down by occiput must be pushed up before forceps can be applied.

insertion of the blade, the distal part of the blade will dig into the side of the baby's head and it will not be possible to lock the handles. The tip must be kept pointed at the sacrum for as long as possible, which means that the guiding hand has to be inserted well into the vagina until the tip has passed round the occiput.

If forceps delivery is not possible the legs may be swung out and up in a Burns Marshall manoeuvre, keeping the vulva completely covered with the other hand. It is essential that the baby's legs should be kept vertically in the air and the weight taken off the cervical spine. Hyperextension of the neck with the body being held over the mother's abdomen will occlude the vertebral arteries and can lead to necrosis of the cervical cord. Excess weight on the cervical spine will either have the same effect or dislocate the baby's neck. The operator's vulval hand can then be opened slowly to allow first the baby's face and then the remainder of the head to deliver. The Mauriceau–Smellie–Veit manoeuvre is favoured by some obstetricians for routine delivery of the head. The middle finger of one hand in the mouth, and the second and fourth fingers on the malar eminences promote flexion and descent, while counterpressure is applied to the occiput with the middle finger of the other hand. Traction on the cervical spine should be avoided as it causes fetal trauma and extension of the head.

Problems

Shoulder dystocia rarely occurs without extended arms; this has usually been caused by traction on the fetus early in the delivery. The body is pulled down leaving the arms behind, rather than the uterus pushing down the whole fetus in a flexed attitude. Often the arms can be brought down as already described but lack of success means that Løvset's manoeuvre will be required. The baby must be held by the thighs—never by the trunk—and the operator must wrap the legs in a towel so that they do not slip when gripped. The baby is rotated so that first one then the other shoulder delivers under the symphysis pubis, always keeping the back upwards. Gentle traction on the delivered hand across the baby's chest may assist the rotation to deliver the second shoulder.

Should the head not enter the pelvis after the shoulders have delivered, the baby's body must be turned sideways and suprapubic pressure used to flex the head and push it into the pelvis. This may be helped by the vaginal hand inserting a finger into the baby's mouth to flex it. Both these actions also make the head descend if it has entered the pelvis but is still not low enough to apply forceps.

Continued failure of the head to engage is the sole indication for symphysiotomy. The technique is described by Philpott (1980) and Gebbie (1982), although the latter points out that, in a mature baby, if the head is not going to fit through the pelvis the buttocks too should be obstructed. With proper predelivery assessment the technique will never be necessary, nor should such extreme measures as replacing the body of the baby and proceeding to caesarean section, as described by Iffy et al (1986). Such potential disasters emphasise the importance of delivery suites having the facilities available to make rapid assessment in unbooked or unsuspected breech presentations (Davis & Brunfield 1984).

KEY POINT

- Suboptimal progress of breech labour at any stage is best managed by caesarean section.

UMBILICAL CORD PRESENTATION AND PROLAPSE

Umbilical cord presentation occurs about once in every 300 deliveries. Cord presentation is when the cord lies below the level of the presenting part, and it is said to have prolapsed following rupture of the membranes and its release into the vagina.

Sometimes a malpresentation of the cord can be identified on ultrasound scan, but more often it is found on vaginal examination when, if the fetus is alive, it becomes an obstetric emergency.

This malpresentation is often associated with a condition in which the presenting part of the fetus is incompletely filling the pelvis, thus allowing room for the umbilical cord to pass between it and the pelvic wall. Thus it should be suspected with a high head, polyhydramnios, a footling or flexed breech, transverse lie and a small fetus, either premature or one of a multiple pregnancy.

Diagnosis

The diagnosis is usually made on vaginal examination following rupture of the membranes. Absence of cord pulsations does not mean that the fetus is not alive, as spasm of the cord vessels may make pulsations difficult to feel. The cord should be handled as little as possible. If it has prolapsed through the introitus, it should be gently replaced in the vagina. The baby's condition should be checked by auscultation, or if necessary a doptone fetal heart detector or ultrasound. If the fetus has not already died it is in imminent danger of doing so, either by spasm of the vessels in the cord exposed to the cooling air or more likely due to compression of the cord against the pelvic wall. On the rare occasions that the diagnosis is made in the second stage of labour, a forceps or vacuum delivery is indicated. In all other cases the mother should be placed in a head-down position so as to dislodge the presenting pole from the pelvis to avoid cord compression. If the uterus is contracting, a tocolytic may be given. The hand of the examiner should be kept in the vagina to prevent further prolapse of the cord and its compression, and arrangements should be made as quickly as possible by others in the department for immediate caesarean section. Occasionally, the cord can be replaced into the uterus and, if this resolves the problem, labour can be allowed to continue (Barrett 1991).

The essence of good management is anticipation. Prophylactic measures such as the admission to hospital of patients with unstable and transverse lie in the last three weeks of pregnancy, the avoidance of artificially rupturing the membranes before the fetal pole has become deeply engaged in the pelvis, and early vaginal examination following spontaneous rupture of the membranes will all help to reduce the mortality and morbidity for the fetus.

CAESAREAN SECTION FOR ABNORMAL POSITIONS AND PRESENTATIONS

Abdominal delivery for fetal malposition or malpresentation often takes place at the end of a long labour and may technically be more difficult than with a normal presentation. Although there is no need to use any of the more complicated extraperitoneal approaches which used to be suggested, there should always be someone experienced scrubbed up in theatre; the operating table must be tilted laterally or a simple wedge inserted under the mother's right buttock and a paediatrician skilled in neonatal resuscitation should be present.

Occipito-posterior positions

However high the head feels on vaginal examination, at caesarean section it can be difficult to extricate from the pelvis and an assistant must be ready to push it up vaginally. Just before commencing the operation, it is important to repeat a vaginal examination in case the head has rotated and descended during preparations for surgery. Check on which side the baby's back lies, as this will facilitate rotation of the head during the delivery. It must be assumed that the lower segment of the uterus will be thin and may tear readily. If there is little amniotic fluid and the fetus is held into the pelvis by the contracting uterus, it may be necessary to give a tocolytic drug to facilitate delivery, realising that uterine contraction after delivery may be somewhat slower. The surgeon should aim to insert a hand around the side of the baby's head and deliver it slowly out of the pelvis, above the level of the uterine incision, and rotate it to the occipito-anterior position before bringing it anteriorly through the uterine incision. In the case of a direct occipito-posterior position, it may be easier to deliver the face first through the uterine incision. Tears arise because the chin catches on the upper edge of the wound and as the face, followed by the brow, the vertex, and finally the occiput deliver, the lower edge is stretched to allow passage of these large diameters and often splits. Such lacerations are never easy to repair and occasionally involve the base of the bladder. The same comments apply to face and brow presentations, where the diameters may be even larger and, especially with the brow, the labour may have become obstructed, leading to excess thinning of the lower segment and occasionally a constriction ring.

Transverse lie

When the membranes are intact the operator has the choice of looking for the baby's head and steering it quickly into the incision as the uterus clamps down when the amniotic fluid rushes out. In practice, a limb often appears in the incision: usually this is an arm. It should be replaced quickly, a leg grasped and the baby extracted as a breech. Many operators choose a breech delivery as a first option, pushing the membranes in front of the operating hand, finding a limb, palpating its lower end to make certain it is a foot and withdrawing it through the incision just as the amniotic fluid starts to escape.

With a transverse lie and already ruptured membranes, the lower segment of the uterus may be so narrow that a conventional incision would not be large enough for any baby. Tocolysis has been suggested to facilitate delivery although it has not yet been proven to be effective (David et al 1998). The anaesthetist should be asked to give a rapid dose of a uterine relaxant for two or three minutes (Maduska 1981). A midline uterine incision may be needed. Jovanovic (1985) has made the point that if the uterine incision is enlarged by cutting rather than tearing, with the extremes of the incision pointing upwards rather than laterally, then not only will the aperture be larger but any extension will go upwards rather than downwards and be easier to repair. Should these measures not be successful the operator has no choice but to enlarge the incision vertically from its middle point, making an inverted T incision. To avoid the possibility of this, many obstetricians regard transverse lie with ruptured membranes as an indication for a midline uterine incision. Here, the bladder should be pushed down and the incision brought as far as possible into the lower segment (a De Lee incision) and only extended upwards as needed.

In all cases the inside of the uterus must be inspected to exclude an abnormality such as a small septum or a fibroid which might have caused the transverse lie. This is carefully noted in the patient's records for future reference, along with inspection of the ovaries and tubes, to rule out other tumours which may have had the same effect.

Premature breech

If the baby is very small the lower segment may not have formed. Although Haesslein & Goodlin (1979) proposed solving this problem by using a vertical incision, most other workers do not agree with them. Westgren et al (1982) advocated a bolus of uterine relaxant such as terbutaline just before opening the uterus, although Westgren later modified this, suggesting that the lower segment should be carefully examined and in some cases a vertical incision performed (Westgren et al 1985a). Hobel & Oakes (1980) suggested that halothane at the induction of anaesthesia was best for all small section babies. Schutterman & Grimes (1983), reviewing 416 breeches of all gestations allocated randomly to transverse or low vertical incisions, found no advantages for low vertical incisions.

It would appear that the normal lower segment transverse incision, with an added uterine relaxant in some cases, is satisfactory for breech section. Whatever incision is used the baby must be delivered as gently as with the vaginal approach: forceps are essential for the aftercoming head. In order that no part of the baby is caught in the abdominal wound the incision should be sufficiently big to take the beak of a large Doyen retractor.

Mature breech

Section for mature breech should produce no technical difficulties but forceps should be available for controlling delivery of the aftercoming head. The point about not hyperextending or placing too much traction on the cervical spine applies with equal force.

KEY POINT

- Caesarean section for abnormal lie or presentation requires special attention to the uterine incision and technique of delivery.

THE NEWBORN BABY

All babies born after abnormal presentations or positions require a thorough paediatric examination even if the delivery was spontaneous and however well they may appear at the time. The unusual moulding caused by the abnormal position of the head or the speed of this moulding may cause intracranial lesions. Some will have had operative vaginal deliveries which, however easy they may seem to the attendant, are more traumatic for the fetus. Above all, there is always the suspicion that the malpresentation or the malposition has been due to some abnormality in the fetus. This is especially so in the case of the breech baby. Many of these will be premature and paediatric assessment will be routine in any case.

In the mature breech, it should be assumed until proved otherwise that some inherent defect in the baby prevented it from turning to the cephalic presentation in utero.

Above all, it is important to be aware that not all neonatal deficiencies are due to the mode of delivery or to incorrect obstetrical management in labour. Illingworth in 1985 was the first to stress that most cases of cerebral palsy or mental subnormality follow a normal pregnancy and delivery: to ascribe brain damage solely to events occurring during labour is too simplistic.

Abnormal presentations and positions will always be found in obstetrical practice. Labour ward routines must be constantly reviewed and agreed guidelines produced so as to counteract the adverse effects of abnormal presentations.

KEY POINTS

- Failure to adopt the cephalic presentation may be seen as failure of the fetus to achieve its first developmental milestone. Developmental impairment may be a cause rather than a result of breech birth.
- Vacuum extraction causes less maternal trauma than forceps delivery, but is associated with an increase in neonatal cephalohaematomata and retinal haemorrhages.
- Occipito-posterior face and persistent brow presentations are managed by caesarean section
- Non-longitudinal lie may be corrected by external cephalic version in early labour or prior to labour induction. If external version is contraindicated or unsuccessful, caesarean section is needed.
- For malpresentation or abnormal lie of the second twin, the choice lies between external cephalic version, caesarean section, and (rarely) internal version and breech extraction.

- External cephalic version for term breech presentation reduces the risk of breech birth and caesarean section.
- Caesarean section is increasingly being used for breech delivery. Data from the Term Breech Trial should help to inform future policy.
- Suboptimal progress of breech labour at any stage is best managed by caesarean section.
- The possibility of cord prolapse must be kept in mind in obstetric situations known to be associated with this risk.
- Caesarean section for abnormal lie or presentation requires special attention to the uterine incision and technique of delivery.

REFERENCES

Acker DB, Sachs BP, Friedman EA 1986 Risk factors for shoulder dystocia in the average-weight infant. Obstet Gynecol 67:614–618

Anderson ABM 1981 Second thoughts on stopping labour. In: Studd J (ed) Progress in obstetrics and gynaecology, vol 1. Churchill Livingstone, Edinburgh, pp 125–138

Andrews CM, Andrews EC 1983 Nursing, maternal postures, and fetal position. Nurs Res 32:336–341

Barrett JM 1991 Funic reduction for the management of umbilical cord prolapse. Am J Obstet Gynecol 165:654–657

Ben-Rafael Z, Seidman DS, Recabi K, Bider D, Mashiach S 1991 Uterine anomalies. A retrospective, matched-control study. J Reprod Med 36:723–727

Besinger R, Compton A, Hayashi R 1987 The presence of fetal breathing movements as a predictor of outcome in preterm labour. Am J Obstet Gynecol 157:753–757

Bingham P, Lilford RJ 1987 Management of the selected term breech presentation: assessment of the risks of selected vaginal delivery versus caesarean section for all cases. Obstet Gynecol 69:965–977

Bodmer B, Benjamin A, McLean FH, Usher RH 1986 Has caesarean section reduced the risks of delivery in the preterm breech presentation? Am J Obstet Gynecol 154:244–250

Bottoms SF, Hirsch VJ, Sokol RJ 1987 Medical management of arrest disorders of labor: a current overview. Am J Obstet Gynecol 156:935–939

Brosset A 1956 The value of prophylactic external version in cases of breech presentation. Acta Obstet Gynecol Scand 35:555–562

Cally E, Walkinshaw S, Chia P, Manasse PR, Atlay RD 1993 Undiagnosed breech. Br J Obstet Gynecol 100:531–535

Cheng M, Hannah M 1993 Breech delivery at term. Obstet Gynecol 82:605–618

Coats PM, Chan KK, Wilkins M, Beard RJ 1980 A comparison between midline and mediolateral episiotomies. Br J Obstet Gynaecol 87:408–412

Crawford JS 1985 Lumbar epidural analgesia for labour and delivery: a personal view. In: Studd J (ed) The management of labour. Blackwell Scientific Publications, Oxford, pp 226–234

Crowley P 1999 Prophylactic corticosteroids for preterm birth (Cochrane Review). In: The Cochrane Library, Issue 4. Update Software, Oxford

Cruikshank DP, Cruikshank JE 1981 Face and brow presentation: a review. Clinical Obstetrics and Gynecology 24:333–351

Danielian PJ, Wang J, Hall MH 1996 Long term outcome by method of delivery of fetuses in breech presentation at term: population based follow up. BMJ 312:1451–1453

David M, Schouli J, Plischek S, Halle H, Lichtenegger W 1998 Nitroglycerine for intraoperative uterine relaxation during Caesarean section (translation). Z Geburtshilfe Neonatol 202:168–171

Davis RO, Brunfield CG 1984 The use of real-time ultrasound in the management of obstetric emergencies. Clin Obstet Gynecol 27:68–77

Department of Health 1989 Report on Confidential Enquiries into Maternal Deaths in England and Wales, 1982–84. Her Majesty's Stationery Office, London

DeRosa J, Anderle LJ 1991 External cephalic version of term singleton breech presentations with tocolysis: a retrospective study in a community hospital. J Am Osteopath Assoc 91:351–352

Drew JH, McKenzie J, Kelly E, Beischer NA 1991 Second twin: quality of survival if born by breech extraction following internal podalic version. Aust NZ J Obstet Gynaecol 31:111–114

Edwards RL, Nicholson HO 1969 The management of the unstable lie in late pregnancy. J Obstet Gynaecol Br Commonwealth 76:713–718

Elkins VH 1982 Procedure for turning breech. In: Enkin M, Chalmers I (eds) Effectiveness and satisfaction in antenatal care. Spastic International Medical Publishers, London, p 216

Faber-Nijholt R, Huisjes HJ, Touwen BCL, Fidler VJ 1983 Neurological follow-up of 281 children born in breech presentation: a controlled study. BMJ 286:9–12

Ferguson JE, Dyson DC 1991 Intrapartum external cephalic version after previous cesarean section. Am J Obstet Gynecol 165:370–372

Fianu S, Vaclavinkova V 1978 The site of placental attachment as a factor in the aetiology of breech presentation. Acta Obstet Gynecol Scand 57:371–372

Flamm BL, Fried MW, Lonky NM, Giles WS 1991 External cephalic version after previous cesarean section. Am J Obstet Gynecol 165:370–372

Fortunato SJ, Mercer LJ, Guzick DS 1988 External cephalic version with tocolysis: factors associated with success. Obstet Gynecol 72:59–62

Friedman EA, Sachtleben MR, Bresky PA 1977 Dysfunctional labor. Am J Obstet Gynecol 127:779–783

Garel M, Lelong N, Marchand A, Kaminski M 1990 Psychological consequences of caesarean childbirth: a four-year follow-up study. Early Hum Dev 21:105–114

Gebbie D 1982 Symphysiotomy. Clin Obstet Gynaecol 9:663–683

Gifford DS, Morton SC, Kahn K 1995 A meta-analysis of infant outcomes after breech delivery. Obstet Gynecol 85:1047–1054

Gilstrap LC, Hauth JC, Toussaint S 1984 Cesarean section: changing incidence and indications. Obstet Gynecol 63:205–208

Goeke SE, Nageotte MP, Garite T, Towers CV, Dorchester W 1989 Management of the non-vertex second twin: primary cesarean section, external version, or primary breech extraction. Am J Obstet Gynecol 161:111–114

Goldenberg RL, Nelson KG 1984 The unanticipated breech presentation in labor. Clin Obstet Gynecol 27:95–105

Gordon B, Mackrodt C, Fern E, Truesdale A, Ayers S, Grant A 1998 The Ipswich Childbirth Study. 1. A randomised evaluation of two stage postpartum perineal repair leaving the skin unsutured. Br J Obstet Gynaecol 105:435–440

Grant A 1999 Elective versus selective Caesarean section for delivery of the small baby (Cochrane Review). In: The Cochrane Library, Issue 4. Update Software, Oxford

Green JF, McLean F, Smith LP, Usher R 1982 Has an increased cesarean section rate for term breech delivery reduced the incidence of birth asphyxia, trauma, and death? Am J Obstet Gynecol 142:643–648

Haesslein HC, Goodlin RC 1979 Delivery of the tiny newborn. Am J Obstet Gynecol 134:192–197

Hannah ME, Hannah WJ, Hewson SA, Hodnett ED, Saigal S, Willan AR, for the Term Breech Trial Collaborative Group 2000 Planned caesarean section versus planned vaginal birth for breech presentation at term: a randomised multicentre trial. Lancet 356:1375–1383

Hanss JW 1990 The efficacy of external cephalic version and its impact on the breech experience. Am J Obstet Gynecol 162:1459–1463

Heritage CK, Cunningham MD 1987 Association of elective repeat cesarean delivery and persistent pulmonary hypertension of the newborn. Am J Obstet Gynecol 152:627–629

Hobel CJ, Oakes GK 1980 Special considerations in the management of preterm labor. Clin Obstet Gynecol 23:147–164

Hofmeyr GJ 1983 Effect of external cephalic version in late pregnancy on breech presentation and caesarean section rate: a controlled trial. Br J Obstet Gynaecol 90:392–399

Hofmeyr GJ 1989 Breech presentation and abnormal lie in late pregnancy. In: Chalmers I, Enkin MW, Keirse MJNC (eds) Effective care in pregnancy and childbirth. Oxford University Press, Oxford, pp 653–665

Hofmeyr GJ 1991 External cephalic version at term: how high are the stakes? Br J Obstet Gynaecol 98:1–3

Hofmeyr GJ 1999a External cephalic version for breech presentation before term (Cochrane Review). In: The Cochrane Library, Issue 4. Update Software, Oxford

Hofmeyr GJ 1999b External cephalic version facilitation for breech presentation at term (Cochrane Review). In: The Cochrane Library, Issue 4. Update Software, Oxford

Hofmeyr GJ, Hannah ME 2001 Planned Caesarean section for term breech delivery (Cochrane Review). In: The Cochrane Library, Issue 1. Update Software, Oxford

Hofmeyr GJ, Kulier R 1999a Hands/knees posture in late pregnancy or labour for fetal malposition (lateral or posterior) (Cochrane Review). In: The Cochrane Library, Issue 4. Update Software, Oxford

Hofmeyr GJ, Kulier R 1999b External cephalic version for breech presentation at term (Cochrane Review). In: The Cochrane Library, Issue 4. Update Software, Oxford

Hofmeyr GJ, Kulier R 1999c Cephalic version by postural management for breech presentation (Cochrane Review). In: The Cochrane Library, Issue 4. Update Software, Oxford

Hofmeyr GJ, Sonnendecker EWW 1983 Cardiotocographic changes after external cephalic version. Br J Obstet Gynaecol 90:914–918

Hofmeyr GJ, Sadan O, Myer IG, Galal KC, Simko G 1986 External cephalic version and spontaneous version rates: ethnic and other determinants. Br J Obstet Gynaecol 93:13–16

Iffy L, Apuzzio JJ, Cohen-Addad N, Zwolska-Demczuk B, Francis-Lane M, Olenczak J 1986 Abdominal rescue after entrapment of the aftercoming head. Am J Obstet Gynecol 154:623–624

Illingworth RS 1985 A paediatrician asks—why is it called birth injury? Br J Obstet Gynaecol 92:122–130

Johanson RB, Menon BKV 1999a Vacuum extraction versus forceps for assisted vaginal delivery (Cochrane Review). In: The Cochrane Library, Issue 4. Update Software, Oxford

Johanson R, Menon V 1999b Soft versus rigid vacuum extractor cups for assisted vaginal delivery (Cochrane Review). In: The Cochrane Library, Issue 4. Update Software, Oxford

Jovanovic R 1985 Incisions of the pregnant uterus and delivery of low-birth weight infants. Am J Obstet Gynecol 152:971–974

Karp LE, Doney JR, McCarthy T, Meis PJ, Hall M 1979 The premature breech: trial of labor or Cesarean section? Obstet Gynecol 53:88–92

Kettle C, Johanson RB 1999a Continuous versus interrupted sutures for perineal repair (Cochrane Review). In: The Cochrane Library, Issue 4. Update Software, Oxford

Kettle C, Johanson RB 1999b Absorbable synthetic versus catgut suture material for perineal repair (Cochrane Review). In: The Cochrane Library, Issue 4. Update Software, Oxford

Kirkinen P, Ylostalo P 1982 Ultrasonic examination before external version of breech presentation. Gynecol Obstet Invest 13:90–97

Kornman MT, Kimball KT, Reeves KO 1995 Preterm external cephalic version in an outpatient environment. Am J Obstet Gynecol 172:1741

Lange IR, Manning FA, Morrison I, Chamberlain PF, Harman CR 1985 Cord prolapse: is antenatal diagnosis possible? Am J Obstet Gynecol 151:1083–1085

Laros RK, Flanagan TA, Kilpatrick SJ 1995 Management of term breech presentation: a protocol of external cephalic version and selective trial of labour. Am J Obstet Gynecol 172:1916–1925

Lau TK, Lo KWK, Wan D, Rogers MS 1997 Predictors of successful external cephalic version at term: a prospective study. Br J Obstet Gynaecol 104:798–802

Lowe B 1987 Fear of failure: a place for the trial of instrumental delivery. Br J Obstet Gynaecol 94:60–66

Maduska AL 1981 Inhalation analgesia and general anesthesia. Clin Obstet Gynecol 24:619–633

Mahomed K, Philipsen T, Secher NJ 1991 External cephalic version at term: a randomised control trial using tocolysis. Br J Obstet Gynaecol 98:8–13

Marchick R 1988 Antepartum external cephalic version with tocolysis: a study of term singleton breech presentations. Am J Obstet Gynecol 158:1339–1346

Michalas SP 1991 Outcome of pregnancy in women with uterine malformation, evaluation of 62 cases. Int J Obstet Gynecol 35:215–219

Moessinger AC, Blaes WA, Marone PA, Polsen DC 1982 Umbilical cord length as an index of fetal activity: experimental study and clinical implications. Pediatr Res 16:109–112

Moore R 1970 Evolution. Life Nature Library. Time–Life International (Nederland), NV, p 165

Morgan B 1972 The descent of woman. Souvenir Press, London, pp 21–42

Myerscough PR 1982 Occipitoposterior positions of the vertex. In: Munro Kerr's Operative obstetrics, 10th edn. Baillière Tindall, London, pp 50–60

O'Connell P, Keane A 1985 The term breech: subsequent growth and development. In: Clinch J, Matthews T (eds) Perinatal medicine. MTP Press, Lancaster, p 219

Parry-Jones E 1968 Barton's forceps: its use in transverse position of the fetal head. J Obstet Gynaecol Br Commonwealth 75:892–901

Phelan JP, Stine LE, Edwards NB, Clark SL, Horenstein J 1985 The role of external version in the intrapartum management of the transverse lie presentation. Am J Obstet Gynecol 151:724–726

Phillips RD, Freeman M 1974 The management of the persistent occiput posterior position. Obstet Gynecol 43:171–177

Philpott RH 1980 Obstructed labour. Clin Obstet Gynecol 7:601–619

Pluta M, Schmidt S, Giffei JM, Saling E 1981 Die Ausere wendung de Feten aus beckenendlage Schadellage in Terminnale unter Tokolyse. Z Geburtshilfe Perinatale 1985:207–215

Rannay B 1973 The gentle art of external cephalic version. Am J Obstet Gynecol 116:239–248

Reading AE, Sledmere CM, Cox DN, Campbell S 1982 How women view postepisiotomy pain. BMJ 284:243–246

Robertson IS 1984 Breech presentation associated with anticonvulsant drugs. J Obstet Gynecol 4:174–177

Sandberg EC 1985 The Zavanelli maneuver: a potentially revolutionary method for the resolution of shoulder dystocia. Am J Obstet Gynecol 152:479–484

Schachter M, Kogan S, Blickstein I 1994 External cephalic version after previous cesarean section—a clinical dilemma. Int J Gynaecol Obstet 45:17–20

Scheer K, Nubar J 1976 Variation of fetal presentation with gestational age. Am J Obstet Gynecol 125:269–270

Schutterman EB, Grimes DA 1983 Comparative safety of the low transverse versus the low vertical uterine incision for cesarean delivery of breech infants. Obstet Gynecol 61:593–597

Soernes T, Bakke T 1986 The length of human umbilical cord in vertex and breech presentation. Am J Obstet Gynecol 154:1086–1087

Stevenson CS 1950 The principle cause of breech presentation in single term pregnancies. Am J Obstet Gynecol 60:41–53

Stevenson CS 1951 Certain concepts in the handling of breech and transverse presentations in late pregnancy. Am J Obstet Gynecol 62:488–505

Stewart DB 1984a The pelvis as a passageway. I. Evolution and adaptations. Br J Obstet Gynaecol 91:611–617

Stewart DB 1984b The pelvis as a passageway. II. The modern human pelvis. Br J Obstet Gynaecol 91:618–623

Tan GW, Jen SW, Tan SL, Salmon YM 1989 A prospective randomised control trial of external cephalic version comparing two methods of tocolysis with a non tocolytic group. Singapore Med J 31:155–158

Tatum RK, Orr JW, Soong S, Huddleston JF 1985 Vaginal breech delivery of selected infants weighing more than 2000 grams: a retrospective analysis of seven years' experience. Am J Obstet Gynecol 152:145–155

Tchabo JG, Tomai T 1992 Selected intrapartum external cephalic version of the second twin. Obstet Gynecol 79:421–423

Thorp JM Jr, Jenkins T, Watson W 1991 Utility of Leopold manoeuvres in screening for malpresentation. Obstet Gynecol 78:394–399

Thunedborg P, Fischer-Rasmussen W, Tollund L 1991 The benefit of external cephalic version with tocolysis as a routine procedure in late pregnancy. Eur J Obstet Gynecol Reprod Biol 42:23–27

Tompkins P 1946 An enquiry into the cause of breech presentation. Am J Obstet Gynecol 51:595–602

Torgrim S, Bakke T 1986 The length of the human umbilical cord in vertex and breech presentations. Am J Obstet Gynecol 154:1086–1087

Van De Pavert R, Gravenhorst JB, Keirse MJNC 1990 Value of external version in breech presentation at term. Ned Tijdschr Geneesk 134:2245–2248

Westgren M, Grundsell H, Ingemarsson I, Muhlow A, Svenningsen NW 1981 Hyperextension of the fetal head in breech presentation: a study with long-term follow-up. Br J Obstet Gynaecol 88:101–104

Westgren M, Ingemarsson I, Ahlstrom H, Lindroth N, Svenningsen NW 1982 Delivery and long-term outcome of very low birthweight infants. Acta Obstet Gynecol Scand 61:25–30

Westgren LMR, Songster G, Paul RH 1985a Preterm breech delivery: another retrospective study. Obstet Gynecol 66:481–484

Westgren M, Edvall H, Nordstrom L, Svalenius E, Ranstam J 1985b Spontaneous cephalic version of breech presentation in the last trimester. Br J Obstet Gynaecol 92:19–22

Wigglesworth JS, Husemeyer RP 1977 Intracranial birth trauma in vaginal breech delivery: the continued importance of injury to the occipital bone. Br J Obstet Gynaecol 84:684–691

Yudkin PL, Redman CWG 1986 Caesarean section dissected, 1978–1983. Br J Obstet Gynaecol 93:135–144

35

Induction and augmentation of labour

Michael S. Rogers

The contribution of the author of the equivalent chapter in the second edition, on which this chapter draws extensively, is gratefully acknowledged.

INTRODUCTION

The terms induction and augmentation of labour are frequently confused because of their methodological similarities: i.e. the use of oxytocin and amniotomy. They are different interventions in the normal process of parturition.

Induction involves the timing of labour and delivery being brought forward, as with elective caesarean section.

Augmentation of labour is where the process of labour, having begun spontaneously, is accelerated by administering oxytocic agents or by amniotomy according to active management principles (Philpott & Castle 1972a, 1972b, O'Driscoll et al 1984). This is, therefore, more akin to emergency caesarean or operative vaginal delivery in terms of obstetric intervention.

The essential differences between induction and augmentation, therefore, relate to the intention of the obstetrician and to the timing of the onset of labour (before or after the intervention). Inevitably there are grey areas where the timing of the onset of labour is in doubt. These are centred around the latent phase of labour and include false labour; delayed latent phase and failed induction. Obstetrics is not always a precise science, but obstetricians are experienced at making decisions under conditions of uncertainty. This approach avoids having to define when labour starts, merely determining that a particular woman (for induction) needs to be delivered within the next few days and that this will not happen if they are left alone. All other instances of oxytocin use or amniotomy can then be classified as augmentation. Following this philosophical approach, the performance of amniotomy or administration of oxytocin after cervical ripening by prostaglandins is considered as part of the process of induction, except in situations where the active phase of labour has started.

Labour is composed of a relatively long latent phase followed by a short and probably irreversible active phase. The major events of the latent phase are:

1. the progression of uterine contractility from an inactive to a vigorously active state
2. cervical ripening
3. activation of fetal membranes.

Although a latent phase probably occurs in all labours, some women are not aware of it. Confusion often arises because of the relationship between uterine contractions and labour. In general the absence of perceived uterine contractions is considered to equate with the woman not being in labour, whereas the presence of (painful) uterine contractions usually equates with labour. There are, however, instances where a woman reaches full dilatation of the cervix without any uterine contractions being apparent to her, and more frequent occurrences where obvious uterine activity is present but no cervical changes are apparent. The myometrium, like all muscular tissue, requires continual stimulation for it to retain its tone and ability to contract. Not surprisingly, therefore, uterine activity can be recorded throughout pregnancy, and even in the non-pregnant state. The mechanism governing the process of cervical ripening, which is a necessary prelude to labour, is still not fully understood, but is thought to involve several hormonal interactions including oestrogens, progesterone, prostaglandins and nitric oxide (NO). Around the time of labour there are considerable morphological, hormonal and biochemical changes that must occur for the process to function normally. These are all interrelated and presumably occur in a defined sequence in the normal woman who labours and delivers spontaneously at term. Out of sequence changes may occur in pathological conditions such as trauma, infection or maternal medical diseases, resulting in labour that is dysfunctional or begins preterm.

Nitric oxide (NO) is an important element in controlling uterine and cervical functions during the transition from pregnancy to the latent phase of labour. NO acts with progesterone to regulate uterine quiescence and cervical rigidity. NO is produced by NO synthase, the expression of which is progesterone-dependent. During pregnancy NO synthase expression is upregulated in the uterus and downregulated in the cervix. This situation reverses at term. A decrease in NO production in the uterus contributes to the initiation of labour, whereas in the cervix NO is a final metabolic mediator of cervical ripening. Local application of NO donors can induce cervical ripening (Chwalisz & Garfield 1998).

Oestrogen and progesterone, the two principal hormones associated with reproductive processes, are both involved in the timing and progress of labour. The precipitous fall in progesterone concentration around term was initially thought to stimulate labour directly. This is true in most mammals but not in humans and other primates. Progesterone is still thought to play an important role in the onset of labour as it is necessary for myometrial relaxation throughout pregnancy. Interruption of secretion or antagonism of progesterone at any time throughout the antepartum period may result in preterm labour. Oestrogen is necessary for the priming of uterine muscle to increase contractility and sensitivity to oxytocic agents. Uterine activity during labour (when oestrogen predominates) is inhibited by adrenaline, whereas it is stimulated in the antenatal period (when progesterone predominates). This relationship explains the association between stress and the onset of preterm labour, and the beneficial effect of a husband's or friend's presence on dysfunctional labour. Oestrogen is also involved in the morphologic changes in the cervix that occur prior to labour onset, and it has been suggested as an alternative to prostaglandins for pre-induction cervical ripening.

Labour is more likely to occur the more advanced the pregnancy. Figure 35.1 shows the probability of labour occurring and the cumulative probability of delivery at different gestational ages. This figure is generated from data concerning 7721 deliveries in our unit between January and December 1996, when most post-dates pregnancies were managed conservatively until 42 completed weeks of gestation. Approximately 50% of women had had early ultrasound examination performed. The date of a woman's last menstrual period (LMP) is the best predictor of the date of confinement (Anderson et al 1981) and is not improved by ultrasound where the LMP date is certain. Between 25% and 45% of women, however, are unsure or totally unaware of their LMP date (Warsof et al 1983). In these cases, early ultrasound examination provides the most accurate form of gestational assessment. In cases where the first contact is in advanced pregnancy, an average of gestational ages calculated from a number of clinical observations can provide an estimate as accurate as that from a certain LMP (Anderson et al 1981). In Figure 35.1, it is apparent that 45% of women reach their estimated delivery date without going into labour. A further 30% will deliver within the next week leaving 15% with pregnancies that go beyond 41 completed weeks of gestation.

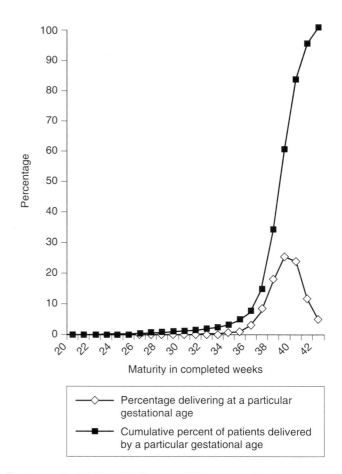

Fig. 35.1 Probability of delivery at different gestational ages.

If Royal College of Obstetricians and Gynaecologists (RCOG) guidelines (1998) to deliver all babies by 41 weeks are followed, most of these 15% will require induction of labour (some will have elective caesarean delivery and others will labour spontaneously on the day of admission for induction). If, however, induction is deferred for a further week, two-thirds of these women will labour spontaneously in uncomplicated prolonged pregnancy. The interval from the expected day of delivery to the spontaneous onset of labour is correlated with parity and cervical score (greater than 294 days) (Ingemarsson & Heden 1989). In a study confined to women who had had a routine ultrasonic scan in weeks 16–18 for the purpose of dating, the duration beyond 294 days to spontaneous onset of labour varied little for nulliparas with scores greater than two and for multiparas regardless of score (Ingemarsson & Heden 1989). Even nulliparous women with a poor score (less than three) had spontaneous onset of labour and delivery within a mean of 9.8 days, and 50.0% of all multiparous women and 43.9% of all nulliparous women gave birth within three days. About 90% of all women gave birth within seven days. They concluded that 'in post-term women dated with a second-trimester ultrasonic scan, the cervical scores are in general more favorable than previously reported in series not dated with early scans. The post-term group is also much smaller, and the time interval from entry into the post-term period to spontaneous onset of labour is shorter.'

INDUCTION OF LABOUR

Induction of labour involves the artificial initiation of uterine contractions prior to their spontaneous onset, leading to progressive dilatation and effacement of the cervix and delivery of the baby. The term is only applicable to pregnancies at or beyond the legal definition of fetal viability (24 weeks in the UK). Medical recommendation for induction of labour should only be made if its associated risks are perceived to be lower than those associated with continuation of pregnancy or with an elective caesarean delivery. Where the risks are similar, it is currently accepted practise to allow women the choice of induction or of waiting for the spontaneous onset of labour.

Indications

Fetal indications

Elective delivery for fetal indications assumes that the chances of neonatal intact survival are greater than those of a fetus which remains in utero. Certain obstetric complications such as rhesus incompatibility, diabetes mellitus and proteinuric pregnancy induced hypertension (PIH) carry clear-cut risks to fetal survival, whereas in other epidemiological indications such as postmaturity, impaired glucose tolerance and non-proteinuric PIH, perinatal mortality is uncommon.

The inaccessibility of the fetus to clinical examination and assessment makes quantification of the risks of remaining in utero difficult. Estimation of the risks of morbidity and mortality after delivery may be no more precise. The increasing willingness of obstetricians to confer with their neonatal colleagues is greatly welcomed, but ultimately the decision is a matter of judgement based on the assessment of several uncertainties. It is a matter of balance. In the majority of pregnancies the balance remains firmly tipped against interference and remains so until the spontaneous onset of labour at term. In some instances the risks in utero may be seen to be gradually rising and delivery may be contemplated at an appropriate moment. In the previous edition of this textbook, Prof. Calder wrote 'The radical obstetrician favours early intervention in the belief that it is better to deliver the offspring before it has been seriously compromised. A conservative colleague will favour delaying intervention until evidence of fetal compromise is clearly seen, which may never happen.' Since then we have mostly become what he referred to as radical obstetricians, exemplified by the current RCOG recommendations on induction for post-maturity.

Fetal surveillance. The past two decades have witnessed increased sophistication in the methods of assessment of fetal condition. Cardiotocography (CTG) may give valuable information about the fetal condition at any particular moment but has limited predictive ability for long-term in utero survival. Similarly, Doppler ultrasound can demonstrate changes in blood flow to and within the feto-placental unit, allowing more informed decision-making regarding delivery of the compromised fetus. In general, however, neither of these modalities of fetal assess-

ment is likely to lead to a decision to induce labour, as abnormalities usually indicate that the fetus will not tolerate labour and, therefore, lead instead to a decision for elective caesarean delivery. Their use, particularly CTG, has become concentrated on the provision of reassurance to the obstetrician that the infant is not only well but also it is likely to tolerate the process of labour. Despite this, fetal heart rate patterns revert to normal in about 60% of cases where an abnormality prompted induction, and if the woman is very keen on a vaginal birth, a closely monitored induction may be offered.

Neonatal risk assessment. Although developments in diagnostic ultrasound have allowed more precise measurement of fetal growth and estimation of birthweight, the most important contribution of ultrasound has been in the accurate assessment of gestational age. The prediction of fetal lung maturity from gestational age has largely removed the need for amniocentesis to allow measurement of liquor phospholipids as an assessment of the likely risks of respiratory distress syndrome in the neonate.

Improvements in paediatric skills and neonatal care facilities have clearly influenced decisions regarding elective preterm delivery. The availability of the highest level of neonatal intensive care often tips the balance in favour of delivery where previously a conservative approach would have been obligatory, with considerable risk of intrauterine death. The frequent use of prophylactic antenatal steroids in high-risk pregnancies and the availability of synthetic surfactant have also improved the prospects for survival. In the absence of such facilities there is little merit in delivering a grossly immature infant with little prospect of survival.

Rhesus disease. Maternal rhesus isoimmunisation illustrates many of the matters considered already. The risks of this complication are almost all directed towards the fetus. Haemolysis of fetal red blood cells may lead to progressive anaemia, cardiac failure and eventually to hydrops fetalis. The earlier these complications appear the greater is the likelihood that intervention will be required to prevent fetal death in utero. Such intervention may be labour induction if it is judged that the fetus is sufficiently mature; otherwise blood transfusion of the fetus is required. The outcome of each case depends on the race between declining haemoglobin concentration and advancing fetal maturation.

Diabetes Mellitus. Maternal diabetes confers major hazards on the offspring. Poor control of the maternal blood glucose level increases the risks of fetal and maternal complications, leading to increased rates of perinatal death and morbidity. Sudden fetal demise in utero during the last weeks of gestation is less common nowadays because of improvements in diabetic control, but induction of labour remains an important weapon in the battle to achieve a successful outcome to these pregnancies.

Combined maternal and fetal indications

Pregnancy-induced hypertention. In England and Wales hypertensive diseases rank second only to pulmonary embolus as a cause of maternal death. The commonest mode of death is cerebral haemorrhage. Cerebral oedema or infarction, pulmonary oedema, and hepatic necrosis are also primary causes of death. Liver damage and fluid overload are frequently associated, and they are likely to contribute significantly to many of the deaths. Heart failure is rarely encountered in young, otherwise healthy women, regardless of the severity of disease. Circulatory collapse most often occurs during labour or a few hours after delivery in elderly multiparae whose hypertension is difficult to control. From the list of causes of maternal death in PIH it is apparent that the disease affects many organ systems including the kidney, liver and central nervous system. Additional complications, which may lead to death, include disseminated intravascular coagulopathy (DIC) and placental abruption. Preterm delivery may be necessary to interrupt the cascade of changes, which lead to eclampsia. The fetus in cases of severe PIH is also often compromised by poor placental function, which may lead to intrauterine growth restriction and intrauterine death.

Prelabour rupture of the membranes. When the membranes have ruptured spontaneously before the onset of labour, controlled trials have shown no difference in outcome whether induction was immediate or delayed, or whether prostaglandins were used or not, whatever the favourability of the cervix (Chung et al 1992, Hannah et al 1996). Although Hannah et al (1996) show an increase in morbidity (infection) with delayed induction, and higher maternal satisfaction with immediate induction.

Epidemiological indications

The basic tenet of modern obstetric practice is the prevention of fetal morbidity and mortality by timely intervention. Most obstetricians would be classified as radical nowadays as the majority of interventions such as induction are performed because of greater perceived risks to the fetus on the basis of epidemiological evidence.

Post-maturity. Policy decisions regarding routine induction for post-dates pregnancy have been reviewed in recent years following the more extensive use of ultrasound for dating pregnancy. This has not only resulted in the expected due date (EDD) being calculated more accurately than before. It has also become apparent that fetal growth does not plateau at 40 weeks as previously determined from studies, which included women with uncertain LMP dates; rather it continues in a linear fashion in the majority of fetuses where placental function remains normal (Westin 1977). For these patients, there is no fetal risk from placental insufficiency, but continued growth will increase the risk of obstructed labour. In those where growth does not remain linear, some degree of placental ineffectiveness may be present, and induction is warranted for fetal risk. The probability of failed induction must be balanced against these factors when making the decision on timing of induction. However, there is now good evidence that induction of labour should be offered routinely to all women whose pregnancies continue beyond 41 weeks' gestation. Induction during this period is associated with beneficial outcome in terms of reduced caesarean section rate, reduced operative vaginal delivery, reduced chance of fetal distress, meconium staining, macrosomia, and reduced risk of fetal and neonatal death (Crowley 1995).

Maternal indications

It is rare nowadays to have to consider labour induction purely in the maternal interest. Nevertheless some maternal diseases such as valvular disorders of the heart, hypertension, renal disease, liver disease and certain autoimmune disorders may, especially if deteriorating, require consideration to be given to delivery in the maternal interest. Malignant conditions present a particularly taxing challenge.

Few maternal diseases are actually improved during pregnancy; in general the extra burden of pregnancy hastens their progression. The existence of such conditions is often recognised before pregnancy but commonly only come to light or indeed may arise *de novo* during the course of pregnancy.

The process of ending the pregnancy may in itself pose an added risk, but as a general, if not invariable rule, when such a disease is threatening a mother's life during pregnancy, it is to her benefit to have the pregnancy removed from the clinical picture. In the past, women with serious medical conditions were often strongly counselled not to embark on pregnancy at all or if they did conceive, therapeutic abortion was immediately advised. This is now less common for two reasons. First, the likely course of the disease states concerned and the effects of pregnancy on them are better understood. Secondly, the methods of management in pregnancy have been steadily improved.

It remains true that the earlier a pregnancy is terminated, the safer it will be for the mother concerned, but it is now more possible to intervene at any stage of gestation if the need to do so becomes apparent. Formerly the pregnancy had to continue for at least 36 weeks to stand a good chance of success; now, thanks to advances in neonatal care, it has a good chance of an intact survival after only 28 weeks and of survival with some morbidity from even earlier. In addition, in years gone by, the dangers from methods of pregnancy interruption rose steeply after the first trimester and they did not begin to decline until the natural course of pregnancy was almost complete. Therefore, there was a window, or perhaps more aptly a closed door, between 12 and 36 weeks during which interruption carried greater hazards, and this encouraged the view that early abortion might be best.

The advent of prostaglandins has brought the ability to induce labour throughout gestation. Therefore, a mother with a serious disease may now more often be allowed to embark on a pregnancy on the understanding that if her condition deteriorates dangerously the pregnancy may need to be interrupted. These women should not be forbidden the chance to reproduce on the grounds of uncertain deleterious effects. We can now more often put the question to the test without incurring unacceptable risks.

Social induction

Induction of labour is sometimes performed for the convenience of the parents in the absence of any definite medical indication (wrongly described as social induction). Induction of labour under such circumstances must be justified and any decision should be taken on an individual basis after fully informing the woman of the potential disadvantages.

Induction may also be indicated for logistic reasons when hospital access is restricted by geography or politics. Induction rates in Rhodesia (now Zimbabwe) exceeded 30% during the latter years of White rule while evening curfew was in force. Similarly, high rates of induction prevailed amongst Protestants in Belfast, where travel to the Royal Victoria Infirmary involved a trip down the Catholic Falls Road.

Induction rates

The foregoing may help to explain the reasons why induction of labour has been such a controversial procedure in recent times. The rate of induction varies widely in different countries and units, and between individual obstetricians within the same unit. Rates between 10% and 25% are common in industrialised countries. Variations in induction rate depend largely on the different obstetrician's perceptions of fetal risk amongst those with uncertain risk such as non-proteinuric PIH or glucose intolerance, as well as on the prevalence of such conditions. Obstetricians have argued bitterly about the appropriate use of induction, and there is no agreement or evidence to suggest an ideal rate.

Cervical status

Bishop score. Induction of labour can be achieved by a variety of physical and biochemical stimuli designed to effect changes in the uterine cervix, cause the myometrium to contract, or both. The favourability, or ripeness of the cervix is of critical importance to the probability of successful induction (especially in nulliparae) and should be assessed prior to induction by means of the Bishop score (Bishop 1964) or one of its modifications (Hughey et al 1976; Table 35.1). Different modifications have been put forward attempting to increase the prediction of successful labour induction. Although subjectivity and inter-observer error limit the scoring system, its advantage lies in its simplicity and practicability. Further studies on cervical assessment using transvaginal ultrasound have failed to demonstrate any improvement in the prediction of induction outcome, whether it was compared with Bishop's score (Paterson-Brown et al 1991) or used as an adjunct to the scoring system (Watson et al 1996).

Scores of less than 5 are considered unfavourable for induction (unripe); scores of 5 and above are considered favourable for induction (ripe).

Fibronectin. Onco-fetal fibronectin (onf-FN) is a special form of the glycoprotein fibronectin. Its presence in cervical secretions has been shown to correlate with cervical ripening (Ekman et al 1995) and it can predict the outcome of induced labour (Ahner et al 1995). A fast-reacting cervical swab test is available for qualitative detection of onf-FN in cervical secretions (Adeza Chemicals, Tokyo). This is a solid-phase immunological assay where the specimen is mixed with an antihuman fibronectin–gold colloid conjugate and passes through a membrane containing a monoclonal antibody (FDC-6) specific to onf-FN. A positive result is determined by observing a visible pink spot in the membrane within five minutes.

Recent literature has established the relationship between the presence of onf-FN in cervical secretions and preterm delivery (Bartnicki et al 1996, Greenhagen et al 1996, Leeson et al 1996, Rizzo et al 1996, Chien et al 1997). The method can be used to predict preterm delivery amongst women with threatened preterm labour or cervical incompetence. The same predictive value for the onset of labour is equally applicable in term pregnancy (Garite et al 1996), although this has little clinical utility, as there is an association between the presence of onf-FN and higher Bishop scores (Blanch et al 1996). Of greater clinical importance is that the presence of onf-FN has a predictive value for successful cervical ripening. In cases with an unfavourable cervix (Bishop Score <5) there is a significant association between the response to prostaglandin and the presence of onf-FN in the cervical secretions. A negative test can help to identify those likely to respond poorly and therefore function as an adjunct to the Bishop scoring. A negative test in association with other risk factors may indicate elective caesarean delivery as an alternative to a prolonged attempt at induction with uncertain outcome. Conversely, a positive onf-FN test suggests the response to prostaglandin E_2 (PGE$_2$) will be good regardless of the initial Bishop score (Tam et al in press).

Methods of induction

The unfavourable cervix

Dinoprostone. If the cervix is unfavourable (Bishop score <5), it is advisable to attempt cervical ripening with prostaglandins prior to commitment to delivery by amniotomy. The use of prostaglandins for ripening the cervix and for induction of labour results in a decreased need for analgesia in labour, fewer cases undelivered within 12 to 24 hours, decreased operative delivery and decreased incidence of postpartum haemorrhage when compared with oxytocin alone. Prostaglandin use is associated with an increased incidence of gastrointestinal side-effects (up to 50% of cases) and of uterine hypertonus (up to 7% of cases) (Keirse 1995a). The response to prostaglandins is dependent on the preparation used. Uterine hyperstimulation can occur if the dosage used is too high, or if absorption is too rapid. Vaginal pessaries are the simplest formulation to apply but the outcome is unpredictable (Lyndrup 1996). If the first dose is ineffective a second dose is usually administered six hours later. There is often a delay of 8–12 hours between PGE$_2$ administration and the onset of labour. This second dose will, therefore, be unnecessary in some circumstances and it may lead to uterine hyperstimulation. Intracervical gel preparations give a more reliable response but they are dependent on accurate placement within the cervix. Inserting the gel into the extra-amniotic space can lead to hyperstimulation, whereas

Table 35.1 Modified Bishop scoring system

Cervical state	Score			
	0	1	2	3
Dilatation (cm)	closed	1–2	3–4	5+
Length (cm)	3	2	1	0
Consistency	firm	medium	soft	
Position	posterior	middle	anterior	
Station of head	−3	−2	−1	0

spillage into the vagina will reduce efficacy. Slow release preparations control the rate of dinoprostone release, and can be easily removed in cases of hyperstimulation.

Prostaglandins can be administered orally, parenterally, vaginally, into the cervix or the extra-amniotic space. Oral and parenteral administration have become unpopular in recent years because of high rates of gastrointestinal side-effects (nausea, vomiting, diarrhoea) and pyrexia. Intracervical gel and intravaginal preparations have fewer systemic side-effects compared with these other routes of administration. However, the rate of release of the PGE_2 may be affected by the pH of the vagina (Johnson et al 1992). The most commonly used preparations are currently intravaginal tablets or pessaries containing 3 mg dinoprostone (Prostin E2, Upjohn) or intracervical gel containing 1–2 mg in a single use syringe system (Prostin E2, Upjohn). Recent studies have shown that intracervical gel has a higher failure rate (10% v. 3%) than intravaginal preparations, as well as being more difficult to administer and less efficient at ripening the cervix (Hales et al 1994, Seeras 1995, Nuutila & Kajanoja 1996). Intravaginal PGE_2 (either gel or tablets) is marginally superior to intracervical PGE_2 gel with higher successful induction rates and decreased need for oxytocin (although several studies have not demonstrated any difference). Plasma levels of prostaglandins are higher with vaginal gel compared with vaginal tablets. In nulliparae, an initial dose of 2 mg may be given, followed by further 1 mg doses at six hourly intervals to a maximum of 4 mg. In parous women, an initial dose of 1 mg, followed by further 1 mg doses to a maximum of 3 mg should be given (Manufacturer's Recommendations). There is no apparent advantage to using more frequent dosage intervals than six hourly, or of increasing the total dose above 3 mg. There is minimal (and probably no) benefit in prolonging an attempt beyond three or four doses.

Slow release intravaginal inserts are also available (Propess, Ferring Pharmaceuticals; Cervadil, Forrest Pharmaceuticals). Propess is a polymer-based vaginal insert containing 10 mg dinoprostone, which is released continuously over a 12-hour period. The main advantage of these sustained release preparations is that the insert can be removed from the vagina if uterine hypertonus or fetal distress occur. Comparison with placebo indicates that it is a safe and effective induction agent (Rayburn et al 1992, Witter et al 1992), but the preparation is expensive and there are few trials comparing its use with vaginal PGE_2 gel (Smith et al 1994).

Misoprostol. Misoprostol (Cytotec, Searle), a methyl ester of prostaglandin E_1, is much cheaper and more easily stored than other prostaglandins. It was originally marketed as a duodenal ulcer therapy and is now frequently taken to counteract the gastrointestinal effects of non-steroidal anti-inflammatory drugs (NSAIDs). Mariani-Neto and colleagues (1987) were the first to report the use of oral misoprostol for induction of labour following intrauterine death.

Misoprostol is more cost effective than comparable commercial dinoprostone prostaglandin preparations for labour induction in those with an unfavourable cervix. Misoprostol has also proved more efficient in stimulating labour without

the use of oxytocin and it has produced speedier deliveries compared with the dinoprostone agents. Several trials have shown it to be efficacious, but questions still remain as to the safest and most effective dose. It has been used in regimens ranging from a single 50 μg or 100 μg dose to repeated 25–50 μg doses. All these studies show misoprostol to be an effective induction agent compared with currently available prostaglandin preparations. There are consistent reductions in induction–delivery intervals, but sometimes at the risk of increased rates of uterine hypertonus. A vaginal dose of 50 μg four-hourly to a maximum of five doses has been shown to be more effective for induction of labour and cervical ripening, and with a lower incidence of adverse side-effects, compared with PGE_2 intracervical gel (Wing et al 1995). Liu and colleagues (1999) have recently reported that a single dose of 50 μg administered intra-cervically achieved successful induction in over 90% of cases regardless of Bishop score. The limited information on lower dosage regimens (25 μg three-hourly) suggests that they may be as effective as other prostaglandins, without increased uterine hyperstimulation.

Although misoprostol appears to be a highly effective, inexpensive and convenient agent for labour induction, concerns still exist regarding its safety. A recent meta-analysis concluded that intravaginal misoprostol causes an increased incidence of uterine tachysystole (>5 contractions per 10 minutes for at least 20 minutes), uterine hypersystole/hypertonus (a contraction of two minutes or more) but no statistically significant increase in adverse fetal outcome (Sanchez-Ramos et al 1997). The possibility of uterine rupture as a rare complication of labour induction with misoprostol must also be considered. Further trials of its use under controlled conditions are needed before it can be recommended for routine use.

The favourable cervix

If the cervix is favourable no one method of induction stands out as being superior to the others in terms of efficacy. However, satisfaction of the woman is higher and rates of analgesia usage, postpartum haemorrhage and neonatal jaundice are lower with prostaglandins than with oxytocin (Kennedy et al 1982, Mahmood et al 1995). Up to 88% of women with a favourable cervix will labour within 24 hours after amniotomy alone (Booth & Kurdizak 1970). Despite this, most obstetricians favour combined induction by amniotomy and oxytocin infusion because of the shorter induction–delivery interval, reduced operative delivery rates and a reduction in postpartum haemorrhage (Keirse 1995b). Amniotomy combined with early oxytocin infusion results in shorter induction to delivery interval than amniotomy alone, primarily because of a shortening of the latent phase (Moldin & Sundell 1996).

Amniotomy. Amniotomy, resulting in drainage of amniotic fluid, may result in stimulation of uterine activity by a combination of uterine decompression and local prostaglandin release. It is particularly useful in the grand multigravid with a favourable cervix where there is a risk of hyperstimulation if uterine stimulants such as exogenous prostaglandins or oxytocin are used. Amniotomy should be performed initially, after careful assessment to minimise the risk of cord prolapse, and only followed by oxytocin infusion after a period of 2–4 hours if no uterine activity ensues. Amniotomy is not without its dangers, which include umbilical cord prolapse (0.5%), particularly in association with a high head or polyhydramnios, and infection if delivery does not follow within 24 hours.

Oxytocin.   Oxytocin, a polypeptide produced in the posterior pituitary gland, is the chemical substance most widely used for labour induction and augmentation. Oxytocin stimulates receptors in the myometrium directly causing uterine contractions. The response to oxytocin depends on pre-existing myometrial activity and the sensitivity of the uterine corpus and cervix. The number of oxytocin receptors and their activity slowly increase after 20 weeks' gestation until the middle of the third trimester and then remains stable until term when it increases dramatically.

The first preparations of oxytocin were crude pituitary extracts of widely varying potency. Unpredictable absorption from intramuscular injection sometimes led to catastrophes from violent and uncontrolled uterine stimulation. Following the isolation of pure oxytocin, its chemical characterisation (DuVigneaud et al 1953) and its subsequent commercial synthesis (Boissonas et al 1955), different routes of administration were used including intranasal, sublingual and buccal oxytocin. These have been replaced almost entirely now by intravenous administration using controlled infusion apparatus, which provides for the greatest efficiency in stimulating uterine contraction, while minimising the risks of hyperstimulation. The sensitivity of the pregnant uterus to oxytocin varies widely between individuals and at differing stages of pregnancy. The risk of hyperstimulation is, therefore, still real and uterine response to oxytocin must be carefully monitored; titrating the infusion rate against contraction frequency and labour progress. The solution of oxytocin should not be too dilute (ideally 20 iu/l) as prolonged use can lead to water intoxication and hyponatraemia because of its antidiuretic hormone action.

Administration should be via an infusion pump, beginning at a low rate of 1–4 mU/min in case of hypersensitivity, and then be increased at 30 minute intervals, doubling the dose each time until a maximum of 32 mU/min (ACOG 1987) is achieved or regular contractions are occurring of adequate duration (30–45 seconds) and frequency (3–4 contractions every 10 minutes). It is rarely necessary to go above this maximum dose. There is no benefit in using intervals of less than 30 minutes. Longer intervals reduce the incidence of uterine hypertonus, decrease the maximum and total dose of oxytocin, and decrease the rate of caesarean section for CTG abnormalities, with no adverse effect on induction–delivery intervals (Irons et al 1993, Orhue 1993). It has been suggested that no benefit accrues from using high maximum infusion rates of oxytocin. A maximum rate of 12 mU/minute has been suggested, and several studies have shown that normal progress is usually achieved at rates below this (Steer et al 1985). Pulsatile infusion regimens, in which boluses of oxytocin are given at 20–30 minute intervals have been suggested to be more physiological, and more logical in view of the half-life of oxytocin and its receptor occupancy in labour. It is possible that such regimens require

less oxytocin overall, with reduced risk of hyperstimulation, but so far there is little evidence to suggest they have any great advantage over those currently used (Keirse 1995c, Reid & Helewa 1995).

Multiparous women tend to be more sensitive to exogenous oxytocin than do the nulliparous. For this reason many obstetricians administer oxytocin in a more dilute solution when inducing labour in multiparous women, or wait for spontaneous uterine activity to occur following amniotomy.

Other methods of cervical ripening and labour induction

Donald (1972), in a historical review of labour induction, described various mechanical and chemical assaults with a wide spectrum of success and failure. The stimulation of uterine contractions by mechanical interference such as passing balloons or bougies through the cervix or performing a digital transcervical membrane sweep long preceded our knowledge of the existence of prostaglandins and understanding of their role in the onset of labour.

Membrane sweep.   A membrane sweep is, of course, only possible in patients with a ripe cervix and, therefore, it may only be coincidental that labour occurs shortly afterwards. Although membrane sweeping increases the chance of delivery within one week, there is no significant increase in the proportion of women delivering within 48 hours. However, a recent randomised trial has suggested that sweeping of the membranes can reduce the incidence of post-dates pregnancy (El-Torkey & Grant 1992).

Mechanical dilators.   Hygroscopic absorption can be used mechanically to expand relatively slender devices (laminaria tent, Dilapan), which can be placed into the endocervical canal of the unfavourable cervix. In prospective studies, pre-induction cervical ripening with these dilators seems to be as efficacious as the use of prostaglandins, but they have not been shown to shorten the length of labour nor lower the caesarean delivery rate (Gilson et al 1996). Use of mechanical dilators reduces the need to monitor the uterus and fetus during cervical ripening, with consequent financial savings. There is no good evidence that sexual intercourse improves cervical ripeness (Keirse 1995d).

Castor oil.   Indirect stimulation of uterine activity by using enemas or laxatives has been part of midwifery practice since ancient times. In general, these methods are frowned on currently as they are, for the most part, ineffective and unpleasant. Castor oil is still used in China as a method of labour induction, however. By binding the oil with egg white the local effects on the bowel are eliminated, allowing absorption of the active ingredient ricinoleic acid, which has been shown to stimulate prostaglandin production (Wang & Xu 1992), which then in turn stimulates uterine activity. The efficacy in terms of improvement in Bishop score, need for oxytocin augmentation and time from start of induction to vaginal delivery is significantly less than for misoprostol (Wang et al 1997a). However, the incidence of uterine tachysystole was also much less than with misoprostol (3% v. 16.7%). Mitri and colleagues (1987) have reported a higher incidence of fetal meconium passage amongst women who had self-medicated with castor oil but not amongst women using other laxatives and enemas.

Antiprogesterones. Mifepristone, a progesterone antagonist, causes softening and dilatation of the cervix in early pregnancy and an increase in uterine activity. It is theoretically attractive for use as an adjunct in cervical priming and labour induction. In a recent study, 200 mg of mifepristone was significantly more likely to result in a favourable cervix than placebo (Elliott et al 1998). Frydman and colleagues compared two doses of 200 mg of mifepristone to a placebo in a double-blind study of 120 pregnant women with indications for delivery between 37.5 and 41.4 weeks' gestation and a Bishop score of four or less. If not in labour on day four of the study, prostaglandin suppositories were given to mature the cervix, or, if already favourable, combined induction by amniotomy and oxytocin infusion was performed. The study demonstrated significant differences in the rate of spontaneous labour (54% v. 18%), mean interval to the onset of labour (51.7 hours v. 74.5 hours), and the total amount of oxytocin in vaginally delivered patients (2.0 IU v. 4.7 IU). No significant maternal or fetal complications were observed (Frydman et al 1992).

Nitric oxide donors. Nitric oxide donors have been found to ripen the cervix, and may be useful induction agents in the future. Pretreatment with isosorbide mononitrate to ripen the cervix before first-trimester termination of pregnancy is associated with fewer side-effects than gemeprost treatment and adequately decreases cervical resistance. The use of nitric oxide donors in ripening of the cervix at term remains to be evaluated.

Extra-amniotic saline. While prostaglandins are currently the most popular method of inducing cervical ripening they are both expensive and unstable if improperly stored. They are also prone to variable absorption leading to unpredictable patient response, uterine hypertonus and gastrointestinal side-effects such as nausea, vomiting and diarrhoea. Mawire and colleagues (1999) in Zimbabwe have shown that using extra-amniotic infusion of normal saline through a Foley catheter inserted through the cervix produces comparable cervical ripening results to infusion of prostaglandins. This technique is associated with a lower incidence of hypertonus, no gastrointestinal side-effects and is six times cheaper than using $PGF_{2\alpha}$. Restricting the maximum volume of infusion fluid to 1.5 l and using sterile isotonic saline solution with aseptic technique minimises the risks of fluid overload and infection. This method is, therefore, attractive in poorer-settings although the financial gain has only been compared with the use of $PGF_{2\alpha}$, and not the much cheaper prostaglandin analogue misoprostol.

Relaxin. The use of relaxin has been proposed as an alternative method of cervical ripening. MacLennan et al (1986) found that a 2 mg dose of pure porcine relaxin administered vaginally significantly improved cervical scores when compared with controls. Brennand et al (1997), however, using recombinant human relaxin administered as an intravaginal gel, failed to demonstrate any effect on cervical ripening.

Timing of induction

Elective delivery, either by caesarean section or by labour induction, is the one area in which obstetricians can achieve a degree of control over their workload out of normal office hours. By initiating the induction process early in the morning amongst women with a favourable cervix, the majority of these women will deliver before midnight. Those with an unfavourable cervix should be admitted for cervical ripening the day before induction is planned. The common practice of giving PGE_2 for cervical ripening in the evening before induction the following morning should be audited carefully in individual obstetric units. It should always be remembered that patients for induction are, by definition, a high-risk group. Even where induction is by maternal request the process of induction must be considered to imply a certain risk as well as the indication. The administration of PGE_2 in these patients can be considered as a stress test and appropriate monitoring of the fetal condition should, therefore, be applied.

Failed induction

The process of labour induction can be considered to have failed where the active phase is not achieved in an appropriate time despite apparently adequate stimulation of uterine activity. The acceptable length of time spent attempting to establish labour by artificial means will obviously depend on the clinical circumstances. If induction is being performed for maternal disease such as pre-eclampsia, the rate of deterioration in the mother's or fetus' condition may require intervention after a relatively short attempt. Conversely, where the indication is epidemiological such as postmaturity, a full trial of induction can be allowed, subject to reassuring fetal surveillance. The incidence of failed induction is dependent on the cervical status at the time the process is commenced and the methods of induction used. The judicious use of prostaglandin for cervical ripening prior to commitment to delivery by performing artificial membrane rupture has considerably reduced the probability of failed induction occurring.

Induction with a uterine scar

The induction of labour in a patient who has had a previous caesarean delivery requires careful consideration. Current literature suggests that the induced labour carries no additional risk to spontaneous labour in women who have had a previous caesarean delivery (Chez 1995). However, if there is a high risk of failed induction (unfavourable cervix, negative cervical fibronectin) it would seem prudent to avoid the risks of inducing uterine hypertonus by opting for elective caesarean delivery. As with trial of scar in spontaneous labour, induction is inadvisable if there are two or more previous caesarian deliveries or if there is known cephalo-pelvic disproportion.

Fetal surveillance following induction

There are no trials which indicate an appropriate level of fetal surveillance during induction. Continuous cardiotocography is recommended by the RCOG whenever an oxytocin infusion is used (Spencer & Ward 1993). If prostaglandins are used for

KEY POINTS: RECOMMENDATIONS FOR INDUCTION

The following recommendations regarding labour induction have been made by the RCOG (1998):

- Women should always be informed of the benefits and risks associated with the policies of induction of labour and expectant management, and their preferences regarding these policies should be respected.
- Induction should be recommended when delivery confers clear benefit to the woman or the baby greater than if the pregnancy continues. This includes prolonged pregnancy (more than 41 weeks' gestation), although accurate dating of gestational age is essential.
- Social induction should only take place after the woman has been fully informed about the risks.
- When induction of labour is undertaken in a case of previous caesarean section, it is important that the decision and subsequent events are under the close supervision of staff at consultant level.
- If the cervix is unfavourable, vaginal prostaglandins should be used to effect ripening. PGE_2 intravaginal gel is the prostaglandin of choice and should be used at 6-hourly intervals. An initial dose of 2 mg may be used in nulliparae but the total dose should not exceed 4 mg. The initial dose in multigravidae should be 1 mg.
- If prelabour rupture of the membranes has occurred, induction with prostaglandins, or oxytocin alone, are equally effective.
- If the cervix is ripe, induction should be by amniotomy, followed by intravenous oxytocin via a controlled infusion pump.
- Oxytocin infusions should be given in the smallest possible volume, by an accurate infusion pump, commencing at a rate of 1 mU/min, increased at intervals of not less than 30 minutes until there are three good contractions every 10 minutes, usually up to maximum rate of 12 mU/min. The total dose of oxytocin should not exceed five units.
- New methods of induction, such as the use of nitric oxide donors, mifepristone, misoprostol, sustained release prostaglandins and pulsatile oxytocin infusions may have benefits, but require further research.

In addition to these can be added:
- Fetal well-being should be confirmed prior to attempting cervical ripening with prostaglandins.
- Self-medication with castor oil should be discouraged as this may lead to exposure of the fetus to undue stress at a time when no surveillance is possible.
- In situations where the availability of adequate fetal surveillance is restricted, the use of physical methods of cervical ripening such as laminaria tents or Foley catheters (with saline infusion) can be considered as these do not tend to cause uterine stimulation.

cervical ripening, it would seem prudent to perform cardiotocography before administration, and when contractions ensue. If there are other risk factors, e.g. fetal growth restriction, continuous CTG should be performed throughout the induction process. It is arguable whether such precautions are necessary after membrane sweeping or nipple stimulation. However, it would seem prudent to ascertain as far as possible that the fetus is in good health before it is submitted to any induced uterine contractions. Unsupervised nipple stimulation or self-medication with castor oil should therefore be discouraged as this may lead to fetal exposure to undue stress at a time when no surveillance is possible.

The 4th Annual Report of the Confidential Enquiry into Stillbirth and Deaths in Infancy (CESDI) cited induction of labour as a contributory cause in 54 cases (CESDI 1997). The main problems identified are shown in Table 35.2.

Table 35.2 Problems identified with induction of labour leading to stillbirth or death in infancy

Inadequate monitoring and supervision in high-risk cases
Lack of monitoring after prostaglandin induction
The use of prostaglandins in higher than recommended doses and for too long
Repeated doses of prostaglandins (often without examination) causing hypertonus
Use of oxytocin for too long despite lack of progress in labour
Use of oxytocin despite evidence of good progress in labour
Use of oxytocin despite clear signs of cephalopelvic disproportion or fetal compromise.

AUGMENTATION OF LABOUR

The virtual elimination of the unfavourable cervix by judicious use of prostaglandins or other ripening methods allows more precise assessment of the factors that lead to abdominal delivery, by removing failed induction from the cause list. For example, Magann et al (1999) were able to determine that the odds ratio for non-Caucasian race leading to abdominal delivery in their unit was 4.7 (95% confidence: 1.6, 15).

The latent phase

The latent phase of labour is the period between the onset of regular contractions and the beginning of the active phase of labour. This is a grey area for both the beginning and the end of the latent phase are difficult to define. As indicated earlier, uterine contractions occur throughout pregnancy and therefore the definition of the onset of labour must include some recognisable change, which is known to precede the process of delivery. Proponents of active management of labour have therefore proposed that gross (measurable) changes in the cervix should accompany regular uterine activity before a diagnosis of labour can be made. Such changes include effacement (reduction in length) and dilatation of the cervix. The end of the latent phase and beginning of the active phase have been defined as full effacement with 3 cm dilatation (World Health Organisation) or 4 cm dilatation with or without full effacement (American College of Obstetricians and Gynecologists).

Delay in latent phase

When a woman is admitted with regular painful uterine contractions, with an uneffaced cervix, sedation or pain relief should be given if required. Sometimes women in this situation are told that they are not in labour yet which can cause great distress if they are in a lot of pain. Instead a proper explanation should be given and effective pain relief offered. Normally however, at term, uterine activity will continue, and cervical effacement will occur over the next 4–8 hours. If progress is slow because of irregular or weak uterine activity, intravenous oxytocin may be commenced. Failure to reach the active phase within 8–12 hours of admission is considered a delayed latent phase. Whether a further four hours of labour should be allowed or termination of labour by caesarean section should be considered will depend on the degree of cervical change, the conditions of the mother and fetus and the desire of the parents to achieve vaginal delivery.

False labour

False labour can be defined as the presence of regular painful uterine contractions, which are not associated with cervical changes. Threatened preterm labour and failed induction can be considered varieties of false labour. False labour occurs frequently at term, contractions ceasing following sedation of the patient.

The active phase

As indicated above, the definition of the beginning of the active phase varies around the world. Once the active phase has started, however, some obstetricians would consider that the mean rate of cervical dilatation should be 1 cm per hour in a nulliparous woman with the fifteenth percentile being 0.5 cm per hour. Augmentation of women progressing at less than 1 cm per hour results in augmentation in up to 50%, as reported in most studies of active management. This figure approximates to the rate of dilatation amongst the slowest 10% of a group of nulliparous African women who pro-

gressed to normal vaginal delivery, without augmentation by oxytocin (Philpott & Castle 1972a). By drawing a line corresponding to 1 cm per hour (alert line) on the partogram (Fig. 35.2), commencing at the first recording of cervical dilatation in the active phase, subsequent progress can be divided into normal (to the left of the alert line; Fig. 35.3) and abnormal (to the right). If progress is to the right of the alert line labour should be augmented by amniotomy (if not already done) and oxytocin infusion. A further line, drawn parallel to the alert line but four hours later, is known as the action line. Crossing of the action line indicates that a decision should be made by the most senior person responsible for the patient and present in the hospital.

The place of amniotomy

Amniotomy is often performed as part of active management protocols and should not be considered as necessarily part of the augmentation process. The benefits of amniotomy are as follows:

- The character of amniotic fluid can be examined, particularly with reference to the presence of meconium or blood. Moderate to thick meconium staining can lead to meconium aspiration syndrome (MAS) in the newborn. Saline amnioinfusion has proved a useful tool for preventing MAS (Wang & Rogers 1997b).
- It provides direct access to the fetal scalp for the purpose of fetal surveillance using electrodes or for scalp blood sampling.
- Amniotomy has a potent labour-promoting effect in slow labour by encouraging application of the presenting part to the cervix and partial decompression of the uterine cavity. It also stimulates the release of endogenous prostaglandins from the amnion and the decidua, which sensitises the myometrium to the action of endogenous or exogenous oxytocin.

Amniotomy is not without its downside, however. Prolonged labour following amniotomy is associated with

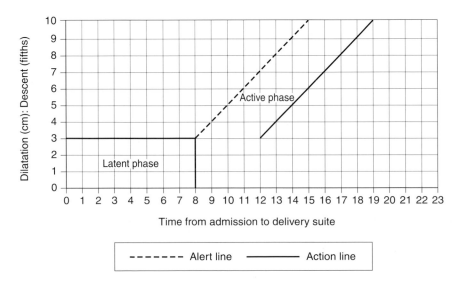

Fig. 35.2   Partogram showing alert line and action line for augmentation of labour.

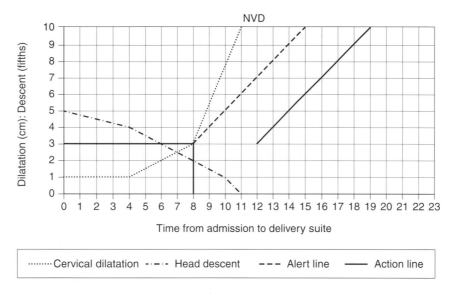

Fig. 35.3 Spontaneous normal labour (NVD, normal vaginal delivery).

ascending infection, particularly if frequent vaginal examinations are performed. Prolonged membrane rupture may also lead to oligohydramnios and encourage cord compression during contractions. Saline amnioinfusion can also be used to correct this deficiency and prevent variable decelerations in the fetal heart rate, reducing operative intervention for fetal distress. The optimal timing of amniotomy in labour is when uterine contractions are well established and the active phase of labour has commenced. If performed when the presenting part is not engaged, or where there is excessive amniotic fluid, there is a risk of umbilical cord prolapse.

The place of oxytocin

Augmentation of labour with oxytocin is advised when progress, determined by cervical effacement or dilatation falls significantly behind the expected rate. For the latent phase the expectation is that progress into the active phase will occur within eight hours of the diagnosis of labour. For the active phase, commencing at 3 cm dilatation and full efface-ment the expectation is for progress of at least 0.5 cm per hour; proponents of active management of labour favour 1 cm/hr.

As with labour induction, the administration of oxytocin should be controlled carefully using an infusion pump with electronic control, since reliance on gravity-feed can result in dangerous fluctuations in dose rate. A paediatric infusion set ensures precise regulation. The decision to commence oxy-tocin infusion in the active phase of labour should be based on failure to progress in labour and not on an impression (usually by the midwife) that the contractions are weak. Contractions can be effective in achieving full dilatation within a short period of time even where the patient has no pain whatsoever. The patient response to the pain of labour is highly individual, and is influenced both by anxiety and by cultural factors. Chinese women tend to be very stoical with regard to labour pain whereas many African societies encourage mothers to express themselves freely. Support from a partner, relative or friend during labour has been shown to lower anxiety and to increase the efficiency of uter-ine activity. With the almost universal use of CTG during labour, attendants frequently use the tocograph to assess the need for augmentation. Care needs to be taken when dealing with very thin or very obese patients as the tocograph is a motion sensor and may therefore suggest hypertonic or hypotonic contractions respectively, when contractions are in fact normal. If the tocograph is to be used in this fashion, duration and frequency measurements are the most reliable unless intrauterine pressure monitoring is being used.

The recording of amniotic fluid pressure by means of an intrauterine catheter connected to a pressure recorder has gradually declined in popularity in recent years, although most fetal monitors are still sold with this facility. There are a number of clinical situations where intrauterine pressure monitoring is still useful:

- where augmentation is contemplated in the presence of a uterine scar
- where progress is slow despite apparently adequate con-traction duration
- where progress is slow despite frequent uterine activity
- where progress is slow despite maximum oxytocin dose.

Each of the latter three situations will probably respond to commencing or increasing oxytocin administration but the obstetrician does not wish to risk hyperstimulation with its deleterious effect on uterine perfusion and fetal well-being. Use of an intrauterine pressure monitor will reassure the obstetric attendants that this is not the case and may allow the mother to proceed to normal delivery rather than undergo caesarean section for failure to progress.

The diagnosis of dystocia is currently a leading indication for caesarean delivery in the United States. The American College has defined active-phase labour arrest (caesarean section indicated for dystocia) as no cervical change beyond 4 cm dilatation, over a 2-hour period, despite a sustained contraction pattern of ≥200 Montevideo units in 10 minutes (Cowan et al 1994). Despite this, caesarean section is performed for the indication of dystocia two to three times more frequently than in European countries (Notzon et al 1994).

The rate of caesarean section amongst women with active phase augmentation is of secondary importance as it is difficult to define failure in these circumstances. The primary reason for augmentation is to accelerate labour in order to protect the mother and fetus from the undesirable consequences of prolonged labour, not just to prevent abdominal delivery.

Results of augmentation

The results of labour augmentation should be judged in terms of progress, not correction of the pattern of uterine activity, although these will normally accompany one another. Once oxytocin infusion has been commenced, cervical dilatation should resume the expected rate of at least 1 cm/h for a nulliparous woman (Fig. 35.4). If this rate of dilatation is not achieved within two hours, the American College advises caesarean section with the indication being active phase labour arrest. There is now evidence that waiting a longer period of time (at least a further two hours) for augmentation to become effective will result in at least 50% of these women ultimately delivering vaginally (Rouse et al 1999). If the rate of dilatation accelerates to ≥1 cm/h in response to oxytocin infusion but then decelerates subsequently, this is known as secondary arrest of labour (Fig. 35.5); this, in the presence of adequate contractions, almost always indicates obstruction. No further increase in oxytocin dosage is indicated for the treatment of secondary arrest as this may lead to hypertonus, which is dangerous for the fetus and will lead at least to a difficult operative vaginal delivery. Another labour pattern that should arouse suspicion is where cervical dilatation accelerates under the influence of oxytocin, but only to 1 cm/h (Fig. 35.6). This pattern is often observed in association with the occiput-posterior position where borderline dystocia exists

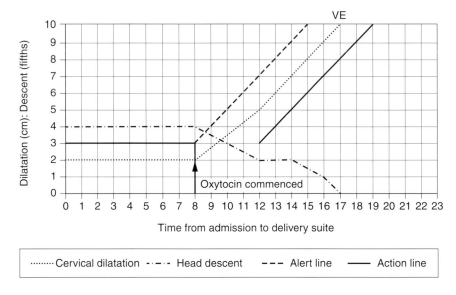

Fig. 35.4   Prolonged latent phase.

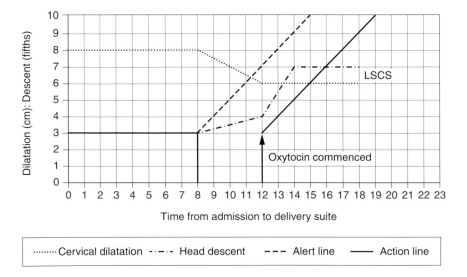

Fig. 35.5   Secondary arrest.

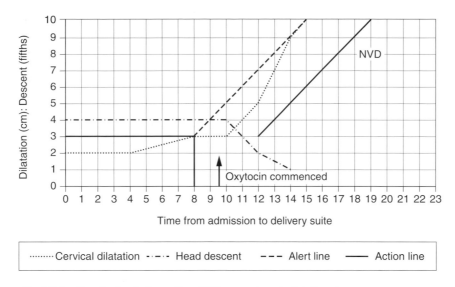

Fig. 35.6 Hypotonic uterine action (NVD, normal vaginal delivery).

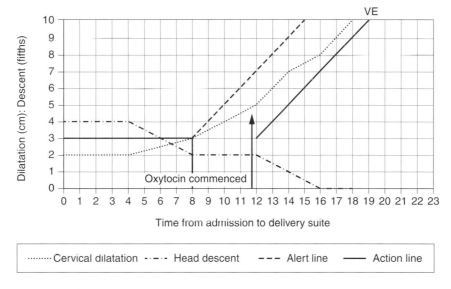

Fig. 35.7 Occiput-posterior.

(Fig. 35.7). Consequently, such cases frequently require operative vaginal delivery for prolonged second stage and there is a high risk of shoulder dystocia (Cheung et al 1990).

Active management

Active management of labour is a package of labour interventions that, as implemented at the National Maternity Hospital in Dublin, is associated with a lower rate of caesarean delivery than that observed in most other developed countries. Thornton & Lilford (1994) reviewed the evidence that the active management package reduces rates of caesarean and operative vaginal delivery amongst nulliparous women. There had been no randomised trials of the active management at that time but they concluded that 'delivery units should endeavour to provide continuous professional support in labour, but routine use of amniotomy and early oxytocin is not recommended'. This article prompted a scathing response from O'Driscoll to

the effect that the true purpose of active management had been misunderstood (O'Driscoll 1994): 'The purpose is to enhance the experience of childbirth for mothers, particularly first time mothers, whose need is greatest ... every expectant mother ... was given two assurances: that labour would not last longer than 12 hours and that a sympathetic nurse-midwife would afford personal attention throughout. The rate of caesarean section was not a motivating factor.' At that time, in fact, caesarean rates on both sides of the Irish Sea were similarly low. The discrepancy in rates observed nowadays is due to caesarean rates in the UK and USA rising (the principal indication being dystocia) while those in Dublin have remained around 5%, due to the continued strict adherence to the principal's of active management. Since then a number of trials have been published. Frigoletto and colleagues (1995) randomly assigned 1934 low-risk, nulliparous women to active management of labour or to a usual-care group. The components of active management were customised childbirth classes; strict criteria for the diagnosis of labour; standardised management of labour, including early amniotomy and treatment with high-dose oxytocin for failure to progress adequately in labour and one-to-one nursing. There was no difference between groups in the rate of caesarean section (active management, 19.5%; usual care, 19.4%). The median duration of labour was shortened by 2.7 hours by active management (from 8.9 to 6.2 hours), and the rate of maternal fever was lower (7% v. 11%). The percentage of women in whom labour lasted longer than 12 hours was three times higher in the usual-care group than in the active-management group (26% v. 9%). They concluded that active management did not reduce the rate of caesarean section in nulliparous women but was associated with a shorter duration of labour and less maternal fever. Similarly, Rogers and colleagues (1997) randomly assigned 405 low-risk term nulliparous patients to either an active management of labour (n = 200) or their usual care control protocol (n = 205). The caesarean section rate in the active management group was lower than that of controls (7.5% v. 11.7%) but not significantly so (p = 0.36). The median length of labour in the active management group was shortened by 1.7 hours (9.7 hours vs. 11.4 hours) and a greater proportion of active management patients were delivered within 12 hours (75% vs. 58%). The control groups in both of these trials would also have been managed with oxytocin in arrest situations so it is not surprising that no significant differences were observed in caesarean section rate. The results do suggest however, that maternal morbidity can be reduced by this approach. Much larger trials will be required to demonstrate any improvement in neonatal morbidity.

Epidural

Epidural analgesia is the most efficient method for pain relief during labour, but it can interfere with the normal process of labour. The incidence of instrumental delivery, caesarean section, malrotation and prolonged labour are all increased. The incidence of instrumental delivery and caesarean section, and the need for oxytocin can be reduced among multiparous women by using a lower dosage of bupivacaine (0.125%) combined with sufentanil (10 µg) in epidural analgesia instead of the higher standard dosage of bupivacaine (0.25%) with adrenaline (Olofsson et al 1998). Alexander and colleagues have suggested that where epidural analgesia is used, guidelines for the management of the active phase of labour should be modified.

Alternative methods of augmentation

Ambulation

Lupe & Gross, in 1986, reviewed the evidence that ambulation during labour was beneficial to the mother. They were unable to conclude that maternal ambulation or maintenance of an upright maternal posture could speed labour progress or improve fetal outcome. However, it was clear that ambulation in labour was not harmful to either the mother or fetus and that it resulted in greater maternal comfort and tolerance of labour with decreased use of anaesthesia and analgesia (Lupe & Gross 1986).

The association of ambulation in labour with operative delivery was examined recently in a low-risk sample of women who received no medical interventions (epidural anaesthesia, oxytocin induction or augmentation) that precluded mobility in labour. Women who walked around for a significant amount of time during labour had half the rate of operative delivery compared with those who did not (2.7% v. 5.5%) (Albers et al 1997).

Emotional support

Maternal anxiety is a common feature of pregnancy and childbirth. Animal and human studies have shown that conditions that arouse anxiety can prolong labour and have a deleterious effect on the fetus. It is likely, therefore, that factors that lessen maternal anxiety will have a beneficial effect. The presence of a supportive companion during labour has been found to reduce the duration of labour and the requirement for oxytocin augmentation. Madi and colleagues recently reported a randomised controlled trial, performed in Botswana to determine the effectiveness of the presence of a female relative as a labour companion (Madi et al 1999). The presence of a female relative was shown to be associated with fewer amniotomies to augment labour (30% v. 54%), less intrapartum analgesia (53% v. 73%), less oxytocin (13% v. 30%), and a higher rate of spontaneous vaginal delivery (91% v. 71%) compared with those without family member support. They concluded that the presence of a female relative as a labour companion is a low-cost, preventative intervention that is consistent with the traditional cultural practices in Botswana.

In many Western countries the husband has adopted this support role. Social support is effective for assisting mothers, particularly first-time mothers, to cope with the stress of labour. An empirical link between the husband's presence at birth and positive obstetric outcomes has been reported (Henneborn & Cogan 1975), but no randomised trials have been performed. Cultural differences need to be taken into account before advocating the routine presence of the spouse during labour as it may not always be beneficial (Yim 1997). In a retrospective controlled study Herman and colleagues observed that, where the husband was present, labour was shorter, and the incidence both of fetal distress and caesarean section was lower, despite more induced deliveries and similar rates of oxytocin augmentation (Herman et al 1997). In addition to the role played by husbands or other companions, continuous support from caregivers (nurses, midwives or lay people) can also reduce the requirements for pain relief and the incidence of both operative vaginal and caesarean delivery (Hodnett 1999). The mechanism which produces this improvement is unknown, but it may involve changes in the sensitivity of uterine muscle to endogenous oxytocin secretion. There is no supporting evidence for the suggestion that actual levels of oxytocin secretion are altered by such emotional support.

Acupuncture

Acupuncture has been shown to have a beneficial effect on the duration of labour, reducing the median duration of the first stage by 40% (p < 0.0001) by significantly reducing the need for augmentation with oxytocin (85% v. 15%, p = 0.01) (Zeisler et al 1998).

Water immersion

The use of warm water immersion for relaxation during labour is being used worldwide, despite an absence of research into the effects on progress or on the fetus. Only one prospective, randomised, controlled study has been performed (Schorn et al 1993). 93 term subjects in active labour, with intact membranes, utilised a tub in labour along with other pain relief measures such as ambulation, rest, showers, and analgesics. Water immersion did not alter the rate of cervical dilatation, change the contraction pattern, length of labour, or influence the use of analgesia.

The second stage

Full dilatation of the cervix preludes the onset of the second stage of labour. Full dilatation does not always equate with vaginal delivery. Labour can still become obstructed if the pelvic outlet is contracted or if there is fetal malpresentation. Fetal distress can also occur, particularly where there is cord entanglement around the neck, which may tighten as the fetus descends through the birth canal. The optimal length of the second stage has been the subject of considerable controversy in recent years. The duration of the second stage and the incidence of operative intervention are lower in nulliparous than multiparous women but they rise with the use of epidural analgesia. Multiparous women using epidural analgesia behave in a similar manner to nulliparous women without epidurals. Despite the longer second stages observed in women using epidural analgesia there appears to be no significant increase in fetal morbidity (Paterson et al 1992).

Advocates for limiting the length of the second stage point out that the fetal pH declines rapidly with strenuous maternal effort. In the presence of epidural analgesia however, maternal effort is often less effective and there is evidence that a longer second stage is acceptable. Recent work in our unit on lipid peroxidation in the fetus has confirmed that oxygen radical activity is directly related to length of second stage amongst patients without epidural, but that there is no rise in the presence of epidural, even with second stage lengths exceeding two hours (Mongelli et al 1997).

KEY POINTS: RECOMMENDATIONS FOR AUGMENTATION

- Efforts to identify abnormal labour patterns using the partogram and to correct them by oxytocin augmentation, may reduce the need for a caesarean delivery.
- Caesarean deliveries for dystocia should not be performed in the latent phase of labour, or in the active phase of labour unless adequate uterine activity has been achieved.
- Women should receive emotional support during labour from either their spouse or a close female friend or relative, and ideally a dedicated midwife.
- Regardless of the oxytocin regimen used for augmentation of labour, administration should be by trained personnel capable of responding to complications.

- A doctor capable of performing caesarean delivery should be readily available in all cases augmented by oxytocin.
- Where epidural analgesia is used, guidelines for the management of the active phase of labour should be modified to reflect any effect on uterine contractions.
- Women with epidural analgesia should not begin expulsive efforts until the head is visible at the vulva and no specific time limit need to be set for the length of second stage.
- Progress in the second stage of labour in those without epidural should be also monitored carefully and delivery expedited if signs of fetal distress are present (thick meconium, fetal bradycardia or deceleration pattern).

REFERENCES

Ahner R, Egarter C, Kiss H, Heinzl K, Zeillinger R, Schatten C, Dormeier A, Husslein P 1995 Fetal fibronectin as a selection criterion for induction of term labour. Am J Obstet Gynecol 173:1513–1517

Albers LL, Anderson D, Cragin L, Daniels SM, Hunter C, Sedler KD, Teaf D 1997 The relationship of ambulation in labour to operative delivery. J Nurse-Midwifery 42:4–8

American College of Obstetricians and Gynecologists. Induction and augmentation of labour. ACOG Technical Bulletin 1987, Number 110

Anderson HF, Johnson TRB, Barclay ML, Flora JD 1981 Gestational age assessment I. Analysis of individual clinical observations. Obstet Gynecol 139:173–177

Bartnicki J, Casal D, Kreaden MS, Saling E, Vetter K 1996 Fetal fibronectin in vaginal specimens predicts preterm delivery and very-low-birth-weight infants. Am J Obstet Gynecol 174:971–4

Bishop EH 1964 Pelvic scoring for elective induction. Obstet Gynecol 24:266–268

Blanch G, Olah KS, Walkinshaw S 1996 The presence of fetal fibronectin in the cervicovaginal secretions of women at term—its role in the assessment of women before labour induction and in the investigation of the physiologic mechanisms of labour. Am J Obstet Gynecol 174:262–266

Boissonas RA, Guttmann S, Jaquenand PA, Waller TP 1955 A new synthesis of oxytocin. Helvetica Chimica Acta 38:1491–1495

Booth JH, Kurdizak VB 1970 Elective induction of labour: a controlled study. Can Med Assoc J 103:245–248

Brennand JE, Calder AA, Leitch CR, Greer IA, Chou MM, MacKenzie IZ 1997 Recombinant human relaxin as a cervical ripening agent. Br J Obstet Gynaecol 104:775–780

Cheung TH, Leung A, Chang A 1990 Macrosomic babies. Aust NZ J Obstet Gynaecol 30:319–322

Chez RA 1995 Cervical ripening and labour induction after previous caesarean delivery (Review). Clin Obstet Gynecol 38:287–292

Chien PF, Khan KS, Ogston S, Owen P 1997 The diagnostic accuracy of cervico-vaginal fetal fibronectin in predicting preterm delivery: an overview. Br J Obstet Gynaecol 104:436–444

Chung T, Rogers MS, Gordon H, Chang AMZ 1992 Pre-labour rupture of the membranes at term and unfavourable cervix; a randomised placebo-controlled trial on early intervention with intra-vaginal prostaglandin E2 gel. Aust NZ J Obstet Gynaecol 32:25–27

Chwalisz K, Garfield RE 1998 Role of nitric oxide in the uterus and cervix: implications for the management of labour. J Perinat Med 26:448–457

Confidential Enquiry into Stillbirths and Deaths in Infancy. 4th Annual Report 1 January–31 December 1995. The Maternal and Child Health Research Consortium, London: 1997

Cowan RK, Kinch RAH, Ellis B, Anderson R 1994 Trial of labour following caesarean delivery. Obstet Gynecol 83:933–938

Crowley P 1995 Elective induction of labour at 41+ weeks gestation. [revised 5 May 1994] In: Enkin MW, Keirse MJNC, Renfrew MJ,

Neilson JP, Crowther C (eds) Pregnancy and Childbirth Module. In: The Cochrane Pregnancy and Childbirth Database [database on disk and CD: ROM]. The Cochrane Collaboration; Issue 2. Update Software, Oxford

Donald I 1972 A review of procedures in induction of labour. The case of prostaglandin E2 and F2α. In obstetrics and gynaecology. Symposia Specialists, Miami, 5–11

DuVigneaud V, Ressler C, Trippet S 1953 The sequence of amino acid in oxytocin with a proposal for the structure of oxytocin. J Biol Chem 205:949–955

Ekman G, Granstrom L, Malmstrom A, Sennstrom M, Svensson J 1995 Cervical fetal fibronectin correlates to cervical ripening. Acta Obstet Gynecol Scand 74:698–701

Elliott CL, Brennand JE, Calder AA 1998 The effects of mifepristone on cervical ripening and labour induction in primigravidae. Obstet Gynecol 92:804–809

El-Torkey M, Grant JM 1992 Sweeping of the membranes is an effective method of induction of labour in prolonged pregnancy: a report of a randomized trial. Br J Obstet Gynaecol 99:455–458

Frigoletto FD Jr, Lieberman E, Lang JM, Cohen A, Barss V, Ringer S, Datta S 1995 A clinical trial of active management of labour. New Engl J Med 333:745–750

Frydman R, Lelaidier C, Baton-Saint-Mleux C, Fernadez H, Vial M, Bourget P 1992 Labour induction in women at term with mifepristone (RU486): a double-blind, randomized, placebo-controlled study. Obstet Gynecol 80:972–975

Garite TJ, Casal D, Garcia-Alonso A et al 1996 Fetal fibronectin: a new tool for the prediction of successful induction of labour. Am J Obstet Gynecol 175:1516–1521

Gilson GJ, Russell DJ, Izquierdo LA et al 1996 A prospective randomized evaluation of a hygroscopic cervical dilator, dilapan, in the preinduction ripening of patients undergoing induction of labour. Am J Obstet Gynecol 175:145–149

Greenhagen JB, Van Wagoner J, Dudley D et al 1996 Value of fetal fibronectin as a predictor of preterm delivery for a low-risk population. Am J Obstet Gynecol 175:1054–1056

Hales KA, Raybum WF, Tumbull GL, Christensen HD, Patatanian E 1994 Double-blind comparison of intracervical and intravaginal prostaglandin E2 for cervical ripening and induction of labour. Am J Obstet Gynecol 171:1087–1091

Hannah ME, Ohlsson A, Farine D et al 1996 Induction of labour compared with expectant management for prelabour rupture of the membranes at term. TERMPROM Study Group. N Engl J Med 334:1005–1010

Henneborn W, Cogan R 1975 The effect of husband participation of reported pain and probability of medication during labour and birth. J Psychosomatic Res 19:215–222

Herman R, Hodek B, Ivicevic-Bakulic T, Kosec V, Kraljevic Z, Fures R 1997 [The effect of the presence of the husband during childbirth]. [Serbo-Croatian (Roman)] Lijecnicki Vjesnik. 119:231–232

Hodnett ED 1999 Caregiver support for women during childbirth. [Topic Review] In: The Cochrane Database of Systematic Reviews. 3: The Cochrane Collaboration; Oxford

Hughey MJ, McElin TW, Bird CC 1976 An evaluation of preinduction scoring systems. Obstet Gynecol 48:635

Ingemarsson I, Heden L 1989 Cervical score and onset of spontaneous labour in prolonged pregnancy dated by second-trimester ultrasonic scan. Obstet Gynecol. 74:102–105

Irons DW, Thomton S, Davison JM, Baylis PH 1993 Oxytocin infusion regimens: time for standardisation? Br J Obstet Gynaecol 100:786–787

Johnson TA, Greer IA, Kelly RW, Calder AA 1992 The effects of pH on release of PGE2 from vaginal and endocervical preparations for induction of labour: an in-vitro study. Br J Obstet Gynaecol 99:877–880

Keirse MJNC Any prostaglandin (by any route) vs oxytocin (any route) for induction of labour. [Revised 22 April 1993]. In: Enkin MW, Keirse MJNC, Renfrew MJ, Neilson JP, Crowther C (eds) 1995a Pregnancy and Childbirth Module. In: The Cochrane Pregnancy and Childbirth Database [database on disk and CD:ROM]. The Cochrane Collaboration; Issue 2. Update Software, Oxford

Keirse MJNC 1995b Amniotomy plus early vs late oxytocin infusion for induction of labour. In: Enkin MW, Keirse MJNC, Renfrew MJ, Neilson JP, Crowther C (eds) Pregnancy and Childbirth Module. In: The Cochrane Pregnancy and Childbirth Database [database on disk and CD:ROM]. The Cochrane Collaboration; Issue 2. Update Software, Oxford

Keirse MJNC Pulsatile oxytocin for induction of labour. In: Enkin MW, Keirse MJNC, Renfrew MJ, Neilson JP, Crowther C (eds) 1995c Pregnancy and Childbirth Module. In: The Cochrane Database of Systematic Reviews [database on disk and CD:ROM]. The Cochrane Collaboration; Issue 2. Update Software, Oxford

Keirse MJNC 1995d Sexual intercourse for cervical ripening/labour induction. [revised 03 April 1992]. In: Enkin MW, Keirse MJNC, Renfrew MJ, Neilson JP, Crowther C (eds) Pregnancy and Childbirth Module. In: The Cochrane Pregnancy and Childbirth Database [database on disk and CD:ROM]. The Cochrane Collaboration, Issue 2. Update Software, Oxford

Kennedy JH, Stewart P, Barlow DH, Hillam E, Calder AA 1982 Induction of labour: a comparison of a single PGE2 vaginal tablet with amniotomy and intravenous oxytocin. Br J Obstet Gynaecol 89:704–707

Leeson SC, Maresh MJ, Martindale EA et al 1996 Detection of fetal fibronectin as a predictor of preterm delivery in high risk asymptomatic pregnancies. Br J Obstet Gynaecol 103:48–53

Liu HS, Chu TY, Chang YK, Yu MH, Chen WH 1999 Intracervical misoprostol as an effective method of labour induction at term. Int J Gynecol Obstet 64:49–53

Lupe PJ, Gross TL 1986 Maternal upright posture and mobility in labour—a review. Obstet Gynecol 67:727–734

Lyndrup J 1996 Prostaglandins and induction of labour. Eur J Obstet Gynecol Reprod Biol 64:1–2

MacLennan AH, Green RC, Grant P, Nicolson R 1986 Ripening of the human cervix and induction of labour with intracervical purified porcine relaxin. Obstet Gynecol 68:598–601

Madi BC, Sandall J, Bennett R, MacLeod C 1999 Effects of female relative support in labour: a randomized controlled trial. Birth 26:4–8

Magann EF, Chauhan SP, Mobley JA, Klausen JH, Martin JN, Morrison JC Jr 1999 Risk actors for secondary arrest of labour among women >41 weeks' gestation with an unfavourable cervix undergoing membrane sweeping for cervical ripening. Int J Obstet Gynecol 65:1–5

Mahmood TA, Rayner A, Smith NC, Beat I 1995 A randomized prospective trial comparing single dose prostaglandin E2 vaginal gel with forewater amniotomy for induction of labour. Eur J Obstet Gynecol Reprod Biol 58:111–117

Mariani-Neto C, Leao EJ, Baretto EM, Kenj G, De Aquino MM 1987 Use of misoprostol for labour induction in stilbirths. Rev Paul Med 105:325–328

Mawire CJ, Chipato T, Rusakaniko S 1999 Extra-amniotic saline infusion versus extra-amniotic prostaglandin F2α for cervical ripening and induction of labour. Int J Gynecol Obstet 64:35–41

Mitri F, Hofmeyr GJ, van Gelderen CJ 1987 Meconium during labour—self medication and other associations. South African Med J 71:431–433

Moldin PG, Sundell G 1996 Induction of labour: a randomised clinical trial of amniotomy versus amniotomy with oxytocin infusion. Br J Obstet Gynaecol 103:306–312

Mongelli M, Wang CC, Wang W, Pang CPC, Rogers MS 1997 Oxygen free radical activity in the second stage of labour. Acta Obstet Gynaecol Scand 76:765–768

Notzon FC, Cnattingius S, Bergsjo P, Cole S, Taffel S, Irgens L, Daltveit AK 1994 Caesarean section delivery in the 1980s: international comparison by indication. Am J Obstet Gynecol 170:495–504

Nuutila M, Kajanoja P 1996 Local administration of prostaglandin E2 for cervical ripening and labour induction: the appropriate route and dose. Acta Obstet Gynecol Scand 75:135–138

O'Driscoll K, Foley M, MacDonald D 1984 Active management of labour as an alternative to caesarean section for dystocia. Obstet Gynecol 63:485–490

O'Driscoll K 1994 Active management of labour. BMJ 309:1015

Olofsson C, Ekblom A, Ekman-Ordeberg G, Irestedt L 1998 Obstetric outcome following epidural analgesia with bupivacaine-adrenaline 0.25% or bupivacaine 0.125% with sufentanil—a prospective randomized controlled study in 1000 parturients. Acta Anaesthesiol Scand 42:284–292

Orhue AA 1993 A randomized trial of 30-min and 15-min oxytocin infusion regimen for induction of labour at term in women of low parity. Int J Gynaecol Obstet 40:219–225

Paterson CM, Saunders NS, Wadsworth J 1992 The characteristics of the second stage of labour in 25,069 singleton deliveries in the North West Thames Health Region, 1988. Br J Obstet Gynaecol 99:377–380

Paterson-Brown S, Fisk NM, Edmonds DK, Rodeck CH 1991 Preinduction cervical assessment by Bishop's score and transvaginal ultrasound. Eur J Obstet Gynecol Repro Biol 40:17

Philpott RH, Castle WM 1972a Cervicographs in the management of labour in primagravidae. I. The alert line for detecting abnormal labour. J Obstet Gynaecol Br Commonw 79:592–598

Philpott RH, Castle WM 1972b Cervicographs in the management of labour in primagravidae. II. The action line and treatment of abnormal labour. J Obstet Gynaecol Br Commonw 79:599–602

Rayburn WF, Wapner RJ, Barss VA et al 1992 An intravaginal controlled-release prostaglandin E_2 pessary for cervical ripening and initiation of labour at term. Obstet Gynecol 79:374–379

RCOG Guideline No 16; 1998. Induction of Labour

Reid GJ, Helewa ME 1995 A trial of pulsatile versus continuous oxytocin administration for the induction of labour. J Perinatol 15:364–366

Rizzo G, Capponi A, Arduini D, Lorido C, Romanini C 1996 The value of fetal fibronectin in cervical and vaginal secretions and of ultrasonographic examination of the uterine cervix in predicting premature delivery for patients with preterm labour and intact membranes. Am J Obstet Gynecol 175:1146–1151

Rogers R, Gilson GJ, Miller AC, Izquierdo LE, Curet LB, Qualls CR 1997 Active management of labour: does it make a difference? Am J Obstet Gynecol 177:599–605

Rouse DJ, Owen J, Hauth JC 1999 Active-phase labour arrest: oxytocin augmentation for at least 4 hours. Obstet Gynecol 93:323–328

Sanchez-Ramos L, Kaunitz AM, Wears RL, Delke I, Gaudier FL 1997 Misoprostol for cervical ripening and labour induction: a meta-analysis. Obstet Gynecol 89:633–642

Schorn MN, McAllister JL, Blanco JD 1993 Water immersion and the effect on labour. J Nurse-Midwifery 38:336–342

Seeras RC 1995 Induction of labour utilizing vaginal vs intracervical prostaglandin E_2. Int J Gynaecol Obstet 48:163–167

Smith CV, Rayburn WF, Miller AM 1994 Intravaginal prostaglandin E_2 for cervical ripening and initiation of labour. Comparison of a multidose gel and single, controlled-release pessary. J Reprod Med 39:381–384

Spencer JAD, Ward RHT 1993 Intrapartum Fetal Surveillance. RCOG Press, London

Steer PJ, Carter MC, Choong K, Hanna M, Gordon AJ, Pradham P 1985 A multicentre prospective randomised controlled trial of induction of labour with an automatic closed-loop feedback controlled oxytocin infusion system. Br J Obstet Gynaecol 92:1127–1133

Tam WH, Tai S, Rogers MS Prediction of cervical response to prostaglandin E2 using onco-fetal fibronectin. Acta Obstet Gynaecol Scand (in press)

Thornton JG, Lilford RJ 1994 Active management of labour: current knowledge and research issues. BMJ 309:366–369

Wang Q, Xu Y 1992 Investigation of maternal peripheral plasma concentration of PG in induction of labour by nutrition food inductive drug. Chung-Kuo I Hsueh Yuan Hdueh Pao Acta Academiae Medicinae Sinicae 14:433–436

Wang L, Shi C, Yang G 1997a Comparison of misoprostol and ricinus oil meal for cervical ripening and labour induction. Chung-Hua Fu Chan Ko Tsa Chih 32:666–668

Wang CC, Rogers MS 1997b Lipid peroxidation in cord blood: A randomised sequential pairs study of prophylactic saline amnioinfusion for intrapartum oligohydramnios. Br J Obstet Gynaecol 104:1145–1151

Warsof SL, Pearce JM, Campbell S 1983 The present place of routine ultrasound screening. Clin Obstet Gynaecol 10:445–458

Watson WJ, Stevens D, Welter S, Day D 1996 Factor predicting successful labour induction. Obstet Gynecol 88:990–992

Westin B 1977 Gravidogram and fetal growth. Comparison with biochemical supervision. Acta Obstet Gynecol Scand 56:273–282

Wing DA, Rahall A, Jones MM, Goodwin TM, Paul RH 1995 Misoprostol: an effective agent for cervical ripening and labour induction. Am J Obstet Gynecol 172:1811–1816

Witter FR, Rocco LE, Johnson TRB 1992 A randomized trial of prostaglandin E_2 in a controlled-release vaginal pessary for cervical ripening at term. Am J Obstet Gynecol 166:830–834

Yim IW 1997 The effect of the husband's presence during labour in Hong Kong. J Clin Nursing 6:169–170

Zeisler H, Tempfer C, Mayerhofer K, Barrada M, Husslein P 1998 Influence of acupuncture on duration of labour. Gynecol Obstet Invest 46:22–25

36

Operative vaginal delivery

Allan M.Z. Chang, T.K. Lau

The contribution of the author of the equivalent chapter in the second edition, on which this chapter draws extensively, is gratefully acknowledged.

Material in this chapter contains contributions from the second edition and we are grateful to the previous author for the work done.

FORCEPS DELIVERY

Historical background

By the seventeenth century, many instruments had been devised to bring forth the tardy child. Midwives commonly used a variety of household utensils including pot hooks and ladles while the man-midwives used purpose-designed hooks, knives and tongs, none of which were intended to deliver a live baby.

With the advent of the obstetric forceps, live births from obstructed labour became a practical possibility and it is not surprising that their inventors tried to keep the instruments a closely guarded Chamberlen family secret; this they succeeded in doing for three generations. The forceps were probably devised by Peter, who delivered Queen Anne. Dr Peter's son Hugh tried to sell the secret to Mauriceau in Paris in 1670 but he failed to accomplish the test which Mauriceau set him—the delivery of a rhachitic dwarf. Hugh, physician to King Charles the Second, fell out of favour and in 1690 left the country for Amsterdam where he sold the secret to Roger van Roonhuyze. In fact it seems that Hugh had sold him but one of the pair of blades. Evidently the secret leaked out or was unravelled in several places in the first half of the eighteenth century. These mechanical aids to delivery were so successful that they gained ground in an atmosphere and philosophy of medicine that was antimechanical. The addi-

tion of a pelvic curve to the blades was first advocated by Smellie in 1762, a concept which was also described by Johnson (1769) in Edinburgh and Levret (1751) in France.

To improve the mechanical advantage of the forceps when delivering a high head, modifications of the shank and handles were made that facilitated traction in the correct axis of the birth canal. The most successful axis traction rods were devised by Neville of Dublin in 1886 as an attachment that could be combined with various types of long forceps then in use. In particular they became wedded to the Barnes forceps and the virtually indestructible Neville–Barnes instruments are, a century later, still in use (albeit without the traction rods) in many units without thought for the original design and purpose of the instrument.

In 1929 Das catalogued over 600 different obstetric forceps. His classic work and those of Laufe (1968) and Hubbard (2000), together with the references previously cited, provide stimulating and thought-provoking reading for the modern obstetrician.

Choice of instrument in modern practice

Different instruments work better in different hands. The only essential rules in the choice of forceps are that they should be appropriate to the task and that the operator should be experienced in their use. It is possible to undertake all forceps deliveries using two, or at most three, instruments. For outlet forceps delivery a short-shanked light forceps of the Wrigley type is the most suitable (Fig. 36.1). For mid-cavity forceps when the sagittal suture is in the anteroposterior diameter, an instrument with a longer shank is needed (Fig. 36.1); it should be as light in weight as possible and should have dimensions appropriate to modern practice. For forceps rotation, if such manoeuvres are undertaken, Kielland's forceps are most widely used. For delivery of the aftercoming head in breech presentation the conventional long-shanked forceps are suitable but the Piper forceps, in which the pelvic curve is set behind the long axis, are widely used.

Terminology

The definitions of certain terms used to describe forceps deliveries vary greatly from author to author; this makes comparison of data difficult. It should be noted that the classification of forceps depends on the status of the fetal presenting part when the instrument is applied rather than on the physical type of instrument used. This is based on the assumption that different types of forceps application will be associated with different degrees of maternal and fetal risks.

A *high-forceps* delivery is one in which the fetal head is not engaged and on vaginal examination the vertex is well above the level of the ischial spines. The hazards of such a procedure are so great that it should hardly ever be contemplated in modern obstetric practice, except in surroundings where a caesarean section cannot be performed and where the operator is highly experienced in vaginal operative delivery. The former situation is now getting rarer while the latter are becoming extinct.

A *mid-forceps* delivery is performed when the head is in the mid pelvic cavity with the vertex at or near the level of the ischial spines. Internal rotation of the head is often incomplete and this will need to be corrected before traction can be applied. The management of such cases is one of the most controversial current issues.

A *low-forceps* delivery usually refers to those cases in which the head is at or near the pelvic floor, or even visible at the introitus, although perineal distension does not occur with contractions.

Outlet forceps refer to when the vertex has reached the pelvic floor, the sagittal suture is in the anteroposterior diameter and only maternal soft tissues are impeding the delivery of the head.

This classification system is similar to that of the American College of Obstetricians and Gynaecologist (ACOG) 1988 definition (Table 36.1), which has detailed descriptions

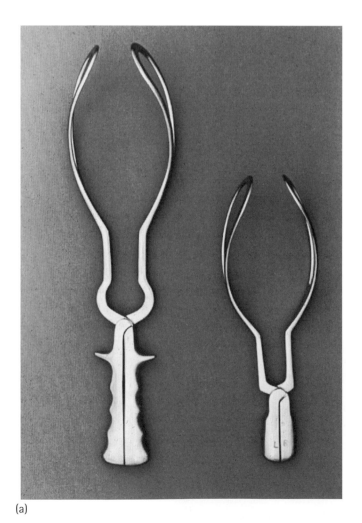
(a)

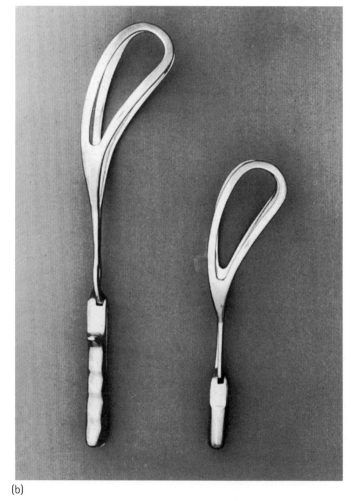
(b)

Fig. 36.1 Anderson's long forceps (left) and Wrigley's forceps (right) compared. (a) Plan; (b) elevation. From Hibbard (1988) with permission.

Table 36.1 Classification of forceps delivery[a]

Type of procedure	Criteria
Outlet forceps	1. Scalp is visible at the introitus without separating labia 2. Fetal skull has reached pelvic floor 3. Sagittal suture is in anteroposterior diameter or right or left occiput anterior or posterior position 4. Fetal head is at or on perineum 5. Rotation does not exceed 45°
Low forceps	Leading point of fetal skull is at station ≥+2 cm and not on the pelvic floor a. Rotation ≤ 45° (left or right occiput anterior, or left or right occiput posterior to occiput posterior) b. Rotation >45°
Midforceps	Station above +2 cm but head engaged
High	Not included in the classification

[a] Adapted from the American College of Obstetricians and Gynecologists. Obstetric forceps. ACOG Committee Opinion 71. Washington DC: ACOG, 1989

of diagnostic criteria based on the station of the presenting part and the rotation of the fetal position (ACOG 1994). Hagadorn-Freathy et al (1991) reported that this classification system has led to a clearer stratification of risks among different types of operation than the old system. It should be noted that the ACOG classification system does not include the definition of high forceps, implying that high forceps has no place in modern obstetrics.

Since no single classification has been universally agreed, it is of paramount importance that all relevant physical findings are clearly documented in the medical notes so that useful comparison could be performed. A pre-coded proforma inviting entries in all appropriate aspects of the delivery can simplify the process of ensuring that no relevant information remains unrecorded.

Indications

The need to expedite vaginal delivery may arise because of poor progress of labour or because of some maternal or fetal emergency. Conditions which limit a woman's ability to push (e.g. neurological disorders with weakness) or require avoidance of prolonged straining (e.g. cardiac disease, eclampsia) are uncommon, but they would indicate a forceps delivery. More common indications are maternal or fetal distress, the latter often a consequence of the former.

Delay in the second stage

It used to be customary to apply arbitrary time limits for the duration of the second stage of labour. These are not particularly useful, especially as it is usually uncertain when the second stage actually began. Of far more importance is the progress, judged by serial assessment of the descent of the presenting part, and the position and attitude of the head. Expulsive forces may be insufficient to maintain progressive

labour because they are inherently weak or because there is undue resistance to descent of the head caused by cephalopelvic disproportion or by soft-tissue obstruction. Disproportion is a relative concept which may be a result of a relatively large head, a relatively small or misshapen pelvis, or positional disproportion caused by malpresentation so that a larger fetal head diameter presents.

There are no absolute criteria for intervention when progress is unduly slow, providing there are no other acute complicating factors. Too early interference may involve the operator in an unnecessarily difficult operative delivery, perhaps with the need for rotation of the head. With a little more patience some further progress could have been achieved, followed by an easier forceps delivery. However, unnecessary waiting increases the physical and mental discomfort for the mother and the risk of hypoxia and trauma for the baby. An outlet forceps delivery carries no significant risk for the mother or baby and it should be freely employed when there is delay because of relative rigidity of the maternal soft tissues or when maternal expulsive efforts are inadequate because of exhaustion, non-cooperation, or lack of the bearing-down reflex associated with epidural anaesthesia.

Specific maternal and fetal indications

Although there are certain clear-cut conditions which in themselves indicate the need for urgent delivery, more commonly intelligent anticipation of maternal or fetal deterioration, particularly in cases of prolonged labour, leads to obstetric intervention.

Maternal compromise. *Maternal obstetric indications* include eclampsia, severe pre-eclampsia and intrapartum haemorrhage. *Intercurrent illness*, such as severe cardiac or pulmonary disease, may be an indication for early recourse to forceps delivery if progress is not rapid, to minimise physical strain.

Maternal distress to former generations of obstetricians meant a mother exhausted physically and mentally, dehydrated and ketotic, with a raised pulse rate and often mildly pyrexial. To allow such a situation to develop in modern obstetric practice is indefensible. However, the term is still used but it refers to circumstances where progress is slow and further encouragement of the mother is to no avail.

Fetal compromise. There are some clearly recognised and defined complications in the second stage, such as umbilical cord prolapse and premature separation of the placenta, in which early delivery, usually by forceps, is imperative.

More commonly, there is gradually accumulating evidence of fetal distress—a clinical concept implying progressive fetal hypoxia and acidaemia—for which no specific cause is identified although in many cases there are defined risk factors, such as maternal age, hypertension, prolonged pregnancy and intrauterine growth restriction. Other altering factors include the passage of meconium-stained amniotic fluid, fetal bradycardia and late deceleration patterns on a cardiotocograph. However, as in the first stage of labour, action based on fetal heart rate patterns alone will lead to many unnecessary interventions and unless the pattern is truly alarming, or delivery is likely to be achieved quickly and easily by episiotomy and outlet forceps delivery, fetal blood sampling may be performed before deciding on the need for, and mode of, delivery.

Alternative methods of management

Since indications for forceps delivery are rarely, if ever, absolute, other options need to be considered.

Wait

When the head is in the mid-cavity and incompletely rotated, temporising may result in some further progress and avoid the need for rotation as well as bringing the head lower in the pelvis. There is of course no case for waiting if there is arrest of progress.

Encourage stronger uterine action

The initiation of, or further increase in the dosage of, syntocinon in the second stage of labour must be used with caution because a delay in second stage may represent underlying cephalopelvic disproportion. The use of syntocinon under this situation may result in further impaction of presenting fetal part and if caesarean section is ultimately needed, displacement and delivery of the head may be more difficult. Clearly, careful selection of cases for such a form of management is vital if both fetal and maternal trauma is to be avoided.

Caesarean section

Abandonment of mid-forceps operations, especially those involving rotation of the fetal head, has gained favour in recent years, not only because of the attitudes expressed by O'Driscoll & Meagher (1980) but because of increasing concern with defensive obstetrics occasioned by attitudes to litigation in the event of misfortune. The risks of caesarean section are clear and relatively well quantified. The risks of forceps delivery from the mid-cavity are not and, in spite of an extensive literature, judgement continues to be based on common sense rather than statistical analyses of often dubious validity. From the published literature, including the review by Cohen & Friedman (1983), it is evident that judgement is confounded by many factors, including the following:

- there have been no prospective or controlled trials
- varying definitions have been used; indications for forceps delivery vary and series may or may not include rotations performed by various means
- management policies include varying degrees of conservatism
- it is difficult to be certain whether many fetal complications and condition at birth are propter hoc or post hoc, cause or effect
- distinction is not made between operations performed by skilled and unskilled obstetricians
- the availability of senior assistance or facilities for immediate caesarean section in case of undue difficulty is a relevant factor.

Many of these problems are highlighted by the provocative papers of Cardozo et al (1982) and Chiswick & James (1979) and the extensive correspondence which followed them.

On the basis of available evidence there does not appear to be a case for absolute abandonment of mid-cavity forceps delivery, even if it involves rotation, in favour of caesarean section. However, the following general guidelines should be followed to ensure that these potentially dangerous operations can be relatively safe for mother and baby and the longer-term sequelae of caesarean section can be minimised:

1. Caesarean section should generally be carried out if there is confirmed evidence of fetal asphyxia and the head has not reached the pelvic floor, so that there is still soft-tissue resistance to be overcome. Reassessment in the operating theatre immediately prior to section is often advisable as the situation may have changed in the interim.
2. Caesarean section is indicated in mid-cavity arrest in multigravidae, with or without malpresentation, as this nearly always indicates disproportion of a degree that would make vaginal delivery dangerous.
3. If mid-forceps delivery is contemplated, senior staff should always be directly involved in assessment and supervision of the delivery. If for any reason senior assistance is not immediately available or advice is available only by telephone, caesarean section is likely to be a preferable option.
4. Application of forceps before full cervical dilatation should be obsolete.
5. Adequate anaesthesia must be established. This usually means epidural or spinal anaesthesia—pudendal nerve block and local infiltration are inadequate for rotation or mid-cavity forceps delivery.

Vacuum extractor

The advantages and disadvantages of the vacuum extractor (ventouse) are discussed later in this chapter. Forceps and the vacuum extractor, rather than rivalling each other, should be regarded as complementary in varying circumstances and their use kept for the appropriate occasion.

Prerequisites

There are certain fundamental rules which must be fulfilled before forceps delivery is attempted, irrespective of an apparent urgency to deliver the baby. Indeed an emergency situation is just the time when discipline and adherence to well established principles are most required.

1. The cervix must be fully dilated.
2. The fetal head must be engaged.
3. The membranes must be ruptured.
4. The position and station of the head must be identified with certainty and the head must be in a suitable position for delivery, with prior rotation if necessary.
5. There must be no major cephalopelvic disproportion.
6. There must be adequate facilities for neonatal resuscitation and special care.
7. The bladder must be emptied, if necessary by catheterisation.
8. There should be adequate anaesthesia.

Technique

Occipito-anterior forceps delivery

The first essential for safe delivery of the baby is that the forceps blades should lie in a correct relationship to the fetal head. To this end, careful reassessment and rehearsal of the position of the blades are a desirable preliminary. The blades are designated left and right. The left blade is that which is applied on the left side of the mother's pelvis and the handle is held in the operator's left hand. The blade fits comfortably into the slightly cupped right hand of the operator (Fig. 36.2).

There are three phases to the operation—application of the blades, adjustment and articulation, and traction.

Application of the blades. The left blade is selected and the handle is held between the finger and thumb of the left hand. The blade rests in the cupped right hand and the handle is approximately parallel with the right inguinal ligament (Fig. 36.3). Only two fingers of the right hand need to be inserted into the vagina to guide the tip of the blade into position alongside the fetal head as the handle is swept round in an arc. Only minimal force should be necessary and grasping the handle of the forceps like a joystick is quite unneces-

sary. If application and manipulation are not possible with a finger and thumb grasp, something is wrong and the situation should be reassessed. The right blade is applied in like manner, using the fingers of the left hand to guide the blade.

Adjustment and articulation. With proper application and positioning the forceps blades should come together and lock easily but some minor adjustments may be necessary. Optimally the blades should ultimately grasp the head at right angles to the submentovertical diameter. If the head is a few degrees off the anteroposterior diameter of the pelvis, the forceps should be applied in correct relationship to the head rather than the pelvis.

The positioning is checked by feeling the lambdoid suture 2 cm from the shank of the forceps and the symmetry of the forceps in relation to the suture lines and fontanelles.

If the blades do not lock easily, undue manipulation is likely to be traumatic to mother and baby. Removal and reassessment are indicated.

Traction. Traction is best applied by the fingers placed between the shanks of the forceps (Fig. 36.4). The use only of fingers imposes some limit to the degree of traction force which can be applied, gives a better feel of the direction of traction and avoids any risk of head compression from gripping the handles. The traction force is also limited if the forearm is kept in a flexed position.

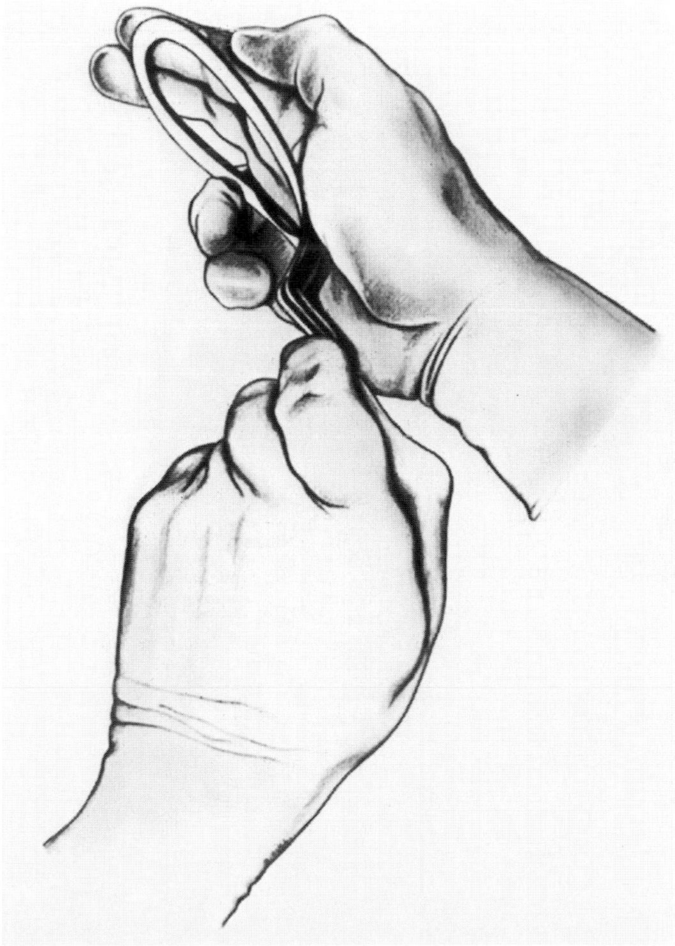

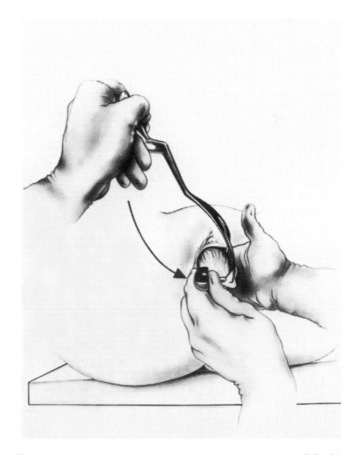

Fig. 36.2 Identification of the left blade of the forceps. The blade fits comfortably into the right hand and the fingers guard the tip. From Hibbard (1988) with permission.

Fig. 36.3 Insertion of the left blade. The handle starts parallel with the inguinal ligament on the opposite side. From Hibbard (1988) with permission.

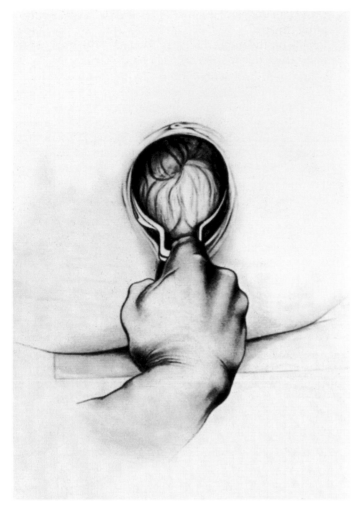

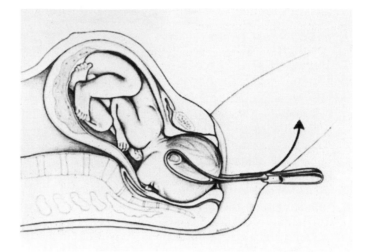

Fig. 36.5 The direction of traction follows the axis of the birth canal, reproducing the normal mechanism of labour. From Hibbard (1988) with permission.

Fig. 36.4 Traction. Note the initial direction of traction which is related to the station of the head in the birth canal. The traction force is applied via the index finger between the shanks of the forceps. From Hibbard (1988) with permission.

The aim of traction is to augment the natural forces. The direction of traction should be in the axis of the birth canal, altering the angle as the head descends (Fig. 36.5). Traction is applied synchronously with uterine contractions. There should always be some descent of the head during traction, even though it retreats in the intervening period. Lack of descent suggests a degree of disproportion incompatible with safe vaginal delivery.

When the head is distending the perineum and the biparietal diameter is at the level of the ischial tuberosities, an episiotomy is performed. Crowning and delivery of the head are achieved in a controlled manner by swinging the handles of the forceps upwards so that the head extends (Fig. 36.6). The blades are removed and delivery is completed in the normal manner, followed by inspection of the birth canal for lacerations and repair of the episiotomy.

Forceps delivery for cephalic malpresentations
The clinical features and general management of occipito-posterior and transverse positions are discussed elsewhere

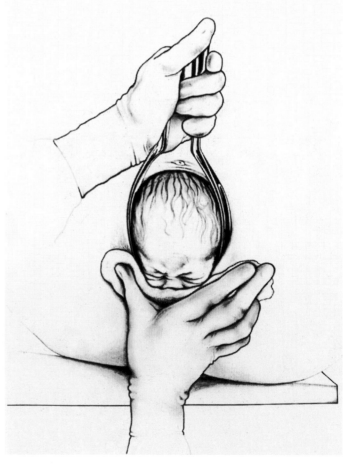

Fig. 36.6 Completion of delivery of the head by extension. The handles of the forceps are almost vertical. From Hibbard (1988) with permission.

(see Ch. 34). In summary, with delay associated with these malpositions the options are:

1. Caesarean section.
2. Manual rotation and forceps delivery.
3. Forceps rotation and delivery.
4. With occipito-posterior position, delivery as an occipito-posterior.
5. Delivery using vacuum extractor.

The choice of operative procedure depends not only on the clinical conditions, but also on the skills and training of the operator. All such deliveries are potentially hazardous, and increasing difficulty is related to, for example, the duration of the 7–10 cm dilatation interval (Davidson et al 1976; Fig. 36.7). Therefore, such procedures must always be undertaken or supervised by the most senior person available and they are often best carried out as a trial of forceps in the operating theatre with facilities immediately available for caesarean section if conditions prove unfavourable.

Manual rotation is the least popular option and it may lead to unexpected and unwanted problems. To facilitate rotation it is usually necessary to disimpact the head by pushing it upward. This increases the risk of cord prolapse and it may leave the head at a higher level after rotation, so making subsequent forceps application more difficult and more hazardous. Undue displacement may even result in the head being above the pelvic brim. Further, to have the occiput anterior when the head is high in the pelvic cavity is unanatomical and is contrary to the normal mechanism of labour. One of the basic rules of assisted delivery is to endeavour to mimic the normal mechanism of labour as closely as possible.

If forceps rotation has been considered to be the treatment option, the following essential preliminaries must be met:

1. Assemble the full team, including anaesthetist and paediatrician.
2. Ascertain that conditions are as previously assessed and that vaginal delivery is likely to be successful.

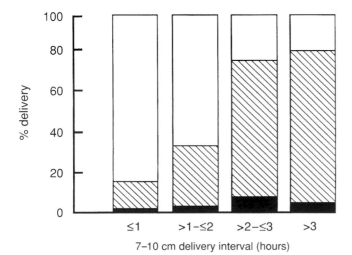

Fig. 36.7 Facility of forceps delivery related to the 7–10 cm cervical dilatation period (occipito-anterior presentations). ■ = difficult; ◳ = moderate; □ = easy. After Davidson et al (1976).

3. Decide on the place of delivery, i.e. delivery room or operating theatre.
4. Decide on the method of pain relief with the patient and anaesthetist. Epidural analgesia is preferred.

Kielland's forceps. Of the many types of forceps designed for rotation of the head only two have found wide favour over a long period. Kielland's forceps have been particularly popular in Europe, while Barton's forceps have had most support in America. The use of the former will be described. Those readers who wish to make a detailed study of Barton's forceps and their modifications are referred particularly to the monograph by Parry Jones (1972).

The two main features of the instrument are:

1. The axis of the blades is parallel to that of the handle, which simplifies the application of rotation (Fig. 36.8).
2. It has a sliding lock (Fig. 36.9), which permits satisfactory cephalic application even in cases of gross asynclitism (Parry Jones 1952).

In inappropriate unskilled hands Kielland's forceps are potentially dangerous, and specialist training and continuing practice are required for their safe use. Hence there has been a growing tendency to abandon mid-cavity rotation in favour of caesarean section. In some working circumstances, the vacuum extractor may be a satisfactory or even desirable alternative, with less risk of trauma since the vacuum extractor does not reduce the already limited available pelvic space. However, there is a greater risk of failure.

Application of Kielland's forceps. The aim is to obtain correct cephalic application with the concavity of the pelvic curve of the forceps directed towards the occiput. To aid orientation there is a raised knob on the upper surface of each finger lug and these should point in the direction of the occiput.

The anterior (superior) blade is always applied first—i.e. the left blade for a right occipito-lateral position and the right blade for a left occipito-lateral position. There are several ways to apply Kielland's forceps, but only the wandering method, which is the most popular option, is described here. The ultimate anterior blade, whether it be right or left, is inserted in the standard manner along the side wall of the pelvis, and it is then wandered by swinging it round to a correct cephalic relationship as insertion proceeds (Fig. 36.10). It is usually advised that it is easier to wander the blade from insertion over the forehead and this has the advantage that during the early part of insertion the pelvic curve of the blade matches the curve of the birth canal.

The application of the posterior blade is often more difficult probably because of obstruction by the sacral promontory (Fig. 36.11). Half of the right hand is introduced into the hollow of the sacrum and is used to facilitate direct application of the blade, which often drops into position with minimal pressure. If the sacral promontory is a problem, it is important for any manipulation to be carried out gently while the soft tissues are guarded by the operator's fingers. Sometimes in cases of difficulty a slightly oblique introduction and wandering application may be helpful.

Readers interested in a more detailed description on the

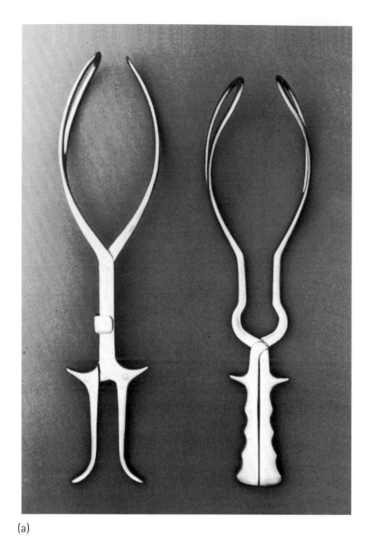

(a)

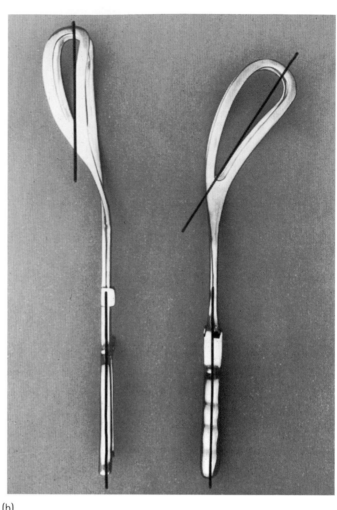

(b)

Fig. 36.8 Kielland's forceps (left) and Anderson's forceps (right) compared. (a) Plan; (b) elevation. Note that in the Kielland's forceps the axes of the blades and handles are parallel. From Hibbard (1988) with permission.

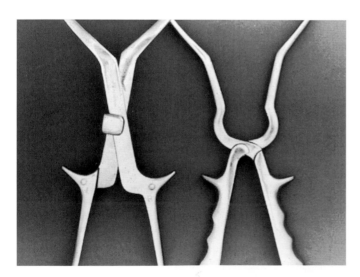

Fig. 36.9 The locks of Kielland's (left) and conventional forceps (right) compared. The sliding lock of the Kielland's forceps facilitates application when there is asymmetric moulding of the head. From Hibbard (1988) with permission.

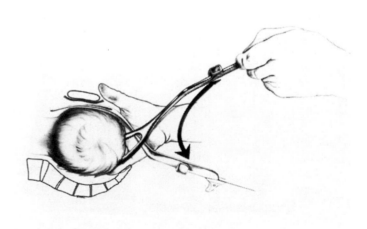

Fig. 36.10 Wandering method of application of the anterior blade. Insertion is started as with a conventional forceps application, swinging the blade round to a correct cephalic application as insertion proceeds. From Hibbard (1988) with permission.

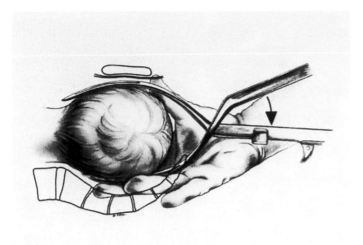

Fig. 36.11 Direct application of the posterior blade. From Hibbard (1988) with permission

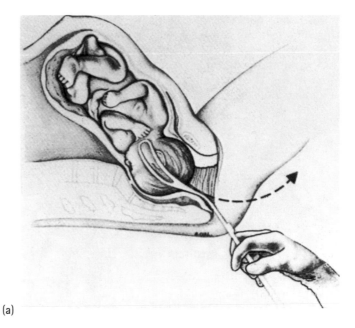

(a)

use of rotational forceps should refer to textbooks on operative vaginal deliveries.

Traction and rotation. Accepting that the desirable objective is to mimic the normal mechanism of labour as closely as possible, traction force in the exact direction of the handles should be applied first and if there is advancement of the head this can be continued without any external rotating force; the head will rotate spontaneously as it descends through the birth canal.

It must be recognised that, because of the design of the forceps, the direction of traction is more posteriorly than with conventional forceps and an early generous episiotomy is required. Also, if the woman is in the lithotomy position, effective traction is difficult with the operator in a standing position or sitting on a normal operating stool. Although Kielland (1916) advocated tilting the bed to facilitate traction a better alternative is for the operator to sit on a low footstool or even kneel.

Delivery is completed in the conventional manner, avoiding compression of the handles and using only the finger lugs to exert traction force (Fig. 36.12).

If the head does not descend readily during the initial traction attempt the situation should be reappraised, with the alternative options of rotation in the mid-cavity or caesarean section.

Mid-cavity rotation must be carried out with gentleness and sensitivity. Slight upward dislodgement of the head, especially with a funnel-shaped pelvis, may facilitate rotation. Only the finger lugs should be used for applying rotational pressure. Traction and rotational forces should not be applied at the same time.

Forceps delivery as an occipito-posterior

The management of delay in second stage of labour associated with occipito-posterior position usually requires correction of the malpresentation before applying traction, but in some cases forceps delivery as an occipito-posterior may be

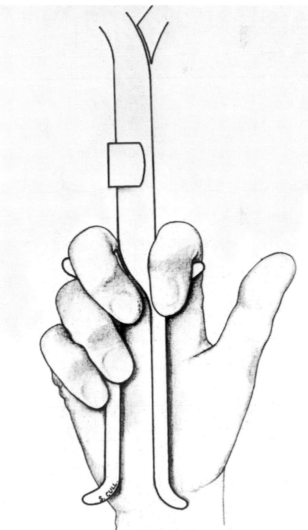

(b)

Fig. 36.12 (a) The direction of traction with Kielland's forceps. (b) The traction force is applied via the finger lugs and not by grasping the handles. From Hibbard (1988) with permission.

justified and preferable. Particular circumstances in which this option should be considered include a satisfactory bony pelvic outlet, as with an anthropoid pelvis (which favours occipito-posterior positions) and delay caused by soft-tissue obstruction. The head must be below the level of the ischial spines and the position must be directly occipito-posterior (occipito-sacral).

The forceps are applied in the conventional manner, with correct pelvic application, taking care not to place the blades too far anteriorly in relation to the head as they may then slip off. A generous episiotomy is usually required and traction is directed posteriorly until the glabella is under the apex of the pubic arch. The handles of the forceps are then swung upwards so that the head is delivered by flexion.

Side effects and complications

The major complication of forceps delivery is maternal and fetal traumatic injury. Some of the complications are inevitable, although their frequency and severity can be aggravated by errors of judgement and inexperience.

Maternal complications

There is a risk of extension of the episiotomy and additional vaginal lacerations occurring during application of the blades and during traction, particularly if forceps of unsuitable design are used. Any additional trauma makes suturing more difficult and increases the risk of painful scars and dyspareunia. The cervix is particularly susceptible to damage during rotational deliveries, either during the application of the blades or during the rotation. Lateral lacerations may extend upwards into the lower uterine segment, with rupture of the uterine artery or main branches. Damage anteriorly can involve the bladder, with production of a vesicocervical or vesicovaginal fistula. Associated traumatic haemorrhage may be severe. In any cases of doubt concerning trauma, full exploration in operating theatre conditions is obligatory. Attempts at semi-blind suturing in the delivery room without adequate exposure and assistance are only likely to compound the problem.

Retention of urine and urinary tract infection are known complications of forceps delivery. In particular a careful watch should be kept to avoid retention with overflow if epidural analgesia has been used. Any difficult delivery should be followed by catheterization, and if haematuria is revealed special precautions are necessary. Gross haematuria suggests the possibility of tearing and fistula formation, and detailed examination is required. Lesser degrees of haematuria are indicative of bruising and devitalisation. This may be associated with tissue necrosis and the risk of late fistula formation when tissue breakdown occurs. In all cases of haematuria, continuous bladder drainage should be instituted and continued for some days after the urine has been microscopically clear of blood.

When labour has been prolonged and difficult there is an added element of maternal tissue bruising with devitalisation and risk of sepsis, which is likely to increase the problems arising from any operative trauma.

Anaesthetic complications are discussed in Chapter 32.

Fetal injury

The infant is at particular risk of intracranial trauma and haemorrhage if forceps are abused, particularly if they are misapplied so that there is not a true cephalic fit. Forceps of unsatisfactory design may lead to undue compression or may slip, causing facial abrasion.

Compression distortion injuries result in tears of the tentorium and rupture of the bridging veins. Rupture of the great vein of Galen leads to bleeding into the posterior fossa with compression of the brain stem, but supratentorial haemorrhages are more common.

Skull fractures are usually linear and not of lasting consequence. Depressed fractures, which may follow forceps delivery, are very uncommon but they can result in subdural or subarachnoid haemorrhage.

Cephalohaematomas are seen most commonly over the parietal bone.

Facial nerve palsy is caused by pressure at the point where the nerve emerges from the stylomastoid foramen or as it passes over the mandibular ramus. The lesion is a lower motor neurone one, with paresis of the whole of the affected side of the face. Uncommonly, temporal bone fracture results in seventh nerve injury; the lesion is an upper motor neurone one and involves the lower two-thirds of the face. Although the occurrence of neonatal facial nerve palsy is commonly associated with the use of obstetric forceps, up to 30% of babies with facial nerve palsy were delivered spontaneously (Levine et al 1984). A more recent study has shown that only 13% of 61 babies with persisting facial palsy had been delivered by forceps. This suggests that most cases of traumatic facial palsy recover spontaneously, whereas those cases that persist had an intrauterine rather than traumatic aetiology (a sort of intrauterine Bell's palsy) (Laing et al 1996).

Failed forceps delivery

The term failed forceps implies that a forceps delivery was initiated in the delivery room in the belief that it could be completed successfully but that it had to be abandoned in favour of caesarean section, either because of failure in application of the instrument, or more commonly after unsuccessful traction. This term should also include cases in which vaginal delivery has been achieved, but only after a second attempt by a more experienced operator. The commonest contributory factors to failed forceps deliveries are unrecognised malpresentation or cephalopelvic disproportion.

Trial of forceps

Trial of forceps refers to an attempt at forceps delivery with all staff and equipment ready for immediate abdominal delivery in the anticipation that undue difficulty may be encountered which necessitates the abandonment of the procedure in favour of abdominal delivery. Trials of forceps are usually performed when a certain degree of cephalopelvic disproportion is suspected. There is no evidence that perinatal outcome is worsened by a properly conducted trial of forceps, although the neonatal morbidity is higher after unexpected failed forceps delivery (Lowe 1987, Revah et al 1997).

THE VACUUM EXTRACTOR (VENTOUSE)

The vacuum extractor has virtually replaced the forceps in many countries of northern Europe and Africa. Its has also been increasingly used in Britain and the USA (Curtin & Park 1999). The vacuum extractor is simple and easy to use; it does not increase the effective diameter of the presenting part, and it promotes autorotation in cases with malposition.

Indications

First stage

Vacuum extraction performed before full dilatation should be considered as an exception rather than the norm. It should only be performed when there is an urgent need to deliver the fetus before full cervical dilatation such as the presence of terminal fetal bradycardia with prolapsed cord, and when there is a clear advantage in using the vacuum extractor over immediate caesarean section (Bird 1982). Such procedure should only be attempted where there is no obvious cephalopelvic disproportion, and the operator must be very skilled in the use of the instrument.

Second stage

The indications for vacuum extraction in the second stage of labour closely resemble those for forceps delivery i.e. delay in the second stage, maternal compromise and severe fetal compromise. Vacuum extraction might, therefore, be considered as an alternative to forceps delivery, but there are some special points that require further discussion.

It is a common belief that the use of vacuum extractor requires more preparation time than forceps and, therefore, it is not suitable for fetal distress. However, this difference in the hands of skilled operators is marginal, if the additional analgesic requirement for forceps delivery is taken into account, and, therefore, it is of no clinical importance in the vast majority of cases. Another useful function of the vacuum extractor is to help the woman whom the obstetrician does not wish to have a long or fatiguing second stage, such as a mother with heart disease or raised blood pressure. Here the efforts of the second stage can be shortened very readily with a vacuum extractor. The obstetrician will be pulling with the woman's own contractions so that she can be making some small effort and does have the satisfaction of delivering her baby vaginally, although the real effort is by the obstetrician.

Vacuum extraction is particularly useful as an alternative to rotational forceps in the presence of malposition, such as occipital-transverse or posterior. The application of a vacuum cup followed by traction allows the fetal head to descend in the birth canal along the path of least resistance, and allows 'auto-rotation' of the fetal head to the occipital anterior position.

The vacuum extractor is used occasionally in other situations. For instance, if the baby is not too immature, it can be used to deliver the second twin when the fetal head is high and the cervix appears not completely dilated, should the need for immediate delivery arise. It is an ideal instrument in these circumstances although such a situation is rare, and few operators are skilled in this procedure.

Contraindications

The vacuum extractor is contraindicated for any presentation other than cephalic. Hence it should not be used on a face, brow or breech presentation, or when the fetus is in a transverse lie. If the fetus is immature (under 34 weeks' gestation), the likelihood of developing a cephalohaematoma rises sharply so that this instrument would be better avoided. Should the obstetrician think that any reasonable degree of cephalopelvic disproportion is present, the vacuum extractor should not be used for it will not overcome a mechanical block.

The apparatus

The essential elements of all vacuum extractors are the cup, which is to be applied to the fetal head, a vacuum generator and the connecting tubings.

Many obstetricians in the Western world use metal cups, either the Malmstrom's equipment (1957) or its major modifications put forward by Bird (1969). Some prefer to use a soft cup made from pliable silicone or plastic. More recently, a disposable plastic Bird-type cup, complete with a hand operated integral vacuum pump has been introduced. It avoids the need for a power supply or complicated assembly procedure. One version also incorporates a traction meter which allows the obstetrician to apply an accurately judged traction force.

Metal cups are of toughened steel, chromium-plated and shaped like a flattened hemisphere. They are 40, 50 or 60 mm in diameter and one uses the largest fits. The edge is curved in so that the rim has a smaller diameter than the cavity of the hemisphere a little higher up. Thus, if it is placed against the fetal scalp and air is evacuated from the cavity, the scalp is sucked in to fill the space of the hemisphere; the chignon, so produced, has a greater diameter above the rim than the rim itself, and traction can be applied to the overhang (Fig. 36.13).

The soft cups are mostly 60 mm in diameter. The silastic model is a trumpet-shaped cup of silicone elastomer (Fig. 36.14); a plastic cup (Mityvac) comes with its own hand

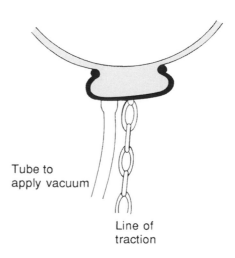

Tube to apply vacuum

Line of traction

Fig. 36.13 The chignon produced on the scalp.

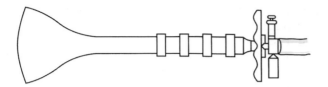

Fig. 36.14   A silastic cup.

pump as a kit for action. The Silc cup of silicone rubber is said to have improved adherence to the fetal scalp (Fig. 36.15). A new version comes with an integral cord traction system. The CMI cup, made of malleable plastic, comes with its own reusable pistol grip hand pump and it is said to produce less trauma to the fetal head (Fig. 36.16). Johanson & Menon (1999a) in a systematic review of five trials found that, compared to rigid metal cup, soft cups were significantly more likely to fail in achieving vaginal delivery (13.0% v. 8.3%), but they were associated with less scalp injury. There was no difference between the two groups in terms of maternal injury. The soft cups in general have bigger traction stems that limit the manoeuvrability in the maternal pelvis to achieve proper placement when the fetal head is deflexed or asynclitic. This probably accounts for the higher failure rate with the soft cup.

The cup of a vacuum extraction is connected to a pump through a thick-walled rubber tube through which air is evacuated. A vacuum can be achieved by a hand or more commonly electrical pump. The more sophisticated mechanical pumps can compensate for small gas leakage in the equipment and automatically maintain a constant preset negative pressure.

Technique

The vacuum extractor system should be checked to be in good condition before application. A cup of the most appropriate size is chosen. Generally this should be one of the

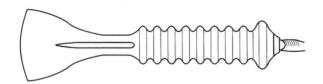

Fig. 36.15   A Silc cup.

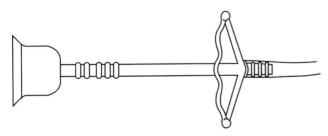

Fig. 36.16   A CMI cup.

larger cups (50 or 60 mm diameter) with which a larger size of chignon can be achieved. The aim of cup application is to place the cup symmetrically over the sagittal suture centred at about 3 cm anterior to the posterior fontanelle (Fig. 36.17). This usually means that the cup will have to be placed as far back as possible in the vagina if the fetus is in an occipital-posterior position. Such an application, when traction is subsequently applied, will maintain normal flexion of the fetal head. On the other hand, when traction is applied to a cup placed in another location of the fetal head, it may result in either extension of the fetal neck or the creation of asynclitism, leading to a more difficult procedure and a higher failure rate (Fig. 36.18).

Negative pressure of 0.8 kg/cm² is applied when the correct position of the cup is achieved and no maternal tissue is included. With an electrical pump, evacuation of the air can be done more efficiently. The final negative pressure can be

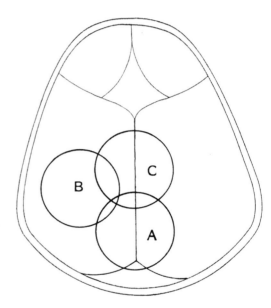

Fig. 36.17   The cap should ideally be as far back as possible over the bregma (A). If it is off the midline (B) it allows an asymmetrical pull and so larger diameters of the fetal head engage. If it is further forward than the bregma (C) the head is deflexed.

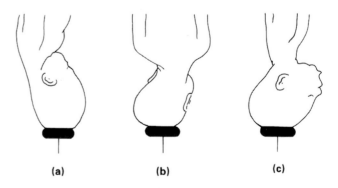

Fig. 36.18   The consequences of applications shown in Figure 36.17 are: (a) good application—good flexion; (b) off the midline—asynclitism; (c) too far forward—deflexion.

achieved as quickly as possible without jeopardising the strength of the chignon, and there is no need for the so-called stepwise increase in creating the vacuum force.

Once the cup has been attached to the scalp by the vacuum force, its position must be carefully checked again to ensure that there is no inclusion of maternal tissue. Traction should be applied only after a proper chignon is formed, which usually takes two minutes. This means that the vacuum extractor is usually ready for use with the next uterine contraction. The principle of vacuum extraction is that the line of traction force should follow the curved pelvic axis, which represents the pathway of least resistance to the fetal head when it descends (Fig. 36.19). Traction should also be synchronised with uterine contraction and maternal effort. If the fetal head is not in the occipital-anterior position, it will automatically rotate as it descends in the pelvis, so that its diameters engage advantageously with the various diameters of the maternal pelvis. This is the vacuum extractor's great advantage, that the head can follow its own pattern of rotation (auto-rotation).

Oblique traction should be avoided because it will increase the chance of cup dislodgement. Traction perpendicular to the fetal head is usually applied with the operator's right hand on the handle. Appropriate concomitant downward force on the cap may be applied by the left hand so as to generate a resultant force which follows the pelvic axis (Fig. 36.20). The index finger of the left hand should be placed on the cup near the periphery so that slip or dislodgement of cup can be detected early. As the head crowns, the negative pressure should be released and the cup detached. Sufficient time should be given to allow normal external rotation of the fetal head before any attempt to deliver the rest of the fetus.

Care should be taken not to dislodge the cup during traction. If the cup dislodges, the reason should be sought and corrected during reapplication of the cup. There should not be a reapplication of a dislodged cup unless a technical and correctable cause can be identified. Cup dislodgement should not be regarded as a safety mechanism of the instrument in avoiding excessive traction force, but as a warning sign of possible cephalopelvic disproportion. Delivery by vacuum extraction should be considered to have failed if no cause could be found for cup dislodgement, or if the cup comes off twice, and another method to achieve delivery should be used.

Even without cup dislodgement, the operator should be willing to abandon the procedure if there is no progress with each traction. Although there is no universally agreed maximum number of traction attempts, delivery of the fetal head should usually occur after three or four traction events and a total application time of 15 minutes or less. If vaginal delivery is not achieved by then, an alternative method should be considered.

Failed vacuum extraction

In experienced hands, the failure rate of the vacuum extractor has been reported to be 0.5% with the Bird cup and 3.2% with the Malmstrom classical cup (Bird 1982). However, higher failure rates of about 10% were reported in randomised trials (Johanson & Menon 1999b). The failure rates are overall higher when soft cups are used (Johanson & Menon 1999a).

The chance of failure increases if the cup is improperly placed, or if the operator applies traction oblique to the fetal head or not in the axis of the birth canal. A large oedematous caput, which is a characteristic feature of a long and difficult

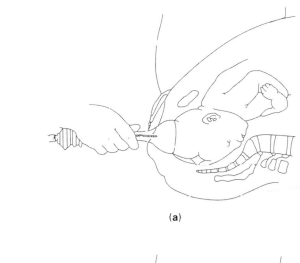

(a)

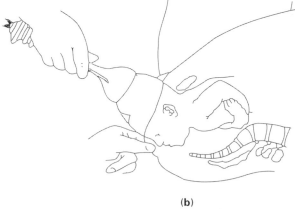

(b)

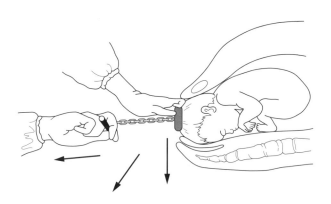

Fig. 36.19 (a) Application of silastic cap. (b) Delivering the head; note change of angle of traction.

Fig. 36.20 Direction of traction force at different stages of descent when using vacuum extraction.

labour, will interfere with the formation of a secure chignon. In that situation, the vacuum cup will not grip well and will dislodge with only limited traction effort. Faulty equipment may also lead to inadequate suction pressure and more dislodgement.

Failure is more common among the new operators. Neophyte operators may be timid and fail to exert sufficient traction, and therefore fail to achieve delivery. Similar to the use of forceps, the success of vacuum extraction depends to a great extent on the skill and experience of the operator. It is important for all operators to practise vacuum extraction under supervision and on easy cases first, and only embark on mid-cavity deliveries when the necessary experience has been obtained.

Side effects and complications

Maternal complications caused by vacuum extraction are uncommon. If a fold of vaginal or cervical tissue is sucked in between the cup and the fetal head without being noticed, it can then be damaged, leading to haemorrhage. Other perineal trauma may happen but is usually less severe than that of forceps delivery.

Fetal complications include superficial scalp abrasions, cephalohaematomas, subgaleal haematomas and intracranial haemorrhage.

The chignon is always present after a vacuum extraction, and it is usually more profound if the metal cup is used. It usually disappears within a few days and has no harmful effect. Superficial abrasions or lacerations occur in about 12% of vacuum extraction, and these also have no long-term significance.

Cephalohaematomas are collections of blood beneath the periosteum of the skull bones caused by the rupture of one of the emissary veins. It complicates about 6% of vacuum extractions. The extent of a cephalohaematoma is limited by the attachment of the periosteum to a single bone. These haematomas usually resolve over one to two weeks, and occasionally lead to transient jaundice.

Subgaleal (or subaponeurotic) haematoma is a rare but potentially fatal complication. The incidence is 0.64% (Ng et al 1995). Because of the voluminous subgaleal space, a significant amount of blood may accumulate. If undetected, or if not managed properly, the baby may suffer from hypovolaemic shock and die.

These fetal soft-tissue complications may occur even after an apparently simple and uncomplicated vacuum extraction, although they are more common after prolonged and difficult procedures, or after dislodgement of the cup.

Intracranial haemorrhage is a much more serious complication, with an estimated incidence of 0.35% (Plauché 1979). However, this is not necessarily a causal relationship. Towner et al (1999), based on a review of 583 340 deliveries, showed a similar incidence of intracranial haemorrhage among infants delivered by vacuum extraction, forceps, or caesarean section during labour, while the incidence is significantly lower among those delivered either spontaneously or by caesarean section before labour. These findings suggest that the common risk factor for haemorrhage is abnormal labour rather than instrumentation. Generally, vacuum extraction does not cause fetal hypoxia or long-term neurological or intellectual impairment.

Comparison of vacuum extraction with the use of forceps

Vacuum extraction is simple to use and, generally speaking, can be practised by less skilled people than can forceps delivery. In many parts of the underdeveloped world, midwives are perfectly competent with vacuum extraction deliveries whereas they have not been appropriately trained to be able to use forceps. The application of forceps requires a greater knowledge of fetal and pelvic anatomy and a greater familiarity with pelvic examinations. If used inappropriately or by inexperienced operators, forceps are potentially more dangerous and more likely to result in major maternal and fetal damages.

The vacuum extractor occupies less space at the side wall of the pelvis than do forceps and so it does not add to any potential disproportion. Traction on a vacuum extractor encourages the fetal head to follow its own mechanisms in the pelvis for rotation. This contrasts with the use of forceps where the head is gripped in place and rotation is in the control of the operator. It is not difficult to imagine that forceps rotation will be associated with more complications.

The disadvantages of the vacuum extractor compared with forceps are that the equipment is more complex and so more likely to go wrong and that it requires maintenance whereas little can happen to two blades of a pair of forceps. The vacuum extractor is also a little less portable than forceps.

Vacuum extraction can be performed with the help of little extra pain relief. Often it can be done without any additional analgesia since the application of the cup is not much more painful for the woman than is a vaginal examination. Putting on forceps is a more difficult art, particularly if the head is in mid-cavity, and a more extensive regional block is required than for a vacuum extraction.

In general, the use of one instrument could be replaced by another with the following exceptions. A vacuum extractor could be used, but not forceps, when the exact position of presenting part is unsure, before full cervical dilatation or when there is malposition unless rotational forceps are going to be used. A vacuum extractor, on the other hand, should not be used in any fetal presentation other than cephalic in premature fetuses, or when fetal coagulopathy is suspected.

In a systematic review of 10 randomised trials, Johanson & Menon (1999b) reported that the vacuum extractor is associated with a significantly higher failure rate (11.6% v. 7.2%), but that despite this, the overall caesarean section rate is lower (1.9% v. 3.5%). The higher overall caesarean section rate in the forceps groups was possibly due to more cases with contraindications for that instrument. Therefore, the use of these two instruments should be considered as complementary rather than competitive. The review also showed that the vacuum extractor is associated with a significantly lower incidence of maternal traumatic morbidity (9.8% v. 20.3%), use of general or regional anaesthesia, or severe pain after delivery. The vacuum extractor on the other hand is associated with a significantly higher incidence of cephalohaematoma (1.0% v. 0.4%) and retinal haemorrhage (48.7% v. 33.5%), but these had no demonstrable long-term significance. The use of forceps was also associated with a higher prevalence of occult anal sphincter defects (82% v. 48%) five years after randomised intervention (Sultan et al 1998).

In summary, it appears that the vacuum extraction offers an immediate benefit of reducing severe maternal injuries on the expense of a higher incidence of fetal haemotoma, which in general carries no long-term morbidity.

The vacuum extractor should be used in parallel with forceps rather than in competition. Skills in the management of delivery with both sets of equipment should be gained in training and kept bright by constant repetition in practice.

DESTRUCTIVE OPERATIONS

Fetal destructive procedures are intended for use to achieve vaginal delivery in otherwise impossible situations. There is virtually no place for such procedures in modern obstetrics for they are associated with an unacceptable level of maternal traumatic morbidity, and they are now considered unjustifiable because of the availability of a safe alternative method of delivery i.e. caesarean section. The general lack of operators experienced in such procedures also makes these procedures highly dangerous. Some of the commoner occasionally used procedures are discussed below.

Decapitation was the standard treatment for neglected labour with shoulder presentation. As a result of long labour, the lower uterine segment was often dangerously stretched and the fetus died in utero. Such a scenario should not occur in modern obstetrics. Even if it does, a caesarean section would be safer for the mother.

Craniotomy was used to reduce the size of the fetal head to achieve vaginal delivery in women with obstructed labour caused by cephalopelvic disproportion. The procedure was associated with serious traumatic morbidity to the genital tract, and was often traumatic psychologically to the operator and the woman. Situations necessitating the use of craniotomy no longer arise in modern obstetric care as pregnancies with cephalopelvic disproportion should be delivered by caesarean section before such complications arise.

Drainage of cerebrospinal fluid can enable vaginal delivery of fetuses with severe hydrocephalus, which otherwise would result in obstruction. Hydrocephalus itself usually would not preclude vaginal delivery unless it is severe and the pregnancy is close to term. Since the effect of prenatal drainage on future fetal development is unknown, such cases should be delivered by caesarean section rather than drainage. Drainage may have a role if the fetal prognosis is unlike to be altered, such as in those with fatal chromosomal abnormalities.

SHOULDER DYSTOCIA

Introduction

Shoulder dystocia means difficulty in delivery of the shoulder. It has been defined as 'a condition in which special manoeuvres are required to deliver the shoulders in addition to downward traction and episiotomy' (Resnik 1980), 'the arrest of spontaneous delivery due to impaction of the anterior shoulder against the symphysis pubis' (Benedetti et al 1989) or 'a head–body delivery time greater than 60 seconds' (Spong et al 1995). The true incidence of shoulder dystocia is difficult to estimate because of wide variations in the definition used but reported figures range between 0.2 to 2.1% of all vaginal deliveries (Gherman & Goodwin 1998). Based on his observation over a 15-year period, Hopwood (1982) reported a rising incidence of shoulder dystocia from 0.2% to 1.1% although a further review by Sandmire & O'Halloin (1988) could not confirm such a trend.

The commonest form of shoulder dystocia is a unilateral dystocia where the posterior shoulder has entered the pelvis but the anterior shoulder is stuck above the symphysis pubis (Gibb 1995). It is important to realise that in this case the shoulder is still above the pelvic inlet and, therefore, forceful direct downward traction alone will not solve the problem and it may lead to further impaction of the shoulder and injury to the brachial plexus.

Complications

Shoulder dystocia is a serious obstetric complication associated with significant perinatal and maternal mortality and morbidity. The major maternal risks are postpartum haemorrhage and soft-tissue trauma, including cervicovaginal lacerations, extensive perineal damage, and uterine rupture (Gherman & Goodwin 1998).

Neonatal complications include mortality, asphyxia, neurological and orthopaedic damage. Although the perinatal mortality rate associated with shoulder dystocia has been frequently quoted in reviews to be between 19 and 289 per 1000 (Wagner et al 1999), a much lower figure of below 1% was reported in more recent series (Gherman et al 1998, Sandmire & O'Halloin 1988). Analysis of the Confidential Enquiry into Stillbirths and Deaths in Infancy (CESDI) registry of England, Wales and North Ireland between 1994 and 1995 showed that there were 56 stillbirths and neonatal deaths attributed to shoulder dystocia alone among 1 400 000 births (Hope et al 1998). The perinatal loss rate in this report would be at the most 0.57 per 100 cases of shoulder dystocia, assuming a vaginal delivery rate of 70% and the incidence of shoulder dystocia as 1% of all vaginal deliveries. This much lower incidence of perinatal mortality associated with shoulder dystocia in recent years may be, at least partly, as a result of improvement in clinical management of this obstetric emergency.

Neonatal morbidity has been reported to complicate 24.9% (Gherman et al 1998) to 42% (Gross et al 1987) of cases of shoulder dystocia. Respiratory arrest and asphyxia is a common complication of shoulder dystocia and it can be rapidly fatal. The median head-to-body delivery time interval among the 56 deaths caused by shoulder dystocia, mentioned above in the CESDI report, was only five minutes. The commonest traumatic morbidity is brachial plexus injury (16.8%), followed by clavicular fractures (9.5%) and humeral fractures (4.2%) (Gherman et al 1998). Most brachial plexus injuries are temporary with only 5–8% having persistent nerve injury by one year (Gherman & Goodwin 1998). Orthopaedic injuries usually heal without long-term morbidity. It has been suggested that permanent brachial plexus injury should be used as the major criterion for judging the consequences and the effectiveness of interventions for shoulder dystocia. It should be noted though that these traumatic injuries are not necessarily a result of shoulder dystocia. Although Erb's palsy is usually considered to be specifically associated with shoulder dystocia, no perinatal risk factors could be identified in about one-third of the Erb's palsies, which mostly likely have arisen in utero (Peleg et al 1997).

Risk factors, prediction and prevention

Among the numerous antenatal and intrapartum factors that have been reported to be associated with the occurrence of shoulder dystocia, macrosomia stands out as the most important one (Johnstone & Myerscough 1998). The risk of shoulder dystocia was 11.4% for babies weighing 4200 g or more (Blickstein et al 1998), and it was 22% for babies 4500 g or more (Berard et al 1998). Other important independent risk factors include maternal diabetes and previous shoulder dystocia. Although maternal obesity, excessive weight gain during pregnancy, previous big baby, postdate pregnancy and prolonged second stage of labour have all been found to be associated with shoulder dystocia, such effects are possibly through their influence on fetal weight.

Unfortunately, the sensitivity and specificity of using risk factors to predict the occurrence of shoulder dystocia and, more importantly, its complications, have been disappointing. Even considering macrosomia, which is the most important risk factor, 50–60% of shoulder dystocias occur in infants weighing less than 4000 g, and most babies weighing more than 4000 g deliver normally. So far, there is insufficient evidence to justify interventions such as induction of labour (Gonen et al 1997) or caesarean section in fetuses estimated to be macrosomic. For example, Rouse et al (1996) estimated that 3695 caesarean deliveries would have to be performed to prevent one case of permanent brachial plexus injury with a policy of elective caesarean section when estimated fetal weight was 4500 g or above, or 2345 caesarean section if a 4000 g policy was adopted. The failure of these prediction models are at least due to the following two reasons. Firstly, the low incidence of shoulder dystocia of around 1% results in unacceptably high false-positive rate. Secondly, the lack of precision in predicting, before the birth of a baby, its actual weight, which is the most important risk factor of shoulder dystocia. The positive predictive value of antenatal ultrasonographic diagnosis of macrosomia has been found to be only 50–60% (Gonen et al 1997). It appears, therefore, that there is insufficient evidence at present to justify interventions in pregnancies with a single risk factor (Gherman & Goodwin 1998).

However, the use of prophylactic caesarean section in the presence of two or more independent risk factors, in particular the combination of maternal diabetes and macrosomia, is more controversial. The reported incidence of shoulder dystocia in the presence of maternal diabetes and fetal macrosomia (>4000 g) ranges between 17% and 73% (Acker et al 1985,

Keller et al 1991). Conway & Langer (1998) showed that, by using a threshold of 4250 g at 37 to 38 weeks for elective caesarean section and 90th centile or beyond as the threshold for induction of labour, they were able to reduce the rate of shoulder dystocia from 2.4% to 1.1% at the cost of increasing the caesarean section rate from 21.7% to 25.1% among the diabetic mothers, although there was no effect on the rate of brachial plexus palsy. Rouse et al (1996) estimated that approximately 789 elective caesarean sections would be necessary to prevent a case of permanent brachial plexus palsy among the diabetic mothers if a 4000 g policy was adopted. Whether this intervention–benefit ratio justifies prophylactic abdominal delivery is debatable.

Management

Shoulder dystocia is an uncommon, mostly unpredictable but serious and rapidly fatal condition. Among 56 cases of shoulder dystocia reported to the CESDI mentioned above, the midwife was the lead professional in 56% of cases when the fetal head was delivered (Hope et al 1998). In the same study, the mean time interval between delivery of the head and the rest of the body was found to be only five minutes. Therefore, it is of paramount importance that all health care professionals, including all obstetricians and midwives, who are involved in the management of labour and delivery, must be familiar with the management of shoulder dystocia from the first day of their duty.

Shoulder dystocia should be recognised when the usual traction fails to deliver the fetal shoulder. Many manoeuvres have been described for the management of shoulder dystocia, but only the most commonly used are described below (Fig. 36.21).

General measures

Each delivery suite should have an agreed management protocol for this complication. The operator must stay calm, and must resist the temptation to use undue traction force on the fetal head. The first step in the management is to summon assistants, who should include extra midwives, obstetrician, neonatologists, and preferably an anaesthetist (Fig. 36.21a). One or more of the following manoeuvres should be used to deliver the baby. After delivery, both the mother and the newborn should be examined carefully to exclude traumatic complications.

Episiotomy

A generous episiotomy should be performed to create more space posteriorly to facilitate the delivery.

Suprapubic pressure

Oblique suprapubic pressure is applied by an assistant to free the anterior shoulder while the operator applies downward traction in an attempt to accomplish the delivery (Fig. 36.21c). In other words, the assistant attempts to push the bisacromial diameter from a direct anteroposterior direction to a more oblique orientation from which the entry into the pelvic inlet should be easier. The use of suprapubic pressure probably is quite safe, although Lee (1987) has reported that

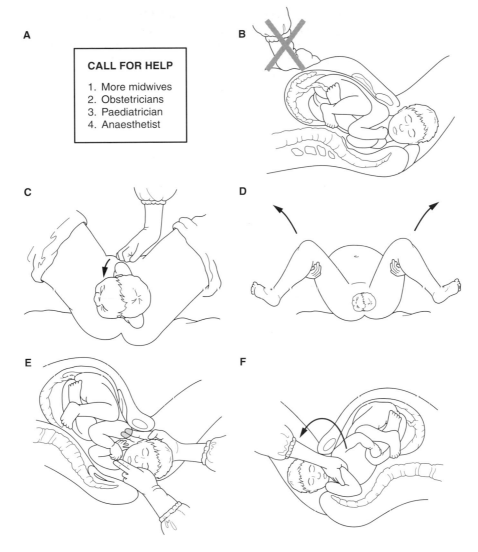

A

CALL FOR HELP

1. More midwives
2. Obstetricians
3. Paediatrician
4. Anaesthetist

B

C

D

E

F

Fig. 36.21 Common manoeuveres for shoulder dystocia. a) summon assistance; b) fundal pressure should never be used; c) suprapubic pressure; d) McRobert's manoeuvre; e) Wood's manoeuvre; f) posterior arm extraction.

five out of six cases of brachial plexus palsy were associated with the use of this manoeuvre. This complication was likely a result of excessive traction being applied at the same time as suprapubic pressure. Therefore, the operator should be extremely careful when employing this manoeuvre.

McRobert's manoeuvre

McRobert's manoeuvre involves the exaggerated flexion of the patient's leg at both the hip and knee joints (Fig. 36.21d). Although this does not change the pelvic dimensions, it causes a significant cephalad rotation of the pelvis, and a significant increase in the mean angle of inclination between the symphysis pubis and the sacral promontory (Gherman et al 2000). This leads to the rotation of the symphysis pubis superiorly, thus freeing the impacted shoulder. Gonik et al (1989) demonstrated in their model that the use of McRobert's manoeuvre reduced the forces for shoulder extraction, brachial plexus stretching, and the incidence of clavicular fracture.

Direct fetal manipulative manoeuvres

With Wood's manoeuvre (Fig. 36.21e), the operator inserts his hand into the posterior vagina and exerts pressure with two fingers on the anterior surface of the posterior shoulder. By so doing, the posterior shoulder should rotate obliquely followed by a corresponding rotation of the anterior shoulder, thus accomplishing delivery much like turning a screw. With the modified Wood's manoeuvre, the fingers are placed in the posterior aspect of the posterior shoulder, which should promote adduction of the shoulder resulting in a smaller transverse diameter across the shoulders.

Posterior arm extraction (Fig. 36.21f) is usually attempted when the above mentioned manoeuvres have failed. There is not much room but the operator tries to insert a hand up the vagina in front of the baby to reach the antecubital fossa of the posterior arm. Once identified, the operator flexes the arm, then gently brings down and delivers the arm by sweeping it across the fetal chest. If the posterior arm is successfully delivered, the rest of the fetal body will usually follow without difficulty.

Cephalic replacement or the Zavanelli manoeuvre is a technique in which the fetal head is replaced into the vagina followed by caesarean delivery as soon as possible. Sandberg (1999) in his review of all reported cases over a 12-year period found that the procedure was successful in 91% of cases. Although Sandberg (1999) noted no significant maternal or fetal complication, hysterectomy was required in two of the 59 cases reported by O'Leary (1993). At present, there is insufficient data to define the exact role of cephalic replacement in the management of shoulder dystocia.

Although these manoeuvres involve direct manipulation of the fetus, they are not associated with any increase in neonatal traumatic morbidity (Gherman et al 1998). On the contrary, these fetal manipulative manoeuvres enable the avoidance of excessive traction force on the fetus, which is the major source of fetal traumatic morbidity.

Symphysiotomy

Although originally described for the management of cephalopelvic disproportion, the successful use of symphysiotomy in relieving shoulder dystocia has been reported (Goodwin et al 1997). However, all women subsequently had urinary tract injury or incontinence, and all babies in this series had sustained severe neurological injury and died. Although these fetal complications were most likely related to shoulder dystocia rather than symphysiotomy, this procedure in general should not be used in developed countries because most obstetricians lack experience in performing the operation.

Fundal pressure

The use of fundal pressure should be abandoned (Fig. 36.21b); it is associated with a very high rate of complication (77%) and it is strongly associated with orthopaedic and neurological damage (Gross et al 1987). There is also no logic behind the use of fundal pressure which only causes further impaction of the shoulder above the pubic symphysis.

Conclusion

Shoulder dystocia is an uncommon, largely unpredictable and catastrophic complication. All health care professionals who perform any deliveries at all should be taught and be familiar with its management. All obstetric units should have a clear set of routines and order of procedure (i.e. guideline or protocol) for the management of shoulder dystocia, so that these cases can be managed promptly with appropriate manoeuvres without delay, in order to minimise fetal and maternal complications. However, it must be realised that fetal or maternal damage is not always preventable even when shoulder dystocia is properly managed, and that some of the coexisting damage such as Erb's palsy might have occurred in utero (Gherman et al 1997).

KEY POINTS

- Forceps and vacuum extractor are complementary instruments.
- If either instrument could be used, vacuum extractor should be the one of first choice.
- Most conditions necessitating the use of destructive operation should be preventable.
- There is insufficient evidence to justify, for the purpose of preventing shoulder dystocia related injuries, the use of routine caesarean section or induction of labour in pregnancies with a diagnosis of fetal macrosomia.
- Every individual who may deliver any baby must be trained in the management of shoulder dystocia.

REFERENCES

Acker DB, Sachs BP, Friedman EA 1985 Risk factors for shoulder dystocia. Obstet Gynecol 66:762–768

ACOG technical bulletin 1994 Operative vaginal delivery. Int J Gynaecol Obstet 47:179–185

Benedetti TJ 1989 Added complications of shoulder dystocia. Contemp Obstet Gynecol 33:150–161

Berard J, Dufour P, Vinatier D, Subtil D, Vanderstichele S, Monnier JC, Puech F 1998 Fetal macrosomia: risk factors and outcome. A study of the outcome concerning 100 cases > 4500 g. Eur J Obstet Gynecol 77:51–59

Bird GC 1969 Modifications of Malmstrom's vacuum extractor. Br Med J 111:526

Bird GC 1982 The use of the vacuum extractor. Clinical Obstetrics and Gynecology 9:641–661

Blickstein I, Ben-Arie A, Hagay ZJ 1998 Antepartum risks of shoulder dystocia and brachial plexus injury for infants weighing 4200 g or more. Gynecol Obstet Invest 45:77–80

Cardozo LD, Gibb D, Studd JWW et al 1982 Predictive value of cervimetric labour patterns in primigravidae. Br J Obstet Gynaecol 89:33–38

Chiswick ML, James DK 1979 Kielland's forceps: association with neonatal morbidity and mortality. Br Med J 1:7–9

Cohen WR, Friedman EA 1983 Management of labor. University Park Press, Baltimore

Conway DL, Langer O 1998 Elective delivery of infants with macrosomia in diabetic women: Reduced shoulder dystocia versus increased cesarean deliveries. Am J Obstet Gynecol 178:922–925

Curtin SC, Park MM 1999 Trends in the attendant, place, and timing of births, and in the use of obstetric interventions: United States, 1987–97. Natl Vital Stat Rep 47:1–12

Das K 1929 The obstetric forceps: its history and evolution. The Art Press, Calcutta

Davidson AC, Weaver JB, Davies P, Pearson JF 1976 The relation between ease of forceps delivery and speed of cervical dilatation. Br J Obstet Gynaecol 83:279–283

Gherman RB, Goodwin TM, Ouzounian JG, Miller DA, Paul RH 1997 Brachial plexus palsy associated with cesarean section: an in utero injury? Am J Obstet Gynecol 177:1162–1164

Gherman RB, Goodwin TM 1998 Shoulder dystocia. Curr Opin Obstet Gynecol 10:459–463

Gherman RB, Ouzounian JG, Goodwin TM 1998 Obstetric maneuvers for shoulder dystocia and associated fetal morbidity. Am J Obstet Gynecol 178:1126–1130

Gherman RB, Tramont J, Muffley P, Goodwin TM 2000 Analysis of McRoberts' maneuver by x-ray pelvimetry. Obstet Gynecol 95:43–47

Gibb D 1995 Clinical focus: shoulder dystocia. The obstetrics. Clinical focus 1:49–54

Gonen O, Rosen DJD, Dolfin Z, Tepper R, Marknov S, Fejgin MD 1997

Induction of labor versus expectant management in macrosomia: a randomised study. Obstet Gynecol 89:913–917

Gonik B, Allen R, Sorab J 1989 Objective evaluation of the shoulder dystocia phenomenon: effect of maternal pelvic orientation on force reduction. Obstet Gynecol 74:44–48

Goodwin TM, Banks E, Millar LK, Phelan JP 1997 Catastrophic shoulder dystocia and emergency symphysiotomy. Am J Obstet Gynecol 177:463–464

Gross SJ, Shime J, Farine D 1987 Shoulder dystocia: predictors and outcome. A five-year review. Am J Obstet Gynecol 156:334–336

Hagadorn-Freathy AS, Yeomans ER, Hankins GDV 1991 Validation of the 1988 ACOG forceps classification system. Obstet Gynecol 77:356–360

Hibbard BM 1988 Principles of obstetrics. Butterworths, London

Hibbard BM 2000 The obstetric forceps. Butterworths, London

Hope P, Bresline S, Lamont L et al 1998 Fatal shoulder dystocia: a review of 56 cases reported to the Confidential Enquiry into Stillbirths and Deaths in Infancy. Br J Obstet Gynaecol 105:1256–1261

Hopwood HG 1982 Shoulder dystocia: fifteen years' experience in a community hospital. Am J Obstet Gynecol 144:162–166

Johanson R, Menon V 1999a Soft versus rigid vacuum extractor cups for assisted vaginal delivery (Cochrane Review). In: The Cochrane Library. Update Software, Oxford

Johanson RB, Menon BKV 1999b Vacuum extraction versus forceps for assisted vaginal delivery (Cochrane Review). In: The Cochrane Library, Update Software, Oxford

Johnson RW 1769 A new system of midwifery founded on practical observations, London

Johnstone FD, Myerscough PR 1998 Shoulder dystocia. Br J Obstet Gynaecol 105:811–815

Keller JD, Lopez-Zeno JA, Dooley SL, Socol ML 1991 Shoulder dystocia and birth trauma in gestational diabetes: A five-year experience. Am J Obstet Gynecol 165:928–930

Kielland C 1916 The application of forceps to the unrotated head. Monatsschrift für Geburtshilffe und Gynakologie 43:48–78

Laing J, Hamson D, Jones B, Laing C 1996 Is permanent congenital facial palsy caused by birth trauma? Arch Dis Child 74:56–58

Laufe LE 1968 Obstetric forceps. Harper and Row, New York

Lee CY 1987 Shoulder dystocia. Clin Obstet Gynecol 30:77–82

Levine MG, Holroyde J, Woods Jr JR, Siddiqi TA, Scott M, Miodovnik M 1984 Birth Trauma: Incidence and predisposing factors. Obstet Gynecol 63:792–795

Levret A 1751 Suite des observations sur les causes et les accidens de plusieurs accouchemens laboreux. Delaguette, Paris

Lowe B 1987 Fear of failure: a place for the trial of instrumental delivery. Br J Obstet Gynaecol 94:60–66

Ng PC, Siu YK, Lewindon PJ 1995 Subaponeurotic haemorrhage in the 1990s: a 3-year surveillance. Acta Paediatr 84:1065–1069

O'Driscoll K, Meagher D 1980 Active management of labour. Saunders, London

O'Leary JA 1993 Cephalic replacement for shoulder dystocia: Present status and future role of the Zavanelli maneuver. Obstet Gynecol 82:847–850

Parry Jones E 1952 Kielland's forceps. Butterworths, London

Parry Jones E 1972 Barton's forceps. Sector, London

Plauché WC 1979 Fetal cranial injuries related to delivery with the Malmstrom vacuum extractor. Obstet Gynecol 53:750–757

Peleg D, Hasnin J, Shalev E 1997 Fractured clavicle and Erb's palsy unrelated to birth trauma. Am J Obstet Gynecol 177:1038–1040

Resnik R 1980 Management of shoulder girdle dystocia. Clin Obstet Gynecol 23:559–564

Revah A, Ezra Y, Farine D, Ritchie K 1997 Failed trial of vacuum or forceps — maternal and fetal outcome. Am J Obstet Gynecol 176:200–204

Rouse DJ, Owen J, Goldenberg RL, Cliver SP 1996 The effectiveness and costs of elective cesarean delivery for fetal macrosomia diagnosed by ultrasound. JAMA 276:1480–1486

Sandberg EC 1999 The Zavanelli maneuver: 12 years of recorded experience. Obstet Gynecol 93:312–317

Sandmire HF, O'Halloin TJ 1988 Shoulder dystocia: its incidence and associated risk factors. Int J Gynaecol Obstet 26:65–73

Spong CY, Beall M, Rodrigues M, Ross MG 1995 An Objective definition of shoulder dystocia: prolonged head-to-body delivery intervals and/or the use of ancillary obstetric maneuvers. Obstet Gynecol 86:433–436

Sultan AH, Johanson RB, Carter JE 1998 Occult and sphincter trauma following randomised forceps and vacuum delivery. Int J Gynaecol Obstet 61:113–119

Towner D, Castro MA, Eby-Wilkens E, Gilbert WM 1999 Effect of mode of delivery in nulliparous women on neonatal intracranial injury. N Engl J Med 341:1709–1714

Wagner RK, Nielsen PE, Gonik B 1999 Shoulder dystocia. Obstet Gynecol Clin North Am 26:371–383

37

Caesarean section

Geoffrey Chamberlain

The contribution of the author of the equivalent chapter in the second edition, on which this chapter draws extensively, is gratefully acknowledged.

HISTORY AND EVOLUTION

The origins of the name *caesarean section* have always fascinated obstetricians. *Section* is fairly obvious, coming from *sectio*, the Latin verb to cut. Caesarean has nothing to do with Julius Caesar. It goes back long before him to 715 BC when Numa Pompilus, then King of Rome, brought in a law which forbade the burial of a pregnant woman unless her child had been removed from the abdomen and buried separately. Thus *Lex Regis de Inferendo Mortis* became the practice and turned into *Lex Caesarea* in about 200 BC where the Kings became Caesars. At this time the operation was only performed postmortem. Julius Caesar could not have been so delivered for his mother, *Aurelia*, was still alive during the Gallish Wars and also was present in the Forum on the day that Julius Cesar was assassinated on 15th March 44 BC. However, early historians felt that such a forceful person as Julius Caesar had to be born in an extraordinary way.

An alternative explanation, which has reasonable credence, is that the name comes from the Latin verb *cedere* meaning to cut and so a caesarean section would mean cutting out of the baby. Most obstetricians prefer to harp back to the former explanation, which personalises the operation.

Although there are isolated caesarean sections done in prehistory and the Dark Ages, it was not until the sixteenth century that real records of caesarean sections begin. The first recorded successful section was done not by a doctor but by Jacob Nufe, a swinegelder, who lived in Sigerhausen in Switzerland. Performed the first caesarean section on a live woman who survived the operation. In 1588 his wife had a prolonged and obstructed labour; after some days Nufer used his swine gelding instruments to cut the baby out. It was alleged that Mrs Nufer had subsequent pregnancies so she herself survived. This is difficult to believe for the uterus and abdominal wall were not closed, but were left open. Several recorded cases occurred in the early seventeenth century; and the first recorded operation in the UK was by Smith, an Edinburgh surgeon on 29th June 1737. Unfortunately both the mother and child died. A midwife, Mary Donally did a successful caesarean section with the survival of the mother and child, at 1738 at Charlemaunt in Ireland. After 12 days of labour, the woman could not deliver and Mary Donally performed a section. It is said that she held the wound together with her fingers while neighbours went to fetch silk and a tailor's needle with which she sutured the wound.

Few sections were performed in the next fifty years until after the arrival of general anaesthesia from Edinburgh.

James Young Simpson used it first in 1851; thence caesarean sections took off. Up to the last quarter of the nineteenth century, maternal mortality was excessively high. In 1878 Lapage reported that no women operated upon in Paris between 1799 and 1877 survived. The uterine wound was usually left unsutured which was thought necessary to allow the lochia to escape. In 1876 Porro described a technique of removing the uterus and ovaries, which reduced the maternal mortality but it was not until 1882 that Sanger described a satisfactory technique of suturing the classical uterine incision, using two rows of sutures. This, together with the introduction of safer general anaesthesia and antiseptic techniques, contributed to declining maternal mortality.

The first recorded transverse lower uterine segment caesarean section is credited to Frank in 1906; Munro Kerr, who first used it in 1911, championed the lower segment operation in the UK. Extraperitoneal approaches were tried, but they were very complicated and often became inadvertently converted to intraperitoneal ones during the course of the operation. The operation did not survive because of the success of the simpler transperitoneal lower segment approach.

Many variations of the caesarean section operation have been described, and each surgeon eventually settles on a technique which suits him- or herself. The description given in this chapter includes practical hints and techniques that the author has found useful, but he recognises that many useful alternatives exist and are equally effective in other obstetricians' hands.

The evolution of caesarean section during the twentieth century as a relatively safe procedure, largely because of improved anaesthetic techniques and antiseptic procedures, have revolutionised obstetric practice. Many vaginal procedures such as internal version, destructive operations and symphysiotomy have become obsolete. The spectre of obstructed labour leading to fetal death and maternal mutilation or death, is still prevalent in many parts of the developing world, but it has been eliminated for women with access to adiquate medical facilities.

In recent years, however, the use of caesarean section has become increasingly controversial. Uncertainty exists about the relative risks and benefits of the operation (Chamberlain 1993) as the indications are progressively widened, and concern is expressed among health professionals and consumers about its increasing use. Increases have varied considerably between centres and countries (Stephenson et al 1993). A large increase in caesarean sections in the USA after 1965 appeared to be justified by improved perinatal mortality rates, yet similar perinatal improvements occurred in Dublin with minimal increase in caesarean sections (Bottoms et al 1980).

Detailed accounts of the indications for caesarean section will be found in the chapters dealing with the relevant complications of pregnancy. This chapter will deal in principle with the process of decision-making preceding caesarean section, discuss the indications with an emphasis on those relative indications that may account for differences in caesarean section rates, and describe the operation itself.

INDICATIONS

There are few absolute indications for a caesarean section. On the maternal side extreme degrees of cephalopelvic disproportion, which can follow childhood rickets or osteomalacia; a fetal indication would be cord prolapse in mid labour and a fetomaternal absolute indication is central placenta praevia.

The rest have relative degrees of ranking and often are multiple. They too may be divided into maternal, fetal and combined indications. Many are controversial indications, which accounts for large differences in caesarean section rates between obstetricians with differing policies. Commonly, more than one indication is considered. Such clustering by medical staff may be understandable but often it is illogical.

Commonly reported indications given for caesarian section are as follows:

- Maternal indications
  - Uterine haemorrhage
  - Uterine rupture
  - Eclampsia
  - Fulminating pre-eclampsia
  - Pelvic space-occupying tumour
  - Previous pelvic surgery
  - Prevent maternal effort
  - Previous caesarean section
  - Extra uterine pregnancy
  - Maternal preferences
- Fetal indications
  - Fetal distress
  - Prolapsed cord
  - Brow presentation
  - Breech presentation
  - Multiple pregnancy
  - Fetal anomaly
  - Maternal HIV infection
  - Maternal herpes genitalis
- Fetomaternal indications
  - Arrested labour

Maternal indications

Maternal indications include situations:

- In which prompt delivery is needed to safeguard the mother's health
- When labour is contraindicated
- When safe vaginal delivery is unlikely.

Life-threatening uterine haemorrhage

Whatever the cause of the haemorrhage, prompt delivery may be needed to limit blood loss. The commonest of these causes used to be central placenta praevia but most women with these in the UK are now diagnosed using antenatal ultrasound resulting in elective surgery to bypass the danger zone. Abruption of the placenta is often managed by a section soon after the first signs of separation of a normally sited placenta when the fetus is alive and sufficiently mature.

Uterine rupture

This can vary in severity from dehiscence of a lower segment transverse uterine scar with minimal bleeding and a live fetus still in the uterine cavity, to rupture of a previous classical operation scar with expulsion of the dead fetus and placenta into the peritoneal cavity accompanied by a life threatening blood loss. The need for abdominal operation must be urgently assessed and acted upon.

Placenta praevia

Major placenta praevia has become an absolute indication for caesarean section. The place of caesarean section for minor placenta praevia is controversial especially when the marginal implantation is anterior. Here, the descending fetal head can compress the separated placental bed against the back of the symphysis pubis. Many successful vaginal deliveries have been recorded but no randomised trials have been reported.

Eclampsia or imminent eclampsia

Caesarean section may be needed unless rapid vaginal delivery is feasible.

Pre-eclampsia

Whilst this is usually a late pregnancy condition, when it comes early and it can start as early as 24 weeks, it is more serious particularly if it does not improve with conservative management (Ch. 31). As well as the hazards of raised blood pressure, the haematological and hepatic aspects of pre-eclampsia are increasingly dangerous to the mother. Hence, preterm deteriorating severe pre-eclampsia is a common indication for caesarean section.

Previous classical caesarean section

Classical caesarean section is probably best followed by caesarean section in subsequent pregnancies, done preferably before the onset of labour, because of the higher risk and serious nature of upper uterine segment scar rupture. In a recent UK survey, 95% of consultants responded that they would not allow trial of scar following a classical caesarean section (Roberts et al 1994). It is still unclear from the smaller number of cases reported whether lower segment vertical midline incisions encroaching on the upper segment, or transverse incisions placed in the upper segment because of a poorly formed lower segment, should be managed as classical incisions.

Previous lower segment caesarean section

Repeat caesarean section has been a major contributor to the rising incidence of caesarean sections in the Western world (Yudkin & Redman 1986). Attempts to predict successful vaginal delivery after caesarean section depend upon the likelihood of scar dehiscence. This rests on the basis of the indication for the previous operation, the number of previous caesarean sections, and assessment of pelvic size (Hofmeyr 1989). For example, previous lower segment caesarean section for failure to progress in labour or cephalopelvic disproportion is associated with only a slightly lower rate of successful vaginal delivery than when the previous caesarean section was for other indications (Impey & O'Herlihy 1999).

Interestingly the risk of scar dehiscence is considerably lower, probably because the original uterine incision was usually placed in a well-formed lower segment following prolonged labour (Hofmeyr 1989). The reported results for trials of labour following more than one caesarean section are similar to those reported for one previous caesarean section.

Overall, scar dehiscence occurs unpredictably in 0.5–2% of women who have a trial of lower segment scar. Of greater importance than the incidence is the fact that in a maternity unit with ready recourse to caesarean section, these episodes are seldom associated with serious sequelae for mother or infant. The relative risks and benefits have not been determined by randomised studies comparing elective repeat caesarean section with trial of scar in women without current indications for caesarean section. The evidence from prospective cohort studies and decision analysis studies, though obviously subject to bias, is in favour of such a trial. The maternal and fetal condition and the progress of labour must be monitored closely. Gentle lower abdominal palpitation will often give guidance as to the state of the uterine scar. Prompt caesarean section must be performed if deterioration or suspicion of dehiscence of any of these occurs. Obstetricians used to take the opportunity to check the integrity of the uterine scar digitally by vaginal examination after placental separation. Since no action used to be taken on the findings, this practice is no longer recommended.

Gross pelvic contraction

The use of X-ray pelvimetry to predict cephalopelvic disproportion has been shown to be insufficiently accurate to be useful (Hofmeyr 1989). This is not surprising for pelvic size is only one of several factors determining successful delivery when the head-to-pelvis fit is imperfect. In all but the most extreme cases of pelvic contraction, cephalopelvic disproportion should only be diagnosed after a trial of labour using a partogram. Imaging pelvimetry by X-ray or computed tomography (CT) scan should be reserved for cases in which specific pelvic inadequacy is suspected after pelvic fracture as happens in a previous severe roll over accident.

Previous urinary incontinence surgery

Vaginal delivery is considered to constitute a risk to the integrity of such repairs. It is hard to assess beforehand, and a bias seems to exist towards protecting any repair operation done previously by the surgeon himself.

Extrauterine pregnancy

This is a surprisingly difficult condition to diagnose but fortunately it is rare. Even ultrasound examination may be misleading, as omentum stretched over the gestational sac can give the appearance of uterine wall. Extrauterine pregnancy must be suspected if the fetal lie is bizarre and if attempts at version are unsuccessful. A lateral abdominal X-ray typically shows fetal parts overlying the mother's spine.

The fetus must be delivered by laparotomy. The placenta is often attached to bowel, omentum or the broad ligament; attempted removal causes much blood loss and damage to underlying tissues. It is usually wiser to leave the placenta in place. Ligate and cut the cord close to the placental insertion and close the abdomen. A repeat laparotomy done later in life often shows complete reabsorption with no adhesions.

Pelvic space-occupying lesions

These include entrapped ovarian tumours and low-lying uterine fibromyomas. If they would interfere with rotation and descent of the fetal head, delivery must bypass them. Do not be tempted to do a myomectomy at the same time. It is too bloody. The only exception is when myomectomy is necessary to allow proper closure of the uterine incision.

Cervical carcinoma

Vaginal delivery is considered to constitute a risk for haemorrhage or dissemination of invasive cervical carcinoma. Classical caesarean section has been recommended, followed by Werthiem hysterectomy at the same surgery if the degree of malignancy is appropriate. Premalignant conditions of the cervix tend to regress after vaginal delivery and are not an indication for caesarean section.

Associated medical illness

In cases of serious maternal compromise such as severe cardiac, respiratory, musculoskeletal or neurological illness, the relative risks of labour compared with surgery need to be weighed up in the light of the specific circumstances of each case. Bearing-down efforts may be contraindicated in many situations such as severe hypertension or a known cerebral aneurysm. It is usually preferable to avoid such pushing by the use of effective regional analgesia and assisted vaginal delivery rather than caesarean section.

Maternal preference

The reason for caesarean section request from the mother may vary from a morbid fear of labour to simple convenience. It can be argued that the mother has the right to informed choice of the method of delivery, including the right to accept the increased risks to herself of caesarean section; labour and vaginal delivery may have benefits for the fetus. What some may consider to be an unnecessary caesarean section, could also be seen as an infringement of the rights of the fetus, particularly when caesarean section is requested before full term. In the absence of information from clinical trials on which to base decisions, most obstetricians are discouraging caesarean section by choice when there is no medical indication, explaining the increased risk to the mother and possible adverse effects for the fetus. This question is discussed further by Chamberlain (1993).

Fetal indications

Fetal indications for caesarean section include:

- The need for prompt delivery
- The need to avoid labour
- The need to avoid vaginal delivery.

Fetal distress

This used to be a clinical diagnosis based on the passage of meconium, violent fetal movements and changes in the fetal heart sounds heard through the mother's abdomen. In the UK this changed during the 1970s to include signals from electronic heart monitoring and fetal blood sampling. Randomised trials of electronic fetal heart rate (FHR) monitoring during labour compared with intermittent auscultation have shown an associated doubling of the caesarean section rate for fetal distress when FHR monitoring was complemented by selective fetal blood sampling, and a four times increase when it was not (Neilson 1993). The only discernible improvement in neonatal outcome was a reduction in neonatal convulsions in certain trials (MacDonald et al 1985). These occurred in labours which were prolonged or had been stimulated with oxytocics, and the long-term outcomes were good. There is no evidence that electronic FHR monitoring used during an uncomplicated normal labour improves neonatal outcome. There is also little or no evidence that the large increase in caesarean sections for suspected fetal distress in recent years has had any effect on the incidence of cerebral palsy (Ch. 45). In a randomised comparison, the rate of caesarean section for fetal distress in labours with FHR monitoring alone was twice that which occurred when FHR monitoring was supplemented with fetal electrocardiogram (ECG) waveform analysis (Westgate et al 1992).

FHR monitoring is inherently imprecise. There is a particular problem with the over-diagnosis of fetal hypoxia. Before labour, non-reactive FHR patterns may be associated with fetal distress, but more often they are not. During labour, early and variable FHR decelerations usually reflect an appropriate vagal response to fetal head compression or umbilical cord compression. Even late decelerations may still be reflecting an appropriate fetal response to no more than mild hypoxia during uterine contractions. Consequently, many FHR patterns create diagnostic uncertainty and the understandable tendency is to expedite delivery just in case fetal distress is indeed present.

The number of unnecessary caesarean sections for suspected fetal distress in labour can be reduced by several methods. Fetal scalp blood pH measurement, or newer techniques such as fetal ECG waveform analysis may be used to confirm the true diagnosis of fetal hypoxia. Intrauterine resuscitation may be used; either the mother is placed in the lateral position and oxygen is administered by facemask, or excessive uterine contractions are inhibited by reducing oxytocic administration or administering a beta-adrenergic agent. Early or variable decelerations can be abolished in the majority of cases by saline amnioinfusion, with significant reduction in the rate of caesarean section (Hofmeyr 1992a). Meconium staining of the amniotic fluid is sometimes associated with fetal distress, but the association is too weak to justify caesarean section.

Prolapse of the umbilical cord

Caesarean section is needed in such a case unless prompt vaginal delivery is feasible, or the baby is dead. Palpation of the cord for pulsation is a poor indicator of whether the fetus is alive, and it may aggravate spasm of the cord vessels. Instead, auscultation for the fetal heart beat, with confirmation by Doppler detection or ultrasound is performed if immediately available. Methods described to reduce compression of the cord between the presenting part and the pelvis while preparing for caesarean section include the Sims' or knee–elbow position, stopping oxytocic administration, tocolysis and digital elevation of the presenting part by an assistant pressing up *per vaginam*. With the woman in a hospital and appropriate management, it is unusual for fetal death to occur after this diagnosis has been made. The same is not true if the woman is outside a unit capable of swift caesarean section. Occasionally, replacing the cord into the uterus (funic replacement) by digital manipulation will avoid the need for caesarean section, but this is usually unsuccessful; as one loop is replaced another slips down.

Fetal bleeding

Rarely, if the blood vessels servicing a villamentous placental lobule run over the internal os of the cervix, membrane rupture can be followed by a tear of the exposed fetal vessels. Fetal blood is then lost and, with the small blood volume, a small loss can be serious. A sudden change in FHR immediately after membranes rupture with blood loss indicates the need for an immediate caesarean section. Methods of detecting fetal haemoglobin do exist but they are usually not immediately available because of the rarity of this condition.

Brow of face presentation

For brow presentation, a short trial of labour is rarely worthwhile but delivery may occasionally occur when the baby is small, the pelvis is unusually large, or conversion to vertex or mento-anterior face presentation occurs during labour. In the great majority of cases, caesarean section is needed. A mento-posterior face presentation might deliver vaginally if long anterior rotation takes place but it too is best managed by caesarean delivery.

Transverse or oblique lie

Transverse or oblique lie may be corrected in the majority of cases by external version during labour or immediately prior to the induction of labour, provided the membranes are intact (Hofmeyr 1993). For persistent non-longitudinal lie in labour, there is no option other than caesarean section.

Breech presentation

The method of delivery for persistent breech presentation remains problematical. Neonatal outcome is worse after breech than cephalic delivery by any route, but this discrepancy may be because of pre-existing fetal problems that have caused the breech presentation rather than harm during breech delivery (Hytten 1982). Randomised trials of vaginal versus caesarean delivery for frank (Collea et al 1980) and non-frank (Gimovsky et al 1983) breech presentations failed to show any difference in perinatal outcome. Large retrospective studies have suggested a poorer perinatal outcome following vaginal rather than abdominal breech delivery, and some have argued in favour of routine caesarean section for breech presentation at term (Thorpe-Beeston et al 1992).

Those who do not agree with surgical delivery of all breeches allow vaginal delivery provided that the fetus is estimated to weigh between 1500 and 3750 g, is a frank or complete breech presentation (the combined diameters of thighs and trunk will then exceed those of the aftercoming head), does not have an extended neck or cord completely encircling the neck on ultrasound examination, is well grown and without evidence of distress. Most importantly labour progresses favourably assessed with a partogram. The baby presenting by the breech who is going to deliver vaginally should descend readily into the pelvis, reaching the level of the ischial spines by the time the cervix is 6 cm dilated, and the pelvic floor when the cervix is fully dilated.

The use of caesarean section for breech presentations estimated to weigh below 1500 g is controversial (Crowley & Hawkins 1980), particularly when viability is uncertain. Evidence from randomised trials to guide management is lacking but a well planned multicentre randomised study had to be abandoned for lack of recruitment. A survey of consultants in England and Wales, showed that 76% of respondents reported routinely using caesarean section for uncomplicated preterm breech delivery, 35% considered that there is sufficient evidence to support this policy, and overall 71% reported that their management was affected by medico-legal considerations (Penn & Steer 1991). This does not prove anything but it is the way medical opinion is heading.

This move is likely to be encouraged by the results of the largest prospective randomised control trial of elective versus selective caesarean for term breech presentation ever performed, reported recently in the Lancet (Hannah et al 2000). Over 2000 women were randomised. Not only was universal elective caesarean associated with a four-fold lower perinatal mortality and morbidity, maternal morbidity was no greater than with planned vaginal birth.

In Chapter 34, there is convincing evidence that breech presentation at delivery and caesarean section may be reduced by external cephalic version at term (Hofmeyr 1993).

Multiple pregnancy

Caesarean section may be indicated in multiple pregnancy when other diverse factors are present such as extreme prematurity (estimated fetal weight below 1000 g), discordant fetal growth, single amniotic sac, conjoined twins and higher order multiple pregnancies (triplets or more). The increasing use of caesarean section for a second twin who does not deliver spontaneously is another facet of this fear of legal enquiry. Internal podalic version for transverse lie, breech extraction for a breech presentation and forceps or vacuum extraction for a cephalic presentation are all easy but rapidly becoming under-used ways of dealing with this problem.

Macrosomia

It has been suggested that the risk of shoulder dystocia can be reduced by the use of elective caesarean section when the fetus is estimated to weigh more than 4500 g, or in diabetic women more than 4000 g. Such a policy would however result in an unacceptably high rate of caesarean sections, and many cases of shoulder dystocia would be missed (Hofmeyr 1992b). The only feasible way of addressing the problem of shoulder dystocia at present is by ensuring that all birth attendants are skilled in its management (Ch. 36).

Fetal anomaly

Fetal anomaly is not an indication for caesarean section *per se* unless the nature of the anomaly is such that vaginal delivery could cause injury or impair the chance of a neonatal surgical correction. A difficult ethical dilemma arises if the baby has an anomaly with little chance of survival, and it is undeliverable vaginally, but it is still alive at the time of decision. This can happen with thanophoric dwarfs and grossly hydropic babies. Destructive operations are so rarely done in the Western world that the surgeon could easily do much damage to the mother's genitourinary tract. Therefore, a caesarean section, with a large uterine incision, would be safer for the mother. A more commonly seen problem is gross hydrocephaly. The choice lies between caesarean section with a large uterine or even a classical incision, or tapping the cerebrospinal fluid (CSF) with a needle so permitting vaginal delivery. The choice must include parental views.

Fetal thrombocytopenia

Maternal autoimmune thrombocytopenia is associated with an unpredictable risk of fetal thrombocytopenia. Suggested management policies include routine caesarean section or selective caesarean section when the fetal platelet count from scalp blood sampling or cordocentesis is below 25 000 per ml. However, most recent studies show such a low rate of fetal and neonatal morbidity that routine caesarean section is not justified (see Ch. 20).

Maternal HIV infections

HIV infection is sweeping both the developed and developing world. The subject is considered in Chapter 23 and here are considered ways of reducing fetal infection. While the major management of spread of infection from mother to baby lies in antiretrovirals; other methods include reducing breast-feeding and delivery by caesarean section. The former is difficult in many parts of the world where bottle-feeding is unsafe because of unsterile water and breast-feeding is also a major method of contraception. Data on caesarean section usage from the European Collaborative Study (1999) shows strongly that the operation helps to reduce transmission. In this study, among the 170 women randomly allocated for a caesarean section only three babies were infected whilst 21 of the 200 mothers randomised for vaginal delivery had an infected baby. Further, meta-analysis of 15 other prospective studies showed an adjusted odds ratio of infection when an elective caesarean section was performed was 0.45 (0.33–0.56) (Johnson 1999). While this is a useful weapon in our armamentorium against HIV in developed countries, the same may not apply were facilities for safe caesarean section do not exist. Very recently, policy has been swinging back to allowing a vaginal birth in women with a very low or undetectable viral load, and a normal CD4 count, as the risk of vertical transmission in such cases is very low.

Other infections

Active genital herpes simplex infection carries a significant risk of serious neonatal infection which may be reduced by caesarean section if performed before rupture of the membranes. Use of acyclovir to mother and baby is an alternative.

Group B haemolytic streptococcal infection is a common inhabitant of the vagina (Van Oppen & Feldman 1993) but the incidence of serious neonatal infection is considered too low to justify caesarean section, provided that intravenous penicillin is given for at least four hours during labour (or the baby treated postnatally if the labour is shorter than four hours). Similarly, the risk of neonatal laryngeal papillomas is considered too small to justify caesarean section for maternal human papillomavirus infection.

Fetomaternal indications

Fetomaternal indications for caesarean section are mostly related to disproportion.

Arrested progress in labour

The term cephalopelvic disproportion is best avoided as an indication for caesarean section, for two reasons. Firstly, it is often difficult to distinguish between true cephalopelvic disproportion and inefficient uterine action as the cause of the arrested progress of labour. Secondly, the term cephalopelvic disproportion suggests an absolute obstruction, and this may bias the mother and her obstetrician against trial of vaginal delivery in a subsequent pregnancy.

The best way to manage any mother in whom there is doubt about the fit of the fetal head in her pelvis is a trial of labour. This is best conducted by skilled observers who are capable and willing to do a caesarean section if the trial is deemed to have failed.

THE CHOICE

The choice between vaginal and abdominal delivery is a complex one involving often more than one factor.

The relative risks to the mother

These may be physical or emotional, immediate and remote. Despite remarkable improvements in safety, caesarean section is associated with an increased risk of maternal death, probably between two- and fivefold. Puerperal complications such as sepsis are increased (see Ch. 41), and caesarean section may be associated with increased postnatal emotional morbidity (Boyce & Todd 1992); it can also complicate the management of subsequent pregnancies. Special attention needs to be given to the potential long-term risks of caesarean section in women in developing countries living far from medical help who may not be able to seek care in the next pregnancy.

The relative risks to the fetus

Caesarean section is usually considered safe for the fetus. Possible adverse effects may be the lack of the preparation for adaptation to extrauterine life that occurs during labour as a result of the outpouring of catecholamines, or the early separation from the mother with reduced chance of successful breast feeding; these are at present poorly understood, but they need to be considered. Iatrogenic prematurity, though greatly reduced for women with access to early pregnancy ultrasound examination, also needs to be eliminated.

The likelihood of successful vaginal delivery

The risks to the mother of intrapartum emergency caesarean section may be as much as twice that of elective caesarean section. Hence, when the likelihood of successful vaginal delivery is small, elective caesarean section may be a safer option than trial of labour from the immediate risks to the mother (Lilford et al 1990).

The urgency of the need for delivery

If the mother is in strong labour, the dilatation of the cervix and the likelihood of an imminent delivery are important in decision-making between caesarean section and assisted vaginal delivery. The ripeness of the cervix is a measure of the readiness of the myometrium to contract if stimulated.

The preference of the mother

As well as the mother's wish to avoid the pain of labour and the advantages of a planned delivery of the baby, more recently has been reported evidence of the damage done to the pelvic floor at the vaginal delivery (Ryhammer et al 1995), particularly if forceps are used. Soltan et al (1993) showed occult defects of the pelvic floor with 35% of women recently delivered *per vaginam*. Of these women 13% were still incontinent of faeces and flatus eight weeks after delivery. All had no apparent anal sphincter damage at the time of the vaginal delivery. The involuntary loss of urine after vaginal delivery can be as high as 36% immediately after giving birth, dropping to 8% some years after delivery. However, this problem increases with the number of deliveries, possibly because of an increased uretheral mobility and lack of support so decreasing the closing pressure (Peschers et al 1997).

In a paper exercise among women obstetricians in the London region, Al Mufti et al (1997) showed that a third would wish to have an elective caesarean section even for an uncomplicated pregnancy at term, with 88% of them giving the reason as fear of pelvic floor damage. This study was only a theoretical one (by questionnaire) and the response rate was not good, but it represented a wave of feeling amongst expert women who know about their pelvic floor.

The report Changing Childbirth (Cumberledge 1993) encourages women 'to decide for themselves the type of care they wished ... the place of delivery and the degree of intervention'. The Audit Commission (1997) considered that the maternity services needed to become more 'women centred'.

We have not come to the end of this debate but amongst the other concerns of obstetricians are the manpower implications of a massively increasing caesarean section rate. Obstetricians, anaesthetists and skilled midwives could be tied up in theatre doing elective caesarean sections for a larger part of the day when we are short of such skilled staff. The costs of the maternity unit too would increase by about £700 per caesarean delivery, an estimated extra £5 million a year for the whole country (Audit Commission 1997).

Perhaps the answer will only come after a full comparison of the long and short-term implications of caesarean section and of vaginal birth. After these have been honestly imparted (and translated fully) to the woman, the uptake of caesarean section may then reflect more the views of women and less the bias in medical practice.

MAKING A DECISION

The decision about a caesarean section can be complicated by the interests of the mother and the fetus being contradictory, and value judgements about the different priorities need to be made. Many of the recent increases in caesarean section rates are a result of indications such as suspected fetal distress and breech presentation, for which the overall benefit to the fetus is uncertain while the increased risk to the mother is certain. The following principles may help the decision-making process:

- It is important not to choose caesarean section as an easy option on the basis of a nebulous cluster of several features of the pregnancy which seem suboptimal. Rather, evaluate each potential indication critically, and choose caesarean section only if a clearly defined indication is present. It can be useful to break down the decision into stages: Is this the optimal time for delivery? Is caesarean section preferable for the mother? Is caesarean section preferable for the fetus?

- Valid information about relative risks and benefits in specific circumstances is often scarce. Wherever possible, rely upon objective information such as that from randomised trials rather than subjective impressions. Try to assess the risk to the individual woman against a trial population into which she would fit, e.g. developed world approaches may not be appropriate in the developing world.

- Every effort should be made to guard against the understandable tendency to choose the option less likely to result in litigation rather than the one more likely to be in the true interests of mother and baby (Savage & Francome 1993).

- Some decisions will inevitably in retrospect appear to have been wrong. It is important to acknowledge to ourselves and to the parents that our knowledge is incomplete and we are not able to predict every eventuality. We should not promise perfection. Having made the best possible decision in the light of available information, we and the parents must accept the consequences of the decision.

BEFORE THE SURGERY

Preoperative counselling

The woman and her partner should be advised carefully about the details and implications of this operation. Many women regard giving birth as an important life event and they will view caesarean section as a personal failure. Stress the positive aspects of how the woman played her part during the long antenatal months and will do so in the subsequent care of her child after delivery. Discuss anaesthetic options considering regional anaesthesia and the partner's presence during the caesarean birth. Find out whether the parents have any special requests regarding the birth and their attitudes to donor blood transfusions. The option of sterilisation should have been discussed during the antenatal period. If not, it should be made clear that a last-minute decision is not wise, as sterilisation can be performed at a later date. If any uncertainty exists, the decision should be postponed.

Written consent to the operation is signed by the mother. Informed consent implies the discussion of possible complications of the surgery such as haemorrhage requiring hysterectomy, and anaesthetic complications. A difficult issue to be faced individually is the problem of extra anxieties created by too detailed description of potential complications as part of the informed consent process.

Preparation for surgery

Before surgery, there are a number of things which must be carried out.

- The woman's fitness for surgery should be ascertained, including the results of appropriate special investigations. Because of the risks of haemorrhage two units of donor blood should be available in the operating theatre (about one-third of all women who have caesarean section lose more than 500 ml blood).
- Neither starvation nor any of several medications commonly used is completely effective in achieving an empty, non-acidic stomach during labour (Johnson et al 1989). Particulate antacids are probably contraindicated. The use of antacids or gastroprokinetic agents should not create a false sense of security. The risk of gastric content aspiration should be minimised by the application of effective cricoid pressure by a competent assistant from the time of induction of general anaesthesia until the correct placement of the endotracheal tube has been confirmed and the cuff inflated.
- Pubic hair shaving causes skin abrasion which may promote infection. Clipping of pubic hair intruding upon the proposed line of incision is preferable.
- Effective emptying of the urinary bladder should be ensured prior to surgery, usually by means of an indwelling urinary catheter.
- Paediatricians should be advised of any anticipated neonatal problem and one should be in the operating theatre at the birth if possible.
- There is unequivocal evidence from a large number of randomised trials that the use of prophylactic antibiotics is associated with a clinically important reduction in infectious morbidity after either emergency or elective caesarean section (Smaill 1993). The added benefit of prophylactic antibiotic therapy for longer than one day is uncertain. Details of antibiotic prophylaxis are given in Chapter 41 on puerperal sepsis.
- The use of prophylactic low-dose heparin in other surgical disciplines has been shown to reduce the risk of pulmonary embolism, and it is probably of value prophylacticly in caesarean section; its use does not appear to be associated with increased blood loss at operation. The evidence available is, therefore, in favour of the use of heparin prophylaxis, probably routinely but certainly for those with known risk factors for increased clotting. Calcium heparin may be used, 5000 units subcutaneously 8 hourly, just after any epidural required has been inserted (see Ch. 42).

THE OPERATION

Choice of anaesthesia

General anaesthesia carries certain specific risks, particularly aspiration of gastric contents and failed intubation. Attempts to minimise the depressant effect of anaesthetic agents on the newborn have sometimes resulted in a mother being paralysed but aware of the operation in the early stages. Regional and general anaesthesia for caesarean section are considered in Chapter 28.

Local field anaesthesia into nerves T_{12} to L_2 where they emerge from behind the rib tips plus a field block of the abdominal wall can be used in an emergency, when there is no anaesthetist available. It is slow and sometimes incomplete but it can be done by the solitary obstetrician.

Preparation in theatre

Once in theatre, the following must be carried out.

- Ensure that any drugs which may be needed, such as oxytocin, syntometrine, ergometrine, prostaglandin F_2 alpha and a beta-adrenergic agent such as hexoprenaline (Ipradol) are available in theatre.
- Position the mother on the table with 15 degrees of left lateral tilt. There is clear evidence that the fetal condition is improved by this simple manoeuvre (Pearson & Rees 1989). The use of 5 degrees of reverse Trendellenburg's position has been shown to reduce the incidence of venous air emboli diagnosed with precordial Doppler monitoring.
- Oxygen should be given to the mother at 100% concentration until the delivery of the infant.
- Check that the fetal heart is still audible particularly when caesarean section is performed for fetal distress. Fetal death may have occurred between leaving the ward and the time the operation is to be commenced.
- Ensure the indication is still valid. For example, if the caesarean section is for failure to progress in labour, a vaginal examination should be performed in theatre to check that unexpected progress has not taken place. A breech presentation should be reconfirmed by palpation or even ultrasound for spontaneous version may occur even during labour.
- Palpate the position of the fetus. It is important to know the orientation of the occiput so that it can be rotated anteriorly during delivery.
- When regional analgesia is used, ask the mother whether she wishes to hold and put the baby to breast immediately after delivery, and arrange her gown and sterile drapes appropriately.

The approach

Transverse abdominal incisions

Compared with vertical incisions, the Pfannenstiel (low transverse) skin incision may be a little slower to perform, but it is more familiar to most obstetricians today (Fig. 37.1). It may be more liable to haematoma formation and it is hard to enlarge if extended access is required, except by cutting into rectus muscle. These limitations are generally accepted in view of its excellent functional and cosmetic results.

Vertical abdominal incisions

A classical caesarean section (vertical uterine scar) needs a vertical abdominal incision unless the uterus is small (very preterm). If the lower segment is expected to be unapproachable because of fibroids or extensive intra-abdominal adhesions, a midline or paramedian abdominal wall incision is preferable to allow a vertical myometrial cut once the intraabdominal situation is clear. In classical caesarean sections, for a transverse lie, a paramedian incision is preferable because of the ease of extension above the umbilicus and its relatively better healing.

The parietal peritoneum

Enter the parietal peritoneum as high up as possible, taking care not to injure an unexpectedly high bladder, particularly in cases of obstructed labour or previous caesarean section. Try to palpate any bladder wall present and then enter the abdominal cavity at least an inch above that upper border.

Uterine incisions

The transverse lower uterine segment incision

Ensure that the lower segment is wide enough to allow an adequate transverse incision to accommodate the baby without lateral extension into the leash of uterine vessels. Check that a fetal pole is present in the lower segment or can be made to enter it. If this cannot be done, use a midline vertical incision. Correct any rotation of the uterus, which is commonly to the right. Open the loosely adherent visceral peritoneum covering the lower uterine segment transversely (Fig. 37.2). Separate the peritoneum digitally from the lower seg-

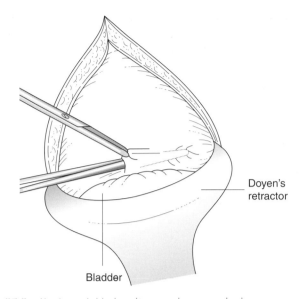

Fig. 37.2 The loose fold of peritoneum between the lower segment of the uterus and the bladder is opened and the underlying tissues separated.

ment, and displace it inferiorly, together with the bladder (Fig. 37.3). Whatever the urgency of the operation, this downward displacement of the bladder is an essential step to avoid bladder damage. When dislocated downward, hold the bladder below the operation field, tucked beneath the Doyen's retractor.

Incise the myometrium of the lower uterine segment with a scalpel transversely in the midline, 1–2 cm below the junction with the upper segment, using gentle featherweight strokes of the scalpel (Fig. 37.4). If membranes are intact and

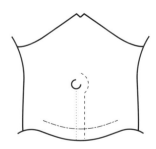

------- Pfanensteil for lower segment caesarian section

Midline for classical caesarian section

- - - - - Paramedian for classical caesarian section

Fig. 37.1 Abdominal wall incisions for caesarean section.

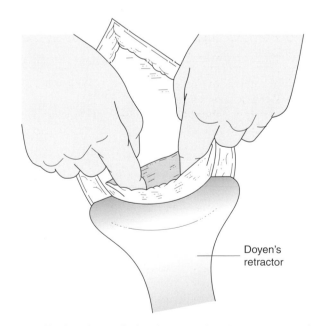

Fig. 37.3 The loosely attached peritoneum of the lower segment of the uterus is carefully separated so the bladder can be pushed down out of the operative field. Then the retractor is advanced to hold it down.

609

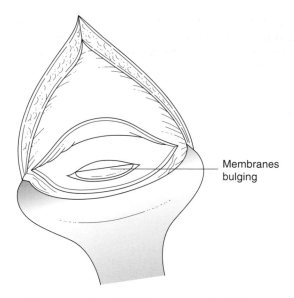

Fig. 37.4 The myometrium of the lower segment is lightly divided around the midline for 4 cm until the membranes bulge through the wound.

The classical uterine incision

If the placenta is anterior, map its borders with ultrasound preoperatively. Ensure adequate access to the upper uterine segment by a medium or preferably a paramedian abdominal incision. Correct any rotation of the uterus and incise the upper segment vertically in the midline; this will often rupture the membranes (Fig. 37.6). Extend the incision sufficiently for delivery of the fetus, using a scalpel or large pair of

liquor volume normal, the shiny fetal membranes will bulge outward. If possible, complete the myometrial incision without rupturing them. Extend the incision laterally with slight upward curvature, using curved scissors, protecting the baby with a finger deep to the blade of the scissors, and cut first towards and then away from the surgeon. Alternatively, use the index finger of each hand to split the myometrium laterally (Fig. 37.5). If it is a repeat lower segment operation, take care the tissues do not tear. Once the membranes rupture, the uterus begins to contract down, and the baby should be delivered without undue delay. Always remember to remove the Doyen's retractor before starting to deliver the baby.

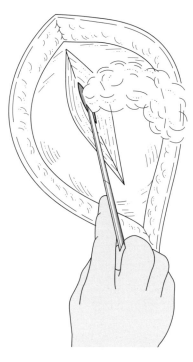

Fig. 37.6 The vertical incision of a classical caesarean section. Note the thickness of the myometrium in the body of the uterus compared with that of the lower segment in Figure 37.5.

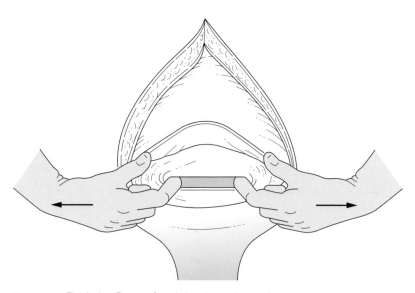

Fig. 37.5 The index finger of each hand may be used to enlarge the incision in the myometrium made in Figure 37.4.

scissors. The site of the placenta should be known from previous ultrasound. If it is under the uterine entry incision, separate any underlying placenta in the direction of its nearest margin. Deliver the fetus by the legs or head, whichever presents, taking care not to allow an arm to prolapse.

Some operators like to use a very low vertical incision involving the lower segment (De Lee approach) if the baby is expected to be very small. Beware, for this can easily extend downwards into the vagina with much blood loss and a difficult repair.

Delivery of the baby

When using the transverse lower segment incision, too hasty a delivery of the head is a common cause of tearing of the lower uterine segment at one or other end of the incision. To avoid this, the position of the head in the uterus must be brought up to above the level of the uterine incision and then the occiput rotated anteriorly before any attempt is made to deliver the head through the uterine incision. If operating from the patient's right side, insert the left hand between the lower uterine segment and the fetal head, gently elevating the head from the mother's pelvis. Resistance to such an elevation of the head can be the result of contraction of the uterus about the fetus, particularly in the presence of obstructed labour or ruptured membranes. Avoid the use of force and let some air into the lower uterus below the head; this will go in with a loud sucking noise and helps to remove the negative retention pressure. If necessary, the resistance can be overcome by intravenous administration of a beta-adrenergic agent. Very occasionally a deeply engaged head may need to be disengaged by upwards pressure at a vaginal examination by an assistant.

As the head is elevated, lift the fingers nearest the fetal occiput ahead of the other fingers; this will help to rotate the occiput anteriorly. Once the head is above the level of the uterine incision and the occiput is anterior, use four fingertips of the right hand, palm upward, to displace the lower edge of the uterine incision posteriorly, the assistant should apply fundal pressure while the surgeon guides the head through the incision with the fingertips of the right hand, while the fingers themselves remain outside the uterus. The uterine incision is thus minimally distended by the head alone in a well-flexed occipito-anterior position. If meconium is present, suck out on the baby's airway immediately the face is born. The assistant continues fundal pressure and the surgeon carefully guides the shoulders through the uterine incision. If regional analgesia is being used, dry and hand the baby wrapped in a warm blanket to the mother as soon as breathing is established and put to the breast if requested, taking care to avoid the baby cooling. If there is difficulty in delivery of the head, some surgeons prefer to use Wrigley's Outlet obstetric forceps. The soft vacuum extractor cup can also been used.

Delivery of placenta and membranes

Once the anterior shoulder has been delivered, administer oxytocin by slow intravenous injection or infusion. If possible avoid routine manual removal of the placenta, which can be associated with a risk of increased blood loss and postoperative endometriosis (McCurdy et al 1992). While awaiting placental separation, secure the midpoint of the lower edge of the uterine incision with a broad haemostatic Green–Armytage forceps. Reinsert the Doyen's retractor only after identifying the lower edge of the uterine incision, as the retractor can easily cover it. If that happened the posterior uterine wall could be mistaken for the lower wound edge and suturing to close the uterus would involve the incorrect layer. Control any actively bleeding points of the uterine wound with similar forceps.

Deliver the placenta and membranes by cord traction once the uterus has contracted firmly. Remove and replace any forceps in place on the uterine wound edge as the membranes are peeled off the underlying uterine wall. Gently explore the uterine cavity manually to exclude retained placental tissue, membrane or clot. If labour had not commenced, wear an extra glove for this intrauterine examination. Check the cervix digitally from above and if needed, dilate it to allow free drainage of blood. Then the outer glove is discarded.

Closure

Closure of the uterus

Closure of the uterus is with two layers of continuous sutures. Make sure the first stitch is well beyond the lateral edge of the incision to ensure haemostasis (Fig. 37.7). A single-layer interrupted suture closes the transverse incision. A second continuous suture buries the first layer ensuring the wound is watertight. The loose peritoneal fold of uterovesical peritoneum is then closed.

A feature of the classical incision is marked retraction of the superficial layers of the myometrium, which may make it difficult to bring together. Two or more layers of interrupted

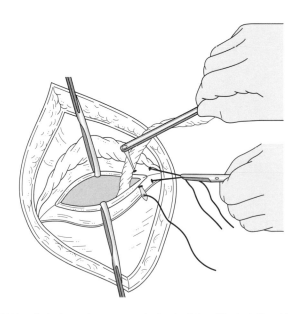

Fig. 37.7 Suturing a transverse uterine incision. Start at the side away from the surgeon and ensure that the first-lateral suture is well beyond the lateral point of the incision.

or continuous sutures are needed for the uterus is thick here. Sometimes a series of full thickness tension sutures are required as well (Fig. 37.8).

Abdominal closure

Check the adnexae for disease before closure. When using regional analgesia, the questionable benefit of palpating upper abdominal organs in asymptomatic women needs to be weighed against the discomfort this causes. If any doubt exists about the effectiveness of haemostasis, drain the relevant area.

Doubt has been cast on the value of abdominal wall peritoneal closure, as spontaneous reperitonisation has been shown to occur when the peritoneum is left unsutured and time is saved at the operation. Secure closure of the sheath, however, is important; a suction drain can be used from under the sheath for it sometimes oozes. If a continuous suture is used, a knot is tied after the first and again after the second stitch to avoid the possibility of unravelling as tension is placed on the continuous suture. Catgut is gradually being phased out because of the tissue reaction produced, and synthetic absorbable polyamide acid sutures are usually adequate. A non-absorbable suture such as nylon should be used for vertical abdominal incisions in the presence of obesity or maternal conditions associated with poor wound healing. Nylon 2/0 mattress sutures may be used for the skin if the approach was vertical, or continuous subcuticular polyamide suture material for transverse incisions.

SPECIAL PROBLEMS

Delivery for malpresentation

If one foot or both feet are presenting, get a firm hold of the posterior foot. If that cannot be done, grasp both feet, and gently extract the leg or legs followed by the breech. Make sure that a fetal hand is not delivered in error. For frank breech

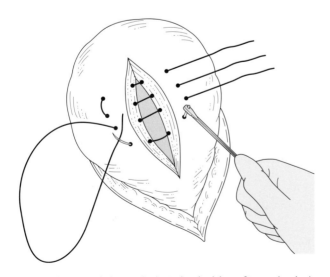

Fig. 37.8 Closure of the vertical uterine incision after a classical caesarean section. Stay sutures to relieve the tension are usually needed.

presentation, use the technique described for cephalic presentation. When delivering the aftercoming head of a breech baby, it is important to maintain flexion of the head using the Mauriceau–Smellie–Veit manoeuvre or obstetric forceps.

If there is a transverse lie, correction to a longitudinal lie may have been possible before opening the uterus. If not, use a vertical uterine incision and insert a hand after opening the uterus to bring out of the incision either the head or more likely one or both feet, whichever is most accessible, and proceed as already described. Tocolysis is advisable if any manipulation of the fetal position is needed.

Placenta praevia

If the diagnosis is in doubt, it should be confirmed by careful vaginal examination under anaesthesia immediately prior to surgery. Careful preoperative localisation of the placental margin with ultrasound is helpful in planning the approach to the uterine cavity. If this is done in each case, a classical incision is often not needed.

If the placenta covers the lower uterine segment anteriorly, the uterine wall will be very vascular and the delivery should be completed quickly and efficiently to minimise blood loss. Keeping in mind the relationship of the nearest placental margin to the proposed incision, open the myometrium as usual without incising the placenta. Separate the placenta from the uterine wall in the direction of the nearest margin, keep the placental edge out of the way, and swiftly bring the presenting part of the baby out through the uterine wound. This will in effect compress the placenta and its bed so reducing immediate blood loss. Occasionally it may be necessary to cut through the placenta to reach the baby. In this case clamp the umbilical cord as soon as it is accessible in case fetal placental vessels have been divided.

Place as many broad Green–Armytage haemostatic clamps at each angle and around the uterine wound edge as needed to obtain haemostasis (usually four are needed). After removal of the placenta, take particular care to ensure that the lower segment placental site is not bleeding actively, undersewing bleeding points if necessary, before closing the uterus.

The use of tocolysis during caesarean section

The possibility that tocolysis may inhibit third-stage contraction of the uterus has not been systematically studied. In practice there has not been any noticeable difference in the response of the uterus to oxytocin infusion following tocolysis in the dosage described. Glyceryl trinitrate sublingual spray may also be an effective tocolytic to facilitate intrauterine manipulations during delivery (Greenspoon & Kovacic 1991).

Tocolysis may be used as follows.

- Always have a beta-adrenergic agent available in theatre.
- Contraction of the uterus, following either prolonged labour or incision and escape of liquor, may make the delivery of the baby difficult.
- Effective relaxation of the uterus can be achieved within 30 seconds by administering a beta-adrenergic agent

such as hexoprenaline (Ipradol) 5 µg intravenously. Halothane, is an alternative which causes uterine relaxation in high doses.

- Give the tocolytic routinely one minute before incising the myometrium if there is:
  - significant prematurity
  - malpresentation
  - multiple pregnancy.

- At a caesarean section for advanced or prolonged labour, have the tocolytic drawn up ready to administer.
- If the baby's head cannot be lifted from the pelvis with ease, administer the tocolytic, wait 30 seconds, then proceed with the delivery.
- For any unanticipated difficulty with delivery, consider prompt tocolysis.

Excessive haemorrhage

If bleeding from the uterine cavity is excessive, do not close the uterus before the bleeding has been controlled, usually by undersewing bleeding points with figure-of-eight 2/0 polyamide sutures. Control bleeding from any severed branches of the uterine artery at the angles of the incision by means of full thickness myometrial suture placed parallel to and above and below the incision. If uterine contraction is inadequate, give i.v. Ergometrine and commence an infusion of oxytocin (20 units in 1 litre normal saline). If this is not effective, consider giving prostaglandin F$_2$ alpha 1 mg diluted to 10 ml slowly directly into the myometrium taking care to avoid intravascular injection. If bleeding continues, a Brace suture may work (Ch. 39), if not ligate one or both internal iliac arteries with absorbable sutures close to the bifurcations of the common ileac arteries, after displacing the ureters medially (van Gelderen 1975). If all else fails, do not delay in resorting to hysterectomy as a life-saving procedure.

Sterilisation

Sterilisation at the time of caesarean section has been shown to be associated with an increased failure rate. A possible explanation is that during pregnancy the Fallopian tubes are oedematous and more friable. So using clips or ligation techniques designed for use in the non-pregnant woman may cut into the tube with proximal sinus formation. If sterilisation must be done at this time, use a ligation and separation technique. It is usually better, however, to perform a laparoscopy sterilisation six weeks after the caesarean section.

POSTOPERATIVE CARE

Adequate analgesia and routine observations including vaginal blood loss should be ensured. Women who have undergone caesarean section need extra help and encouragement to manage their babies and establish breast-feeding. Hospital routines should be established which minimise the separation of babies from mothers except at the mother's request. Early mobilisation of the mother should be actively encouraged

remembering the temporary leg weakness after regional anaesthesia if she goes to the lavatory.

During a straightforward caesarean section, the bowel is not exposed particularly if the uterus is not externalised, so paralytic ileus is rarely a problem. It is not necessary to limit oral fluids after caesarean section, and once oral fluids are being well tolerated and the woman's condition is stable, the intravenous infusion can be discontinued and food gradually introduced. A small study has shown no significant difference in gastrointestinal function between women allowed to drink immediately postoperatively and those starved for 24 hours (Guedj et al 1991).

Postoperative care should include careful temperature monitoring, as puerperal sepsis is considerably more common following caesarean section than following vaginal delivery (see Ch. 41).

POSTOPERATIVE COMPLICATIONS

Potential postoperative complications of caesarean section are:

- Bleeding
- Infection
- Deep vein thrombosis
- Bladder damage
- Small bowel ileus.

Bleeding

As has been indicated before, the caesarean section is a bloody operation, about 350 to 500 ml are lost at most operations and over a third have lost an amount of blood to bring them into the definition of a primary postpartum haemorrhage. This mostly comes from the large veins in the lower segment or the larger sinuses of the myometrium. As has been indicated, excessive bleeding can occur if the uterine wound extends out into the leash of blood vessels at the side. Haematomas of the uterus at the scar are common after caesarean section but they are usually localised. However, if the broad ligament is involved, blood can track out into the loose tissues and hence to the retroperioneal space. A woman can lose two litres from her circulation into this area. The primary treatment of haemorrhage is the correct insertion of the sutures lateral to the edge of the lower segment caesarean section uterine wound to make sure that one has caught the uterine arteries and veins lateral to the incision. If ooze occurs after the operation is completed it is by far best to treat it conservatively. Transfuse the woman with blood and await resolution, which usually occurs. Rarely is surgical reintervention helpful.

Infection

Infection of the uterine wound or the abdominal wall incision can occur, particularly if the caesarean section was done in labour and the membranes have been ruptured for some time. It is best treated by appropriate antibiotics if swabs can be cultured or by broad spectrum ones if they cannot. It usually responds well and there is no need to intervene surgically. Should the infection be of the abdominal wall wound, local heat is helpful and secondary suture may be required if the skin and subcutaneous tissues gape.

Deep vein thrombosis

This is more common after caesarean section than after vaginal delivery. The trauma and the hypercoagulability of the blood lead to deep vein thrombosis. Further, low-grade infection can spread in the uterine veins to the sidewalls of the pelvis where deep vein thrombosis forms on the iliac veins. This is more dangerous than the phlebothrombosis in the leg at the soleal veins. In the pelvic veins, thrombophlebitis forms and such clots are more friable and are more likely to break off, moving towards the pulmonary circulation. Most of the deaths from pulmonary thrombosis after a caesarean section occur after the first week following puerperium, after the woman has left hospital (Confidential Enquiry into Maternal Death 1996).

The diagnosis of pelvic sidewall thrombosis is hard to make. It is usually associated with a dull ache in the lower abdomen, an offensive vaginal discharge and ill-defined tenderness on either side of the uterus. The temperature is raised and the pulse often is elevated more than one would expect for that degree of pyrexia.

Treatment is with antibiotics and anticoagulation to try to prevent further clotting occurring and thus increasing the risk of pulmonary embolism. This is dealt with fully in Chapter 41.

Bladder damage

Damage to the bladder is best avoided by draining the organ before surgery and leaving an indwelling catheter *in situ* during the operation. Careful dissection and displacement of the bladder before the myometrium is incised removes that organ from the operation field (Fig. 37.3). Sometimes the bladder is hitched high by old fibrosis and it may be damaged when making an incision into the lower segment of the uterus. Provided this is recognised there is no great harm. The incision of the bladder can be localised and dissection at the back of the bladder wall can now be made easily from the uterus. The bladder is then repaired in two layers of continuous sutures, the second one burying the first. If all is well, one can then proceed to the lower segment caesarean section and deliver the baby. After the operation, if there has been any bladder damage it would be wise to continue urinary drainage for five days and give appropriate antibiotics for that time. The bladder heals well and since the damage is at the dome of the bladder, ureteric function and urethral control is not affected. If the bladder does not heal well, a fistula may follow and this then needs separate repair.

Paralitic ileus

The incision of a caesarean section is usually low in the abdomen and the uterus itself acts to prevent the small bowel intruding into the wound; one no longer puts in large lengths of gauze roll to pack off intestinal contents and the incidence of paralitic ileus has reduced from the days when one used to pack off formally. If ileus does occur, gastric suction and parenteral fluids should be given until bowel sounds are heard easily.

INCREASING RATES

From the beginning of the twentieth century caesarean section rates in all Western countries have been increasing. This is not a recent phenomenon, a senior obstetrician in 1922 wrote to the British Medical Journal:

> 'The art and science of midwifery have either been lost by the younger generation in this country or will certainly be lost if this mad rage for caesarean section is continued'.

At that time, caesarean sections were performed in 3% of deliveries. After this, the rate rose gradually until the 1970s (Fig. 37.9). A big increase occurred in 1976–1978, following the *Jordan v. Whitehead* case where an experienced obstetrician had attempted a vaginal rotation at forceps delivery, had failed and moved to caesarean section. Afterwards with a brain damaged baby, Mrs Whitehead sued the obstetrician and, in a celebrated case, won her case for damages. Although this was reversed at a higher court later the damage had been done for, as always, the first day of the case when the prosecution lays out its contentions had all the press publicity. When obstetricians of all grades saw that their helpful attempts to avoid caesarean section would be met with legal onslaught, they said publicly that they would no longer do mid-cavity forceps deliveries and rotations but would go straight to caesarean section. This had a profound effect on the profession which shows on Figure 37.9.

A plateau was reached in the caesarean section rate in the 1980s at about 10% but since the 1990s this has been gradually moving up with a sharp increase in the last three or four years. The second increase may be a result of the mother's own wishes, discussed on p 604.

Of all the indications listed earlier most are unchanged in importance but a few are responsible for slight changes in caesarean usage.

Fulminating pre-eclampsia
Here we are more prepared to intervene earlier than we were ten years ago on less mature babies. Results of neonatal care

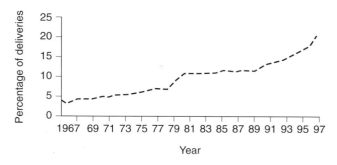

Fig. 37.9 The caesarean section rate of the last thirty years in England and Wales.

are so good that one is prepared to advise stopping a pregnancy at 30 weeks or even at lower gestation if the preeclamptic process is getting worse. This accounts for a small increase.

Previous caesarean sections

The old adage of 'Once a caesar always a caesar' is no longer true. Even in the USA now, more vaginal births are taking place after caesarean sections. As indicated previously, in UK probably two-thirds of women with a previous caesarean section are now allowed to proceed into normal labour and about two-thirds of those deliver. Still, however, habits of the previous generation of obstetricians, teachers of the current generation, die hard.

Fetal distress

This is now being diagnosed far more readily, sometimes perhaps even unnecessarily. In large parts of the world a fetal heart rate monitor alone is used to provide indication of the state of the fetus. This is not a good screening test (see Ch. 27). Unless it is backed up with fetal blood sampling to measure the acid–base state of the fetal circulating blood; it is not in itself enough to diagnose fetal hypoxia on cardiotocograph (CTG) changes except in extreme cases. Despite this, CTG is used alone and some of the increase in caesarean section rates lies at the door of this false diagnosis.

Breech presentation

As is outlined earlier in this chapter, there is often little benefit in delivering a baby presenting by the breech by caesarean section but the idea has entered the minds of both mothers and medical professionals. The fear of litigation drives the latter into performing defensive caesarean sections for breech presentation.

Maternal HIV infection

Undoubtedly this indication will rise but it occurs in so few pregnancies in the UK that it is not a major reason for the increase in rates.

The UK is not alone in these increased caesarean section rates, it is happening throughout the world as shown in Figure 37.10. The rates which were exceeding the UK in the US are now starting to level off there and they have even slightly reduced to about 20%. The Netherlands, always a conservative obstetrical country, is getting equally good results with an only slowly increasing rate whereas in South America the rate of caesarean sections in Chile has now gone up to 40% (Belezan et al 1999). In other countries in South America it even exceeds this. Analysis shows this increase to be principally among the affluent population and not the deprived.

It would seem then that the major reasons in the UK for the sharply increased caesarean section rate are a fear of litigation and an increase in maternal preference. In a survey performed by Francome & Savage (1993) anxiety about legal procedures was attributed by consultant obstetricians in 46.8% of cases as the reason for increased caesarean section

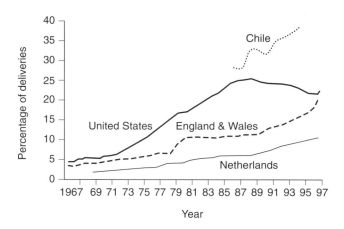

Fig. 37.10 The caesarean section rate of the last thirty years in some selected countries.

rates; this was far higher than any other single attributed cause. To rush to caesarean section will lead to a deskilling of middle grade and senior obstetricians in dealing with problems such as vaginal breech delivery. Hence, this will lead in a few years to a cohort of obstetricians who cannot do anything else but caesarean section when they run into problems. Undoubtedly, the unpleasant publicity the national press raised in the *Jordan v. Whitehead* case bit hard into professional attitudes. In the survey by Francome and Savage quoted above, the other major reasons giving for the rise were that 'Better care has improved survival' (22%) and 'The improved safety of the operation including anaesthesia' (18.7%).

In the UK various bodies have set up groups to assess the rapid increase in caesarean section rates. The Royal College of Obstetricians and Gynaecologists is doing this currently and the House of Commons Health Committee did in a previous year. The rate of caesarean sections could be reduced by:

- Operating only when a clear-cut indication exists.
- Performing external cephalic version at term for breech presentation.
- Performing external cephalic version just before induction or in early labour for transverse or oblique lie.
- Evolving a protocol for vaginal breech delivery in selected cases.
- Allowing carefully monitored trial of previous caesarean section scar whenever no clear contraindication exists.
- Diagnosing cephalopelvic disproportion only after an adequate trial of labour.
- Avoiding electronic FHR monitoring in uncomplicated labours.
- Confirming suspected fetal distress at FHR with fetal blood sampling.
- Managing variable or early FHR decelerations with amnioinfusion.
- Proper discussion with women requesting surgery as a preference.

Long-term solutions would include changes in the medico-legal system so that compensation would be provided without having to attribute blame and go to a long legal case before getting damages. Better understanding of true fetal distress could be taught and wider publicity given to the lack of benefit of caesarean section for twins. Further measures would include explaining the operation to women requesting surgery to avoid vaginal birth. Undoubtedly the greater involvement of consultants on the labour ward can do this so that more experienced doctors are looking after cases than occurs at the moment.

CONCLUSION

Caesarean section has become a prominent feature of obstetrical practice. Better anaesthetic care and attention to details of postoperative problems has improved safety enormously. However, there are still disadvantages to the operation and these should be borne in mind by both mothers and professionals. The rate has increased rapidly in the Western world and deserves attention from obstetricians.

A technique for the operation is critically described and the special needs of women having a caesarean section are outlined.

ACKNOWLEDGEMENT

The diagrams illustrating the operation are taken from the great Victor Barney (with permission) and so show his favourite neddle – the Periden. this needle is not used commonly now, but the techniques are.

KEY POINTS

- Caesarean section is a helpful method of delivery in an emergency or to prevent one.
- It should be used if vaginal delivery is considered to be harmful to mother or baby.
- Principle reasons for this are obstruction to the passage of the baby, lack of coordinated uterine action and fetal hypoxia.
- Other important reasons are maternal bleeding and avoiding maternal over-exhaustion.
- In actuality, fear of litigation and maternal preferences are driving the rates upward.

REFERENCES

Al Mufti R, McCarthy A, Fisk N 1997 Survey of obstetricians personal preferences and discretionary practice. Eur J Obstet Gynaecol 169:936–940

Audit Commission 1997 First Class Delivery. Audit Commission Publications, London

Belezan J, Althabe F, Barros F, Alexander S 1999 Rates and implications of caesarean sections in South America. Br Med J 319:1397–1402

Bottoms SF, Rosen MG, Sokol RJ 1980 The increase in the caesarean birth rate. N Engl J Med 302:559

Boyce PM, Todd AL 1992 Increased risk of postnatal depression after emergency caesarean section. Med J Australia 156:172–174

Chamberlain G 1993 What is the correct caesarean section rate? Br J Obstet Gynaecol 100:403–404

Collea J, Chein C, Quilligan E 1980 The randomized management of term frank breech presentation: a study of 208 cases. Am J Obstet Gynecol 137:235–244

Confidential Enquiry into Maternal Deaths in UK 1996 Department of Health, London

Crowley P, Hawkins DS 1980 Premature breech delivery—the caesarean section debate. J Obstet Gynaecol 1:2–6

Cumberledge J 1993 Changing Childbirth. HMSO, London

European Collaborative Study 1999 Elective caesarean section versus vaginal delivery in preventing vertical HIV-1 transmission. Lancet 353: 1035–1039

Gimovsky M, Wallace R, Schifrin B, Paul R 1983 Randomized management of the non-frank breech presentation at term: a preliminary report. Am J Obstet Gynecol 146:34–40

Francome C, Savage W, Churchill H, Lewison H 1993 Caesarean birth in Britain. Middlesex University Press, London

Greenspoon JS, Kovacic A 1991 Breech extraction facilitated by glyceryl trinitrate sublingual spray. Lancet 338:124–125

Guedj P, Eldor J, Stark M 1991 Immediate postoperative oral hydration after caesarean section. Asia Oceanea J Obstet Gynaecol 17:125–129

Hannah M, Hannah W, Hewson S, Hodnett S, Willan A 2000 Planned caesarean section versus planned vaginal birth for breech presentation at term. Lancet 356: 1375–1383

Hofmeyr GJ 1989 Suspected feto-pelvic disproportion. In: Chalmers I, Enkin M, Keirse M JNC (eds) Effective care in pregnancy and childbirth. Oxford University Press, Oxford, pp 493–498

Hofmeyr GJ 1992a Amnioinfusion: a question of benefits and risks. (Commentary). British J Obstet Gynaecol 99:449–451

Hofmeyr GJ 1992b Breech presentation and shoulder dystocia in childbirth. Curr Opin Obstet Gynecol 4:807–812

Hofmeyr GJ 1993 External cephalic version at term. Fetal and Maternal Medicine Review 5:213–222

Hytten F 1982 Breech presentation: is it a bad omen? Br J Obstet Gynaecol 89:879–880

Impey I, O'Herlehy C 1999 Vaginal delivery after caesarean section for cepholpelvic disproportion. Contemp Rev Obstet Gynaecol 11:175–180

Johnson C, Keirse MJNC, Enkin M, Chalmers I 1989 Nutrition and hydration in labour. In: Chalmers I, Enkin M, Keirse MJNC (eds) Effective care in pregnancy and childbirth. Oxford University Press, Oxford, pp 827–832

Johnson F 1999 HIV, pregnancy and the antivirals. Contemp Rev Obstet Gynaecol 11:229–234

Lilford RJ, Van Coeverden De Groot HA, Moore PJ, Bingham P 1990 The relative risks of caesarean section (intrapartum and elective) and vaginal delivery: a detailed analysis to exclude the effects of medical disorders and other acute pre-existing physiological disturbances. Br J Obstet Gynaecol 97:883–892

McCurdy CM, Magann EF, McCurdy CJ, Saltzman AK 1992 The effect of placental management at cesarean delivery on operative blood loss. Am J Obstet Gynecol 167:1363–1366

MacDonald D, Grant A, Sheridan-Pereira M, Boylan P, Chalmers I 1985 The Dublin randomised trial of intrapartum fetal heart monitoring. Am J Obstet Gynecol 152:524–539

Neilson JP 1993 Cardiotocography during labour. Br Med J 1:528–529

Pearson J, Rees G 1989 Technique of caesarean section. In: Chalmers I, Enkin M, Keirse MJNC (eds) Effective care in pregnancy and childbirth. Oxford University Press, Oxford, pp 1234–1245

Penn ZJ, Steer PJ 1991 How obstetricians manage the problem of preterm delivery with special reference to the preterm breech. Br J Obstet Gynaecol 98:531–534

Peschers U, Schaer G, Delancy J 1997 Pelvic floor function before and after childbirth. Br J Obstet Gynaecol 104:1004–1008

Ryhammer A, Bek K, Laurberg S 1995 Multiple deliveries increase the risk of permanent incontinence of faeces and urine. Dis Colon Rectum 38:1206–1209

Roberts LJ, Beardsworth SA, Trew G 1994 Labour following caesarean section: current practice in the United Kingdom. Br J Obstet Gynaecol 101:153–155

Savage W, Francome C 1993 British caesarean section rates: have we reached a plateau? Br J Obstet Gynaecol 100:493–496

Smaill F 1993 Prophylactic antibiotics in caesarean section (all trials), review no 03690; prophylactic antibiotics for elective caesarean section, review no 03775; 1-day vs 3–5 day courses of antibiotics for caesarean section, review no 03250. In: Enkin MW, Keirse MJNC, Renfrew MJ, Neilson JP (eds) Pregnancy and childbirth module. Cochrane database of systematic reviews. Update Software, Oxford

Stephenson PA, Bakoula C, Hemminiki E et al 1993 Patterns of use of obstetrical interventions in 12 countries. Paediatr Perinat Epidemiol 7:45–56

Soltan A, Kahn M, Hudson C et al 1993 Anal sphincter disruption during vaginal delivery. N Engl J Med 329:1905–1911

Thorpe-Beeston J, Banfield P, Saunders N 1992 Outcome of breech delivery at term. Br Med J 305: 746–747

Van Gelderen CJ 1975 Internal iliac artery ligation in obstetrics and gynaecology. South African Med J 49:1997–2000

Van Oppen C, Feldman R 1993 Antibiotic prophylaxis of neonatal group B streptococcal infections. Br Med J 1:531–532

Westgate J, Harris M, Curnow JSH, Greene KR 1992 Randomised trial of cardiotocography alone or with ST waveform analysis for intrapartum fetal heart rate monitoring. Lancet 340:194–198

Yudkin PL, Redman CWG 1986 Caesarean sections dissected 1978–1983. Br J Obstet Gynaecol 93:135–144

38

Postpartum haemorrhage and abnormalities of the third stage of labour

William Thompson, M. Ann Harper

Material in this chapter contains contributions from the first and second editions and we are grateful to the previous authors for the work done.

'There are but two things which have much effect on me in a labour, haemorrhage and convulsions'
William Hunter 1718–83

INTRODUCTION

Postpartum haemorrhage is a major cause of maternal mortality. In developing countries, over 125 000 or approximately 28% of maternal deaths each year are caused by postpartum haemorrhage; the risk is approximately 1 in 1000 deliveries (Drife 1997). In developed countries such as the United Kingdom, the risk is approximately 1 in 100 000 deliveries. Obstetric haemorrhage is often a contributing factor to other causes of direct maternal death and a cause of postpartum morbidity in survivors. The number of maternal deaths from obstetric haemorrhage has decreased greatly since the report of the Confidential Enquiry into Maternal Deaths in England and Wales, covering the triennium 1952–1954, which reported 188 deaths from haemorrhage,

compared with 12 deaths in the whole of the United Kingdom in the triennium 1994–1996 (Department of Health 1998). The antenatal diagnosis of placenta praevia by ultrasound scan, the routine use of oxytocics for the third stage of labour, improvements in intensive care, anaesthesia, management of massive haemorrhage, the availability of blood transfusion and better antibiotics, and less anaemia in pregnant women have all contributed to the reduction in mortality. Nevertheless, obstetric haemorrhage remains one of the leading causes of maternal death in the United Kingdom and there has been no significant reduction in mortality in recent years (Table 38.1).

Each Confidential Enquiry into Maternal Deaths in the United Kingdom identifies avoidable factors and substandard care in the majority of cases reported. These factors include

Table 38.1 Number and causes of deaths from haemorrhage and rates per million maternities; United Kingdom 1985–1996 (Department of Health 1998)

Triennium	Placental abruption	Placenta praevia	Postpartum haemorrhage	Total	Rate per million maternities
1985–1987	4	0	6	10	4.5
1988–1990	6	5	11	22	9.2
1991–1993	3	4	8	15	6.4
1994–1996	4	3	5	12	5.5

delay or failure to recognise the extent of blood loss or to appreciate the frightening speed with which obstetric haemorrhage can become life threatening. This is particularly so in cases of placenta praevia. There is also delay or failure to take appropriate action to involve senior staff, especially consultant obstetricians, anaesthetists and haematologists at an early stage.

Risk factors for postpartum haemorrhage include maternal obesity, antepartum haemorrhage, prolonged labour, large baby, multiple pregnancy, and increased maternal age, although in the UK not grand multiparity (Drife 1997). A previous history of postpartum haemorrhage carries a significant risk of recurrence. Postpartum haemorrhage is more likely to occur after operative delivery or emergency caesarean section, and placenta praevia, particularly in patients with a previous uterine scar, may be associated with uncontrollable uterine haemorrhage at delivery (Department of Health 1998). Women who have a known coagulation disorder or significant anaemia are at particular risk of the effects of haemorrhage as are also those who refuse blood transfusion for religious or other reasons. When the risk of obstetric haemorrhage can be anticipated, it should be prepared for as far as possible. All the above factors should be taken into account and, after appropriate discussion with the woman, delivery should be booked in a suitably equipped unit. The consultant obstetrician should be directly involved in the management of labour and delivery. Venous access with two large-bore cannulae should be set up and at least four units of cross-matched blood should be available in the delivery ward. Oxytocic drugs should be used in the third stage. Most importantly, at caesarean section for placenta praevia, an experienced operator is essential and must be readily available (Department of Health 1998).

Postpartum haemorrhage, however, is usually unpredictable and this is relevant to discussions with all women about the place of delivery, especially if they are intending to deliver at home or in small maternity units without immediate access to blood transfusion services.

PRIMARY POSTPARTUM HAEMORRHAGE

Definition

Primary postpartum haemorrhage is traditionally defined as a blood loss of 500 ml or more occurring within 24 hours of delivery of the baby. Its incidence is about 5% of deliveries.

This definition is limited by the fact that blood loss, particularly after delivery, is difficult to estimate accurately: clinical estimates of blood loss tend to underestimate the true volume of blood loss by between 34% and 50% (Prendiville & Elbourne 1989). It may be better at the time to consider factors which have more clinical relevance, such as a fall in haematocrit or the need for blood transfusion (Roberts 1995).

Concentration on the amount of revealed blood loss may distract attention from the fact that many serious postpartum haemorrhages are associated with concealed bleeding. Such bleeding may be concealed in the uterine cavity (as retained clot), in the myometrium (after placental abruption), in the broad ligament or the peritoneal cavity (both after uterine rupture), or in the paravaginal or paravulval tissue spaces. Also, persistent moderate blood loss may go unnoticed for some time and soon result in significant total haemorrhage.

Most primary postpartum haemorrhage occurs within the first 4 hours after delivery of the baby. During this time women are usually under supervision by midwives or doctors. Bleeding that is delayed and occurs when the birth attendants are no longer with a patient can go unrecognised and thus has its own particular danger. It is wise to continue regular observation of general condition, blood pressure, pulse rate, abdominal signs, the size and consistency of the uterus and the amount of vaginal loss in the first 12–24 hours postpartum. Equally, it is important to look for paravaginal or vulval haematoma formation in any woman who complains of excessive pain after delivery.

Causes

The main causes of primary postpartum haemorrhage are:

- uterine atony; this accounts for about 90% of cases
- genital tract trauma
- partially retained placenta & fragments
- placenta praevia and accreta
- coagulation disorders.

A reference to Table 38.2 will help focus on the main factors underlying the causation of the bleeding.

Prevention

Active management of the third stage of labour comprises early cord clamping, giving prophylactic oxytocic drugs before delivery of the placenta, and controlled cord traction

Table 38.2 The four Ts—mnemonic for the main causes of primary postpartum haemorrhage

- Tone
- Trauma
- Tissue
- Thrombin

using the Brandt–Andrews method of placental extraction. Routine prophylactic use of an oxytocic drug to assist contraction of the uterus following delivery of the baby and controlled cord traction to effect delivery of the placenta is effective in reducing the risk of postpartum haemorrhage, although early cord clamping is not (Prendiville & Elbourne 1989).

Use of oxytocics

Bleeding from the placental bed following separation of the placenta is mainly controlled by compression of the vessels through retraction and contraction of the uterine muscle fibres. Normal coagulation is also important but is a secondary factor. The prophylactic use of oxytocic drugs reduces the risk of postpartum haemorrhage by 30–40% (Prendiville et al 1988) and also hastens placental separation. The drug most commonly used is Syntometrine: a 1 ml ampoule contains a combination of 5 IU oxytocin and 0.5 mg ergometrine. Oxytocin is faster acting than ergometrine and causes exaggerated physiological uterine contractions that expel the placenta from the upper uterine segment before the tonic action of ergometrine becomes effective. This combination of drugs reduces the incidence of a separated but retained placenta. Syntometrine is administered by deep intramuscular injection in the mother's thigh with crowning of the head, the delivery of the anterior shoulder or just after delivery of the baby. There are few contraindications to the use of Syntometrine but it should be used with caution in hypertensive patients; asthma and cardiac disease are also regarded as relative contraindications. Syntometrine commonly causes nausea and vomiting and is unstable if stored at high ambient temperatures or in light (El-Refaey et al 1997).

Oxytocin (10 IU intravenously or intramuscularly) is almost as effective (McDonald et al 1993), causes less nausea and vomiting, and is more stable in hot climates. Injectable prostaglandins are effective uterotonic agents in the control of intractable postpartum haemorrhage but cannot be recommended for routine prophylactic use as they are expensive and there are concerns about their safety (Gulmezoglu 1999).

Oral misoprostol 400 or 600 µg given after delivery of the baby is effective in the prevention of postpartum haemorrhage, has few side effects and may be given to women with hypertension (El-Refaey et al 1997). It is easily stored and does not require the use of sterile syringes and needles so may prove to be a particularly useful drug in developing countries. Further trials are required. In April 1998, the WHO commenced recruitment to a large multicentre international trial of oral misoprostol (600 µg) compared with oxytocin 10 IU.

Active management of the third stage of labour

Physiologically, the uterus should contract soon after delivery of the baby. The placenta will then separate from the uterine wall and is spontaneously expelled, a process that can take up to half an hour. Separation of the placenta is evidenced by a show of blood, lengthening of the cord and a firmly contracted uterus that rises up in the abdomen and assumes a more globular shape with greater mobility. With the active management of the third stage, in which oxytocin and ergometrine have been administered during birth, this process is hastened and in most cases is complete within 10 minutes following delivery of the infant. After separation, delivery of the placenta can be painlessly effected by the Brandt–Andrews technique of controlled cord traction. The cord is re-clamped near the vulva and steadied with the right hand while the left hand is used to press on the abdomen to push the contracted uterine fundus upwards. This will confirm if the placenta has separated, since the cord will not be drawn back into the vagina following the upward movement of the uterus. A combined movement is made of downward and backward traction on the cord and upward displacement of the uterus provided that the latter is firmly contracted. If the placenta does not descend, it may still be partially attached to the uterus or trapped in a tightly contracted lower uterine segment. In such cases the procedure of controlled cord traction can be repeated at intervals of several minutes. If the bladder is obviously distended, catheterisation should be performed. If the uterus is firmly contracted and controlled traction on the cord still fails to deliver the placenta, it can be deemed to be retained after 20–30 minutes have elapsed and manual removal should then be employed. This procedure may have to be undertaken earlier if the patient develops significant bleeding.

ABNORMALITIES OF THE THIRD STAGE OF LABOUR

Retained placenta

The possible explanations for retained placenta are abnormal uterine contractions resulting in a constriction ring or, rarely, a morbidly adherent placenta. The patient who has a retained placenta may be shocked, having had a postpartum haemorrhage; adequate resuscitative measures must be commenced before attempting manual removal. These should include giving blood if the patient is bleeding and the administration of a second dose of oxytocic to encourage uterine contractions and placental separation. A syntocinon infusion should also be set up. Evidence available from randomised controlled trials indicates that there is no advantage in the intraumbilical cord injection of saline with or without oxytocin to encourage placental separation, and this method is not recommended (Carroli & Bergel 2000).

Technique of manual removal

Manual removal should be performed using an aseptic surgical technique and adequate analgesia (either regional or general anaesthesia). The patient is placed in the lithotomy position. One hand is placed on the abdomen to encourage the uterus to contract and a last attempt is made with the Brandt–Andrews method of controlled cord traction. If this fails, the abdominal hand should steady the uterus, pressing down onto the vaginal hand. The fingers of the vaginal hand are brought into the shape of a cone and the hand follows the umbilical cord into the uterine cavity. If a constriction ring is present at the lower uterine segment it can be overcome by firm upward pressure so as to allow the entire hand to enter the upper segment. An assessment is made of the degree of adherence of the placenta and the site of attachment. The lower edge of the placenta is then located and the fingers are inserted into the placental bed; at all times the external hand on the abdomen exerts firm counterpressure. With sweeping movements using the ulnar border of the hand as far as possible, the placenta is stripped from the wall of the uterus. It is important that the procedure is carried out gently and methodically; uterine perforation is a rare but serious complication of this procedure. When there is total separation of the placenta it is removed and an intravenous oxytocic (preferably Syntometrine, unless contraindicated) is administered to promote uterine contraction. An oxytocin infusion may then be continued for a few hours to maintain uterine contraction.

Following a manual removal a careful check of the birth canal is made to exclude tears and it is mandatory to undertake a careful inspection of the removed placenta to confirm that it is complete. The patient is given a course of antibiotics to prevent infection.

Placenta accreta

In most cases the placenta separates spontaneously from its implantation site some minutes after delivery of the baby. Occasionally, the placenta may be morbidly adherent to the wall of the uterus, either wholly or partially. In such cases a plane of cleavage will not be found and the risk of uterine rupture is increased. The term placenta accreta describes any implantation of the placenta in which there is an abnormally firm adherence to the uterine wall. Partial or total absence of the decidua basalis results in a direct attachment of the placental villi to the myometrium. The villi may invade the myometrium (placenta increta) or even penetrate the full thickness of the myometrium (placenta percreta), in some cases involving adjacent pelvic structures. The abnormal adherence may involve all of the cotyledons (total placenta accreta) or only some (partial placenta accreta). The incidence of the condition has been reported as 1 in 2500 deliveries (Read et al 1980). The aetiological factor leading to abnormal adherence of the placenta is defective decidual formation. This situation is commoner after a placental implantation in the lower uterine segment or over a previous caesarean section scar or other uterine incision, e.g. myomectomy. The condition has also been associated with previous uterine curettage and high parity (Fox 1972).

The management of placenta accreta will depend on the site of implantation, the depth of penetration and the extent of the placental involvement. It may be possible to diagnose the condition antenatally by ultrasonic scan; the absence of a sonolucent area at the placental bed is consistent with the diagnosis (Cox et al 1988). If a single cotyledon is involved it may be possible to tear it from the uterine wall; the risk of uterine rupture is always present. Excessive bleeding from the placental bed will occur but this may be controlled with oxytocics. Cases managed in this way require careful follow-up as there is an increased risk of secondary postpartum haemorrhage and a placental polyp may form as a long-term sequel.

When there is total placenta accreta or a large part of the placental bed is involved, the placenta will be retained and manual removal will not succeed as a plane of cleavage between the placenta and the uterine wall cannot be developed. Leaving the placenta in place is inadvisable because of the risks of infection and haemorrhage (Gibb et al 1994). Experienced senior obstetric and anaesthetic staff should be involved in the management of this dangerous condition. The safest treatment is surgical control of haemorrhage, usually by prompt hysterectomy. Appropriate antibiotic cover should be given.

Acute uterine inversion

Acute uterine inversion is a rare obstetric complication but is of extreme importance because of the threat it poses to the life of the mother. The reported incidence varies from 1 in 20–25 000 deliveries in large studies from India (Das 1940) and the Middle East (Fahmy 1977) to approximately 1 in 2000 deliveries (Watson et al 1980). Uterine inversion may be described as of first, second, third or fourth degree:

1 The inverted uterine fundus extends to the level of the cervical os.
2 The inverted uterine fundus extends through the cervical os but not to the introitus.
3 The fundus extends to the introitus.
4 The inverted uterus and cervix extend below the introitus with associated vaginal inversion.

Alternatively, uterine inversion may be described as complete or incomplete depending on whether the fundus has passed through the cervix (Wendel & Cox 1995). Acute inversion occurs during the first 24 hours postpartum and is the most common type (Brar et al 1989). Incomplete uterine inversion may be associated with a constriction ring and go undetected for some time, resulting in subacute inversion which presents after 24 hours but within 4 weeks of delivery or chronic inversion which presents after 4 weeks.

Uterine inversion is traditionally thought to arise most commonly as a result of mismanagement of the third stage of labour, particularly Credé's method of expelling the placenta when the uterus is relaxed, inadvertent fundal pressure when the uterus is poorly contracted or cord traction with an unseparated placenta. Often, however, acute inversion of the uterus occurs spontaneously after delivery of the infant; primiparity, oxytocin use, and macrosomia are risk factors and a fundally inserted placenta is found in the majority of cases (Brar et al 1989). Other predisposing factors include an unusually short umbilical cord or a sudden rise in the intra-abdominal pressure (by the patient coughing or vomiting) when the uterus is atonic. Certain obstetric conditions such as a morbidly adherent placenta and uterine abnormalities may also predispose to uterine inversion. It can also occur during manual removal of the placenta.

Acute uterine inversion may present with pain, haemorrhage or sudden collapse; the degree of shock may be inconsistent with the visible blood loss. The shock is thought to be neurogenic, resulting from the anatomical stretching of the infundibulopelvic ligaments and compression of the ovaries within the inverted uterus, which is in spasm. Shock may also be associated with postpartum haemorrhage in the presence of uterine atony and placental separation. More commonly, bleeding is not excessive because the inverted uterus will retract and constrict the uterine vessels.

Uterine inversion should be suspected in any woman with unexplained shock during or following the third stage of labour. The differential diagnosis includes pulmonary or amniotic fluid embolism, uterine rupture or myocardial infarction. The most obvious finding is the absence on abdominal palpation of the uterine fundus and the appearance of a fleshy mass at or outside the introitus. In incomplete inversion, the diagnosis may not be evident and a prompt vaginal examination should be performed to confirm or exclude the diagnosis. The other condition that can simulate inversion is a submucous fibromyoma projecting through the external os. In this case the uterus will be easily palpable in the abdomen.

In this condition, prevention is better than cure, and mismanagement of the third stage should be avoided. The use of Syntometrine with delivery of the anterior shoulder should ensure that the uterus contracts. Cord traction should not be performed until the signs of placental separation are apparent. The uterus should always be protected during cord traction by pressing with the other hand on the abdomen suprapubically and pushing the contracted uterus upwards. Credé's manoeuvre should be avoided.

Once the diagnosis of acute inversion is made, the sooner steps are taken to correct the problem the better. The longer the uterus remains inverted, the more oedematous and difficult to replace it will become, therefore an immediate attempt should be made to reposition the uterus manually. If the placenta is adherent, removal should not be attempted until the uterus has been replaced. The majority of cases will be associated with maternal collapse and immediate anti-shock measures also need to be commenced. These include the siting of large intravenous cannulae and ensuring the availability of blood and blood products. Correction of maternal shock may not be successful until the inversion has been corrected. The first line of management is to attempt to replace the uterus manually under suitable local or regional analgesia. The operator's hand is placed within the vagina and strong upward pressure is exerted to place the uterine ligaments on the stretch. Sustained pressure is maintained for 3–5 minutes and the fundus will usually recede upwards as the cervical ring widens. It is then pushed upwards with the clenched fist. The placenta, if still attached to the uterus, is manually removed after the inversion has been replaced. Tocolytic agents such as ritodrine (Clark 1984), magnesium sulphate (Grossman 1981) or terbutaline (Cantanzarite et al 1986)

can be used to relax the uterus during manual replacement. General anaesthesia with halothane has also been recommended to relax the uterus (Datta 1991) but may cause severe hypotension and refractory atony; it is associated with an increased maternal mortality and is probably best avoided (Abouleish et al 1995).

If manual replacement fails to correct the inversion, the hydrostatic method originally described by O'Sullivan (1945) may be attempted. The method consists of occlusion of the vaginal introitus by the operator's hand and infusing a large volume of warm saline under a head of pressure to distend the vagina and subsequently to push the fundus back to its original position. The container of saline should be held about 1 metre above the patient and be connected to one or two tubes placed into the posterior vaginal fornix; a considerable amount of saline may be required to replace the uterus. The main difficulty with this technique is developing an adequate seal at the introitus to allow the generation of hydrostatic pressure high enough to overcome the cervical constriction. A Silastic ventouse cup of suitable size inserted into the vagina produces a better seal (Ogueh & Ayida 1997); intravenous fluid at body temperature is administered through an intravenous giving set attached to the Silastic cup. The surgeon's hand in the vagina will help to maintain the seal between the vagina and the cup.

If the uterus cannot be replaced by vaginal manipulation, usually because of a tight constriction ring, a laparotomy must be performed. The site of the inverted fundus is identified. Allis forceps are placed within the dimple and gentle upward traction is exerted on the clamps with a further placement of the forceps on the advancing fundus. The process is repeated until the procedure is complete (Huntington et al 1928). If the constriction ring still prohibits repositioning, Haultain's technique is employed (Haultain 1901, Oxorn 1986). This involves incising the cervical ring posteriorly with a longitudinal incision; this facilitates uterine replacement. After replacement the uterus is repaired in two layers.

Following successful replacement of the uterus, ergometrine or syntocinon should be given to maintain uterine tone and prevent reinversion. Appropriate antibiotic cover should also be given.

MANAGEMENT OF PRIMARY POSTPARTUM HAEMORRHAGE

Risk management

Massive postpartum haemorrhage usually occurs within the first hour or so of delivery. It can rapidly become life threatening and there is often a short but critical window of opportunity where prompt and effective action can make the difference between life and death. Delay in instituting appropriate and effective treatment is a major factor in the associated morbidity and mortality (Bonnar 2000). Massive life-threatening haemorrhage is a relatively rare event in UK maternity units and inexperienced staff may not always appreciate the speed at which acute torrential haemorrhage can cause critical shock. Also, bleeding may be concealed or persistent insidious loss of smaller amounts of blood may go unrecognised until the patient suddenly de-compensates and develops hypovolaemic shock. Meticulous regular and frequent observation of vital signs and vaginal blood loss after delivery is most important. All staff should be alert to the signs of significant haemorrhage and be able to take appropriate action.

The Report on Confidential Enquiries into Maternal Deaths in the United Kingdom 1994–1996 (Department of Health 1998) emphasises that every maternity unit should have a risk management system in place with well-rehearsed guidelines which should be implemented as soon as a significant obstetric haemorrhage is suspected or recognised. Key recommendations of this Report relevant to the management of major haemorrhage were that:

- Each unit should identify a lead professional to develop and update guidelines.
- Local multidisciplinary guidelines for the management of obstetric haemorrhage should be developed.
- Guidelines should be prominently displayed in all antenatal, postnatal and labour wards and Accident and Emergency departments, and given to all new members of staff.
- Implementation of the guidelines should be subject to regular audit.
- Each maternal death or case of severe morbidity due to obstetric haemorrhage should be discussed at multidisciplinary audit meetings.
- Drills for cases of massive obstetric haemorrhage should be rehearsed regularly.
- Good communication between the labour ward and the blood bank is essential to ensure that large quantities of blood can be delivered to the labour ward without delay—ideally the labour ward and the blood bank should be on the same site.
- Placenta praevia, particularly in patients with a previous uterine scar, may be associated with uncontrollable haemorrhage at delivery and caesarean hysterectomy may be necessary. A very experienced operator is essential and a consultant must be readily available.
- Any pregnant (or recently delivered) woman admitted to an Accident or Emergency department should be seen by the duty obstetrician.

As well as undergoing regular training, staff should be encouraged to attend critical care courses such as ALSO (Advanced Life Support in Obstetrics) and MOE&T (Management of Obstetric Emergencies and Trauma) courses where emergency skills are taught.

Guidelines

An example of a locally developed management protocol for massive haemorrhage based on those published in *Maternal Mortality—The Way Forward* (1992) and the Report on Confidential Enquiries into Maternal Deaths in the United Kingdom 1998–1990 (Department of Health 1994) is reproduced in Figure 38.1. Such guidelines may be easily adapted to reflect local circumstances and should be regularly reviewed, updated and rehearsed.

Definition of massive obstetric haemorrhage

Massive obstetric haemorrhage implies the loss of very large amounts of blood from the genital tract with potentially life-threatening consequences. Different definitions have been proposed. Blood loss in excess of 1000 or 1500 ml from the genital tract (Walker et al 1994, Jouppila 1995), blood loss requiring immediate transfusion or transfusion of more than 10 units of blood within 24 hours, the replacement of the patient's total blood volume or 50% of the circulating blood volume in less than 3 hours or more than 150 ml per minute have all been suggested (Bonnar 2000). This variety of definitions causes problems in auditing and estimating the true incidence of massive haemorrhage. Accurate measurement of blood loss is difficult, the amount is often underestimated and in some situations, e.g. ruptured uterus, significant bleeding may be concealed. Major postpartum haemorrhage in excess of 1000 ml occurs after 1.3% of deliveries in the UK (Stones et al 1993.

Response to blood loss

In normal pregnancy, increased red cell mass, plasma volume and cardiac output provide a compensatory reserve for blood loss at delivery. Marked increases in the levels of blood coagulation factors during pregnancy and the haemostatic effect of sustained uterine contraction on the placental bed after delivery minimise postpartum blood loss. The physiological changes that occur after birth result in a reduced circulating blood volume, increased peripheral resistance, and haemoconcentration.

The homeostatic response to blood loss is intense sympathetic activity. This causes peripheral vasoconstriction and an increase in the rate and force of cardiac contraction, which maintains cardiac output and blood pressure. Selective vasoconstriction redistributes blood flow to maintain circulation to vital organs. Increased secretion of stress-related hormones—antidiuretic hormone, cortisol, aldosterone and catecholamines—reduces renal blood flow and urinary output. With continued uncorrected haemorrhage, compensatory mechanisms become inadequate to maintain tissue perfusion and oxygenation, resulting in cell damage and deterioration of organ function. Capillaries dilate and leak, peripheral vascular tone is lost, and blood pressure falls further. Resuscitation becomes more difficult and endothelial injury may trigger disseminated intravascular coagulation. Metabolic acidosis develops as tissue perfusion decreases and ultimately leads to organ failure and death. Successive Maternal Mortality Reports repeatedly identify delay in instituting resuscitative measures, and procrastination in decision-making, to be the most important avoidable factors in maternal deaths due to haemorrhage.

The signs and symptoms of haemorrhage are well known (Table 38.3). Palpitations, weakness, sweating, pallor, hypotension, oliguria, restlessness, air hunger, collapse and anuria progressively follow initial tachycardia. Young pregnant or recently delivered women without medical problems can maintain their blood pressure remarkably well for some time and may appear deceptively well in the face of consider-

Call for help
1. Summon most experienced resident staff: obstetrician, anaesthetist and senior midwife
2. Alert porters, blood transfusion laboratory staff and duty haematologist
3. Assign one midwife to observations and record keeping
4. Inform consultant obstetrician, consultant anaesthetist, and consultant haematologist
5. Prepare theatre

Restore circulating blood volume
1. Put in at least two large-bore (14 gauge) peripheral intravenous lines
2. Take 20–25 ml of blood for crossmatching, FBP, U&E and coagulation screen
3. Give the following fluids as appropriate—use fluid warmer and pressure infusion
   a. Hartmann's solution—rapid infusion of 2 litres, followed by Gelfusion—up to 1.5 litres
   b. Transfuse crossmatched blood as soon as available
   c. If no crossmatched blood and blood is essential, give ABO and RhD-compatible blood
   d. Uncrossmatched O Rh-negative blood should only be used as a last resort

Correct coagulopathy
1. Give 1 unit of fresh frozen plasma and change blood filter for every 4 units of blood transfused
2. Check coagulation screen at intervals as a guide
3. If the platelet count is less than 50×10^9/l, give platelet concentrates (use special giving set provided)
4. If severe bleeding continues and fibrinogen is less than 1.0 g/dl, give cryoprecipitate
5. Correct coagulopathy before embarking on major surgery

Monitor
1. Insert a self-retaining urinary catheter to monitor hourly urinary output
2. Consider insertion of central venous pressure line to monitor fluid replacement (anaesthetist)
3. Consider insertion of arterial line to monitor arterial pressure and blood gases (anaesthetist)
4. Assign one midwife to observations and record keeping:
   a. pulse
   b. blood pressure (DINAMAP/arterial BP)
   c. maternal heart rate (ECG)
   d. maternal oxygen concentration (pulse oximeter)
   e. central venous pressure
   f. urine output (hourly)
   g. amount and type of fluids the patient has received
   h. amount and type of drugs the patient has received

Stop the bleeding
1. Postpartum: rub up a contraction
2. Give syntometrine 1 amp i.v. or oxytocin 5–10 units i.v.
3. Set up i.v. infusion of 40 units of syntocinon in 1 litre Hartmann's solution at 150–250 ml/h
4. Under appropriate anaesthesia, exclude damage to the genital tract and retained placental tissue

If massive haemorrhage continues
1. Consultant obstetrician and consultant anaesthetist should be present
2. Commence bimanual compression of the uterus
3. Carboprost 250 µg by deep intramuscular or direct myometrial injection—may be repeated after 90 minutes
4. Uterine packing or balloon tamponade
5. Ligation of uterine arteries, internal iliac arteries, and ovarian arteries (vascular surgeon)
6. Arterial embolisation if resources and experience available
7. Hysterectomy

Fig. 38.1 Guidelines for the management of massive obstetric haemorrhage.

Table 38.3 The clinical picture in haemorrhagic shock and expected response to volume replacement (American College of Obstetricians and Gynaecologists 1997)

| Clinical sign | Primary shock | | Secondary shock |
	Early	Late	
Mental state	Alert and anxious	Confused	Coma
General appearance	Normal and warm	Pale and cold	Cyanotic and cold
Blood pressure	Slightly hypotensive	Moderately hypotensive	Markedly hypotensive
Respiratory system	Slight tachypnoea	Tachypnoea Cyanosis	Tachypnoea
Urinary output	30–60 ml/h	<30 ml/h	Anuria
Effect of fluid challenge on:			
Blood pressure	Increased	Slightly increased	No response
Urinary output	Increased	Slightly increased	No response

able blood loss before suddenly de-compensating and developing hypovolaemic shock. Tachycardia is a significant sign. The effects of blood loss will depend to some extent on the initial blood volume and haemoglobin concentration; underestimation of blood loss is common. The mortality rate increases with maternal age, especially in those aged 35 and over, who may be less able to withstand the effects of haemorrhage (Department of Health 1994).

Clinical management

The immediate management of haemorrhage is essentially the same irrespective of the cause or amount of blood loss. The circulating blood volume must be restored and maintained and the source of bleeding must be identified and dealt with promptly.

The first step is to palpate the abdomen and check that the uterus is well contracted. If not, a contraction should be rubbed up, the bladder emptied, and an indwelling catheter left in place so that urinary output can be monitored. An intravenous injection of ergometrine 0.5 mg or Syntometrine 1 ampoule should be given (unless contraindicated), and intravenous oxytocin (40 units oxytocin in 1 litre of Hartmann's solution) infused at a rate of 150–250 ml/h.

Adequate venous access should be established quickly to restore and maintain circulating blood volume. *An obstetric haemorrhage emergency trolley* set up in the labour ward with all the basic equipment and drugs for initiating resuscitation may be useful. At least two large-bore intravenous cannulae, preferably 14 gauge, should be inserted into suitable sites without delay; compensatory peripheral vascular shutdown occurs to maintain blood pressure and it can rapidly become very difficult to gain satisfactory venous access. The expertise of an anaesthetist can be life saving in this situation.

It may become difficult to crossmatch blood after a large blood transfusion because of replacement with donor red cells, therefore at least 20–25 ml of blood should be taken as soon as possible and sent urgently to the appropriate laboratory for:

- crossmatching at least 6 units of packed red cells (at least 10 ml clotted blood)

- haemoglobin, packed cell volume and platelet count (4 ml EDTA blood)
- coagulation screening tests, activated partial thromboplastin time, thrombin time, prothrombin time and fibrinogen D-dimers (5 ml clotted blood)
- baseline urea and electrolytes (5 ml clotted blood).

The Royal College of Obstetricians and Gynaecologists recommend that uncrossmatched blood should be available within 10 minutes and crossmatched blood within 30 minutes (Royal College of Obstetricians and Gynaecologists 1994). The blood transfusion laboratory staff should be informed immediately of the situation and the possible urgent need for very large amounts of blood and blood products. The hospital porters should be informed of the emergency situation. A consultant haematologist should be involved at an early stage. The blood transfusion laboratory staff should be involved in the development of unit protocols and guidelines, and in rehearsal emergency drills. Some blood transfusion laboratories have their own internal procedures in place to deal with requests arising from massive haemorrhage; the laboratory should also be informed once the emergency is over.

A recurring factor in Maternal Mortality Reports is delay in calling senior staff, possibly owing to inexperience, ignorance, underestimation of blood loss or bravado. The most senior resident obstetrician and resident anaesthetist should be summoned and the on-call consultant obstetrician and anaesthetist informed immediately. The midwife in charge should also be informed immediately and should allocate extra staff to help.

Fluid replacement should be commenced immediately. Crystalloid solutions such as Hartmann's solution or 0.9% saline should be infused rapidly to restore systolic blood pressure (although saline is best avoided in patients with pre-eclampsia or liver disease). Glucose-containing solutions are less effective as less fluid is retained in the intravascular space. If the patient remains hypotensive and hypovolaemic after rapid infusion of two litres of crystalloid, and blood is not yet available, a colloid such as Gelfusion may be commenced, although large volumes (>1500 ml in 24 h) may affect haemostatic function (Bonnar 2000). Dextran interferes with crossmatching and affects platelet function; it should therefore be avoided (Drugs and Therapeutics Bulletin 1992). Colloid solutions including modified fluid gelatin (Gelfusion, Haemaccel), hydroxyethyl starch (Hespan), dextran and human albumin are more expensive than crystalloids, and do not improve survival (Schierhout & Roberts 1998). Infusion of human albumin may be associated with an increased mortality risk in critically ill patients (Cochrane Injuries Group Albumin reviewers 1998). The Committee on Safety of Medicines concluded that further clinical trials are needed to clarify this issue and recommended that patients should be monitored carefully if albumin is used to correct hypovolaemia as there is a risk of hypervolaemia and cardiovascular overload (Woodman 1999).

Accurate records of fluid input and output should be kept. It is difficult to keep track of events when massive haemorrhage occurs. One midwife should be assigned to keep records of patient observations, fluid input and output, and any drugs administered. Standard observations of pulse, blood pressure and temperature should be continued at intervals dictated by the condition of the patient. Oxygen should be given by facemask at a flow rate of 10–15 litres per minute and a pulse oximeter attached to monitor oxygen saturation. Continuous ECG monitoring should be carried out. An indwelling urinary catheter is essential to assess urinary output, which is a useful indicator of tissue perfusion. An output of 30–60 ml/h indicates adequate volume replacement. If urine output is less than 30 ml/h despite apparently adequate volume replacement, a better method is required. Once initial resuscitation is under way, a central venous line should be put up to help assess the intravascular compartment and determine the need for further fluid replacement. If there are cardiac or respiratory problems (e.g. coexisting cardiac disease, severe pre-eclampsia or adult respiratory distress syndrome), it is preferable to measure the pulmonary capillary wedge pressure with a Swan–Ganz catheter but this should normally only be inserted in the intensive care unit. An arterial line may be used to monitor blood pressure and blood gases. Invasive monitoring techniques can have serious complications and should be used only when absolutely necessary, preferably with the involvement of an experienced anaesthetist; great care and attention needs to be taken if coagulopathy is present.

Blood transfusion provides volume replacement and oxygen-carrying capacity. Six units of packed red cells is the minimum amount that should be ordered initially; 10–20 units are often used and sometimes massive blood transfusion of over 100 units of blood may be required. Good communication is essential: laboratory staff, porters and the consultant haematologist should all be informed of the urgency of the situation as early as possible so that the required amount of blood and blood products can be supplied. Concentrated stored red cells are generally used; fresh whole blood is not available in the United Kingdom because plasma and platelets are removed from donated whole blood for separate use. The patient's blood group, rhesus type and antibody status are usually determined during pregnancy, which facilitates rapid crossmatching of blood. Type-specific ABO compatible blood without antibody screening carries a slightly higher risk of haemolytic transfusion reaction but may be used in an emergency until fully crossmatched blood is ready. Uncrossmatched O Rh-negative blood is usually available in all labour wards and may be used in cases of dire emergency. Blood must be infused through a separate intravenous line from crystalloids, and no other infusion solutions or drugs should be added to any blood or blood product as clotting may occur. A blood filter and suitable approved blood warmer should be used and a rapid infusion pressure system is recommended. It is also important to keep the patient warm, as hypothermia will exacerbate poor peripheral perfusion, acidosis and the development of coagulopathy.

Coagulopathy

In major haemorrhage, replacement of lost blood by concentrated stored red cells and large amounts of crystalloid will result in a dilutional coagulopathy. Stored packed red cells available for transfusion contain negligible amounts of platelets and clotting factors. Dilutional coagulopathy is likely to occur once 80% of the original blood volume has been replaced and is manifest by prolonged bleeding and oozing from puncture sites and wounds or incisions, bruising, and poor or no clot formation. Fresh frozen plasma contains all the clotting factors and at least two units of fresh frozen plasma should be transfused for every six units of red cells, guided by results of coagulation studies, which should be carried out at frequent intervals. While waiting for laboratory results, a quick guide to the coagulation state may be obtained at the bedside by taking some blood into a plain glass tube and observing the clotting time, the quality of the clot and whether the clot breaks down quickly, suggesting active fibrinolysis. If the platelet count falls below 50×10^9/l, platelets should be transfused (see Ch. 20). Blood transfusion giving sets and blood filters are unsuitable for platelet transfusion. The blood transfusion laboratory often supplies a special giving set.

Acute disseminated intravascular coagulation may occur with amniotic fluid embolism or in association with placental abruption or severe pre-eclampsia. In this situation, the thrombin clotting time will be excessively prolonged, fibrinogen decreased, and fibrin degradation products such as D-dimer raised. Cryoprecipitate, which contains more fibrinogen than fresh frozen plasma, may be given if the fibrinogen level is less than 1.0 g/dl, or pure recombinant fibrinogen may be given if available (see Ch. 20).

As soon as resuscitation is under way steps must be taken to identify the cause and stop the bleeding. Delay can be fatal—blood and fluid replacement is slow in comparison to the huge amounts of blood that can be lost in minutes or even seconds in some cases of obstetric haemorrhage. It is essential to keep ahead of the blood loss. The decision to undertake surgery should not be delayed although the patient should be resuscitated and coagulopathy corrected as far as possible before any major surgical procedure is undertaken. When attempting to control severe haemorrhage by surgical means, it may be impossible to control the bleeding and keep pace with the amount of coagulation factors required. Temporary measures to staunch the haemorrhage by pressure on the aorta, by ligation of the uterine vessels or by large packs in the case of severe pelvic venous haemorrhage, may allow time to correct coagulation factors with beneficial effects on the permanent arrest of bleeding (Rennie & Cardozo 1998).

Occasionally patients have known coagulation disorders caused by liver disease, autoimmune disease or inherited vascular, platelet or coagulation factor deficiencies, or come to delivery while anticoagulated for medical reasons, usually with heparin. These situations can usually be anticipated and special care should be taken to avoid haemorrhage.

Uterine atony

Uterine atony, when the contraction and retraction of the uterus, so vital for haemostasis after delivery, fails to occur, is the commonest cause of postpartum haemorrhage. The uterus remains soft, boggy and relaxed; it either completely fails to contract or does not maintain its contraction. Possible causes include retained placenta or blood clot, uterine overdistension by multiple pregnancy, large fetus or polyhydramnios, impairment of contractile and retractile function by uterine fibroids or placenta praevia, or diffuse bleeding into the myometrium during placental abruption.

The first step is to rub up a contraction. If the uterus remains atonic or repeatedly relaxes despite attempts to rub up contractions, check that the bladder is empty and oxytocics have been given. A second intravenous injection of ergometrine may be given unless contraindicated. Venous access with two large-bore cannulae should be established and blood taken for crossmatching. An oxytocin infusion of 40 units of syntocinon in 1 litre of Hartmann's solution at 150–250 ml/h should be in place. Retained products of conception may be the cause of atony. If the placenta is undelivered, active management of the third stage is performed. If this fails, manual removal may be required. Once delivered, the placenta and membranes should be examined carefully to see whether they are complete. If equipment is available in the labour ward, an ultrasound scan will indicate whether the uterine cavity is empty. If retained products are suspected, the uterine cavity must be explored and any pieces of placenta, membranes or blood clot removed. The uterus may be explored immediately if effective epidural analgesia is in place. If not, epidural and spinal anaesthetics are relatively contraindicated in the presence of major haemorrhage with cardiovascular instability or possible coagulopathy; a general anaesthetic may be given, remembering that drugs used in general anaesthesia, particularly halothane, contribute to uterine relaxation.

Carboprost (15-methyl prostaglandin $F_{2\alpha}$ tromethamine) 250 μg given by intramuscular injection stimulates myometrial contraction and may be used if conventional treatment fails (Oleen & Mariano 1990). The dose may be repeated after 90 minutes if required. This interval may be reduced to not less than 15 minutes. The total dose should not exceed 2 mg (8 doses). Prostaglandin $F_{2\alpha}$ causes a rise in heart rate, blood pressure, cardiac output and pulmonary vascular resistance; side effects include diarrhoea, vomiting, pyrexia, flushing, headache, hypertension, bronchospasm and fall in Po_2 from intrapulmonary shunting, therefore it should be used very cautiously in women with pre-eclampsia or a history of cardiac problems or asthma. Other prostaglandin products have also been used to treat atonic uterine haemorrhage by intramuscular or intravenous injection, by direct injection or infusion into the myometrium or uterine cavity, or by placing pessaries in the uterus or vagina. Prostaglandin E_2 (dinoprostone) is primarily a vasodilator and may produce severe hypotension.

Bimanual compression may be employed if uterine atony persists or to control bleeding while waiting for drugs to act or while preparing for hysterectomy. The uterus is compressed between the operator's vaginal hand, pushing the uterus upwards and stretching the uterine arteries, and the abdominal hand. The aorta may be compressed against the sacral promontory.

Hysterectomy is the definitive treatment for persistent uterine atony. Depending on the circumstances, subtotal hysterectomy may be a better option than total hysterectomy. The decision should be made by a consultant obstetrician and should not be delayed as prompt action may be life saving. Depending on the situation, this should only be done when all available conservative measures have been tried first.

Uterine packing is still a useful technique in appropriate circumstances (Maier 1993). Haemorrhage is controlled by applying pressure to the bleeding source until the uterus regains its ability to maintain contraction and retraction and adequate blood coagulation has been restored; this may be particularly useful in dealing with haemorrhage from a placental bed in the lower uterine segment, which has less muscle than the upper part of the uterus. Other sources of bleeding, such as uterine perforation or rupture, should be excluded first. Under adequate analgesia or anaesthesia, the uterus, starting from the fundus, should be packed as tightly as possible with lengths of gauze (dry or soaked in cold or hot saline or in povidone–iodine) tied together; the vagina should be packed as well. The anterior and posterior lips of the cervix may be steadied using ring forceps during the procedure. Oxytocics should be used. Broad-spectrum antibiotic cover should be given and an indwelling catheter left in the bladder. If bleeding is successfully controlled, the pack should be removed after 24–36 hours with facilities for resorting to immediate surgery if necessary. Successful cases of balloon tamponade using multiple Foley catheters or a Sengstaken–Blakemore tube inserted into the uterus and inflated have also been described (Katesmark et al 1994, DeLoor & vanDam 1996).

Successful arterial embolisation, usually by the internal iliac arteries, has been reported in cases of persistent bleeding after hysterectomy, where hysterectomy was contraindicated, or bleeding from cervical or vaginal lacerations. This technique can only be carried out in specialist centres by an experienced angiographic radiologist (Drife 1997). There are risks of infection, vascular injury, radiation exposure and sciatic nerve injury; collateral circulation preserves tissue viability and uterine function.

Finally, oversewing the uterus with Vicryl or Dexon, passed through the anterior and posterior lower segment and tied at the fundus (the Brace suture), may be effective and avoid the need for hysterectomy (B-Lynch et al 1997; see below).

Lower genital tract trauma

If the uterus is well contracted and the placenta has been delivered and appears complete, the most likely cause of persistent bleeding is genital tract trauma. Episiotomy, vaginal or cervical tears, vulval, vaginal or broad ligament haematoma, and ruptured uterus may be the source of bleeding. Rarely, ruptured liver, especially in severe pre-eclampsia, ruptured splenic artery aneurysm or some other intra-abdominal catastrophe may be the cause.

First, the lower genital tract should be properly inspected; this requires good relaxation, good light and good assistance. The source of bleeding should be identified and repaired. The patient should be placed in the lithotomy position. Effective regional analgesia or general anaesthesia is required to undertake a thorough assessment of the genital tract. A digital exploration of the lower uterine segment is performed to exclude a rupture. Persistent bleeding from this source necessitates laparotomy to repair the lesion and arrest the haemorrhage. The lower genital tract is then inspected. Proper exposure of the cervix and upper vagina is essential and the operator will require assistance. Two large retractors are inserted into the vagina to separate the walls laterally. A pair of obstetric forceps with the blades at 180° to their usual orientation can provide large and readily available retraction. Ring forceps are then placed on the anterior and posterior edges of the cervix which is pulled down and carefully inspected. It is most important to examine the lateral margins of the cervix which are a common site of a laceration and the source of the bleeding. If present, a laceration is promptly repaired with figure-of-eight sutures; the highest suture must be placed above the apex of the tear. If an episiotomy has been performed, the upper limit of this wound is inspected and care is taken to identify any extension into the upper vagina. The wall of the vagina and underlying tissues are repaired with deep figure-of-eight sutures to close the defect and ensure haemostasis.

Uterine rupture

Rupture of a previous caesarean section scar is the commonest cause of uterine rupture in the developed world. A previous lower segment scar carries a 0.25–0.5% risk of rupture, compared with a vertical (classical) scar where the risk of rupture is 3–4% (Ritchie 1971). Previous scar rupture carries a much higher risk of recurrent rupture (Ch. 37). Other factors predisposing to uterine rupture are a history of myomectomy, external cephalic version, operative vaginal delivery, trauma, use of oxytocics, high parity and obstructed labour, particularly in developing countries. Uterine rupture may be incomplete or complete, where rupture extends through all layers of the uterine wall and serosa. If rupture occurs before delivery, signs and symptoms usually include abdominal pain, vaginal bleeding, fetal heart rate abnormality and easy palpation of fetal parts through the abdominal wall as the fetus is partially or completely extruded from the uterus.

Treatment is resuscitation and immediate delivery, usually by caesarean section followed by repair of the uterus. If rupture is not diagnosed until after delivery, it may be suspected by signs of collapse or hypovolaemic shock associated with some vaginal bleeding and lower abdominal pain, and there may be a relevant history. Shoulder tip pain from haemoperitoneum may be present. If uterine rupture and intraperitoneal bleeding is suspected, an abdominal ultrasound scan may demonstrate the presence of intraperitoneal fluid. Vaginal examination with palpation of the lower uterine segment may reveal the defect in the uterine wall. Such an examination should not, however, be performed routinely, as it may cause a rupture where none previously existed, and it has not been shown to be effective in revealing occult ruptures.

Laparotomy should be performed by a consultant. Various surgical techniques designed to control uterine haemorrhage caused by atony or rupture without resorting to hysterectomy have been described. Excessive bleeding from the placental bed at caesarean section may be controlled with figure-of-eight sutures and oxytocics (generally, getting the uterus to contract is a much more effective way to control bleeding than local suturing). Ligation of the arterial supply to the uterus may control haemorrhage sufficiently to avoid hysterectomy. Bilateral mass ligation of the uterine arteries and veins at caesarean section by placing a suture to include 2–3 cm of myometrium at a level 2–3 cm below the uterine incision, with careful attention to avoid inadvertent ligation of the ureter, is the most straightforward technique and was successful in all but 10 of 265 cases of bleeding at caesarean section over a 30-year period (O'Leary 1995). Stepwise uterine devascularisation was successful in a series of 103 patients (AbdRabbo 1994). The sequence described was:

1. unilateral uterine vessel ligation, at the upper part of the lower uterine segment
2. bilateral uterine vessel ligation
3. low uterine vessel ligation, to include the cervicovaginal branches after mobilisation of the bladder and taking care to avoid the ureters
4. unilateral ovarian vessel ligation
5. bilateral ovarian vessel ligation.

Bilateral internal iliac or hypogastric artery ligation is successful in preventing hysterectomy in 42–50% of patients at best; complications include damage to other pelvic vessels, ureteric damage and considerable operative morbidity (Clark et al 1985, Gilstrap & Ramin 1994). These procedures should only be attempted by a surgeon of considerable experience, possibly a vascular surgeon.

The success of these procedures in the short term to control bleeding and in the long term to preserve uterine function may depend on the collateral circulation, the skill of the surgeon and the presence of other complications. Large compression sutures placed across the uterine body with inversion of the fundus (Schnarwyler et al 1996) and the B-Lynch technique, which compresses the uterus by a belt and braces type of suture without inverting the fundus (B-Lynch et al 1997), have been used to control haemorrhage from the atonic uterus which has failed to respond to medical therapy. Considerations of age, parity and the wishes of the patient are important when deciding whether to attempt conservative surgery. Time is not on the surgeon's side and prompt hysterectomy may be a life-saving procedure. Hysterectomy may be total or subtotal depending on individual circumstances.

Long-term complications

Patients who have massive haemorrhage may develop renal, liver or pituitary failure and will generally require transfer to renal or intensive care units. Improvements in intensive care have led to longer survival but some patients may succumb to adult respiratory distress syndrome. Long-term sequelae include renal failure and Sheehan's syndrome (avascular necrosis of the pituitary gland characterised by failure of lactation followed by amenorrhoea, hypothyroidism and adrenocortical insufficiency).

WOMEN WHO REFUSE BLOOD TRANSFUSION

A few women do not accept blood transfusion because of specific personal or religious beliefs: members of the Jehovah's Witnesses believe that the Bible forbids the consumption of blood or blood products. Specific recommendations for the management of women who are likely to refuse blood transfusion even in the face of life-threatening haemorrhage are detailed in the 1991–1993 Confidential Enquiry into Maternal Deaths (Department of Health 1996), where it is estimated that the death rate from haemorrhage in such women would be approximately 1 in 1000 compared with an expected incidence of less than 1 in 100 000 maternities in the UK. Such patients should be identified at an early stage during pregnancy. Appropriate documented discussion should take place to make sure that they are fully informed about the risks of refusing blood transfusion in the event of massive haemorrhage and to establish their precise wishes if this situation should occur. Many hospitals have a Jehovah's Witnesses Hospital Liaison Committee who may be involved in discussions, and there are usually specific operation consent forms for Jehovah's Witnesses.

Every effort should be made to avoid the occurrence of obstetric haemorrhage and to minimise its effects. This includes antenatal prevention of anaemia by supplementary haematinics throughout pregnancy (the use of erythropoeitin has also been suggested), ultrasound identification of the placental site, close supervision of the management of labour by experienced senior staff including the consultant obstetrician, and prompt action if haemorrhage should occur. The threshold for intervention should be lower than in other patients. Careful attention to maintaining blood volume, anaesthetic procedures and surgical technique to minimise blood loss, the use of drugs such as aprotinin or intravenous antifibrinolytics to reduce blood loss during surgery, or desmopressin to reduce acute bleeding may be helpful. In some cases it may be possible to salvage the patient's own blood and re-infuse it directly via a closed circuit (Spence 1995). In cases with a high risk of haemorrhage, a unit of blood can be taken each week for up to six weeks before a planned delivery and used for autologous transfusion.

OTHER CAUSES OF COLLAPSE WITHIN 24 HOURS OF DELIVERY

A diagnosis of significant haemorrhage is usually obvious by the extent of revealed blood loss. However in some cases of haemorrhage, for example resulting from uterine rupture, most of the blood loss may be concealed and, conversely, not all cases of postpartum collapse or apparent shock with hypotension are caused by haemorrhage. Other conditions that may result in a similar clinical picture are listed in Table 38.4.

These conditions should be borne in mind as they require specific therapeutic measures; inappropriate resuscitation involving the intravenous infusion of large volumes of fluid could seriously harm patients with these conditions. A history of hypertension or pre-eclampsia, previous thromboembolic disease, cardiac disease, diabetes, factors such as prolonged rupture of the membranes predisposing to infection or administration of general anaesthesia during labour, delivery or third stage may be relevant in making the correct diagnosis. Symptoms of chest pain or breathlessness are also significant.

Table 38.4   Causes of postpartum collapse

- Massive postpartum haemorrhage
- Amniotic fluid embolism
- Pulmonary embolism
- Acute cardiac failure in a patient with existing valvular disease or cardiomyopathy
- Mendelson's syndrome (pneumonitis due to inhalation of gastric contents)
- Pneumothorax
- Eclampsia
- Septicaemia
- Hypoglycaemia
- Cardiovascular accident
- Myocardial infarction

AMNIOTIC FLUID EMBOLISM

Amniotic fluid embolism is rare; it occurs in 1:20 000 deliveries (Gilbert & Danielsen 1999) to 1:80 000 deliveries (Garland & Thompson 1983) but has a high maternal and perinatal mortality rate. The true incidence and mortality rate is difficult to establish. The maternal mortality rate has been reported as 61%, with intact neurological survival rate of 15%, and a perinatal mortality rate of 79% of undelivered fetuses (Clark et al 1995). In another series (Gilbert & Danielsen 1999), maternal mortality was 26.4%. Amniotic fluid embolism was the third commonest cause of direct maternal death in the UK in the triennium 1994–1996 (Department of Health 1998): there were 17 deaths from amniotic fluid embolism compared with 10 in 1991–1993, 11 proven and one diagnosed on clinical grounds in 1998–1990, and nine in 1985–1987. Amniotic fluid and particulate matter escape into the maternal circulation to cause an anaphylactic reaction and the diagnosis is ultimately confirmed by the histological finding of fetal squames or hair in the maternal lungs at autopsy. In the 1991–1993

Confidential Enquiry into Maternal Deaths (1996) it was accepted that a diagnosis of amniotic fluid embolism could be made if the clinical presentation of sudden collapse followed rapidly by cyanosis and then by the development of coagulopathy and bleeding was present and no other explanation could be found. This may partly account for the increased incidence of amniotic fluid embolism in the 1994–1996 Report.

Amniotic fluid embolism may occur during labour (70%), during caesarean section (19%) or immediately postpartum (11%). It characteristically presents with sudden cardiovascular and respiratory collapse followed by the development of coagulopathy; subsequent deterioration and death may occur very rapidly. Predisposing causes remain obscure. Amniotic fluid embolism is rare under the age of 25; the incidence increases with increasing maternal age. The use of oxytocic drugs is thought to be a risk factor, yet in the 1994–1996 triennium in the UK, nine of the women who died as a result of amniotic fluid embolism had not received either prostaglandin or oxytocin. However, only one case occurred in a woman of low parity with a straightforward pregnancy. It was suggested that mortality from amniotic fluid embolism could be reduced by avoiding uterine overstimulation, by prompt diagnosis of obstructed labour, and by better treatment of women who survive long enough to be transferred to intensive care.

The diagnosis is essentially clinical and there is no specific treatment. Management consists of basic life support; respiratory support with endotracheal intubation, mechanical ventilation with 100% oxygen and positive end-expiratory pressure is likely to be required. Massive haemorrhage resulting from coagulopathy should be anticipated and managed as outlined earlier in this chapter. Immediate delivery, usually by caesarean section under general anaesthesia, should be performed. It may be worth giving adrenaline, hydrocortisone or piriton, although there is no evidence for or against their use. Left ventricular failure is a feature of the condition, and cardiac inotropes guided by invasive monitoring may be of benefit (Clark 1990). Cardiac arrest is likely and resuscitation should be attempted. The patient will usually require transfer to an intensive care unit if and when her condition allows this.

SECONDARY POSTPARTUM HAEMORRHAGE

Secondary postpartum haemorrhage is defined as any sudden loss of blood (regardless of volume) from the genital tract occurring after the first 24 hours postpartum and within 6 weeks of delivery. The reported incidence ranges from 0.5% to 1.5%. Most secondary postpartum haemorrhage results from retained and often infected products of conception. Tissue remaining in the uterus forms a favourable medium for bacteria. Rarely, secondary postpartum haemorrhage may result from a submucous fibromyoma or a choriocarcinoma. The bleeding may be preceded by an offensive and/or persistently red lochia, subinvolution of the uterus and a low-grade pyrexia. The condition is most commonly seen 5–15 days postpartum. Most women with secondary postpartum haemorrhage have not lost sufficient blood to become

shocked. An ultrasound scan should be performed—if the uterine cavity is empty and there is no evidence of infection conservative management may be employed. In all cases, a high vaginal swab should be taken for culture. The patient should be treated with antibiotics effective against aerobic and anaerobic organisms. If the ultrasound scan shows the presence of retained products within the uterine cavity (Fig. 38.2) then evacuation of the uterus should be undertaken under general anaesthesia. It should be remembered that nearly all postpartum uteri will show high-level echoes in the endometrial cavity because of retained clot and placental fragments; an endometrial diameter of up to 2 cm is probably

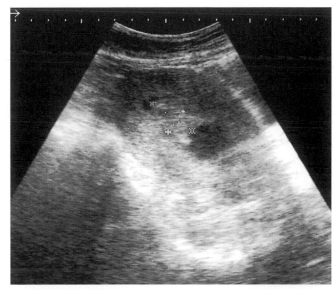

(a)

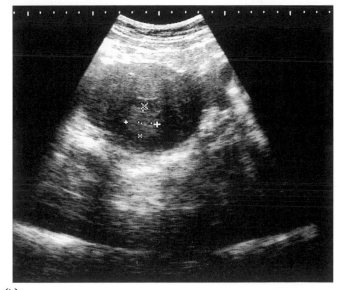

(b)

Fig. 38.2 Longitudinal (a) and transverse (b) ultrasound scans of the uterus showing retained products of conception; the patient was 9 days postpartum and presented with secondary postpartum haemorrhage.

normal. Inexperienced sonographers often report such clot as retained products of conception, leading to an unnecessary evacuation of the uterus with all its attendant risks. It is therefore important that scans are undertaken by appropriately experienced staff. Evacuation of the uterus requires care as the postpartum uterus is soft and the risk of perforation is high. It should be undertaken by a senior obstetrician. Any tissues obtained should be sent for histological examination. If there is clinical evidence of sepsis (pyrexia, offensive discharge, lower abdominal pain and uterine tenderness) evacuation of retained products should be delayed for 12–24 hours, if the patient's condition permits, to allow appropriate broad-spectrum intravenous antibiotics to be given and reduce the risk of septicaemia following curettage. On rare occasions, secondary postpartum haemorrhage may be severe and cause shock. Bleeding may originate from blood vessels on the placental bed or from a healing caesarean section scar. Oxytocic drugs are rarely effective in dealing with this problem. Uterine packing may occasionally be of benefit. In exceptional cases with persistent secondary postpartum haemorrhage it may be necessary to undertake uterine artery ligation or hysterectomy.

KEY POINTS

- Postpartum haemorrhage is a leading cause of maternal mortality.
- Causes: uterine atony (90%), genital tract trauma, coagulopathy.
- Routine oxytocics and controlled cord traction in third stage are effective preventive measures.
- Maternity units should have well-rehearsed protocols for the management of massive haemorrhage.
- A contraction should be rubbed up and large-bore venous access sited. Appropriate resuscitation, including blood transfusion and treatment of coagulopathy, should be commenced.
- Senior obstetricians and anaesthetists should be directly involved in management.
- Uterine atony should be treated by oxytocic drugs and carboprost; retained products and genital tract trauma should be excluded.
- Conservative methods of controlling haemorrhage may be appropriate in some cases, but early resort to hysterectomy may be life-saving.

REFERENCES

AbdRabbo SA 1994 Stepwise uterine devascularisation: A novel technique for management of uncontrollable postpartum haemorrhage with preservation of the uterus. Am J Obstet Gynecol 171:694–700

Abouleish E, Ali V, Joumaa B et al 1995 Anaesthetic management of acute puerperal uterine inversion. Br J Anaesth 75:486–487

American College of Obstetricians and Gynaecologists 1997 Hemorrhagic shock. ACOG Educational Bulletin, no. 235

B-Lynch C, Coker A, Lawal AH, Abu J, Cowen MJ 1997 The B-Lynch surgical technique for the control of massive postpartum haemorrhage: an alternative to hysterectomy? Five cases reported. Br J Obstet Gynaecol 104:372–375

Bonnar J 2000 Massive obstetric haemorrhage. In: Thompson W, TambyRaja RL (eds) Emergencies in obstetrics and gynaecology. Bailliere-Tindall, London, ch 1, pp. 1–18

Brar HS, Greenspoon JS, Platt LD, Paul RH 1989 Acute puerperal uterine inversion. J Reprod Med 34:173–177

Carroli G, Bergel E 2000 Umbilical vein injection for management of retained placenta (Cochrane Review). In: The Cochrane Library, Issue 1. Update Software, Oxford

Catanzarite VA, Moffitt KD, Baker ML et al 1986 New approach to the management of acute puerperal uterine inversion. Obstet Gynecology 68 (suppl): 7–10

Clark SL 1984 Use of ritodrine in uterine inversion. Am J Obstet Gynecol 151:705

Clark SL 1990 New concepts of amniotic fluid embolism: a review. Obstet Gynecol Surv 45:360–368

Clark SL, Phelan JP, Yeh SY, Bruce SR, Paul RH 1985 Hypogastric artery ligation for obstetric haemorrhage. Obstet Gynecol 66:353–356

Clark SL, Hankins GDV, Dudley DA, Dildy GA, Porter TF 1995 Amniotic fluid embolism: Analysis of the national registry. Am J Obstet Gynecol 172:1158–1169

Cochrane Injuries Group Albumin reviewers 1998 Human albumin administration in critically ill patients: systematic review of randomised controlled trials. Br Med J 317:235–240

Cox SM, Carpenter RJ, Cotton DB 1988 Placenta percreta: ultrasound diagnosis and conservative surgical management. Obstet Gynecol 71:454–456

Das P 1940 Inversion of the uterus. J Obstet Gynaecol Br Empire 47:525–548

Datta S 1991 Anaesthesia and obstetric management of high-risk pregnancy. Mosby Year Book, St. Louis

DeLoor JA, vanDam PA 1996 Foley catheters for uncontrollable obstetric or gynecological haemorrhage. Obstet Gynecol 88:737

Department of Health 1994 Report on Confidential Enquiries into Maternal Deaths in the United Kingdom 1988–1990. HMSO, London

Department of Health 1996 Report on Confidential Enquiries into Maternal Deaths in the United Kingdom 1991–1993. HMSO, London

Department of Health 1998 Why mothers die. Report on Confidential Enquiries into Maternal Deaths in the United Kingdom 1994–1996. HMSO, London

Drife J 1997 Management of primary postpartum haemorrhage. Br J Obstet Gynaecol 104:275–277

Drugs and Therapeutics Bulletin 1992 The management of postpartum haemorrhage. Drug Ther Bull 30:89–92

El-Refaey H, O'Brien P, Morafa W, Walder J, Rodeck C 1997 Use of oral misoprostol in the prevention of postpartum haemorrhage. Br J Obstet Gynaecol 104:336–339

Fahmy M 1977 Acute inversion of the uterus. Int J Surg 62:100

Fox H 1972 Placenta accreta 1945–1969. Obstet Gynecol Surv 27:475

Garland I, Thompson W 1983 Diagnosis of amniotic fluid embolism using antiserum to human keratin. J Clin Pathol 36:625

Gibb DMF, Soothill PW, Ward KJ 1994 Conservative management of placenta accreta. Br J Obstet Gynaecol 101:79–80

Gilbert WM, Danielsen B 1999 Amniotic fluid embolism: decreased mortality in population-based study. Obstet Gynecol 93(6):973–977

Gilstrap LC, Ramin SM 1994 Postpartum haemorrhage. Clin Obstet Gynecol 37:824–830

Grossman RA 1981 Magnesium sulphate for uterine inversion. J Reprod Med 26:261–262

Gulmezoglu AM 1999 Prostaglandins for prevention of postpartum haemorrhage (Cochrane Review). In: The Cochrane Library, Issue 3. Update Software, Oxford

Haultain FWN 1901 The treatment of chronic uterine inversion by abdominal hysterotomy with a successful case. Br Med J ii:974

Huntington JL, Irving FC, Kellogg FS 1928 Abdominal reposition in acute inversion of the puerperal uterus. Am J Obstet Gynecol 15:34–40

Jouppila P 1995 Postpartum haemorrhage. Curr Opin Obstet Gynecol 7:446–450

Katesmark M, Brown R, Raju KS 1994 Successful use of a Sengstaken–Blakemore tube to control massive postpartum haemorrhage. Br J Obstet Gynaecol 101:259–260

McDonald S, Prendiville W, Blair E 1993 Randomised controlled trial of oxytocin alone versus oxytocin and ergometrine in active management of third stage of labour. Br Med J 307:1167–1171

Maier RC 1993 Control of postpartum haemorrhage with uterine packing. Am J Obstet Gynecol 169:317–323

Ogueh O, Ayida G 1997 Acute uterine inversion: a new technique of hydrostatic replacement. Br J Obstet Gynaecol 104(8):951–952

Oleen MA, Mariano JP 1990 Controlling refractory atonic postpartum haemorrhage with Hemabate sterile solution. Am J Obstet Gynecol 162:205–208

O'Leary JA 1995 Uterine artery ligation in the control of postcaesarean haemorrhage. J Reprod Med 40:189–193

O'Sullivan JV 1945 Acute inversion of the uterus. Br Med J 2:282–283

Oxorn H 1986 Human labor and birth. Appleton Century Crofts,

Prendiville WJ, Elbourne D 1989 Care during the third stage of labour. In: Chalmers I, Enkin M, Keirse MJNC (eds) Effective care in pregnancy and childbirth. Oxford University Press, Oxford, pp 1145–1169

Prendiville WJ, Elbourne D, Chalmers I 1988 The effects of routine oxytocic administration in the management of the third stage of labour: an overview of the evidence from controlled trials. Br J Obstet Gynaecol 95:3–16

Read JA, Cotton DB, Miller FC 1980 Placenta accreta: changing clinical aspects and outcome. Obstet Gynecol 56:31

Rennie J, Cardozo L 1998 The seven surgeons of King's: a fable by Aesop. Br J Obstet Gynaecol 105:1241

Ritchie EH 1971 Pregnancy after rupture of the pregnant uterus. J Obstet Gynaecol Br Commonwealth 78:642–648

Roberts WE 1995 Emergent obstetric management of postpartum haemorrhage. Obstet Gynecol Clin North Am 22:283–302

Royal College of Obstetricians and Gynaecologists 1994 Deriving standards from the Maternal Mortality reports. RCOG, London

Schierhout G, Roberts I 1998 Fluid resuscitation with colloid or crystalloid solutions in critically ill patients: a systematic review of randomised trials. Br Med J 316:961–964

Schnarwyler B, Passweg D, von Castelberg B 1996 Erfolgreiche Behandlung eine medikamentos refraktaren Uterusatonie durch Funduskompressionsnahte. Geburtshilfe Fraunheilkundl 56:151–153

Spence RK 1995 Surgical red cell blood transfusion practice policies. Blood management policies for Jehovah's Witnesses. Am J Surg 170(6A, suppl):14–15

Stones RW, Paterson CM, Saunders NStG 1993 Risk factors for major obstetric haemorrhage. Eur J Obstet Gynecol Reprod Biol 48:15–18

Walker ID, Walker JJ, Colvin BT, Letsky EA, Rivers R, Stevens R 1994 Investigation and management of haematological disorders in pregnancy. J Clin Pathol 47:100 108

Watson P, Besch N, Bowes WA 1980 Management of acute and subacute puerperal inversion of the uterus. Obstet Gynecol 55:12

Wendel PJ, Cox SM 1995 Emergent obstetric management of uterine inversion. Obstet Gynecol Clin North Am 22(2):261–274

Woodman R 1999 Doctors advised to take special care with human albumin. Br Med J 318:1643

Section 6
THE PUERPERIUM

39

The physiology of the puerperium

Frank Hytten

INTRODUCTION

That period in a woman's life which follows childbirth may be one of the most physiologically dramatic she will face. In pregnancy the body is subject to physiological turmoil on a scale not otherwise experienced in healthy adult life. No system escapes; there are huge changes in cardiovascular, respiratory and renal function, and widespread metabolic upheaval most evident in the grossly altered composition of the blood. Hytten & Leitch (1971) commented that

> It is reasonable to assume that, in health, the body maintains in its fluid environment the amounts and concentrations of the substances it needs for maximum efficiency of function; that is the purpose of homeostasis. If that is so then the greatly altered amounts and concentrations which are characteristic of pregnancy cannot reasonably be assumed to be equally advantageous to the mother's metabolism. The most plausible explanation is that they represent changes which allow maximum efficiency of

fetal growth and metabolism. The fetus, using hormones as manipulators, overrides and resets the mother's homeostatic mechanisms in its own interests; it is the price of viviparity.

After months adapting to fetal demands, the baby is born and the mother finds herself without a fetus but still physiologically pregnant. How she extricates herself from that situation, the winding down process which returns her to a non-pregnant state, is the physiology of the puerperium.

The widely accepted length of the puerperium is 6 weeks, but whether the figure derives from the ubiquitous use of 40 days to delineate that and many other aspects of medical, social and religious customs is unclear (Hytten 1995). It certainly has no basis in physiology; some pregnancy changes revert within minutes or hours of birth, others take days or weeks, and some never return to the situation prior to the first pregnancy.

Two major pitfalls await those studying the literature in this field. One is that many papers, almost all in the early literature, fail to state the precise time after delivery when observations were made, and where rapid changes are occurring such findings are uninterpretable. The second is that clinical management is seldom described; it is almost always taken for granted and yet major changes have occurred in the past century, for example in time of ambulation, in diet and in the use of drugs, which can profoundly affect physiological behaviour. It is to be hoped that any future studies will avoid those defects.

What follows is based on a recent extensive review of the literature (Hytten 1995) and readers are referred to *The Clinical Physiology of the Puerperium* (1995) for details of documentation.

THE RECOVERY OF PELVIC ORGANS AND TISSUES

The uterus

When the baby has been born and the placenta expelled with a substantial proportion of the uterine lining, the 1 kg uterus must contract within a few minutes from a sac enclosing a volume of some 4.5 litres to one with no more than a nominal cavity; it is a remarkable achievement. Physiologically, the immediate priority is to prevent blood loss from the mass of blood vessels torn across when the placenta separates; this is met both by compression of the vessels by myometrial contraction and by enhanced blood-clotting activity (see below).

At a time when maternal death in the puerperium was commonplace, many uteri from autopsies must have been available for measurement, but few data have been published. In round figures it is probable that the average uterus has fallen in weight to 500 g by the end of the first week, and to 300 g after 2 weeks, reaching a non-pregnant weight after about 4 weeks. It seems certain that the nulliparous uterine size is never regained and there is a steady rise in the size of the non-pregnant uterus with increasing parity from an average of less than 50 g before the first pregnancy to more than 100 g after five or six pregnancies. The few ultrasound studies published suggest a steady fall in overall uterine length from about 18 cm after delivery to about 12 cm after a week, but with a shallower decline in anteroposterior diameter and myometrial thickness (Fig. 39.1). Despite popular belief, there is general agreement that breast feeding has no perceptible effect on the speed of uterine involution. Ultrasound studies have also shown that the normal non-pregnant situation in which the uterine cavity is no more than a potential space may not be achieved for at least 4 or 5 weeks; evidence of fluid, even gas, in the cavity is common.

It would appear that involution of the myometrium involves no loss of myometrial cells; associated with a conspicuous increase in protease activity they simply contract in size from a length in late pregnancy of some 500–800 μm to less than 100 μm. There is a parallel reduction in collagen and elastin content.

Myometrial function. While the myometrium is making arrangements to diminish itself, it must continue to contract, at least for a time, both to prevent blood loss from the torn vessels of the placental bed, and to expel the detritus of

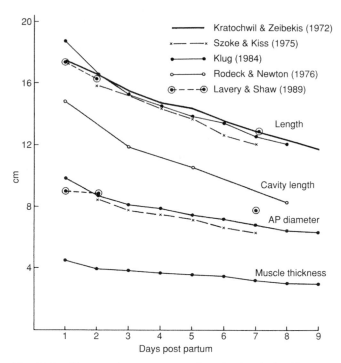

Fig. 39.1 Ultrasound measurement of uterine involution (for references see Hytten 1995).

endometrium and any remaining fragments of membranes and placenta. The pattern of contractions appears to be relatively uncoordinated. Uterine capillary blood flow, as indicated by the clearance of tracers from the myometrium, is considerably raised in the first few days of the puerperium. At the same time overall uterine blood flow is falling, Doppler ultrasound showing evidence of continuously increasing vascular resistance.

The endometrium. The decidua is, as its name denotes, the endometrium shed after parturition. There are three recognised layers: a surface, or zona compacta; a densely vascularised middle layer with glands, or zona spongiosa; and a zona basalis. As a general rule it is reckoned that the top two zones, compacta and spongiosa, which together form the zona functionalis, are shed after parturition; apart from the placental site, the basal zone remains to give rise to the new endometrium. The reality is more complex and more variable. In places a thick layer of decidua may be retained, in others only a few layers of cells, and in places the myometrium is almost bare. The new endometrium grows from the remaining gland stubs, and the mucosal surface, albeit thin, is complete within 14 days. A feature of the immediate puerperium, lasting for about 10 days, is a conspicuous infiltration of polymorphonuclear leucocytes and lymphocytes, after which a plasma cell and lymphocyte infiltration remains until about 60 days.

An exception to this general picture is the placental site, which takes much longer to recover; some evidence of the uteroplacental vasculature remains almost indefinitely. The arteries, after their initial clamping by myometrial contraction, become obliterated by an endarteritis and hyalinised within a week; the veins thrombose and become organised.

The terminal portions of the vessels, which form the bulk of the tissue in the raised placental site so characteristic of the recently emptied uterus, become necrotic and slough, but the hyalinised remains probably persist and provide clear evidence of a previous pregnancy. Although there may be some endometrial growth across the surface of the raised placental site, the definitive covering proceeds from the periphery of the site deep to the raised area, causing a considerable bulk of tissue consisting largely of necrotic vessel ends and some decidua to be shed. Thus, although a relatively normal endometrium may have returned by the conventional period of 6 weeks, and even early secretory characteristics have been observed by 7 weeks, some residua of pregnancy such as plasma cell infiltration and hyalinised decidua may persist for more than 20 weeks.

The cervix is generally damaged to some extent by birth; it remains open, sufficient to admit two fingers, for a few days, but by the end of the first week the os is closing. The damage, which is sufficiently common to be regarded as normal, is generally slight with lacerations, bruising, and ectopic columnar epithelium (ectropion) most usual, particularly in primiparae. In a small proportion of women some residual damage is still evident at 6–8 weeks. Cervical mucus is relatively sparse and electron microscopy shows a dense mesh of material and a high cellularity, with almost no interstitial spaces which would allow the passage of sperm, a condition that may remain for several months in breast feeding women.

Lochia. The lochial discharge consists of blood from the placental site together with the detritus of necrotic decidua and any trophoblastic remains. It begins as frank blood; when bleeding stops it remains red for a few days from disintegrating clot (lochia rubra), after which it becomes brownish pink (lochia serosa) and eventually yellow/white (lochia alba). For a phenomenon so universally recognised, the dearth of numerical information about it is remarkable.

Fallopian tubes

The considerable literature on changes in the tubes is confused. Some investigators have described a rapid increase within the first 10 days to a high secretory epithelium with well-formed vigorous cilia, while others have found a decline in the height and activity of the epithelium to that found in postmenopausal women. It seems certain that the finding of a proliferating epithelium was caused by the previous use of oestrogens to suppress lactation, but most papers do not give that information, and oestrogens are hardly ever used now for suppression of milk production.

The vagina

During the first few days after parturition the vagina appears as a capacious, smooth-walled passage, after which there is a gradual reduction in size with rugae appearing after 3 or 4 weeks. Histologically, there is progressive thinning to six or seven layers of cells by the end of 2 weeks, with no sign of cellular activity or glycogen storage, so that the epithelium resembles that of a postmenopausal vagina. Proliferative activity returns after 4–6 weeks and presumably depends on ovarian activity.

The pelvic floor

Some degree of pelvic floor damage is probably inevitable during a vaginal delivery. There is evidence of pelvic floor stretching and some pudendal nerve damage, even in women delivered by caesarean section if they had been in labour. This can be shown by magnetic resonance imaging. Defects can be classified by their site (Fig. 39.2). The damage is characteristic of a first delivery and does not usually progress with subsequent childbirth. The anal sphincter is also often subject to damage. There is usually some temporary functional impairment, but even without apparent injury long-term changes have been noted including anterior sphincter thinning and lateral external sphincter thickening.

(a) (b)

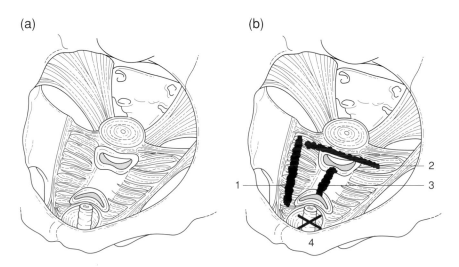

Fig. 39.2 The anopelvic fascia in (a) a nulliparous woman, (b) a multiparous woman. The supports of the vagina may be damaged and lead to prolapse years later. They can be classified as: (1) lateral (paravaginal); (2) transverse; (3) central; (4) distal (pubocervical). (From Quinn & Roberts 1999.)

The pelvic joints

Relaxation of the pelvic joints, particularly the symphysis pubis, is characteristic of pregnancy. Early radiographic studies suggested that there is a longitudinal and horizontal extension of the pelvis which has not completely reverted after 2 years. In particular, pregnancy seems to have a permanent effect on symphyseal separation.

THE RESUMPTION OF OVARIAN ACTIVITY

In pregnancy, cyclical ovarian activity is suppressed by the high plasma concentrations of placental steroids which reduce pituitary levels of both LH and FSH to about 1% of normal. Oestrogen levels fall rapidly after delivery to reach their lowest levels by about the end of the first postpartum week. Progesterone concentration also falls rapidly; where the corpus luteum has been removed at caesarean section, it has been found to reach zero in less than 24 hours.

Without the support of pregnancy the ovaries become physiologically quiescent, and the resumption of normal pituitary–ovarian mechanisms depends on whether or not the mother breast-feeds (see Ch. 40).

CHANGES OF BODY WEIGHT AND COMPOSITION

By the end of pregnancy the maternal body has undergone major structural modifications which have added considerably to body weight, and in the puerperium much of that added weight is lost.

Total body weight

To determine the pattern of weight loss after childbirth by the daily measurement of body weight during the puerperium would seem to be an undemanding exercise, but there are many difficulties. What, for example, should be the starting point? Clearly it is necessary to wait until the products of conception have been removed, but at that point the woman may be in considerable water deficit after a long dehydrating labour, or carrying a water excess as a result of infusions. Furthermore, there will have been a variable loss of blood. Thereafter, when should subsequent weights be taken? The standard design would be with an empty bladder before breakfast, but many women have difficulty with micturition in the early puerperium, and some will be confined to bed. Many studies took place at a time when large doses of oestrogen were given to suppress lactation and that is likely to have had a major effect on subsequent water loss. With the practice of allowing women home within a few days of delivery, a series of weights for, say, the first 10 days of the puerperium may represent a highly selected population of women who for one reason or another remained in hospital.

In what was probably the most satisfactory published study (Dennis & Bytheway 1965), of over 400 Scottish women, most of those difficulties were avoided or taken into account. Figure 39.3 shows the mean weight changes during the first 6 days postpartum for 178 normal women who were not given oestrogen to suppress lactation. In primiparae with

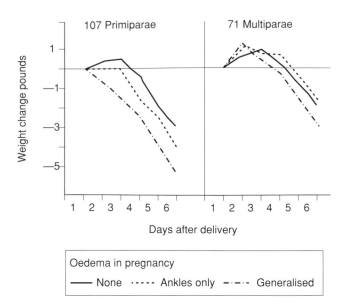

Fig. 39.3 Body weight changes in the puerperium in three oedema groups (from the data of Dennis & Bytheway 1965).

no recorded oedema in pregnancy, and in most parous women, body weight rose until the third or fourth day postpartum by an average of as much as 454 g, but from the fourth day there was a steady weight loss in all groups. The pattern was considerably modified if the woman had exhibited oedema in pregnancy. In primiparae who had oedema there was no postpartum weight gain, and in those where the oedema had been recorded as generalised, weight loss began on average immediately after delivery. For multiparae, oedema appeared to have much less effect; all groups initially gained weight postpartum, but those in whom generalised oedema had been noted began to lose weight earlier, from the second day. When oestrogen was given to suppress lactation, the onset of weight loss was postponed for a day and the rate of loss was reduced. Women who had experienced a heavy blood loss at delivery tended to gain slightly more weight during the first two or three days, presumably as a result of retaining water for compensatory expansion of their circulating volume. Younger women tended to gain more weight than older women, and fatter women gained more than thinner women. The tendency to gain weight in the early puerperium is greatest in young multiparae of average body build, a group with the best reproductive performance, which suggests that the pattern is physiological. Weight loss continues, but at a diminishing rate, until at least 10 weeks after delivery and tends to be greater in those women who continue breast feeding. Why weight should be gained in the immediate puerperium is unclear; water retention is the most plausible explanation although how and where it is stored has not been investigated.

While the more recent studies of weight change after delivery all suggest that weight rises temporarily, the findings are in conspicuous contrast to those reported in the older literature, where an immediate and continuous weight loss was reported, one comprehensive review giving an average weight loss of 8.1 kg during the first 10 days. The explanation may lie in the clinical management of the puerperium characteristic of the early decades of the twentieth century: food intake was restricted during the first few days and there was much emphasis on emptying the bowels. Moreover the strict confinement to bed which characterised puerperal management may have allowed a more rapid removal of dependent oedema.

After the first three or four days the immediate loss of weight in the first few weeks of the puerperium is largely the result of the contracting blood volume, the loss of accumulated extracellular water, and the involution of the uterus. The large accumulation of depot fat by the average woman in pregnancy takes longer to go and the physiological pattern of its disappearance is less clear, if only because puerperal changes inevitably overlap with the many other influences on body weight associated with everyday living.

Body composition

There are few data available on the two major components of the body lost in the first few weeks of the puerperium, extracellular water and body fat, largely because the techniques of measurement are so difficult. Total body water has returned to an early pregnancy value by about 6 weeks postpartum, due to a loss (which has yet to be confirmed) of extracellular water. Oedema, which is evident in pregnancy both as dependent oedema and as the widespread increase in hydration of connective tissue ground substance, disappears postpartum but there is no information about either the speed or pattern of change. The net gain of weight following pregnancy, averaging almost 2 kg at 6 weeks postpartum, appears to be fat accumulated predominantly in the subcutaneous depots of the abdomen and thighs. During lactation, lipid mobilisation increases much more in the femoral than the abdominal region, suggesting that the adipose tissue in different regions may have specialised functions. Whether the substantial quantity of depot fat stored in pregnancy is ever completely lost is a contentious issue.

On theoretical grounds it might be supposed that an energy store laid down as a buffer against possible privation in late pregnancy when the fetus is growing most rapidly, or as a subsidy for the large energy demands of lactation, might not be used in Western women who suffer no lack of food and often do not breast-feed. On the other hand if, as seems likely, fat storage is promoted by the high progesterone concentrations of pregnancy, then the removal of that stimulus might lead to a return to the prepregnancy situation. Many physicians believe that a net accumulation of body fat with each pregnancy produces a stepwise progression to obesity in parous women, but epidemiological evidence is against such a view and indicates that middle-aged multiparae carry no more than an extra one or two kilograms compared to their nulliparous counterparts. Only in a small minority of women does there appear to be a progressive gain in body weight associated with childbearing, and even in that group it is often difficult to discover whether their excess weight was aquired in the course of their pregnancies or between pregnancies. This is an important question to resolve, but it is a particularly difficult field to study because of so many confounding variables, not least the fact that many women deliberately manipulate their body weight. The true physiological pattern of events may never be known.

NUTRITION

Energy metabolism

The specific energy needs of the puerperium are complex and very variable. Any nutritional changes which might result from the winding down of pregnancy and are related specifically to the puerperal state will be submerged by the needs of milk production and the physical exertion associated with caring for a young infant. There is the further complication of the energy subsidy available from the breakdown of the depot fat accumulated in pregnancy. The literature is almost exclusively orientated towards the requirements of lactation.

There is convincing evidence that the maternal basal or resting metabolic rate (RMR) is reduced during pregnancy, a saving that makes a major contribution to the extra energy needs of pregnancy. When that pregnancy effect disappears in the puerperium is not known. The general opinion is that the puerperal state, as such, has no more than a marginal effect, if any, on RMR. More surprisingly, it would appear that there is little difference between lactating and non-lactating women, which is difficult to understand when milk production, a costly activity, must proceed throughout the 24 hours. Could it be that the underlying maternal RMR remains depressed, perhaps at the pregnancy level, as long as the woman is producing milk, so that the underlying RMR, together with the cost of milk production, roughly equates with the usual RMR of the non-lactating woman? There is also evidence of enhanced metabolic efficiency in lactating women; for example, they show a much smaller rise in metabolic rate in response to a meal, or to an infusion of noradrenaline, although an increase in general metabolic efficiency has been disputed. There can be no doubt that the average cost of established lactation is of the order of 500–700 kcal per day, and that must be found by some combination of increased energy intake, including a contribution from depot fat, reduced physical activity, and increased metabolic efficiency. The last words have not been written on this aspect of puerperal energy metabolism.

As with energy, any nutrient requirements specific to the puerperal state are swamped by the needs of milk production. A comprehensive discussion of nutrient requirements, and nutrient intakes, related to lactation have been provided by the US Institute of Medicine (IOM 1991). The usual point is made that the average intakes of individual nutrients frequently fall short of the recommended dietary allowances (RDAs) published by such official bodies as the World Health Organization, but RDAs have little to do with the physiological needs of the individual and will not be discussed.

Alimentary function

Alterations to *appetite* and the *sensation of taste* are well recognised in pregnancy, but when they revert to normal in the puerperium is not known; there is only anecdotal evidence that pica disappears abruptly after delivery. The sodium and calcium concentrations in *saliva* are depressed in pregnancy and return to normal within the first week postpartum. The relaxation of the *oesophageal sphincter* and its accompanying symptom of heartburn, which is so characteristic of pregnancy, probably reverts to normal rapidly, perhaps within 24 hours. The many methods of measuring motility in the *stomach* have given a confused picture, but there is little convincing evidence of a change in pregnancy. On the other hand there is good evidence that motility is considerably depressed in labour and that depression may continue for the first two or three days postpartum. In general it would appear that gastric acid production is at normal non-pregnant levels in the puerperium, with perhaps a slight surge during the first few days, but for women with depressed acid production in pregnancy there may be a return to normal during the first week. There are few physiological data for *liver* function in the postpartum period, but since liver function appears generally to be unchanged in pregnancy, postpartum changes would not be expected. The most studied of the liver function tests has been the clearance of the injected dye bromsulphthalein (BSP), which in the normal person is rapidly removed from the blood by the liver, conjugated, and excreted in the bile. It is generally agreed that, for a number of reasons, clearance is slower in pregnancy, but it returns rapidly to normal within the first postpartum week. The *gallbladder* empties poorly in pregnancy and a number of studies have shown that this sluggishness returns only slowly to normal over a period of perhaps months.

Among the confusing phenomena of pregnancy are the large changes in nutrient concentration in blood; water-soluble nutrients tend to fall, lipid nutrients to rise. The mechanisms behind these changes and their biological significance are not understood, but the speed with which levels return to non-pregnant values might offer useful clues. Unfortunately the data are seldom sufficiently detailed to be helpful. Almost all the data for *proteins* refer to studies made when paper electrophoresis became popular; the more elaborate modern methods of protein separation have not been used in puerperal studies. Total protein, which is relatively meaningless and largely a reflection of albumin, is considerably reduced in late pregnancy and appears to fall further in the first few days of the puerperium before returning to non-pregnant levels within the first two or three weeks. The pattern for albumin is the same; colloid osmotic pressure, which closely reflects albumin concentration, follows suit. The three or four groups of proteins separated by paper electrophoresis which are labelled *globulins* conceal many individual proteins whose behaviour may differ from the overall pattern, but for what it is worth the evidence suggests that, apart from the gamma fraction, they are all raised in late pregnancy, rise further in the first few days of the puerperium, perhaps in part because of acute phase proteins, and then decline to normal levels within 6 weeks. Gamma globulin, again a collection of many proteins which may behave in different ways, is reduced in pregnancy and remains at depressed levels even at 6 weeks postpartum. There are very few data on the behaviour of free amino acids, whose pattern is considerably modified in pregnancy. While it seems likely that a normal non-pregnant pattern is restored by 2 months after delivery, there may be large

individual differences. For example, in one case report it was found that while levels of some amino acids such as glutamic acid and ornithine returned rapidly to normal within 4 weeks, others such as glycine and proline had high postpartum values which did not return to normal until after 14 weeks.

For plasma and serum *lipids* the picture is blurred; this results in part from changes in laboratory methods, in part from lack of standardisation of conditions of sampling, and in part from ill-defined and heterogeneous groups of subjects. For example, lactation seems to have a major influence on plasma lipids, yet it is often not possible to know whether the women were breast feeding. The level of *triglyceride* is characteristically high in late pregnancy, and a somewhat inconsistent literature suggests that it is probably reduced to about half that level within the first two postpartum weeks and then declines more slowly to reach a non-pregnant value after 6 weeks. A major influence on the speed with which triglyceride levels return to non-pregnant values is lactation; the fall is rapid in breast feeding women and much slower in those who are not lactating. The effect is still apparent after 6 weeks. The proportions associated with high-density lipoprotein (HDL) and very low-density lipoprotein (VLDL) appear to decline similarly in the two groups, but there is consistent evidence that the low-density fraction (LDL) remains elevated during lactation. Two mechanisms probably contribute to the postpartum fall in triglyceride levels: there is a rapid rise in the activity of hepatic lipoprotein lipase (LPL) previously suppressed by oestrogen, and a fall in the oestrogen-induced hepatic synthesis of VLDL triglyceride.

Most published information on *cholesterol* refers only to total cholesterol, with little information on ester cholesterol or fractions associated with various lipoprotein fractions. Plasma cholesterol is characteristically high in late pregnancy and the return to non-pregnant values is slow, probably taking more than 8 weeks; there is some, not very convincing evidence that the fall may be more rapid in lactating women. VLDL cholesterol, which is raised in late pregnancy, falls throughout the puerperium to reach non-pregnant values by 6 or 7 weeks. LDL cholesterol tends to increase slightly but may be higher in women who are not lactating. HDL cholesterol increases, to a greater extent in those who are lactating, to reach non-pregnant values by about 6 weeks. *Phospholipid* concentrations rise in parallel with cholesterol in pregnancy, and fall in a similarly sluggish fashion postpartum. There is little information about phospholipid fractions. The measurement of non-esterified *fatty acids* (NEFA), or free fatty acids (FFA), is technically very difficult because of their lability; levels rise continuously during fasting and are extremely sensitive to many other influences such as exertion, emotional stress, venous stasis, and even the presence of an indwelling needle. NEFA levels rise in late pregnancy as lipolysis begins in the accumulated depot fat, and oxytocin provokes a further considerable increase in labour. In the first two or three days postpartum, NEFA levels fall quickly to a level that is probably below the normal non-pregnant value, after which there is a rise to normal by about 6 weeks.

Many studies of *vitamin* levels in blood during pregnancy

agree that there is a progressive fall in the water-soluble group, and a rise in most of the fat-soluble vitamins. Much discussion has been provoked about the meaning of these changes, in particular whether the falling levels of such vitamins as folate, ascorbic acid and riboflavin indicate a dietary inadequacy which supports a need for supplements. Curiously, few studies continued into the puerperium where the return, or otherwise, to non-pregnant values might have settled the question, and the puerperal data are so inadequate that no more than a tentative statement is possible. *Vitamin A* (retinol) is unusual in remaining well below non-pregnant values throughout pregnancy, and it is generally agreed that there is a conspicuous increase within the first 24 hours postpartum which continues for up to 6 weeks. *Carotene* (the chemical description is seldom more explicit) follows the more usual pattern for fat-soluble nutrients in having considerably raised values in pregnancy which fall within 24 hours of delivery. *Vitamin E*, a mixture of tocopherols, behaves like most lipids in having raised values in pregnancy; these fall progressively from early in the puerperium. *Thiamin* (vitamin B_1), *riboflavin* (vitamin B_2) and *piridoxyl* (vitamin B_6) have been examined only by means of tests to determine status, and then in the laboratories of a vitamin manufacturer. Status for all three was claimed to worsen in the puerperium although it remained adequate. *Folic acid* is perhaps the most studied of the water-soluble vitamins because of its importance in haematopoiesis, and because overt deficiency, with megaloblastic anaemia, is a recognised complication of pregnancy. There are few useful data for the puerperium, but some evidence that levels fall in the immediate puerperium followed by a gradual rise towards non-pregnant values after several months. Where plasma volume has been measured simultaneously it would appear that the total folate in the circulation changes very little. *Vitamin B_{12}*, *cyanocobalamin*, is known to fall progressively in pregnancy, but there are surprisingly few data for the puerperium. What evidence there is suggests a rapid rise in the first few days postpartum followed by a continuing increase for some weeks to non-pregnant values. *Vitamin C*, ascorbic acid, falls progressively in pregnancy even in women on a diet with a high vitamin C content, but the few postpartum studies do not agree on what happens in the puerperium: some suggest a continuing fall in the immediate puerperium; others, where the possibility of supplementation cannot be excluded, suggest a rise. The results are so variable that no simple conclusion is justified.

Information about mineral salts is uneven, with some cations receiving a great deal of attention and many receiving none. *Sodium* is consistently reduced in pregnancy and is a major contributor to the fall in plasma osmolality. Its return to normal values postpartum occurs rapidly within the first week. *Potassium* levels show a substantial rise in the first few days of the puerperium, falling back to non-pregnant values after a few weeks. That early puerperal surge is consistent with the large amount of tissue destruction occurring as the uterus and other pelvic tissues involute and excess red cells are disposed of. *Zinc* levels are also reduced in pregnancy but probably begin to rise before delivery with a rapid return to non-pregnant values within the first postpartum week. Plasma *copper* content increases in pregnancy from the oestrogen-induced rise in the level of the copper-containing enzyme caeruloplasmin; there is a rapid drop postpartum. *Nickel* concentration in serum is reduced in pregnancy, but there is a massive rise between the second and third stages of labour which returns to a non-pregnant value within an hour of delivery. Neither the source of the nickel, nor the significance of the changes is known. One of the most striking physiological changes in pregnancy is the early abrupt fall in plasma *osmolality* by about 10 mOsm/kg, caused mostly by sodium and attendant anions; this is associated with complex changes in osmoregulation. Normal non-pregnant values are reached rapidly in the puerperium, within the first week, but detailed data are lacking.

CALCIUM METABOLISM

The pregnant woman, with raised circulating levels of both vitamin D and parathyroid hormone, greatly increases her absorption of calcium and phosphate, and she shows a remarkable capacity to preserve the integrity of her own skeleton while supplying substantial quantities of calcium to her fetus. In the quite different physiological circumstances of the puerperium, the production of milk also requires the mother to provide large quantities of calcium to the infant while again attempting to conserve her own bone structure.

Vitamin D
The plasma level of the major active form of vitamin D, dihydroxycholecalciferol, doubles during pregnancy, in part because of placental production. The generally agreed pattern of change in the puerperium is that the plasma level of vitamin D drops sharply in the immediate puerperium, as would be expected from the loss of the placental source, and probably reaches the normal non-pregnant value within the first four weeks. Thereafter there are no convincing changes, nor any consistent difference between women who are lactating and those who are not.

Plasma or serum calcium
Plasma levels fall in pregnancy; this is almost entirely, if not entirely, the result of a fall in the protein-bound fraction following the fall in albumin concentration. The return to non-pregnant values follows the recovery of albumin levels and may take several weeks. Lactation appears to make no difference to the pattern of change.

Plasma or serum phosphate
Inorganic phosphate remains at normal non-pregnant levels in pregnancy, and probably in the puerperium, except for women who are lactating, in whom values are consistently higher. That difference is still evident even at 12 months postpartum in women who are only partially breast feeding.

Parathyroid hormone (PTH)
The pattern of change is unclear in an inconsistent literature, but the somewhat raised concentration characteristic of

pregnancy tends to fall slowly after delivery, except in lactating women where it remains elevated. *Parathyroid hormone-related protein (PTHrP)* is also elevated during lactation and is significantly associated with the bone loss that occurs.

Calcitonin

There is probably no change either in pregnancy or postpartum.

The overall effects of these changes can be summarised as follows: there is no dispute about the fact that lactation is associated with loss of bone mineral, the large calcium need being met by increased bone resorption and decreased urinary excretion but not by increased intestinal absorption. Three other biochemical indices confirm that effect. There is increased excretion of hydroxyproline derived from the degradation of collagen, plasma alkaline phosphatase is increased, and there is a raised serum osteocalcin, a bone-specific polypeptide which is elevated during periods of increased bone turnover. There is increased bone formation and a recovery of lost bone between 2 and 6 months after lactation stops with conspicuously increased renal conservation of calcium and a large increase in PTH, but without a change in plasma calcium.

Women cannot be assumed to have returned to the normal range of calcium biochemistry for at least 6 months after the cessation of lactation.

CARBOHYDRATE METABOLISM

In early pregnancy the fasting concentration of glucose in plasma falls to a new homeostatic level some 0.05 mmol/l (10 mg/100 ml) below the normal non-pregnant value, associated with an increasing resistance to the action of insulin, the basis of which is uncertain. The plasma insulin response to a carbohydrate meal increases continuously as pregnancy progresses while there is a progressive apparent 'deterioration' of glucose homeostasis: plasma glucose levels rise higher and remain elevated for longer, and many women progress to a state that would ordinarily be regarded as diabetic, while a few develop unequivocal diabetes. It is usual to investigate such women postpartum to see whether carbohydrate tolerance has returned to normal, and it is therefore of considerable clinical importance to determine how rapidly the pregnancy-induced changes disappear. For plasma glucose there is some confusion about the pattern of change in the first 24 hours, perhaps because of such circumstances as the length of fasting enforced by labour and the use of intravenous infusions. There is no dispute, however, about the fact that for about the first 5 postpartum days plasma glucose is below the level of late pregnancy. It is not clear when normal non-pregnant values are re-established. Fasting plasma insulin falls rapidly postpartum and a normal non-pregnant value is probably reached within 2 or 3 days. Lactation appears to make no difference, but it is worth noting that plasma insulin may show a marked, but brief peak in association with suckling.

Although the fasting concentrations of plasma glucose and insulin fall rapidly in the puerperium, the response to an oral glucose load does not return to the non-pregnant pattern for some time. While the metabolic response to an intravenous load of glucose returns to non-pregnant values within a day or two of delivery, as does the insulin response to an oral glucose load, glucose homeostasis following an oral load remains at the pregnancy level of relative inefficiency for at least 5 days. A protein meal, or more effectively an amino acid infusion, leads to a release of insulin from the pancreas; in pregnancy that response is not modified, but it is considerably attenuated in the early puerperium and the effect may last for more than 6 weeks.

BLOOD VOLUME AND HAEMATOLOGY

At the end of a normal pregnancy, the blood volume is enormously expanded to service the greatly increased circulation to the uterus, kidneys and other sites; plasma volume is increased by an average of about 50%, and the red cell mass by about 20–25%. Some blood is, of course, shed at parturition, but most of the pregnancy excess must be dispersed in other ways. The published evidence is sparse because of the technical and ethical difficulties associated with repeated measurements in the puerperium.

Plasma volume. Most studies agree that plasma volume falls in the first 24 hours, even in the first hour, by some 15 or 20% of the prepartum value, but all show great variation which may or may not represent physiological instability, with rises and falls up to 3 days postpartum.

Red cell mass, so called in spite of being expressed as a volume because the term *red cell volume* traditionally refers to the size of a single cell, can be estimated either by derivation from plasma volume plus the haematocrit, or by direct labelling of red cells. Only the latter method gives reliable results postpartum, and the few studies made agree that there is a rapid fall of some 200–250 ml in the first few hours. That figure agrees well with the directly measured loss.

In summarising a very unsatisfactory literature, all that can be said is that the red cell mass appears to return to a non-pregnant level rapidly, perhaps within 24 hours, whereas plasma volume subsides more slowly, even increasing somewhat in the first day or two of the puerperium, and may not reach its non-pregnant level until the end of the first postpartum week. That pattern of change would result in increasing haemodilution during the first few days of the puerperium, which is supported by haematological data.

Haemoglobin concentration falls to its lowest point on about the fourth day of the puerperium, after which it rises progressively to reach normal non-pregnant values at between 4 and 6 weeks. A similar pattern occurs, but at a higher level, if the woman has been given supplemental iron during pregnancy, but the eventual non-pregnant values are the same (Fig. 39.4). The concentration is appreciably lower in the immediate puerperium if the woman has been given intravenous fluids in labour. The *red cell count* and *packed cell volume (haematocrit)* follow parallel patterns of change.

Red cell characteristics. The mean cell volume (MCV),

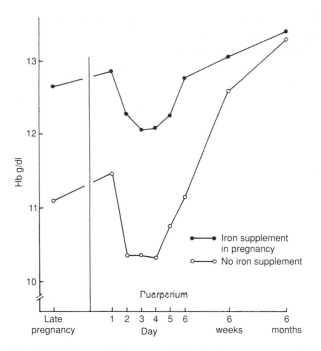

Fig. 39.4 Haemoglobin concentration in the puerperium: the effect of iron supplementation in pregnancy (from the data of Taylor et al 1981).

mean cell haemoglobin (MCH) and mean cell haemoglobin concentration (MCHC) are all appreciably raised if supplemental iron has been given, an effect that remains for up to 6 weeks postpartum although it has gone by 6 months.

The erythrocyte sedimentation rate (ESR) is considerably and variably raised in pregnancy, perhaps as a result of raised fibrinogen concentration; it is further increased in the first week postpartum and would appear to have returned to normal by about 4 weeks.

Iron metabolism. In healthy pregnancy, serum iron falls in line with most nutrients in blood, and an increased concentration of the protein transferrin (iron-binding capacity) is induced by oestrogen, so that the percentage saturation of iron-binding capacity is particularly low. These indices have now been largely replaced by the measurement of plasma ferritin, the iron storage glycoprotein which reflects storage iron. *Serum iron* remains low postpartum, perhaps for as long as 6 weeks, but most studies suggest that normal non-pregnant values are reached by 2 months. *Serum transferrin* falls rapidly postpartum and normal values are reached within the first month; saturation of iron-binding capacity is back to normal by the end of the first week. *Plasma ferritin* shows enormous individual variation, but in general levels rise quickly within the first postpartum week, with iron-supplemented women showing a much more pronounced increase. The rise probably continues for at least 6 weeks. It is by no means certain that ferritin provides a useful guide to iron storage in the puerperium.

In summary, haemoglobin concentration and such indices as serum iron, or even plasma ferritin, are valueless in the first days after parturition and the clinician needs some useful guidelines to assess the haematological status of individual women; at present there seem to be none.

Leucocytes. A considerable polymorphonuclear leucocytosis associated with labour has long been recognised; that increase slowly subsides during the first postpartum week. There is also a conspicuous rise in the number of eosinophils, centred on about the fourth postpartum day and lasting until about the end of the week. As polymorphonuclear leucocytes increase in the first days of the puerperium, there is a proportional, but probably not an absolute, fall in the number of lymphocytes.

Haemostasis and fibrinolysis

In late pregnancy the haemostatic mechanism appears to be altered towards an enhanced capacity to form fibrin and a diminished ability to lyse it, resulting in a hypercoagulability ready to meet the demand for haemostatic components at delivery. It is analogous to a motor car standing with its engine running at high speed, and the brakes off, ready for an instant getaway. When the placenta is torn from the uterine wall at parturition it leaves a wound of some 300 cm^2 with perhaps 100 severed arcuate arteries which until that moment had been delivering more than half a litre of blood per minutes; this is massive trauma by any standards and requires a massive haemostatic response. The primary and most important first step is physical compression of the torn vessels by myometrial contraction, but repair by normal haemostatic mechanisms must quickly follow. Once the job of repairing the damaged surface has been done it is important that the temporary state of hypercoagulability, and the inevitably associated danger of thromboembolic disease, should be reversed. There is an immediate shortening of the clotting time after delivery of the placenta, seen in the uterine blood even as the placenta is separating, with sharp increases in clotting factors VIII and V, and a decrease in fibrinogen. After delivery, factor VIII activity remains high and the number of circulating platelets increases. The level of tissue plasminogen activator, produced by the placenta, is particularly high in labour so that the brake on fibrinolysis is abruptly released on placental separation. The sudden increase in fibrin formation is thus associated with a greatly enhanced potential for fibrinolysis, and there is a rapid increase in fibrin/fibrinogen degradation products (FDP), particularly in uterine blood, within a few minutes of placental separation.

The result of the haemostatic frenzy accompanying placental separation is that the placental bed is quickly covered by a carpet of fibrin mesh which has been estimated to have used up to 10% of the circulating fibrinogen. The concentration of plasma fibrinogen therefore falls abruptly immediately postpartum but recovers to the high values associated with late pregnancy within about 24 hours.

In the later puerperium fibrinogen values return to non-pregnant levels by 6 weeks but the pattern of change, both for fibrinogen and other coagulation factors, is variable and a matter of some dispute. These complex data are discussed by Hytten (1995). There is also disagreement about whether or not there is a decrease in platelet numbers during pregnancy but little doubt that there is a considerable fall at the time of placental separation; the latter is caused by platelet consumption associated with the massive haemostatic activity at that time. This is followed by a conspicuous rise in numbers, accompanied by increased adhesiveness, during the first postpartum week. Fibrinolytic activity has probably returned to normal within a few hours of parturition. While plasminogen remains at above non-pregnant values for two or three weeks postpartum, increases in plasminogen activators and probable decreases in plasminogen inhibitors appear to be transitory. There is some evidence that plasmin inhibitory activity may be raised in the immediate puerperium. If the behaviour of some of the components of the chain leading to fibrinolysis is uncertain, there is no dispute about the rise in FDP within an hour of delivery which continues for several days; it has returned to non-pregnant values within 5 weeks.

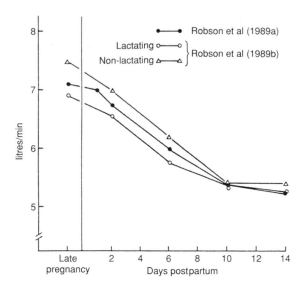

Fig. 39.5 Cardiac output in the puerperium measured at the aorta (for references see Hytten 1995).

THE CARDIOVASCULAR SYSTEM

Almost all measurements related to cardiovascular function, from pulse rate and blood pressure to cardiac output and regional blood flow, are particularly sensitive to the conditions under which they are made; anxiety, pain and even quite trivial changes of posture or muscular activity can cause major alterations. While that is a problem at any time, it is a particular impediment in the puerperium where the excitement and perhaps anxiety associated with a new baby, perineal pain and general restlessness make the achievement of standard conditions unusually difficult. In these circumstances it is hardly surprising that wide individual variation is a common feature of published studies.

The heart is increased in size during pregnancy, with a larger left ventricular mass and ventricular wall thickness, and greater aortic, pulmonary and mitral valve areas. These dimensions return progressively and slowly to non-pregnant values over at least 24 weeks, although there is some evidence that a complete return may not occur. Heart sounds that are changed in pregnancy return more quickly: the first sound, which is considerably louder in pregnancy, has returned to normal by 2–4 weeks, and its splitting by 4 weeks. The third sound, audible in late pregnancy, usually disappears by 8 days, and a systolic ejection murmur, present in most pregnant women, has usually gone in a week but may linger for up to 4 weeks.

Cardiac output remains at almost the high late pregnancy level during the first 24 hours postpartum, after which there is a steady decline until the tenth day when near non-pregnant values are reached; breast feeding does not appear to influence the pattern. Cardiac output continues to fall very slowly beyond the immediate puerperium and the eventual non-pregnant value is probably not reached until after 6 months. Figure 39.5 shows the immediate pattern of change.

Increased cardiac output in pregnancy is brought about both by an increase in heart rate and by a proportionally slightly smaller increase in stroke volume. In the puerperium heart rate changes parallel the pattern of change in cardiac

output, remaining at the raised pregnancy level during the first 24 hours before falling to a non-pregnant value by about 2 weeks. Stroke volume lags behind; it remains raised for at least 48 hours and then continues to fall until at least 24 weeks, so that the prolonged decline in cardiac output is due to a continuing reduction in stroke volume after the heart rate has stabilised at 2 weeks.

Intravascular hydrodynamics. Published data on arterial blood pressure is confusing and contradictory. At the end of pregnancy, brachial blood pressure in the average normotensive woman is not convincingly different from that when she is not pregnant. There appears to be a slight progressive rise in both diastolic and systolic pressures during the first four days postpartum, with afternoon pressures systematically somewhat higher than those in the morning; it is probable that normal non-pregnant values are reached by the end of the first week. Blood flow velocity measured in large arteries shows no change in the common carotid or middle cerebral arteries; in the femoral artery, however, where it is greatly reduced in late pregnancy, there is a substantial increase after one week and that continues until beyond 6 weeks. Total peripheral vascular resistance is characteristically low in pregnancy; during the first two postpartum days it remains low but as the cardiac output falls peripheral resistance rises rapidly although it does not appear to return to prepregnant values for perhaps 6 months. Venous pressure is greatly affected in pregnancy by mechanical obstruction and veins below the level of the inferior vena cava show large pressure rises; the effect is reversed immediately after delivery.

There are few data for peripheral blood flow. Increased blood flow is most noticeable in the extremities, particularly the hands where palmar erythema is common. Blood flow decreases postpartum, mostly within one week, but there is a further slow decline for several months; palmar erythema has usually disappeared within a few days.

RESPIRATION

Lung volumes and capacities. There are few data, largely because classical methods of study are unsuitable for the puerperal woman and there has been little interest in the subject since the advent of modern techniques. Such evidence as there is suggests that vital capacity, inspiratory capacity, expiratory reserve volume and residual volume return to non-pregnant values within about 2 weeks.

Anatomical changes. In pregnancy there are major changes in the anatomy of the chest: the transverse diameter increases as the lower ribs flare out, the subcostal angle increases and the diaphragm rises. Those changes appear to have reversed within a few weeks, but it is a frequent complaint of women that their waistline, as determined by the lower rib cage, is permanently increased by childbearing.

Respiratory function. Tidal volume, which is increased by about 40% by late pregnancy, returns only slowly to a normal non-pregnant value after perhaps 6 weeks. Respiratory rate, on the other hand, which does not alter in pregnancy, increases in the immediate puerperium by about one per minute before returning to normal after several weeks. Alveolar ventilation, which is greatly enhanced in pregnancy, returns very slowly to non-pregnant values and has been recorded as still 30% above normal at 6 weeks postpartum.

Gas distribution in the lungs. The greatly increased alveolar ventilation in pregnancy makes for considerably more efficient mixing of gas, but that reverts to a non-pregnant state within 48 hours of delivery. By contrast, gas transfer to pulmonary blood deteriorates in pregnancy and there are no data about the speed of recovery postpartum. The transfer of carbon dioxide from the blood to the alveoli is much more efficient in pregnancy, and that effect disappears within the first postpartum week.

THE URINARY SYSTEM

Anatomical changes. The kidney increases considerably in size during pregnancy; to a large extent this is because of an expanded vascular volume consequent on the greatly increased renal blood flow. That has begun to reverse within 48 hours of delivery and is complete by 6 weeks. The most obvious and almost universal change in the urinary tract in pregnancy is dilatation of the calyces, renal pelvis and ureters, almost certainly as a result of mechanical compression at the level of the pelvic brim. There are relatively few data about the pattern of recovery postpartum. It seems likely that for most women dilatation of the upper urinary tracts has disappeared within the first two weeks, although for some return to normal is slower or may never occur. The bladder is markedly hypotonic in pregnancy and that remains, with decreased bladder sensation and an increased capacity for at least the first postpartum week, with a return to normal in the subsequent few weeks. The bladder also enters the puerperium bruised and battered by the jostling it receives in childbirth, but mucosal oedema and submucosal bleeding probably disappear within a few days. There is some evidence that a first vaginal delivery results in reduced urethral length and decreased closing pressure, a change which may be permanent.

Renal haemodynamics. One of the best recognised pregnancy changes in renal function is the conspicuous increase in both renal plasma flow and glomerular filtration rate. The pattern of recovery postpartum is unknown, except that normal non-pregnant values have been regained by 6–8 weeks.

Osmoregulation. The remarkable abrupt drop in the osmolality of body fluids in early pregnancy by 10 mosmol/kg requires the resetting of osmoreceptors, with perhaps the primary change being an equivalent reduction in the osmotic threshold for thirst which may be provoked by hCG. There is a return to normal within 2 weeks.

Reabsorption of nutrients. Glycosuria, which is both variable and intermittent, is characteristic of normal pregnancy and disappears quickly, within a few days postpartum. Lactosuria is also common in pregnancy and has been found in all postpartum women during the first week of the puerperium; it tends to persist in lactating women and to disappear in those who do not breast-feed. Both amino acids and folate are excreted in large amounts in pregnancy; excretion has reverted to normal non-pregnant values by 6 weeks postpartum, but the pattern of change is not known.

THE ENDOCRINE SYSTEM

Few aspects of endocrine physiology remain undisturbed by pregnancy. These are considered in Chapters 6 and 25. The changes associated with lactation are dealt with in Chapter 40, while the hormones associated with calcium and carbohydrate metabolism are described above.

Growth hormone. The secretion of pituitary growth hormone is inhibited in pregnancy, and the response to provocative stimuli reduced, caused both by the overwhelming presence of hPL and, perhaps, by growth hormone from the placenta. When normal postpartum production is resumed is not known, but it appears to have recovered by 6 weeks.

The thyroid gland. There is little unanimity about changes of thyroid function and iodine metabolism in pregnancy, and that is reflected in the puerperium. The size of the thyroid gland has generally been found to increase in pregnancy although this appears not to occur in populations with a high iodine intake; where it does enlarge, the return to a prepregnant size is slow and probably takes more than 6 months. Renal clearance of iodine is considerably raised in pregnancy and takes several weeks to return to normal, but the reduced plasma inorganic iodine has returned to the normal non-pregnant range by 2 weeks. Whether thyroid-stimulating hormone (TSH) is increased in pregnancy is uncertain, but where high levels were found they remained high for at least a week postpartum.

Thyroxine-binding globulin (TBG) is raised in pregnancy as an effect of oestrogen, and falls to normal levels within about 2 weeks. As a result of the raised TBG, thyroxine (T_4) levels are raised in pregnancy but fall to non-pregnant values by 2–4 weeks. Free T_4 remains at normal levels, but the free throxine index, which is reduced in pregnancy, has risen to normal values by 4 weeks postpartum. Triiodothyronine (T_3) is, like T_4, in higher than normal concentration during pregnancy, but returns to normal by 4 weeks; reverse T_3, which occurs in relatively high concentration in pregnancy, has reached non-pregnant values within 2 days of delivery. Free T_3, which is somewhat depressed in pregnancy, remains below normal levels for at least 2 weeks postpartum.

The pituitary–adrenal axis. Corticotrophin-releasing factor (CRF) is produced by the placenta with a consequent increase in the plasma levels of corticotrophin (ACTH) and associated hormones. After delivery there is a rapid decline, within 24 hours or less, of corticotrophin, beta-endorphin and beta-lipoprotein. Cortisol levels fall more slowly and may not reach non-pregnant values until 2–3 weeks postpartum; aldosterone, also considerably raised in pregnancy, returns to normal within 2 weeks.

Long-term effects. With the rapid return of most hormones to non-pregnant values, it is of particular interest that in some respects the hormonal environment may be permanently changed by pregnancy. For example, serum oestriol has been found to be raised for more than a year after delivery, and dehydroepiandrosterone (DHA) and its sulphate reduced for as long as 13 years.

KEY POINTS

- The huge and widespread physiological changes which the mother makes for the benefit of her fetus must be reversed after delivery, and the restitution of non-pregnant normality represents the physiology of the puerperium.
- That definition cannot include a simple time for completion, such as 6 weeks; some changes are reversed within minutes of childbirth, some take days or weeks, some may never return to nulliparous normality.
- Some changes, such as weight loss, may be affected by clinical management; others, such as the rapidly shifting haematological pattern and unstable glucose homeostasis, may cause clinical confusion.
- Here is a rich, relatively unexplored, field for research.

REFERENCES

Dennis KJ, Bytheway WR 1965 Changes in body weight after delivery. J Obstet Gynaecol Br Commonwealth 72:94–102

Hytten FE 1995 The clinical physiology of the puerperium. Farrand Press, London

Hytten FE, Leitch I 1971 The physiology of human pregnancy, 2nd edn. Blackwell Scientific, Oxford

IOM (Institute of Medicine) 1991 Nutrition during lactation. Food and nutrition board. National Academy Press, Washington, D.C.

Quinn M, Roberts A 1999 The anatomy of prolapse and incontinence. Contemporary Reviews in Obstetrics and Gynaecology 11:281–288

Taylor DJ, Phillips P, Lind T 1981 Puerperal haematological indices. Br J Obstet Gynaecol 88:601–606

40

Lactation

P.W. Howie

INTRODUCTION

Lactation is a physiological process which is common to all mammals and this is strong evidence of its evolutionary importance. Despite its central place in the natural reproductive cycle, many women find breast feeding a difficult skill to learn and the human species is the only one in which lactation has been widely replaced by artificial feeding. Within the time scale of human evolution, this change from breast to bottle feeding is relatively recent, and the true clinical and social implications of the change are only now becoming apparent. This chapter will consider how knowledge of the anatomy and the physiology of lactation can underpin an understanding of the maternal adaptions to breast feeding and its substantial effects on infant health; in addition, some of the steps that can be taken to promote effective breast feeding will also be discussed.

THE BREAST

Anatomy

The breast extends from the second to the sixth rib and from the sternum to the mid axillary line with a tail extending into the axilla. It overlies the pectoralis major, serratus anterior and external oblique muscles. The main constituents of the breast are the glandular cells with their associated ducts, a very variable quantity of adipose tissue, connective tissue, blood vessels, nerves and lymphatics (Fig. 40.1). The gland lies in the superficial fascia of the thorax under its overlying skin. The lactiferous ducts lead to the nipple and dilate to form sinuses immediately below the surface of the areola. The nipple is surrounded by the areola, a pigmented area of varying size which darkens during pregnancy. The areola contains sebaceous glands, which hypertrophy and become prominent during pregnancy, called Montgomery's tubercles. The areola is richly supplied with sensory nerves, which are important during suckling. Throughout pregnancy the areola is relatively insensitive to touch but sensitivity increases greatly immediately after delivery. This change ensures that the suckling of the infant sends a stream of afferent neural impulses to the hypothalamus to control not only the process of lactation itself but also other important maternal adaptations, which are discussed later.

The glandular tissue of the breast is derived from the ectoderm and is arranged in 15–20 ductal–lobular–alveolar systems (Fig. 40.1). The alveolar or secreting cells are grouped in grape-like bunches around the ductules, which join to form the main ducts leading to the nipple (Gardner & Dodds 1976). The alveolar cells are cuboidal cells in the resting breast, which develop full secretory features during lactation. The alveolar cells are surrounded by oxytocin-sensitive contractile myoepithelial cells, which play an important part in milk ejection. The ducts are lined by contractile longitudinal cells which, during the milk ejection reflex, open the ducts widely to assist milk flow (McNeilly 1977).

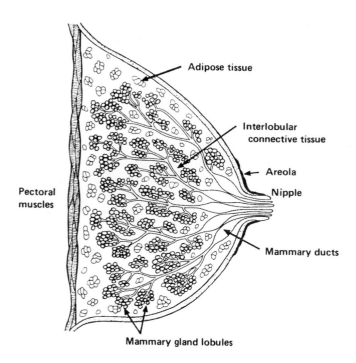

Fig. 40.1 Structure of the breast during lactation. Reproduced from Gardner & Dodds (1976) with permission.

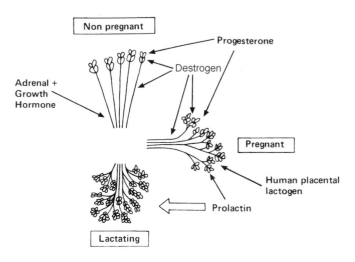

Fig. 40.2 Endocrine requirements for breast development and lactogenesis in the human. Lobulo-alveolar and ductal development appear to be steroid dependent with an undetermined role of prolactin or placental lactogen during pregnancy. Prolactin is essential for lactogenesis. Reproduced from McNeilly (1977) with permission.

Growth and development

In the adult breast, four phases of mammary growth and development can be recognised. These are the resting phase, the development phase during pregnancy, the milk-secreting phase during lactation, and the involutionary phase.

The human species is unusual in that a major degree of breast development occurs at puberty prior to pregnancy.

It seems likely that the reason for this is that the erotic significance of the female breast plays an important part in the attraction of male to female that is essential for human reproduction. At puberty, the milk ducts leading from the nipple branch and sprout and form a modest degree of alveolar development. The control of human breast development is not fully understood and current concepts come mainly from animal experiments in which ovaries, pituitary and adrenal are removed, followed by the replacement of hormones both individually and in combination. These experiments suggest that mammary growth and development are under the control of multiple hormones. At present it seems likely that proliferation of the ducts is primarily dependent upon oestrogen in conjunction with glucocorticoids and growth hormone (Fig. 40.2). On the other hand, alveolar growth is stimulated by progesterone in the oestrogen-primed breast but it may also require prolactin, prednisolone and other growth promoting factors.

Once the adult breast has developed it requires only minimal stimulation by the appropriate hormones to begin milk secretion. As little as 14 days' exposure to conjugated oestro-gens followed by stimulation of prolactin secretion can lead to the establishment of milk production. This sensitivity to endocrine stimuli has been used to encourage lactation in women who wish to suckle adopted infants.

During early pregnancy there is a sharp increase in both ductal and alveolar elements of the mammary gland due to hyperplasia, while during later pregnancy, there is alveolar cell hypertrophy and the initiation of secretory activity. These changes during pregnancy are probably dependent upon the lactogenic hormones, prolactin and human placental lactogen, with placental oestrogens and progesterone playing an important modulatory role. During human pregnancy, full milk production is inhibited by the high concentrations of progesterone (and possibly oestrogen) from the placenta and the copious milk production of established lactation does not occur until after parturition (McNeilly 1977).

INITIATION AND MAINTENANCE OF LACTATION

Lactogenesis

Following parturition, there is a progressive rise in the volume of milk secreted by the breast; this is maintained in mothers who suckle their infants. During the first 30 hours after parturition, the early milk or colostrum has high concentrations of protein relative to the concentration of lactose (Fig. 40.3). During the next three days, the concentrations of lactose increase sharply under the influence of prolactin stimulation and, in order to maintain ionic equilibrium, water is drawn into the breast causing an increase in milk volume (Kulski & Hartmann 1981). At the same time, the concentrations of milk proteins fall because of a dilution effect, although the absolute amounts of the individual proteins remain constant or rise slowly (Hartmann & Prosser 1984).

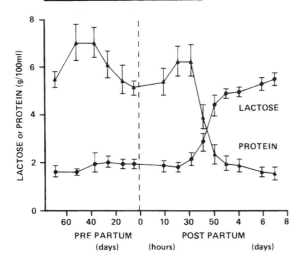

INITIATION OF HUMAN LACTATION

Fig. 40.3 Changes in lactose and protein concentrations in mammary secretions during the postpartum period, showing the sharp rise in lactose and the fall in protein concentration due to dilution. Reproduced from Kulski & Hartmann (1981) with permission.

After this phase of transitional milk formation, a relatively stable phase of mature milk production is reached at about day five, after which there is a slow but steady increase in milk volume to a peak around three weeks postpartum.

Galactopoiesis

Mothers who do not suckle their infants secrete some milk and this may persist for 3–4 weeks postpartum. The suckling stimulus, which releases both prolactin and oxytocin, is essential for the maintenance of lactation and these reflexes are discussed below. Provided that the breast is emptied regularly by sucking, lactation can be maintained for long periods and in some communities will continue for two years or more.

Most studies have estimated that after lactation is established, the average daily volume of milk production in a healthy well nourished mother is of the order of 750–800 ml/day (Whitehead et al 1980). Mothers who are feeding twins produce twice as much milk as mothers feeding singletons, strongly suggesting that suckling, which is doubled in the case of twins, is the key to milk production.

The influence of maternal diet on milk production has not been clearly defined and only small differences have been observed between Swedish and Ethiopian mothers and British and Gambian mothers (Hartmann & Prosser 1984). It may be that babies of poorly nourished mothers have to suckle more intensively and for longer to achieve an adequate milk supply.

Prolactin and milk production

Prolactin is a long-chain polypeptide hormone which is secreted from the anterior pituitary gland in response to suckling and it is essential for successful lactation.

The suckling stimulus of the baby sends afferent impulses to the hypothalamus, leading to a surge of prolactin release. Prolactin release is controlled by prolactin inhibitory factors secreted into the pituitary portal blood system; dopamine is generally considered to be the most important. The suckling-induced burst of prolactin secretion from the pituitary may be induced by the inhibition of dopamine release from the hypothalamus, although the mechanisms for control of dopamine release are not fully understood (Fig. 40.4).

In response to suckling, prolactin levels rise quickly to reach a peak about 30 minutes after the baby is put to the breast and then progressively decline to reach presuckling levels after about 120 minutes (Whitehead et al 1980). Areolar stimulation is essential for prolactin release—the Humalactor, a breast pump which empties the breast by negative pressure, does not stimulate the nipple to release prolactin (Fig. 40.5). Basal prolactin levels are high in the immediate postpartum period and progressively decline after the sixth postpartum week at a rate that is dependent upon suckling frequency and duration (Howie et al 1980). The peak levels of prolactin achieved in response to suckling also decline progressively over time.

Prolactin has a diurnal variation, being higher during hours of sleep, and it has been shown that prolactin responses to suckling are higher in the evening hours compared with those achieved earlier in the same day. These considerations suggest that prolactin production is increased by frequent suckling at regular intervals throughout the 24 hours, including the night time, and that feeding practices that encourage such suckling patterns will produce optimal milk volumes. The relationship between prolactin and milk volume is complex.

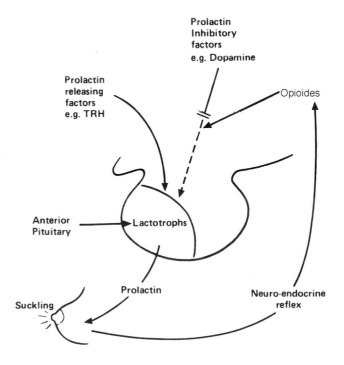

Fig. 40.4 Prolactin release is mainly under the control of prolactin inhibitory factors (dopamine) but can also be stimulated by prolactin-releasing factors (TRH, Hyrotropin-releasing hormone). Suckling may release prolactin by an opiate-mediated inhibitor of dopamine.

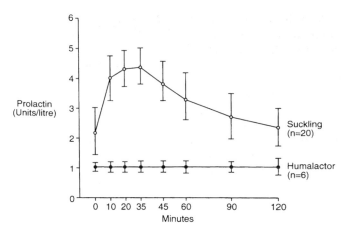

Fig. 40.5 Prolactin release in response to normal suckling and Humalactor. The Humalactor does not stimulate the nipple directly and fails to achieve effective prolactin release. Adapted from Howie et al (1980).

The action of prolactin is to bind to receptors on the alveolar milk-secreting cells of the breast. Prolactin appears to act at multiple sites to stimulate the synthesis of several milk components, including casein, lactalbumin (which may regulate lactose synthesis), fatty acids and other constituents. It appears that prolactin interaction with the plasma membrane of the alveolar cells sets in motion a series of intracellular events that lead to the synthesis and secretion of all milk components (Neville & Berga 1983).

The importance of prolactin to lactogenesis can be demonstrated clinically: the administration in the early puerperium of bromocriptine, a dopamine agonist, rapidly reduces prolactin levels and abolishes milk production (Rolland & Schellekens 1973). There is conflicting evidence about the exact quantitative relationship between prolactin levels and milk production. On the one hand there is no correlation between prolactin levels and milk production in the early puerperium (Howie et al 1980) and mothers who have had pituitary surgery can breast-feed successfully despite having prolactin levels just above the non-pregnant range. On the other hand, dopamine receptor-blocking drugs, such as metoclopramide and sulpride, raise prolactin levels and appear to improve milk production, especially in mothers with failing lactation (Ylikorkala et al 1982). It seems that at least basal levels of prolactin are required for milk production but that above a certain threshold the absolute levels of prolactin do not by themselves dictate the volume of milk produced.

Oxytocin and the milk-ejection reflex

The milk-ejection reflex is responsible for transferring milk from the secreting glands of the breast to the baby. The milk-ejection reflex mimics the prolactin reflex in some respects, insofar as both are initiated by suckling and mediated by afferent neural impulses from the areola to the hypothalamus. They are, however, quite separate physiologically and they have important differences.

The milk-ejection reflex is mediated by the hormone oxytocin, an octapeptide synthesised in specialised magnocellular neurones in the supraoptic and paraventricular nuclei of the hypothalamus. The neuroendocrine reflex leading to oxytocin release can be initiated not just by the suckling of the infant, but also by the mother handling the baby, hearing its cry or even just thinking of feeding. In one mother who was feeding twins, it was noted that regular spontaneous letdown could occur even in the absence of suckling (McNeilly et al 1983). At two weeks postpartum, let-down occurred at 30 minute intervals, increasing to four-hourly intervals at four months postpartum. It is of interest that the frequency of these let-down reflexes has close parallels with the observed nursing frequency in traditional hunter-gathering communities such as the !Kung in the Kalahari desert. Frequent suckling may have been the true norm for the human species until relatively recent times.

In animal studies, a burst of electrical activity in oxytocic neurones can be measured 10–15 seconds prior to milk ejection, indicating that nerve depolarisation is the stimulus for oxytocin release. In contrast to prolactin, oxytocin is released in short bursts (Fig. 40.6) lasting less than a minute, and frequently the largest release of oxytocin occurs in response to the cry of the baby before feeding begins (McNeilly et al 1983). This understanding of the prefeeding release of oxytocin may explain, at least in part, why rooming-in of mother and baby is associated with successful breast-feeding.

The action of oxytocin is to bind to specific receptors on the myoepithelial cells of the breast, thereby causing them to contract. These myoepithelial cells are placed around the milk-secreting cells of the mammary gland and longitudinally in the walls of milk ducts. When the milk-ejection reflex occurs, the contraction of the myoepithelial cells around the alveoli expels the milk into the ducts (McNeilly 1977). The flow of milk to the nipple is facilitated by the wide opening of the ducts, which is induced by contraction of the longitudinal oxytocin-sensitive cells in the duct walls. When the milk-ejection reflex is well established, a mother may be aware of milk being spontaneously ejected from one breast while she suckles her baby on the other.

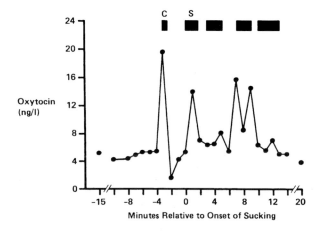

Fig. 40.6 Release of oxytocin in response to an infant's cry (C) and to suckling episodes (S), showing the importance of the presuckling stimuli in stimulating the let-down reflex. Reproduced from McNeilly et al (1983) with permission.

The milk-ejection reflex is very sensitive to emotional stress and the adverse effects of threatening or discouraging remarks to the nursing mother may act in this way. Inhibition of oxytocin release may occur, and catecholamines released by stress may cause constriction of the mammary vessels and prevent oxytocin access to the myoepithelial cells.

It is clear that the milk-ejection reflex is complementary to the prolactin reflex, and both pathways are required for successful lactation. Various studies have suggested that pharmacological stimulation of both the oxytocin and the prolactin (Ylikorkala et al 1982) pathways can improve lactation, although their place in clinical practice is likely to remain very small.

Infant sucking and milk transfer

In addition to milk secretion and ejection by the mother, effective sucking by the infant is also an important part of successful breast feeding. It is now clear that effective removal of the milk during sucking is a very important stimulus for the maintenance of milk production. In contrast to bottle-feeding, where the baby obtains the milk by negative pressure, breast feeding involves milking of the cisterns of the breast, which lie deep to the nipple. To do this, the baby must take the whole nipple into its mouth and place its tongue under the adjacent areola. A baby properly fixed in this way will milk the cisterns with its tongue and, aided by the milk-ejection reflex, will establish a good milk flow. One of the most important aspects in the clinical management of breast feeding is to ensure that the baby is properly fixed. This can be assisted by encouraging the rooting reflex of the baby with the smell and feel of the nipple round its mouth. This makes the baby open its mouth widely and fix properly on the breast.

Detailed observation of babies during breast feeding have shown two distinct sucking patterns, which have been described as nutritive and non-nutritive sucking. Nutritive sucking is characterised by a continuous stream of strong, slow sucks while non-nutritive sucking shows an alternation of rapid shallow bursts of sucking with rests (Drewett & Woolridge 1979). Nutritive sucking occurs predominantly at the beginning of the feed and is increasingly replaced by non-nutritive sucking as the feed progresses. As a result of the changing sucking pattern, the greatest proportion of milk transfer occurs in the early part of the feed (Lucas et al 1979). Patterns of sucking and milk transfer vary substantially among individual mothers. Therefore, it is inappropriate to manage breast feeding on the basis of arbitrary time schedules, and the duration of a feed should be determined by the infant's response.

Table 40.1 Proper fixing of the baby's mouth on the areola enables successful breast feeding by stimulating the following:

- Effective sucking movements from the baby
- Frequent neural impulses to the maternal anterior and posterior pituitary glands
- Prolactin secretion to promote milk production
- Oxytocin release to induce milk let-down
- Efficient milk flow from mother to baby
- Reduced risk of cracked and painful nipples

The physiological function of non-nutritive sucking is not clearly understood. It may be that the baby derives comfort from the close mother–infant contact, but the additional sucking may also be responsible for additional prolactin release and the regulation of maternal fertility and energy balance, which are discussed later.

Mechanisms of milk secretion

A number of separate pathways are involved in the synthesis and secretion of milk products by the mammary alveolar cells. These are summarised below; a more detailed description has been given by Neville & Berga (1983).

Exocytosis

Many of the major components of milk, including lactose, proteins, calcium and phosphate, are packaged into secretory vesicles and secreted by exocytosis. The amino acid sequences of the milk proteins are coded in the nuclear DNA and transcribed into messenger RNA (mRNA), which moves into the cytoplasm. Protein synthesis occurs by translation of the mRNA, and the protein molecules are then transferred to the Golgi system for further processing into secretory vesicles. These vesicles subsequently move to the apex of the cell and they are discharged by the process of exocytosis into the alveolar lumina.

Secretion of ions and water

According to one hypothesis the major milk sugar, lactose, is synthesised when the membrane-bound enzyme, galactosyltransferase, interacts with the protein alpha-lactalbumin within the Golgi system. The Golgi system is impermeable to lactose so that an osmotic gradient is set up, which attracts water into the alveolar cell. Electrolytes follow the water according to their electrochemical gradients. Chloride, however, is out of equilibrium with its concentration in the cytoplasm, and it is postulated that there must be an active transport mechanism to move chloride back into the cell.

Lipid secretion

Lipid secretion is controlled by a different mechanism from the one responsible for lactose and protein synthesis. The lipids in breast milk are mainly triglycerides and they are synthesised in the cytoplasm and smooth endoplasmic reticulum of the alveolar cells. The triglycerides coalesce to form fat droplets which migrate to the apex of the cell; they are secreted by a mechanism which does not involve the Golgi apparatus.

Secretion of immunoglobulins

Immunoglobulin A is the principal immune protein in milk and with some other proteins it can combine with specific receptors on the alveolar basement membrane before being internalised in a secretory vesicle and transported to the apex of the cell for secretion into the lumen.

Paracellular pathway

Some substances may pass between the gaps in the alveolar cells into the milk, and this may be the pathway by which leucocytes and other cells enter the milk. During pregnancy and involution of the breasts, these gaps are relatively leaky but during full lactation the junctions between alveolar cells are much tighter and less permeable.

BREAST MILK

Constituents

The composition of milk varies greatly among species, suggesting that evolution has developed specific milks suited to the needs of the young of each species (Hartmann & Prosser 1984). Studies of human milk composition also show that the concentrations of the various constituents are not constant. The constituents vary from one mother to another and, in any one mother, the milk content varies between one feed and another on the same day and even between the beginning and the end of the same feed. Probably the most important variable is the length of time postpartum, suggesting that the milk content adapts to meet the needs of the infant at any particular stage of development.

These considerations suggest that mother's milk is adapted to meet the needs of the young in a sensitive way which cannot be matched by artificial feeds. It also means that any statements about milk composition merely reflect an average value, around which there is considerable individual variation (Jelliffe and Jelliffe 1978).

The composition of mature human milk is used as a guide for the preparation of artificial feeds; the recommended figures for some of the major constituents are shown in Table 40.2.

Carbohydrates

Human milk contains one of the highest concentrations of carbohydrate of any mammal, mainly in the form of lactose. The dramatic rise in the synthesis of lactose in the first few days after delivery is one of the main features of the transition from colostrum to mature milk. The intestinal enzyme lactase, which is responsible for the hydrolysis and subsequent absorption of lactose, develops late in fetal life so that any intestinal inflammation that interferes with lactase function will lead to lactose intolerance and diarrhoea. When lactose is digested it yields a mixture of galactose and glucose so lactose is not considered to be an essential sugar. The reason for the high lactose content in human milk is not clear, but it may be important in controlling stool acidity and the characteristics of the intestinal flora.

Protein

The total protein content of human milk is much lower than that of cows' milk, and about 40% is in the form of casein. This means that the curds formed in human milk are much softer, more floculent and more easily digestible for the intestinal tract. The remaining proteins are called whey proteins; they represent a mixture of soluble proteins left after the casein curd has formed. Many of these soluble proteins, such as the immunoglobulins, lactoferrin and lysozyme, are important for the anti-infective qualities of human milk and these are discussed below.

Human milk contains high concentrations of alpha-lactalbumin and, although it has been proposed as a regulator of lactose synthesis, a direct correlation between lactose and alpha-lactalbumin levels has yet to be established (Kulski & Hartmann 1981).

Fat

Lipid, which appears mainly as triglycerides, is the most variable constituent of human milk, the highest concentrations appearing in the hind-milk as milk fat globules. Fat is the major source of energy in human milk so that the estimated calorific value of 75 kcal/100 ml (315 kJ/100 ml) is at best only an approximation. The fat content of human milk is also important as the carrier of the fat-soluble vitamins A, D, E and K and of the essential fatty acids. Deficiency of vitamin D can lead to rickets, while that of vitamin K may lead to haemorrhagic disease of the newborn.

Minerals

Compared with cows' milk, human milk has low concentrations of sodium, chloride, iron and some other minerals. The low levels of sodium and chloride are advantageous in infants with diarrhoea because milks with a high solute load can aggravate dehydration. The concentration of iron is low (0.5 μmol/ml) in human milk and some clinicians advise iron supplements in breast fed babies. There is a much higher absorption of iron from breast milk (>75%) compared with cows' milk (30%) or iron-supplemented infant formula (10%) and, although the reason for the greater bioavailability of iron from breast milk is not known, its binding to lactoferrin in human milk may be responsible.

Nutritional adequacy

The nutritional adequacy of breast milk is a matter of controversy. Most authorities, including the Health Departments in the UK, recommend that breast milk alone is sufficient to meet infants' nutritional needs until between four and six months of age. In practice most UK mothers introduce supplementary foods before this and a World Health Organisation (WHO) Survey in 1981 involving 27 different socioeconomic groups throughout the world showed that this was generally true. On the other hand, studies of well nourished mothers from the USA and Australia have shown that some mothers can adequately sustain their babies on breast milk alone for longer than this. By eight months, however, faltering in growth will occur on breast milk alone and supplements are needed. Breast milk can, however, make a

Table 40.2 Comparison of the constituents of human and cow's milk

Constituent	Human milk	Cow's milk
Energy (kcal/100 ml)	75	66
Protein (g/100 ml)	1.1	3.5
Fat (g/100 ml)	4.5	3.7
Lactose (g/100 ml)	6.8	4.9
Sodium (mEq/l)	7	22

major contribution to infant nutrition well into infancy in combination with weaning foods. The nutritional adequacy of breast milk is very variable, depending upon the success of milk production; clinical decisions must be made for individuals on the basis of the infant's progress.

Mammary function during weaning

Breast milk contains a natural inhibitor so that, if her milk is not being removed on a regular basis, the mother will lose secretory activity from her breasts. Thus, during the process of weaning, when there is a reduction in suckling, the milk supply will progressively decline. When weaning is abrupt the concentrations of potassium, glucose and lactose decrease while those of sodium, chloride and protein increase. During gradual weaning the changes are similar but they occur over a longer period of time. If conception occurs during lactation, the rising levels of placental steroids inhibit milk secretion and this overrides the positive stimulus of the infants' sucking.

Following the cessation of regular sucking the mammary gland quickly ceases secretory activity and enters a phase of regression. The milk in the ducts and alveoli is resorbed and, although there is a decrease in parenchymal elements, the breast does not return to its prenatal state as many alveoli persist.

Anti-infective properties

Breast milk contains a number of proteins with antimicrobial activity. The anti-infective properties of breast milk are an important protection for the breast feeding infant, especially in areas with infected water supplies, and the antimicrobial proteins may also protect the breasts against infection and abscess formation (Hartmann & Prosser 1984).

Lactoferrin

Lactoferrin is an iron-binding glycoprotein that inhibits bacterial growth non-specifically. *Escherichia coli* have a high

requirement for free iron; lactoferrin, with its high affinity for iron, may restrict the growth of pathogenic iron-dependent bacteria. The action of lactoferrin may be low in the stomach as little iron is protein-bound in an acidic environment. In the proximal duodenum, however, bicarbonate secretion will favour the binding of iron to lactoferrin and enhance its bacteriostatic action in the intestinal tract.

Lysozyme

Lysozyme is a cationic protein that is present in concentrations of 30–40 mg/100 ml of human milk. Its bactericidal activity is mediated by its ability to cleave proteoglycans in the cell walls of a number of Gram-positive and Gram-negative bacteria. The activity is promoted by other milk components, especially IgA. Lysozyme is stable in the gut because active material is present in the faeces of breast fed babies.

Immunoglobulins

The major immunoglobulin in breast milk is IgA, with smaller amounts of IgM and IgG. The concentration of IgA is particularly high in colostrum and, although its concentration falls to about 2 mg/ml in mature milk, the daily yield remains relatively constant. The IgA in breast milk is poorly absorbed and persists in the infant's gastrointestinal tract to protect against infection. The high concentration of IgA in colostrum enables it to enter the proteoglycan lining of the gastrointestinal tract and this may provide initial surface protection (Whitehead et al 1980).

Specific IgA antibodies, mostly against gastrointestinal pathogens, are also present in human milk. The mechanism of their formation is illustrated in Figure 40.7. It is suggested that if the mother meets a potential pathogen in her own gastrointestinal tract, the antigen is taken up by the gut-associ-

Table 40.3 breast feeding has been adapted by evolution to provide the following:

- The ideal nutrition for human infants
- Immune protection against infection
- Warmth and comfort to the baby
- A natural period of postpartum infertility
- Efficient use of energy resources

Table 40.4 The health benefits associated with breast feeding include the following:

- Reduced neonatal morbidity and mortality from gastrointestinal disease
- Protection against respiratory illnesses in childhood
- Lower risk of necrotising enterocolitis in preterm infants
- Improved development of cognitive function and visual acuity
- A lower incidence of premenopausal breast cancer
- Possible protection against longer term obesity and cardiovascular disease

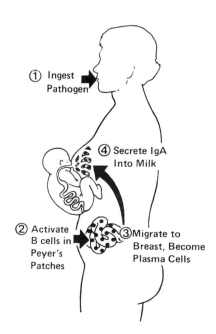

Fig. 40.7 Pathways involved in the secretion of IgA in breast milk by the enteromammary circulation. Figure kindly provided by Professor R.V. Short, Monash University, Australia.

ated lymphoid tissue (GALT) in the Peyer's patches of her terminal ileum. Plasma cells are formed which migrate to the breast where specific IgA is secreted into the breast milk. In this way, the mother is able to give her baby specific protection against pathogens endemic in her environment. This remarkable interaction between mother and baby is, of course, a mechanism that cannot be replicated by artificial feeds.

Other anti-infective factors

Human milk contains a growth factor for *Lactobacillus bifidus* which facilitates colonisation with this organism, which competes with intestinal pathogens. Breast milk also contains cells in the form of macrophages and leucocytes, small amounts of complement and lactoperoxidases; their importance as anti-infective agents *in vivo* has not been defined. The clinical importance of these anti-infective properties will be discussed in a later section.

MATERNAL ADAPTATIONS DURING LACTATION

During lactation, three physiological maternal adaptations take place, all of which have important practical implications. These are:

- the natural inhibition of the mother's fertility
- changes in maternal energy utilisation which enable her to use her calories more efficiently
- regulation of calcium metabolism.

Fertility after childbirth

Because of the importance of breast milk to the nursing infant, it is not surprising that maternal fertility is suppressed during lactation. In this way the baby is not prematurely displaced from the breast by a new sibling, because breast milk tends to decline during another pregnancy. There is also good evidence that both maternal and child health are improved by adequate birth intervals, therefore, it is important to understand and support the natural interbirth intervals induced by breast feeding.

Postpartum fertility in bottle- and breast feeding mothers

Mothers who do not breast-feed have an early resumption of menstruation, ovulation and the potential for fertility. On the basis of basal body temperature rises, the earliest that ovulation has been observed after delivery is four weeks, although it is unusual before five weeks and more commonly delayed until 8–10 weeks postpartum (Howie et al 1982a). Most non-lactating mothers will have resumed ovulation and menstruation by 15 weeks postpartum. The first postpartum cycle in bottle-feeding mothers is frequently anovular (80%) or associated with an inadequate luteal phase (McNeilly et al 1982). By the third cycle normal ovulation and luteal activity have been restored. In non-lactating women who use no contraception, 50% will have conceived by about 6–7 months postpartum (Berman et al 1972). In contrast, breast feeding

women experience a period of lactational amenorrhoea and reduced fertility. The duration of lactational amenorrhoea varies greatly among different populations and among women within the same population. In many developing countries, lactational amenorrhoea may last for two years or more, whereas in developed countries menstruation and fertility may be delayed only for a few weeks (Howie & McNeilly 1982B). During the greatest part of lactational amenorrhoea, ovulation is suppressed and conception cannot occur. In the four weeks prior to the end of lactational amenorrhoea, ovarian activity will return and 30–70% of these cycles will be ovulatory. The longer the period of lactational amenorrhoea, the greater the chance of ovulation in the cycle prior to first menstruation (Howie & McNeilly 1982b). The number of women conceiving during lactational amenorrhoea in the first six months after birth is less than 2% but rises with the passage of time (Kennedy et al 1989B). After the return of menstrual cycles during lactation, the potential for fertility increases, but it does not return to normal because many of the cycles are either anovular or associated with inadequate luteal function (McNeilly et al 1982). On a global scale, lactational amenorrhoea is of great importance for fertility rates in countries where contraceptive usage is low. It has been estimated that in some developing countries breast feeding prevents more pregnancies than all other methods of family planning combined (Howie & McNeilly 1982B).

Endocrine changes after delivery

The normal endocrine control of ovarian function and how it may be modified by suckling are summarised in Figure 40.8. In response to the pulse generator in the hypothalamus, gonadotrophin-releasing hormone (GnRH) is released into the hypophyseal portal blood system. This provokes a pulsatile release of luteinizing hormone (LH) from the anterior pituitary which, in combination with follicle-stimulating hormone (FSH), stimulates follicle development and oestradiol secretion in the ovary. The oestradiol promotes further follicle growth and by positive feedback stimulates the preovulatory LH surge and ovulation (McNeilly et al 1985).

During pregnancy, the high levels of placental steroids suppress the pituitary secretion of both LH and FSH to about 1% of normal. After delivery, oestrogen and progesterone levels fall and, in bottle-feeding mothers, plasma FSH and LH rise to early follicular phase levels by about three weeks postpartum to stimulate ovarian activity.

The mechanisms that lead to the suppression of ovarian activity during lactation are not fully understood but inhibition may occur in two ways (for a review see McNeilly et al 1994). In the first place, suckling induces changes in the sensitivity of the hypothalamic-pituitary axis to oestrogen, making it more sensitive to the negative feedback effects of ovarian steroids and less sensitive to positive feedback. As a result, there is inhibition of GnRH, leading to diminished or inappropriate secretion of LH. When there is sufficient gonadotrophin to stimulate a small follicle during lactation, oestrogens inhibit further pulsatile LH release from the pituitary because of the changed sensitivity to feedback and prevent further follicle development. As the suckling stimulus

ENDOCRINE CONTROL. I

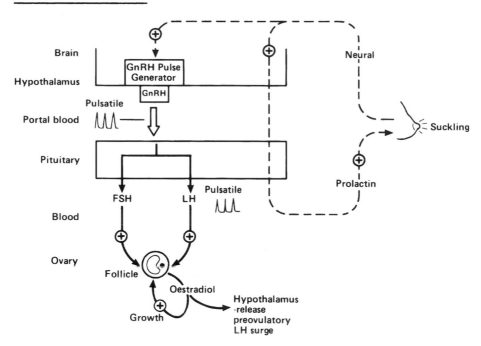

Fig. 40.8 Schematic diagram of the hypothalamic control of gonadotrophin secretion. Gonadotrophin releasing hormone (GnRH) pulses from the hypothalamus induce luteinising hormone (LH) pulses from the pituitary which control follicle development and ovulation. Suckling, either through a direct neural input or by increased prolactin secretion, alters LH pulse secretion through an action on the GnRH pulse generator. (FSH, follicle stimulating hormone) Reproduced from McNeilly et al (1985) with permission.

declines, there is progressive recovery of gonadotrophin levels and menstrual cycles may return during lactation. Many of the cycles remain abnormal, being either anovular or having inadequate luteal phases, and these may be due to suboptimal gonadotrophin stimulation (McNeilly et al 1985).

In the second place, the prolactin that is released during suckling may contribute to ovarian inhibition during lactation. Prolactin may have a direct inhibitory effect on the ovary or may, through a short-loop feedback effect, contribute to the reduced gonadotrophin secretion from the pituitary (McNeilly et al 1994). At present there is no direct evidence that prolactin plays a part in ovarian inhibition during lactation and its exact role has yet to be defined.

Contraceptive effect of breast feeding

In countries where contraceptive usage is low, breast feeding makes an important contribution to birth-spacing and completed family size. It is clearly important not to change breast feeding practices in countries with low contraceptive usage without fully appreciating their implications for fertility. In Africa, Asia and Latin America, contraceptive usage would have to increase sharply to keep fertility rates at their present levels if the average duration of lactational amenorrhoea was to fall (Howie 1992).

breast feeding, although having an important influence on fertility at a population level, is often regarded as an unreliable method of contraception for individual women. In

1988, an interdisciplinary group met in Bellagio, Italy and produced a consensus on how breast feeding could serve as a safe and effective family planning method (Kennedy et al 1989). The guidelines depend upon the evidence that a mother who is still amenorrhoeic and fully breast feeding has more than 98% protection from pregnancy during the first six months postpartum. These guidelines (Fig. 40.9) have been described as the Lactation Amenorrhoea Method (LAM), and a number of studies have shown their validity within a variety of cultural settings (World Health Organisation 1999). The length of lactational amenorrhoea is the most important marker of continuing protection against returning fertility and, although it does not give complete protection against conception, lactational amenorrhoea is a culturally acceptable method for spacing pregnancies for many individuals, especially in traditional communities.

Maternal energy requirements during lactation

For lactating mothers the daily calorie intake recommended by WHO is 2700 kcal/day for the first 6 months and 2950 kcal/day from six months onwards. This figure is reached by the arithmetic calculation of 2200 kcal/day for normal non-lactating non-pregnancy requirements plus an additional 500 kcal/day for the overall energy cost of the milk. Assuming an average milk volume, the average calorie value of breast milk is 750 kcal/day, which is supplemented from the maternal fat stores laid down during pregnancy to the

Ask the mother:

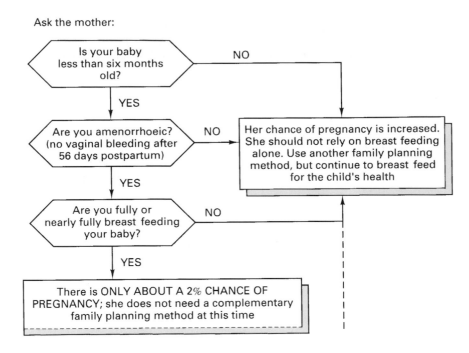

Fig. 40.9 Diagrammatic representation of the application of the lactational amenorrhoea method of fertility control for breast feeding mothers.

tune of 250 kcal/day. At the end of six months it is assumed that the available fat stores will have been used up and an additional dietary supplement of 250 kcal/day will be required.

Observational studies on healthy lactating women in developed countries have shown that their actual calorie intakes based on measured portions of food do not reach the theoretical recommendations. For example, Whitehead et al (1981) reported 2300 kcal/day in mothers who had no limitation on food availability and successfully breast fed their babies (Whitehead et al 1981). In developing countries the gap between theoretical and actual food intake is even greater. Prentice et al (1981) found that Gambian mothers took 1773 kcal/day in the dry season and 1474 kcal/day in the less plentiful wet season and, despite the calorie shortfall, breast fed their babies successfully for prolonged periods (Prentice et al 1981).

One possible reason for this discrepancy between the theoretical and actual energy requirements of nursing mothers is an increase in energy efficiency during lactation. Animal studies have shown that lactation is associated with an inhibition of non-shivering thermogenesis, leading to storage of all available dietary calories to be used in milk formation. In the mouse this is achieved by physiological inhibition of brown-fat cells which, in the non-lactating state, can burn off excess calories. In this way the lactating animal becomes more energy-efficient. Recent studies have shown that similar adaptations takes place in nursing mothers although the biological mechanism in the human probably does not occur through brown fat. Compared with the bottle-feeding mother, the lactating mother shows an increased sensitivity to insulin and changes in resting metabolic rate may also be important.

Although the biological mechanisms have not been fully defined, it is clear that nursing itself conserves maternal energy resources for the benefit of the sucking infant.

This concept of maternal energy adaptation during lactation has two potential implications. Firstly, it means that a mother who eats according to the WHO recommendations may fail to lose weight in the postpartum period. Secondly, mothers who bottle-feed in developing countries will lose the energy-sparing effect and society will have to provide more calories to meet the needs of the mother–infant pair. Further research is required to define the biological mechanism and practical implications of this physiological adaptation in nursing mothers.

Calcium balance and bone metabolism

During the third trimester of pregnancy and lactation, calcium is transferred from mother to baby at a rate of 200–250 mg per day for mineralisation of the fetal skeleton. In addition, the breast feeding mother has low circlating oestrogen levels as a result of ovarian suppression, raising theoretical concerns about bone health in lactating women. Recent research, however, suggests that these demands for calcium are met by adaptive changes, which include increased absorption of dietary calcium, greater renal tubal reabsorption of calcium and mobilisation of maternal bone with subsequent repletion at weaning.

There is no evidence that these changes in calcium balance during lactation carry any long-term risk of osteoporosis and fractures nor that supplementation with calcium modifies the natural adaptive process (Prentice et al 1995).

CLINICAL EFFECTS OF BREAST FEEDING

There has been a recent surge in the amount of research investigating the short and long-term effects of infant feeding on health and development. Many of the necessary studies have long time frames and it may be some years before the full range of benefits are completely understood.

Effects on infant mortality

In non-industrialised countries, breast feeding is a matter of life and death for newborn babies and infants. The World Health Organisation estimates that 1.5 million deaths per annum could be prevented if women were encouraged to breast-feed their infants exclusively for six months and partially until two years of age (World Health Organisation 1992). The benefits are greatest in those settings where clean water supplies cannot be guaranteed and adequate supplies of infant formula cannot be provided.

The principal cause of excess deaths among non-breast fed infants is diarrhoeal disease, although other factors, such as acute respiratory infection, also play a part. Overall, breast feeding offers about a twofold reduction in mortality in non-industrialised countries, and it is vital that effective steps are taken to promote and protect breast feeding rates in these settings.

Gastrointestinal infection

Even in industrialised countries, there is now strong evidence that breast feeding has a protective effect against infantile gastrointestinal illness. Studies have used different methodologies but typical results from a longitudinal study, which corrected for confounding variables, are shown in Figure 40.10. Babies who were bottle fed from birth or weaned at an early stage had gastrointestinal illness rates of 5–8 times greater than those who were fully or partially breast fed for 13 weeks (Howie et al 1990). A meta-analysis of all comparative studies from developed countries shows a significant

and important protective effect, which leads to reduced disease rates, lower hospital admission and less use of financial resources. When studies have examined the protective effect of breast feeding against specific organisms, the clearest benefits have been shown against *E. coli*, giardia, salmonella and campylobacter but less clearly against rotavirus diarrhoea (Golding et al 1997a).

Non-gastrointestinal infections

Respiratory infections are the commonest cause of morbidity amongst infants and exact a huge toll of infant deaths in non-industrialised countries. The evidence that breast feeding protects against respiratory infection in infants is less clear-cut than with gastrointestinal disease. The balance of evidence, however, suggests that a small, but nevertheless important, degree of protection does occur, particularly against lower rather than upper respiratory tract infections (Golding et al 1997b).

In respect of acute and chronic otitis media, there is consistent evidence of protection with extended duration of breast feeding (Golding et al 1997b). Other infections which are reduced by breast feeding include haemophilus B meningitis, neonatal sepsis and urinary tract infection (Golding et al 1997b).

Interesting new information is emerging that breast feeding in infancy may have important long-term protective effects against recurrent chest infections in older children (Wilson et al 1998). In addition to the effect of breast or formula feeding, there are important confounding effects that increase the risk of childhood wheeze when solids are introduced prematurely. This work suggests that the issue of infant feeding should not be seen only in the narrow, and often emotional, debate of breast versus bottle but in the wider context of a good start to a lifetime of healthy eating.

HIV infection

There is now clear evidence that HIV infection can be transferred from mother to child through breast milk. This risk is particularly high in mothers with overt clinical symptoms, and in the early weeks of the baby's life. Mothers who are known to be HIV positive should be advised to bottle-feed in those countries such as the UK where infant formula can be given as a safe alternative to breast milk. In less developed countries, this advice may not be appropriate because the risks of not breast feeding may be greater than those of HIV transmission. Furthermore, in a setting where breast feeding is the norm, the decision to formula feed may be tantamount to a declaration of HIV status and social exclusion. Policies have to be sensitive and relevant to local circumstances.

Allergic disease

Although there is a widespread belief that breast feeding protects against asthma, eczema and allergy, the evidence to support this is inconsistent. It is clear that a family history of allergic disorders is crucially important and not all studies

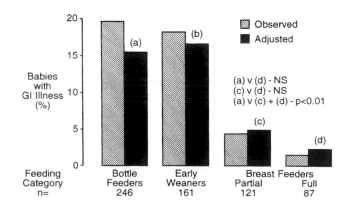

Fig. 40.10 Rates of gastrointestinal illness during the first 13 weeks of life according to infant feeding method (bottle fed from birth; early weaning before 13 weeks; partial and full breast feeding for 13 weeks). Adapted from Howie et al (1990).

have taken this sufficiently into account (British Paediatric Association 1994). Babies who are breast fed are less likely to be given solid food at an early stage, and avoiding early solids may be more important than breast feeding itself in reducing the risk of allergy. Advice on infant feeding to reduce the risk of allergy should be focussed mainly on those with a strong family history.

Other illnesses

A number of published reports suggest that breast feeding may have protective effects for a number of clinical conditions. In some of these conditions, there is, as yet, relatively little information but further research may confirm important health benefit.

Necrotising enterocolitis

This condition occurs in premature babies and there is good evidence that breast milk helps to reduce its incidence and severity (Lucas & Cole 1990). It has been estimated that giving breast milk to preterm babies will save 100 lives per year in the UK (Lucas & Cole 1990). Every effort should be made to encourage mothers to provide breast milk for their own preterm babies. Because of the need to quarantine milk against the risk of HIV transmission, many breast milk banks were closed in the 1980s but some centres are making strenuous efforts to reopen them in order to meet the needs of vulnerable preterm babies.

Insulin dependent diabetes mellitus (IDDM)

Recent evidence has suggested that exposure to bovine human albumin through infant feeding could trigger the auto-immune process leading to juvenile onset diabetes (British Paediatric Association 1994). Some studies have shown an association between formula feeding and IDDM, but not all reports have confirmed this. Further work is needed to define the role of breast feeding, but it seems plausible that the method of early infant feeding has an important role in early onset diabetes.

Haemorrhagic disease of the newborn

breast fed babies are at greater risk of this disorder, but it can be prevented by the appropriate use of vitamin K supplementation.

Neoplastic disease

There have been isolated reports that breast feeding is associated with reduced levels of childhood cancer, particularly lymphoma, but more work is required to establish the strength and importance of these associations (British Paediatric Association 1994).

There is, however, considerable evidence to show that breast feeding is associated with a small, but important, reduction in premenopausal breast cancer among lactating mothers (UK National Case-Control Study Group 1993). The protection increases with duration of breast feeding but it does not extend to offer any protection against the commoner postmenopausal breast cancer. There is also some evidence of reduced ovarian and endometrial cancer although there is

controversy over aspects of study design in the reports that have considered these topics.

Heart and vascular disease

One of the most interesting concepts to emerge in recent years is that early infant feeding may play a part in programming individuals for or against the development of illnesses in later life. For example, recent work suggests that breast feeding may protect against obesity, hypertension and adversely high cholesterol levels and low-density lipoprotein to high-density lipoprotein (LDL/HDL) ratios (Ravelli et al 2000). All of these factors are markers for maturity onset diabetes, cardiac and vascular disease and long-term cohort studies are required to establish the validity and importance of such associations. This possibility should prove to be a fruitful area for future research and may have profound, and as yet unrecognised, implications for community health.

breast feeding and neurological development

Studies which have compared IQ development have consistently shown higher scores among breast fed than bottle-fed children (Golding et al 1997c). Similarly, a comparative study, with long-term follow-up, found that preterm babies who had received breast milk had better intellectual development than those who did not. In addition to IQ, there is evidence of behavioural effects, such as fewer speech difficulties in children under five years who were breast fed (Golding et al 1997c). Although these reports are consistent and they show that the effects are related to the duration of breast feeding, they have been criticised on the grounds that they cannot correct for potential confounding variables, especially parental IQ, parenting skills and other factors that could influence development.

Nevertheless, there are also associations between breast feeding and improved visual acuity, an outcome which will be less influenced by parental behaviour. Also, the presence of long-chain polyunsaturated fatty acids in breast, but not formula, milk give biological plausibility for a true difference because they play a part in neurological development.

It is not possible to mount randomised controlled trials for breast and bottle feeding so it is difficult to fully resolve the issue as to whether breast milk has a true independent effect on neurological development. On the other hand, the evidence is compatible with a real and important health benefit. It is appropriate that health professionals should provide prospective parents with a balanced view of the available information so that they can make the infant feeding choices they deem best for their own child.

COST EFFECTS OF BREAST FEEDING

The Department of Health in the UK has estimated that the NHS would have saved £35 million in 1995 had all babies been breast fed, on the basis of the reduced incidence of gastrointestinal illness. Similarly, in the US, the costs per never breast fed baby have been estimated at between $331–$475 during the first year of life (Ball & Wright 1999). In developing countries, the discontinuation of breast feeding would have even more far reaching economic effects.

For the individual parents, breast feeding leads to savings on the expense of formula although the economic need to return to work is frequently cited as a reason for choosing to bottle feed.

CHOICE OF INFANT FEEDING

One of the common criticisms made by prospective parents is that those who choose to artificially feed their infants are made to feel guilty by their attending health professionals. It is most important that information and advice is given in a non-judgmental fashion and that parents are supported fully once they have made their decision.

Every five years, there is a national study of infant feeding rates in the UK, the last being conducted in 1995 (Foster et al 1997). After falling to their lowest levels in the late 1960s and 1970s, breast feeding rates rose steadily in the UK during the 1980s but they have remained relatively unchanged over the past ten years (Foster et al 1997).

Overall, the initial breast feeding rate in the UK is between 50–65%, being higher in England and Wales than in Scotland and Northern Ireland. In all UK countries, however, there is a rapid fall in breast feeding rates during the first four months with only about half the mothers continuing to breast-feed at that time. Many factors are associated with the choice to initiate breast feeding and the ability to sustain it. Most importantly these include social class, maternal age and previous breast feeding experience (Fig. 40.11).

Choice of infant feeding is very strongly influenced by the cultural environment. Mothers who choose to formula feed will often do so because it is the norm among their family and friends. In addition, they can share the responsibility for feeding and they gain confidence from seeing that the baby is getting enough. There is also a common perception that bottle fed babies gain weight more steadily and settle into all-night sleeping more quickly.

The UK has one of the lowest breast feeding rates in Europe and compares poorly with such as the Scandinavian countries, where breast feeding initiation and continuation rates to four months are in excess of 90%. The Health Departments in the UK have established the promotion of breast feeding as a health priority because of the potential short and long-term health gains both for the individuals and for the community.

MANAGEMENT OF BREAST FEEDING

Despite the many advantages of breast feeding, there is evidence of its decline in many countries although this is not universal.

WHO/UNICEF have made a joint statement outlining 'Ten steps to successful breast feeding'. (Six of these are relevant to the development of personnel properly equipped to help new mothers.)

1. Have a written breast feeding policy.

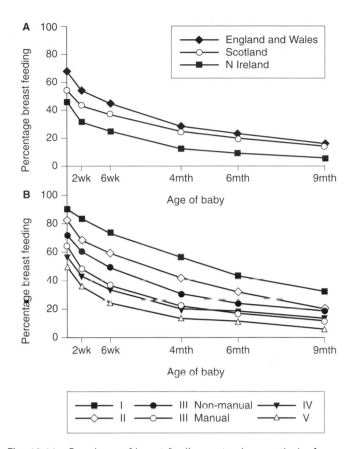

Fig. 40.11 Prevalence of breast feeding up to nine months by **A** country and **B** social class in the United Kingdom 1995 (adapted from Infant Feeding, 1995, Office for National Statistics).

2. Train all staff.
3. Inform all pregnant women about the benefits and management of breast feeding.
4. Help mothers to initiate breast feeding within half an hour of birth.
5. Show mothers how to breast-feed.
6. Foster the establishment of breast feeding support groups.
7. Practice 24-hour rooming-in.
8. Encourage breast feeding on demand.
9. Give newborn infants no other food or drink, unless medically indicated.
10. Use no artificial teats.

These ten steps are used as the basis on which the award of baby-friendly status is awarded to hospitals or communities. All of the ten steps have an evidence base to support their inclusion and the relevant information has been published by WHO/UNICEF (World Health Organisation 1998).

A major complaint from many mothers is the conflicting advice that they receive from health professionals. The details of how to manage breast feeding is beyond the scope of this chapter but there are now several texts on best practice. It is essential that all who attend new mothers should understand the mechanisms and management of successful breast feeding (Sikorski and Renfrew 2000).

FORMULA FEEDING

Mothers who choose to formula feed require the same care and attention as breast feeding mothers. Most mothers who initially choose to breast-feed will move to formula at some stage so all mothers should be shown how to prepare feeds correctly and to observe the necessary standards to minimise the risk of infections. Mothers should be encouraged not to change formula and, whether bottle or breast feeding, to delay introducing solids until the recommended time of four months of age.

SUMMARY

Lactation is an important part of natural human reproduction. Efforts by modern civilisation to replace lactation by artificial substitutes do not detract from its physiological relevance or its practical importance.

The primary function of lactation is to nourish the infant and human milk is the ideal, and best adapted, food for the human baby. Far reaching immediate and long-term health benefits occur as a consequence of breast feeding, and the full range and extent of these are only now being uncovered by new research.

Important secondary features of breast feeding are birth spacing, energy sparing effects and the adaptations to calcium balance. Infant feeding policies have important financial consequences, both for the community and the individual, which are especially relevant in developing countries.

Policies related to the initiation and maintenance of breast feeding, the appropriate use of supplements, contraceptive advice to nursing mothers and maternal diet must all be based on a sound understanding of the physiology of lactation.

The promotion of breast feeding is a stated health priority in the UK and the baby-friendly initiative is a practical approach towards meeting this important goal.

KEY POINTS

- Lactation is a finely adapted mechanism to ensure the optimum nutrition of human infants.
- Good fixing is a key to successful breast feeding by stimulating prolactin and oxytocin release and promoting good milk flow.
- Important consequences of successful breast feeding are the protective health benefits for both the baby and mother.
- Secondary effects of breast feeding are uterine involution, a natural period of infertility and efficient use of energy.
- The 10 steps to successful breast feeding have been developed to promote increased initiation and continuation rates.
- Infant feeding has important social and psychological effects and all mothers must be fully supported in their individual choice.

REFERENCES

Ball T, Wright A 1999 Health care costs of formula feeding in the first year of life. Pediatrics 103:870–876

Berman ML, Hanson K, Hillman IL 1972 Effect of breast feeding on postpartum menstruation, ovulation and pregnancy in Alaskan Eskimos. Am J Obstet Gynecol 114:524–534

Drewett RF, Woolridge M 1979 Suckling patterns of human babies on the breast. Early Hum Dev 3/4:315–320

Foster K, Lader D, Cheesbrough S 1997 In Infant Feeding. The Stationery Office, London

Gardner DL, Dodds TC 1976 Human Histology. Churchill Livingstone, Edinburgh

Golding J, Emmett PM, Rogers IS 1997a Gastroenteritis, diarrhoea and breast feeding. Early Hum Dev 49(suppl):83–103

Golding J, Emmett PM, Rogers IS 1997b Does breast feeding protect against non-gastric infections? Early Hum Dev 49(suppl):105–120

Golding J, Rogers IS, Emmett PM 1997c Association between breast feeding, child development and behaviour. Early Human Dev 49(suppl):175–184

Hartmann PE, Prosser CG 1984 Physiological basis of longitudinal changes in human milk yield and composition. Federal Proc 43:2448–2453

Howie PW, McNeilly AS, McArdle T, Smart L, Houston M 1980 The relationship between suckling induced prolactin response and lactogenesis. J Clin Endocrinol Metab 50:670–673

Howie PW, McNeilly AS, Houston MJ, Cook A, Boyle H 1982a Fertility after childbirth: postpartum ovulation and menstruation in bottle and breast feeding mothers. Clin Endocrinol 17:323–332

Howie PW, McNeilly AS 1982b Effect of breast feeding patterns on human birth intervals. J Reprod Fertil 65:545–557

Howie PW, Forsyth JS, Ogston SA, Florey CD 1990 Protective effect of breast feeding against infection. Br Med J 300:11–16

Howie PW 1992 Natural family planning. Br Med Bull 49:182–199

Jelliffe DB, Jelliffe EFP 1978 Human milk in the modern world. Oxford University Press, Oxford

Kennedy RI, Rivera R, McNeilly AS 1989 Consensus statement on the use of breastfeeding as a family planning method. Contraception 39:477–496

Kulski JK, Hartmann PE 1981 Changes in human milk composition during the initiation of lactation. Aust J Exp Biol Med Sci 59:101–104

Lucas A, Lucas PJ, Baum JD 1979 Pattern of milk flow in breast-fed infants. Lancet ii:57–58

Lucas A, Cole TJ 1990 Breast milk and neonatal necrotising enterocolitis. Lancet 336:1519–1523

McNeilly AS, Howie PW, Houston MJ, Cook A, Boyle H 1982 Fertility after childbirth: adequacy of post-partum luteal phases. Clin Endocrinol 17:609–615

McNeilly AS 1977 Physiology of Lactation. J Biosoc Sci suppl 4:5–21

McNeilly AS, Robinson IC, Houston MJ, Howie PW 1983 Release of oxytocin and prolactin in response to suckling. Br Med J 286:257–259

McNeilly AS, Glasier A, Howie PW 1985 Endocrine control of lactational infertility. In: Dobbing J (ed) Maternal nutrition and lactational infertility. Nestle Nutrition Workshop Series vol 9. Raven, New York, pp 1–5

McNeilly AS, Tay CCK, Glasier A 1994 Physiological mechanisms underlying lactational amenorrhoea. Ann NY Acad Sci 709:145–155

Neville MC, Berga SE 1983 Cellular and molecular aspects of the hormone control of mammary control. In: Neville MC, Neifert MR (eds) Physiology, nutrition and breast feeding. Plenum, New York, pp 141–156

Prentice AM, Whitehead RG, Roberts SB, Paul AA 1981 Long-term energy balance in child-bearing Gambian women. Am J Clin Nutr 34:2790–2799

Prentice A, Jargon L, Cole T, Stirling D, Dibba B, Fairweather-Tait S 1995 Calcium requirements of lactating Gambian mothers; effect of a calcium supplement in breastmilk calcium concentrations, maternal bone mineral content and urinary calcium excretion. Am J Clin Nutr 62:58–67

Ravelli ACJ, Van der Meulen JHP, Osmond C, Barker DJP, Beker OP 2000 Infant feeding and adult glucose tolerance, lipid profile, blood pressure and obesity. Arch Dis Child 82:248–252

Rolland R, Schellekens LA 1973 A new approach to the inhibition of puerperal lactation. J Obst Gynaecol Br Commonw 80:945–951

Sikorski J, Renfrew M 2000 Support for breast feeding mothers (Cochran review). In: The Cochran Library, Issue 2. Update Software, Oxford

Standing Committee on Nutrition of the British Paediatric Association. Is breast feeding beneficial in the UK? Arch Dis Child 1994; 71:376–380

United Kingdom National Case-Control Study Group. Breast feeding and risk of breast cancer in young women. Br Med J 1993; 307:17–20

Watson DL 1980 Immunological functions of the mammary gland and its secretion—comparative review. Aust J Biol Sci 33:403–422

Whitehead RG, Paul AA, Rowland MGM 1980 Lactation in Cambridge and the Gambia. Topics in Paeds 2:2203

Whitehead RG, Paul AA, Black AE, Wiles SJ 1981 Recommended dietary amounts of energy for pregnancy and lactation in the United Kingdom. In: Torun B, Young VR, Rand WM (eds) Protein energy requirements of developing countries: evaluation of new data. United National University, Tokyo, pp 259–265

Wilson AC, Forsyth JS, Greene SA, Irvine L, Hau C, Howie PW 1998 Relation of infant diet to childhood health; seven years of follow-up of cohort of children in Dundee infant feeding study. Br Med J 316:21–25

World Health Organisation Contemporary patterns of breast feeding. Report on the WHO collaborative study on breast feeding. WHO, Geneva, 1981

World Health Organisation Breast feeding: the technical basis and recommendations for action. Sacchen RJ (ed) WHO, Geneva, 1993

World Health Organisation 1998 Evidence for the ten steps to successful breast feeding. Division of Child Health and Development. WHO, Geneva

World Health Organisation Multinational study of breast feeding and lactational amenorrhoea 111 Pregnancy during breast feeding. Fertil Steril 1999; 72:431–440

Ylikorkala O, Kaupilla A, Kivinen S, Viinikka L 1982 Sulpiride improves inadequate lactation. Br Med J 285:249–251

41

Puerperal sepsis

Philip J. Steer

This chapter is based on the chapters in the previous editions and the current author wishes to acknowledge their contribution. All errors are, however, his own.

HISTORY

Today, the idea that hospitals are dangerous places in which to be is widely appreciated. The concept of nosocomial (iatrogenically acquired) infection is also familiar, not least because of the publicity given to multidrug resistant *Staphylococcus aureus* (MRSA). It is something of a shock to be reminded that such awareness has not always been present. Alexander Gordon's 'Treatise on the Epidemic Puerperal Fever of Aberdeen', published in 1795, was the earliest report that puerperal fever was contagious. It is remarkable that, long before the recognition of microorganisms, he was able to deduce that hand washing reduced the spread of disease. Unfortunately, Gordon's insights were greeted with hostility and he had to leave Aberdeen to become a naval surgeon.

Oliver Wendell Holmes (1809–1894) was more successful. He received a medical degree from Harvard Medical School in 1836 and began to practice medicine in Boston, Massachusetts. From 1847 to 1882 he taught at Harvard Medical School. Holmes' essay 'The Contagiousness of Puerperal Fever' (1843) advanced the use of aseptic techniques in obstetrics and surgery. Perhaps surprisingly, Holmes was better known in his day as a popular novelist, rather than as a physician.

Ignaz Semmelweis, working in the Obstetric Clinic in Vienna in the nineteenth century, is probably the best known of the campaigners against puerperal sepsis. He concluded that students in his hospital were transmitting contamination from the postmortem room to the delivery ward, where they attended women in labour. He deduced this by comparing the higher rate of infection in the obstetrical division with that of the pupil midwives, who trained on mannequins rather than cadavers. By making his students wash their hands in carbolic, he reduced the rate of sepsis, and the prevailing maternity mortality rates of 18% dropped to 1.27% (similar to that in the midwives' division). In March and August of 1848 no woman died of childbirth in his division. The younger medical men in Vienna recognised the significance of Semmelweis' discovery but his superior, on the other hand, did not and was critical. Semmelweis had to leave Vienna. He worked for the next six years at the St Rochus Hospital in Pest. An epidemic of puerperal fever had broken out in the obstetrics department, and, at his request, Semmelweis was put in charge of the department. His measures promptly reduced the mortality rate, and in his years there it averaged only 0.85%. In Prague and Vienna, meantime, the rate was still high, ranging from 10 to 15%.

In 1855 Semmelweis was appointed professor of obstetrics at the University of Pest. His ideas were accepted in Hungary, and the government addressed a circular to all district authorities ordering the introduction of his prophylactic methods. Vienna remained hostile towards him, and the editor of the Wiener Medizinische Wochenschrift wrote that it was time to 'stop the nonsense about the chlorine hand wash'.

In 1861 Semmelweis published his principal work, Die Ätiologie, der Begriff und die Prophylaxis des Kindbettfiebers ('Aetiology, Understanding and Prevention of Childbed Fever'). He sent it to many prominent obstetricians, but most disagreed with his theory. He addressed several open letters to professors of medicine in other countries, but to little effect. At a conference of German physicians and natural scientists, most of the speakers, including the pathologist Rudolf Virchow, rejected his doctrine. The years of controversy gradually undermined his spirit. In 1865 he suffered a breakdown and he was taken to a mental hospital, where he died. Ironically, his illness and death were caused by the infection of a wound on his right hand, apparently the result of an operation he had performed before being taken ill. He died of the same disease against which he had struggled all his professional life.

However, eventually asepsis and antisepsis were accepted, because of the outstanding work of scientists such as Pasteur and Koch and clinicians such as Lister and Simpson. The next breakthroughs were the introduction of Prontosil (a sulphonamide) in the 1930s and penicillin in the 1940s. After being static for almost a hundred years, maternal mortality finally began to drop, to reach such a low level today that it would have been almost unimaginable 70 years ago. Despite this, maternal deaths still occur from puerperal sepsis. In the Confidential Enquiry into Maternal Deaths from 1994 through 1996 (Anonymous 1998), there were 16 deaths caused by genital tract sepsis, a similar number to those which occurred in the previous triennium. Of these, five early onset and one late onset (six weeks) cases were positively identified as being due to β haemolytic streptococcus group A, one to group B, and one unspecified group. Other bacteria identified included one case each of enterococcus and *Escherichia coli*. The comment was made that 'Puerperal sepsis is not a disease of the past, and GPs and midwives must be aware of the signs and be prepared to institute immediate treatment and referral of any recently delivered woman with a fever or offensive vaginal discharge.'

MICROBIOLOGY

In the nineteenth and first half of the twentieth century, it is likely that streptococcus Lancefield group A was the main cause of puerperal sepsis. Although the discovery and development of antibiotics in the mid twentieth century had a major impact, it is likely that this streptococcus had been declining in virulence for some time. This was probably part of a natural cycle, whereby human populations build up their inherited resistance to specific microorganisms, only to find their place taken by more virulent strains. However, more recently, there is evidence that the streptococcus has been making a comeback (Holm 1996, Kent et al 1999). Streptococci are gram-positive cocci which appear in short twisted chains (hence their name).

Beta-haemolytic streptococcus group A

Group A streptococci (GAS) produce over 20 extracellular products, including streptokinase (produced by all β haemolytic strains), streptodornase (a deoxyribonuclease that depolymerises (uncoils) DNA molecules), and hyaluronidase (splits hyaluronic acid, an important component of connective tissue, and helps in the spread of GAS through the tissues). It also produces three pyrogenic exotoxins. The exotoxins have been associated with streptococcal toxic shock syndrome. Diphosphopyridine nucleotidase provides GAS with the ability to kill leucocytes; haemolysins give all haemolytic streptococci their characteristic ability to lyse the cells in blood agar culture media. Streptolysin is of interest because of the antibody that it induces. Antistreptolysin O can be titred, a high titre meaning a recent infection. Streptolysin S is elaborated in the presence of serum and is responsible for the haemolysis seen on agar plates. It is not antigenic.

Because serological tests do not distinguish reliably between current and recent infection, diagnosis is dependent on culture and more recently, on a rapid diagnostic test for GAS based on the identification of a cell wall antigen and detected by latex agglutination or other method. This gives a result in 10–60 minutes instead of the two days required for a culture. Its sensitivity is 60–85% and specificity 90–95%.

For all streptococci, there is a large reservoir of the organism in the form of chronic carriers. Carriage develops after infection. Carriers usually have relatively small bacterial loads. They are at little risk for acute disease or sequelae but are probably the most common source of infection for others. The distinction between colonization and infection is however less clear for GAS than for the other groups. Infection can be acquired from carriers by poor hygiene in maternity wards. For example, an outbreak of GAS puerperal sepsis from the communal use of bidets that were not properly cleaned has been reported (Gordon et al 1994). Eight women were affected, as were three of their babies.

The streptococcal Toxic Shock Syndrome is a fulminant, invasive group form of GAS infection. It is characterised by shock, bacteraemia, respiratory and multi-organ failure. Death occurs in about 30% of patients. Bacteraemia occurs frequently in patients with severe GAS infections. Complications include necrotising fasciitis, a progressive infection of the subcutaneous tissue with destruction of fascia and fat, and myositis. Necrotising fasciitis can start with infection of perineal tears or episiotomies and pictures of such a case have been published by Ammari et al (1986). It can also start in the abdominal wound following caesarean section. Such infections are often reported in the Press as 'the flesh eating killer bug', which dramatically describes the effect it has on the patient. It responds poorly to antibiotics and treatment consists of urgent and very extensive tissue debridement. Once the wound has healed, skin grafting is often necessary.

The main treatment for streptococcal infection remains high dose intravenous penicillin.

Beta-haemolytic streptococcus group B

The β haemolytic streptococcus group B (GBS) bacterium is widely carried in the large intestine, and about 20 to 30% of the female population are carriers during their reproductive years. The rate of carriage is higher in women of African ethnic origin. In carriers, the vagina becomes intermittently colonised. Detection of carriage is often fortuitous, with the organism being discovered at the time of routine urine or vaginal or rectal swab cultures taken for other reasons. Detection is by culture, although the culture media routinely used detects only about 60% of the carriers. Special culture media for enhanced detection are available, but they are too expensive for routine use at present. Methods for direct immunological detection are being developed, which will be much quicker and probably less expensive.

The main problem with this organism is that it can cause early (1–10 days after birth, usually presenting with septicaemia and respiratory disease) and late onset (6–12 weeks, usually presenting with meningitis) infections in the newborn, which have a 5–20% fatality rate, the rate being higher with early onset disease. About 10% of babies born to carrier mothers become infected, so it has been calculated that about 75 babies per year in the UK die of the disease, and about 40 (10% of the survivors) are handicapped.

The following clinical risk factors increase the risk of infection in the newborn of carriers at least three-fold:

- Preterm labour
- Prelabour rupture of membranes
- Prolonged rupture of membranes (more than 18 to 24 hours before delivery)
- Pyrexia (38°C or higher) during labour

A previous baby infected with GBS is associated with a 10-fold increased risk of a subsequent child being infected. Colonisation combined with one or more clinical risk factors increases the risk at least 12-fold.

Seventy-five per cent of early-onset GBS disease and 90% of resultant deaths follow deliveries with one or more of these risk factors. About half of the babies born to mothers colonised with GBS at the time of delivery will become colonised themselves but of these, only around 1 in 200 will develop GBS disease.

Many studies have shown that the chance of a baby developing early-onset GBS infection can be reduced by over 70% (and the number of fatalities by 75–80%) by adopting the following measures (Boyer & Gotoff 1986, 1998, Gotoff & Boyer 1997).

Women at increased risk should be offered intravenous penicillin (or alternative if allergic) immediately at the onset of labour or rupture of membranes. For women in labour, the recommended doses of penicillin G are 3 g (or 5 mU) intravenously initially and then 1.5 g (or 2.5 mU) at four-hourly intervals until delivery. For women who are allergic to penicillin, the recommended doses of clindamycin are 900 mg intravenously every eight hours until delivery. Intravenous antibiotics should be given for at least four hours prior to delivery whenever possible. Babies born when the mother has not received at least four hours of intravenous antibiotics should be investigated and commenced on antibiotics until it has been established the baby is not infected. It should be noted in this context that it is not possible to eradicate carrier status in most women and therefore antibiotic treatment before the onset of labour is not recommended. Although routine screening at 36–37 weeks is currently being advocated by some groups in the USA (for example, see www.groupbstrep.org), it is currently not being recommended in the UK, mainly on the grounds of cost and logistics. For further information there are several excellent websites; the UK Group B Strep support group can be found at www.gbss.org.uk.

CLINICAL PRESENTATION AND MANAGEMENT

Until the late 1960s, puerperal sepsis was a notifiable disease in the UK because of its association with streptococcal infec-

tion. Now, however, febrile morbidity is more likely to indicate a wide range of puerperal infections, and not just streptococcal disease. The definition of febrile morbidity in the UK is a temperature of 38°C or higher on any two of the first 10 days postpartum except in the first 24 hours. This definition is based on the traditional criteria for notifiable puerperal sepsis. In the USA, the threshold temperature is 100°F (equivalent to 37.8°C). These numbers are obviously selected because they are convenient round numbers, rather than for any scientific reason. Excluding the first 24 hours takes account of the high incidence of non-infective pyrexia in labour especially, in modern practice, that relates to the use of epidurals (Macaulay et al 1992a, 1992b).

A major cause of puerperal sepsis used to be caesarean section, with incidences of sepsis following section quoted as high as 36% (Sweet & Ledger 1973) compared with less than 1% for vaginal deliveries. However, following the widespread introduction of prophylactic antibiotic administration at the time of caesarean, this rate is now much lower. In the most recent Cochrane review (Smaill & Hofmeyr 2000), 66 trials were included. The use of prophylactic antibiotics in women undergoing caesarean section substantially reduced the incidence of subsequent episodes of fever, endometritis, wound infection, urinary tract infection and other serious infections. The reduction in the risk of endometritis with antibiotics was similar across different patient groups. The reviewers concluded that the reduction of endometritis by two-thirds to three-quarters justifies a policy of administering prophylactic antibiotics to all women undergoing elective or non-elective caesarean section. As regards the best antibiotic to use, both ampicillin and first generation cephalosporins were shown to have similar efficacy (Hopkins & Smaill 2000). Multiple dose regimens for prophylaxis appear to offer no added benefit over a single dose regimen; systemic or lavage routes of administration appear to have no difference in effect. There does not appear to be added benefit in utilising a more broad-spectrum agent or a multiple dose regimen.

Diagnosis

The diagnoses causing puerperal sepsis are outlined in Table 41.1.

Endometritis

Endometritis is usually polymicrobial with a mixture of aerobic and anaerobic organisms. A particularly high fever within the first 24 hours after delivery may indicate a serious acute onset infection; Gram-negative sepsis, GBS disease, clostridial sepsis, or toxic shock syndrome should all be considered. Risk factors for endometritis include caesarean section, chorioamnionitis, prolonged rupture of membranes or premature labour, multiple vaginal examinations, retained products of conception and low socioeconomic status.

Infection confined to the uterus may present with either local or systemic signs and symptoms. Pyrexia of significant degree is frequent in either case, and may be associated with tachycardia and rigors. General complaints such as headache, malaise, nausea and feverishness are common. Complaints of abdominal pain are usual. The uterus is tender

Table 41.1 Puerperal sepsis

Site of infection	Typical microorganisms
Endometritis	Usually *mixed flora* from the vagina, occasionally *group A or B streptococci*, rarely *Clostridium welchii*
Pelvic abscess	As above, plus *Escherichia coli* or *Bacteroides*
Septic pelvic thrombophlebitis	As above, plus *Proteus* or *anaerobic cocci*
Wound infection	As above, plus *staphylococci, streptococci groups C, F & G, enterococci*
Pulmonary atelectasis	*Staphylococcus, pneumococcus, mycoplasma, Klebsiella*
Cystitis and/or Pyelonephritis	*Escherichia coli, Group B or D streptococci, Proteus, Klebsiella, Enterobacter, Pseudomonas*
Mastitis	*Staphylococcus aureus*

to palpation, and it is softer and larger than normal, with delay in the process of involution. There may be evidence of localised peritoneal irritation. Vaginal examination may reveal traumatic damage to the cervix or even to the lower uterine segment. There may be evidence, palpable on bimanual examination, of extrauterine spread of infection. The lochia may be profuse and malodorous, or less commonly, scanty and inoffensive. If the cervix is open, the uterine cavity should be palpated for evidence of trauma, and for retained portions of placenta and membranes.

Ultrasound examination of the uterine cavity has the advantages that it is painless, more sensitive and specific, and not limited by inaccessibility. If it is available, it should be used as a routine. It should be borne in mind however that there are commonly clots remaining in the uterus even after caesarean delivery, and these will show up as high level echoes on scan. Provided they are not more than 3 cm in diameter, they can probably be disregarded. Also, when the placenta is expelled, there are always chorionic villi remaining in the endometrium. These normally degenerate and are passed with the lochia. Consequently, tissue obtained when the uterus is surgically evacuated will nearly always contain degenerating chorionic villi, and their presence alone on histological examination does not indicate significant retained products. The diagnosis of significant retained products therefore remains a clinical one. Secondary postpartum haemorrhage is much more likely to be caused by infection than retained products, and antibiotic therapy is the first line of management, provided there is no clear clinical evidence of retained products. Even if evacuation of the uterus is decided upon, it will be safer after 24 hours of antibiotic therapy, as instrumentation in the presence of active sepsis can cause septicaemia.

Appropriate cultures are essential before starting any treatment. Blood cultures should always be taken if the mother's temperature exceeds 39°C. Contrary to traditional wisdom, if the temperature is fluctuating, one does not need to wait until there is a high temperature before taking the

blood culture. Repeating the cultures several times is often necessary. An intrauterine swab taken through a speculum is also important.

Treatment should begin as soon as the cultures are taken, without waiting for results. There is no consensus on the safest and most effective antibiotic regimens, only that they must have a broad spectrum. Antibiotics are usually continued for four or five days, and for 24 to 48 hours after defervescence. A typical regime would include Gentamicin (2 mg/kg i.v. loading dose, followed by 1.5 mg/kg i.v. every eight hours) plus Ampicillin 2 g i.v. every four to six hours, or Clindamycin (900 mg i.v. every eight hours). Newer single-agent regimens (second- or third-generation cephalosporins, semisynthetic penicillins) include Cefoxitin 1–2 g i.v. every six to eight hours. If there is no response to a single regimen treatment (maximum temperature not dropping within 48 hours of initiation of therapy), triple-agent therapy with ampicillin and gentamicin and clindamycin can be tried next.

Pelvic abscess

This should be suspected if the patient develops a pelvic mass or has persistent fever and pain despite therapy for aerobic bacteria. If they occur, they often develop five or more days after delivery. Therapy for anaerobic bacteria (i.v. metronidazole) must be added. Surgical or percutaneous drainage should be considered if there is clinical and ultrasound evidence of a localised collection.

Septic pelvic thrombophlebitis

Symptoms include spiking fevers with or without pain despite antibiotic therapy. The patient may have a tender palpable mass. The diagnosis may be aided by ultrasound, computed tomography (CT) scan, or even magnetic resonance imaging (MRI). However, if doubt about the diagnosis remains, a trial of heparin therapy is often appropriate. Rapid improvement of symptoms after beginning intravenous heparin is diagnostic.

Wound infection

Presentation includes fever; a tender, erythematous, or fluctuant incision; drainage of pus or blood. It most commonly presents after the fifth postoperative day. Risk factors include having an intrapartum caesarean section, wound haematomas, placement of open drains, obesity, and diabetes. Treatment includes ensuring proper drainage (which may require laying the incision open, at least in part) and antibiotic therapy. This should be with a broad spectrum antibiotic plus metronidazole to cover the Gram-negative anaerobes which are commonly implicated. The antibiotic may need to be changed when sensitivities are available for organisms cultured from the site. Prevention involves careful operative technique to avoid haematoma formation, the avoidance of dead space during closure and intraoperative antibiotic prophylaxis (as discussed previously).

Pulmonary atelectasis

Fever usually begins within 48 hours. Patients may have poor inspiratory effort, dullness to percussion, rales, or decreased breath sounds. Pulmonary infection occurs with increased frequency in patients who receive general anaesthetics or have an abdominal delivery. Narcotic analgesics may also predispose to atelectasis. Treatment involves the use of broad spectrum antibiotics and physiotherapy.

Cystitis and pyelonephritis

These infections are usually accompanied by fever, malaise, suprapubic tenderness, and pyuria; there is flank pain and costovertebral angle tenderness if the kidneys are involved. Risk factors include occult bacteriuria, bladder trauma, and catheterisation. The role of catheterisation in causation is important. Only between 1 and 5% of patients with single, short-term catheterisation develop bacteriuria, but this rises to 50% after repeated catheterisation. It is important to maintain a good fluid intake and make sure antibiotic therapy is targeted according to the sensitivities of cultured organisms. However, therapy should not be changed if it appears to be producing a good response, as the cultured organism is not invariably the major infecting agent.

Mastitis

This diagnosis is suggested by fever and a swollen, tender breast. Typically it occurs three to four weeks after delivery. Cracked nipples associated with breast feeding, and contact with a carrier of *Staphylococcus aureus* are the two prime risk factors. Antibiotic therapy should be commenced promptly, and needs to be effective against penicillinase-producing staphylococci. Flucloxacillin is the usual first choice. The milk flow should be maintained by expressing the milk, as proliferation of staphylococcus occurs most readily in stagnant collections of milk. Analgesics are commonly required to allow expression, which is otherwise too painful. Breast feeding from the affected breast can continue so long as the nipples are not cracked, because the infant will not be affected by ingested staphylococcus (which will be digested). If there is a suggestion of abscess formation, then incision and drainage may well be necessary. In the UK, it is now common practice for such surgery to be carried out by a general surgeon rather than an obstetrician.

Clinical procedure for making the diagnosis

The clinical features of puerperal sepsis will depend on the nature of the infecting organism, the site of primary infection and the rapidity and extent of spread. In all cases the history of the antecedent pregnancy and the circumstances and course of labour should be carefully reviewed. Possible risk factors should be noted as they will have a bearing on the organisms that can be anticipated. The nature of any prior administration of antibiotics must be established as this will dictate both the investigations and treatment.

Examination is directed at detecting the source and location of the infection, as well as ruling out any other cause for the pyrexia, some of which are not infective (for example, deep vein thrombosis, see Ch. 42). Physical examination of the pyrexial postpartum woman must therefore always include the following:

1. *Head, neck and spine*. Look for evidence of anaemia, jaundice, lymphadenopathy and throat infection. Neck stiffness should also be checked for, especially if a spinal or epidural anaesthetic has been administered.
2. *Breasts*. Look for engorgement and inflammatory changes, and possible abscess formation.
3. *Heart and lungs*. Look for evidence of valvular disease in the former, and of pneumonia or collapse in the latter. This is especially important if the patient has been given an inhalational anaesthetic.
4. *Abdomen*. The abdomen must be generally examined, noting the presence of free fluid, enlargement of liver and spleen, and any abnormal masses. Particular note must be taken of uterine size and tenderness, renal angle tenderness and the presence or absence of signs of peritonitis. The presence or absence of bowel sounds should be recorded.
5. *Pelvis*. A pelvic examination must be performed in all cases. The lochia should be checked for colour, consistency and unpleasant odour. The external genitalia must be inspected, and infected lacerations sought in the lower tract. Bimanual palpation of the uterus and parametrial tissues must be done. The size of the uterus and the degree of tenderness should be noted. The pouch of Douglas must be carefully examined, as this is a common site for abscess formation.
6. *Limbs*. The legs should be checked carefully for evidence of thrombosis or thrombophlebitis. The clinical signs are both misleading and non-specific. If there is any suspicion of thrombosis or embolism, specific investigations such as Doppler flow studies or venography must be instituted immediately.

Investigations

Blood count

If the patient is anaemic, she may require haematinic or even transfusion therapy to enable her to mount the best possible defence against infection. The leucocyte count will give an indication as to the efficacy of the immune response, and the trend of repeated counts will map the progress of the infection. A low platelet count may be the first intimation of complications such as septicaemia or disseminated intravascular coagulation.

Urine culture

A clean-catch (mid-stream) specimen of urine should always be sent for microscopy and culture. Urinary tract infection may mimic uterine sepsis closely, and in any event it may coincide with the latter condition. It is important to be aware of its presence, as urinary infection may require different treatment from uterine sepsis as regards both the agent to administer and the duration of treatment.

Pelvic ultrasound

Pelvic ultrasound, preferably using both a vaginal probe and an abdominal sector-scanning probe, is of great value in locating collections of pus, in affording guidance in the sampling of fluid collections and in investigating the presence of retained products of conception within the uterus. If it is available, the colour-flow Doppler scanner will also enable a precise diagnosis and localisation of venous thrombosis to be made.

Blood urea and electrolyte estimation

It is a good idea to have an initial measurement of these indices as renal failure may ensue later in the course of the disease, and a basis for comparison is then available.

Chest X-ray

Lung pathology, such as infection or collapse, is always a possibility, particularly after inhalational anaesthesia, and it may be the primary cause for the pyrexia. Lung complications, the result of septic or non-septic embolism, may also complicate puerperal sepsis. The early signs of adult respiratory distress syndrome may be noted in cases of septicaemia.

Microbiology

Appropriate cultures should be taken, according to the suspected site of infection.

Localised disease

Perineum, vulva, vagina and cervix

Infections in the perineum and vagina are usually secondary to tears or to episiotomy. They tend to remain local and cause little general disturbance, although there may be a mild pyrexia. Symptoms consist of discomfort, pain and discharge at the site of the infection. A common predisposing factor is delayed suturing of perineal tears and episiotomies. Wounds which have for any reason not been sutured within 2–4 hours should be left to heal by second intention. An approach the author has found useful is to suture only the perineal skin, with interrupted non-absorbable sutures, to allow drainage into the vagina and between the sutures, but minimise the dead space that has to heal by granulation. Such an approach is also appropriate for the resuturing of perineal repairs that have broken down, provided the local infection is not too severe and that antibiotic therapy is given. It is more comfortable for the woman than having to sit on a completely open wound. Prior to suturing, the wound must be adequately debrided under local or even general anaesthesia (depending on the degree of pain); any dead tissue or remaining suture material must be removed. When a woman presents with local sepsis, on examination the wounds will appear reddened and oedematous. The sutures will have cut through the tissues, and there will be a disagreeable discharge. Local suppuration may occur and rarely there may be an associated ischio-rectal abscess, palpable as a fluctuant mass through the lateral vaginal fornix. In the latter case, more radical surgery is likely to be necessary to ensure adequate drainage.

Epidemiological considerations

Notification of puerperal sepsis is no longer required as the disease has to a large extent lost its epidemic nature, and it is seldom necessary to trace contacts and close hospitals in an effort to contain spread. Many maternity hospitals still have separate wards for patients with postpartum infection, but the practice of isolation is tending to disappear. However, provided they are not understaffed, and have the facilities for coping with serious illness, isolation wards do provide a satisfactory method of dealing with puerperal infection. It is not a bad thing for patients with wound sepsis to be segregated from others with clean wounds, provided they are not made to feel that their dismissal from the company of their peers is because of some deficiency on their part. If β haemolytic GAS is cultured, then isolation is mandatory.

General care

As in any illness, the general care of the patient is important. Adequate fluid and caloric intake must be ensured, by intravenous infusion if necessary. Anaemia if present should be corrected, and repeated checks of haemoglobin, leucocyte and platelet counts should be requested. Pain must be treated with adequate dosage of analgesic agents, and sources of distress such as a distended urinary bladder or distended bowel must be attended to. Urinary retention is a frequent concomitant to pelvic infection, especially if there has been abscess formation, and the placing of an indwelling catheter will not only relieve the discomfort, but also provide the means of accurate measurement of the urinary output.

Systemic infection from a pelvic source

Blanco et al (1981) found the incidence of bacteraemia to be 7.5 per 1000 obstetric admissions. There were 123 patients with puerperal endoparametritis, of whom 99 (80.5%) had delivered by caesarean section. Bacteraemia had occurred in 3% of patients who had had a caesarean section as opposed to 0.1% of those who had delivered vaginally. None of the patients in this study developed septic shock or died, and most responded to the initial antibiotic therapy (penicillin and an aminoglycoside). Therefore, although bacteraemia is not rare in patients with puerperal sepsis, with prompt treatment the prognosis appears to be good in this group of relatively young and healthy people who constitute the obstetric population.

The picture is different when the bacteraemia is associated with hypotension, and the condition is characterised as septic shock. Septic shock is fortunately infrequent. When it does occur in obstetric patients, the majority arise in the puerperium (Lee et al 1988), and it is much more common after caesarean section than after vaginal delivery. Septic shock, endotoxic shock and bacterial shock are synonyms for the same condition—inadequate tissue perfusion related to inappropriate vasodilatation and circulatory maldistribution secondary to the release of vasoactive mediators. The classic causative organism is *Escherichia coli* and other members of the Gram-negative *Enterobacteraciae*, including the *Klebsiella–Enterobacter–Serratio* group, *Proteus mirabilis* and *Pseudomonas aeruginosa*, but septic shock has occurred in association with streptococci (groups D, B and A) and *Staphylococcus aureus* (Lee et al 1988). Anaerobic streptococci and *Bacteroides* species have also been incriminated. The condition is a response to the release of a lipopolysaccharide endotoxin (lipid A) after lysis of the bacterial cell wall. The endotoxin results in enhanced coagulation and fibrinolysis, and the release of inflammatory mediators such as hydrogen peroxide and free radicals. Practically all systems in the body suffer some degree of damage.

The clinical features are primarily those of infection associated with hypotension and (usually) oliguria, not attributable to hypovolaemia. A history of a prior operative procedure should increase suspicion of the condition. The complications include pulmonary oedema, adult respiratory distress syndrome, disseminated intravascular coagulation, renal failure and thromboembolism.

Management is complex, and is best undertaken in an intensive care facility. Aspects that will require therapy include:

1. Fluid balance. The fluid balance must be corrected rapidly but such correction requires the control afforded by knowledge of the pulmonary capillary wedge pressure, or at the minimum, of the central venous pressure. The urine output must also always be recorded. Blood is used to replace blood loss, and thereafter crystalloid solutions are administered.
2. Respiratory support. The lungs are almost always involved, sometimes severely. A considerable proportion of these patients will require mechanical ventilation. This becomes essential if the arterial blood Pco_2 exceeds 8.0 kPa or the Po_2 is less than 8.0 kPa.
3. Circulatory support. If the response to fluid replacement is not satisfactory, inotropic agents such as dopamine or dobutamine will have to be used, as obstetric patients with septic shock tend to have depressed myocardial function (Lee et al 1988).
4. Renal failure. Kidney function must be monitored, and haemodialysis resorted to sooner rather than later.
5. Infection control. There is no hope of saving the patient unless the infection is eradicated. Intensive antibiotic therapy must continue, and surgical removal of septic foci may be called for, including, on occasion, hysterectomy and even oophorectomy.
6. Corticosteroids. The value of corticosteroid administration has not been established after many years and innumerable trials. Many intensive therapists nonetheless recommend their use.

Tetanus

Fortunately this condition is almost never seen in the developed world, but Yadav et al (1991) writing from Chandigarh in India described 50 cases with a 52% mortality. Death was most often caused by respiratory complications. Prevention is much easier than treatment, and immunisation during pregnancy should be recommended to patients who have not been immunised previously. Treatment involves supportive therapy including mechanical ventilation until the disease has run its course.

PREVENTION

Basic hygiene, including hand washing, should never be forgotten. However, this must be part of a total strategy to prevent cross-infection. Simply encouraging traditional birth attendants to wash their hands more failed to reduce the incidence of puerperal sepsis in one recent trial in Bangladesh (Goodburn et al 2000). Instead, other factors, such as pre-existing infection, long labour and insertion of hands into the vagina were found to be highly significant, and attention to factors such as these needs to be included in a comprehensive strategy for infection prevention and outbreak control. The involvement of appropriately trained infection control nurses whenever there is an outbreak, or in the development of policy, is essential.

Some simple techniques such as the use of chlorhexidine for cleaning the vagina are probably worthwhile. It seemed promising when initially studied (Kollee et al 1989) and was supported subsequently by prospective randomised double blind studies on over 6000 women (Burman et al 1992, Adriaanse et al 1995, Stray-Pedersen et al 1999). These studies showed a statistically significant reduction in the incidence of neonatal infection with GBS, and several also showed significant reductions in overall maternal and neonatal septic morbidity. However, one trial of over 1000 women has failed to show such an improvement in outcome (Rouse et al 1997), once again suggesting that prevention of sepsis requires an overall strategy and not just simple specific interventions.

A number of factors influence febrile morbidity in relation to caesarean section, of which haemostasis and prophylactic antibiotics have already been mentioned. Delivery of the placenta by controlled cord traction is to be preferred to routine manual removal, as it is associated with a much lower incidence of postpartum endometritis (McCurdy et al 1992, Lasley et al 1997).

KEY POINTS

- Puerperal sepsis is still a significant cause of maternal morbidity and mortality.
- A systematic search for infection should be carried out on any woman with a temperature of more than 38°C for two days at any time after the second day of the puerperium, or more than 39°C at any time.
- Beta-haemolytic streptococcus group A is the main cause of fatal maternal puerperal sepsis and is associated with necrotising fasciitis; it must be treated vigorously and the patient isolated.
- Beta-haemolytic streptococcus group B is a major cause of neonatal mortality and carriers should be treated with intravenous penicillin during labour.
- Prophylactic antibiotics for all caesarean sections are strongly recommended.

REFERENCES

Adriaanse AH, Kollee LA, Muytjens HL, Nijhuis JG, de Haan AF, Eskes TK 1995 Randomized study of vaginal chlorhexidine disinfection during labor to prevent vertical transmission of group B streptococci. Eur J Obstet Gynecol Reprod Biol 61:135–141

Ammari NN, Hasweh YG, Hassan AA, Karyoute S 1986 Post-partum necrotizing fasciitis. Case report. Br J Obstet Gynaecol 93:82–83

Anonymous 1998 Report on Confidential Enquiries into Maternal Deaths in the United Kingdom 1994–1996. The Stationery Office, London,

Blanco JD, Gibbs RS, Castaneda YS 1981 Bacteremia in obstetrics: clinical course. Obstet Gynecol 58:621–625

Boyer KM, Gotoff SP 1986 Prevention of early-onset neonatal group B streptococcal disease with selective intrapartum chemoprophylaxis. N Engl J Med 314:1665–1669

Boyer KM, Gotoff SP 1998 Alternative algorithms for prevention of perinatal group B streptococcal infections. Pediatr Infect Dis J 17:973–979

Burman LG, Christensen P, Christensen K, Fryklund B, Helgesson AM, Svenningsen NW et al 1992 Prevention of excess neonatal morbidity associated with group B streptococci by vaginal chlorhexidine disinfection during labour. The Swedish Chlorhexidine Study Group. Lancet 340:65–69

Goodburn EA, Chowdhury M, Gazi R, Marshall T, Graham W 2000 Training traditional birth attendants in clean delivery does not prevent postpartum infection. Health Policy Plan 15:394–399

Gordon G, Dale BA, Lochhead D 1994 An outbreak of group A haemolytic streptococcal puerperal sepsis spread by the communal use of bidets. Br J Obstet Gynaecol 101:447–448

Gotoff SP, Boyer KM 1997 Prevention of early-onset neonatal group B streptococcal disease. Pediatrics 99:866–869

Holm SE 1996. Invasive group A streptococcal infections. N Engl J Med 335:590–591

Hopkins L, Smaill F 2000 Antibiotic prophylaxis regimens and drugs for cesarean section. Cochrane Database Syst Rev CD001136

Kent AS, Haider Z, Beynon JL 1999 Puerperal sepsis: a disease of the past? Br J Obstet Gynaecol 106:1314–1315

Kollee LA, Speyer I, van Kuijck MA, Koopman R, Dony JM, Bakker JH et al 1989 Prevention of group B streptococci transmission during delivery by vaginal application of chlorhexidine gel. Eur J Obstet Gynecol Reprod Biol 31:47–51

Lasley DS, Eblen A, Yancey MK, Duff P 1997 The effect of placental removal method on the incidence of postcesarean infections. Am J Obstet Gynecol 176:1250–1254

Lee W, Clark SL, Cotton DB, Gonik B, Phelan J, Faro S et al 1988 Septic shock during pregnancy. Am J Obstet Gynecol 159:410–416

Macaulay JH, Bond K, Steer PJ 1992a Epidural analgesia in labor and fetal hyperthermia. Obstet Gynecol 80:665–669

Macaulay JH, Randall NR, Bond K, Steer PJ 1992b Continuous monitoring of fetal temperature by non-invasive probe and its relationship to maternal temperature, fetal heart rate, and cord arterial oxygen and pH. Obstet Gynecol 79:469–474

McCurdy CM Jr, Magann EF, McCurdy CJ, Saltzman AK 1992 The effect of placental management at cesarean delivery on operative blood loss. Am J Obstet Gynecol 167:1363–1367

Rouse DJ, Hauth JC, Andrews WW, Mills BB, Maher JE 1997 Chlorhexidine vaginal irrigation for the prevention of peripartal infection: a placebo-controlled randomized clinical trial. Am J Obstet Gynecol 176:617–622

Smaill F, Hofmeyr GJ 2000 Antibiotic prophylaxis for cesarean section. Cochrane Database Syst Rev CD000933

Stray-Pedersen B, Bergan T, Hafstad A, Normann E, Grogaard J, Vangdal M 1999 Vaginal disinfection with chlorhexidine during childbirth. Int J Antimicrob Agents 12:245–251

Sweet RL, Ledger WJ 1973 Puerperal infectious morbidity: a two-year review. Am J Obstet Gynecol 117:1093–1100

Yadav YR, Yadav S, Kala PC 1991 Puerperal tetanus. J Indian Med Assoc 89:336–337

42

Venous thrombosis and pulmonary embolism

John Bonnar

INTRODUCTFION

Since 1985, pulmonary thromboembolism has been the leading cause of maternal death in the United Kingdom. The Report of the Confidential Enquiries into Maternal Deaths (1998), entitled *Why Mothers Die*, reported 48 deaths from thrombosis or thromboembolism (Department of Health 1998). Pulmonary embolism accounted for 36% of direct deaths and exceeded the combined deaths from hypertension (20), haemorrhage (12) and sepsis (14). Table 42.1 shows the causes of direct maternal deaths since 1979 and the increase in deaths from pulmonary embolism. (The Confidential Enquiries are the longest running audit of obstetric care and are aimed at reducing mortality through identifying avoidable factors or suboptimal care.) Pulmonary embolism can occur without warning in women at low risk but in the main the complication arises in the presence of multiple risk factors. The Confidential Enquiries have emphasised that in many cases care was suboptimal: mainly a failure to appreciate the significance of risk factors, failure to give adequate prophylaxis and a failure of diagnosis and treatment when venous thromboembolism occurred. Wider use of thromboprophylaxis and better investigation of symptoms are urgently recommended (Royal College of Obstetricians & Gynaecologists 1995).

The risk factors for venous thrombosis include both genetic and acquired conditions. Inherited thrombophilia is now recognised as an important risk factor for venous thrombosis arising in pregnancy, the puerperium and with oral contraception. Current evidence suggests that genetic

Table 42.1 Causes of direct maternal deaths (1979–1996)

Years	Thromboembolism	Hypertension	Haemorrhage	Sepsis
1979–1981	23 (12.9%)	36 (20.2%)	14 (7.9%)	8 (4.5%)
1982–1984	25 (18.1%)	25 (18.1%)	9 (6.5%)	2 (1.4%)
1985–1987	32 (23.0%)	27 (19.4%)	10 (7.2%)	6 (4.3%)
1988–1990	33 (22.8%)	27 (18.6%)	22 (15.2%)	7 (4.8%)
1991–1993	35 (27.1%)	20 (15.5%)	15 (11.6%)	9 (7.0%)
1994–1996	48 (35.8%)	20 (14.9%)	12 (8.9%)	14 (10.4%)

factors account for 50% of venous thrombotic events arising in pregnancy. Major advances have occurred in identifying the gene mutations in coagulation and fibrinolytic proteins which predispose to venous thrombosis (Bonnar et al 1998, Greer 1999). This new information, in conjunction with the knowledge on acquired risk factors derived from the Confidential Enquiries, provides a rational basis for recognising high-risk patients and using effective prophylactic treatment. Currently this would seem to be the only feasible approach to reducing deaths from pulmonary embolism as most patients with fatal pulmonary embolism die within two hours, before diagnosis and treatment is possible. The puerperium is the time of greatest risk, particularly in patients delivered by caesarean section. All women undergoing caesarean section should be considered for prophylaxis against thromboembolism.

EPIDEMIOLOGY

While we have accurate data on fatal pulmonary embolism from the Confidential Enquiries, less information is available on the incidence of non-fatal thromboembolic complications in pregnancy. The diagnosis of deep vein thrombosis is important as pulmonary embolism has been shown to arise in 16% of patients with untreated deep vein thrombosis, resulting in a 13% mortality (Villa Santa 1965). The mortality rate of deep vein thrombosis was reduced to 0.7% with accurate diagnosis and antithrombotic therapy. The incidence of deep vein thrombosis during pregnancy based on clinical diagnosis is not reliably known, but is estimated to lie between 0.05% and 1.8%. Following vaginal delivery it is between 0.08% and 1.2%, and the incidence is up to 3% following caesarean section (Greer 1996). National hospital data from Scotland between 1983 and 1992 based on objective diagnosis found an incidence of antenatal deep vein thrombosis of 0.615 per 1000 maternities in women under the age of 35 years and 1.216 per 1000 maternities over the age of 35 years. The incidence of pulmonary embolism was 0.108 per 1000 maternities under 35 years and 0.405 per 1000 maternities over 35 years (Macklon & Greer 1996).

A Glasgow study of 72 000 pregnancies reported an incidence of deep vein thrombosis of 0.71 per 1000 deliveries and an incidence of pulmonary embolism of 0.15 per 1000 deliveries (McColl et al 1997). If the Scottish data is calculated in women years, the incidence of thrombotic events during pregnancy was 0.97 per 1000 pregnant women years and, postpartum, 7.19 per 1000 women years. This represents a 2.5-fold increase in the risk of thrombotic events during pregnancy and a 20-fold increase in the puerperium relative to non-pregnant women of the same age. Table 42.2 from the Confidential Enquiries analysed 159 deaths from pulmonary embolism over the 15 years between 1982 and 1996; 73 deaths occurred during pregnancy and 82 deaths in the puerperium with one death recorded during labour. Again, using pregnant women years, the incidence of fatal pulmonary embolism is 7–8 times higher in the puerperium than during pregnancy. Caesarean section is associated with 70% of deaths from fatal pulmonary embolism in the puerperium. Clearly, the puerperium is the time of greatest risk for venous thrombosis and pulmonary embolism; postpartum thromboprophlaxis for women identified as being at increased risk could have a major impact in reducing venous thrombosis and fatal pulmonary embolism.

PATHOGENESIS

The major factors predisposing to venous thrombosis were described in the mid nineteenth century by Virchow (1860) who postulated the triad of venous stasis, hypercoagulability and vascular injury. The physiology of pregnancy results in increased venous distensibility which is apparent from the first trimester. In addition, the pressure of the pregnant uterus impedes venous return from the lower limbs with a greater effect on the left side due to the anatomical arrangement of the common iliac vessels. Using duplex Doppler ultrasound, a marked decrease in blood flow velocity has been shown during pregnancy and for 6 weeks following delivery (Macklon & Greer 1997, Macklon et al 1997). The reduced flow velocity is much greater in the left common femoral vein than in the right, which explains why around 85% of deep vein thrombosis during pregnancy occurs in the left leg compared with 55% in the non-pregnant (Linghagen et al 1986, McColl et al 1997).

In contrast with the non-pregnant, the majority of deep vein thromboses in pregnancy involve the ileofemoral segment, which is more likely to embolise. The rates of venous insufficiency are also much higher following deep vein thrombosis in pregnancy than observed in women outside pregnancy. A report from Sweden showed that 65% of women with deep vein thrombosis in pregnancy developed

Table 42.2 Maternal deaths from pulmonary embolism

Years	Total	After abortion or during pregnancy	Death in labour	After vaginal delivery	After caesarean section
1982–1984	29	13	0	4	12
1985–1987	30	17	0	6	7
1988–1990	24	13	0	3	8
1991–1993	30	12	1	4	13
1994–1996	46[a]	18	0	10	15
	159	73	1	27	55

[a] Includes 3 deaths for which details were not available.

venous insufficiency in the affected leg within 3–10 years of the event despite appropriate anticoagulant therapy (Linghagen et al 1986).

Normal pregnancy involves major changes in the blood coagulation and fibrinolytic systems with an increased concentration of coagulation factors I, VII, VIII, IX, X, XII, von Willebrand factor antigen and ristocetin co-factor activity, the functional assessment of von Willebrand factor (Greer 1997). During pregnancy, acquired resistance to the endogenous anticoagulant activated protein C appears to develop and in the second half of pregnancy a marked reduction occurs in protein S, the co-factor for protein C (Clark et al 1998). Fibrinolytic activity shows progressive impairment during pregnancy with a rapid return to normal following delivery. The impairment of fibrinolysis appears to be due mainly to the production of plasminogen activator inhibitor type 2 by the placenta.

The changes in coagulation and fibrinolysis appear to be physiological developments to protect the integrity of the maternal and fetal circulations and also to provide a physiological preparation for the haemostatic challenge that arises during placental separation and delivery. Damage to the endothelium in the uteroplacental vasculature occurs during normal delivery, and additional damage to pelvic vessels will arise during operative delivery, especially caesarean section. Pregnancy and delivery therefore provides all the predisposing factors of Virchow's triad of venous stasis, hypercoagulability and vascular damage.

INHERITED THROMBOPHILIA IN PREGNANCY

Inherited thrombophilia is the term applied to the genetic conditions that increase the risk of venous thrombosis. The hypercoagulable state of pregnancy presents special problems for the woman with inherited or acquired thrombophilia. The identified main causes of inherited thrombophilia are deficiencies of antithrombin, protein C and protein S and the presence of factor V Leiden, the prothrombin gene variant, and homozygosity for the thermolabile variant of methylenetetrahydrofolate reductase (MTHFR). Factor V Leiden manifests as resistance to activated protein C and is the most common inherited defect underlying venous thromboembolism. Resistance to activated protein C also occurs with other defects in the factor V molecule and antiphospholipid syndrome. In pregnancy, an acquired resistance to activated protein C develops, probably as a result of the increases in factor V and factor VIII (Greer 1997).

In a recent study in the West of Scotland, 75 women who had suffered an objectively confirmed episode of venous thromboembolism during pregnancy or in the puerperium were screened for thrombophilia including antithrombin and protein C activities, total and free protein S antigens, IgG and IgM anticardiolipin antibodies and lupus anticoagulant (McColl et al 2000). Polymerase chain reaction was used to determine the presence or absence of the factor V Leiden, prothrombin 20210 G→A mutations, and C677T mutations in the MTHFR gene. The prevalence of these abnormalities was compared with the general population. The population incidence of clotting abnormalities is: antithrombin deficiency type 1, 1 in 5000, type 2, 3 in 2000, factor V Leiden 2.2%, prothrombin mutation 20210A 2.2% and the MTHFR mutation (homozygous C677T) 12%. In pregnant women who had suffered venous thromboembolism the odds ratio of increased incidence for antithrombin deficiency type 1 was 282 and type 2 was 28, for factor V Leiden 4.5 and for prothrombin mutation 4.4; the homozygous C→T mutation in the MTHFR gene did not have an increased frequency (odds ratio 0.45). This study concluded that both the factor V Leiden and the prothrombin mutation are associated with maternal venous thromboembolism but that the MTHFR mutation does not identify women at increased risk of maternal venous thrombosis. Since the odds ratio for the prothrombin mutation is similar to factor V Leiden, routine population screening for this mutation is not indicated. However, based on these findings it was recommended that women with a personal or strong family history of venous thromboembolism should be screened for the prothrombin mutation in addition to screening for other thrombophilias (McColl et al 2000). Ideally this should be carried out before pregnancy to allow time to plan pregnancy management with joint consultation between the haematologist and the obstetrician. Women with a history of recurrent fetal loss, fetal growth restriction, severe pre-eclampsia and placental abruption should also be screened for inherited and acquired thrombophilia (Bonnar et al 1998, McColl et al 1999).

Inherited thrombophilia frequently appears to be a multiple gene disorder with more than one gene defect occurring within thrombophilic families. The risk of venous thromboembolism with underlying thrombophilia will depend on the thrombophilic defect, history of thrombotic events and acquired risk factors. Clinical thrombosis usually results from an interaction between congenital and acquired risk factors. Pregnancy and the puerperium often trigger the first thrombotic event in women with deficiencies of antithrombin, protein C and protein S. Occurrence rates of venous thrombosis of 32–40% have been reported in Europe for pregnant women with antithrombin deficiency (Greer 1999, McColl et al 1999). For pregnant women with abnormalities of the protein C and protein S system the risk is substantially lower and postpartum thrombosis is more common than antepartum thrombosis. The risk of thrombosis in pregnancy is 3–10% for protein C deficiency and 0–6% for protein S deficiency. In postpartum women the risk for protein C deficiency is 7–19% and for protein S deficiency 7–22%. These studies, however, are based on investigations in women with venous thromboembolism and do not reflect the risk of thrombosis in previously symptom-free women with the mutations. In the West of Scotland study of 72 000 pregnancies, the risk of venous thromboembolism in pregnancy was 1 in 437 for factor V Leiden, 1 in 113 for protein C deficiency, 1 in 2.8 for type 1 (quantitative) antithrombin deficiency, and 1 in 42 for type 2 (qualitative) antithrombin deficiency (McColl et al 1997).

ACQUIRED RISK FACTORS IN OBSTETRICS

The Confidential Enquiries indicated that when thromboembolism results in a maternal death the following risk factors are important:

- inherited or acquired thrombophilia
- operative delivery
- over 35 years
- obesity
- restricted activity
- previous venous thrombosis
- hypertension in pregnancy
- surgical procedure during pregnancy
- sickle cell anaemia
- dehydration.

Operative delivery. The increased risk of thromboembolism after caesarean section is clearly shown in Table 42.2. The frequency of fatal pulmonary embolism during these years was on average more than 10 times greater after caesarean section than after vaginal delivery.

Age and parity. The risk of fatal pulmonary embolism increases more sharply with advancing age (especially in women aged 35 years or more) than with increasing parity.

Hospitalisation and restricted activity. Women admitted to hospital with complications such as hypertension and placenta praevia are at an increased risk, most likely because of restricted activity.

Obesity (exceeding 76 kg). Obesity is an important factor in the development of thromboembolism. Approximately 1 in 5 women dying of pulmonary embolism are obese.

Surgical procedures during pregnancy. Operations such as ovarian cystectomy and appendectomy increase the risk of thrombosis.

History of deep vein thrombosis or pulmonary embolism in association with pregnancy, surgery or the contraceptive pill. Women with a previous history of deep vein thrombosis or pulmonary embolism must be regarded as especially at risk during pregnancy, whether or not underlying thrombophilia has been detected.

CLINICAL FEATURES AND DIAGNOSIS

The clinical diagnosis of deep vein thrombosis during pregnancy is unreliable: fewer than half of all cases of deep vein thrombosis involving major proximal veins are identified clinically. When present, venous thrombosis will almost invariably cause more symptoms in one leg than the other, usually in the left leg. The diagnosis of deep vein thrombosis is almost certain when physical signs such as definite tenderness or induration of the calf muscle, leg oedema and increased skin temperature are present. The role of clinical evaluation is to identify the patient at risk, and objective methods should be used to confirm the diagnosis. During pregnancy duplex Doppler ultrasound is the recommended method for the diagnosis of deep vein thrombosis. Ultrasound examination has the benefit of being non-invasive and has a high sensitivity and specificity for the ileofemoral segment and the proximal veins. The method is less accurate for the diagnosis of minor calf vein thrombosis. Ascending phlebography will also provide an accurate and precise diagnosis and lateral views of the calf will detect thrombi in the soleal veins. When contrast phlebography is used during pregnancy a large measure of protection to the fetus can be provided by shielding the mother's abdomen with a lead apron.

The clinical diagnosis of pulmonary thromboembolism is likewise unreliable and autopsy findings have indicated that only about one-third are diagnosed clinically (Palla et al 1995). The symptoms and signs of pulmonary embolism are associated predominantly with the cardiovascular and respiratory systems. The effects vary from clinically silent to sudden death and depend on the size of the embolus and the preceding health of the patient. Most pregnant women with ileofemoral thrombosis show evidence on lung scanning of small symptomless pulmonary emboli. These small emboli are usually cleared from the pulmonary circulation by the potent fibrinolytic activity in the lung vasculature. The most common clinical features of acute pulmonary embolism are dyspnoea, tachypnoea, pleuritic chest pain, haemoptysis, hypotension and tachycardia. The classic symptoms of massive pulmonary embolism are severe chest pain, air hunger and sudden collapse. Predominant clinical signs are cyanosis, rapid breathing and jugular vein distension. Isolated dyspnoea without cyanosis can also be the presenting feature.

When there is a clinical suspicion of pulmonary embolism the initial assessment should include a chest radiograph, electrocardiography (ECG) and arterial blood gases. The two most common findings in the plain chest radiograph are the presence of a consolidation or infiltration and an elevated hemidiaphragm on the affected side. In late pregnancy elevation of the diaphragm is a normal feature. The ECG changes include rhythm disturbance, QRS abnormalities and ST segment and T-wave alterations. The ECG may be normal except for a sinus tachycardia. While not specific in diagnosing pulmonary embolism, the ECG is useful for excluding acute myocardial infarction which may be confused with massive pulmonary embolism.

Ventilation/perfusion lung scanning

The ventilation/perfusion lung scan (V/Q scan) is the primary investigation in the evaluation of suspected pulmonary embolism. V/Q scanning should be performed within 24 hours as scans can revert to normal within a few days. The perfusion phase is normally performed first. A normal perfusion scan in a previously healthy woman will almost certainly exclude any clinically significant pulmonary embolism and the ventilation scan can be omitted, thereby reducing the radiation dose. Perfusion scanning is performed by the intravenous injection of technetium-99m-labelled macroaggregates of albumin or human albumin microspheres. The radiation to the fetus can be minimised by reducing the technetium-99m dose from 3 millicuries to 1 or 2 millicuries without affecting the quality of the scan.

Pulmonary angiography

Pulmonary angiography is also a definitive method for diagnosing pulmonary embolism but is invasive and carries some risk. Where other investigations have failed to provide a firm diagnosis pulmonary angiography should be considered if cardiovascular collapse or hypotension is present.

Magnetic resonance imaging (MRI)

MRI has the advantage of direct imaging of thrombi in the pulmonary arteries and the large veins. The lack of ionising radiation makes MRI attractive for use in pregnancy.

In the investigation of suspected pulmonary embolism duplex Doppler ultrasound and V/Q scanning are recommended and will usually provide a diagnosis. If these are negative in the presence of a high degree of clinical suspicion, treatment with anticoagulant therapy should be considered, and the tests repeated after an interval of one week. If the repeat investigations are negative, treatment can be discontinued.

D-dimer

The measurement of plasma D-dimer, a breakdown product of cross-linked fibrin, has been used in non-pregnant patients as a biochemical method of detecting venous thromboembolism. The levels of D-dimer are usually raised in normal pregnancy, and increased levels are found in the puerperium and with complications such as pre-eclampsia. This being so, D-dimer is of doubtful diagnostic value during pregnancy or the puerperium.

Screening for inherited thrombophilia

Screening for inherited thrombophilia is indicated in women who present with venous thromboembolism associated with pregnancy or the oral contraceptive pill. About 50% of such women will be found to have a thrombophilic defect.

Screening for inherited thrombophilia is also recommended in women with recurrent pregnancy loss in the second and third trimester and in women with recurrent early onset pre-eclampsia or recurrent intrauterine growth restriction. Control trials are needed to assess the effectiveness of antithrombotic intervention in patients with recurrent pregnancy loss and inherited thrombophilia (Greer 1999).

The routine screening of all pregnant women for congenital thrombophilia is not recommended, because most identified will not have a history of thrombosis and will therefore not be at substantially increased risk. Likewise, the value of screening for inherited thrombophilia in women with recurrent first-trimester miscarriage is doubtful although they should be screened for acquired thrombophilia due to antiphospholipid antibodies and activation of the coagulation system.

ANTICOAGULANT THERAPY IN PREGNANCY

Both unfractionated heparin and low molecular weight heparin (LMWH) do not cross the placenta and thus do not carry a risk of teratogenesis or fetal haemorrhage. Heparin is not secreted in breast milk and can be used during lactation. The disadvantages of heparin treatment are the need for parenteral administration and complications such as heparin-induced thrombocytopenia, allergy and, with prolonged use, osteoporosis can occur. LMWH has been shown to be safe and effective in non-pregnant women and is associated with fewer side effects than unfractionated heparin in the treatment of acute leg vein thrombosis and pulmonary embolism (Hull et al 1992, Simmoneau et al 1997). Outpatient treatment with LMWH is now the preferred management of deep vein thrombosis in non-pregnant subjects. LMWH for the immediate management of thromboembolic disease in pregnancy has been reported (Thomson et al 1998).

Coumarin derivatives such as warfarin should be avoided during pregnancy; the drug crosses the placenta, and warfarin embryopathy may occur in 4–5% of fetuses exposed to the drug between 6 and 9 weeks of gestation (Bates & Ginsberg 1997). Warfarin embryopathy can be avoided by substitution of heparin for warfarin during the first trimester. Central nervous system abnormalities have also been reported with warfarin exposure in the fetus, most likely caused by spontaneous intracerebral bleeding during pregnancy. The fetal liver is immature and concentrations of vitamin K dependent coagulation factors are low in the fetus. Warfarin therapy in the optimal range for the mother will result in excessive anticoagulation in the fetus. Warfarin, if used in pregnancy, should be avoided after 36 weeks' gestation because of the risk of haemorrhage in both mother and baby. Oral anticoagulant therapy should be avoided if at all possible during pregnancy. Women who are taking long-term oral anticoagulant prophylaxis should be informed of the risks of fetal complications if they become pregnant. They should be advised to avoid pregnancy and to contact their family doctor immediately if pregnancy is likely. Self-administered heparin can be substituted for warfarin as soon as possible after conception and before 6 weeks' gestation.

MANAGEMENT

While the objective diagnosis of venous thromboembolism during pregnancy is crucial, treatment should be commenced on clinical grounds if objective tests cannot be performed quickly. Extensive clinical experience has established heparin to be the safest anticoagulant to use during pregnancy. Immediate treatment of venous thromboembolism with heparin is important to reduce the morbidity and mortality from pulmonary embolism and arrest the extension of deep vein thrombosis, so reducing long-term morbidity from post-thrombotic venous insufficiency.

Intravenous unfractionated heparin is the recommended treatment in antenatal venous thromboembolism. An intravenous bolus of 5000 IU or 75 IU/kg bodyweight should be given slowly over 3–5 minutes followed by 15–25 IU/kg/h by continuous intravenous infusion to prolong the activated partial thromboplastin time to a therapeutic ratio of 1.5–2.5 times the control value. Intermittent bolus injections should not be used because of the increased risk of bleeding. The precise duration of the initial treatment must be tailored to the individual but the objective is to maintain full anticoagulation until active thrombosis has been arrested, thrombi in the leg veins have been firmly attached to the vessel wall and the process of organisation has begun. This usually requires intravenous therapy for 5–10 days. Acute treatment with unfractionated heparin can also be given by subcutaneous injection into the flank of the anterior abdominal wall; dosage of subcutaneous heparin of 10 000–15 000 IU at 12-hourly intervals will usually provide adequate anticoagulation.

In late pregnancy heparin resistance occurs, most likely due to increased physiological activation of the coagulation system and raised levels of factor VIII and fibrinogen. If available, assessment of the anti-Xa level to monitor the dose of heparin is recommended and will allow better control of heparin dosage. Therapeutic treatment with heparin should be continued for at least 6 weeks, following which prophylactic subcutaneous heparin should be continued with stopping or reduction of heparin during labour and delivery. Patients usually have no difficulty in learning to self-administer subcutaneous heparin into the lateral aspect of the anterior abdominal wall. The injection site should not be rubbed or massaged. Subcutaneous heparin is best avoided in the arms and legs as pain and bruising are more likely in these areas.

LMWH is used increasingly in pregnant women and its pharmacokinetic profile is under investigation. Experience has been gained with enoxaparin and tinzaparin for treatment of antenatal venous thromboembolism. Enoxaparin is given at a dose of 1 mg/kg subcutaneously 12-hourly. With tinzaparin the dosage is 175 IU/kg once daily by subcutaneous injection. Until further experience is published, treatment is best monitored by measuring anti-Xa activity and the recommended therapeutic range is between 0.35 and 1.0 IU/ml at 2–3 hours after injection. As with standard heparin, LMWH is reduced or discontinued for labour and delivery.

If a woman is anticoagulated during labour, epidural or spinal anaesthesia should be avoided because of the risk of haematoma formation during insertion and removal of the indwelling cannula. If heparin has been discontinued for 12 hours and the platelet count and APTT are normal, epidural or spinal anaesthesia should not be associated with any increased risk of bleeding. Similar precautions are recommended in the use of LMWH, and the insertion and removal of a cannula for epidural or spinal anaesthesia should be delayed until 12 hours after LMWH has been administered (Bonnar et al 1999).

Anticoagulant prophylaxis should resume within 4–8 hours following delivery, using either subcutaneous standard heparin or LMWH. The puerperium is the time of greatest risk; if standard heparin is used, 5000–10 000 units every 12 hours is advisable. Warfarin therapy can begin postpartum with 7 mg on the first and second days and 5 mg on the third day. Both heparin and warfarin are safe for nursing mothers to use. Heparin can be discontinued when the International Normalised Ratio (INR) has increased to a therapeutic range of 2.0–3.0 for two consecutive days. Warfarin therapy should be continued for at least 3 months. If there is a severe underlying thrombophilic problem such as antiphospholipid antibody syndrome, the INR should be maintained at between 3.0 and 3.5. Following 3 months of anticoagulant treatment the patient should be referred for thrombophilia screening tests if these have not previously been carried out. If the mother has inherited thrombophilia the child has a 50% chance of being affected. In symptomatic families with inherited thrombophilia, screening tests before puberty are recommended (Bonnar et al 1998). This allows time to discuss with young women the possible risks of oral contraceptives and pregnancy before sexual activity begins. The mother should also be advised that screening for thrombophilia should be done at an even earlier age if the child experiences any major illness or injury.

Vena cava filters

The vena cava may be completely ligated or partially occluded with a variety of Teflon clips. Inferior vena cava filters have been used successfully during pregnancy and placement above the level of the renal vessels is recommended (Narayan et al 1992). Indications for use are similar to those in the non-pregnant patient and include contraindication to anticoagulant therapy, complications of anticoagulation (such as heparin-induced thrombocytopenia) and recurrent pulmonary embolism in patients with adequate anticoagulation.

Fibrinolytic agents

Recent surgery or delivery is a contraindication to thrombolytic therapy. Pulmonary emboli are lysed more rapidly with streptokinase or recombinant tissue plasminogen activator than with conventional anticoagulation, and these agents should be considered in massive pulmonary embolism during pregnancy. The treatment can result in placental bleeding and abruption. Thrombolysis should be avoided if delivery is imminent or within one week of childbirth as severe haemorrhage from the placental site is to be expected. Likewise, extensive bleeding will occur from any genital tract lacerations or episiotomy wounds.

Pulmonary embolectomy

Pulmonary embolectomy should be considered in pregnant women with massive pulmonary embolism who fail to respond to medical treatment within 1–2 hours. The use of cardiopulmonary bypass has improved the results of the surgical approach to massive thromboembolism. The decision must be based upon the clinical and haemodynamic state of the patient as well as the ready availability of the surgical team and required facilities. If the patient survives long enough to be put on cardiopulmonary bypass, embolectomy is likely to be successful.

THROMBOPROPHYLAXIS IN PREGNANCY AND THE PUERPERIUM

If maternal mortality from pulmonary embolism is to be reduced, thromboprophylaxis is required for women at increased risk of venous thromboembolism. No randomised control trials to determine optimal management have been carried out. Advice is therefore based on observational studies and expert opinion. Given the lack of randomised controlled trials of antithrombotic prophylaxis in pregnancy, the need for prophylactic therapy in women with a previous history of a single episode of deep vein thrombosis with no additional risk factors has been questioned. This approach would reserve prophylaxis for women with additional risk factors such as inherited or acquired thrombophilia, post-thrombotic venous insufficiency and recurrent thrombosis. However, previous deep vein thrombosis is a proven risk factor for further thrombosis and we are still at an early stage in determining all the genetic mutations which predispose to venous thrombosis. At present, because maternal deaths from pulmonary embolism are increasing and 50% of these deaths occur antenatally, probably a safer approach is to advise thromboprophylaxis in women with a previous thrombosis, particularly where this occurred during pregnancy, even when current screening tests for both inherited and acquired thrombophilia are negative. Controlled trials are required in this area to guide management, and some are already in progress (for example, the APPLE trial).

In assessing the thrombotic risk in the individual patient, acquired risk factors as well as genetic predisposition should be considered. A personal and family history of venous thrombosis would be a major factor in the decision. The issues of prophylaxis and its risks should be discussed with the patient before or during early pregnancy and a management policy based on the individual assessment agreed and recorded. Close liaison between the haematologist and obstetrician is recommended and each hospital should have agreed guidelines for the management of women at an increased risk of venous thromboembolism during pregnancy. In 1995 the Royal College of Obstetricians and Gynaecologists (RCOG) published recommendations for prophylaxis against thromboembolism in obstetrics and gynaecology (Royal College of Obstetricians & Gynaecologists 1995). The next Report of the Confidential Enquiry should indicate if these recommendations have had any effect in reducing maternal mortality from thromboembolism. Recommendations for the antenatal management of women at risk of venous thromboembolism are shown in Table 42.3. These are based on the author's experience and a recent major review from Glasgow where there has been a long-standing research programme in venous thromboembolism in pregnancy (McColl et al 1997, Bonnar et al 1998, Clark et al 1998, McColl et al 1999).

Based on a combination of inherited and acquired risk factors, women are classified as being at very high risk, high risk, moderate risk or low risk of venous thromboembolism.

Women at very high risk

The group at very high risk includes patients currently on anticoagulants for a previous episode of venous thromboembolism (irrespective of the presence or absence of underlying thrombophilia), venous thromboembolism in the current pregnancy, and patients with antithrombin deficiency with type 1 or certain type 2 defects. In this group, anticoagulants should be commenced or continued throughout pregnancy. In women who are already on anticoagulants, treatment should be changed to heparin before the sixth week of pregnancy. In women who are not already on anticoagulants, heparin should be commenced as soon as pregnancy is confirmed and continued throughout pregnancy and for at least 3 months following delivery.

In this group adjusted-dose heparin is used in conjunction with the use of anti-embolic stockings throughout pregnancy and the postpartum period. Adjusted-dose heparin can be given as standard heparin or LMWH to achieve a peak anti-Xa activity of 0.35–1.00 IU/ml 3–4 hours after injection. This will usually require a dose of 7500–12 500 IU of standard heparin twice daily during the first half of pregnancy and 10 000–15 000 IU twice daily in the second half of pregnancy. LMWH can be given according to bodyweight. Suggested dosage regimens for LMWH are enoxaparin 40 mg 12-hourly, tinzaparin 10 000 IU daily. In women with a bodyweight of less than 50 kg, satisfactory heparin levels can be achieved with lower doses of standard heparin or LMWH. Likewise, if renal function is impaired, a lower dose of heparin will be required.

Women at high risk

Women at high risk are those who have had a previous thromboembolism but are not on anticoagulant therapy, protein C deficiency plus a family history of thromboembolism, homozygous factor V Leiden, prothrombin mutation and combined thrombophilia. In this group thromboprophylaxis is introduced 4–6 weeks before the gestational age of the event in a previous pregnancy, or from 20–24 weeks of gestation in the others. Anticoagulation may be given earlier if additional risk factors for venous thromboembolism are present. Heparin prophylaxis may be given as standard heparin 7500 IU 12-hourly until 30 weeks and 10 000 IU 12-hourly

Table 42.3 Risk assessment and prophylaxis for venous thromboembolism (VTE) in pregnancy (McColl et al 1999)

Group	Patients	Management
Very high risk	Antithrombin deficiency. Previous VTE on anticoagulants. VTE in current pregnancy	Adjusted-dose heparin, TED stockings
High risk	Protein C deficiency and family history of VTE. Homozygous factor V Leiden. Prothrombin mutation. Combined thrombophilia. Previous VTE not on treatment	Fixed-dose heparin from 20–24 weeks or 4–6 weeks before gestation of previous event. Postpartum anticoagulation for 12 weeks
Moderate risk	Family history of VTE and heterozygous factor V Leiden, prothrombin mutation, or protein S deficiency	Antenatal TED stockings. Monitor for other VTE risks. Postpartum anticoagulation for 6 weeks
Low risk	No personal or family history of VTE and heterozygous factor V Leiden or prothrombin mutation	Monitor for additional risk for VTE

for the remainder of the pregnancy. Once-daily LMWH may be given as enoxaparin 40 mg daily or tinzaparin 4500–7500 IU per day. Postpartum anticoagulation should be continued for 12 weeks together with the use of anti-embolism stockings.

Women at moderate risk

Those women at moderate risk include patients with heterozygous factor V Leiden, prothrombin mutations, or protein S deficiency and a family history of venous thromboembolism. Anti-embolism stockings are recommended in the antenatal period. Anticoagulation is given for 6 weeks during the puerperium, starting with heparin 4–8 hours after delivery and continuing with warfarin. Anticoagulation is used in late pregnancy if additional risk factors such as age, obesity or restricted activity are present.

Women at relatively low risk

Patients at relatively low risk are those with factor V Leiden or prothrombin mutations who have no personal or family history of venous thromboembolism. These patients may be detected as a result of a routine screening for thrombophilia. If no other risk factors for venous thromboembolism during pregnancy are present, such as pre-eclampsia or caesarean section, these patients are not offered antenatal thromboprophylaxis but are reviewed regularly to determine if additional thrombotic risk factors have developed during pregnancy.

Management of labour and delivery

In women at increased risk of venous thromboembolism, the additional risk of caesarean section makes spontaneous labour and delivery preferable. In general, women can continue on heparin prophylaxis and discontinue the treatment at the onset of labour, with heparin prophylaxis being resumed 4–8 hours after delivery.

In a patient receiving therapeutic heparin the infusion should be stopped for labour and delivery. Heparin activity should fall to safe levels within one hour. A protamine sulphate infusion can be used if needed to neutralise the heparin activity. The dose of protamine sulphate is calculated from the formula

plasma heparin activity (IU/ml) × plasma volume (50 ml per kg bodyweight) × 0.01

e.g. a woman with a heparin activity of 0.8 IU/ml and weighing 70 kg would require $0.8 \times (50 \times 70) \times 0.01 = 28$ mg protamine sulphate. If a woman fully anticoagulated on warfarin starts labour she should be given fresh frozen plasma (FFP) to return the prothrombin time to normal. The baby should be given FFP and vitamin K on delivery and screened by ultrasound for any signs of haemorrhage in the head and abdomen.

Women who have been on antenatal standard heparin may have epidural or spinal anaesthesia providing their coagulation and platelet count is normal. LMWH does not prolong the activated partial thromboplastin time to the same extent as standard heparin. Monitoring the effect of LMWH requires an anti-Xa assay which is not widely available. Peak levels of anti-Xa occur 2–4 hours after subcutaneous LMWH or standard heparin is administered. The optimal time for insertion and removal of a spinal or epidural catheter would be at least 12 hours after the last dose (Bonnar et al 1999).

Women with antithrombin deficiency are at very high risk for venous thromboembolism and in this group the use of antithrombin concentrate should be considered in order to increase the antithrombin levels to normal for labour and delivery. Increasing the plasma antithrombin activity to 80–120% is recommended on the day of delivery by infusion of 0.6–0.7 U antithrombin concentrate per kg maternal weight. This allows the heparin level to be reduced or discontinued (Walker 1998).

THROMBOPROPHYLAXIS AND CAESAREAN SECTION

Approximately two-thirds of the postpartum deaths from thromboembolism in the years 1982–1996 in the UK followed delivery by caesarean section. Over this period the national caesarean section rate was approximately 14%. Because of the high risk associated with caesarean section, the Report of the Confidential Enquiry published in 1998 included the recommendations of the RCOG on prophylaxis against thromboembolism (RCOG 1995, Department of Health 1998). The recommendations from the RCOG are based on the data from the Confidential Enquiries and observational studies, and as yet there have been no randomised control trials on thromboprophylaxis in pregnancy.

The recommended risk assessment for patients undergoing caesarean section is as follows:

Low risk – early mobilisation and hydration:

- elective caesarean section – uncomplicated pregnancy and no other risk factors.

Moderate risk – consider one of a variety of prophylactic measures:

- age >35 years
- obesity (>80 kg)
- para 4 or more
- gross varicose veins
- current infection
- pre-eclampsia
- immobility prior to surgery (>4 days)
- major current illness, e.g. heart or lung disease, cancer, inflammatory bowel disease, nephrotic syndrome
- emergency caesarean section.

High risk – heparin prophylaxis with or without leg stockings:

- a patient with 3 or more moderate risk factors from above
- extended major pelvic or abdominal surgery, e.g. caesarean hysterectomy
- patients with a personal or family history of deep vein thrombosis, pulmonary embolism or thrombophilia, paralysis of lower limbs

- patient with antiphospholipid antibody (cardiolipin antibody or lupus anticoagulant).

This remains a useful risk assessment profile which can be a basis for guidelines. Some obstetric units have incorporated the risk assessment profile in the obstetric chart so that it is used when the patient is admitted for caesarean section. Patients in the moderate and high-risk categories should receive prophylaxis with standard heparin in a dose of 5000 units 12-hourly by subcutaneous injection or LMWH as a single daily dose starting during the operation if the patient has regional anaesthesia. Treatment should be given for a minimum of 5 days and can be self-administered.

In the patient with inherited thrombophilia as listed in Table 42.3, anticoagulation should be continued in the postpartum period for at least 6–12 weeks. In this group oral anticoagulants can be commenced 1–2 days following delivery and the heparin discontinued once the International Normalised Ratio (INR) has been in the therapeutic range for 4 consecutive days. Anticoagulant therapy in the patient undergoing caesarean section is likely to increase the risk of wound haematomas; care should be taken to ensure that subcutaneous heparin is injected subcutaneously in the flank as far away as possible from the wound.

CARDIAC PROSTHETIC VALVES

Women with cardiac prosthetic valves who are on long-term anticoagulant therapy require careful counselling about pregnancy and fetal risks. The best method of maintaining adequate anticoagulation of women with mechanical heart valves during pregnancy remains controversial. Clinicians responsible for these women should be aware of the increased risk of thrombosis in pregnancy and the hazards of treatment so that an informed decision can be agreed with the patient. The patient should be fully informed of the benefits and risks of the anticoagulant options available so that both the expectant mother and the clinician can embark on a mutually agreed treatment plan.

The occurrence of valve thrombosis is a serious and life-threatening event for both mother and baby. Retrospective studies of women with prosthetic heart valves during pregnancy have reported a higher thromboembolic risk with heparin than oral anticoagulants. In the main, the thromboembolic events occurring with heparin therapy were associated with suboptimal or undetermined levels of anticoagulation. A review in this area concluded that the reported risk of valve thrombosis and other embolic events with pregnancy could be explained by a combination of inadequate heparin dosing, control and reporting (Ginsberg & Barron 1994). Studies which have been quoted in support of the inadequacy of heparin in preventing valve thrombosis have been using low-dose heparin 5000 units twice daily, which is known to be inadequate for preventing thrombosis during pregnancy and is associated with undetectable levels of heparin in pregnancy.

In a recent review of anticoagulation in women with prosthetic heart valves it was recommended that laboratories using the APTT ratio to control heparin therapy must calibrate their therapeutic range to be equivalent to an antifactor-Xa level of 0.3–0.7 IU/ml (Sadler et al 2000). Frequent monitoring to maintain an APTT ratio of 1.5–2.0 has been associated with a good maternal and fetal outcome, but a higher level of anticoagulation with a mid-interval APTT ratio of 2.0–2.5 may be safer. Careful studies are needed to determine the optimal level of heparinisation in pregnant women with mechanical heart valves.

LMWH has a half life 2–4 times longer than standard heparin and a bioavailability of 93–95% compared with around 30% for standard heparin. The risk of heparin-induced thrombocytopenia, allergic reactions and osteoporosis also appears to be reduced.

This is a controversial subject. Recently, Sadler et al (2000) reported experience from Auckland for the years 1972–1992 and reported a fetal loss rate of 70% with warfarin compared with 25% with heparin, but a rate of 29% (4/14) thromboembolic complications in women on heparin compared with zero in warfarin treated women. There is some evidence that heparin is a safer option throughout pregnancy in women with mechanical heart valves and avoids the hazards for the fetus which arise with warfarin but this may be at the expense of the mother. In women on warfarin anticoagulation, subcutaneous standard heparin in doses of 7500–12 500 IU every 12 hours should replace the warfarin before the sixth week of pregnancy. The dose should be adjusted to achieve a mid-interval APTT ratio of 2.0–2.5. Initially the APTT ratio should be checked daily until the patient is consistently within the therapeutic range and thereafter at 1–2-week intervals for the duration of the pregnancy. If difficulty arises in maintaining a target APTT ratio during the third trimester the anti-Xa assays can be used for monitoring heparin activity (Frewin & Chisholm 1998). The matter is considered also in Chapter 17. A national register is recommended to document prospectively the use of heparins and other antithrombotic measures to determine the most effective way to ensure good maternal and fetal outcome (Frewin & Chisholm 1998).

CONCLUSIONS

Our first priority must be to bring proven prophylactic methods to obstetric patients who are at increased risk of thromboembolic complications. No method is likely to be 100% effective but present evidence indicates that both standard heparin and LMWH confer a high degree of protection (perhaps as much as 60%) against venous thrombosis and can be used by the woman herself throughout pregnancy.

The time of greatest danger is the immediate puerperium, particularly in the patient who has been delivered by caesarean section. Prophylaxis with low-dose heparin or LMWH should be given to all mothers in the moderate or high risk category for thromboembolic complications. This includes all women undergoing emergency caesarean section. In addition to reducing the number of maternal deaths from pulmonary embolism, the judicious use of prophylactic methods should also decrease the incidence of deep vein thrombosis and the postphlebitic syndrome.

Major advances have occurred in identifying women at

increased risk of venous thrombosis in pregnancy as a result of both inherited and acquired risk factors and it is now essential for obstetricians to understand this subject. Every woman with a personal or family history of venous thromboembolism should be screened for both inherited and acquired thrombophilia. In addition to increasing the risk of venous thrombosis in pregnancy, inherited and acquired thrombophilia may be partly responsible for recurrent fetal death and intrauterine growth restriction. Wider use of thromboprophylaxis and thorough investigation of symptoms of venous thromboembolism are urgently required. All women undergoing caesarean section should be assessed for prophylaxis against thromboembolism.

KEY POINTS

- Pulmonary embolism has been the leading cause of maternal death in the UK for over a decade, accounting for a third of deaths; it outrates the deaths from hypertension, haemorrhage and sepsis combined.
- Genetic factors are associated with half of venous thrombotic deaths in pregnancy.
- Acquired factors relate to operative deliveries, changes in blood coagulation and fibrinolytic systems, reduced venous flow from leg to pelvis, restricted activity, obesity and a past history of relevant deep vein thromboses.
- Early diagnosis and treatment of peripheral thromboses using prompt anticoagulation reduces the rate of pulmonary embolism.
- Prophylactic anticoagulation is needed for those with high-risk factors for thrombosis.

REFERENCES

Bates SM, Ginsberg JS 1997 Anticoagulants in pregnancy: fetal defects. In: Greer IA (ed) Baillière's Clinical obstetrics and gynaecology. Thromboembolic disease in obstetrics and gynaecology. Baillière Tindall, London, pp 479–488

Bonnar J, Green R, Norris L 1998 Inherited thrombophilia and pregnancy: the obstetric perspective. Semin Thromb Hemost 24(suppl 1):49–53

Bonnar J, Norris LA, Greene R 1999 Low molecular weight heparin for thromboprophylaxis during Caesarean section. Thromb Res 96:317–322

Clark P, Brennand J, Conkie JA et al 1998 Activated protein C sensitivity, protein C, protein S and coagulation in normal pregnancy. Thromb Haemost 79:1166–1170

Department of Health, Welsh Office, Scottish Home and Health Department and Department of Health and Social Services, Northern Ireland 1998 Confidential Enquiries into Maternal Deaths in the United Kingdom 1994–1996. Stationery Office, London

Frewin R, Chisholm M 1998 Anticoagulation of women with prosthetic heart valves during pregnancy. Br J Obstet Gynaecol 105:683–686

Ginsberg JS, Barron WM 1995 Pregnancy and prosthetic heart valves. Lancet 344:1170–1172

Greer IA 1996 Special case of venous thromboembolism in pregnancy. In: Tooke JE, Lowe GDO (eds) A textbook of vascular medicine. Edward Arnold, London, pp 538–561

Greer IA 1997 Epidemiology, risk factors and prophylaxis of venous thromboembolism in obstetrics and gynaecology. Baillières Clin Obstet Gynaecol 11:403–430

Greer IA 1999 Thrombosis in pregnancy: maternal and fetal issues. Lancet 353:1258–1265

Hull RD, Raskob GE, Pineo GF et al 1992 Subcutaneous low-molecular weight heparin compared with continuous intravenous heparin in the treatment of proximal-vein thrombosis. N Engl J Med 326:975–982

Linghagen A, Bergqvist A, Bergqvist D, Hallbrook T 1986 Late venous function in the leg after deep venous thrombosis occurring in relation to pregnancy. Br J Obstet Gynaecol 93:348–352

McColl MD, Ramsay JE, Tait RC et al 1997 Risk factors for pregnancy associated venous thromboembolism. Thromb Haemost 78:1183–1188

McColl MD, Walker ID, Greet IA 1999 The role of inherited thrombophilia in venous thromboembolism associated with pregnancy. Br J Obstet Gynaecol 106:756–766

McColl MD, Ellison J, Reid F et al 2000 Prothrombin 20210G— A MTHFR C677T mutations in women with venous thromboembolism associated with pregnancy. Br J Obstet Gynaecol 107:565–569

Macklon NS, Greer IA 1996 Venous thromboembolic disease in obstetrics and gynaecology: the Scottish experience. Scott Med J 41:83–86

Macklon NS, Greer IA 1997 The deep venous system in the puerperium: an ultrasound study. Br J Obstet Gynaecol 104:198–200

Macklon NS, Greer IA, Bowman AW 1997 An ultrasound of gestational and postural changes in the deep venous system of the leg in pregnancy. Br J Obstet Gynaecol 104:191–197

Narayan H, Cullimore J, Krarup K et al 1992 Experience with the cardial inferior cava filter as prophylaxis against pulmonary embolism in pregnant women with extensive deep venous thrombosis. Br J Obstet Gynaecol 99:637–640

Palla A, Petruzzelli S, Donnamaria V, Giuntini C 1995 The role of suspicion in the diagnosis of pulmonary embolism. Chest 107 (suppl):215–245

Royal College of Obstetricians and Gynaecologists 1995 Report on the RCOG Working Party on Prophylaxis against thromboembolism in Gynaecology and Obstetrics. RCOG, London

Sadler L, McCowan L, White H, Steward A, Bracken M, North R 2000 Pregnancy outcomes and cardiac complications in women with mechanical, bioprosthetic and homograft valves. Br J Obstet Gynaecol 107:245–253

Simmoneau G, Sors H, Charbonnier B et al 1997 A comparison of low molecular weight heparin with unfractionated heparin for acute pulmonary embolism. N Engl J Med 337:663–669

Thomson AJ, Walker ID, Greer IA 1998 Low molecular weight heparin for the immediate management of thromboembolic disease in pregnancy. Lancet 352:1904

Villa Santa U 1965 Thromboembolic disease in pregnancy. Am J Obstet Gynecol 93:142–146

Virchow R 1860 Cited in: Cellular pathology as based on physiological and pathological histology. Churchill Livingstone, Edinburgh, pp 197–203

Walker ID 1998 Inherited coagulation disorders and thrombophilia and pregnancy. In: Bonnar J (ed) Recent advances in obstetrics and gynaecology. Churchill Livingstone, Edinburgh, pp 35–64

43

The newborn

Terence Stephenson, Helen Budge

This chapter contains contributions from previous editions and we are grateful to the previous authors for their work.

ADJUSTMENTS AT BIRTH

Lung expansion and the onset of breathing

Once the infant emerges from the birth canal and the umbilical cord is occluded, the infant's immediate priority is to establish an alternative oxygen supply. To do this, he or she needs to fill their lungs with air and to breathe regularly at an appropriate rate and depth.

At the time of birth, the infant's sensory system is well in advance of the motor system, so the brain will record a myriad of new sensations as, during birth, the infant is handled, head, trunk and limbs drop into novel positions and there is a dramatic fall in environmental temperature. These sensations are such that the majority of babies gasp at birth without additional stimulus. If the gasp occurs while the airway is clear, then the gas–liquid interface moves down the respiratory tree as the lungs fill with air. In healthy infants, the first inspiratory gasps can generate intrathoracic pressures of over 100 cmH$_2$O (Milner & Vyas 1982). The formation of the functional residual capacity depends on a number of factors, including diaphragmatic tone and the presence of surfactant. Usually, functional residual capacity is established to 70% of its final volume within a few gasps. Sometimes, despite gasps, little or no air is retained. Only when the lungs are filled with air will tidal ventilation begin and only then will the infant have established an independent oxygen supply. Most healthy infants achieve this by 1–2 minutes (Fig. 43.1). Asphyxiated, sedated and premature infants may have problems with the initial gasps and the establishment and maintenance of a functional residual capacity. Infants born by caesarean section have lower gas exchange levels during the second minute after birth compared to infants born vaginally.

The closure of the fetal channels

Upon clamping the umbilical cord, venous return from the placenta stops abruptly, the ductus venosus collapses, the pressure in the right atrium falls and the foramen ovale closes. The mechanical effect of the lungs expanding and filling with air causes a fall in pulmonary vascular resistance, the pulmonary blood flow increases, and the increased pulmonary venous return causes a rise in the left atrial pressure which further contributes to the closure of the foramen ovale (Fig. 43.2). The mechanical effect of lung inflation on the pulmonary vasculature is reinforced by the falling pCO$_2$, rising pH and rising pO$_2$, all of which favour pulmonary vasodilatation. Hormonal changes may also influence pulmonary vascular resistance and, in addition, nitric oxide has a direct relaxant effect on the endothelium (De Marco et al 1996).

With the fall in pulmonary pressure, the flow through the ductus arteriosus reverses so that oxygenated blood traverses the duct. The oxygen acts on the muscle in the duct wall causing it to contract, a mechanism which involves prostaglandins. Drugs inhibiting the synthesis of prostaglandins may cause the duct to close, whereas an infusion of prostaglandin E$_1$ can keep the ductus open. Prostaglandin inhibitor drugs given to mothers, particularly during the second trimester, can cause intrauterine closure of the ductus, compromising the fetus and causing persistent pulmonary

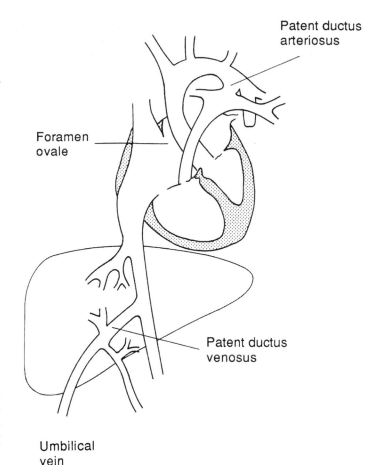

Fig. 43.2 The fetal channels.

hypertension. Indomethacin, a prostaglandin synthetase inhibitor, is used to close a persistent patent ductus in preterm infants. Prostaglandin E$_1$ infusions are used to keep the ductus open in selected infants with congenital heart defects (those with duct-dependent pulmonary or systemic blood flow such as severe pulmonary stenosis or coarctation of the aorta respectively) until surgical intervention.

The ductus closes physiologically by vasoconstriction within a matter of minutes and over the next few weeks it closes anatomically by involution and is replaced by a fibrous cord. However, if an episode of hypoxia occurs before anatomical duct closure, it may reopen. With the closure of the fetal channels, the chambers of the heart, which previously worked in parallel begin to work in series. If one ventricle is hypoplastic, the other will no longer be able to maintain both circulations and acute circulatory problems are precipitated.

Colour, tone and blood pressure

With birth, pulmonary arterial blood pressure falls and systemic pressure rises and, after the initial gasps, the infant's blood rapidly becomes well oxygenated. Birth is a stressful experience and peripheral vasomotor control has been largely untried. Thus, during the first hours of life, the limbs and trunk of normal, healthy infants can appear to be mottled or

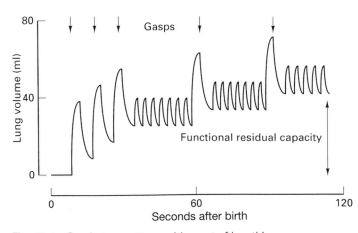

Fig. 43.1 Respiratory patterns with onset of breathing.

may have a striking harlequin pattern, and many infants have acrocyanosis (peripheral cyanotic discolouration of the hands and feet) for some time after birth. Circulating catecholamine levels after delivery are high and, together with an increase in muscular tone, the newborn infant is usually wide awake and ready to suckle.

Temperature control

It is a cold world for the infant. In utero, the fetus is bathed in amniotic fluid at 37°C. The fetus generates heat from its own metabolism and, in accordance with the second law of thermodynamics, there has to be a heat gradient down which the fetus can lose heat to its mother. This results in the fetus having a core temperature about 1°C higher than that of the mother. At birth, there is evaporation from the wet skin and the infant loses heat rapidly. Heat loss by convection is inversely associated with the environmental temperature and ventilation of the delivery room. These mechanisms of heat loss have to be reduced to a minimum if a significant fall in body temperature is to be avoided. Drying with a warm towel, followed by swaddling in a warm wrap by the mother is ideal. Even with these precautions, an infant's rectal temperature often falls after birth and then rises slowly over the first hours of life. This subsequent rise is associated, in the term infant, with the production of large amounts of heat from brown adipose tissue as independent existence is established.

The term infant has a limited capacity to control body temperature. Thus on exposure to cold he may reduce surface heat losses by vasoconstriction and increase body heat production by up to two-fold using thermogenesis in brown adipose tissue. Even so, because of an infant's body weight to surface area ratio, if he is taken from a warm cot, undressed and prepared for a bath in a warm room at 25°C, he will not be able to maintain body temperature. In a hot environment a baby can sweat a little but this capacity is limited so he is also vulnerable in hot environments. Infants have always been dependent on their parents for protection and this is particularly important with respect to body warmth in the first days of life. Cuddling and swaddling are not just comforting but are also important for sensing and maintaining the baby's temperature.

RESUSCITATION

The healthy term infant usually gasps within 60 s of birth, stimulated by the fall in po_2 that accompanies delivery and obstruction of the umbilical vessels. An infant will need active resuscitation if he fails to gasp, initiate and maintain a functional residual capacity, establish effective rhythmical respiration or independent systemic circulation. The phrase birth asphyxia has been widely, but inappropriately, used to indicate a baby in poor condition at birth. In many babies such poor condition is secondary to an insult in pregnancy before labour (MacLennan 1999), and the already damaged fetus exhibits problems during labour, thus intrapartum malfunction is a sign of damage rather than the cause.

Asphyxia embraces the concepts of both decreased oxygen in the blood (hypoxaemia) and decreased blood supply to the organs (ischaemia). However, at a cellular level, a result in both cases is decreased oxygen delivery to the tissues. The terms fetal and neonatal hypoxia should, therefore, supersede the often misleading asphyxia with its simplistic connotations of strangulation by an umbilical cord tight around the neck. Lastly, hypoxic ischaemic encephalopathy (HIE), literally encephalopathy as a result of inadequate oxygen supply and perfusion, should be used to describe the clinical manifestations of fetal or neonatal hypoxia in the newborn infant, again rather than the misnomer birth asphyxia, HIE also describes the infant's encephalopathy as distinct from that caused by toxins, bilirubin, infectious agents and errors of metabolism. HIE can be graded I (mild) to III (severe) and this helps predict outcome (American College of Obstetricians and Gynecologists Committee 1998).

Failure of initial gasp

Infants may fail to gasp or establish regular respiration as a result of fetal hypoxia, whatever its cause, although infants who cry immediately at birth can also have been irreversibly damaged by intrauterine hypoxia. Risk factors for fetal hypoxia include maternal sedation and anaesthesia, prolonged labour and decreased placental or umbilical blood flow.

Fetal hypoxia may be acute or prolonged. In prolonged hypoxia, the infant's energy resources, particularly glycogen, are depleted, there is an associated acidosis and gradually widespread damage evolves which may or may not be reversible. In contrast, the infant may have suffered total acute hypoxia, as may occur with cord prolapse when the oxygen supply is suddenly obstructed. Depending on the nature of the insult, infants differ both in their response to birth and in their recovery during resuscitation (Fig. 43.3) and there are often other complicating factors. Babies experiencing trauma during delivery may be suffering as much from shock (hypotension) and acidosis as from hypoxia, and this may be complicated further by aspiration of meconium into the respiratory tract.

Failure to establish functional residual capacity

Although the infant may gasp on delivery, air entry may be impeded by airway obstruction. Most commonly, this can result from aspiration of meconium, maternal blood or amniotic fluid and mechanical aspiration of the airway will become an emergency intervention (Gregory et al 1974). Mechanical insufflation of the infant's lungs without prior clearing of the airway is inappropriate and probably inadequate in these circumstances. Alternatively, the infant may gasp but fail to gain adequate inflation of the lungs as a consequence of decreased tone of the respiratory muscles resulting from fetal hypoxia, transplacental passage of respiratory depressants, or poor pulmonary compliance as manifested by the surfactant-deficient preterm infant. Other causes of ineffectual gasp at delivery are shown in Table 43.1.

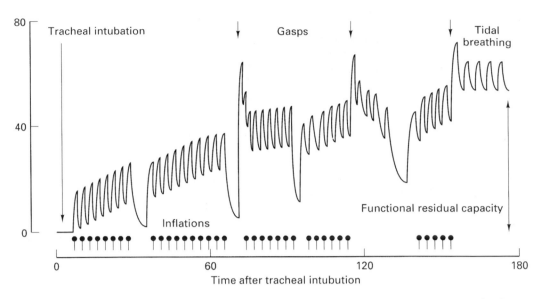

Fig. 43.3 Diagrammatic representation of the establishment of the functional residual capacity (FRC) during artificial ventilation of an asphyxiated infant. Only when the FRC had formed, partly with inflations and partly after gasps, did the infant begin spontaneous breathing.

Table 43.1 Reasons why gasps may not draw air into the lungs

Airway obstruction
  Aspirated meconium or blood
  Large or floppy tongue
  Laryngeal spasm or stenosis
  Tracheal atresia
  Choanal atresia
Deformed thoracic cage
  Thoracic dystrophy
  Diaphragmatic paralysis
Thoracic cage filled with:
  Pleural effusions
  Bowel and liver (diaphragmatic hernia)
  Pneumothorax
  Haematomas
Pulmonary hypoplasia
  Secondary to severe oligohydramnios
  (renal agenesis, chronic amniotic leak)
  Associated with diaphragmatic hernia

Failure to establish tidal breathing

Occasionally, despite the establishment of a patent airway and functional residual capacity, the infant fails to establish regular tidal breathing. This can result simply from the presence of an endotracheal tube or the hypocarbia of inadvertent mechanical hyperventilation. However, it may result from severe asphyxia, profound sedation, significant neurological abnormality or extreme prematurity.

Persistent pallor and cyanosis

Pallor may be caused by hypovolaemia and shock, sometimes from bleeding, or by acidosis resulting from hypoxia. Persistent cyanosis may be the result of ineffective oxygen delivery and the resuscitation technique and equipment should be speedily checked. With adequate oxygen delivery, persistent fetal circulation (persistent pulmonary circulation of the newborn) or severe congenital heart disease should be considered.

Anticipation of the need for resuscitation

There are a number of identified maternal, fetal and intrapartum circumstances which are associated with an increased probability that the newborn will require resuscitation:

- preterm delivery
- fetal distress
- meconium-stained liquor
- severe intrauterine growth restriction
- significant fetal anomaly or rhesus disease
- multiple pregnancy
- maternal insulin-dependent diabetes
- placenta praevia
- emergency caesarean section
- vaginal breech delivery.

The majority of these infants have at least one or more of these risk factors. Prior identification of such infants should prompt the presence at the birth of staff skilled in advanced neonatal life support

Nevertheless, for a significant number of infants, the need for resuscitation will not have been anticipated (Peliowski & Finer 1992). Hence, a professional trained in the basic skills of resuscitation should be in attendance at every delivery and advanced life support personnel should be readily available (European Resuscitation Council 1998, ILCOR Advisory Statement 1999). Local guidelines should highlight risk factors and indicate how to call appropriate staff to the birth.

Equipment and environment

In order to allow effective resuscitation in both foreseen and unforeseen circumstances, standardised resuscitation equipment and drugs should be immediately available and in working order. Attention should be paid to the environmental temperature, with a local heat source and an ambient delivery room temperature of 25°C at the time of birth.

Assessment

A procedure must be adopted whereby vital signs are simultaneously evaluated and appropriate intervention instituted. Assessment and management are thus integrated. At the delivery of the infant, the cord is clamped and cut and the baby placed in warm towels as quickly as possible. If risk factors are present, the infant should be placed on a dry, warm surface under a radiant heat source in a good light and examined closely. The first priority, regardless of initial clinical condition, is to dry the infant, remove the wet towels and place in a warmed wrap to prevent catastrophic rapid cooling. Cold stress is not only associated with adverse outcomes but may inhibit the response to resuscitation. There is some evidence of the neuroprotective role of moderate cranial cooling to protect against the effects of birth asphyxia in animal models but this should not be tried outside the context of controlled studies. After the initial gasp, the healthy infant will establish regular respirations, a pink colour and a heart rate greater than 100 beats per minute. On initial assessment, therefore, observation of the infant's respiratory pattern, colour of the trunk (acrocyanosis of the peripheries is common and does not require life support measures) and estimation of the heart rate by palpation of the umbilical cord at the abdominal junction or auscultation of the heart is made.

The newborn infant in the moments after delivery can be assigned to one of four groups using the variables in Table 43.2.

Rapid recognition of these features guides the timing and nature of intervention (European Resuscitation Council 1998, ILCOR Advisory Statement 1999; Table 43.3) with the aim of expanding the chest, oxygenating the baby and restoring the heart rate.

Table 43.2 Assessment of the newborn

Respiration	Colour	Heart rate
Breathing	Pink	Heart rate >100 bpm
Apnoeic or gasping	Blue	Heart rate >100 bpm
Apnoeic	Blue or pale	Heart rate <100 bpm (but >60 bpm)
Apnoeic	White	Heart rate <60 bpm

Techniques of resuscitation

Stimulation

The cold extrauterine world usually provides adequate stimulation to provoke the initial large negative pressure of the first gasps. Should the response be weak or absent, other simple but powerful stimuli may be delivered. Tactile stimulation is provided by drying the infant at delivery and by tapping the soles of the feet. Oxygen blown onto the nasal mucosa, for example, may work when handling does not and has the added advantage of ensuring that if the baby gasps, an oxygen-rich mixture is inhaled. The infant may also gasp during clearing of the airway. If all this had failed, and artificial ventilation is required, the first inflation often provokes an inspiratory effort, a reflex response which contributes considerably to the success of the procedure (Milner et al 1984).

Airway patency

Airway patency is obviously required for effective ventilation (both spontaneous and artificial) and is achieved by positioning and, where necessary, clearing secretions. The optimal position for the newborn infant's airway to avoid obstruction from the soft tissues of the naso- and oropharynx is described as neutral. The infant is placed supine with the mandible perpendicular to the horizontal surface on which she has been laid. Where present, airway secretions are removed using gentle low pressure suction to clear the mouth and pharynx, if necessary under direct vision using a laryngoscope. The use of mouth suction devices for clearing pharyngeal mucus or meconium has been superseded because of the risk of the

Table 43.3 Resuscitation interventions by clinical assessment

Respirations	Breathing	Apnoeic or grunting	Apnoeic	Apnoeic
Colour	Pink	Blue	Blue or pale	White
Heart rate (HR)	>100 bpm	>100 bpm	>60 bpm but <100 bpm	<60 bpm
Resuscitation measures	• Dry • Warm • Place with mother • Observe	• Stimulate • Airway (positioning; clear with suction) • Oxygen • Reassess—if fails to respond or heart rate falling, proceed to respiratory support	• Airway (positioning; clear with suction) • Respiratory support (facemask and bag) with oxygen • Reassess • Intubate at 2 minutes if absent spontaneous effective respirations or HR <100 bpm	• Intubation • Pulmonary inflations • Reassess—if HR <60 bpm after 30 s commence cardiac compressions at 120 per min (3 : 1 with inflations) • Reassess—ET position, O_2 supply • Optimise respiratory and cardiac support • Reassess—if HR <60 bpm, establish vascular access via umbilical vein, consider resuscitation drugs

attendant ingesting infected material and readily available mechanical suction should be available at all deliveries. Injudicious suction of the lower pharynx can cause laryngeal spasm or bradycardia from vagal stimulation and should be avoided.

The airway of the infant who has liquor stained with meconium should be aspirated as soon as the head is delivered; the airway should then be visualised. If any meconium is seen around the vocal cords or in the trachea, a suction catheter should be inserted through the cords under direct vision and the meconium aspirated using a suction pressure of −70 mmHg. Positive pressure ventilation is avoided until as much meconium has been removed as possible. Repeated suctioning can be continued for up to two minutes provided the heart rate remains above 60 beats per minute, but if the baby is severely hypoxic, positive pressure ventilation through an endotracheal tube should be commenced at one minute (ILCOR Advisory Statement 1999).

Oxygenation

To deliver oxygen to the infant it is necessary to fill the lungs with gas. For the majority, it is probable that air is all that is necessary, although there are currently insufficient data to support the use of unsupplemented room air alone (Ramji et al 1993, ILCOR Advisory Statement 1999) where oxygen is available.

Oxygenated gas, provided by facemask, can be inspired by the infant's own ventilatory effort or delivered by positive pressure from an oxygen-filled resuscitation bag, either via a close-fitting facemask or endotracheal tube. Resuscitation bags have a simple blow-off valve to prevent the inadvertent use of excessive pressures which may result in pneumothoraces. If the infant is resuscitated with oxygen and respiratory support withdrawn once effective respiration has commenced, the oxygen may be absorbed from the lungs should the infant subsequently become apnoeic and the secondary atelectasis may be difficult to reverse. Hence, it is established practice to let the infant briefly breathe air through an endotracheal tube before removing it, so that some nitrogen remains in the lung.

Facemask and bag

A facemask and bag are perfectly adequate for most babies who fail to breathe and is the initial method of choice. The mask should be of an appropriate size to seal around the mouth and nose without overlapping the eyes or chin. It has the advantage of being simple to apply, readily available and relatively safe. The first breaths are given at long inflation times to facilitate the establishment of a functional residual capacity (Vyas et al 1981) and subsequent inflations sufficient to produce chest rise are given at a rate of 40–60 breaths per minute. Equipment is used that limits the pressure of gas delivery to below 30 cmH$_2$O so that the stomach does not become distended with gas. If an emergency arises away from a delivery room, mouth-to-mouth resuscitation can be effective using only sufficient inflation pressure to produce a gentle rise of the chest, that is, only the pressure that can be generated by the cheeks. Forceful inflation by the attendant can cause a pneumothorax and even surgical emphysema.

Tracheal intubation

When bag and facemask ventilation is prolonged or unsuccessful or if meconium is present in the respiratory tract, tracheal intubation by the oral route should be performed. This is the most certain way for experienced staff to resuscitate the baby and expand the lungs. Inflation of the lungs by positive pressure ventilation via endotracheal tube is confirmed by chest rise and is more reliable than auscultation of breath sounds (confirmed as isolated to both axillae compared with over the stomach).

External cardiac compressions

Establishment of adequate oxygenation with ventilation will be all that is required for cardiac function to return to normal in the majority of infants and is the priority. A small number of infants fail to respond to these measures alone: chest compressions are indicated if the heart rate is absent or a heart rate below 60 beats per minute persists despite 30 seconds of effective ventilation. The infant is placed on a firm horizontal surface and his or her chest is compressed by one-third of its anterioposterior diameter (2–3 cm) using two fingers placed perpendicular to the chest on the lower one-third of the sternum (just below the inter-nipple line). Alternatively, two thumbs may be similarly positioned on the sternum with the fingers encircling the thorax. The chest is compressed in a ratio of 3 compressions to 1 pulmonary inflation to achieve an overall rate of 100 cardiac compressions each minute.

Medications

In the event of failure to respond to resuscitation measures, evidence for reversible aetiologies is sought (Table 43.4). On rare occasions, effective ventilation and external cardiac massage fail to establish and maintain a heart rate greater than 60 beats per minute, whereupon cannulation of the umbilical vein may be performed and pharmacological agents delivered. Adrenaline (epinephrine) at 0.01–0.03 mg/kg, volume expansion with 10 ml/kg of normal saline or 4.5% human albumin solution and 1 mmol/kg of 4.2% sodium bicarbonate may be appropriate. Evidence of hypoglycaemia should be sought and, if present, glucose given.

Table 43.4 Failure to respond to resuscitation measures

Poor or absent chest movement
  Airway obstruction from soft tissues, secretions or meconium
  Poor seal with facemask
  Malpositioning of endotracheal tube in oesophagus
  Disconnected oxygen supply
  Inadequate inflation pressure
  Pneumothorax
  Diaphragmatic hernia
  Pulmonary hypoplasia
Persistent pallor or cyanosis
  Hypovolaemia
  Acidosis from hypoxia or hypovolaemia
  Primary cardiac disease

Special circumstances

Maternal analgesics and anxiolytics. Certain drugs (in particular benzodiazepines, barbiturates and opioids) administered to the mother during late pregnancy or labour may, via transplacental passage, manifest as respiratory depression in the newborn infant. The degree of maternal sedation may not be predictive of the effect on the infant. Such infants may require respiratory support and, where the respiratory depressant is thought to be an opiate, may benefit from administration of naloxone once vital signs have been corrected using the techniques above (European Resuscitation Council 1998, ILCOR Advisory Statement 1999). Naloxone should not be used as a sole agent without respiratory support and subsequent observation, as late respiratory collapse may result if its duration of action proves too short to negate that of the respiratory depressant. It should not be given to infants of mothers with a history of chronic opiate use as it may precipitate acute withdrawal.

Prematurity. Lung maturity largely determines whether an infant survives the first 24 hours and does not necessarily correspond to gestation. Some advocate intubation and ventilation at birth of all infants under 28 weeks' gestation to assist them in the formation of a functional residual capacity. Such a policy may not be beneficial compared to the expectant approach whereby premature infants with respiratory distress receive early respiratory support when required. Observation for signs of respiratory distress is made although colour should be interpreted with caution as it may be a poor guide to Pao_2. Infants may look pink with a low Pao_2 (because of the predominance of fetal haemoglobin with high oxygen affinity) or blue with a normal Pao_2 (because of their relative polycythaemia).

Gastroschisis. Deliveries of infants with gastroschisis should be attended by a paediatrician and the infant resuscitated with the whole lower body being placed in a sterile clear plastic bag to allow visual assessment and reduce fluid losses. As infants are at risk of profound hypovolaemia and hypothermia resulting from evaporative losses from the exposed bowel, particular attention should be paid to normalising their circulating volume and temperature and providing any necessary respiratory support before surgical management.

When to resuscitate

The decision when to resuscitate is difficult and is dependent on clinical judgement. If an infant has a congenital abnormality incompatible with life (such as anencephaly, renal agenesis or profound multiple anomalies) active resuscitation will not be appropriate. Nonetheless, antenatal diagnoses should not be assumed to be infallible and should always be confirmed by the attendance of an informed paediatrician.

At the limits of viability, an experienced neonatologist will wish to have established a common understanding with the parents and to assess known determinants of outcome, in particular the history of this pregnancy, the baby's size, gestational age, respiratory effort and condition at birth including bruising. Local guidelines may be in place that suggest that cardiac stimulant drugs may not be useful at the limits of viability.

The Royal College of Paediatrics and Child Health consider that there are a number of instances in which withholding or withdrawing some therapies from the newborn might reasonably be considered:

- the *no chance* situation where the disease is of such severity that treatment only delays death without alleviating suffering
- the *no purpose* situation where the degree of impairment will be too great
- the *unbearable* situation where the addition of further treatments for progressive and irreversible illness is more than can be borne.

When there is doubt, or when further time is required to make an informed choice, resuscitation should be performed. The additional information gained of the infant's response to resuscitation may help in making decisions, together with further clinical information and discussion with parents. Agreement can then be made about whether and when to withdraw support. Such situations are emotionally demanding, owing to the parents' tragedy and concerns of staff and timing cannot be solely dependent on biological factors (Stephenson & Barbor 1995). Full documentation of these decisions should be made in the infant's record at the time and signed by the senior neonatologist. Some neonatologists would also request written parental consent in these circumstances. If there is doubt or time is needed to make an informed choice, resuscitation should be continued.

When to discontinue resuscitation attempts

Despite advanced life support measures some infants will fail to establish a circulation. The outcome of the resuscitation of these infants experiencing prolonged cardiorespiratory arrest is poor and it is thought reasonable to discontinue advanced life support if spontaneous circulation cannot be established after 15–20 minutes of resuscitation (European Resuscitation Council 1998, ILCOR Advisory Statement 1999).

Documentation of resuscitation

When active resuscitation measures are no longer in progress, thorough examination of the infant should be performed and clear, detailed annotation of the clinical condition of the infant at each stage of the resuscitation, the management instituted and any response, should be made.

It is common practice to have scoring systems for the assessment and resuscitation of the newborn. Whilst there are advantages in such uniformity, one cannot assume that all infants in need of resuscitation have similar problems and that all assessment criteria have the same meaning irrespective of these problems. An internationally respected and understood method for documentation of such assessment is the Apgar score (Table 43.5). In essence, it is a numerical interpretation of the infant's heart rate, respiratory efforts,

Table 43.5 The Apgar score

Factors	Score		
	0	1	2
Heart rate	Absent	Slow, <100 bpm	>100 bpm
Respiratory effort	Absent	Slow, irregular	Good, crying
Muscle tone	Flaccid	Some limb flexion	Active movement
Reflex irritability	No response	Cry	Vigorous cry
Colour	Blue, pale	Body pink, limbs blue	Completely pink

colour, responsiveness and tone. It is customary to record the score at one and five minutes but further assessment is also recorded once stabilisation is achieved following resuscitation. Such scores are not used to dictate resuscitation interventions, which must not be delayed, but provide a common score to enable international data comparison when correctly recorded and interpreted. Whereas early Apgar scores indicate the effectiveness of resuscitation and say little about ultimate outcome, a low Apgar score beyond 15 minutes is predictive of a poor neurological prognosis (Marlow 1992).

EXAMINATION OF THE NEWBORN

Immediate scrutiny

The newborn is examined under three sets of circumstances:

1. immediately at birth
2. as a routine check within 48 hours, although there is some debate regarding the cost/benefit of an early repeat examination
3. when necessary if a problem arises.

Having made the transition from intrauterine to extrauterine existence, the newborn infant is closely inspected for reassurance that no abnormalities are present. The person attending the delivery should be able to identify any major problems present. Occasionally this may be difficult but parents can reasonably expect their attendants to be as truthful as possible in as sympathetic a manner as possible.

Inspection of the infant yields the most valuable information. The infant's head, eyes, ears, limbs, back, digits and movements are observed. Inspection of the external genitalia is usually sufficient to determine the infant's gender. Fused labia are often an isolated anomaly but may be a feature of masculinising syndromes. It is sometimes difficult to determine the sex from the external genitalia at the time of birth and further examination and tests are required. These will assign a definitive and lifelong gender within a week at most and choosing a neutral name is not helpful.

In addition, the delivery room attendant should consider oesophageal atresia in infants with copious oral secretions after delivery and in those with a history of polyhydramnios. Passage of a firm gastric tube and the aspiration of acid stomach contents after birth can exclude the presence of this anomaly. Rectal agenesis may be obvious at a glance; in others the anal dimple is present and the problem escapes detection. Routine recording of the infant's rectal temperature ensures that rectal agenesis (except in the very rare cases of high membranes) is recognised early. Taking the rectal temperature is not without risk, but properly performed it is safe and highlights the need to keep the infant warm. Clinical signs of respiratory distress, apathy or irritability may be apparent on initial examination and need urgent assessment.

Vitamin K

It is recommended that all infants be given vitamin K as prophylaxis against haemorrhagic disease of the newborn (VonKries 1991). This can be administered by the oral or intramuscular route. Babies are more at risk if they are given a single dose of oral vitamin K rather than parenteral vitamin K, if they are breast fed, or if they have liver disease (McNinch & Tripp 1991). Some epidemiological studies have shown a statistical association between neonatal vitamin K injection and subsequent risk of malignancy. However, this has not been confirmed by subsequent studies and while the risk of haemorrhagic disease is certain, that of cancer is not (Hull 1993).

Oral administration of vitamin K is thought to be as effective as intramuscular administration in preventing the classic presentation of vitamin K deficient bleeding but late vitamin K deficiency in breast fed infants should be addressed by repeated administration of oral vitamin K. Our present policy in Nottingham is to give intramuscular vitamin K only to infants on the neonatal unit (birthweight >1.5 kg, 1 mg; birthweight <1.5 kg, 0.5 mg). This injection is never given on the labour suite because of the danger of inadvertent administration of ergometrine. All other infants receive 1 mg vitamin K orally. Further 0.5 mg doses are given to breast fed infants at one and four weeks after birth. In all cases, vitamin K prophylaxis is discussed with the family of the infant, administered with informed parental consent and supported with written documentation and health visitor support to maximise compliance to later oral doses.

Routine examination

A detailed routine examination of all infants should be performed in the neonatal period. Although the ideal postnatal age for this is a matter of debate, it is commonly performed within 48 hours of birth, in the presence of the parents, and should be entered into the infant's parent-held records. Examination of the newborn is primarily a surveillance procedure aimed at identifying problems that need further attention. In some it is secondary prevention—the early identification of a disorder to minimise its expression, e.g. dislocated hips. In others, it is concerned with tertiary prevention—recognising a handicap so that care and support can be provided, thus reducing the accumulating problems which add to the child's and the family's disability. Before approaching the parent and baby, the doctor should know the name and sex of the infant, the past obstetric history and whether there have been any previous fetal or neonatal deaths of siblings. Most information is again obtained by inspection and much may be achieved without waking, and before undressing, the baby. The sequence of the newborn examination needs to be, by the infant's nature, opportunistic, but formal inspection of the infant must be made:

- colour (cyanosis, anaemia, polycythaemia, jaundice)
- respiratory rate and pattern (tachypnoea, respiratory distress or depression)
- skull shape and fontanelles (is there a third fontanelle?)
- facial asymmetry (facial nerve palsy)
- clavicles (trauma)
- heart murmur
- equal breath sounds (diaphragmatic hernia)
- brachial and femoral pulses (coarctation of aorta)
- abdomen (organomegaly, masses)
- hernial orifices
- genitalia
- spine and arms
- hips: Ortolani and Barlow tests
- eyes:
  — both present behind eyelids?
  — red reflexes
- weight and head circumference
- tone, cry, alertness
- suck, palate.

Any concerns and questions of the parents should be honestly addressed and the examination sensitively discussed. The infant's weight and occipitofrontal circumference should be measured and annotated in comparison to population centiles with postnatal age corrected for gestation.

Specific anomalies and minor problems

Superficial lesions. Parents often welcome reassurance about a variety of minor matters. Red marks over the eyes, bridge of nose and nape of neck (stork bites, salmon patches) usually disappear without trace within a year. White pimples in the glands on the butterfly area of the face (milia) can be prominent but also disappear in time. Cysts on the gums (ranula) disperse spontaneously. Breast development with small amounts of milk secretion occurs in 90% of term infants, boys and girls alike, and reflects the mother's rather than the infant's hormonal status. In most infants, after initial swelling, the breast tissue gradually disappears over a period of weeks. Girls may also have a mucous plug in the vagina or a little bleeding which has no significance; the latter follows withdrawal from the high oestrogen milieu of the uterus.

Babies develop a surprisingly wide range of rashes. Neonatal urticaria (erythema toxicum) can be very florid,

with a widespread fluctuating maculopapular rash that is most marked on the second day. It does not appear to distress the infant and requires no treatment. A different rash, characterised by red macular patches and superficial clear vesicles (miliaria) may be evident. It has been called a heat rash and may be precipitated by a warm humid atmosphere.

Dysmorphic features. While some congenital structural abnormalities may be in themselves of minor significance, they may provide clues to problems elsewhere. Minor and isolated dysmorphisms are common, often familial and may not be associated with underlying abnormality. They may manifest an association with an underlying disorder or syndrome. Occasionally the facial features of Down's syndrome (trisomy 21) are hard to recognise in the first days of life (Stephenson & Wallace 1995; Table 43.6). Hypotonia and hyperextensibility are characteristic features and often help in the decision of whether to investigate further. Single palmar creases (simian creases) occur in a minority of normal individuals and are sometimes, though not invariably, a feature of Down's syndrome. Infants with Turner's syndrome (XO) may pass undetected but webbing of the neck, oedema of the feet or abnormal nails all indicate the need for further enquiry. Large fontanelles and wide sutures are not uncommon and usually have no significance if the head circumference is normal. However, a third fontanelle is found in some chromosome abnormalities, for example in Down's syndrome infants.

In the newborn period, with superficial changes in appearance after delivery, dysmorphic features may not be recognised and, with the anxiety of parents and staff to establish the normality of the infant, they may be overlooked. If a child has dysmorphic features, it is important to document them precisely and, if there is doubt, expert advice should be sought. The significance of all examination findings and any concerns and questions should be sensitively discussed with the parents. If any abnormalities are found, this information should be shared with the parents at once, and a diagnosis established as soon as possible. Efforts to conceal the discovery of, for example the stigmata of Down's syndrome often increase rather than decrease anxiety. They also diminish subsequent confidence in medical advice.

External ear and palate anomalies. Accessory auricles are usually isolated abnormalities but may also be asso-

Table 43.6 Percentage of Down's syndrome infants with dysmorphic features (reproduced with permission from Stephenson & Wallace 1995)

Feature	Percentage
Flat facial profile	90%
Hypotonia	80%
Hyperflexibility of joints	80%
Excess skin on back of neck	80%
Slanted palpebral fissures	80%
Anomalous auricles	60%
Clinodactyly of fifth finger	50%
Single palmar crease	45%

ciated with inner ear problems and deafness, and with syndromes involving hypoplasia of the mandible or maxilla. Abnormally formed ears are a feature of many dysmorphic syndromes and are often associated with renal abnormalities for, during embryogenesis, the ears develop at a similar gestation as the kidneys. All infants with accessory auricles, any malformation of the external ear, cleft lip or palate, a family history of deafness, and all preterm infants should receive hearing screening in the neonatal period. This policy targets an at-risk subgroup in which deafness is much more common and allows early (within the first 6 months of life) fitting of hearing aids.

Although cleft lip is easily identified, cleft palate can be missed if the infant is reluctant to cry. Hard palatal defects may be felt or palpation may reveal a submucous cleft with an intact mucosal covering. In the newborn period, attention should be paid to the establishment of feeding and this can usually be achieved with the assistance of specialist liaison staff and specially designed teats.

Spinal abnormalities. Spinal dysraphisms form a spectrum of congenital anomalies in the normal closure of the posterior elements of the spine. Major spinal anomalies are often detected on antenatal ultrasound scan and, in these cases, antenatal discussions regarding perinatal management and prognosis will have been commenced by an experienced paediatrician. When infants with spinal defects present unexpectedly, they should be resuscitated and, once stable, a sterile dressing placed over the defect. The infant should be swaddled by the mother as a routine, with the attendance of a paediatrician requested for assessment, discussion and transfer to the neonatal unit to permit further evaluation and appropriate treatment. Infants with spina bifida benefit from an early multidisciplinary approach to their management.

Birth trauma

Fortunately, serious birth trauma has become more rare. The incidence per 1000 live births between 1985 and 1990 was 5 for clavicular fracture, 0.6 for facial nerve injury and 1 for brachial plexus injury (Perlow et al 1996). Multiple perinatal variables are statistically significantly associated with birth injuries:

- primiparity
- instrumental delivery
- difficult caesarean section
- malpresentation (arm, brow, face, breech)
- macrosomia
- shoulder dystocia
- preterm delivery.

Multiple logistic regression analysis, however, shows that the feasibility of the obstetrician predicting these injuries is limited (Jakobovits 1996). The most serious long-term injuries are those involving the head or spine. Subgaleal or subaponeurotic haemorrhage can lead to life-threatening hypovolaemia and a coagulopathy should be sought. Extradural haemorrhage is less common than subdural haematoma and is the most serious complication of neonatal immune thrombocytopenia (caused by maternal platelet antibodies) and haemorrhagic disease of the newborn (vitamin K deficiency).

Although blood in the subarachnoid space is a very common finding in the neonate, and its incidence increases with prematurity, it is rarely of clinical significance. In contrast, intraventricular haemorrhage and intracerebral haemorrhage are very infrequent in term infants (Medlock & Hanigan 1997). Cervical cord injury can occur with or without vertebral fracture. Parietal linear fractures are the most common skull fracture but plain radiographs miss 20% (Harpold et al 1998). Fractures not related to birth trauma are also very rare in term infants but have been reported in 1% of preterm infants (Amir et al 1998). Some sites of birth trauma are given in Table 43.7.

Table 43.7 Sites of birth trauma

Scalp
Caput
Chignon
Electrode mark
Cephalohaematoma
Subaponeurotic haemorrhage
Skull
Moulding
Fractures
Subdural haematoma
Face
Bruising
Seventh nerve palsy
Brachial plexus
Upper: Erb's palsy
Lower: Klumpke's paralysis
Fractures
Skull
Clavicle
Cervical spine
Limbs
Soft tissue injuries
Minor (buttocks, scrotum)
Major (visceral tear)

Cardiac anomalies

Congenital heart diseases are the commonest congenital abnormalities with an incidence of 0.6% of live births. Although many are minor abnormalities requiring no treatment, those that present with symptoms in the neonatal period are often severe, associated with other extracardiac anomalies, and have a high morbidity and mortality. Positive detection on routine antenatal ultrasonography at 20 weeks is valuable but may not reveal up to 50% of those anomalies that present in the newborn period as, in particular, it does not detect Fallot's tetralogy or transposition of the great arteries which form the majority of severe congenital heart defects presenting in the time after birth.

One-third of infants with congenital heart disease present with central cyanosis which, unlike that from respiratory causes, does not improve with administration of 100% inspired oxygen. Causes of structural congenital heart disease presenting with cyanosis in the neonatal period include:

- transposition of the great arteries (TGA)
- tricuspid atresia
- pulmonary atresia and severe pulmonary stenosis
- total anomalous pulmonary venous drainage (TAPVD) with obstruction
- Epstein's anomaly with atrial right to left shunt
- atrioventricular septal defect
- tetralogy of Fallot.

Central cyanosis, peripheral collapse (prolonged capillary refill time and pallor) and signs of heart failure (tachycardia, tachypnoea, difficulty with feeding, excess sweating, an enlarged liver) all indicate the possibility of an underlying heart problem. Examination of the pulses may point to a patent ductus arteriosus (full and bounding) or coarctation of the aorta (absent femoral pulses) but is unreliable as the femoral pulses are often palpable at the first neonatal check in infants with coarctation because the ductus arteriosus has not yet closed. In addition to those who become symptomatic, many infants are found to have a heart murmur at auscultation during routine neonatal examination. Haemodynamic benign murmurs may be heard in over half of normal healthy infants. The presence of a heart murmur is always a matter of concern to parents in an otherwise healthy infant and may be difficult to interpret but many murmurs subsequently disappear by 72 hours, and most by six weeks, of life. Conversely, in infants with severe defects, no murmurs may be heard in the first days of life as right-sided cardiac pressures are relatively high and there is little gradient for shunting between left and right.

An asymptomatic infant with normal femoral pulses and characteristics of an innocent murmur (Table 43.8) may be reviewed at discharge and at four weeks of age. Nevertheless, the parents of all infants with a murmur should be told of the warning signs that would dictate earlier review: dusky or pale episodes, slow feeding, excessive sweating, breathlessness and poor weight gain. In the presence of other clinical signs, further investigation may be considered with chest radiography, electrocardiography and echocardiography.

Dislocated hips

About 2% of infants have unstable hips on testing at birth but in many the signs will resolve without treatment. However, in 10% of this group there will be signs of dislocation and a further 10% show evidence of subluxation or dysplasia. Current policy recommends that all infants should be examined soon after birth, as intervention, by splinting the hips in abduction, is more successful if started early. Anyone performing this examination must be well practised in the pro-

cedures. Experience can be gained initially on models and then increased by examining infants under expert guidance. The more experienced the clinician, the higher the detection rate. Even so, the diagnosis can be missed. The hips of those at high risk of dislocation (family history, breech delivery) should be examined by ultrasound (Clarke et al 1985).

FEEDING

Once the infant has gained independent existence an alternative source of nutrition must be established. Most infants root and suckle soon after birth but the volume they take is small, for little is usually available and colostrum itself has relatively little energy content. Nevertheless, the experience is a first important step both in the infant's nutrition and in the induction of lactation, as well as an occasion for the emotional meeting of mother and child. The breast fed baby must then await the establishment of lactation when infant and mother together determine the supply and demand.

Breast feeding

Breast feeding does not appear to be entirely instinctive and has to be learnt. It is more likely to be established when there has been an information programme before delivery, when mistaken notions about the effects of breast feeding have been discussed and when the mother has a source of advice and support. The atmosphere in the postnatal ward and home is key. It helps if both mother and baby are relaxed, if the baby suckles early, and if mother and infant have free and easy contact. Fixed schedules and unnecessary supplementary feeds can interfere. With support and encouragement, most mothers who wish to are able to breast feed. Although there are very few absolute contraindications to breast feeding, the method is not recommended in developed countries if the mother is infected with HIV or is suffering a severe illness, galactosaemia or phenylketonuria. Only rarely do drugs given to the mother pass to the infant in significant amounts (*British National Formulary* 1999) but some exceptions are given in Table 43.9.

In the UK it is currently recommended that breast feeding should be continued for four months before a weaning diet is introduced. By four months of age, the infant's ability to digest, metabolise and excrete a wider range of substances

Table 43.8 Characteristic features of an innocent murmur

Short
Soft
Systolic
Symptom-free
Audible over small area of the chest, without radiation
Second heart sound normal
Absence of other cardiovascular signs
Varies with respiration

Table 43.9 Some drugs unsuitable for administration to breast feeding mothers (see *British National Formulary* for advice)

Chloramphenicol	High-dose aspirin
Gancyclovir	Indomethacin
Tetracyclines	Gold salts
Oestrogens and androgens	Doxepin
Antineoplastics, radioactive drugs	Lithium
Immunosuppressants	Amiodarone
Atropine	Iodine/iodides
Ergotamine	High-dose vitamins A and D
Phenindione	

has increased, head control has developed and developmental progress towards chewing is beginning. However, milk remains a good food for a growing infant and breast milk will complete the diet. In the developing world continued breast feeding brings with it many additional benefits (such as contraception) and is a major factor in the survival and future well-being of infants and toddlers.

Despite information campaigns and initiatives, many mothers elect not to breast feed and many others stop soon after they leave hospital, bottle feeding artificial formula milk to their infants. On enquiry, these mothers cite a variety of reasons such as insufficient milk, painful breasts, a desire to return to work and the baby rejecting the breast but these are undoubtedly only a crude index of underlying social attitudes within some communities. Many investigators have found a protective effect of breast feeding against gastrointestinal infection, and breast feeding for only 12 weeks confers significant protection against gastrointestinal illnesses beyond the period of breast feeding itself (Howie et al 1990).

Bottle feeding

Although modern food technology can produce many different milk formulations, it is not entirely certain what the primary objectives and optimal characteristics of artificial formula should be. Instinctively, it may seem that artificial infant formula should be comprised of the same constituents as human milk. National and international advisory bodies have recommended that infant formulas used as the sole feed should resemble as far as possible the constituents of human milk, although some formulas, regarded by parents as standard, may contain entirely vegetable-based proteins and oils with glucose syrup and mineral additives. Human milk also appears able to provide some nutrients in bioavailable forms that are more difficult to mimic than by mere concentration of minerals provided per millilitre of milk. In addition, infant formula milks may not contain many other substances (for example, complex proteins and, in some cases, long chain polyunsaturated fatty acids) that are found in human milk. The presence and role of some of these are currently under evaluation but it appears that their simple addition to artificial formulas may not yet have provided an exact equivalent to the milk of the mother (Lucas et al 1999).

The preparation and delivery of formula milk requires clean equipment and water. Feeds from powdered milk must be correctly prepared as their correct calorie and electrolyte concentrations depend on measurement by carefully levelled scoop. Inadvertent errors produce potentially hazardous feeds with concentrations of electrolytes that are too low or too high. Special formula milks are available for selected infants who have specific requirements. Breast milk fortifiers and alternative formulas may have a role in promoting the postnatal growth of the very low birthweight infant and elemental feeds are available for babies with particular enteropathies.

Swallowing, digesting and evacuation

A total of 10% of an infant's body weight at birth is formed by adipose tissue of which half is fat, stored as triacylglycerol, which can provide sufficient calories to sustain the infant for some weeks after birth. Thus, there is no great urgency for the bowel to become fully functional in the first hours of life. Indeed it has to develop and grow to accommodate its increasing workload.

In utero, the fetus swallows amniotic fluid containing some protein but suckling is more of a physiological challenge for the newborn infant as it is vital that milk is not aspirated into the air-filled lungs. Coordinated sucking and swallowing requires protective bulbar reflexes that are only achieved in the human infant by 35 weeks' gestation, coincident with significant increases in circulating concentrations of intestinal regulatory polypeptides (gastrin, motilin, neurotensin) which occur in response to milk feeds. Therefore, unlike other systems that mature earlier in gestation and can function adequately, although not perfectly, following extremely preterm delivery (e.g. the kidney and endocrine pancreas), the gastrointestinal system cannot support independent oral nutrition until well into the final trimester. After birth, the bowel must not only accommodate a larger volume, digesting disaccharides, fats and many complex proteins, but it must also adjust to colonisation with bacteria.

By the end of the first trimester, the neuromuscular development of the human gut is largely complete. Circular and longitudinal muscle are present in both small and large bowel and the autonomic neural plexuses are identifiable. These structures, necessary for peristalsis, are morphologically mature long before enteral feeding is required or coordinated sucking and swallowing are possible. The preterm human infant passes an average of one stool per day from as early as 25 weeks' gestation, even if not enterally fed. This suggests that there is an intrinsic pattern of large bowel motor activity that can function in a coordinated propulsive fashion. This does not usually lead to defaecation in utero. Indeed, meconium-stained liquor is only rarely seen before 34 weeks. However, the incidence of meconium staining of the amniotic fluid rises towards term, reaching more than 30% by 42 weeks' gestation. This is probably the result of maturation of a defaecatory reflex in the fetus and is not associated with hypoxia unless the fetal heart rate pattern is abnormal.

The newborn infant has no voluntary control over evacuation and defaecation probably occurs as a reflex response to rectal load. Milk feeds entrain the intrinsic activity of the colon and induce regular defaecation at a frequency determined by the volume of the products of digestion that reach the rectum; the more feeds, the more stools. Although the amount of stool varies, the water content remains within a narrow range (around 70%) consistent with the water-reabsorptive function of the colon. After the first week of life, stool volume falls although milk intake continues to increase, partly owing to further maturation of the water-conserving capacity of the gut.

Babies often defaecate for the first time during delivery but, if not, usually do so within the first day of life; 95% of infants pass meconium by 24 hours and 98% by 48 hours. Delayed passage of meconium raises the possibility of anal atresia, Hirschsprung's disease or meconium ileus in cystic fibrosis.

Renal function

Infants micturate regularly in utero, making a considerable contribution to the amniotic fluid. Thus infants with obstructive problems of the urinary tract experience oligohydramnios, postural deformations and lung hypoplasia. The kidneys receive a relatively small proportion of cardiac output in utero (2–3%) compared to postnatal life and the placenta performs many of the functions that the kidneys assume in postnatal life. After birth, the kidney takes up its key role in fluid and electrolyte balance and excretion of chemical waste. During labour and immediately after birth, there are large surges of antidiuretic hormone, renin, cortisol and angiotensin II, resulting in renal vasoconstriction and salt and water retention. In early postnatal life, renal vascular resistance falls and renal blood flow increases until the kidneys receive approximately 20% of cardiac output. The initial low renal blood flow may be beneficial in a term infant who usually has little fluid intake in the first days of postnatal life, particularly if breast fed. The glomerular filtration rate is also lower in the first two days of postnatal life than later in the first week resulting in a limited ability to excrete a water load. The subsequent increase in glomerular filtration rate results in a rapid postnatal increase in the ability to excrete a water load. Postnatally, there is a rapid increase in the maximum urine osmolality attainable, from around 500–600 mOsm/kg H_2O in the first two weeks of postnatal life to greater than 1000 mOsm/kg H_2O after six to eight weeks. The increase in concentrating ability can be influenced by protein intake and antidiuretic hormone secretion which rises in response to haemorrhage, diuretics or hypertonic saline.

Hypoglycaemia

Prolonged symptomatic hypoglycaemia is associated with an adverse neurodevelopmental outcome and, although there is debate between some clinicians about its precise definition, a blood glucose concentration above 2.6 mmol/l is generally held to be desirable. Although hypoglycaemia may have been anticipated in those infants at most risk (the preterm, intrauterine growth restricted and those born to diabetic mothers) it can also occasionally occur in infants without any clinically obvious predisposing factors (Aynsley-Green & Soltesz 1986). In addition, perinatal asphyxia, sepsis and hypothermia may contribute. Although most infants remain asymptomatic, apnoeas, poor feeding, hypotonia, pallor, irritability, tremor or jitters, seizures, lethargy or hypothermia may be manifestations of hypoglycaemia. The finding on bedside heelprick testing should be confirmed by analysis of a venous sample analysed by the laboratory while normoglycaemia is achieved by provision of substrate. This may be possible with enteral milk feeds but, in those unable to feed, or those who are symptomatic, intravenous glucose infusion should be initiated. The cause of the hypoglycaemia (Table 43.10) should be considered and evidence of infection or polycythaemia actively sought. Investigation for metabolic causes is required if hypoglycaemia persists.

Table 43.10 Causes of neonatal hypoglycaemia

Insulin level	Cause
Transient hypoglycaemia	
Normal insulin levels (lack of substrate)	Small for gestational age (SGA)
	Intrauterine hypoxia
	Inadequate glucose supply
	Sepsis
	Hypothermia
High insulin levels	Maternal diabetes
	Maternal glucose infusions
	Idiopathic transient hyperinsulinaemia (often SGA)
	Beckwith–Wiedemann syndrome (macroglossia–exophthalmos)
	Maternal drugs (e.g. ritodrine)
	Erythroblastosis fetalis
Persistent hypoglycaemia	
Normal or low insulin levels	Congenital hypopituitarism
	Cortisol deficiency
	Glucagon deficiency
	Metabolic disorders (e.g. glycogen storage disease)
High insulin levels	Islet cell tumours (insulinomas)

ROUTINE SCREENING

Many diseases and anomalies present in the newborn period and all infants receive health screening in their routine examination in the first days of life. In addition, specific screening of infants at risk of deafness (those receiving neonatal intensive care and those with a family history, abnormal external ears or periauricular tags) is performed.

Biochemical screening

Many inherited metabolic diseases, of which the great majority are recessive, present in the newborn period. In some cases, this is because the placenta discharged the harmful metabolites; in others it is because milk feeds present a previously unfamiliar nutrient load, such as galactose in lactose and phenylalanine in milk proteins. Disorders such as galactosaemia and phenylketonuria, therefore, only come to light as milk feeding is established. In other babies, for example those with hypothyroidism, it is the accelerated metabolism of independent existence that reveals the disorder. Such disorders may be detected in three ways: (i) by mass screening, (ii) by screening infants at risk by virtue of a family history, and (iii) by biochemical investigation of infants with a cluster of clinical features.

Mass screening is appropriate if the disease is an important problem, the natural history is known and there is a latent period before irreversible damage occurs. There must be an agreed approach with recognised treatment, a suitable acceptable test with few false positives or negatives and adequate resources. Although screening investigations are available for a variety of disorders such as galactosaemia, maple syrup urine disease, tyrosinaemia, homocystinuria, cystic fibrosis and muscular dystrophy, screening is not performed for these in all parts of the UK as not all of the criteria for mass screening programmes can be met. Screening programmes for phenylketonuria and hypothyroidism are agreed to fulfil the desired criteria and are in universal use in the UK. Capillary blood from the infant's heel is collected from the healthy infant by the primary health team at six days of life for the Guthrie test.

Phenylketonuria is a rare condition (affecting about one in 10 000) and is implicated by detection of raised phenylalanine concentrations in heelprick blood from an infant once feeding is established. All positive results require further investigation, as the condition inevitably results in brain damage unless a special and demanding dietary regimen is adopted. Congenital hypothyroidism, caused by agenesis or dyshormonogenesis, has an incidence of one in 4000. The same blood spot is used to assay thyroid-stimulating hormone. A raised level provides an indication for further investigations to define the problem and, where hypothyroidism is confirmed, expedient treatment is required before irreversible damage has occurred. In some regions, measurement of galactosaemia or immunoreactive trypsin (IRT) is also performed. When a significantly high concentration of the latter is present, further investigations to exclude or confirm cystic fibrosis are indicated.

Until recently, these screening tests detected abnormal amounts of amino acids (excess phenylalanine), peptides (excess TSH), sugars (galactosaemia) or enzymes (IRT). However, it is now possible to test the dried blood spot on the Guthrie card for abnormal genes. For example, the polymerase chain reaction can be used to amplify the DNA and the probe for the ΔF508 mutation used to look for the commonest gene defect in cystic fibrosis. Many more examples will follow in the near future and this will lead to ethical dilemmas unless such knowledge leads to clear benefit for the child.

In addition, if there is a known familial risk of an inborn error of metabolism or a history of unexplained infant deaths, it is mandatory to institute appropriate investigations as soon as possible so that, for example, galactosaemia can be diagnosed without exposing the child to galactose, or megavitamin therapy (coenzymes) can be given in an attempt to induce some enzyme systems and so avoid harm in certain inherited metabolic disorders.

ILLNESS IN THE NEWBORN PERIOD

Most infants will be transferred from the delivery room, with their mothers, either to the postnatal wards or, increasingly commonly, to the family home in the community. A variety of disease states may emerge in the time after birth.

Respiratory distress

Some infants who establish regular respiratory effort at birth later develop respiratory distress which manifests as tachypnoea and chest wall recession with or without central cyanosis. Grunting respiration (expiration through a partially closed glottis) provides positive pressure at the end of expiration to avoid collapse of the terminal alveoli. Respiratory distress may result from a myriad of pulmonary pathologies, of which respiratory distress syndrome (RDS) is one; it is of significance that many systemic illnesses may manifest in this manner. Some common aetiologies are listed in Table 43.11. Respiratory distress is worsened by hypothermia and hypoglycaemia which require speedy intervention. The condition is most common in preterm infants, for whom there will be paediatric involvement, but respiratory distress can occur in larger, more mature infants. The midwife or obstetrician should be vigilant as the baby may appear well initially. For the obstetrician involved with an initially apparently well term infant, the most likely causes of respiratory distress are residual fluid in the lung (transient tachypnoea of the newborn) following caesarean section without labour at 36–38 weeks' gestation and infection, especially with group B streptococcus.

Respiratory distress syndrome

Surfactant deficiency combined with immature lung development is the commonest cause of respiratory distress in the preterm infant, although surfactant deficiency may, rarely, cause problems for the infant delivered at term. A chest radiograph reveals air bronchograms with reticulonodular shadowing of the lung fields which are frequently described as having a homogeneous *ground glass* appearance. Respiratory distress syndrome (RDS) was hitherto known as hyaline membrane disease; it results primarily from a relative deficiency of surfactant production from the pulmonary epithelium. Its occurrence is associated with decreased postconceptional age at delivery, perinatal hypoxia and

Table 43.11 Factors causing respiratory distress in the newborn infant

Interstitial pulmonary causes
    Respiratory distress syndrome
    Transient tachypnoea of the newborn
    Pneumonia
    Meconium aspiration
    Milk aspiration
    Pulmonary haemorrhage
    Chronic lung disease
Structural respiratory causes
    Pneumothorax
    Diaphragmatic hernia
    Pulmonary hypoplasia
    Upper airways obstruction (for example in Pierre Robin sequence)
    Cystic adenomatous malformation
    Congenital lobar emphysema
Systemic causes
    Cardiac failure
    Anaemia
    Hypothermia
    Septicaemia
    Acidosis
    Encephalopathy

maternal diabetes. Maternal administration of corticosteroids (which enhance surfactant production), mild intrauterine growth restriction and maternal opiate addiction are protective. RDS is worsened by hypothermia, acidosis and hypoxia and attention should be paid to preventing these causes where possible. Infants requiring intubation benefit from exogenous surfactant therapy early in the illness. In the natural course of RDS, a progressive worsening over the first 72 hours is to be expected with gradual improvement thereafter.

A proportion of the most immature and unwell infants will have persistent respiratory symptoms after their initial illness and progress towards chronic lung disease (hitherto known as bronchopulmonary dysplasia) with typical chest radiograph appearances and oxygen dependence beyond 28 postnatal days. These infants are often the most immature at delivery and chronic lung disease tends to improve with increased age and postnatal growth so that by the EDD chronic lung disease is present in less than 5% of all infants ventilated in the newborn period for RDS.

Transient tachypnoea of the newborn
Transient tachypnoea of the newborn usually occurs in term infants and describes the respiratory distress associated with delayed clearance of pulmonary fluid. The infant rarely requires mechanical ventilation; supportive management with oxygen and minimal handling is all that is usually required. Chest radiography may show air trapping and fluid in the horizontal fissure of the right lung.

Congenital pneumonia
The ubiquitous possibility of pulmonary infection, its manifestation with non-specific symptoms of respiratory distress in the newborn period, the difficulty of its immediate exclusion and the catastrophic consequences of shock and septicaemia ensure that this differential diagnosis remains foremost in the infant with respiratory symptoms. The commonest organisms are group B streptococcus (GBS) and *E. coli*. Our policy is to start intravenous benzyl penicillin in all babies at the onset of signs of respiratory distress as GBS can present early and cannot be excluded on clinical grounds. Support of respiration and circulation may also be indicated in infants and antibiotic chemotherapy is continued until confirmatory evidence (from the clinical course and blood cultures) is available. The antibiotic spectrum can be broadened by the addition of an intravenous aminoglycoside if other factors (prolonged rupture of membranes, maternal fever, maternal antibiotics or clinical amnionitis with offensive liquor) suggest a risk of *E. coli*, *Listeria monocytogenes* or other organisms.

Meconium aspiration
Aspiration of meconium most commonly presents soon after a delivery during which meconium has been passed before birth. Meconium in the airways and lung causes obstruction and pneumonitis. Production of surfactant is inhibited and maximal respiratory support for these infants is sometimes required. Extracorporeal membrane oxygenation (ECMO) is of benefit in severe cases.

Jaundice

It is common for healthy newborn infants to become jaundiced. In a caucasian infant, in good natural light, jaundice of the skin or sclerae may be visible when the serum bilirubin concentration is above 85 μmol/l. However, estimation of the degree of jaundice by visual means is unreliable; if there is doubt, more than a tinge of jaundice is present or the infant is less than 24 hours or more than two weeks of age, plasma bilirubin should be measured. In utero, unconjugated bilirubin is cleared by the placenta but, after birth, excretion requires uptake by the hepatocytes of the newborn's liver and conjugation by glucuronyl transferase. Enzyme induction is required for uptake and conjugation and physiological jaundice may occur in the second to fifth days of life as a result of the relatively low activity of these maturing systems and the increased red cell breakdown of the naturally polycythaemic infant. Although jaundice beginning on the second to fifth day of life is likely to be physiological unconjugated hyperbilirubinaemia, other causes should be considered (Table 43.12). Disorders causing red cell haemolysis (Table 43.13), for example bruising and materno-fetal red cell antigen incompatibility, increase the bilirubin awaiting conjugation resulting in unconjugated hyperbilirubinaemia. Further investigations should be undertaken if the infant is unwell, significantly hyperbilirubinaemic, or more than two weeks or less than 24 hours of age (Table 43.13). Although the majority of jaundiced infants are healthy, some significant disorders may present in this way and the differential diagnosis of rarer causes of hyperbilirubinaemia is beyond the scope of this chapter (Ives 1999).

Treatment of jaundice
Therapeutic strategies are aimed at decreasing the circulating concentration of unconjugated bilirubin to a level that is not

Table 43.12 Factors exacerbating neonatal jaundice

Factors	Examples
Prebirth events	Fetal infection, e.g. rubella
	Blood group incompatibilities, e.g. rhesus, ABO
Birth events	Asphyxia
	Bruising
Postbirth events	Ongoing haemolysis from red cell abnormality or blood group incompatibility
	Delayed passage of meconium
	Dehydration
	Polycythaemia
	Infection (congenital or acquired)
	Breast milk jaundice
Congenital disorders	Galactosaemia
	Hypothyroidism
	Crigler–Najjar syndrome, Dubin–Johnson syndrome, Gilbert's disease
	Cystic fibrosis
Impaired bile secretion	Neonatal cholestatis
	Extrahepatic bilary atresia
	Duodenal and low bile duct obstruction

Table 43.13 Aetiologies of jaundice commencing in the first 24 hours or persisting at two weeks of age

Jaundice commencing in the first 24 hours after birth
  Rhesus haemolytic disease
  ABO incompatibility
  Other blood group incompatibilities
  Congenital spherocytosis
  Congenital infection
  Haemoglobinopathy
Prolonged jaundice
  Persistence of physiological jaundice
  Persistent haemolysis
  Infection
  Extrahepatic bilary atresia
  Neonatal cholestasis
  Neonatal hepatitis
  Hypothyroidism
  Cystic fibrosis
  Drugs
  Metabolic disorders
  Breast milk jaundice

Table 43.14 Side effects of treatment of neonatal jaundice

Treatment	Complication
Phototherapy	Unstable body temperature
	Increased transcutaneous water loss
	Loose stools and increased stool frequency (with increased water loss)
	Skin rashes
Exchange transfusion	Embolism of air or clot
	Thrombosis
	Haemorrhage
	Cardiac arrhythmias
	Hypervolaemia and hypovolaemia
	Hypothermia
	Respiratory distress
	Hypokalaemia, hypocalcaemia, hypomagnesaemia
	Hypoglycaemia
	Acidosis
	Thrombocytopenia
	Infection (bacterial and viral)

thought to place the infant at risk for kernicterus or deafness. Prematurity, low plasma albumin concentrations, the hypoxia, acidosis and hypoglycaemia that may accompany systemic illness and drugs that displace bilirubin from binding to albumin are associated with neurotoxicity at lower plasma bilirubin concentrations. Dehydration and hypoglycaemia should be avoided and phototherapy used early to prevent the devastating, irreversible sequelae of kernicterus while avoiding exchange transfusion if possible.

Unconjugated bilirubin in the skin, when exposed to light from the blue end of the visible spectrum, undergoes photoisomerism to a water-soluble form that can be excreted by the kidneys and is less lipophilic and hence less neurotoxic. Each neonatal service has its own guidelines about when and how to use phototherapy. Generally, phototherapy is instituted if the bilirubin concentration in μmol/l exceeds one-tenth of the infant's birthweight in grams. It is usually well tolerated and most term infants are able to remain with their mothers on the postnatal ward. Exchange transfusion is indicated when the risk from the high plasma concentrations of unconjugated bilirubin outweighs the complications of the therapy. Some side effects of the management of jaundice are detailed in Table 43.14.

Infection

Risk factors for early neonatal infection include:

- prolonged rupture of membranes
- preterm rupture of membranes
- fetal hypoxia
- chorio-amnionitis
- offensive liquor
- maternal infection (especially gastrointestinal and urinary tract)
- colonisation on high vaginal swab with group B streptococcus (GBS)
- previous sibling with GBS.

The most virulent neonatal infection is caused by group B streptococcus. This organism can be found in the vagina of many pregnant women; a much smaller proportion of infants become infected, but there is a high mortality and morbidity for those who are. General poor condition of the affected infant may be obvious from birth but the onset may be insidious. In either case, the signs are non-specific and may mimic hyaline membrane disease. Largely for these reasons, paediatricians have a low threshold for commencing intravenous benzylpenicillin in all babies at the onset of signs of respiratory distress, and broad-spectrum antibiotics in any infant seriously ill at birth. We recommend maternal intravenous, intrapartum antibiotics at least four hours before delivery if there is proven maternal colonisation with GBS or a previous child was infected with GBS to reduce the transmission rate or severity of the illness in the infant.

On occasion, offensive liquor is evident at delivery or there has been prolonged rupture of membranes, in which case the baby should be examined for signs of sepsis.

If the infant is unwell, or there are other problems such as prematurity, grunting respiration or hypoxic–ischaemic encephalopathy, the infant should be transferred to the neonatal unit for a full infection screen including viral and bacterial surface swabs, suprapubic aspiration of urine (ideally under ultrasound guidance), full blood count, blood cultures, chest radiograph and lumbar puncture. Intravenous penicillin and gentamicin should be started immediately after the specimens have been obtained. The combination of a vague flu-like illness in the mother, green liquor, a neonatal rash and, rarely, abscesses on the placenta, implicates *Listeria monocytogenes* as the causative organism and ampicillin and gentamicin form a powerful synergistic therapy.

If the baby is well and at term, our policy is to admit the infant to the neonatal unit and commence antibiotics only if all three of the following conditions are met:

- The mother has a pyrexia at the time of delivery or has been treated with antibiotics prior to delivery.
- The liquor or vaginal discharge before birth was offensive.
- The membranes have been ruptured for more than 24 hours.

For the well baby, in which all three criteria are not met, samples are taken but antibiotics are not commenced unless his condition changes. The infant may accompany his mother to the postnatal ward but should receive four-hourly review with regular temperature and respiratory rate observations.

Manifestations of infections in the newborn period and common causative organisms are given in Table 43.15. Often, however, these warning circumstances or signs are not present in infants who contract infection from the birth canal. If the mother is known to have genital herpes, streptococcal, gonococcal or listeria infections, it is essential that those responsible for the care of the newborn should be informed immediately. Primary herpes cervicitis is an indication for elective caesarean section to protect the infant but this is not necessarily true for a recurrence. Only one-third of asymptomatic women who shed herpes simplex virus in early labour have a recently acquired primary infection. Infants of mothers with a primary infection are ten times more likely to have neonatal herpes infection than babies whose mothers have asymptomatic reactivation of herpes simplex (Brown et al 1991).

Encephalopathy

Some newborn infants exhibit abnormal neurological function. This may be the result of overwhelming systemic or central infection or, more rarely, of structural abnormality of the brain. More commonly, it results from hypoxia or ischaemia or a combination of the two. These may have their aetiology in the antenatal, intrapartum or postnatal periods and are more common in preterm infants, the growth restricted and those with congenital anomalies. Presenting up to 48 hours after birth, infants may manifest a variety of abnormal behaviours and these have been used to compile clinical grading systems (Sarnat & Sarnat 1976, O'Callaghan & Stephenson 1992; Table 43.16) to predict outcome. Over 95% of those with grade I hypoxic–ischaemic encephalopathy (HIE), and 75% of those with grade II, are categorised as normal at later follow-up. However, up to 50% of those with grade III HIE die in the newborn period and only one-fifth of the survivors are found to be without significant sequelae. Therapeutic strategies optimise oxygenation, perfusion, normoglycaemia and fluid balance, aiming for normocarbia as an arterial carbon dioxide tension of less than 3.5 kPa is associated with cerebral vasoconstriction. In infants with severe hypoxic–ischaemic

Table 43.15 Signs and symptoms of infections of the newborn with most common causative organisms

Type	Manifestations	Commonest organisms
Congenital	Seizures Encephalopathy Microcephaly Thrombocytopenia Hepatitis Severe intrauterine growth restriction Sepsis Early jaundice	Listeria Toxoplasmosis Rubella CMV Herpes Parvovirus Hepatitis B GBS HIV
Superficial (usually trivial but can spread to cause systemic infection)	Conjunctivitis	Staph. aureus Gonococcus Chlamydia
	Skin sepsis Paronychia Umbilical infection Oral or perineal candida	Staph. aureus Staph. aureus Staph. aureus Candida albicans
Systemic	Septicaemia	Staphylococci Streptococci Gram negatives
	Meningitis Pneumonia UTI	GBS, E. coli GBS E. coli

Table 43.16 Grades and outcome of hypoxic–ischaemic encephalopathy

	Grade		
	I (mild)	II (moderate)	III (severe)
Conscious level	Hyperalert (staring and irritable)	Lethargic	Stuporose
Muscle tone	Normal	Mildly hypotonic (decreased spontaneous movements)	Flaccid (no spontaneous movements—require ventilation)
Tendon reflexes	Increased	Increased	Decreased/absent
Suck	Weak	Weak/absent (require tube feeding)	Absent
Autonomic function	Increased sympathetic activity	Increased parasympathetic activity	Decreased sympathetic and parasympathetic activity
Seizures	None	Common (most frequent in second 24 h after delivery)	Absent or prolonged and difficult to control

encephalopathy, hypoxic/hypovolaemic effects on the kidneys (acute tubular necrosis), myocardium (ischaemia, depressed contractility, bradycardia) and bowel (necrotising enterocolitis) are anticipated. Prolonged or frequent seizures are treated with pharmacological agents in addition to the above supportive measures and the infant is maintained in the thermoneutral range. Specific therapeutic strategies to diminish cerebral injury following hypoxia and ischaemia, for example by local brain cooling, are undergoing clinical trials. The presence of focal brain injury and ventricular size may be apparent from cranial ultrasound imaging and increased resistance to flow in the middle cerebral arteries on Doppler imaging is associated with a worse outcome. Even in marked encephalopathy, the appearances on cranial ultrasound may not be profoundly abnormal and more detailed information may be obtained from magnetic resonance imaging.

Periventricular haemorrhage

Periventricular haemorrhage occurs mainly in preterm infants with a peak incidence at three days after delivery. Haemorrhage originating from the fragile capillaries of the subependymal germinal matrix may occur into the ventricles and, in those infants most severely affected, is also seen into the brain parenchyma. This may arise from secondary haemorrhage into areas of brain that have undergone venous infarction or by direct extension. It is thought that preterm infants are predisposed to such events as a result of their profusion of fragile capillaries. Factors that produce fluctuations in perfusion (such as fluctuations in blood pressure, oxygen and carbon dioxide) are associated with an increased incidence of periventricular haemorrhage. The outcome of periventricular haemorrhage is partly dependent on its severity and is complicated by associations with significant illness and prematurity. Although most of those who develop small intraventricular haemorrhages will develop no detectable long-term sequelae, the neurodevelopmental outcome of those with the most extensive parenchymal damage is likely to be abnormal and there is a high incidence of cerebral palsy in those who require ventriculoperitoneal shunt insertion for ventricular dilatation.

OUTCOME OF PRETERM BIRTH

Survival

Neonatal mortality and morbidity is highly associated with gestational age and birthweight, and the probability of mortality for the very preterm, very low birthweight infant is high (Fig. 43.4). Accurate, current data are necessary to guide clinicians in advising parents facing preterm birth about their infant's chance of survival. However, the use of studies that report survival of infants admitted for neonatal intensive care significantly overestimates what can be expected for an infant not yet born alive; antenatal, intrapartum and neonatal care in historical studies must be comparable to be of contemporary value.

Data from a population demographically representative of the United Kingdom have been collected from the Trent health region over the three years to December 1997 (Draper

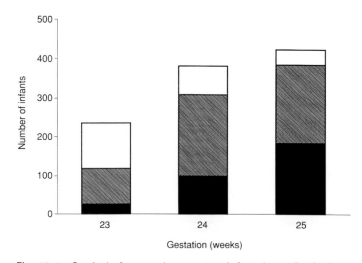

Fig. 43.4 Survival of extremely premature infants born alive in the United Kingdom and Republic of Ireland, March to December 1995 (EPICure Study, personal communication). Filled bars: survival to discharge from neonatal intensive care. Hatched bars: admitted for neonatal intensive care but died before discharge. Open bars: died before admission to intensive care.

et al 1999). This study has reported survival to discharge from neonatal intensive care of infants of 22–32 weeks' gestation, known to be alive at the onset of labour or at the time of the decision to deliver. Of 3760 infants born between these gestations in the study period, nearly 93% were admitted for neonatal intensive care and, of these, approximately 87% survived to discharge. Thus, overall, approximately 80% of babies alive at the onset of labour survived to discharge from neonatal intensive care. Survival was positively associated with gestational age (Fig. 43.5) and at each gestation beyond 24 weeks there was a positive association between survival and birthweight.

After discharge from neonatal intensive care, a small number of infants succumb to the sequelae of preterm birth but, in addition, they have an increased incidence of sudden unexplained death. In the cohort of 314 survivors of neonatal intensive care of less than 26 weeks' gestation collected by the EPICure Investigators, 6 (1.9%) died after discharge (EPICure Study Investigators, personal communication).

Outcome of survivors

Very low birthweight and very preterm survivors have a significant risk of subsequent disability (Fig. 43.6). Infants experiencing preterm birth are more likely to suffer respiratory morbidity and may feed and grow poorly. Neurological disability may be manifest as a severe impairment of movement, hearing, vision or learning, while more subtle problems with behaviour and cognition may only become apparent with increasing postnatal age. Assessment of survivors beyond the neonatal period is therefore necessary to assess both the needs of the individual child and to provide population outcomes for these infants, their parents and their clinicians.

The outcome at 2½ years corrected age of a national population-based study of children born before 26 weeks' gestation has highlighted that these extremely preterm infants

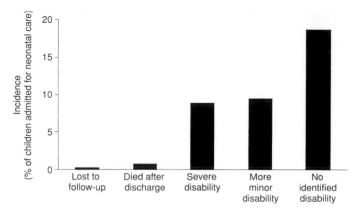

Fig. 43.6 Summary of outcome of national cohort of extremely premature infants (22 weeks' to 26 weeks' gestation) born in the United Kingdom and Republic of Ireland from March to December 1995 surviving to discharge from neonatal intensive care units (EPICure Study, personal communication). Severe disability: for example, movement disorders; severe cerebral palsy, developmental delay, blindness. More minor disability: for example, hearing impairment corrected with aids, lower limb weakness not interfering with walking.

have persistent morbidities and has shown that severe neurodisability is present in just over 30% of survivors from these gestations (Wood & Marlow 1999a,b; Table 43.17). Nevertheless, the majority of survivors of preterm birth have no identified disability and, despite their increase in numbers, there has been no significant rise in the overall rates of disability.

CONCLUSIONS

Although the majority of newborn infants effect the transition from intrauterine to extrauterine existence without difficulty, there will be a number for whom greater attention from health care professionals will be required as a result of, for example, congenital anomaly, the failure to establish

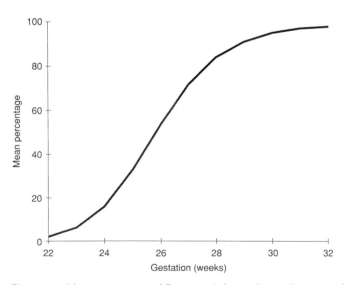

Fig. 43.5 Mean percentage of European infants alive at the onset of labour surviving to discharge from neonatal intensive care (data from Draper et al 1999).

Table 43.17 Health outcomes at 2.5 years of infants born at less than 26 weeks' gestation (data from Wood & Marlow 1999a,b)

Outcome measure	Percentage of survivors
Required home oxygen therapy (beyond one year corrected age)	35.8 (8.4)
Significant developmental delay of DQ <70 (profound delay DQ <50)	29.5 (18.2)
Neuromotor impairment	29.2
More than 3 hospital readmissions by 2.5 years	23.3
Poor growth in weight (<2 SD)	17.2
Poor growth in height (<2 SD)	11.8
Severe neuromotor disability	9.3
Not communicating with speech	6.4
Recurrent non-febrile seizures	5.4
Blind	1.8
Deaf, even with aids	0.4

effective respiration or circulation, or prematurity. As the antenatal prediction of neonatal problems can never be complete, skills in resuscitation and in the early identification of important anomalies and problems form part of the repertoire required for all delivery room attendants. In addition, those attending mother and child require a knowledge of the aetiology and prognosis of common normal findings in newborn infants to provide accurate, contemporary information to the newborn's parents while remaining vigilant for indications of disease or abnormality that may emerge in the time after birth.

KEY POINTS

In the delivery room
- The need for resuscitation cannot always be anticipated. A professional trained in the basic skills of resuscitation should be in attendance at every delivery to initiate resuscitation and summon advanced life support personnel if necessary.
- The timing and nature of resuscitation interventions are guided by the respiration, colour and heart rate of the baby with the aim of expanding the chest, oxygenating the baby and restoring the heart rate.

After birth
- Initial superficial examination for birth injuries, major congenital anomalies, cyanosis or respiratory distress should be performed, with a more detailed examination later.
- A variety of disease states may emerge even in the infant who appears initially healthy. Therefore, all should be vigilant, in particular for the signs of respiratory distress and congenital heart disease.

In general
- Procedures and clinical findings should be documented and discussed with the parents and any concerns and questions honestly addressed.

REFERENCES

American College of Obstetricians and Gynecologists Committee 1998 Inappropriate use of the terms fetal distress and birth asphyxia. Int J Gynaecol Obstet 61:309–310

Amir J, Katz K, Grunebaum M, Yosipovitch Z, Wielunsky E, Reisner SH 1988 Fractures in premature infants. J Pediatr Orthop 8:41–44

Aynsley-Green A, Soltesz G 1986 Metabolic and endocrine disorders. In: Roberton NRC (ed) Textbook of neonatology. Churchill Livingstone, Edinburgh, pp 605–623

Brown Z, Benedetti J, Ashley R et al 1991 Neonatal herpes simplex virus infection in relation to asymptomatic maternal infection at the time of labor. N Engl J Med 324:1247–1252

Clarke NMP, Harcke HT, Mettugh P et al 1985 Real time ultrasound in the diagnosis of congenital dislocation and dysplasia of the hip. J Bone Joint Surg 67B:406–412

DeMarco V, Skimming JW, Ellis TM, Cassin S 1996 Nitric oxide inhalation: effects on the ovine neonatal pulmonary and systemic circulations. Reprod Fertil Dev 8:431–438

Draper ES, Manktelow B, Field DJ, James D 1999 Prediction of survival for preterm births by weight and gestational age: retrospective population based study. BMJ 319:1093–1097

European Resuscitation Council 1998 Recommendations on resuscitation of babies at birth: to be read in conjunction with the International Liaison Committee on Resuscitation Paediatric Working Group advisory statement (April 1997). Resuscitation 37:103–110

Gregory GA, Gooding CA, Phibbs RH, Tookey WH 1974 Meconium aspiration in infants—a prospective study. J Pediatr 85:848–852

Harpold TL, McComb G, Levy ML 1998 Neonatal neurosurgical trauma. Neurosurg Clin N Am 9:141–154

Howie P, Forsyth J, Ogston S, Clark A, Florey CD 1990 Protective effect of breast feeding against infection. BMJ 300:11–16

Hull D 1993 Vitamin K and childhood cancer. The risk of haemorrhagic disease is certain; that of cancer is not. BMJ 305:326–327

ILCOR Advisory Statement 1999 Resuscitation of the newly born infant. An advisory statement from the Paediatric Working Group of the International Liaison Committee on Resuscitation. Circulation 99:1927–1938

Ives NK 1999 Neonatal jaundice. In: Rennie JM, Roberton NRC (eds) Textbook of neonatology. Churchill Livingstone, Edinburgh, pp 715–732

Jakobovits A 1996 Medico-legal aspects of brachial plexus injury: the obstetrician's point of view. Med Law 15:175–182

Lucas A, Stafford M, Morley R et al 1999 Efficacy and safety of long-chain polyunsaturated fatty acid supplementation of infant-formula milk: a randomised trial. Lancet 354:1948–1954

MacLennan A 1999 A template for defining a causal relation between acute intrapartum events and cerebral palsy: international consensus statement. BMJ 319:1054–1059

McNinch AW, Tripp JH 1991 Haemorrhagic disease of the newborn in the British Isles: two year prospective study. BMJ 303:1105–1109

Marlow N 1992 Do we need an Apgar score? Arch Dis Child 67:765–767

Medlock MD, Hanigan WC 1997 Neurologic birth trauma. Clin Perinatol 4:845–857

Milner AD, Vyas H 1982 Lung expansion at birth. J Pediatr 101:879–886

Milner AD, Vyas H, Hopkin IE 1984 Efficacy of face mask resuscitation at birth. BMJ 289:1563–1565

O'Callaghan C, Stephenson T 1992 Pocket paediatrics. Churchill Livingstone, Edinburgh

Peliowski A, Finer NN 1992 Birth asphyxia in the term child. In: Sinclair JC, Bracken MB (eds) Effective care of the newborn infant. Oxford University Press, Oxford, pp 249–273

Perlow JH, Wigton T, Hart J, Strassner HT, Nageotte MP, Wolk BM 1996 Birth trauma—a five year review of incidence and associated perinatal factors. J Reprod Med 41:754–760

Ramji S, Ahuja S, Thirupuram S, Rootwelt T, Rooth G, Saugstad OD 1993 Resuscitation of asphyxic newborn infants with room air or 100% oxygen. Pediatr Res 34:809–812

Sarnat HB, Sarnat MS 1976 Neonatal encephalopathy following fetal distress. A clinical and electroencephalographic study. Arch Neurol 33:696–705

Stephenson T, Barbor P 1995 Ethical dilemmas of diagnosis and intervention. In: Levene M, Lilford R, Bennett M, Punt J (eds) Fetal and neonatal neurology and neurosurgery, 2nd edn. Churchill Livingstone, London, pp 709–718

Stephenson T, Wallace H 1995 Clinical paediatrics for postgraduate examinations. Churchill Livingstone, Edinburgh

VonKries R 1991 Neonatal vitamin K—prophylaxis for all. BMJ 303:1083–1084

Vyas H, Milner AD, Hopkin IE, Boon AW 1981 Physiological responses to prolonged slow-rise inflation in the resuscitation of the asphyxiated newborn infant. J Pediatr 99:635–639

Wood N, Marlow N (on behalf of the EPICure Investigators Group) 1999a Developmental and neurological disability in extremely preterm children at two and a half years. Arch Dis Child 80(suppl 1): P1

Wood N, Marlow N (on behalf of the EPICure Investigators Group) 1999b Nonneurological morbidity among extremely preterm children at two and a half years. Arch Dis Child 80(suppl 1): G98

44

Psychological effects of perinatal death

Gillian Forrest

INTRODUCTION

The loss of a baby in the perinatal period is a traumatic event that has far-reaching consequences for the bereaved parents. Over the past few years, with dramatic improvements in perinatal and infant mortality rates, parents' expectations of the safe delivery of a healthy baby have become very high. When things do go wrong, therefore, they are confronted not only with the loss of their baby but also with the loss of their faith in modern medical care. In addition, as part of societies in developed countries, which have lost their familiarity with death and bereavement, many parents do not even have the comfort of the mourning rituals which have traditionally helped the bereaved to cope. It is important, therefore, for professionals dealing with perinatal death to have an understanding of the bereavement process, and an awareness of the difficulties and dilemmas facing parents so that staff can offer the best possible care.

BEREAVEMENT

Our knowledge of bereavement is based partly on descriptive accounts of patients in psychiatric treatment, and partly on objective studies of groups of bereaved subjects (Parkes & Markus 1998). Normal grief reactions vary between individuals, but there are some common features. At first, there is usually a period of shock or numbness, which may last for hours or days and is more marked after an unexpected death.

This is followed by acute episodes of intense emotional distress with weeping, protestation and anger, with accompanying somatic symptoms of anxiety such as palpitations or choking sensations in the throat. These pangs of grief are precipitated by any reminders of the loss and are accompanied by disturbances of concentration, sleep, appetite and weight, and social withdrawal. In the third phase, irritability and depression are typical. Vivid dreams and hallucinations of the dead person or his voice are quite common. There is an overwhelming need to rehearse the events around the death and this is one aspect of grief work, the process by which we accept the reality of the loss and withdraw from the relationship with the dead person, in order to continue our own life in a positive manner.

Chronic low mood and loss of purpose in life may continue for months or years, while the pangs of grief tend to decrease in intensity and frequency with time (Fig. 44.1). There is an increase in psychosomatic and somatic illness in the year following bereavement; this may be a consequence of the disturbance of the immune system which has been reported (Schleiffer et al 1983). Anniversary reactions with short intensifications of grief symptoms are commonly experienced for some years.

Recovery from bereavement is marked by a return to psychological, social and physical well-being. The enormous individual variations in response mean that it is not possible to provide a specific time scale. However, a successful outcome depends on the individual's personality and life experiences, the circumstances of the death, the relationship he had

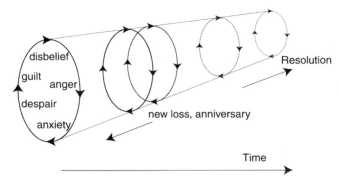

Fig. 44.1 The cycle of grieving.

with the dead person and on the supportive network surrounding him (Raphael 1977).

The style of an individual's grief reaction will be determined by both personality traits and gender, for example, grieving in private or openly expressing emotions.

PERINATAL DEATH

Today, it is widely accepted that losing a baby late in pregnancy or soon after delivery is accompanied by the same sort of grief reaction described above. Since 1970 there has been a great deal of descriptive literature, with some objective studies on management and outcome, and it is now clear that grief after perinatal death is no different, qualitatively, from that following the death of any loved person (Forrest 1989, Zeanah 1989).

There are some special features. Anxiety and anger are frequently described, with blame being directed at the medical or midwifery staff, other members of the family, or at one's self, in the form of guilt. This may result in part from the suddenness of the death and is probably compounded when there is no scientific explanation available to help the parents understand exactly what went wrong (Newton et al 1986). Desperately seeking for a cause for the baby's death is also common. Clearly, it is easier for parents who do have an explanation such as malformations of the baby or extreme prematurity. *Empty arms* is another common and distressing symptom after the phase of numbness has passed and mothers are frequently tormented by hearing their dead baby crying, or feeling fetal movements. Some experience negative or aggressive feelings towards other babies and are fearful of losing control, while others long to hold a baby, any baby, however painful this might be. Many mothers do not expect to lactate once the baby has died, and find the fact that they do very upsetting. Most authors emphasise the great sense of loss of self-esteem experienced by bereaved mothers; they experience failure both as women and as wives or partners.

Most young parents will not have been bereaved before and often experience difficulties coping with the complicated registration and funeral procedures (Forrest et al 1981). Many mothers are unprepared for the emotional turmoil of their grief reaction and of the exacerbation of symptoms that often accompanies the expected date of delivery or the return

of menstruation. They may feel they should be over it after a few weeks. This view may be reinforced by well-meaning friends and relatives and even some medical practitioners, who may advise the couple to go ahead with another pregnancy long before they have sufficiently recovered from their loss to cope with this psychological stress. There is evidence that fathers recover from grief more quickly than mothers (Forrest et al 1982, Boyle 1997) and this in itself may lead to relationship problems, particularly if the couple are not used to sharing their feelings, or if one is blaming the other for the baby's death. Sexual and marital difficulties are common sequelae (Meyer & Lewis 1979), although there is no evidence of an increase in marital breakdown (Boyle 1997).

Another difficult area is the reaction of other young children in the family to the loss of the baby. They may be very confused about what has happened to the baby and even feel responsible for his disappearance (Bowlby 1979). Behavioural changes are common and may take the form of over-activity, naughtiness, regression and school problems, as well as emotional problems (Van Eerdewegh et al 1985, Dyregrov 1991). These reactions are usually fairly short-lived—a few weeks or months is the time noted by most authors—unless the emotional state of the parents is such that there is an absence of normal warmth in family relationships for an extended period (Black & Urbanowicz 1985) or if serious relationship difficulties develop between the mother and the surviving children (Lewis 1983, Bryan 1995).

With miscarriages and stillborn babies there are particular problems in which iatrogenic factors undoubtedly play a part. Professionals and others frequently regard miscarriages as minor setbacks in successful childbearing. For some women, however, they represent a loss as painful as that of a full-term baby (Oakley et al 1984). This is particularly so if there have been difficulties conceiving, previous miscarriages, or if the pregnancy was terminated because of fetal abnormalities (Lloyd & Laurence 1985, Lilford et al 1994). Here there is the double loss of that baby and of the chance of childbearing. A previous termination of pregnancy has been reported by many clinicians as a complicating factor for normal grieving because of the associated guilt and sense of retribution that is experienced by the mothers. If the pregnancy was well advanced, beyond 18 weeks or so, many parents now want to hold a funeral for their baby. At one time this presented administrative difficulties but these can now usually be overcome.

Much has been written about unresolved grief after a stillborn baby, notably by Lewis (1983). He attributes this to the painful emptiness of the experience. There is no real object to mourn, as the baby never lived outside the womb. It is similar to the situation in which someone is missing, believed dead. The problem is accentuated if the stillborn baby is rapidly removed from the delivery room before the parents have a chance to see or hold him or her, no mementoes are kept, and the hospital takes over the funeral arrangements without involving the parents. The attitudes of friends and relations may also contribute to the difficulties. For example, one grieving mother was told: 'You can't have postnatal depression, you haven't got a baby'. For these reasons, successful mourning after stillbirth may be harder to achieve without the guidance of well-informed staff and greater understanding on the part of society in general.

Long-term effects of perinatal death

There have been few studies on the long-term effects of perinatal death.

Nicol et al (1986) followed up 110 women for 6–36 months after a perinatal death. They found that 21% were suffering from a pathological grief reaction, with continuing severe psychological symptoms (depression, anxiety, tiredness, etc.), social adjustment problems and marital difficulties, and a resolve to have no further children. They also found that a poor outcome was associated with a crisis in the pregnancy, and an unsupportive family network.

Boyle (1997) followed up 194 bereaved mothers (80 neonatal deaths, 78 stillbirths and 36 SIDS) at 2, 8, 15 and 30 months after the loss of the baby, and compared them with 203 mothers with a live-born child. The bereaved mothers showed high levels of anxiety and depression two months after the loss, and these symptoms persisted in 14% of the bereaved mothers throughout the study. Vulnerability factors in this group of mothers were perceived non-supportive social networks, difficulties with childrearing and poor socioeconomic circumstances—factors which have been shown to increase the risk of mental health problems in women generally, particularly when associated with major life events.

There have been reports of serious relationship problems with babies conceived too quickly after a loss (Bourne & Lewis 1984). It seems that if the dead child has been incompletely mourned before the start of a new pregnancy, mourning may be postponed until after the delivery of the next baby, when it can reappear as postnatal depression (Lewis 1979). The new baby's identity can become confused with that of the idealised dead baby, causing great emotional problems. He may never be able to live up to his parents' expectations and may also become the focus of any unresolved anger which the parents feel as a result of their loss. The survivor of twins may also be involved in very similar problems if the dead twin is not properly mourned at the time (Bryan 1995). This has been called the replacement baby syndrome. However, Boyle's study (1997) suggests that the risk of this is low, with most mothers showing high levels of anxiety about their next live-born child.

Overall, therefore, it seems that about one in six bereaved families are likely to suffer adverse long-term effects after losing a baby, and unsupported mothers in poor social circumstances are very vulnerable. Good care should therefore aim to try to prevent these long-term sequelae.

CARE

In many countries now, the recommendations for care emphasise the important role of maternity unit staff in dealing with families facing the loss of their baby (Giles P 1970, Kowalski K 1980, Fetus and Newborn Committee, Canadian Pediatric Society 1983, Royal College of Obstetricians and Gynaecologists 1985, Fox et al 1997).

This section brings together the recommendations for care made by individual clinicians and organisations concerned with helping parents cope with perinatal death. It is generally agreed that the key task is to enable parents to overcome their fear of death and dying so that they can experience the painful reality of their loss and allow mourning to begin. This involves encouraging them to have as much contact as possible with their baby, both before and after death. There is widespread agreement by authors that it is particularly important for parents of stillborn babies to see, hold and name their baby.

Intrauterine death and stillbirth

When an intrauterine death is suspected, the fears for the baby's condition should be shared with the parents, together if at all possible, and not denied. If the mother is at the clinic, efforts should be made to contact her partner or a friend, so that she is not left to travel home alone and unsupported. The ultrasonographers in the scanning room have an important role to play when the confirmatory scan is done. They need to be sympathetic to the situation, relaxing any rules to allow the mother to be accompanied by anyone she chooses.

After intrauterine death has been confirmed, most women are very frightened at the prospect of delivering a dead baby, as well as being shocked by their loss. It helps if staff take time to explain carefully what will happen, that adequate pain relief will be available, and what the baby will look like at delivery. This is often successful in overcoming any reluctance the parents may have about seeing or holding their baby. If the baby is very malformed or macerated, it may help to wrap him up first before showing him to the parents. Even so, a few parents will not be able to cope with seeing and holding their baby at the time of delivery. Permission to take a photograph should always be sought; this should be a sympathetic view and not a clinical record. This can be kept in the medical notes for possible use later if necessary. Further opportunities for seeing the baby should be offered to parents over the next few days, as they often change their minds. Photographs, hand and footprints, and other mementoes of the baby are in fact very important, as they provide tangible evidence of the reality of the baby's existence and of his loss. They should be stored in the medical records but be available for parents as keepsakes, if they wish.

If a baby dies in labour, it is good practice to inform the consultant in charge immediately (or very soon if it is the middle of the night). The fact that a senior member of staff has come promptly to try to help the parents from his own experience is nearly always deeply appreciated by parents, and can soften any resentful feelings the couple may have towards the hospital staff. The general practitioner or a senior member of the practice staff should also be telephoned before the mother goes home.

Neonatal death

When the baby lives long enough to be transferred to an intensive care unit, it is again very important that the staff make time to keep parents as fully informed as possible about the baby's condition and encourage them to share in any possible part of the care. Photographs of the baby are very helpful, particularly for the fathers to keep at home, or if the mother is too unwell to visit the unit. In a randomised trial of the use of routine Polaroid photographs of sick babies in the first week of life (Pareira et al 1980), there was a significant increase in visiting by the parents of photographed babies compared with the non-photographed group. When the baby's condition is known to be terminal, it is important to try to involve the parents in the decision to cease life support and then to let them nurse their dying baby in their arms, if possible free from all the equipment that has been necessary until then. Guilt for removing the baby from the life support system has not been reported.

Many parents like to help with the laying-out of the baby's body and this should be encouraged. They often select special clothes or toys to be placed in the coffin with the baby. Some parents will want to involve their other children in this, and they should be supported in doing so, as children seem to cope better when they are included (Black & Urbanowicz 1985).

Enabling the family's contact with the reality of the death of their baby in these ways facilitates their grief reactions. They also need time and privacy to express their grief and this should be provided, however busy the unit.

Aftercare

The choice of site of the aftercare of the mother is important as mothers differ in their requirements at this time. Most want to be on their own, far away from the sound of babies crying; others long to return to familiar faces on the ward, particularly if they have been inpatients before delivery. It is helpful if care can be as flexible as possible in this respect. The mother will also need her partner to remain with her for the first night at least. Ideally, the hospital should provide a couch in her room so that the couple can share their grief together. Help with the suppression of lactation has already been mentioned as an important issue for the mother whose baby has died. If the mother is physically fit to return home immediately and wishes to do so, it is essential to ensure that she has a good supportive network of family, friends and professionals before letting her go; if she is unsupported an extra day or two with sympathetic support in hospital may be preferable.

The autopsy

Consent for autopsy should always be requested after a perinatal death, as it may provide invaluable information about the cause of death and help parents not only with their grief but also assist in the planning of future pregnancies. Most parents do consent although the decision is often painful. As one mother put it: 'She's been through enough; must she be cut up now as well?'. Anxieties may well occur because of media publicity about organs retained for study without parents' knowledge. There are, however, a small number of parents whose religion forbids autopsy and their dilemma needs to be acknowledged to avoid a situation in which they are subjected to inappropriate pressure to consent.

Having consented, parents cherish great hopes that the findings will answer their questions about why their baby died. It is therefore very important for them to receive the results in a form that makes sense to them. The best person to do this is a senior member of staff who can interpret the pathologist's findings. This can be done as part of the follow-up interview for it often takes time to get the full report from the pathology department. Provision of a photocopy of the report is often valued by the parents, provided it is properly explained.

Registration and funeral arrangements

Fundamental to good care is knowledge not only of the bereavement process but also of the legal procedures required when a baby dies or is stillborn. It is also necessary to be familiar with the registration and funeral arrangements in one's own unit or locality. Religious practices vary greatly, and an awareness of these and sensitivity to parents' wishes is crucial. A funeral may involve considerable expense: assisting parents in making difficult choices, helping those in financial straits and encouraging them to attend the funeral are therapeutic aspects of care. The unit should ensure that a suitable individual is available for this task.

Many units have prepared leaflets and videos outlining their own procedures and providing helpful advice on various aspects of losing a baby; these can be very helpful for parents.

Communication

Good care hinges around good communication and parents often comment on communication failures in describing their experiences. Specialist interpreters may be needed to assist with this, and should be available. Staff need to give bereaved parents opportunities for talking together about the loss of their baby and listen sympathetically to their expressions of grief. It is much harder to listen than talk oneself. In addition, staff need to try to help parents in their search for a cause of death; senior obstetric or paediatric staff need to discuss this with the parents. Seeing both parents together not only helps to strengthen their relationship as they share the experience of their baby's loss, but also helps to prevent misunderstandings or inconsistencies in explanation. Arranging for the same members of staff to meet regularly with the parents also helps.

Any information given in the first few days of the loss will probably have to be repeated later as the initial shock of bereavement passes. A follow-up interview a few weeks later seems to be the best way of overcoming this difficulty. Good communication between staff about the loss of the baby is also vital to prevent painful situations, such as an individual being unaware that a baby has died and breezily asking the mother when she is to be delivered. Some known and agreed sticker on the front of the hospital records can prevent this. Communication between hospital and primary health care teams also needs to be good. The primary care team and community midwife should be informed immediately about the baby's loss so that they can contact the family as soon as, or even before, the mother is discharged from hospital. Parents may want the support of their own religious adviser; the hospital needs to check on this and contact the person concerned.

The next pregnancy

The timing of the next pregnancy is important, as has already been discussed, to allow for the dead baby to be mourned first. Our study (Forrest et al 1982) found that pregnancy occurring less than six months after the loss was strongly associated with high depression and anxiety scores at the 14 months' assessment. However, the enormous individual variation in bereavement response means that it is inappropriate to recommend a fixed time interval, and Boyle (1997) found no association between timing of the next pregnancy and mental state. The best advice appears to be to wait a while until the parents have had a chance to say goodbye to the dead baby and until the mother feels emotionally as well as physically strong enough to cope with another pregnancy. The next pregnancy will inevitably be an extremely anxious time and she will need extra support during it and in the first few months after delivery. In terms of minimising complications, a 2-year interval between pregnancies has been found to give the lowest morbidity in the next pregnancy, although older women in particular may not wish to wait this long.

Follow-up

Most mothers will be discharged home within a few days of their baby's death, still too shocked to grasp properly what has happened or why. Careful follow-up is extremely important. Parents should be able to contact by telephone the staff who cared for them after they leave the hospital; some units offer home visits by a worker associated with the delivery team. An appointment should be made for both parents to see the consultant or a senior member of staff about 3–6 weeks later, as soon as the chromosomes and autopsy results are available and some form of perinatal mortality conference has taken place, to cover the following points:

1. to give the parents the opportunity of going over the events involved in the loss of their baby and releasing emotion
2. to allow clarification of why the baby died, if at all possible; the autopsy results should be given to parents in an appropriate form
3. to give obstetric counselling and, in particular, advise about the timing of future pregnancies
4. to make any necessary arrangements for genetic counselling.

Although returning to the maternity unit for these appointments is usually a harrowing prospect for parents, they almost always find it helpful. Perhaps this is because they have moved a step further in their grief by once again facing the painful memories.

Checklists

Some units find it useful to have checklists to ensure that all practical aspects of care have been covered (White et al 1984). Although they can be helpful as *aide-mémoires*, checklists should not replace personal, compassionate contact with bereaved parents.

Care of the family at home

The general practitioner (GP), health visitor and other primary health care workers form the professional supportive network for the family once the mother has been discharged home. These professionals can help by continuing to express concern, informing parents about the symptoms of bereavement and putting them in touch with any local support groups for parents who have lost a child (see Useful Addresses at the end of the chapter). The GP can watch for signs of a pathological grief reaction and refer for specialist help if necessary. These reactions are most likely to take the form of unremitting symptoms of depression, severe anxiety or the appearance of psychosomatic illness. There may also be drug or alcohol abuse.

Anger is another feature of grief reactions and the GP may need to deal with anger focused on the maternity unit. To do so, he needs to have good relationships with the obstetric and paediatric staff and to be fully informed about the course of events that preceded the baby's loss. The parents may also blame the GP, of course. When this happens, it is essential for him to meet the family as soon as possible so that they can air their feelings, and, it is to be hoped, re-establish their relationship. Many parents remain angry simply because they were denied any compassionate response to their situation; no one on the staff said: 'I'm so sorry your baby has died'.

The GP or health visitor will probably be the person the family turn to for help with the reactions of their other children to the baby's death. Parents may need help in allowing their children to vent their feelings about such a painful subject and it must be remembered that young children will use play as a vehicle for expressing their feelings and confusion. Explaining death to children under 5 is also difficult because developmentally they are not yet able to understand the finality of it (Lansdown & Benjamin 1985). Even very simple statements such as 'The baby's gone' or 'We've lost the baby' will be interpreted literally and lead to questions about where to find him, or when a visit can be made. The parents will need to provide more information as the child's capacity for understanding develops.

THE ROLE OF SPECIALIST COUNSELLORS

So far, this chapter has concentrated on the management of normal grief and the prevention of abnormal reactions through the care of the ordinary staff of maternity units and primary health care teams. There is no evidence as yet that the provision of routine bereavement counselling after the loss of a baby is effective (Chambers & Chan 1999). However, about one in six families will show pathological reactions, and all of these are likely to be accompanied by family relationship problems. In such cases, the help of specialist counsellors trained in grief work will be needed to advise on management or to take over the case if necessary. The treatment required is often lengthy; antidepressant drugs and psychiatric surveillance may be necessary for severe depressive symptoms. Child and family psychiatrists may be particularly helpful in dealing with family relationship problems. Specialist counsellors can help to promote normal grieving in parents who are most at risk of pathological reactions, and can also be useful in supporting the staff of the unit through regular staff meetings, case discussions, training sessions and offering advice to self-help groups.

SELF-HELP GROUPS

Self-help can be very effective in providing appropriate support for parents facing many different problems and perinatal bereavement is no exception. In the UK, several national organisations exist (e.g. the Stillbirth and Neonatal Death Society, SANDS, and the Miscarriage Association) and there are often locally based groups as well. SANDS has played a major part in changing attitudes and practices in hospitals and in the community through the production of guidelines for care (Stillbirth and Neonatal Death Society 1995) and has campaigned for the reform of hospital funeral arrangements and registration anomalies. Its support groups are to be found in most parts of the UK. Parents can benefit from sharing their experiences together, discovering that they are not alone in their suffering and that time helps to heal their wounds. However, not everyone can cope with group support and it is not wise to rely entirely on local self-help groups to meet all the needs of bereaved families. While it is invaluable to give parents the telephone number or address of a local contact, this should not replace follow-up by the hospital and general practitioner.

TRAINING

The training of staff in the care of families who have lost their baby or who are faced with the birth of a malformed or handicapped baby deserves as much emphasis as the development of their technical expertise. We have lost our familiarity with death and bereavement at a personal level, and staff need to be informed about the process of mourning as well as being trained in the basic skills of interviewing and counselling. They also need to explore their own feelings about death if they are to understand and help others. A good training programme should therefore combine formal with informal teaching, such as the use of group discussions, videotapes and role-play. In addition, junior staff should be present when senior staff see the parents, even from the first vital visit. They can learn a great deal from watching and listening while more experienced members of staff handle difficult and painful situations.

CONCLUSIONS

Good care does not end with a baby's death; much can be done to help the family cope with their loss and facilitate recovery from bereavement. In this chapter, an attempt has been made to describe parental grief reactions and set out guidelines for care, but successful implementation depends on the attitudes of individual staff members and the importance attached to training in this area.

Effective care has implications for both maternity unit staff and professionals working in the community. Time needs to be spent with parents whose baby dies or is malformed, listening as well as talking. Attention also has to be paid to the details of follow-up in individual cases. The unit may have to review its procedures for postnatal care in order to be able to offer more flexibility; senior members of staff need to play a central role in caring for the parents, sharing their own experience and expertise with junior staff. Attention must be given to the practical aspects of the registration and funeral arrangements for babies and the primary health care team should monitor the bereavement process. Such changes in care improve rapport with grieving families; staff cope better with the painfulness of perinatal death because they feel able to help. Finally, families on the whole emerge from their grief able to continue functioning well, with positive attitudes towards the professionals who shared in the loss of their baby.

USEFUL ADDRESSES

- Miscarriage Association, c/o Clayton Hospital, Northgate, Wakefield, West Yorkshire WF1 3JS. Tel: 01924 200799.
- Stillbirth and Neonatal Death Society (SANDS), 28 Portland Place, London W1 3DE. Tel: 0207 436 5881.
- Twins and Multiple Births Association (TAMBA), Harnott House, 309, Chester Road, Little Sutton, Ellesmere Port CH66 1QQ.

KEY POINTS

1. Perinatal death is accompanied by high levels of psychological distress.
2. This improves over the first year for the majority of parents who have received good care.
3. About one in six mothers has long-term psychological difficulties. Vulnerability factors include lack of a supportive network and adverse socioeconomic circumstances.
4. Good care involves:
   - openness
   - acknowledging parents' grief
   - giving parents information
   - helping them create memories of their baby
   - offering them choices wherever possible
   - involving the family as far as possible
   - helping with registration and funeral arrangements
   - ensuring good communication between professionals
   - carefully planning follow-up
   - arranging special support for vulnerable mothers
   - providing training for staff.

REFERENCES

Black D, Urbanowicz A 1985 Bereaved children—family intervention. In: Stevenson J E (ed) Recent research in developmental psychopathology. Pergamon, Oxford

Bourne S, Lewis E 1984 Pregnancy after stillbirth or neonatal death. Lancet ii:31–33

Bowlby J 1979 Attachment and loss, vol 3. Hogarth, London

Boyle FM 1997 Mothers bereaved by stillbirth, neonatal death or sudden infant death syndrome. Ashgate, Sydney

Bryan EM 1999 The death of a twin. Palliat Med 9(3):187–192

Chambers HM, Chan FY 1999 Support for women/families after perinatal death (Cochrane Review). In: The Cochrane Library, Issue 4. Update Software, Oxford

Dyregrov A 1991 Grief in children: a handbook for adults. Jessica Kingsley, London

Fetus and Newborn Committee, Canadian Pediatric Society 1983 Support for parents experiencing perinatal loss. CMAJ 129:335–339

Forrest GC 1989 Care of the bereaved. In: Chalmers I, Enkin MW, Keirse MJ (eds) Effective care in pregnancy and childbirth. Oxford University Press, Oxford

Forrest GC, Claridge RS, Baum JD 1981 The practical management of perinatal death. BMJ 282:31–33

Forrest GC, Standish E, Baum JD 1982 Support after perinatal death: a study of support and counselling after perinatal bereavement. BMJ 285:1475–1479

Fox R, Pillai M, Porter H, Gill G 1997 The management of late fetal death: a guide to comprehensive care. Br J Obstet Gynaecol 104:4–10

Giles P 1970 Reactions of women to perinatal death. Aust N Z J Obstet Gynaecol 10:207–210

Kowalski K 1980 Managing perinatal loss. Clin Obstet Gynaecol 23:1113–1123

Lansdown R, Benjamin G 1985 The development of the concept of death in children aged 5–9 years. Child Care Health Dev 11:13–20

Lewis E 1979 Inhibition of mourning by pregnancy: psychopathology and management. BMJ 11:27–28

Lewis E 1983 Stillbirth: psychological consequences and strategies of management. Milunsky A, Friedman EA, Gluck L (eds) Advances in perinatal medicine, vol 3. Plenum, New York

Lilford RJ, Stratton P, Godsil S, Prasad A 1994 A randomised trial of routine versus selective counselling in perinatal bereavement from congenital disease. Br J Obstet Gynaecol 101:291–296

Lloyd J, Laurence KM 1985 Sequelae and support after termination of pregnancy for fetal malformation. BMJ 290:907–909

Meyer R, Lewis E 1979 Impact of stillbirth on a marriage. Journal of Family Therapy 1: 361

Newton RW, Bergin R, Knowles D 1986 Parents interviewed after their child's death. Arch Dis Child 61:711–715

Nicol MT, Tompkins JR, Campbell NA, Syme GJ 1986 Maternal grieving response after perinatal death. Med J Aust 144:287–289

Oakley A, McPherson A, Roberts H 1984 Miscarriages. Fontana, London

Pareira GR, Talbot YR, Boatwell WR, Parina PA, Musholt KS 1980 Photographs of sick neonates prior to transport; the effect on parental visiting pattern. Pediatr Res 14:2662–2673

Parkes CM, Markus A 1998 Coping with loss. BMJ Books, London

Raphael B 1977 Preventive intervention with the recently bereaved. Arch Gen Psychiatry 34:1450–1454

Royal College of Obstetricians and Gynaecologists 1985 Report of the RCOG working party on the management of perinatal deaths. RCOG, London

Schleiffer SJ, Keller SE, Camerino M et al 1983 Suppression of lymphocyte stimulation following bereavement. JAMA 250:374–377

Stillbirth and Neonatal Death Society 1995 Pregnancy loss and the death of a baby. Guidelines for professionals. SANDS, London

Van Eerdewegh MM, Clayton P, Van Eerdewegh P 1985 The bereaved child; variables influencing early psychopathology. Br J Psychiatry 147:188–194

White MP, Reynolds B, Evans TJ 1984 Handling of death in special care nurseries and parental grief. BMJ 289:167–169

Zeanah CH 1989 Adaptation following perinatal loss: a critical review. J Am Acad Child Adolesc Psychiatry 28:467–480

45

Obstetrical responsibility for abnormal fetal outcome

Fiona J. Stanley, Eve M. Blair

INTRODUCTION

The responsibility of the obstetric caregiver is to optimise obstetric outcome for both mother and child. This is achieved by predicting or recognising problems and suggesting or implementing prophylactic or remedial strategies. This is only possible however, if the problems, and the factors predicting problems, are recognisable and effective management strategies exist. Obstetric caregivers cannot take sole responsibility for all poor obstetric outcome as they cannot predict every problem, nor, when problems arise, can they always be put right (especially those initiated preconceptionally or early in pregnancy).

PRECONCEPTIONAL CARE

While many preconceptional factors are known to be associated with fetal outcome, obstetric caregivers have little control over the conditions under which reproduction occurs. The profession sometimes attributes falling stillbirth rates and some part of the falling neonatal mortality in developed countries to coincident changes in obstetric care, such as the increasing use of caesarean section (Fig. 45.1) or electronic fetal monitoring. However, changes in other factors are likely to have played a more important role. The increasing variety, availability and acceptability of methods of contraception makes planned parenthood easier, which together with improved general health has helped parents produce children under optimal circumstances. Adverse circumstances include giving birth too young or too old, (the latter can be due to

impaired fertility), poor health or social circumstances, inadequate diet, conceiving while suceptable to rubella or conceiving despite known genetic diseases. Obstetric caregivers have a responsibility to create and use opportunities to provide accurate and timely preconceptional advice concerning the likely pregnancy outcomes for particular couples. This enables prospective parents to make responsible and informed decisions about the appropriateness of conception. Notwithstanding the heroic efforts of the disability lobby which laudably seeks to improve a quality of life once a suboptimal outcome has occurred, the hope of every prospective parent is to deliver a living, healthy and happy child who will

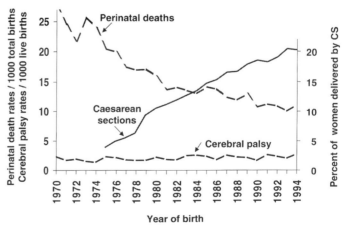

Fig. 45.1 Trends in cerebral palsy, perinatal death and caesarean section rates in Western Australia by year of birth.

709

Table 45.1 Realistic expectations of abnormal obstetric outcomes

Of recognised conceptions:
Miscarriage: 12–18% (varies with means of recognising conception)
Terminations (including ectopic pregnancies): variable (23% USA)
Sum ~33%

Of births (pregnancies lasting longer than 20 weeks' amenorrhoea):[a]
Stillbirth: 0.76%
Neonatal death: 0.48%
Postneonatal death: 0.30%
All infant deaths: 1.54%
Very preterm birth (<32 weeks): 1.57%
Moderately preterm birth (32–36 weeks): 6.65%
All preterm birth: 8.22%
Birth defect: 5%
Cerebral palsy by age 5: 0.2%
Intellectual disability by age 6: 0.8%
School failure: 6% (Zubrick et al 1997)
Mental health problem: 18% (Zubrick et al 1995)

[a]Different categories of abnormal outcome are not all mutually exclusive and are often associated, particularly with very preterm birth.

achieve independence as an adult. It is irresponsible both to prospective parents and to society to encourage inappropriate childbearing by reassurance that reproductive deficits can be overcome with medical assistance. Even with the best medical care, normal outcome cannot be guaranteed as many deaths and disabilities are not avoidable by obstetric care. Table 45.1 shows the proportions of several abnormal outcomes experienced in the developed world with modern medical services.

We can only estimate miscarriage rates when early pregnancy loss can be recognised reliably and recorded on a population basis. Despite this apparent difficulty, the estimated proportions of pregnancies lost before 20 weeks are remarkably constant. During the 1980s in the USA an estimated 35% of recognised conceptions did not reach 20 weeks (Saraiya et al 1999) while in a small study of couples trying to conceive (i.e. no elective terminations of pregnancy), pregnancy loss was estimated at 31.3% (Zinaman et al 1996). Of Western Australian pregnancies surviving to 20 weeks, 1.5% will die before their first birthday, 8% will be delivered before they reach 37 weeks' gestation, and 5% will have a significant birth defect. Of postneonatal survivors, 0.2% (1 in 500) will have cerebral palsy and 0.8% (1 in 125) an intellectual disability. School failure and mental health problems are increasingly being associated with obstetric problems such as low birthweight, very preterm birth and poor intrauterine growth (Whitaker et al 1997, Zubrick et al 2000).

Preconceptional advice is therefore the first responsibility of the obstetric caregiver and is already established as a desirable component of antenatal care (see Ch. 8). However, while preconceptional care is highly desirable, the obstetric caregiver is likely to meet the majority of women only once they have already conceived.

PERINATAL MORTALITY AND PRETERM BIRTH

For gestational durations up to term, perinatal mortality falls as gestation increases (Table 45.2). In term infants in developed countries it is now very low. Despite a generally decreasing perinatal mortality rate in developed countries, very preterm delivery rates have not decreased and may even have increased (Stanley et al 2000). An exception has been reported from France where observed decreases have been attributed to a programme of social interventions (Papiernik 1993). The French interventions have been applied to whole communities, but their results have not been duplicated in randomised trials in other communities (Hodnett 1998). The difficult task of replicating the same social interventions in different communities has not been attempted. It may be that social changes introduced in France have contained effective elements lacking in trials conducted elsewhere. If this is the case, the nature of these elements is not well understood, and manipulation of the social and working conditions of pregnant women may be considered a political rather than an obstetric responsibility.

Reducing the incidence of very preterm delivery should not be considered an end in itself, as it would not necessarily improve fetal outcome. Indeed, some part of the increase in very preterm delivery is iatrogenic. There is a willingness to induce labour and delivery increasingly early in the face of intractable fetal or maternal problems, encouraged by the survival of increasingly immature infants due to the increasing sophistication of neonatal intensive care. The feasibility of earlier delivery to reduce the extent of fetal compromise when intrauterine conditions are unfavourable is likely to be responsible for at least some part of the observed gestation-specific decrease in perinatal mortality. Very preterm delivery may not always therefore be a causal factor in an abnormal outcome; it may be an epiphenomenon of the true cause of an abnormal outcome, such as a co-fetal death (Ch. 15) or severe antepartum haemorrhage (Ch. 14), or it may be a means (natural or medically induced) of optimising outcome given certain conditions, such as severe preeclampsia (Ch. 21), intrauterine infection (Ch. 22) or multiple pregnancy (Ch. 15).

Delivery after more than 42 completed postmenstrual weeks has been reported to occur spontaneously in about 5–15% of births (see Ch. 32), and in the 1980 Western Australian birth cohort was reported in 8% of all births.

Table 45.2 Stillbirth and neonatal mortality rates by gestation of delivery: Western Australia 1980–1993

Gestation of delivery (weeks)	Stillbirth/1000 births	Neonatal mortality/1000 live births
22–27	342 (688/2012)	452 (598/1324)
28–31	125 (349/2785)	64 (156/2436)
32–36	23 (509/22022)	12 (257/21513)
37–41	2.1 (614/288959)	1.7 (502/288345)
>41	2.6 (47/17859)	2.4 (43/17812)

Inaccurate gestational dating and pre-ovulatory periods of greater than 14 days mean that the proportion of post-dates pregnancies overestimates the proportion of prolonged pregnancies (Boyd et al 1988), but pregnancies classified as post dates are at somewhat higher risk of stillbirth and neonatal death (Sims Walther 1989) and Table 45.2. This knowledge is no doubt responsible for inductions reducing the occurrence of post-term deliveries in developed countries. For example, in Western Australia the proportion delivered after more than 42 weeks decreased from 8% in 1980 to 2.9% in 1995. Birth after 41 weeks' gestation is associated with an increased risk of poor perinatal outcome, and therefore appropriate induction of labour may reduce perinatal mortality and poor long-term outcome.

The distribution of apparent causes of all stillbirths and neonatal deaths in infants, born in Western Australia in 1980–1993 is shown in Tables 45.3 and 45.4, separately for births at or before 32 weeks and for births after 32 weeks. It can be seen that the largest groups of stillbirths were unexplained, that is, no sufficient cause of death was recognised. Very few pregnancies in this group had *any* recognised antecedent pathology. Since this is a population-based data set, one must assume that most of the pathologies responsible for these stillbirths were not recognisable

with standard obstetric practice in a developed country and thus are not currently amenable to obstetric care. More than one-third of all neonatal deaths were the result of gross immaturity and, as indicated above, very preterm birth is proving refractory to obstetric intervention. About 60% of neonatal deaths after 32 weeks were attributed to birth defects. The deaths most likely to be amenable to obstetric care are those occurring in the intrapartum period, representing 8.8% of all perinatal deaths: 6.6% (n = 129) of perinatal deaths at or before 32 weeks' gestation and 11.2% (n = 221) of perinatal deaths after 32 weeks' gestation. To this number should be added the 21 deaths occurring more than 28 days after delivery that were attributed to the late effects of intrapartum asphyxia. Table 45.5 subcategorises the causes of death attributed to intrapartum events. In almost half of the intrapartum asphyxial deaths there was no satisfactory explanation for the asphyxia; these may have represented antenatally compromised infants. A further third were born before 26 completed weeks' gestation and their deaths were attributed to an inability to withstand the stresses of delivery as a direct result of immaturity. The intrapartum asphyxial deaths preceded by recognised factors were responsible for much smaller proportions than were attributed to them at the beginning of the twentieth century: for example, Cosbie attributed 41% of perinatal deaths in a Canadian Hospital in 1921 to complications of delivery such as malpresentations (Cosbie 1992). This at least suggests that obstetric procedures to prevent birth asphyxia have improved over the last 75 years. However, there is no valid epidemiological evidence which demonstrates an association between quality of obstetric care and overall perinatal death rates, not least on account of the difficulty of retrospectively assessing quality of care. Using case–control methodologies,

Table 45.3 Causes of stillbirth of ≥400 g birthweight by gestation at delivery: Western Australia 1980–1993

Apparent	Gestation at delivery			
	≤32 weeks		>32 weeks	
	n	%	n	%
Unexplained	467	43.5	666	63.0
Birth defect	187	17.4	129	12.2
Intrapartum	120	11.1	113	10.7
Chorio-amnionitis	50	4.7	6	0.6
Other infection	25	2.3	11	1.0
Major antepartum haemorrhage	96	8.9	55	5.2
Other and unknown	129	12.0	79	7.5
Total	1074	100	1059	100

Table 45.4 Causes of neonatal death of ≥400 g birthweight by gestation at delivery: Western Australia 1980–1993

Apparent cause	Gestation at delivery			
	≤32 weeks		>32 weeks	
	n	%	n	%
Birth defect	125	15.9	462	60.9
Immaturity	538	64.2	17	2.2
Intrapartum	6	0.7	90	11.9
Chorio-amnionitis	104	12.4	3	0.4
Other infection	13	1.6	44	5.8
Major antepartum haemorrhage	13	1.6	22	2.9
Other and unknown	39	4.6	121	15.9
Total	838	100	759	100

Table 45.5 Subcategories of intrapartum causes of perinatal death

	Gestation at delivery in weeks			
	≤32	>32		
Description	n	n	Total n	%
None of the descriptions below	17	148	165	47.1
Death in labour of normally formed non-infected fetus of <26 weeks' gestation	105	0	105	30.0
Intrapartum death following sentinel event[a]	0	14	14	4.0
Obstructed labour	2	28	30	8.6
Cord prolapse @ >32 weeks	0	24	24	6.9
Intrapartum complications of twin delivery	2	2	4	1.1
Unattended birth	3	5	8	2.3
Total	129	221	350[b]	100

[a]A sentinel event is a pathological hypoxic event likely to overcome the protective mechanisms of a normal, healthy fetus, such as a ruptured uterus, placental abruption, amniotic fluid embolism or fetal exsanguination (MacLennan and International Cerebral Palsy Task Force 1999).
[b]Includes those attributed to interapartum events who died more than 28 days after delivery.

Niswander et al 1984) considered the effect of quality of pregnancy care on 53 antepartum stillbirths, and both Niswander et al (1984) and Gaffney et al (1994) considered the effect of intrapartum care on, respectively, 5 intrapartum stillbirths and 62 intrapartum and neonatal deaths that had been attributed to asphyxia. Both studies found increased risks of death associated with obstetric failure to respond appropriately to signs of fetal distress. In both studies controls were randomly selected and therefore had a much lower frequency of signs of fetal distress, but those without signs of fetal distress were included in the group classified as receiving appropriate management of their 'fetal distress', considerably inflating the relative risk (Blair 1994). Nonetheless, both studies demonstrated that the majority of supposedly asphyxial deaths had received care classified as appropriate, and most babies receiving inappropriate care had a normal outcome. Intrapartum asphyxial death can follow an appropriate obstetric response to signs of fetal distress if the first signs of fetal compromise are recognised too late for intervention to be effective, or if the intrapartum clinical signs taken to infer current asphyxia are in fact the first signs of pre-existing damage (Blair 1993). Both these studies also considered cerebral palsy as an outcome and the same criticisms apply to their estimates of the proportion of this outcome attributable to suboptimal obstetric care.

BIRTH DEFECTS

While birth defects are responsible for a very significant proportion of perinatal deaths (24% in the Western Australian 1980–1993 cohort) the majority of children with birth defects survive. Few obstetric interventions would make a difference to the outcome of children with birth defects other than those preventing their conception or birth, i.e. preconceptional genetic counselling (Ch. 8) or early detection and termination of affected fetuses (Ch. 12). Caesarean section before the onset of labour may improve the motor outcome of children with meningomyelocele without severe hydrocephalus or chromosomal anomaly (Luthy et al 1991) but fetal surgery to improve outcome is still at the experimental stage (Simpson 1999).

INTELLECTUAL IMPAIRMENT

There are many possible causes of intellectual impairment. For one-third of Western Australian children with intellectual impairment born in 1967–1976 the aetiology was unknown (Wellesley et al 1991) and the next largest aetiological category was Down's syndrome accounting for a further 14%. The main cause of intellectual impairment for which there is most often considered to be an obstetric responsibility is cerebral palsy.

CEREBRAL PALSY

Cerebral palsy is defined as 'an umbrella term covering a group of non-progressive, but often changing, motor impairment syndromes secondary to lesions or anomalies of the brain arising in the early stages of development' (Mutch et al 1992). These motor impairments are frequently accompanied by intellectual impairments and epilepsy and less frequently by visual and auditory impairments. This definition suggests that there are several aetiological routes to cerebral palsy despite the opinion, popular for much of the twentieth century, that it is primarily the result of birth asphyxia and hence, potentially an obstetric responsibility. Such an opinion sits uneasily with the stable frequency of cerebral palsy over a period of considerable change in obstetric practice (Fig. 45.1) (Stanley et al 2000, Ch. 4). However, as an infant needs to survive the neonatal period to be described as having cerebral palsy, the stable rate of cerebral palsy could reflect a balance between a decreasing perinatal death rate (which may contribute to the number of brain-damaged survivors) and an increasing rate of rescuing survivors from brain damage. The origin of the belief that cerebral palsy was primarily an intrapartum disease has been attributed to a presentation to the Obstetrical Society in London in 1862 by WJ Little, an orthopaedic surgeon, with the title *On the incidence of the abnormal parturition, difficult labour, premature birth and asphyxia neonatorum on the mental and physical condition of the child, especially in relation to deformities* (Little 1958). It was a remarkable paper, discussed further below, which demonstrated an appreciation both that the causes of cerebral palsy could be multifactorial and consist of pathways in which intrapartum events are only the final straw, and that intrapartum events were only one among several possible causes. Unfortunately the paper was very long and perhaps too many drew their conclusions from the title only. However, much recent research is now confirming that cerebral palsy is aetiologically a very heterogeneous condition and that each pathway may involve many factors (Stanley et al 2000).

Cerebral palsy and preconceptional factors

Monogenetic patterns of occurrence of cerebral palsy are rare except in inbred communities, particularly those cultural groups in which consanguinity is common. However, familial recurrence of cerebral palsy, which occurs somewhat more frequently than would be expected by chance, may also result from common or continuing environmental challenges. These are not well understood but there is a general association with several causes of suboptimal maternal health such as pre-existing hypertension, thrombotic disorders and abnormal thyroid or reproductive function. Chronic problems such as these may result in more than one affected child or an increase of other poor obstetric outcomes. There is agreement that the risk of cerebral palsy increases with increasing maternal age, with socioeconomic disadvantage and with poor maternal obstetric history. In the past, and currently in developing countries, maternal rhesus incompatibility (and subsequent kernicterus in the offspring) was the principal risk factor for choreoathetosis. Choreoathetosis has virtually disappeared where appropriate obstetric management with anti-D vaccination is widely used. It is now considered likely that genetically determined vulnerabilities to antenatal, intrapartum or even postnatal factors (Morton et al 1991) play a larger role than hitherto suspected.

Cerebral palsy and pregnancy factors

The importance of early pregnancy factors is suggested by a consistent association of cerebral palsy with congenital malformations both of the central nervous system and of other structures. Congenital malformations were reported in almost 30% of people with moderate and severe cerebral palsy in a population-based series (Palmer et al 1995) but even this may be an underestimate as more subtle cerebral anomalies such as neuronal migration disorders are difficult to detect neurones migrate as an essential part of normal development but occasionally stop at an inappropriate final destination. The origin of the malformations is often unknown, but toxic exposures, such as carbon monoxide, methyl mercury or excessive alcohol, and infectious exposures, particularly toxoplasmosis, rubella and cytomegalovirus, are recognised risk factors for cerebral palsy. The most common cause of cerebral palsy world-wide is severe iodine deficiency (Hetzel & Pandav 1996); these cases should be simply and cheaply preventable.

Cerebral palsy and very preterm birth

The risk of cerebral palsy increases with earlier gestation at delivery, being greatest before 30 weeks of gestation when it is up to 30 times that of full-term infants (Kuban & Leviton 1994). While it is important to remember that two-thirds of cases of cerebral palsy continue to be born at term, because most births occur at term, very preterm births are now making a significant contribution to rates of cerebral palsy (Fig. 45.2). The increased rates of cerebral palsy observed in the 1980s coincided with a marked reduction in neonatal mortality attributed to advances in neonatal care.

Figure 45.3 shows three possible causal pathways that can be constructed that include very preterm birth (VPTB) and cerebral palsy. Path A shows antenatal factor(s) (X), such as placental abruption, ascending intrauterine infection

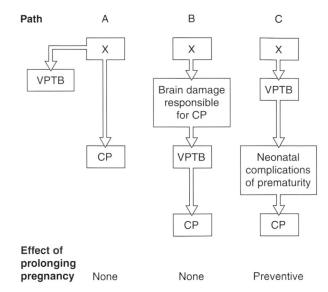

Fig. 45.3 Pathways from antenatal events (X) to cerebral palsy (CP) which include very preterm birth (VPTB).

or a co-fetal death, causing both cerebral palsy and very preterm birth independently. The latter would then be an epiphenomenon, i.e. the very preterm birth does not itself cause the cerebral damage. Path B shows early damage to the cerebral motor cortex triggering early delivery, a possibility suggested by the increased rate of miscarriage of abnormal embryos and fetuses with chromosomal anomalies. In neither of these cases would the cerebral palsy be prevented simply by extending the duration of pregnancy. Path C, on the other hand, illustrates the vulnerability of the very preterm neonate to cerebral haemorrhage or to infarcts, sometimes exacerbated by extrinsic factors, such as hypothermia or birth at some distance from a neonatal intensive care unit. Extrauterine exposures associated with cerebral haemorrhage or infarcts include hypoxia/acidosis, hypoglycaemia, hypothyroxinaemia, sepsis, cerebral blood flow disturbance or circulatory problems. In this case the very preterm birth is a necessary step on the causal pathway that exposes the (antenatally undamaged) very preterm infant to the hazards of extrauterine life. In this case delaying the birth would prevent the cerebral palsy.

Antecedents of very preterm birth include social factors, multiple pregnancy, antepartum haemorrhage, preterm onset of uterine contractions, preterm rupture of membranes, maternal disease (particularly preeclampsia) and fetal conditions such as intrauterine growth restriction, restricted placental blood supply or cardiotocographic changes suggestive of fetal hypoxia. These antecedents are not mutually exclusive. The main distinction to be made is between causes leading to spontaneous preterm delivery (with a higher risk of cerebral palsy) and medical indications for elective very preterm delivery (with a relatively lower risk). Probably the most common reason for elective delivery is preeclampsia.

The decreased risk of cerebral palsy in very preterm births which are delivered electively relative to other very preterm births has been variously attributed to:

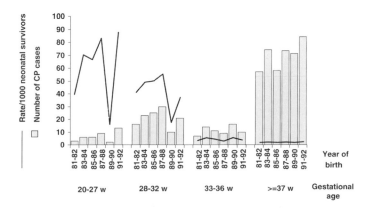

Fig. 45.2 Distribution and rates of cerebral palsy* by gestational age of delivery, Western Australia 1981–1992 (adapted from Stanley et al 2000). *Excludes cerebral palsy from postneonatal causes.

a. a protective effect of preeclampsia or therapies administered for preeclampsia (Nelson & Grether 1995)

b. the optimal conditions under which these deliveries usually occur

c. other reasons for very preterm birth being more potent causes of cerebral palsy (Blair et al 1996).

It is not usually possible to ascertain whether the increased risk of the cerebral palsy relative to term births in those very preterm births who were delivered electively is attributable to the indication for the delivery or to the increased vulnerability of the very preterm neonate. Very preterm births following placental abruptions (with their potential for haemodynamic shock) may be an example of the former and preeclampsia an example of the latter.

Chorio-amnionitis, with or without signs of infection in the mother and almost invariably without signs of fetal infection, is strongly associated with cerebral palsy in both very preterm (Redline et al 1998) and more mature infants (Grether & Nelson 1997). Biological mechanisms have been suggested for its association both with very premature delivery and with fetal neuronal damage mediated by the fetal immunological response. The responsible organisms tend to be those commonly found in vaginal flora, yet only a small proportion of pregnancies develop chorio-amnionitis with only a small proportion of these developing cerebral palsy. The initiators of these causal pathways to cerebral palsy are not known.

The fetal immunological response is immature before 24–26 weeks. If this response is the mechanism by which these infections trigger very preterm labour, the timing of delivery may be determined by the stage of fetal immune competence rather than the time of the original infection. The latter may have predated the onset of labour or even conception.

There is not yet a clear role for obstetric care in cases of spontaneous onset of very preterm labour, as inhibition of delivery when intrauterine infection is present may further compromise the fetus, and chorio-amnionitis is often difficult to detect antenatally. The infection hypothesis suggests that antimicrobial therapy might be a preventive strategy, particularly if there is a window of opportunity between the presence of infection and the fetal immunological response to it. Results of preliminary trials, however, have been equivocal. Such therapy may even be harmful in the short term and there is no evidence concerning its long-term effects on the development of the fetal immune system. In contrast, in cases where very preterm delivery is indicated but can safely be delayed sufficiently there is good evidence that antenatal administration of dexamethasone and delivery in a tertiary care centre reduces the risk of abnormal outcome (Stanley et al. 2000, Ch. 12).

Cerebral palsy and intrauterine growth restriction

Intrauterine growth restriction is also associated with cerebral palsy. The reasons for this association are unclear. The risk of cerebral palsy increases with increasing growth deficit, which suggests that the causal factor may be some aspect of the restriction itself. However, since the degree of growth deficit is determined by the cause and duration of restriction, and

hence also with the gestational age of onset, it may be that a combination of these factors determines the risk of cerebral palsy. Obstetric management consists primarily of balancing the dangers of prematurity against the dangers of leaving the fetus in a hostile environment, but there is currently little agreement or evidence on how to achieve this (Stanley et al 2000, Ch. 12). A trial is in progress to determine the optimal timing and mode of delivery of severely growth-restricted fetuses (GRIT, Study Group 1996) but, in common with other randomised trials of obstetric interventions, it will only be informative about the risks of cerebral palsy if the trial participants are followed up to an age at which cerebral palsy can reliably be recognised. Ideally they should be followed for at least three and preferably for five years.

Several workers have suggested that intrauterine growth restriction may increase fetal vulnerability to the hypoxic stress of labour. It seems plausible that an undernourished fetus with low glycogen reserves might be less able than a normal fetus to withstand the energy demands of acute hypoxic stress. However, this is not supported by the observation that markers of intrapartum hypoxia are less strongly associated with cerebral palsy in infants classified as small for gestational age than in those classified as appropriately grown (Stanley et al 2000, Ch. 8). The underlying reason for these apparent discrepancies may be that there are no reliable clinical methods of recognising or measuring intrapartum stress (Blair 1993).

Cerebral palsy and multiple pregnancy

Multiple pregnancy is associated with cerebral palsy. A twin has a 4.5-fold risk and a triplet an 18-fold risk of cerebral palsy compared with a singleton (Table 45.6). Twins tend to be born earlier in gestation and be more growth restricted

Table 45.6 Risks of cerebral palsy per multiplet (Stanley et al 2000, Ch. 10)

	Relative risk of cerebral palsy	(95% confidence interval)
Compared with singleton		
Risk per twin	4.49	(3.9–5.2)
Risk per triplet	18.21	(10.4–31.9)
Compared with singleton in the same gestational age stratum		
Risk per twin 20–28 weeks	1.94	(1.2–3.2)
Risk per twin 29–32 weeks	1.02	(0.7–1.6)
Risk per twin 33–36 weeks	2.25	(1.4–3.7)
Risk per twin 37–44 weeks	3.04	(1.9–4.9)
Compared with a singleton in the same birthweight stratum		
Risk per twin <1500 g	1.08	(0.8–1.3)
Risk per twin 1500–2499 g	0.83	(0.7–1.1)
Risk per twin ≥2500 g	2.7	1.9–3.8)
Compared with twins whose co-twins survived birth		
Twin with stillborn co-twin	11.44	(7.0–18.8)

than singletons, and since preterm delivery and growth restriction are associated with cerebral palsy, these factors alone would be expected to confer greater risk. Table 45.6 shows that very low birthweight twins and twins born at 29–32 weeks have the same increased risks as singletons of the same birthweight or gestation, though the origins of their increased risks may differ. However, the tendency to preterm delivery and growth restriction accounts only for a part of their excess risk. The majority of twins are born after 32 weeks and are of normal birthweight, and these twins have an increased risk of cerebral palsy compared to singletons in the same gestational and birthweight strata. The antenatal death of a co-twin is a strong risk factor for cerebral palsy (Table 45.6). Co-fetal death is likely to be important only in monochorionic twins, as it is twin–twin transfusion syndrome, unequal sharing of the placenta and shared intra-amniotic space (which may result in cord entanglement, with attendant intrauterine deprivation and asphyxia) and twin–twin entanglement during labour which creates most of the difficulties. However, unexpectedly, given that that these pathological mechanisms are specific to monochorionic (necessarily like-gender) twins, the rates of cerebral palsy are similar in like-gender and unlike-gender twin pairs. This may be because the higher rate of abnormal outcome anticipated in monozygotic twins manifests primarily as mortality.

Alternatively, intrapartum difficulties associated with multiple birth may have been underestimated as a cause of cerebral palsy in studies assuming that this risk affected the second-born twin exclusively. For example, 9 of 11 cases of cerebral palsy with a stillborn co-twin were born first (Stanley et al 2000, Ch. 10). Thus birth order may be determined by fetal survival relative to one's co-twin, which in turn determines cerebral palsy. While the pathological mechanisms of the enhanced risk of cerebral palsy in term and near-term twins are still unclear, it is clear that multiple pregnancies carry a higher risk of abnormal fetal outcomes and that the higher the multiplicity, the greater the risk. This underlines the need to avoid iatrogenic multiple births secondary to infertility management. In Western Australia during the 1980s, the simultaneous replacement of several zygotes after *in vitro* fertilisation contributed to rising rates of multiple pregnancy. In the early 1990s, the rate of triplet pregnancies dropped, perhaps because the growing awareness of the problems associated with multiple pregnancy led the Reproductive Technology Accreditation Committee to recommend that no more than three embryos be replaced in any one cycle (Watson et al 1996). In the UK, it is likely that the regulatory authorities will soon require that only two embryos be replaced.

Cerebral palsy and intrapartum factors

As long ago as the middle of the nineteenth century, WJ Little appreciated that intrapartum problems usually ended in death or unharmed recovery (Little 1958, p. 6) and that impaired survival of abnormal parturition was unusual (Little 1958, pp 5,6). He also noted that vaginal delivery imposed an obligatory hypoxia (Little 1958, p. 7) but the fetus during labour has a greater resistance to hypoxia than the adult (Little 1958, p. 7). Perhaps unexpectedly, he considered that

asphyxia (as denoted by cerebral oedema) was more frequently associated with poor outcome than trauma, despite trauma being considerably less avoidable then than it is today (Little 1958, pp. 8,9). He wrote that the intensity and duration of birth hypoxia could be exacerbated by an unnatural presentation (including breech), a constricted pelvis (as would have resulted from maternal ricketts in those days), instrumental deliveries, external version, premature labour, nuchal cord, cord prolapse and *suffocation from maternal secretions*.

As with perinatal death, public health measures have prevented some of these factors (e.g. ricketts) and the obstetric profession has learnt to manage most of the other factors appropriately. Where these factors remain antecedents of cerebral palsy, the association is now less likely to be causal. For example, Little considered breech *delivery* a causal antecedent in the mid-nineteenth century. While he may well have been correct, the assumption of causality was already being questioned by Freud in 1897. By 1959–1966, the association with breech delivery for births in the USA arose from breech *presentation* and not the *delivery* (Nelson & Ellenberg 1986). The remaining risk was, by the 1960s, associated with those prenatal factors which caused the baby to present by the breech and not with intrapartum factors associated with extracting an infant presenting by breech. If the increased risk did arise from breech *delivery* in Little's day, the change is likely to be the result of the greater availability of caesarean section and more refined techniques for vaginal breech delivery. Maintaining these gains remains of course an obstetric responsibility, but the likelihood of obstetric caregivers failing that responsibility must be kept in perspective. Relatively recently, epidemiological studies have attempted to ascertain cases of cerebral palsy resulting *exclusively* from intrapartum hypoxia. This was done by excluding firstly those with direct evidence of prior damage, using tools such as antenatal cerebral imaging, and then those with antecedent events likely to have caused brain damage before the onset of labour. These studies suggest that, in developed countries, only about 10% of cerebral palsy is now associated exclusively with intrapartum events (Stanley et al 2000, Ch. 9). This may still be an overestimate, however, since antenatal events are more likely to go unrecognised than intrapartum events. Nonetheless, while this is a smaller proportion than was previously attributed to intrapartum events, it is a higher proportion that is attributed to any other individual cause of cerebral palsy (Blair & Stanley 1993).

Birth asphyxia is a poorly defined term relating to a sequence of events occurring during labour and delivery, initiated by hypoxia and culminating in a long-term detrimental effect on outcome. Hypoxia is normal during vaginal delivery and, without sequelae, does not constitute birth asphyxia. Both hypoxia and adverse sequelae are necessary to the concept of asphyxia. The sequence of cellular responses to excessive hypoxia is now being elucidated as a result of investigations in animal models. These experiments indicate that either prolonged partial hypoxia or intermittent hypoxia produces a pattern of cerebral damage more similar to that seen in the child with cerebral palsy than total anoxia, which must be of at least 10–12 minutes, duration to effect lasting damage to a healthy fetus (Myers 1972). However, as Little had foreshadowed, survival reminiscent of cerebral palsy was rare, and death (primarily from the effects of hypoxia on the heart) or total recovery was the norm. This suggests that where hypoxia is a causal factor for cerebral palsy it is likely to be of long standing, perhaps preceding the onset of labour. The ready acceptance that excessive intrapartum hypoxia was the primary cause of cerebral palsy was encouraged by the strong association between cerebral palsy and signs taken to indicate intrapartum asphyxia. These signs consist of abnormal intrapartum measures collectively taken to indicate *fetal distress* (e.g. abnormalities of the fetal heart rate, metabolic acidosis), low Apgar scores, and neonatal encephalopathy. While each of these signs is strongly associated with cerebral palsy and also with experimental asphyxia, none is specific to asphyxia, still less to intrapartum asphxyia. They represent either the response to hypoxia (*fetal distress*), a compromised fetus from any cause (Apgar scores) or a baby neurologically damaged from any cause (neonatal encephalopathy). Each sign could also be the result of factors other than birth asphyxia that may have existed before the onset of labour, such as maternal infection or fetal anomalies of the central nervous system. The criteria that are currently considered most suggestive of birth asphyxia require a coincidence of both types of signs: evidence of excessive fetal hypoxia and evidence of long-lasting detrimental effects, together with an absence of prior causes of cerebral damage and preferably some evidence of a cause of excessive intrapartum hypoxia. Such causes include prolapse of the cord, intrapartum haemorrhage, obstructed labour because of multiple fetuses, malpresentation or cephalo-pelvic disproportion, uterine rupture and maternal shock such as cardiac arrest or acute hypotension (MacLennan and International Cerebral Palsy Task Force 1999).

However, even if hypoxia is not unduly excessive, it seems likely that birth asphyxia may ensue if the fetus is excessively vulnerable to damage by the hypoxia, such that it decompensates in the face of the level of hypoxia normally encountered during labour. It is not certain what factors could be responsible for excessive vulnerability, since any cause of vulnerability is also a potential cause of antepartum cerebral damage. There is no evidence to suggest such a role for preeclampsia in the absence of growth restriction, and even the evidence for growth restriction playing this role is equivocal (see above). There is also no evidence to suggest such a role for multiple pregnancy in the absence of prior haemodynamic insult or mechanical intrapartum difficulties. Placental and placental bed problems are plausible candidates. Placental structural anomalies have been associated with cerebral palsy, but not placental infarcts, and the association with placental evidence of antepartum haemorrhage is equivocal. Increased risk may only be associated with particularly severe haemorrhages, or those occurring at particular gestations. In view of these uncertainties, it is not easy to identify the vulnerable fetus with accuracy.

Recognising the vulnerable fetus

Electronic fetal monitoring (EFM) is now widely used in both the antepartum and intrapartum periods. It was assumed that EFM would allow earlier recognition of abnormal fetal heart rate patterns, enabling timely intervention to avoid birth asphyxia. Randomised trials have not supported this assumption. A systematic review of nine randomised controlled trials of routine intrapartum fetal monitoring including 58,855 pregnant women found no measurable effect on mortality or short-term morbidity, with the consistent exception of reducing the frequency of neonatal seizures: summary odds ratio 0.5 (95% confidence interval 0.3–0.8) (Thacker & Stroup 1998). Only two studies followed participants for a sufficient time to assess neurological abnormalities, and despite the reduction in rate of neonatal seizures, one study found a slight increase in the rate of cerebral palsy and the other much smaller trial of infants less than 1750 g found a considerable increase in rate of cerebral palsy (although in the monitored group the incidence of cerebral palsy correlated positively with the duration of abnormal heart rate). The increased rates of cerebral palsy in the monitored arms could not be accounted for by greater mortality in the auscultated groups. This discrepancy in results between neonatal seizures and cerebral palsy provides a lesson about drawing inferences concerning long-term outcomes from short-term outcomes and underlines the need to follow the participants of randomised controlled trials to an age at which neurological function can be properly assessed. Offsetting any benefit of EFM to the fetus, EFM was associated with a 23% (95% confidence interval 15–31%) increase in the rate of caesarean sections and other operative deliveries. The rate of operative deliveries with EFM may be somewhat reduced by adding qualitative assessment of the ST segment of the fetal electrocardiogram to the fetal heart rate data (Mistry & Neilson 1998).

It was hoped that the biophysical profile might aid the antenatal detection of the vulnerable fetus. An observational study conducted in Canada indicated a 3.5 increase in cerebral palsy in the untested group (Manning et al 1998). However, this was not a randomised trial and the results could not be duplicated in a meta-analysis of four small controlled trials which randomised a total of less than 3000 patients (Alfirevic & Neilson 1999). While no significant differences could be detected for fetal outcomes, there was a statistically significant 3–4-fold increase in induction of labour for abnormal fetal assessment in the arm in which the biophysical profile was assessed.

There is a strong belief that once the vulnerable fetus has been identified caesarean delivery can avoid cerebral palsy. Scheller & Nelson (1994) reviewed the literature and found no randomised controlled trial of caesarean section for any indication in term infants that considered cerebral palsy as an outcome, probably because it is not possible to persuade doctors to allocate randomly mode of delivery (Lumley et al 1985). Observational studies therefore provide the only evidence of effectiveness of caesarean section rendering it very difficult to draw valid conclusions. The two non-randomised, retrospective studies comparing vaginal and caesarean delivery for term breech deliveries showed no differences in cerebral palsy rates. However, as with retrospective studies for preterm infants, it is inevitable that the indications for delivering by caesarean will also be strongly associated with the outcome. Scheller & Nelson concluded that 'caesarean delivery can reduce the risk of adverse childhood neurologic outcome for those born with myelomeningocele and may reduce the rate of brachial plexus palsies and neonatal herpes and HIV infections'. However, there have not been (and are never likely to be) trials, or even retrospective studies, of caesarean delivery for indications such as dystocia, fetal distress or macrosomia. For these indications, the fact that a caesarean delivery was performed may well be retrospectively the best available indicator of the presenting condition, thus totally confounding any attempt to adjust for the presenting condition (the treatment paradox). This is likely to be the reason that case–control studies of cerebral palsy have shown no consistent or statistically significant associations with caesarean delivery for any indication.

A comparison of the frequency of neonatal intracranial injury and serious neonatal morbidity between groups of 1992–1994 Californian births, delivered during labour by different operative methods, demonstrated no significant differences between forceps, vacuum and caesarean modes of delivery (Towner et al 1999). On the assumption that caesarean delivery itself could not be responsible for either of these outcomes, these authors concluded that 'a substantial proportion of the morbidity associated with operative vaginal delivery may be due to an underlying abnormality of labor rather than to the procedure'. However, they did observe an increase in neonatal morbidity if more than one mode of delivery had been attempted. This is consistent with the observation that deliveries described as difficult or precipitous, with a second stage of greater than one hour, or with failed procedures (including repeated or prolonged use of vacuum extraction), were associated with spastic cerebral palsy in a Western Australian study. Evidence of a vacuum extraction was the most common reason for inferring birth trauma to the head, which was also associated with cerebral palsy. The statistically insignificant odds ratio estimated for birth trauma to the head (odds ratio 1.74; 95% confidence interval 0.98–3.1) could be an underestimate if cases and controls with missing data (1.86; 1.1–3.1) had in fact sustained birth trauma to the head (Blair & Stanley 1993).

Thus there is likely to be a proportion of deliveries in which recognisable signs associated with impending disaster, such as a cord prolapse, enable a timely caesarean section and thus the avoidance of cerebral damage. It is obviously an obstetric responsibility to recognise these signs and respond appropriately. The greater part of this proportion is almost certainly being appropriately managed as a component of standard obstetric practice. If this has been the case since before the commencement of any systematic and ongoing registration of cerebral palsy (1954), the frequency of cerebral palsy would not be expected to change as caesarean section rates increase for other indications. For the reasons outlined above concerning the difficulties in timing brain damage and correctly interpreting the significance of intrapartum signs traditionally associated with intrapartum asphyxia, it is not known how often contemporary cases of cerebral palsy could have been avoided by a section or an earlier section. The increase in litigation concerning cases of cerebral palsy makes it tempting to be more liberal with the use of caesarean section in the hope of avoiding such cases, however there are several reasons to believe that this may not have the desired effect.

1. Figure 45.1 shows that increasing caesarean section rates have not been associated with any change in birth prevalence of cerebral palsy.
2. Caesarean section is associated with increased neonatal morbidity (Morrison et al 1995) even in samples restricted to elective repeat sections (Hook et al 1997).
3. Caesarean section entails significant maternal morbidity and may compromise early bonding between mother and child (Boyce & Todd 1992).

The lesson from maternal mortality concerning excessive intervention (Ch. 48) must not be forgotten. Perhaps obstetricians would do well to adopt the serenity prayer adapted thus:

> God, grant me the serenity
> To leave the things I cannot improve upon,
> Courage to change the things I can,
> The wisdom to know the difference
> And a legal system that allows me to act on it.

Obstetric responsibility for cerebral palsy in perspective

Table 45.7 lists several social and medical risk factors that have been associated with cerebral palsy. Connections may plausibly be drawn between many of them. When they can be connected, social factors tend to precede the medical factors, may have cycled through families for generations and unequivocally dominate that significant proportion of cerebral palsy acquired after the neonatal period (Stanley et al 2000), Ch. 11).

Perinatal medicine in the developed world has invested heavily in research for the care of high-risk mothers and babies, resulting in dramatic increases in individual survival. This has given rise to the perinatal paradox (Leviton 1995), an emphasis on late and costly interventions which contrasts starkly with the virtual neglect of the social problems that often initiate the pathways that lead to mothers and babies

Table 45.7 Risk factors associated with cerebral palsy

Social factors	Medical factors
Close child spacing	Child abuse
Consanguinity	Difficult delivery
Delayed childbearing	Infection
Domestic violence	Infertility
Early childbearing	Intrauterine growth restriction
Greed	Maternal abdominal trauma
Lack of education	Maternal morbidities
Overpopulation	Multiple pregnancy
Poor personal hygiene	Nutritional deficiencies
Poor nutrition	Preterm birth
Poverty	Recessive genetic defects
Promiscuity	Reproductive technology
Social isolation	Sexually transmitted disease
Stress	
Substance abuse	
Toxic exposures	
Unemployment	

being at high risk. This has led to increasing numbers of very preterm-born people with disabilities, static rates of very preterm births and static levels of indicators of poor maternal and child health. Considering causal pathways encourages broader thinking about causes and increases the opportunities for prevention. Currently, funding and commitment favours later and more obviously preventative medical interventions rather than earlier social and public health programmes. Obstetric care providers have some justification in thinking that population-based interventions and social legislation are beyond their jurisdiction, but they should be encouraged to think about causal sequences and add their voices to the call for policies to address social conditions such as those listed in Table 45.7

CONCLUSION

Obstetric responsibility for abnormal fetal outcome extends throughout pregnancy and ideally commences in the preconceptional period. It is limited by both knowledge and opportunity but includes maximising personal knowledge and the opportunity for its application. One important opportunity involves fully informing the woman as only she can be responsible for her lifestyle and conduct. Not only may such communication improve fetal outcome, it may also afford the obstetric caregiver protection against litigation (Levinson 1994). Much (ideally all) of that responsibility should be embodied in standard obstetric care. It is therefore appropriate to challenge each aspect of care periodically with the most scientifically valid information available. Through the efforts of the Cochrane Collaboration, the field of pregnancy and childbirth is privileged to have a large number of systematic reviews of the most scientifically rigorous trials pertaining to many aspects of obstetric care. If these are translated into standard obstetric management, they should ensure that obstetric management does improve outcome and does not merely perpetuate misconceptions of earlier practitioners.

KEY POINTS

- Work at two-way communication with each woman.
- Provide accurate and timely preconceptional advice.
- Advise as to realistic expectations of pregnancy outcomes.
- Fully inform the woman about her responsibilities with respect to lifestyle and conduct.
- Incorporate the results of the most scientifically rigourous evaluations of obstetric care into daily practice.
- Demand evaluation of long term as well as immediate outcomes of obstetric practice.
- Do not incorporate novel practices before they have been adequately evaluated, except in the context of well designed research.

REFERENCES

Alfirevic Z, Neilson J 1999 Biophysical profile for fetal assessment in high risk pregnancies (Cochrane Review). In: The Cochrane Library, Issue 3. Update Software, Oxford

Blair E 1993 A research definition for 'birth asphyxia'? Dev Med Child Neurol 35:449–455

Blair E 1994 Cerebral palsy and intrapartum care: Wrong denominator used (letter). BMJ 309:1229

Blair E, Stanley FJ 1993 Aetiological pathways to spastic cerebral palsy. Paediatri Perinat Epidemiol 7:302–317

Blair E, Palmer L, Stanley F 1996 Cerebral palsy in very low birth weight infants, pre-eclampsia and magnesium sulfate (letter). Pediatrics 97:780–781

Boyee PM, Todd L 1992 Increased risk of postnatal depression after emergency caesarean section. Med J Aust 157:172–174

Boyd M, Usher R, McLean FH, Kramer MS Obstetric consequences of postmaturity. Am J Obstet Gynecol 158:334–338

Cosbie W 1992 The obsterical causes and prevention of stillbirth and early infant mortality: reprinted from Can Med J 1923; 13: 877–880. Can Med J 146(7):1203–1207

Gaffney G, Sellers S, Flavell V, Squier M, Johnson A 1994 Case-control study of intrapartum care, cerebral palsy, and perinatal death. BMJ 308:743–750

Grether JK, Nelson KB 1997 Maternal infection and cerebral palsy in infants of normal birth weight. JAMA 278:207–211

GRIT Study Group 1996 When do obstetricians recommend delivery for a high-risk preterm growth-retarded fetus? Growth Restriction Intervention Trial. Eur J Obste Gynecol Reprod Biol 67:121–126

Hetzel B, Pandav C 1996 S.O.S. for a billion—the conquest of iodine deficiency disorders. Oxford University Press, New Delhi

Hodnett ED 1998 Support from caregivers during at risk pregnancy (Cochrane Review). In: The Cochrane library, Issue 2. Update software, Oxford

Hook B, Kiwi R, Amini SB, Fanaroff A, Hack M 1997 Neonatal morbidity after elective repeat cesarean section and trial of labor. Pediatrics 100:348–353

Kuban KCK, Leviton A 1994 Cerebral palsy. N Eng J Med 330:188–195

Levinson 1994 Physician–patient communication: a key to malpractice prevention. JAMA 272:1619–1620

Leviton A 1995 The perinatal paradox (editorial). Am J Public Health 85:906–907

Little WJ 1958 On the influence of abnormal parturition, difficult labours, premature birth, and asphyxia neonatorum, on the mental and physical condition of the child, especially in relation to deformities. Reprinted from Trans Obstet Soc Lond. 1861–62; 3: 293. Cerebral Palsy Bulletin 1:5–36

Lumley J, Lester A, Renon P, Wood C 1985 A failed RCT to determine the best method of delivery for very low birth weight infants. Control Clin Trials 6:120–127

Luthy DA, Wardinsky MD, Shurtleff DB, Hollenback KA, Hickok DE, Nybeng DA, Bonedetti TJ, 1991 Cesarean section before the onset of labor and subsequent motor function in infants with meningomyelocele diagnosed antenatally. N Engl J Med 324: 662–666

MacLennan A and International Cerebral Palsy Task Force 1999 A template for defining a causal relation between acute intrapartum events and cerebral palsy: international consensus statement. BMJ 319:1054–1059

Manning FA, Bondaji N, Harman CR, Casiro O, Menticoglas S, Morrison I, Berck DJ 1998 Fetal assessment based on fetal biophysical profile scoring VIII. The incidence of cerebral palsy in tested and untested perinates. Am J Obstet Gynecol 178(4):696–706

Mistry RT, Neilson JP 1998 Intrapartum fetal ECG plus heart rate recording (Cochrane Review). In: The Cochrane Library Issue 2. Update Software, Oxford

Morrison JJ, Renni JM, Mitton PJ 1995 Neonatal respiratory morbidity and mode of delivery at term: Influence of timing of elective caesarean section. Br J Obstet Gynaecol 102:101–106

Morton DH, Bennett MJ, Seargeant LE, Nichter CA, Kelley RI 1991 Glutaric aciduria type I: common cause of episodic encephalopathy and spastic paralysis in the Amish of Lancaster County, Pennsylvania. Am J Med Genet 41:89–95

Mutch LW, Alberman E, Hagberg B, Kodama K, Perat MV 1992 Cerebral palsy epidemiology: where are we now and where are we going? Dev Med Child Neurol 34:547–555

Myers RE 1972 Two patterns of perinatal brain damage and their conditions of occurrence. Am J Obstet Gynecol 112:246–276

Nelson KB, Ellenberg JH 1986 Antecedents of cerebral palsy. Multivariate analysis of risk. N Engl J Med 315:81–86

Nelson KB, Grether JK 1995 Can magnesium sulfate reduce the risk of cerebral palsy in very low birthweight infants? Pediatrics 95:263–269

Niswander K, Henson G, Elbourne D, Ctialmers I, Redman C, Macfarlane A, Tizard P 1984 Adverse outcome of pregnancy and the quality of obstetric care. Lancet 2:827–830

Palmer L, Blair E, Petterson B, Burton P 1995 Antenatal antecedents of moderate and severe cerebral palsy. Paediatr Perinat Epidemiol 9:171–184

Papiernik E 1993 Prevention of preterm labour and delivery. Baillieres Clin Obstet Gynaecol 7:499–521

Redline R, Wilson-Costello D, Borausti E, Fanaroff AA, Hack M 1998 Placental lesions associated with neurologic impairment and cerebral palsy in very-low-birth-weight infants. Arch Pathol Lab Med 122:1091–1098

Saraiya M, Berg CJ, Shulman H, Green CA, Atrash HK 1999 Estimates of the annual number of clinically recognized pregnancies in the United States, 1981–1991. Am J Epidemiol 149:1025–1029

Scheller JM, Nelson KB 1994 Does cesarean delivery prevent cerebral palsy or other neurologic problems of childhood? (letter) Reply Obstet Gynecol 84:482

Simpson J 1999 Fetal surgery for myelomeningocele. Am J Obstet Gynecol 282:1873–1874

Sims M, Walther F 1989 Neonatal morbidity and mortality and long term outcome of postdate infants. Clin Obstet Gynecol 32(2):285–293

Stanley F, Blair E, Alberman E 2000 Cerebral palsies: epidemiology and causal pathways MacKeith Press, London

Thacker SB, Stroup DF 1998 Continuous electronic fetal monitoring during labour (Cochrane Review). In: The Cochrane Library, Issue 2. Update software, Oxford

Towner D, Castro M, Eby-Wilkens E, Gilbert W 1999 Effect of mode of delivery in nulliparous women on neonatal intracranial injury. N Engl J Med 341:1709–1714

Watson L, Stanley F, Petterson B 1996 Rates of triplet pregnancies in Western Australia may be beginning to fall (letter). BMJ 313:625–626

Wellesley DG, Hockey KA, Stanley F 1991 The aetiology of intellectual disability in Western Australia: a community based study. Dev Med Child Neurol 33:963–973

Whitaker AH, Van Rossem R, Feldman JF 1997 Psychiatric outcomes in low-birth-weight children at 6 years: Relation to neonatal cranial ultrasound abnormalities. Arch Gen Psychiatry 54:847–856

Zinaman M, Clegg E, Brown CC, O'Connor J, Selevan SG 1996 Estimates of human fertility and pregnancy loss. Fertil Steril 65(3):503–509

Zubrick S, Silburn S, Garton A 1995 Western Australian Child Health Survey: Developing health and well being in the nineties Australian Bureau of Statistics and Institute for Child Health Research Perth, Western Australia, p. 35

Zubrick S, Silburn S, Gurrin L, Teoh H, Shepherd C, Carlton J, Lawrence D 1997 Western Australian Child Health Survey: Education, health and competence. Australian Bureau of Statistics and Institute for Child Health Research, Perth, Western Australia, p. 19

Zubrick S, Kurinczuk J, McDermott BM, McKelvey RS, Silburn SR, Davies LC 2000 Fetal growth and subsequent mental health problems in children aged 4 to 13 years. Dev Med Child Neurol 42:14–20

46

Birth rates

Geoffrey Chamberlain

INTRODUCTION

Most countries in the developed world collect data on the numbers of births that take place; they also do a regular census of the population every 10 years. With these data, they can derive birth rates. In July 1837, the registration of live births started in England and Wales; from 1927 data on still-births were also collected. The Population (Statistics) Act 1938 was the beginning of the analysis of these data for statistical purposes and it was from this time that multiple births could first be distinguished in this country. The next Population (Statistics) Act of 1960 required further questions about the father. Data from the countries of the United Kingdom (England, Wales, Scotland and Northern Ireland) are now published regularly by the Registrar General for England and Wales through the Office for National Statistics (ONS) formally the Office of Population, Censuses and Surveys (OPCS), and for Scotland and Northern Ireland respectively by the General Registry Office of Scotland and the Northern Ireland Statistics and Research Agency. National population projections for the UK and its constituent countries are also published regularly in association with the Government Actuary's Department.

Births have to be registered by law under the Births and Deaths Registration Act of 1836. The General Registrar Office and the Local Registrars were established by that Act, which requires a Registrar to inform him- or herself within 42 days of any birth occurring inside the District. It obliged the parents, or failing them the occupier of the tenement in which the birth took place, to provide such information to the local Registrar.

The amount of data collected in the UK has increased so that now details are obtained about:

1. The child
   - date and place of birth
   - sex
   - legitimacy

2. The father
   - date and place of birth
   - occupation
3. The mother
   - date and place of birth.

For legitimate births only, further data are collected about the parents' marriage and the number of children born to the mother. These data are checked locally.

As well as this system of registration performed by parents, the midwife or doctor who attended the birth must notify the District Public Health Consultant (England and Wales) or the Chief Administrative Medical Officer (Scotland and Northern Ireland) within 36 hours of the birth. This and the civil registration system are quite separate and so can act as a check on each other. The District Health Authority (DHA) informs the local Registrar of Births of babies notified. In return, the Registrar returns to the DHA the list of registered babies with their new National Health Service number, a service the Registrars must initiate.

The population of the UK (58.8 million in 1996) is expected to rise slowly to 62.2 million in 2021 and it may decline after 2031. The four countries of the UK had 1996 populations in millions of: England, 49.1; Wales, 2.9; Scotland, 5.1; Northern Ireland, 1.7.

DEFINITIONS

The numbers of births is well known and can be expressed in various ways. The absolute number may be helpful to know so that calculations can be made about the population in coming years (Fig. 46.1); these figures can be refined in demograms (see later). The *Crude Birth Rate* is the number of live births per thousand of the total population (Fig. 46.2). This is a simple mathematical fraction that can be derived from the birth data and the Census returns.

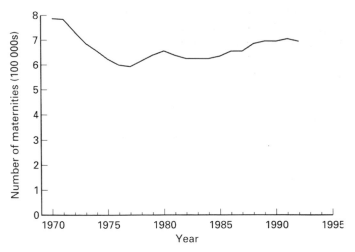

Fig. 46.1 Absolute numbers of women giving birth in England and Wales (1970–1992).

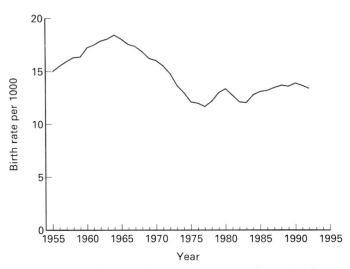

Fig. 46.2 Crude birth rates for England and Wales (1955–1992).

$$\text{Crude Birth Rate} = \frac{\text{Live Births per year} \times 1000}{\text{Mid-year population}}$$

This rate is a simple and unsophisticated measure; the denominator is all the population, which includes men and many women above and below the reproductive age group. This would be more appropriate if it consisted of all those, and only those, who might appear in the numerator as the women who could get pregnant. Hence a more appropriate measure of birth rates could be obtained by looking at the births in relation to the number of women in the reproductive age group, taken nominally as women from age 15 to 44 years (Fig. 46.3) although it makes no allowance for different sized cohorts of women. Thus the *General Fertility Rate* is derived:

$$\begin{array}{c}\text{General}\\\text{Fertility}\\\text{Rate}\end{array} = \frac{\text{Total live births per year} \times 1000}{\text{Women aged 15–44 years in mid-year population}}$$

Another measure used is the *Total Period Fertility Rate.* This is the summation of the fertility rates in any given year

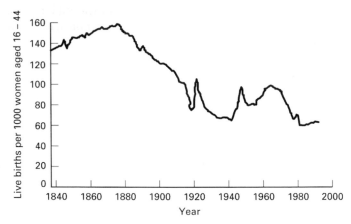

Fig. 46.3 General fertility rate for England and Wales (1838–1992).

by the years the mother has left to an age when it is considered that reproduction will probably stop (conventionally taken as 45 years). The *Total Period Fertility Rate* measures the average number of children that might be expected to be born to a woman if she experienced the age-specific fertility rates of the calendar year in question throughout the rest of her childbearing life (Fig. 46.4).

The *Total Period Fertility Rate* is a more current measure than is that of *Mean Family Size*, which can only be calculated in retrospect when a woman has completed her family. However, *mean family size* is a popular index and often used in the lay press to give the coarse differences between countries. When the completed family size drops below 2.0, replacement of the population has stopped and therefore that society is no longer replacing the numbers who die and it is below *zero population growth*. In UK the *Mean Family Size* is now 1.8 children per woman born in 1975 or later compared

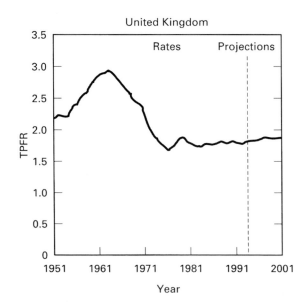

Fig. 46.4 Total period fertility rate (TPFR). Average number of children which would be born per woman if women experienced the age-specific fertility rates of the period in question throughout their childbearing lifespan. Data from Office of Population Censuses and Surveys 1994 Social Trends 24. HMSO, London.

with 2.5 children to each woman born in the mid 1930s. This drop below replacement level is in common with most Western European countries.

WORLD POPULATION CHANGES

Population dynamics express how populations change in countries and between countries. The relation of this to births and deaths can be shown simply as follows:

Births → Population size → Deaths

Migration

At times of economic stability, migration is not a major feature in many countries. although it obviously has a great part to play at times of rapid economic growth, such as immigration to the USA at the beginning of the last century, or emigration from Ireland at the time of the potato famines. Currently international migration into the UK is 50 000 per annum projected to rise to 65 000 per annum in twenty years. There are small but persistent international UK shifts from Scotland and Northern Ireland into England and Wales.

Leaving migration aside, one can then calculate how a country is likely to expand. A good example of straightforward population dynamics would be from the flourishing country of Kenya, the population of which was six million in 1950 and 24 million in 1990. It has a large tourist industry with virtually no migration either in or out. The birth rate is 31 per 1000; the death rate is 15 per 1000. There is, therefore, a natural annual increase of growth of 1.6% and a *Total Family Rate* of 3.9 per woman. From this, one can extrapolate that in about 20 years' time, the population will have approximately doubled.

In most countries in Western Europe, the birth rate is below the death rate. If migration is not a major factor, they have dropped below the point of *zero population growth* and numbers are in decline. In 1798 Thomas Malthus, an economist and pioneer in population studies, published his first edition of 'The Principle of Population as it Effects the Future Improvement of Society' (Malthus 1798). He laid down what he considered were the factors which stabilised populations in the eighteenth century.

- Positive effects on an increased death rate

  Famine
  War
  Disease.

- Negative effects on increased birth rate

  Celibacy
  Restraint.

Malthus' ideas held sway for over a century, during which the three influences which affect death rates were considerably curtailed. At the end of the twentieth century, the effect of reduced disease and death rates have become apparent in the Western world; There are still, however, many diseases, particularly infections such as malaria and HIV that still need to be overcome in the developing world. The effects of famine are often being overcome by agricultural policies, like those in the Punjab in India who are leading the world away from starvation. Despite the campaigns of Korea, Vietnam and the Gulf War, the United Nations claim there have been no real world wars for 50 years and so deaths from this cause are greatly reduced in both the warrior class and the civilians involved in these wars. Hence, reduction in birth rates has now become the major instrument in altering populations in the twenty-first century. In many countries contraception has overtaken celibacy as restraint which influences birth rates and wider family spacing is the desired aim.

WORLD POPULATION CONTROL

World population is growing faster than ever before. Malthus pointed out two centuries ago that population increases at a geometric rate while productivity of food has increases only arithmetically. Were the world population to continue to increase at the present rate, it would grow from six billion people at present to nine billion by 2050 (Fig. 46.5). Growth is uneven between the regions, 90% being in the less developed parts of the world thus increasing their share of the world's population (Asia's went from 55% to 60% within the last fifty years while Africa's increased from 9% to 12%).

World organisations such as the World Health Organisation (WHO) and the World Bank have been attempting to cope with this for many years. Their first emphasis was on prevention of births by the provision of contraception. They were not very sensitive about the ethical ideas of many recipient countries and so, not surprisingly, it was not very popular at first. However, women want help in spacing their families and so now contraception is becoming a more acceptable method of trying to control populations. World population control is very different from family planning (which is when a couple wants to produce the number of children they want at the intervals they want them). World population control is just a general reduction in the number of babies born and it is considered, perhaps unfeelingly, to need less precise tools than family planning.

Scientific advances in the use of oral contraception and intrauterine devices have been embraced by some countries enthusiastically. For example, South Korea offered these techniques openly and backed them up with a safe early termination of pregnancy (TOP) programme. The *Total Fertility Rate* declined from 6 in 1960 to 1.7 in 1990. Other countries, such as India, tried to teach periodic abstinence.

The position of TOP in population control conflicts with the ethical principles of many religions and it is hence considered an anathema in some countries. Not just the Roman Catholic faith, but those of Islam and Hinduism, are ideologically against TOP. It is, however, important to remember that many women who live in countries ruled by these faiths do wish to have access to safe and properly performed TOP. Even in Southern Europe and Saudi Arabia, TOP still takes place for the women who wish it and who can afford it. The provision of safely done procedures would be welcomed by a significant proportion of the populace.

In many places the medical profession, in its paternalistic

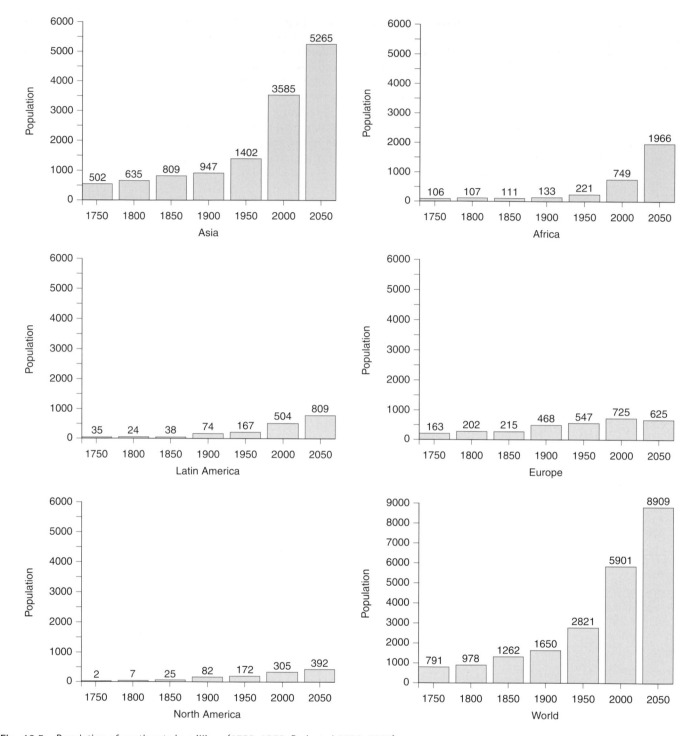

Fig. 46.5 Population of continents in millions (1750–1950. Projected 2000–2050).

fashion, considers that all contraception should be handled through conventional clinics staffed by doctors or trained nurses. This is wishful thinking in many developing countries where such skills are scarce.

Malcolm Potts (2000) considers that the professionals can make a difference by promoting three strategies:

- Promoting the expansion of budgets for family planning in developing countries and provision of adequate contraceptive supplies.

- Ensuring that most family planning procedures are performed by lower level providers other than doctors and nurses.

- Helping society to accept the reality of TOP.

Others would look to other ways of reducing the births. In the developing world large numbers of babies die in infancy: up to 60 per 1000 die in their first year compared with 9 per 1000 in more developed regions. The deaths are often caused by diarrhoeal diseases and reducing this toll would mean that more children live on. With a larger continuing family, women would voluntarily have fewer births.

Some propose solving the population problem by improving the food supply. Undoubtedly by a world effort, more crops could be grown, e.g. irrigation of parts of the Sahara or the breeding of germ resistant foodstuffs. Unfortunately, the *Living Planet Index* which attempts to quantify the effects of human activity on natural eco systems is still showing an unsustainable rate of decline and much would have to be done fairly swiftly to improve this aspect. Undoubtedly the United Nations means well but international agencies and national governments must give stronger leadership to stabilising population growth and integrating this into the larger picture of building an equitable global human ecology. At the moment, priority should be given to reducing the numbers of babies born.

LONGITUDINAL POPULATION CHANGES

The effects of changes in the birth rate can be seen readily in demograms by examining the information from age-specific rates in five-year samples of the population. From this population projections can be derived. Figure 46.6 shows three demograms from the same region, Hong Kong over a 20-year period. In the years since World War II, the birth rate had been going up sharply and so, in the mid 1960s, the Government of Hong Kong began an intensive campaign to promote the use of contraception. The 1971 demogram shows that this had worked, for the effect of contraception was a great reduction in the birth rate. By 1981, this reduced birth rate structure had been sustained. The bulge of children born in the late 1950s was working its way through and was represented by figures showing a bulge of people in their 20s. The implication of this for the provision of facilities for schooling, universities and job opportunities is obvious and demograms

are often used for social planning. Similar demographs for later years will show the population bulge will continue to age. It can be predicted that Hong Kong will require an enlargement in geriatric services from 2010 onwards.

The projection demogram for the UK shows a slight diminution in births since 1965 to the late 1970s and the results of the population bulge in the 1950s and 1960s. The demogram is reasonably straight-sided, as in other developed countries. With improvements in health and better nutrition, an ageing population will soon weigh down the upper end of this demogram in the 2020s. The increased numbers of older people will place increased demand on geriatric and social services over the next 30–40 years, a strain on any social security system.

Data from Western Europe from the Economie Intelligence Unit (1999) confirm a similar trend from 1950 to 2040. The bulge of 1930–1950s births in working through to old age brings problems of support for the aged. As a consolation, it is probable that wars are more likely to be waged when countries have broadbased demographs, with higher rates of 15–25-year-old males then 55–65-year-olds.

BIRTH RATES IN ENGLAND AND WALES

The birth rate in England and Wales shown in Figure 46.3 illustrates trends for the last century. In the Victorian days, the birth rate was high. This was just after the Industrial Revolution, when Britain was an economically rich nation. Birth rates declined from then until the 1920s, when there was the great economic depression. The birth rate of the 1930s was slightly boosted by the threat of war and a recovery in heavy industry. However, the birth rate has stayed at a generally lower level since the Second World War, apart from a temporary bulge shortly after hostilities ceased and men returned to their homes.

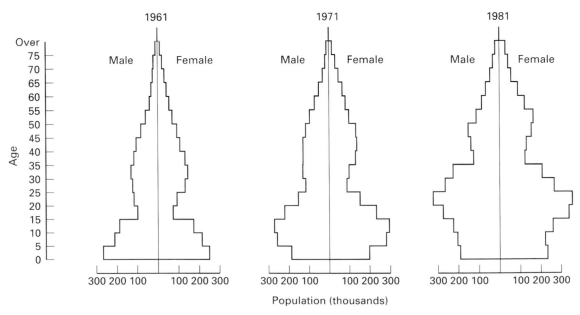

Fig. 46.6   Smoothed-off demogram of Hong Kong in 1961, 1971 and 1981 recording male and female populations in 5-year cohorts.

Examination of the more recent *crude birth rate* data shows that the post-war boom rose to a peak in 1964 when it was about 17 per 1000 and since then it has declined and steadied (Fig. 46.2). There was a minor resurgence in 1980, when the birth rate was about 14 per 1000 but the *total period fertility rate* was only 1.8—still a figure below replacement rates for the population.

FACTORS THAT MODIFY THE BIRTH RATE

Family spacing

Obviously the earlier in life couples start reproducing, the more likely they are to have a larger family. In many parts of Asia and Africa, girls marry at 12 or 13 years of age or they may have a greater exposure to intercourse even if not married; they are consequently more likely to have more babies. Conversely, in countries like Sri Lanka, the mean age of marriage is 28 years and birth rates are dropping fast in that country.

In many parts of the world, breast feeding is the most commonly used method of contraception and so a pregnancy occurs every two or three years during reproductive life. Other methods of pharmaceutical and mechanical contraception are more common in the Western world. Their use, combined with later marriage, has led to a later start in reproduction and a wider spacing of families and so a lower birth rate.

Table 46.1 represents the average number of children born per woman at the current fertility rates in the major

Table 46.1 Total Fertility Rates for some major regions of the World (1998 WHO)

Region	Total fertility rate
Western Europe	1.4
North America	1.9
Latin America	2.7
Asia	2.6
Africa	5.1

regions of the world. It is sharply divided into those areas where contraception is more widely used and those where it is not. Apart from conventional contraception, in many parts of Eastern Europe TOP is considered a method of contraception. This method is unacceptable in the Western world because of the increased rate of serious sequelae.

Seasonal variations

Another inbuilt variant in birth rates is the seasonal pattern throughout the year. In the UK, seasonal variations in birth rate have remained the same for over a century with only minor variations occurring during the years of World Wars I and II. The birth rate in England and Wales is highest from January to March and generally lowest from October to December. Several explanations have been put forward, ranging from the hypothesis that intercourse may be more frequent in the spring, or that the tax year finishes in early April, to the idea that trace elements are entering the diet in different rates at different times of the year. These theories are hard to substantiate for there have been different patterns shown in other parts of the world, such as Australia, where the peak of birth rate is from their spring to autumn (September to March). Further, limited work based on sixteenth-century baptismal data (which bears a strong relation to birth rate data) implies that these trends were in existence long before income tax was invented—though obviously not before intercourse was invented.

Figure 46.7 shows the variation in daily births for England and Wales from 1969 to 1980. It is remarkable for its consistency. A secondary peak in birth rates can be seen in September of each year. This is thought to be associated with the fact that nine months before September was Christmas and New Year with their usual festivities.

Daily variations

A short-term cyclical influence is seen in birth rates when one examines the day of the week on which people are born. Figure 46.8 explores this in a simplified way. The birth ratio is derived by dividing the number of births on any given day

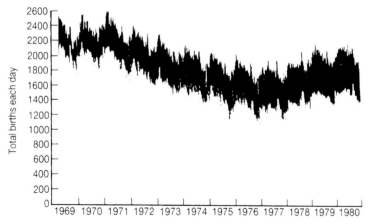

Fig. 46.7 Daily numbers of births for England and Wales (1969–1980).

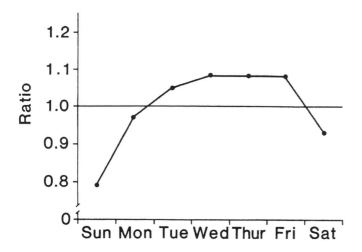

Fig. 46.8 Birth rates in 1980 by day of the week (see text).

of the week by one-seventh of the total number of births, the daily mean. If the distribution were random, the expected number of births on any day would be one-seventh of the total ie: the ratio would be 1.0. Any figures above 1 indicate an increase in the number of expected births that day, while below 1 indicates a deficit in births on that day.

It can be seen that at the weekend there is a deficiency in the number of births: the lowest ratio is on Sunday and the next lowest on Saturday. It is not the purpose of this chapter to pursue the reasons for this but intercourse may be a precipitating factor. Some women may have a lower threshold for the near term uterus contracting spontaneously. It might be that stimulation of the cervix could cause an unusual release of prostaglandins which, while not enough to start labour in most women, could start the process in a woman who is very close to labour and has a low threshold for onset.

It is as probable that in the UK sexual intercourse is more frequent on Friday and Saturday; this might be the stimulus to the release of prostaglandins. This hypothesis is being explored at the moment.

CONCLUSIONS

Examination of birth rates is not a dull, statistical process but one that gives information in a wide range of social and medical fields. A country that keeps proper data about its births and deaths is usually one that has a good health service. If the information is not counted then the people do not count.

ACKNOWLEDGEMENTS

Much of the data are easily available and are constantly being updated from Government sources. The author would like to acknowledge the great help he has had from the following sources:

- McFarland & Mugford Birth Counts (2000)
- Office of Population Censuses and Surveys Birth Statistics (1837–1991).

REFERENCES

Economist Intelligence Unit 1999 Health care Europe 1999 E.I.U.
Malthus TR 1798 'The Principles of Population as it Effects the Future Improvements of Society'. First published anonymously Johnson, St. Paul's Churchyard, London
McFarland A, Mugford M 2000 Birth Counts, the Statistics of Pregnancy and Childbirth. HMSO, London
Office of Population Censuses and Surveys Birth Statistics 1837–1991. Series FM1 nos 13.21. HMSO, London
Potts M 2000 The Most Pressing Issue. J Roy Soc Med 93:1–2

47

Perinatal mortality

Jean Chapple

Material in this chapter contains contributions from the first and second editions and we are grateful to the previous authors for the work done.

INTRODUCTION

Modern technology gives us countless methods of investigating and treating both health and disease. However, many of the procedures carried out by health professionals are ineffective and they do not produce a better state of health for those individuals who have sought clinical help (Enkin et al 1989). In a tax-funded health care system such as the National Health Service (NHS), it is inevitable that interest now focuses on funding good outcomes of health care rather than emphasising the processes (e.g. numbers of operations or other procedures). One of the earliest outcome measures used in the NHS was perinatal mortality. This measure was first proposed in an article published in 1948 (Peller 1948) which suggested combining stillbirth and first week death rates, as the time trends for early neonatal deaths were more like those for stillbirths than other death rates in infancy. This chapter looks at how often and why perinatal deaths occur and discusses whether the perinatal death rate is a good measure of the effectiveness of maternity and neonatal services.

DEFINITIONS

Definitions of live and still birth and perinatal death:

- A **liveborn baby** is a child who breathes or shows signs of life after complete expulsion from its mother, regardless of length of gestation.
- A **stillbirth** is defined in England & Wales as a child issuing forth from its mother after the 24th completed week of pregnancy which did not at any time after being completely expelled from its mother breathe or show any other signs of life. (Section 41 of the Births and Deaths Registration Act 1953, amended 1 October 1991)
- An **early neonatal death** occurs when a child is delivered alive, but who dies before six completed days of life.
- A **neonatal death** is one delivered alive but who dies in the first 28 days. These include early neonatal deaths.
- A **perinatal death** is either a stillbirth or an early neonatal death.

Definitions of mortality rates:

- **Perinatal mortality rate (PNMR)** is calculated from the number of stillbirths and early neonatal deaths (those occurring in the first week of life) per 1000 total births (live and stillbirths).
- **Stillbirth rate** (SR) is the number of stillbirths per 1000 total births (live births and stillbirths).
- **Early neonatal death rate (ENDR)** is the number of

early neonatal deaths (occurring within the first seven days of life) per 1000 live births.

- **Neonatal death rate (NNDR)** is the number of neonatal deaths (occurring within the first 28 days of life) per 1000 live births (including ENDR).
- **Infant mortality rate (IMR)** is the number of deaths under the age of one year following a live birth, per 1000 live births (i.e. including NNDR and ENDR).

Definitions of live births and stillbirths and hence perinatal mortality vary with national policy and with time. All live-born babies must be registered. This categorisation varies greatly from one country to another, as there are different legal definitions excluding live births below defined lower limits of gestational age or birthweight. Laws relating to the timing of registration may also affect whether the child is certified as live or stillborn (Macfarlane & Mugford 2000).

A stillborn baby in the UK must also be registered with the local Registrar of Births and Deaths. The current definition, where a baby is defined as stillborn if it is born dead at or after 24 weeks' gestation came into force on 1 October 1992; prior to this, the cut-off gestational age was 28 weeks. This change in definition has increased the PNMR, as babies dying between 24 completed weeks and 28 weeks are now included in the figures whereas previously they were not. Stillborn babies are defined by the gestation at which they are born, rather than the gestation at which they died, so a papyraceous twin who has died months before its sibling is born should be registered as a stillbirth. In practice, this is not always done.

Individual judgement also plays a part in certification of perinatal deaths (Keirse 1984) and decisions about viability (Fenton et al 1990). Some fetuses are born so early that they are not truly viable but they may still show visible signs of life for a few minutes. The current law in England, Wales and Scotland allows termination of pregnancy for severe fetal malformation at any gestational age. If the termination is carried out after 24 weeks' gestation and the fetus is dead at birth, it should officially be registered as a stillbirth, and the legal forms relating to termination of pregnancy must also be completed. If feticide is not carried out prior to delivery, such a fetus may be live born and die after delivery, and this should again be registered as a live birth and subsequent death, with official disposal of the body, and with completed termination documentation. However, it is not unknown for clinicians to be influenced by perceptions of how the parents will feel about official form filling and financial consequences for the parents with regard to maternity benefit and the cost of burial. This is understandable but technically illegal—the legal cut-off points may be arbitrary but still have the force of law. However, parental grief pays no regard to such legal niceties.

THE COLLECTION OF DATA ABOUT PERINATAL MORTALITY

Different countries have different methods of collecting data about perinatal deaths as well as different definitions. This section deals with the situation in England and Wales.

Greater detail can be found in volume 1 of *Birth Counts* (Macfarlane & Mugford 2000).

Civil registration of births

The industrialisation of society, with the population moving from villages to large cities, led to major changes in the way data on births, deaths and marriages were collected. Authorities could no longer rely on information from parish baptismal and burial records. In 1837, a law was passed to make it a statutory requirement to register all births with the Registrar of Births and Deaths in the locality in England and Wales where the birth had taken place. Registration was required in Scotland in 1855 (Nissel 1987).

Parents are required to give details of the baby and demographic data, such as their own date and place of birth, to the Registrar within 42 days of the birth. Certain details, such as the parity of the mother and the occupation of the father (to determine social class) are requested only for legitimate babies. As over one-third of babies are now born to parents who are not married, this information does not apply to an increasingly large proportion of births. Important information, such as birthweight, gestational age and ethnic group of parents, is completely omitted from initial collection of registration data.

Medical notification of births

An increasing interest in improving maternal and child health at the beginning of the twentieth century led to the introduction of another system of collecting data about births in order to ensure that midwives, health visitors and doctors were aware that a baby had been born and could offer clinical support and advice. The attendant at the birth has to notify the designated medical officer (usually the Director of Public Health) of the local health authority of any birth occurring in that authority, in writing, within 36 hours of birth. This system gives the opportunity to collect information on birthweight, which since 1978 has been statutorily transferred from the notification system to the birth registration system to provide national statistics on birthweight. Birth attendants are also asked to notify the Office for National Statistics (ONS) about congenital malformations noted within 10 days of birth to give a national picture of the birth prevalence of malformations. This requirement started in 1964 in response to the thalidomide tragedy.

Death certification

Stillbirths and neonatal deaths must all be registered. The certificates made out by the Registrar of Births and Deaths include the medical cause of death, certified by the doctor in attendance. Stillbirth certificates act as both a birth and death certificate and the child's name can be included, as well as the birthweight, gestational age and cause of death, which may be certified by a midwife. Since 1986, a neonatal certificate has been issued, which, like a stillbirth certificate, collects data on maternal causes contributing to the death.

Linkage of birth and death certificates

Butler (1967) stated that a prerequisite to the reduction of perinatal mortality is to identify the obstetric and sociological associates of perinatal deaths. Heady & Heasman (1959) first demonstrated that linkage of the information on birth certificates with that on death certificates of infants who subsequently died would allow calculation of death rates by demographic factors collected for babies at birth, such as mother's country of birth and social class.

Some data collected by statute, such as parity of the mother, are for legitimate births only. The proportion of illegitimate births more than doubled between 1976 and 1986 (from 9.2 to 21.4%) and had reached 35.8% by 1996, so such data have less value. Other data, such as place of birth of mother, can no longer be used as an approximation of ethnic group because of the rising number of second- and third-generation children born to immigrant groups. ONS publishes reports on births and deaths for England and Wales from routinely collected data from birth registration and notification. However, there have been problems in collecting timely and compatible data within rapidly changing organizations such as the NHS and ONS. This puts limits on the use of routinely collected national data and has led to increasing interest in more intensive surveys and enquiries.

SURVEYS OF PERINATAL DEATHS

The first of these national studies was done in 1946 (Joint Committee of the RCOG and the Population Investigation Committee 1948) but this was more concerned with examining maternity services in Britain at the time when the NHS was being planned than with looking at causes of death. In 1958 the British Perinatal Mortality study (Butler & Bonham 1963) evaluated nationally how and when British babies were born or died, how often they died and what clinico-pathological features led to their death. The study used a cohort of births between 3 and 9 March 1958 plus deaths in the next three consecutive months. This cohort has been studied long term to look at the effects of prenatal factors in parents on the next generation (Emanuel et al 1992). The detailed first report contained statistical data on factors such as maternal age, parity, place of booking, gestation and birthweight, while the second report (Butler & Alberman 1969) used multivariate analysis of high risk influences on the outcome of pregnancy, such as smoking and sociobiological factors.

A third study was done in 1970 to look at all babies born alive or dead after the 24th week of gestation (Chamberlain et al 1975). This provided basic data in Britain for factors such as low birthweight and placental abnormalities and quantified them. These studies did not look at deaths individually but epidemiologically. A proposed fourth study in 1982 did not occur in England and Wales (Chalmers 1979). By this time, deaths had fallen to a level where it was possible to do a confidential enquiry on each case. A more unified routine data collection system for the far fewer births taking place in Scotland made a Scottish study feasible at this time (McIlwaine et al 1979).

PERINATAL ENQUIRIES

Staff working in maternity services have a long history of investigating deaths through confidential enquiries, a form of external clinical audit (Shaw 1980). In such studies, each death is reviewed individually by a group of clinicians from different disciplines concerned in maternity care, and *avoidable*, *adverse* or *notable* factors which may have contributed to the death are identified. Identification of less than optimal resources and practice can be fed back anonymously to all clinicians to make them rethink how they provide maternity care.

From 1928 onwards, the main concern of obstetricians was for maternal rather than perinatal deaths, as the maternal mortality rate was 4.4 deaths per 1000 total births, or 3000 mothers dying each year. This led to a national confidential enquiry into maternal deaths. The persisting differences in the PNMR between countries and between regions in England and Wales in the 1970s led to interest in applying the methodology of confidential enquiries to perinatal deaths—although, as there were then 10 perinatal deaths for each maternal death, the task was much larger (Chalmers 1979, Chalmers & McIlwaine 1980).

Enquiries instituted in the 1970s were conducted on a regional basis. Some involved interviews with the bereaved parents and the primary care professionals involved (Paediatric Research Unit 1973, Mutch et al 1981, Mersey Region Working Party on Perinatal Mortality 1982, Wood et al 1984). A considerable amount of relevant data are available from statutory returns on births and deaths (Black & Macfarlane 1982, Clarke 1982). However, without good denominator data from detailed information on all births or a proper case-control study, it is impossible to put perinatal deaths in an enquiry into perspective and calculate a relative risk for factors leading to perinatal death (Coggon et al 1993). This is a major problem of current confidential enquiries. Adverse factors occur in the care of mothers and babies who survive as well as those who die. Lack of denominator data to put the risks in perspective makes it impossible to assess the sensitivity and specificity of screening for adverse risk factors. Most screening tests in pregnancy produce a high proportion of false positives, leading to unnecessary clinical intervention, and there is a danger that confidential enquiries may contribute to this. Studies of sudden infant deaths with controls have been undertaken in three regions as a pilot study for the national Confidential Enquiry into Stillbirths and Deaths in Infancy (CESDI) to look at the use of case controls in assessing adverse factors (Fleming et al 2000). Controls are also being used in the 1998–2000 CESDI study of deaths (Project 27/28) in babies born at 27 or 28 weeks' gestation.

The Confidential Enquiry into Stillbirths and Deaths in Infancy

A full national Confidential Enquiry into Stillbirths and Deaths in Infancy (CESDI) 0was instituted in England, Wales and Northern Ireland from 1 January 1993, with assessments of anonymised case notes by multidisciplinary regional panels. Scotland has a separate survey of stillbirths and neonatal deaths (Information and Statistics Division, 1994). Slightly contrary to its name, CESDI covers all deaths from the 20th week of pregnancy to the end of the first year of life, including some late fetal losses as well as all stillbirths (fetuses born dead after 24 weeks). In 1998, perinatal deaths made up 51.5% of the 10 225 rapid reports forms returned to CESDI. Stillbirths made up 63.6% of these perinatal deaths although there has been a steady decrease in the stillbirth rate since the start of CESDI (Confidential Enquiry into Stillbirths and Deaths in Infancy 2000; Table 47.1).

Between 1994 and 1995, confidential assessments by local regional multidisciplinary panels of obstetricians, paediatricians, midwives, general practitioners, pathologists and others focused on an intrapartum group. This included babies who would be expected to have developed beyond the stage when the problems of prematurity might influence their survival. An intrapartum death is defined as the death of a normally formed baby weighing 1.5 kg or more after the onset of labour and before 28 days of life, related to intrapartum events. This group of 873 babies (1 in every 1561 births) represented only 4.3% of CESDI deaths but it was felt to be the group which was most amenable to improvement through feedback of the organisational problems in maternity care identified in the national CESDI reports.

Over 78% of these intrapartum related deaths were criticised for suboptimal care because alternative management 'might' (25%) or 'would reasonably be expected to' (52%) make a difference to the outcome. About 95% of critical comments described failures to act appropriately, to recognise problems or to communicate effectively. The dominant time for suboptimal care was during labour (70% of comments), followed by antepartum (19%) and postpartum (11%), with 22% of the 375 neonatal deaths having suboptimal resusci-

tation (Confidential Enquiry into Stillbirths and Deaths in Infancy 1997).

Other CESDI reports include confidential enquiries on a one in 10 sample of all deaths over 1 kg (excluding post neonatal deaths and major abnormalities), and all deaths of babies of 4 kg or over and reports from focus groups on shoulder dystocia, ruptured uterus, planned home delivery, anaesthetic complications and delays and breech presentation at the onset of labour. (Confidential Enquiry Into Stillbirths and Deaths in Infancy 1998, 1999, 2000).

CESDI provides on overview of the numbers and causes of stillbirth and infant deaths, with detailed enquiries into specific subsets. CESDI has used case control studies where risk factors need to be assessed and focus group work to provide greater detail and overview of rare events. Publishing reports is not enough—CESDI has also undertaken audits on postmortem reporting, cardiotocograph education and resuscitation of premature babies to see if messages from its reports are noted and changes implemented. It has also produced notes for both parents and professionals on postmortem examination, which is essential if the causes of perinatal deaths are to be determined accurately so that action can be taken to prevent future deaths.

TRENDS IN PERINATAL DEATHS

Comparisons of the perinatal mortality rates between Western countries in the 1970s led the Committee on Child Health Services (1976) to refer to the infant mortality rate in the UK as a 'holocaust'. This led to a renewed interest in perinatal mortality and to the regionally based confidential enquiries into such deaths mentioned above. In 1977, the PNMR for England and Wales was 17.0 per 1000 births. By

Table 47.1 Rapid report form returns to CESDI 1993–1998
(Source: Confidential enquiry into Stillbirths and Deaths in Infancy 7th Annual report, 2000
Live births—ONS, Northern Ireland GRO 1998
Deaths—CESDI rapid report forms)

	England, Wales and Northern Ireland											
	1993		1994		1995		1996		1997		1998	
	No.	Rate	No.	Rate	No.	Rate	No.	Rate	No.	Rate	No.	Rate
Legal abortions	–	–	–	–	959	–	1102	–	1299	–	1503	–
Late fetal loss[a]	1495	–	1573	–	1553	–	1659	–	1774	–	1672	–
Stillbirths[a,b]	3726	5.3	3747	5.4	3698	5.5	3688	5.4	3440	5.1	3347	5.0
Perinatal deaths[a,b]	–	–	5897	8.5	5829	8.6	5898	8.7	5503	8.2	5266	7.9
Neonatal deaths[a,c]	2755	4.0	2749	4.0	2714	4.0	2785	4.1	2648	4.0	2494	3.8
Post neonatal deaths[c]	1242	1.8	1199	1.7	1156	1.7	1253	1.9	1257	1.9	1209	1.8
Total rapid report forms	9218		9268		10 080		10 487		10 418		10 225	
Total live births	696 133		688 545		671 861		674 071		666 370		659 762	

[a] (excluding legal abortions)
[b] rate per 1000 live and stillbirth
[c] rate per 1000 live births

1987, it had fallen to 8.9 and by 1997 to 7.0 (8.4 when still-births between 24 and 27 weeks are included). This is similar to trends in other Western countries, which are all beginning to converge at rates of less than 10 per 1000. There are now equal proportions of stillbirths to early neonatal deaths, but this was not always the case; in the 1930s the stillbirth rate was more than double the first week death rate. Stillbirth and early neonatal death rates began to converge in the mid 1950s, reaching the same levels by the mid 1970s.

It is difficult to analyse international trends in causes of perinatal mortality as there have been changes in the international classification of causes of death (World Health Organization 1977) and the way in which deaths are coded.

CAUSES OF PERINATAL DEATHS

Classification of immediate causes

OPCS uses the International Classification of Diseases (ICD) codes to classify disease and injuries for national statistics. Since 1 January 1986, the certifier has been able to record separately the main fetal and maternal conditions leading to stillbirth or neonatal death without giving precedence to one particular condition. However, classification using ICD codes is not easy, and clinicians do not always complete death certificates as fully as they might, so that there is considerable underreporting of specific conditions through the ONS.

Pathological causes of death such as anoxia or prematurity give little precise information on the aetiology of deaths. Baird and his colleagues (1954) in Aberdeen therefore devised a clinical classification with an hierarchical structure—for example, if a baby weighing 1500 g dies shortly after an operative delivery done because of a placental abruption and is found at postmortem to have a tentorial tear, then it seems more logical to attribute the death primarily to placental abruption than to prematurity or birth trauma. This classification was used as the basis of the British Perinatal Mortality Survey in 1958 (Butler & Bonham 1963). A modified version of this clinicopathological approach (Cole et al 1986) is also used for the current national CESDI, as it gives a classification of obstetric factors.

Other recent classifications have tried to relate the classification to the time in pregnancy, delivery or postnatal period when the factor causing eventual death occurred. This then allows health services to focus on preventive action at the appropriate time. Wigglesworth (1980) proposed a classification using a pathophysiological approach which did not need detailed pathological investigation and that shows fetal and neonatal factors. It arranges causes of death in a mutually exclusive hierarchy: congenital malformations, stillbirths occurring before the onset of labour (both pregnancy related), neonatal deaths as a result of immaturity (neonatal period), deaths caused by asphyxial conditions (related to labour and delivery) and other specific causes. This classification of fetal causes of death has been extended and is also used in CESDI assessments (OPCS 1991, Alberman et al 1994).

Both these types of classification need to be used with data on the maturity of the baby at birth. Gestational age is not routinely collected in national statistics. It is considered difficult to categorise accurately, as the dates for calculation of gestational age given by the mother may differ from those calculated from ultrasound readings or they may not be available at all. Birthweight is, therefore, often used as a proxy for gestational age, although this too has its drawbacks if the baby is at the extremes of the birthweight distribution for its gestation.

Immediate causes

The three major determinants of perinatal mortality found in all studies (Chamberlain 1980) are:

1. Congenital anomalies
2. Low birthweight (LBW) and very low birthweight (VLBW)—taken as less than 2500 g and less than 1500 g respectively
3. Hypoxia.

Although perinatal death rates have fallen considerably in the last two decades, the proportions of deaths from specific causes have not changed. This suggests that the fall in mortality is because of overall improvements in general maternal health and in maternity care, rather than particular innovations in diagnosis and treatment of pregnancy complications. Figure 47.1 shows the cause of death of stillbirths notified to CESDI in 1998 using the Wigglesworth and Aberdeen classifications. Seventy per cent were unexplained antepartum fetal deaths, 12% caused by congenital malformation and 9% resulted from intrapartum causes. When the Aberdeen classification was applied to the deaths categorised as unexplained by the Wigglesworth criteria, 69% were still unexplained, 16% caused by antepartum haemorrhage, 7% by maternal disorder and 5% by pre-eclampsia. In the neonatal period, immaturity caused 48.5% of the deaths, congenital malformations 23% and infections 9% (Fig. 47.2). Of the deaths resulting from immaturity, 58% were related to asphyxia before birth, 35% to hyaline membrane disease and 3.8% to intraventricular haemorrhage.

Predisposing causes

It seems likely from the data available that all causes of perinatal mortality are falling in incidence, mainly because predisposing factors are falling in prevalence. These can act at several different stages of pregnancy.

Prepregnancy risk factors

Deaths resulting from lethal congenital malformations are falling because of prenatal diagnosis with termination of affected pregnancies. Some families are aware that they carry genes for severe genetic disease and seek advice prepregnancy. In others, fetal anomaly scanning may reveal structural abnormalities such as spina bifida and allow a fall in perinatal mortality because of their detection (Saari-Kemppainen et al 1990). However, routine scanning has not been shown to reduce mortality and improve outcome from any other cause (Bucher & Schmidt 1993, Ewigman et al 1993).

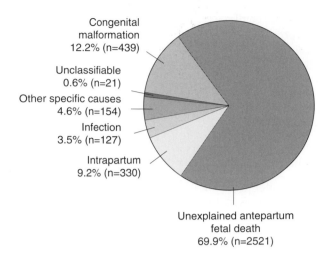

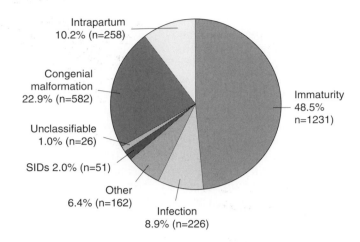

Unexplained deaths by Aberdeen classification	Number	Percent
Antepartum haemorrhage	395	15.7%
Maternal disorder	181	7.2%
Pre-eclampsia	136	5.4%
Mechanical	48	1.9%
Miscellaneous	12	0.5%
Unexplained	1749	69.4%
Total	**2521**	**100.0%**

Source: Confidential Enquiry 2000

Fig. 47.1 Stillbirths (n=3592) in England, Wales and Northern Ireland by Wigglesworth classification – 1998.

Immaturity deaths by Fetal Classification	Number	Percent
Asphyxia before birth	718	58.3%
Hyaline membrane disease	433	35.2%
Intraventricular haemorrhage	47	3.8%
Infection	30	2.4%
Unclassifiable	3	0.2%
Total	**1231**	**100.0%**

Source: Confidential Enquiry 2000

Fig. 47.2 Neonatal deaths (n=2536) in England, Wales and Northern Ireland by Wigglesworth classification – 1998.

Some maternal infections such as rubella and toxoplasmosis may be transmitted vertically from mother to child and cause severe malformation. Although the birth prevalence of severe malformations and deaths from these infections may be falling, it remains to be seen if public health programmes to immunise children against rubella, prevent the spread of toxoplasmosis through personal and food hygiene (RCOG Multidisciplinary Working Group 1992) and to prevent neural tube defects by periconceptional increase in maternal folic acid intake (MRC Vitamin Study Research Group 1991, Czeizel & Dudas 1992, Czeizel 1993) will actually result in primary prevention of malformations.

Maternal ill health or stunted growth may conspire against a normal fetal growth rate or even, as in the case of diabetes, accelerate fetal growth to a dangerous degree. Defects such as abnormal uterine shape may prevent normal placentation, and anomalies of the cervix predispose to incompetence of the internal os and premature delivery.

Advanced maternal age is associated with antepartum haemorrhage (Butler & Alberman 1969), possibly in some cases because fibroids are commoner and may distort the uterus, leading to abnormalities of placentation.

Conceptional risk factors

Random errors of meiotic or early mitotic divisions can lead to fetal chromosomal abnormalities or multiple pregnancy,

both of which are commoner in older mothers. Some trisomies, such as trisomy 18 (Edward's syndrome) and trisomy 13 (Patau's syndrome) are rapidly lethal, often in the middle or third trimester, but others such as trisomy 21 (Down's syndrome) may produce viable fetuses if there is no major structural abnormality such as a congenital heart defect.

Multiple births are exposed to many hazards and they are becoming commoner with increasing use of infertility treatment. Multiple placentation and increased nutritional demands made by two or more fetuses can result in fetal growth restriction. In monozygous twins, cords can become entangled in a single amniotic sac, competition for placental tissues may occur, or one twin may transfuse blood into the other, resulting in a marked size difference between them or the death of one twin. Premature delivery is also very high, especially in higher-order births.

Environmental factors acting in pregnancy

External environment

There are many well-recognised teratogens and other fetal toxins which may play a small part in perinatal mortality in developed countries. These include viral infections such as fetal rubella, cytomegalovirus and toxoplasmosis that may cause minimal symptoms in a pregnant woman if caught during pregnancy, but which can seriously damage a fetus, especially in the first trimester. Other organisms, such as listeriosis, salmonella and parvovirus (fifth disease) can cause death through prematurity with or without intrauterine or neonatal infection.

Altitude plays a part in producing low birthweight— about 30% of babies born in Colorado above 10 000 feet (3050 m) were low birthweight in Lubchencho's classic study (Lubchencho et al 1963) on birthweight distribution for gestational age, compared with 7% in the UK today. This may play a part in perinatal mortality in some countries.

Exposure to occupational or environmental hazards such as radiation or lead can contribute to perinatal mortality. However, the literature is not clear on the magnitude of the risks, mainly because the numbers of births affected have been generally too few to achieve sufficient statistical power for the quantification of the risk (Rosenberg et al 1987, Savitz et al 1989). A retrospective case control study of over 1000 perinatal deaths in Leicester between 1976 and 1982 showed that leather workers were at increased risk of perinatal deaths, particularly from congenital malformations and macerated stillbirths, compared with other manual workers in the same class (Clarke & Mason 1985). The effect of occupational hazards on perinatal mortality may also be mediated through an increased risk of prematurity or low birthweight, both of which have a major influence on the risk of a baby dying. One study has shown a dose-related association between blood lead and risk of preterm delivery (McMichael et al 1986). The risk of preterm delivery and low birthweight was shown to be over 50% higher in the children of women who worked with electrical, metal or leather goods than in other female manual workers and it was more frequent in the children of mothers and fathers employed in manual rather than non-manual jobs in a large study in Scotland between 1981 and 1984 (Sanjose et al 1991).

In utero environment

The effects on the fetus of maternal smoking have been intensively studied and include abnormal placentation (Christianson 1979) and fetal growth restriction (Naeye 1978). The actual contribution made by maternal smoking to the risk of perinatal death is not direct but it appears to depend on the presence of other adverse factors, as smoking reduces fetal growth rate and therefore potentiates other detrimental influences. However, its importance even in a low-risk population is shown by the estimate that, in England and Wales in 1984, 18% of babies of low birthweight were attributable to maternal smoking (Simpson & Armand Smith 1986).

The role of undernutrition and specific dietary constituents is still uncertain (Naismith 1981) but will also vary with the underlying health of the mother.

Complications specific to pregnancy

Hypertension in pregnancy is not only potentially dangerous for the mother (Report on Confidential Enquiries into Maternal Deaths in the UK 1988–90) but it is associated with changes to placental bed blood vessels with a consequent reduction in blood flow and fetal growth restriction. It may also lead to prematurity, either by elective or spontaneous

preterm delivery. Urinary tract infections can also predispose to preterm labour, as may infections of the amniotic sac (Peckham & Marshall 1983).

FETAL GROWTH AND MATURITY

Birthweight is the best predictor of perinatal mortality. ONS statistics for England and Wales in 1996 show that 70% of perinatal deaths occurred in the 7.6% of babies who weighed less than 2500 g at birth. Fifty-three per cent of perinatal deaths occurred in the 1.5% of babies who weighed less than 1500 g at birth.

Most of the factors which contribute to perinatal death do so by influencing fetal growth rate, gestational age or both. The size of any baby is influenced by genetic factors (including the presence of congenital malformations and maternal height and weight), birth order, and ethnic group (Thomson 1983). These are all closely associated with socioeconomic status, as is risk of exposure to environmental health hazards, such as those at work, and personal health behaviour, such as smoking. All these factors produce very robust birthweight distributions which change only slowly with time. There has been virtually no change in the birthweight distribution in England and Wales between 1983 and 1998. The fall in mortality over these years is not caused by a decrease in the proportion of LBW babies, but in improved survival rates, especially in LBW and VLBW babies. However, there is much debate as to whether there are limits to the gestational age and birthweight below which aggressive resuscitation and active treatment should not be instituted, as there is considerable short- and long-term morbidity in survivors (Walker & Patel 1987, Allen et al 1993). The cut-off in improved survival appears to be at 25 weeks' gestation and 750 g birthweight (Hack & Fanaroff 1989).

Growth-restricted babies are at higher risk of perinatal mortality. A study in Sweden showed that growth-restricted babies had four times the PNMR of the general population, even after deaths resulting from congenital malformations were excluded (Wennergren et al 1988). In Ontario, preterm growth-restricted babies had a PNMR of 180 per 1000 (Fitzhardinge & Inwood 1989) and in Baltimore, 86% of perinatal deaths occurred in growth-restricted babies (Callan & Witter 1990).

Intrauterine growth restriction is also associated with an increased risk of perinatal death not only through its link with low birthweight but also through an increased association with major congenital abnormalities. Studies report a birth prevalence of 4.6% to 11% (Butler 1974, Wennergren et al 1988) in small for gestational age (SGA) infants and 31.6% in SGA infants under 1500 g birthweight (Drillien 1974).

DEMOGRAPHIC FACTORS

Some demographic factors will affect overall birthweight distribution, mainly by subtly influencing the birthweight distribution. This includes the proportion of multiple births, as the median birthweight is lower (2960 g at 40 weeks compared with 3480 g for singletons) and the birthweight distribution for multiple births considerably to the left of that for singletons. Even small increases in multiple birth rates will increase the incidence of low birthweight. Increasing use of modern infertility treatments has caused multiple pregnancy rates to rise dramatically since the introduction of *in vitro* fertilisation. In 1980, there were 9.8 multiple pregnancies per 1000 maternities. By 1990, this had risen to 11.6 and by 1998, to 14.4 per 1000. Although birthweight-specific mortality rates for multiple births are lower than those for singletons this does not compensate for their disadvantageous weight distribution.

The distribution of birthweight is also shifted to the left in primiparity and in disadvantaged socioeconomic conditions. There is still great disparity between the PNMR in different social classes in Britain (Fig. 47.3), although the increasing

proportion of babies born to unmarried women has meant that illegitimate babies are now less disadvantaged at birth than they were. Figure 47.4 shows the social class distribution of live births, which is relatively static. Although illegitimate births are increasing, the proportion of births registered solely by the mother is still small but increasing slightly. Hellier (1977) showed that almost a quarter of the reduction in PNMR that occurred in England and Wales between 1953 and 1978 was explained by the demographic changes in maternal age, parity and social class that had occurred.

Babies of women from minority ethnic groups have a higher risk of perinatal death than babies born to indigenous mothers. Routinely collected national statistics do not include the ethnic group of the mother but can be analysed by country of birth although this then aggregates second and subsequent generations of ethnic minority women born in the UK with the White European population). Women born abroad but having their babies in England and Wales in 1996 lost a higher proportion of babies than women born in England and Wales, with perinatal mortality rates of 11.3 per 1000 for women born in India, and 15.8 for women born in Pakistan compared to 8.2 for women born in the United Kingdom (ONS 1997). A minor part may be a result of a difference in birthweight distributions, but the incidence of malformations is also very different. The increased incidence of lethal congenital malformations in British Pakistanis made a large contribution to their perinatal mortality rate of 18 per 1000 in 1984, compared with 12 per 1000 in other ethnic groups: a 50% excess (Balarajan & Botting 1989, Chitty & Winter 1989). Access to and use of maternity services may also affect outcome (Clarke et al 1988).

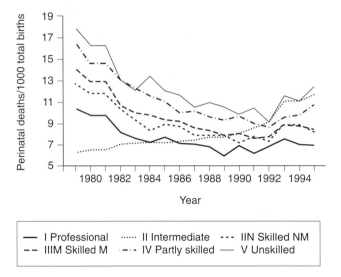

Fig. 47.3 Perinatal mortality by father's social class 1979–1995. Source: ONS Mortality statistics, DH3 series. (The upturn from 1992 results from the change in the definition of stillbirth.)

Cross-sectional and longitudinal birth data

A PNMR is usually calculated from cross-sectional information on the occurrence and rate of perinatal deaths in a given period, usually over a year, so that data do not follow a cohort of women through their reproductive careers. This is

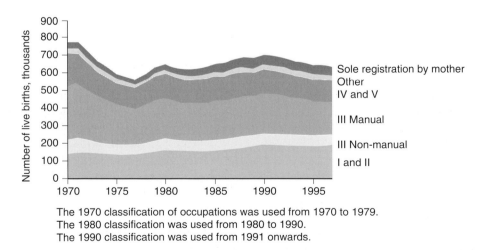

The 1970 classification of occupations was used from 1970 to 1979.
The 1980 classification was used from 1980 to 1990.
The 1990 classification was used from 1991 onwards.

Source: Office for National Statistics Birth Statistics, Series FMI

Fig. 47.4 Numbers of live births by social class of father England and Wales, 1970–1997.

misleading; analysis of data on births and deaths within sibships to the same mother presents different demographic patterns associated with low birthweight and perinatal death, particularly in regard to parity (Roman et al 1978, Bakketeig & Hoffman 1979, 1981). Cross-sectional data suggest a U- or J-shaped pattern of risk with parity, with risk being high in primiparous women, falling in the second pregnancy and then rising with each subsequent pregnancy. Longitudinal studies show that within sibships, average risk seems to fall steadily with increasing parity, with highest risks at all parities in the largest sibships. This may be caused by overrepresentation of highly parous mothers whose previous pregnancies had ended in a miscarriage, fetal or infant death.

Longitudinal studies can also examine the effects of birth interval—close spacing of pregnancy may contribute to an increased risk of perinatal death and there is also a tendency for repeated perinatal death in the same mothers.

ARE PERINATAL MORTALITY RATES A MEASURE OF MATERNITY AND NEONATAL CARE?

There are several factors that make the continued use of a PNMR as a measure of the effectiveness of maternity and neonatal care increasingly unsafe.

Perinatal rates include only deaths in the first week of life. Many babies who would previously have died within this period are now surviving into the late neonatal period, thanks to improved paediatric care, but they still die. There is a strong case for including late neonatal deaths in analyses of deaths occurring around the time of delivery to prevent the postponement of death from artificially lowering perinatal rates.

Place of delivery of premature babies of less than 28 weeks' gestation (on the delivery suite or on a gynaecology ward) may affect classification and hence, figures for perinatal mortality (Fenton et al 1990). The onus of judgement regarding viability and classification is often placed on relatively junior staff. There is a theoretical possibility that there may be pressure on clinical staff to regard a fetus as non-registrable if the clinical performance of their unit is judged on its crude PNMR alone.

Crude comparisons of perinatal mortality, either by hospital or by district of residence, can be highly misleading because of the problems caused by statistics involving very small numbers in numerator data and large denominators—are the figures a result of random variation? Increasingly small numbers and rates of deaths have led ONS to publish rates for combined 3-year periods with 95% and 99% confidence limits to give some idea of the reliability of the crude figure.

Low and very low birthweights are such strong determinants of perinatal survival that any maternity hospital with a neonatal unit, especially one which takes tertiary referrals, will have a high crude perinatal mortality rate simply because of the types of cases it cares for. Evaluating its services on this basis is akin to castigating a geriatric hospital because of its high numbers of deaths—units looking after

high-risk patients have high death rates. Some effort should be made to adjust the PNMR for case mix and referral patterns to get a meaningful result (Clarke et al 1993). Calculating birthweight-specific perinatal rates may help (see Table 47.2), although numbers at individual hospitals will again be very small. Even when this is done, it is difficult to compare the effectiveness of hospital units using PNMR because of the increasingly small subset of perinatal deaths that are amenable to medical intervention (Field et al 1988).

Other outcome or risk assessment scores may be much more useful. Reliable assessment of neonatal care is impossible without correcting for major risk factors, particularly initial disease severity (Tarnow-Modi et al 1990). One robust method of assessing initial neonatal risk, which is more predictive of outcome than birthweight alone, is the clinical risk index for babies (CRIB) score (International Neonatal Network 1993). This includes birthweight, gestational age, congenital malformations, maximum base excess in the first 12 hours, and minimum and maximum appropriate fraction of inspired oxygen in the first 12 hours. On the obstetric side, Buekens (1990) describes six outcome measures influenced by process of care and its quality: maternal and perinatal mortalities, postpartum haemorrhage, the sequelae of obstructed labour, Apgar scores and very early neonatal seizures.

Table 47.2 Birthweight-specific perinatal mortality rates per 1000 total births in England & Wales 1993–1997 (Source: ONS DH3 monitors)

Birthweight group (g)	1993	1994	1995	1996	1997
<1500	319.9	310.6	301.8	306.9	293.3
1500–1999	59.5	55.2	52.9	49.8	50.4
2000–2499	18.6	18.1	17.7	16.4	17.4
2500–2999	5.5	5.5	5.3	5.4	4.9
3000–3499	2.4	2.4	2.4	2.2	2.1
>3500	1.7	2.0	2.2	1.6	1.6
Not stated	28.5	26.2	58.5	81.9	122.1

CONCLUSIONS

While all perinatal deaths are tragic and should not be dismissed lightly, there is concern that death may be preferable to severe long-term impairment and anxiety about the quality of life for some very small babies who would have become part of the perinatal mortality statistics if modern technology had not been used to save them. It is important that in the future as much attention is paid to morbidity arising in the antenatal and perinatal period as has been paid to perinatal mortality in the past.

ACKNOWLEDGEMENTS

We wish to thank Alison Macfarlane from the National Perinatal Epidemiology Unit and Mary Macintosh from CESDI for providing statistics.

REFERENCES

Alberman E, Botting B, Blatchley N, Twidell A 1994 A new hierarchical classification of causes of infant deaths in England and Wales. Arch Dis Child 70:403–409

Allen MC, Donohoe PK, Dusman AE 1993 The limit of viability—neonatal outcome of infants born at 22 to 25 weeks' gestation. N Engl J Med 329:1597–1601

Baird D, Walker J, Thomson AM 1954 The causes and prevention of stillbirths and first week deaths. J Obstet Gynaecol Br Empire 61:433–448

Bakketeig LS, Hoffman HJ 1979 Perinatal mortality by birth order within cohorts based on sibship size. Br Med J 2:693–696

Bakketeig LS, Hoffman HJ 1981 Epidemiology of preterm birth. In: Elder MG, Hendricks CH (eds) Results from a longitudinal study of births in Norway in preterm labour. Butterworths, London

Balarajan R, Botting B 1989 Perinatal mortality in England and Wales: variations by mother's country of birth (1982–1985). Health Trends 21:79–84

Black N, Macfarlane A 1982 Methodological kit: monitoring mortality statistics in a health district. Community Med 4:25–33

Bucher HC, Schmidt JG 1993 Does routine ultrasound scanning improve outcome in pregnancy? Meta-analysis of various outcome measures. Br Med J 307:13–17

Buekens P 1990 Outcome measures of obstetrical and perinatal care. Qual Assur Health Care 2:253–262

Butler NR 1967 Causes and prevention of perinatal mortality. WHO Chronicle 21:43–61

Butler NR 1974 Late postnatal consequences of fetal malnutrition. Current Concepts in Nutrition 2:173–178

Butler NR, Alberman ED (eds) 1969 Perinatal Problems: The Second Report of the 1958 British Perinatal Mortality Survey. Livingstone, Edinburgh

Butler NR, Bonham DG 1963 Perinatal Mortality. The First Report of the 1958 British Perinatal Mortality Survey. Livingstone, Edinburgh

Callan NA, Witter FR 1990 Intrauterine growth retardation: characteristics, risk factors and gestational age. Int J Gynecol Obstet 33:215–220

Chalmers I 1979 Desirability and Feasibility of a 4th National Perinatal Survey: report submitted to the Children's and Reproductive Research Liaison Group's Research Division of the DHSS. National Perinatal Epidemiology Unit

Chalmers I, McIlwaine G (eds) 1980 Perinatal audit and surveillance. Proceedings of the 8th study group. RCOG, London

Chamberlain G 1980 Background to better perinatal health. Lancet i:1–7

Chamberlain R, Chamberlain G, Howlett B, Claireaux A 1975 The first week of life. British births 1970, vol 1. Heinemann Medical, London

Chitty LS, Winter RM 1989 Perinatal mortality in different ethnic groups. Arch Dis Child 64:1036–1041

Christianson RE 1979 Gross difference observed in the placentas of smokers and non-smokers. Am J Epidemiol 110:178–187

Clarke M 1982 Perinatal audit: a tried and tested epidemiological method. Community Med 4:104–107

Clarke M, Mason ES 1985 Leatherwork: a possible hazard to reproduction. Br Med J 290:1235–1237

Clarke M, Clayton DG, Mason ES, MacVicar J 1988 Asian mothers' risk factors for perinatal death—the same or different? A ten year review of Leicestershire perinatal deaths. Br Med J 297:384–387

Clarke M, Mason ES, MacVicar J, Clayton DG 1993 Evaluating perinatal mortality rates: effects of referral and case mix. Br Med J 306:824–827

Coggon D, Rose R, Barker DJP 1993 Epidemiology for the uninitiated. BMJ Publishing Group, London

Cole SK, Hey EN, Thomson AM 1986 Classifying perinatal death: an obstetric approach. Br J Obstet Gynaecol 93:1204–1212

Committee on Child Health Services 1976 Fit for the future. Cmnd 6684 (Court report). HMSO, London

Confidential Enquiry into Stillbirths and Deaths in Infancy 1997. 4th Annual report, 1 January–31 December 1995. Maternal and Child Health Research Consortium, London

Confidential Enquiry into Stillbirths and Deaths in Infancy 1998 5th Annual report Maternal and Child Health Research Consortium, London

Confidential Enquiry into Stillbirths and Deaths in Infancy 1999. 6th Annual report Maternal and Child Health Research Consortium, London

Confidential Enquiry into Stillbirths and Deaths in Infancy 2000. 7th Annual report Maternal and Child Health Research Consortium, London

Czeizel AE 1993 Prevention of congenital abnormalities by periconceptional multivitamin supplementation. Br Med J 306:1645–1648

Czeizel AE, Dudas I 1992 Prevention of the first occurrence of neural tube defects by periconceptional vitamin supplementation. N Engl J Med 327:1832–1835

Drillien CM 1974 Prenatal and perinatal factors in etiology and outcome of low birthweight. Clin Perinatal 1:197–211

Emanuel I, Filakati H, Alberman E, Evans SJW 1992 Intergenerational studies of human birthweight from the 1958 birth cohort. 1. Evidence for a multigenerational effect. Br J Obstet Gynaecol 99:67–74

Enkin M, Keirse JNC, Chalmers I 1989 A guide to effective care in pregnancy and childbirth. Oxford University Press, Oxford

Ewigman BG, Crane JP, Frigoletto FD, Lefevre ML, Bain RP, McNellis D 1993 Effect of ultrasound screening on perinatal outcome. N Engl J Med 329:821–827

Fenton AC, Field DJ, Mason E, Clarke M 1990 Attitudes to viability of preterm infants and their effect on figures for perinatal mortality. Br Med J 300:434–436

Field DJ, Smith H, Mason E, Milner AD 1988 Is perinatal mortality a good indicator of perinatal care? Paediatr Perinat Epidemiol 2:213–219

Fitzhardinge PM, Inwood S 1989 Long term growth in small for date children. Acta Paediatr Suppl 349:27–33

Fleming P, Blair P, Bacon C, Berry J 2000. Sudden unexpected deaths in infancy; The CESDI SUDI Studies 1993–96. The Stationery Office, London

Hack MH, Fanaroff AA 1989 Outcomes of extremely low birth weight infants between 1982 and 1988. N Engl J Med 321:1642–1647

Heady JA, Heasman MA 1959 Social and biological factors in infant mortality. Studies on medical and population subjects No 15. HMSO, London

Hellier J 1977 Perinatal mortality 1950 and 1973. Population Trends 10:13–15

Information and Statistics Division, 1994 The National Health Service in Scotland. Scottish Stillbirth and Neonatal Death Report 1993. Common Services Agency, ISD Publications, Edinburgh

International Neonatal Network 1993 The CRIB (clinical risk index for babies) score: a tool for assessing initial neonatal risk and comparing performance for neonatal intensive care units. Lancet 342:193–198

Joint Committee of the RCOG and the Population Investigation Committee 1948 Maternity in Great Britain. Oxford University Press, London

Keirse MJNC 1984 Perinatal mortality rates do not contain what they purport to contain. Lancet i:1166–1169

Lubchenco LO, Hansman C, Dressler M, Boyd E 1963 Intrauterine growth as estimated from liveborn birthweight data at 24 to 42 weeks of gestation. Pediatrics 32:793–800

Macfarlane A, Mugford M 2000 Birth counts: statistics of pregnancy and childbirth. The Stationery Office, London

Maternal and Child Health Research Consortium 2000 Confidential Enquiry into Stillbirths and Deaths in Infancy 7th Annual report, London

McMichael AJ, Vimpani GV, Robertson EF, Baghurst PA, Clark PD 1986 The Port Pirie cohort study: maternal blood lead and pregnancy outcome. J Epidemiol Community Health 40:18–25

McIlwaine GM, Howat RCL, Dunn F, MacNaughton MC 1979 The Scottish Perinatal Mortality Survey. Br Med J 2:1103–1106

Mersey Region Working Party on Perinatal Mortality 1982

Confidential inquiry into perinatal deaths in the Mersey region. Lancet i:491–494

MRC Vitamin Study Research Group 1991 Prevention of neural tube defects: results of the Medical Research Council Vitamin Study. Lancet 338:131–137

Mutch LMM, Brown NJ, Spiedel BD, Dunn PM 1981 Perinatal mortality and neonatal survival in Avon: 1976–79. Br Med J 282:119–122

Naeye R 1978 Effects of maternal cigarette smoking on the fetus and placentae. British J Obstet Gynaecol 83:732–737

Naismith DJ 1981 Diet during pregnancy—a rationale for prescription. In: Dobbing J (ed) Maternal nutrition in pregnancy. Eating for two? Academic Press, London, pp 21–40

Nissel M 1987 People count; a history of the General Register Office. HMSO, London

ONS 1997 Stillbirths and infant mortality by mother's country of birth, England and Wales, 1996 ONS Monitor DH3 97/3. HMSO, London

OPCS 1990 Mortality statistics. Perinatal and infant: social and biological factors. Review of the Registrar General on Deaths in England and Wales, 1990. Series DH3 No 3. HMSO, London

OPCS 1991 Annual reference volume Series DH6 No 5. Mortality statistics in childhood. HMSO, London

OPCS 1993 Population trends no 74. HMSO, London

Paediatric Research Unit, Royal Devon and Exeter Hospital 1973 A suggested model for inquiries into perinatal and early childhood deaths in a health care district. Children's Research Fund Report

Peckham CS, Marshall WC 1983 Infections in pregnancy. In: Barron SL, Thomson AM (eds) Obstetrical epidemiology. Academic Press, London, pp 209–262

Peller S 1948 Mortality past and future. Popul Stud 1:405–456

RCOG Multidisciplinary Working Group 1992 Prenatal screening for toxoplasmosis in the United Kingdom. RCOG, London

Report on Confidential Enquiries into Maternal Deaths in the UK 1988–90 1994. HMSO, London

Roman E, Doyle P, Beral V, Alberman E, Pharoah P 1978 Fetal loss, gravidity and pregnancy order. Early Hum Dev 2:131–138

Rosenberg MJ, Feldblum PJ, Marshall EG 1987 Occupational influences on reproduction: a review of the recent literature. J Occup Med 29:584–591

Saari-Kemppainen A, Karjalainen O, Ylostalo P, Heinonen OP 1990 Ultrasound screening and perinatal mortality: controlled trial of systematic one-stage screening in pregnancy. Lancet 336:387–391

Sanjose S, Roman E, Beral V 1991 Low birthweight and preterm delivery, Scotland, 1981–1984: effect of parents' occupation. Lancet 338:428–431

Savitz DA, Whelan EA, Kleckner RC 1989 Effect of parents' occupational exposures on risk of stillbirths, preterm delivery, and small for gestational age infants. Am J Epidemiol 129:1201–1218

Shaw CD 1980 Aspects of audit. Br Med J 1:1256

Simpson RJ, Armand Smith NG 1986 Maternal smoking and low birthweight: implications for antenatal care. J Epidemiol Community Health 40:223–227

Tarnow-Modi W, Ogston S, Wilkinson AR et al 1990 Predicting death from initial disease severity in very low birthweight infants: a method for comparing the performance of neonatal units. Br Med J 300:1611–1614

Thomson AM 1983 Fetal growth and size at birth. In: Barron SL, Thomson AM (eds) Obstetrical epidemiology. Academic Press, London, pp 89–142

Walker EM, Patel NB 1987 Mortality and morbidity in infants born between 20 and 28 weeks gestation. Br J Obstet Gynaecol 94:670–674

Wennergren M, Wennergren G, Vilbergsson G 1988 Obstetric characteristics and neonatal performance in a four-year small for gestational age population. Obstet Gynaecol 72:615–620

Wigglesworth JS 1980 Monitoring perinatal mortality—a pathological approach. Lancet ii: 684–686

Wood B, Catford JC, Cogswell JJ 1984 Confidential paediatric enquiry into neonatal deaths in Wessex, 1981 and 1982. Br Med J 288:1206–1208

World Health Organization 1977 Manual of the international statistical classification of diseases, injuries and causes of death, vol 1. WHO, Geneva

48

Maternal mortality

Geoffrey Chamberlain

INTRODUCTION

Today, both maternal and perinatal deaths are rare in the developed world so that standards of obstetric care cannot be measured in terms of mortality rate; these measures are, however, still used where more deaths occur, in developing countries. Until the 1930s, the maternal mortality rate (MMR) was the dominant statistic. The downward trend in death rates from other causes in Britain between the second half of the nineteenth century and the mid 1930s is well known. Figure 48.1 shows the death rate from all causes in women aged 15–44 in England and Wales between 1838 and 1993. It illustrates the steady reduction in death rate, interrupted only by the influenza epidemic of 1920. It is now generally agreed that this decline was largely the result of improvements in social and economic conditions, primarily in hygiene and nutrition, as well as in medical care.

If social and economic improvements were responsible for the fall in the general death rate, the same factors should have produced a fall in MMR. In fact, as Loudon (1987) points out, the fall in maternal deaths should have been even steeper because of advances in obstetric care including antisepsis and asepsis in the 1870s and 1880s; caesarean section soon became a safe technique for some obstetric emergencies. The growing recognition of the importance of antenatal care after 1900 and the improved organisation of the specialty of obstetrics and gynaecology in the 1920s and 1930s together with higher standards of specialist care associated with improvements in the teaching of obstetrics and midwifery to the professionals, should all have led to a fall in maternal mortality—they did not.

Maternal deaths were defined as those occurring in pregnancy, labour or the lying-in period. The latter was not clearly defined before the mid nineteenth century, and some very late deaths were included in reports. It became conven-

tional for registration purposes that the lying-in period lasted 6 months from birth. Maternal deaths used to be classified as puerperal or associated deaths. Puerperal deaths resulted from either puerperal fever (puerperal sepsis) or accidents of childbirth, the latter representing all other deaths, dominated by haemorrhage and toxaemia.

Despite the downward trend in deaths from all other causes shown in Figure 48.1 and the seeming improvements in maternity care, maternal mortality paradoxically did not fall. Instead, it remained on a plateau from the 1850s to the mid 1930s. Figure 48.2 shows the quinquennial MMR in England and Wales between 1850 and 1996. The persisting high MMR became a public and political scandal by the 1920s. It was not confined to England and Wales, for the same trends were seen in Europe, and the rates were even higher in the USA. Even in the Netherlands and Scandinavia,

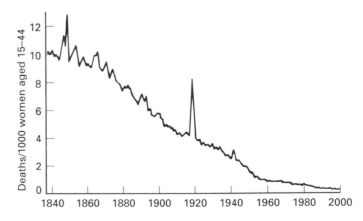

Fig. 48.1   Death rates from all causes in women aged 15–44 in England and Wales from 1838 to 2000.

741

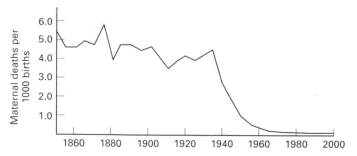

Fig. 48.2 Maternal mortality in England and Wales. Quinquennial rates per 1000 births from 1850 to 1996.

where maternal mortality had always been lower than in Britain, the rates stayed level rather than falling. The trends in maternal mortality over these years and the factors which predisposed to the lack of improvement have been reviewed by Loudon (1992).

In England and Wales, maternal mortality finally began to drop in the 1930s and, when it did, the fall was sudden, profound and sustained, continuing to the present time. There have been few more remarkable statistical changes during the twentieth century. At about the same time the fall occurred in all the developed countries of Western Europe and the USA. There is little doubt that this change was first initiated by the introduction of sulphonamides for the treatment of puerperal infection but after the first few years, this cannot have been the only explanation; other probable factors in the UK include:

- the introduction of the National Blood Transfusion Service
- improved training of doctors and midwives
- improved regulation of obstetrics and midwifery by the respective colleges
- improvement in nutrition and general health of the population.

Figure 48.3 shows the importance of the reduction in deaths from puerperal fever in the overall fall in MMR after 1934. There was little reduction in deaths from accidents of

childbirth between 1911 and 1934, after which a gradual fall began. By contrast, deaths from puerperal fever showed more variation, with peaks of high mortality in 1920, 1930 and 1934, and low rates in 1913 and 1918. After 1934, the reduction in deaths from puerperal fever was rapid, accounting for 78% of the total reduction in maternal deaths in England and Wales between 1934 and 1940. Loudon (1987) argues convincingly that sulphonamides were generally available, widely used and known to be effective by late 1937. The possibility of a simultaneous decline in streptococcal virulence was suggested by several experienced observers, notably Colebrooke (Colebrooke & Kenny 1936), but nevertheless the improvement was caused mainly by the introduction of sulphonamides. The first year with a notable fall in maternal mortality was 1937. From 1940, penicillin and blood transfusion played increasingly important roles in lowering maternal mortality and tended to eclipse the early but vital contribution of the sulphonamides (Fig. 48.3). The persistently high maternal mortality was also partly attributable to poor obstetric care, resulting from poor training or poor clinical application, as well as to social and economic deprivation which adversely influenced the health of the mother and her ability to withstand the stresses of pregnancy and birth. Poor obstetric care was probably the more important: 'Maternal mortality appears to be remarkably resistant to the ill effects of social and economic deprivation, but remarkably sensitive to the good and bad effects of medical intervention' (Loudon 1986).

Between the mid nineteenth century and the 1930s, maternal mortality tended to be higher in the middle and upper social classes than in the working classes. Most births took place at home under the care of midwives or general practitioners, there being a strong association between social class and attendance of doctors. For first pregnancies, 82% of the wives of professional or salaried workers were delivered by doctors, compared with only 35% of the wives of manual workers. These data are from a study conducted by the Population Investigation Committee in 1948; the difference was probably even greater in the 1920s and 1930s. As the vast majority of births were domiciliary, the outcome of home delivery was largely responsible for the national level of maternal mortality.

Excessive obstetric intervention

In the second half of the nineteenth century there was a profound change in obstetric practice. During the preceding 80 or 90 years, practice had been extremely conservative. From the 1870s, however, obstetricians, especially those in general practice, began to intervene in normal labour to an astonishing extent. They took their lead from those who advocated the active use of forceps delivery, usually under general anaesthesia. From the end of the nineteenth century, forceps delivery under chloroform or anaesthesia was used extensively in domiciliary deliveries. This was justified on the grounds that modern women should not be expected to bear the pains of normal labour. There was also widespread disregard of antiseptic practice and little interest in antenatal care.

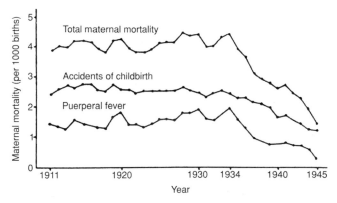

Fig. 48.3 Total maternal morbidity and mortality from puerperal fever and accidents of childbirth in England and Wales from 1911 to 1945. (From Loudon 1987 with permission.)

By contrast, extremely good results were often reported in home confinements conducted by midwives trained by charities. The poor of the great cities were delivered by midwives. The Liverpool Ladies' Charity, for example, reported an MMR of 1.3 per 1000 in over 6000 deliveries, undertaken in the poorest homes in the city (Bickerton 1936). Such good results would have been unlikely if socioeconomic deprivation was a major cause of high maternal mortality.

Important evidence for the significance of good obstetric care came from the Rochdale experiment of the early 1930s. When Dr Andrew Topping was appointed Medical Officer of Health to Rochdale in 1930, the city had the highest maternal mortality in the country, just under 9 per 1000 births. By vigorous reformation of the maternity services, but with no alteration to the diet or living conditions of the poor, the MMR was reduced to 1.7 per 1000 births by 1935, showing that here obstetric care was the decisive factor. The measures introduced were simple. Publicity, with the help of the press, led to a high attendance rate at specially established antenatal clinics; general practitioners were alerted to the serious hazards of interference in labour. Good cooperation was established between midwives, general practitioners and a consultant, recruited especially from Manchester. A puerperal fever ward was opened. When the Rochdale experiment was reviewed (Oxley et al 1935), the previously high MMR could not be attributed to economic disabilities; it had been caused to a greater extent by obstetrical factors working on specific conditions which in many instances had proved preventable.

It would be a mistake, however, to conclude that poverty and malnutrition do not influence maternal mortality. The lesson of the period between 1850 and 1930 is that the persistence of a high MMR resulted from poor obstetric care, with excessive intervention (usually forceps) by poorly trained general practitioner obstetricians at home confinements. In this situation, the better-off who could afford a general practitioner fared worse than the poor, who were looked after by a midwife whose care was likely to be less interventionist. Obstetric care has improved a great deal over the past 50 years and analysis nowadays demonstrates the expected trend, with MMR being lower in social classes I and II and higher in IV and V (Confidential Enquiries into Maternal Deaths 1979–1981).

CONFIDENTIAL MEDICAL ENQUIRY INTO INDIVIDUAL MATERNAL DEATHS

Although the MMR did not begin to fall significantly until 1937, an organisation for recording and publicising the causation of maternal deaths in England and Wales was originally set up in 1928 by the Minister of Health, Neville Chamberlain, when he established a Departmental Committee on Maternal Mortality and Morbidity. In that year alone there were 2920 maternal deaths in relation to 660 267 live births, an MMR of 4.42 per 1000 births or 442 per 100 000. In 1930, the Departmental Committee tried to find a primary avoidable factor in maternal death in its

interim report, published in 1932. The investigation covered 5800 cases and proved so valuable that Medical Officers of Health were asked to continue the enquiries, submitting their confidential reports to the Chief Medical Officer of the Ministry of Health. Summaries of the enquiries appeared in successive annual reports on the State of the Public Health. A primary avoidable factor was considered to be present in 46% of the cases investigated in the first report, and the proportion with avoidable factors altered very little in subsequent years.

The number of deaths diminished markedly from 1937. The diminishing urgency of maternal mortality, combined with other problems during the war years, led to enquiries being conducted in a decreasing proportion of registered maternal deaths. By 1951, reports were received for only about 60% of known deaths. New methods were clearly needed to study preventability in the smaller number of deaths then occurring.

In 1949, maternal mortality was the subject of a discussion at the 12th British Congress on Obstetrics and Gynaecology and reference was made to a method of enquiry sometimes used in the USA—investigation by a local committee of experts, publication of case reports and comments in medical journals. The president of the congress, Sir Eardley Holland, suggested to the Minister of Health the possibility of adopting a similar method in this country. Consultations followed with the Royal College of Obstetricians and Gynaecologists and the Society of Medical Officers of Health, resulting in the adoption of a new system of enquiry involving the family doctor, the Medical Officer of Health, the midwife and the consultant obstetrician. These Confidential Enquiries into Maternal Deaths (CEMD) commenced in 1952 and the findings of the first triennial report (1952–1954) were published in 1957 by Her Majesty's Stationery Office. Triennial reports on these confidential enquiries have been published for the 14 triennia since then. That for 1982–1984 was the last for England and Wales, because reports from 1985 have been published on a UK basis. Previously, Scotland had produced a quinquennial report and Northern Ireland a decennial report.

CEMD in England and Wales from 1952 to 1996

These 14 confidential enquiries have provided an unique monitoring system for maternal mortality during the past 45 years in England and Wales; the latest reports incorporate data from the whole of the UK (England, Wales, Scotland and Northern Ireland). While studies of maternal mortality have been published in many countries, for example by Högberg (1985) on maternal mortality in Sweden, there is no continuing national surveillance organisation for the detailed investigation of every maternal death in any country outside the UK.

Constant rate of fall in maternal mortality

Figure 48.4 is similar to the graph of maternal mortality shown in Figure 48.1, but based on annual rather than quinquennial rates between 1847 and 1982. Figure 48.4 appears to indicate that the main fall in maternal mortality began in 1937 and was at first extremely rapid, particularly

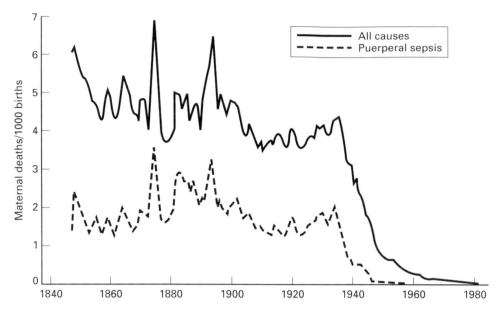

Fig. 48.4 Maternal mortality in England and Wales from 1847 to 1982. (From Confidential Enquiries into Maternal Deaths in England and Wales 1982–1984.)

during the war years and immediately afterwards. When the CEMD commenced in 1952, the death rate was only a fraction of what it had been in 1937 and the fall between 1952 and 1984 looks relatively insignificant. However, such a graph is unduly influenced by the very large number of deaths in the earlier years which must have been potentially avoidable by relatively minor improvements in care. As triennia pass and the MMR falls even lower, the number of potentially avoidable deaths inevitably becomes smaller so that in the latest enquiry covering the years 1994–1996 there were only 268 maternal deaths in the UK among 2 197 640 maternities—a rate of 9 per 100 000 maternities (Fig. 48.5).

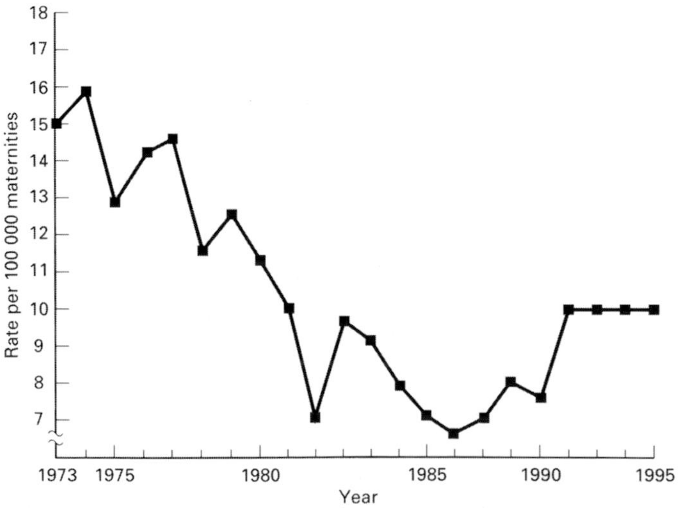

To avoid the bias resulting from the larger number of deaths in earlier years, the changing MMR may be expressed on a semi-logarithmic scale. Figure 48.6 shows MMR

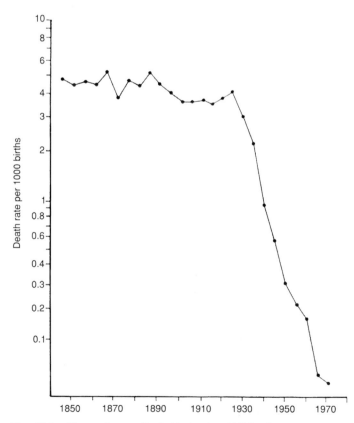

Fig. 48.5 The maternal mortality rate per 100 000 maternities, UK 1973–1996. (Source: Confidential Enquiry into Maternal Deaths in England and Wales 1988–1990.)

Fig. 48.6 Maternal mortality in England and Wales from 1850 to 1970. Quinquennial rates per 1000 births; semilogarithmic graph. (From Loudon 1986 with permission.)

between 1850 and 1970 expressed in this way and reveals that the rate of reduction in MMR has been maintained between 1937 and 1970. In other words, since the MMR first began to fall in England and Wales, the rate of improvement has been constant, approximately halving every 10 years. From over 4000 per million in 1937, the rate has fallen to 122 per million maternities by 1994–1996, so that after almost 50 years MMR has fallen to one-fiftieth of its original level.

The method for conducting the CEMD

Enquiry into known or suspected maternal deaths used to be initiated by the Medical Officer of Health of the town or district. With reorganisation of the National Health Service, this post became that of Area Medical Officer and, in turn, District Medical Officer and then Director of Public Health Services. The enquiry from (MCW97), which has been modified, developed and expanded over the years, is sent to all health staff concerned in the care of the woman— the midwife, general practitioner, health visitor, community physician, consultant obstetrician and any other individual professional involved in the death. Every possible attempt is also made to obtain details of autopsy, including histology.

When all the available local information has been collected, the Consultant in Public Health forwards the partially completed form to the Regional Obstetric Assessor, a senior consultant obstetrician in the region who has been appointed by the Chief Medical Officer. The Regional Anaesthetic Assessor also reviews the enquiry forms of women who have had an anaesthetic. While there have been Regional Assessors in Obstetrics and Anaesthetics since the earliest years of the CEMD, it was only in 1981 that Regional Pathology Assessors joined the team. They also review the MCW97 forms and add their comments and opinions about the autopsy findings. Regional Assessors in Midwifery were later appointed to review any features relevant to midwifery.

The MCW97 form is then sent to the Chief Medical Officer at the Department of Health. The Department's Central Assessors in Obstetrics and Gynaecology, Anaesthetics and Pathology review all facts recorded in each case and act as final arbiters in assessing the main cause of death, any contributing factors and whether or not care was of an acceptable standard. Strict confidentiality is observed at all stages of the CEMD. The identity of the patient is erased from all forms so that the opinion of assessors cannot be related to a named individual. After the completion of and before the publication of each triennial report, all MCW97 forms are destroyed.

For each death, a single main cause is allotted and classified according to the WHO *Manual of the International Classification of Diseases, Injuries and Causes of Death*, 10th revision (ICD 10) (1992). Although deaths are assigned to one main cause, they may be referred to in other chapters; thus, a death assigned to hypertensive diseases of pregnancy, in which haemorrhage and anaesthesia also played a part, might be mentioned in all three chapters, but would only be counted as a death from hypertensive diseases.

KEY POINTS: MECHANISMS OF THE CONFIDENTIAL ENQUIRY INTO MATERNAL DEATH IN THE UK

- Local Director of Public Health Service (DPHS) issues form (MCW97) to doctor or midwife concerned with care of mother.
- Form completed and returned to DPHS.
- After checking, DPHS sends completed form to a Regional Obstetric Assessor (ROA).
- ROA checks it and, if relevant, sends form in turn to Regional Anaesthetic Adviser, Regional Pathological Adviser and Regional Midwifery Adviser.
- MCW97 returned to ROA who double checks it and adds his opinion about suboptimal care.
- Form now sent to CMO at Department of Health.
- Data examined by Committee of Central Assessors in Obstetrics, Anaesthetics, Pathology, Midwifery, Medical Specialities and Statistics who give the final opinion.
- Data clustered and published every three years in a Confidential Enquiry. Last one covered years 1994–1996 and was published in 1998.

CLASSIFICATION OF MATERNAL DEATHS

Until the 1973–1975 triennial report, deaths were coded under the *International Classification of Deaths* (ICD), 8th revision (WHO 1967). Up to that time, deaths classified under the heading of complications of pregnancy, childbirth and the puerperium were classified as true maternal deaths, while deaths with main causes coded elsewhere in the International Classification, in women known to have been pregnant at the time of death or to have been pregnant within 1 year of death, were classified as associated maternal deaths.

ICD 9 (WHO 1975), defined maternal deaths as:

1. *Direct*, resulting from obstetrical complications of the pregnant state (pregnancy, labour and the puerperium), from interventions, omissions, incorrect treatment or from a chain of events resulting from any of the above.
2. *Indirect*, resulting from previous existing disease, or diseases which developed during pregnancy and were not due to direct obstetric causes but aggravated by physiological effects of the pregnancy.
3. *Fortuitous*. Deaths from other causes, which fortuitously occur in pregnancy or the puerperium, are excluded from maternal mortality as internationally defined. These have been defined as fortuitous deaths in the triennial CEMD reports from 1976.

In the 1994–1996 report, direct causes accounted for 134 (45%), indirect for 134 (45%) and fortuitous deaths were 36 (10%).

A further recommendation of ICD 10 is that maternal death should be defined as the death of a woman while pregnant or within 42 days of termination of pregnancy, irrespective of the duration and the site of the pregnancy, from any cause related to or aggravated by the pregnancy or its management, but not from an accidental or incidental cause. This is in line with the definition adopted by the International Federation of Gynaecology and Obstetrics (FIGO). In the CEMD, maternal death had always been defined as one occurring during pregnancy or labour, or as a consequence of pregnancy, within 1 year of delivery or abortion. This wider definition has the advantage of including deaths in which the period of the survival is longer than 42 days but in which pregnancy played an important role.

Late deaths (after 42 days) have been included in all the triennial reports but their presence has been specifically indicated since they were not included within the FIGO definition. There were 72 in 1994–1996. Since the 1979–1981 report, late deaths have been documented separately CEMD in an additional chapter.

KEY POINTS: CLASSIFICATION

Maternal deaths may be:
- direct   45%
- indirect   45%
- fortuitous   10%

See text for definitions

Denominators for calculation of incidence and rates

Historically, MMR was defined as the number of maternal deaths per 1000 total births. Strictly this is not a rate, but a ratio for the denominator is not included in the numerator as it should be in a rate. The numerator of deaths includes those associated with ectopic pregnancy and abortions but the denominator refers to maternities (i.e. women giving birth to viable babies), not to the numbers of all those pregnant. Thus the term ratio is mathematically correct but rate has been used for many years. The CEMD has based mortality rates on the number of maternities. This is the number of mothers delivered as distinct from the number of babies born, the latter being a larger figure because it includes infants from multiple births.

As MMR has fallen, it has proved necessary to express the rate per 10^4, 10^5 and, in the most recent reports, per 10^6 maternities. The change in the reports after 1985 when the total population of the UK was examined did not have a major effect on the resulting statistics. Table 48.1 shows that although the maternal mortality rate per 100 000 ranges from 5.8 to 7.4 in the UK as a whole, the number of births in Northern Ireland, Wales and Scotland is too few to alter the total rate (6.1) much from that of England at 6.2 per 100 000.

To provide realistic denominators for deaths occurring in early pregnancy, such as ectopic pregnancy or abortion, the National Office for Statistics (NOS) data have been used to calculate total pregnancies, a figure including legal and spontaneous abortions, ectopic pregnancies and total maternities (Table 48.2). Many rates have been calculated from this denominator since 1979–1981.

Table 48.1 Direct maternal deaths in CEMD by area of residence: 1985–1990

Area	Total births (n)	Direct deaths (n)	Direct MMR (per 100 000)
UK	4 666 120	284	6.1
England	3 876 169	240	6.2
Wales	228 495	17	7.4
Scotland	396 509	23	5.8
N. Ireland	164 947	4	42.4

Table 48.2 Total maternities and total pregnancies in England and Wales from 1970 to 1993 (from Confidential Enquiries into Maternal Deaths 1993–1996)

Triennium	Total maternities	Total pregnancies
1970–1972	2 222 500	2 732 600
1973–1975	1 851 900	2 366 800
1976–1978	1 781 300	2 275 800
1979–1981	1 910 900	2 437 800
1982–1984	1 905 800	2 427 000
1985–1987	1 987 900	2 439 000
1988–1990	2 073 000	2 886 900
1991–1993	2 045 300	2 000 000

Avoidable factors or substandard care

From 1930, when the Departmental Committee on Maternal Mortality identified a *primary avoidable factor* in some maternal deaths, the annual reports of the Chief Medical Officer up to 1950, and subsequently the triennial reports on the CEMD from 1952 to 1978, have included data about the incidence of avoidable factors. An avoidable factor was considered present if there was a departure from generally accepted standards of satisfactory care, or if the care provided was considered inappropriate in the circumstances. In the 1979–1981 report, the term *substandard care* was substituted for avoidable factors to take into account not only failures in clinical care but also some of the other underlying factors which may have produced a low standard of care for the patient. These included shortage of resources for staffing and facilities, and administrative failure in the maternity services or in backup facilities such as anaesthetic, radiological or pathology services covering multiple sites. It was considered that the term *avoidable factors* had often been misinterpreted as meaning that avoiding these factors would have prevented the death.

In 1952–1954, the incidence of avoidable factors was approximately 45%. By 1976–1978, the incidence had increased to approximately 58%. The latest report does not report substandard care collectively but only in each pathology section; it probably accounted for about 65% of direct deaths. This apparent increase resulted more from changed inclusions in assessment (e.g. lack of equipment or staff) than from deterioration in management.

It has proved more difficult quantitatively to assess the incidence of substandard care since 1979. Apart from those due to pulmonary or amniotic fluid embolism, a high proportion of deaths due to other causes are still associated with substandard care. In the last report, for example, substandard care was evident in 88% of deaths from hypertension and 63% of those from haemorrhage. Considerable further improvement must therefore be possible, even though maternal mortality has now fallen to such a low level.

KEY POINTS: SUBSTANDARD CARE

- Substandard care is management below generally accepted levels of care or inappropriate in the circumstances.
- This can include short staffing, lack of equipment or multiple sites being covered by the same medical personnel.

TRENDS IN CAUSES OF MATERNAL MORTALITY FROM 1970 TO 1984

The numbers of deaths from individual causes in England and Wales from 1970 to 1984 are shown in Table 48.3. Table 48.4 gives rates per million for England and Wales 1973–1984 and the UK 1985–1996. The first triennia were dominated by deaths from hypertensive diseases of pregnancy, pulmonary embolism, haemorrhage and abortion. Bearing in mind the fluctuation in the number of maternities

during the triennia years between 1970 and 1984, the rates shown in Table 48.4 are more reliable indicators of trends than the numbers of deaths in Table 48.3.

There has been a steady reduction in the MMR from hypertensive diseases of pregnancy and from haemorrhage between 1976 and 1984. It may have been easy to improve on previously very poor standards of care. By comparison, the MMR from pulmonary embolism has fallen relatively little over these years. In these years, the reports comment repeatedly on the dangers of home confinement in women with a previous history of haemorrhage, of inadequate anticipation or treatment of the complications of hypertensive disease, on the need for better booking arrangements and for effective flying squad facilities.

The introduction in the 1960s of a combined preparation of oxytocin and ergometrine for intramuscular use must have helped to maintain the reduction in deaths from postpartum haemorrhage over the first six triennia. Table 48.3 shows that deaths from haemorrhage continued to fall between 1976 and 1984, perhaps because of better management, the avoidance of unwanted high-risk pregnancy in women of high parity, and possibly because of better prophylaxis in the second and third stages of labour.

The most dramatic change in the CEMD has been shown in the effects of the Abortion Act (1967) which came into force in 1968. Abortion remained the main cause of death in

Table 48.3 Numbers of direct deaths by cause[a] from 1970 to 1984 in England and Wales (from Confidential Enquiries into Maternal Deaths 1982–84)

Causes	1970–1972	1973–1975	1976–1978	1979–1981	1982–1984
Hypertensive diseases of pregnancy	47	39	29	36	25
Pulmonary embolism	52	33	43	23	25
Abortion	71	27	14	14	11
Haemorrhage	27	21	24	14	9
Anaesthesia	37	22	27	22	18
Ectopic pregnancy	34	19	21	20	10
Amniotic fluid embolism[b]	16	14	11	18	14
Sepsis (excluding abortion)	30	19	15	8	2
Ruptured uterus	13	11	14	4	3
Other direct causes	13	22	19	17	21
Total	340	227	217	176	138

[a] Late deaths were excluded; [b] confirmed histologically.

Table 48.4 Direct maternal death by cause, rates per million estimated pregnancies, England and Wales 1973–1984 and UK 1985–1996

	Pulmonary embolism	Hypertensive disorders of pregnancy	Anaesthesia	Amniotic fluid embolism	Abortion	Ectopic pregnancy	Haemorrhage	Sepsis, excluding abortion	Ruptured uterus	Other direct causes	All deaths
1973–1975	12.8	13.2	10.5	5.4	10.5	7.4	8.1	7.4	4.3	8.5	88.0
1976–1978	18.5	12.5	11.6	4.7	6.0	9.0	10.3	6.5	6.0	8.2	93.4
1979–1981	9.0	14.2	8.7	7.1	5.5	7.9	5.5	3.1	1.6	7.5	70.0
1982–1984	10.0	10.0	7.2	5.6	4.4	4.0	3.6	1.0	1.2	8.4	55.0
1985–1987	9.1	9.4	1.9	3.4	2.3	4.1	3.8	2.3	1.9	7.5	45.6
1988–1990	8.0	8.6	1.0	3.5	2.4	5.2	7.3	2.1	0.7	8.3	47.0
1991–1993	13.0	8.6	3.3	4.3	3.5	3.0	6.5	3.9	NR	NR	40.0
1994–1996	21.8	9.1	0.5	7.7	1.4	4.0	5.5	6.4	NR	NR	43.0

NR not recorded separately

1967–1969. Although there was a marked reduction in deaths from criminal and spontaneous abortion in 1970–1972, abortion was still the main cause of death in that triennium because there was an increase in therapeutic abortion deaths associated with many relatively late abortions and the continuing use of techniques such as morcellation, hysterotomy or hysterectomy. By 1973–1975, legal abortions were more often being performed earlier in pregnancy and more often by simpler vaginal techniques and the abortion MMR fell. By 1982–1984, the death rate from abortion was very low indeed and for the first time there were no deaths from criminal abortion; this has since continued for in the reports right up to 1996 no deaths occurred from illegal abortions in any of the four parts of the United Kingdom. For 15 consecutive years, no death from septic abortion was reported in the UK, while in the worldwide data about a fifth of maternal deaths (20%) are from this cause.

Between 1970 and 1990, there was little improvement in MMR from pulmonary embolism. A slight reduction was seen from hypertensive causes but these and pulmonary embolism were the equal main causes of death in 1990. Although the MMR from hypertensive diseases of pregnancy is lower in the 1990s than in the 1950s, the slow improvement over the 40 years has been disappointing. The contemporary CEMD report highlighted the serious hazards of hypertensive diseases, which can develop insidiously and progress rapidly to a dangerous stage with little warning. Death is still mainly caused by cerebral haemorrhage, probably the result of failure to control severe hypertension, but it can also result from disseminated intravascular coagulation, renal failure or liver necrosis. These complications can all be anticipated by appropriate investigations (repeated platelet counts, performed with measurement of the levels of blood urea, urate, creatinine and transaminases). The establishment of expert teams in each region was suggested, either to advise about management or to take over cases if requested. In the 1988–1990 survey, the authors report surveying UK obstetric units and finding that 9% still had no eclampsia protocol while in 24% there was no intensive care unit on the same site as the unit.

Pulmonary embolism remains a major problem, largely because no effective method has been developed for preventing it or for the early detection of deep vein thrombosis. The triennial reports have repeatedly stressed the importance of an awareness of factors predisposing to pulmonary embolism. The 1982–1984 report drew attention to the hazard of pulmonary embolism in women delivered by elective caesarean section for severe hypertensive diseases of pregnancy. This was re-emphasised in the 1988–1990 report and additional warnings were given about older and fatter mothers. Further, the need for much greater surveillance of antenatal potential thrombotic factors was stressed and the value of prophylactic anticoagulation in pregnancy re-stressed.

In previous reports the scene was dominated by four main causes of death—thrombosis, hypertensive disease, haemorrhage and abortion; the period between 1970 and 1984 saw the emergence of new major causes as the previous four diminished. Thus, in 1979–1981, complications of anaesthesia were the third main cause of death, followed by ectopic pregnancy and amniotic fluid embolism. In 1982–1984, anaesthesia was again the third commonest cause of death followed by amniotic fluid embolism, abortion, ectopic pregnancy and haemorrhage. By 1990, anaesthesia had dropped considerably in the ranking order, leaving ectopic pregnancy as third in frequency.

That deaths from amniotic fluid embolism are of relatively increasing importance is hardly surprising because no advance has been made in its prevention, detection or treatment. The MMR from this cause has remained practically unchanged.

Deaths from genital sepsis include deaths from puerperal sepsis, from sepsis after surgical procedures and from sepsis before or during labour. While the previous huge reduction in deaths from sepsis was impressive, the reduction in the MMR from sepsis between 1970 and 1996 has in fact been equally rapid.

The incidence of ectopic pregnancy has not increased as much in England and Wales as in some European countries. The figures in the CEMD show that deaths following ectopic pregnancy have decreased in absolute numbers but the rank remains about the same because of reductions in the other indices. Since many of the deaths occur very early in pregnancy, improvements may be associated with increasingly sophisticated diagnostic tests, including rapid sensitive assays of β-hCG in urine or blood, improved ultrasound diagnosis including transvaginal scanning (Urquhart & Fisk 1988), and a more rapid recourse to laparoscopic investigation in women with pelvic pain of uncertain origin.

Deaths from ruptured uterus have fallen considerably, perhaps because of increasing awareness of the dangers of excessive uterine stimulation with oxytocic drugs, especially in women previously delivered by caesarean section, or with possible cephalopelvic disproportion in labour.

Other direct deaths, also classified as miscellaneous, show a varying incidence over the triennia, reflecting the difficulty of reliably attributing to this category direct deaths not readily attributed to other causes.

TRENDS IN CAUSES OF MATERNAL MORTALITY SINCE 1990

Two CEMD cover 1990–1996, both of the whole of the United Kingdom, and in each, special aspects of maternal mortality have been examined. Further, from 1993 onwards a NOS computer programme has been used which automatically codes the cause of death. As a result, some 67 deaths not otherwise known to the Enquiry can now be included (10 direct, 40 indirect and 17 fortuitous deaths). The apparent rate of maternal mortality has increased slightly in the last two reports but this follows the adding of the new data. Had they not been included, there would have been 9.9 maternal deaths per 100 000 maternities. Inclusion of these data causes a major increase in indirect deaths.

The reduction in deaths associated with anaesthesia has been sustained in the last two triennial reports of the UK (1991–1993 and 1994–1996). Numbers are small, however, and perhaps they should be set against the general anaesthetics given. There is probably a reduction in the use of general anaesthetic since 1953 as regional (epidural and spinal) blocks are much more frequently used for elective caesarean sections and pudendal blocks for vaginal operative deliveries than in the middle years of the century. Intubation errors are not reported so commonly and the use of H_2 receptor blocking drugs is advised to prevent acid reflux. Pulse oximetry and CO_2 analysis of expired air is strongly recommended. The large number of women who died with adult respiratory distress syndrome is noted even though the main cause of death may have been recorded elsewhere.

The major pathological finding in these years was an increase in deaths from thromboembolism (from 14.5 per 100 000 of maternal deaths in 1988 to 21.8 per 100 000 in 1994). Deaths from amniotic fluid embolism and sepsis also increased, from 4.7 to 7.7 and 3.0 to 6.4 per 100 000 respectively. Among the indirect deaths, cardiac causes increased from 8.9 to 17.7 per 100 000.

The reports from CEMD have become more discursive and examine particular aspects such as psychiatric disease and domestic violence to women. It was notable that only one death was associated with anaesthesia in the latest report and there was a further reduction in deaths from haemorrhage. Moreover, there were fewer deaths in early pregnancy from ectopic pregnancy or spontaneous miscarriage. Many of the changes in the latest report (1994–1996) can be attributed to increased case ascertainment.

An attempt to break down maternal deaths by ethnic origin was made, using ethnic groups derived from the mother's country of birth. This method has many faults, most obviously that in women in the second and third generations in the UK, their grandparents were from other countries but they themselves were born in the UK. It is the best that could be done. It would appear from this analysis that black women have a three times greater risk of maternal mortality than whites, but the numbers are very small.

KEY POINTS: MAJOR CAUSES OF MATERNAL MORTALITY IN THE UK, 1994–1996

Direct
- Hypertensive disease
- Thromboembolism
- Haemorrhage

Indirect
- Heart disease

DEATHS ASSOCIATED WITH CAESAREAN SECTION

There was some information about the total number of caesarean sections performed in the UK in the period covered by each report. The increasing number of caesarean sections in each triennium is clear; the rate has risen from 5.2% in 1970–1972 to 16% in 1996. From these data, the fatality rate per 1000 caesarean sections was calculated and shows a steady rate of improvement.

In 1979–1981 there was concern that, despite a falling fatality rate, the number of caesarean sections had increased so much that the number of deaths was actually increasing; however, the fall in the number of caesarean section deaths since is reassuring and the fatality rate has continued to fall steadily despite the rising caesarean section rate.

When only direct deaths are considered, the caesarean fatality rate over the past eight triennia has fallen faster than the MMR from all causes, until the last two reports when it rose. Further analysis of the 1982–1984 figures showed that the incidence of direct deaths from elective caesarean sections was only 0.09 per 1000 operations; this compares with 0.37 per 1000 for all emergency operations, a fourfold increase. A similar difference was found in the previous triennium, but the 1982–1984 report does not show the reason for the higher mortality rate amongst the emergency group. The conditions for which the operation is performed undoubtedly entail greater risks among women undergoing emergency procedures. It is rarely possible to predict the need for delivery by emergency caesarean section, so attempting to reduce the number by performing more elective operations would merely increase the overall caesarean section rate.

DEATHS ASSOCIATED WITH CARDIAC DISEASE

Maternal death rates associated with cardiac disease are dropping sharply. Table 48.5 shows the more recent position over the last decade. Most of the change is in the acquired heart disease category. In the mid 1950s, 80% of heart disease was rheumatic; in the latest report only those deaths from congenital abnormalities have remained stable. Among the deaths from acquired disease, ischaemic heart disease now accounts for more cases than rheumatic disease. It is a sad reflection that, in some of the Confidential Enquiries into Maternal Deaths, the majority of women with acquired heart disease were judged to have received substandard care. Some had been refused medical advice while others were affected by professional shortcomings. Further, some women who disregarded professional advice may not have been advised sufficiently strongly; when faced with a life-threatening condition, a doctor should not hesitate to say so. Women now want to be better informed, and this is no time for pussyfooting. The doctor should spell out the possible deterioration that can occur. Prepregnancy counselling would be wise in such cases to warn of forthcoming risks and possible unpopular management (e.g. hospital admission). If the woman then entered into pregnancy with known cardiac hazards, she should be seen at a special antenatal clinic with an obste-

Table 48.5   Deaths from heart disease (UK 1985–1996)

	Acquired	Congenital	Total
1985–1987	13 (9)	10	23
1987–1990	9 (5)	9	18
1991–1993	28 (8)	9	37
1994–1996	29 (6)	10	39

Note: in parenthesis, in the acquired deaths column, are those from ischaemic causes.

trician and a cardiologist attending also, so that they may see the woman together and consult on her condition.

Amongst the congenital heart lesions, the full spectrum of conditions expected in this age group was found. The numbers have stayed fairly constant but, since cases of acquired disease are reducing in number, the proportion of congenital heart disease contributing to the total has now increased and is about half the total.

Substandard care occurred in the majority of cases of deaths from acquired heart disease. Much of this involved the professionals who had not recognised the heart condition or had underestimated its effects. It is important that, when a woman presents for the first time in a pregnancy, a careful history and clinical examination should be performed to exclude congenital heart disease. Further, comparatively minor symptoms should be treated with grave respect in anyone with heart disease who is pregnant, e.g. minor pains in the chest in a woman with Marfan's syndrome.

MATERNAL MORTALITY IN DEVELOPING COUNTRIES

While the MMR in the developed countries ranges between 6 and 30 per 100 000 live births, the MMR in developing countries still remains between 100 and 3500 deaths per 100 000 live births. For these countries, the experience of Europe and the USA should be helpful. In general, the present problems of the developing countries are similar to those in the developed countries before 1938. As Walker (1986) pointed out, maternal mortality must rank with some infectious diseases as among the few instances where medical care has achieved a dramatic reduction in mortality rates. In support of the proposal that effective medical care has been more important than improved socioeconomic status in reducing maternal mortality is the report of Kaunitz et al (1984). In a religious community in the USA avoiding medical, obstetric or midwifery care, MMR between 1975 and 1982 was 87 per 10 000 live births—a level over 90 times higher than in the remainder of the state of Indiana and comparable with that in many developing countries. Walker (1986) also pointed out that many maternal deaths in developing countries could be prevented if the number of births to older, high-parity women could be reduced by appropriate family planning.

The status of women in society in many countries of the developing world is considerably inferior to that of men. They are less educated and have less say in the affairs of their family, society and country. This needs to be changed, but change must come form inside the country according to the wishes of the people and not be imposed form the West as a catch-all cure. Until this ideal top-down cure arrives, it is necessary to concentrate on bottom-up improvements in the health of individual women and delivery of services in the field.

Birth rates are high in many developing countries, and one of the major associations with maternal mortality is high parity. The people of Sri Lanka have shown that an increase in literacy among girls led to wider use of contraception, achieving a reduction in family size. This was followed by a drop in maternal mortality. This is attained not only by wider use of family planning but by improved total health, for then fewer children die in infancy and the mother will be reassured that more of her babies would survive childhood. Reduced parity will also be followed not only by an improvement of the woman's health but also by a reduction in the risk of death in childbirth in future generations.

Based upon fecundity and the maternal mortality rate, one can calculate the lifetime risk of a woman of any nationality dying from pregnancy-related causes. This is basically the maternal mortality rate for each delivery multiplied by the number of deliveries. Table 48.6 shows lifetime risk for some developed and developing countries. The range is wide.

Inequalities in maternal death rates have only become apparent in the last 30 years because the problem was largely undocumented before that. Most countries in which maternal mortality rates are high do not keep good data; only since the WHO and the World Bank started their investigations with community level surveys has the enormity of the problem become evident. The probable estimate of 600 000 deaths a year in the world associated with pregnancy and childbirth raised awareness of the problem in a world eager to try and help. However, as well as the medical causes of maternal death shown in Table 48.7, there are multiple social and economic factors including education, background nutrition and distance from medical help. There is a further aspect—the country's own economic and political situation. Many countries are not democratic, and money poured into them will remain in the hands of top government officials and not reach the people who need it (Fig. 48.7); money from poor people in rich countries going to rich people in poor countries. This has proved to be the problem in *Operation 2000*, in which a small number of governments and agencies in the developed world would, in principle, be prepared to cancel their Third World debt if they could be assured that the monies would be received by the people.

Table 48.6 Lifetime risk of maternal death based on maternal mortality and fertility rates per country (data supplied by Maternal Help Around The World)

Countries	Lifetime risk of maternal death (one in . . . .)
Mali	10
Ghana	18
Kenya	20
India	37
South Africa	85
Saudi Arabia	95
Malaysia	270
Cuba	490
Kuwait	820
New Zealand	1600
Poland	2200
Singapore	4090
United Kingdom	5100
Sweden	6000
Switzerland	8200

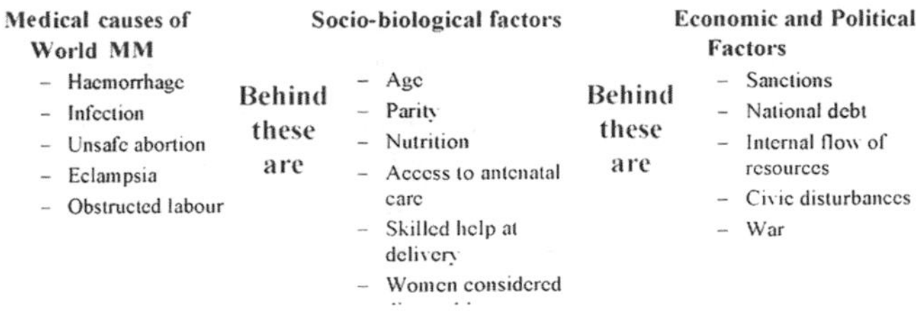

Medical causes of World MM		Socio-biological factors		Economic and Political Factors
– Haemorrhage – Infection – Unsafe abortion – Eclampsia – Obstructed labour	**Behind these are**	– Age – Parity – Nutrition – Access to antenatal care – Skilled help at delivery – Women considered	**Behind these are**	– Sanctions – National debt – Internal flow of resources – Civic disturbances – War

Fig. 48.7 Factors behind the medical causes of maternal mortality.

Table 48.7 Major causes of maternal death in developing countries (from Action for Safe Motherhood)

Haemorrhage	25%
Sepsis	15%
Unsafe abortion	13%
Hypertensive disorders	12%
Obstructed labour	8%
Other	8%
Indirect causes	19%

Attempts to improve maternal health around the world are led by the WHO, the United Nations Fund for Population, and the World Bank. They started at a conference in 1987 in Nairobi on the topic of Safe Motherhood. Since then there have been other conferences in other parts of the world to try to progress this matter, but there seems to have been little effect on the ground. It is a difficult problem for the world to grasp. Little will be gained by trying to bully heads of state or governments into looking after women in pregnancy and childbirth; they must realise themselves how important economically and morally women are in their society and then improvement may occur (Table 48.8). Until then it is necessary to rely upon practical measures, some of which are also shown in Table 48.8 and all of which have varying relevance in different localities. Further, attitudes to the place of women in society often lead to an underrating of the importance of care in childbirth. Changes in education and recognition of women in the governance of countries will improve, and with it maternal mortality will decline.

While improving living conditions is a praiseworthy aim in every country, reducing excessive MMR in developing countries is not likely to be achieved without the provision of effective obstetric care for all pregnant women.

NEAR MISSES

The number of maternal deaths in countries with good data collections systems are comparatively few, and one is now able to learn less from analysis of maternal mortality because of small figure variation. Attempts have been made to look at this problem on a wider scale. Using uniform definitions that are correctly adhered to, one might be able to collect information about the clinical syndromes which would at the extreme have led to death but, thanks to medical care, have not. Thus the near misses could be carefully examined (Table 48.9).

Table 48.9 Conditions that might be considered in an examination of near misses to maternal death

Eclampsia
Deteriorating PIH
Haemorrhage >2000 ml
Uterine rupture
Septicaemia
Pulmonary embolism
Some defined anaesthetic complications
Some defined surgical complications

This would increase the number of cases to be examined by a factor of 100 and would allow a more detailed analysis of the factors behind the pathology which would have led to a death in previous years. Problems with this method consist of persuading a large number of doctors and midwives to agree on the definitions and ensuring that the data are collected in a uniform fashion in all places where deliveries occur. These data must be analysed centrally, fairly swiftly after the events. This can lead to a series of meetings, both peripherally and centrally in a region in the United Kingdom and in similar geographical areas in other parts of the world. A good example was a study in the South East Thames Regional Health Authority in 1997, whose potential efficacy is shown in Table 48.10.

Table 48.8 Steps to reduce maternal mortality

Improvement in women's status
Education
Nutrition
Changing attitudes and practices
Improvement in health service
Antenatal
Delivery
• safe delivery
• improved emergency service
• transport
Contraception

Table 48.10 A practical example of the increased power of an examination of maternal death causes by the regional assay of near misses

Deliveries	24 581
Maternal deaths	5
Severe haemorrhage	246
Severe pre-eclampsia	106
HELLP	8
Eclampsia	10
Severe sepsis	8
Uterine rupture	9
Others (defined)	17
Direct maternal mortality ratio	2 per 100 000
Defined severe morbidity	165 per 100 000
i.e. × 82 increase in cases	

CONCLUSIONS

This has been a brief account of a successful audit made by the health services in the UK and in developed countries in general to overcome the huge problem of maternal mortality. The great improvements brought about in the past 50 years have been illustrated and the factors responsible for the improvement discussed.

In the space available, review of the 15 triennial reports of the CEMD in the 44 years between 1952 and 1996 has been extremely limited. During the period of the enquiries more than 32 million births were registered in England and Wales, and between the introduction of the 1967 Abortion Act in 1968 and the end of 1990, nearly 3 million legal terminations of pregnancy were performed.

Although the rate of improvement in mortality in England and Wales has been almost linear between 1937 and 1988, reaching its lowest level of 7.4 per 10 000 total births in 1988–1990, the continuing high rate of substandard care shows that further improvement can and should be achieved.

ACKNOWLEDGEMENTS

I am grateful to the Comptrollers of Her Majesty's Stationery Office and of the Stationery Office for permission to use tables and figures from the Reports of the Confidential Enquiries into Maternal Deaths.

KEY POINTS

- The time of birth is still a time of increased risk to the mother.
- Many risk factors have been reduced in the Western world by universal antenatal care and by supervision of the birth by professionals—doctors, midwives or trained birth attendants.
- A small number of women still die in association with birth, often leaving a new baby and other children in the family to be brought up. In the Western world, these deaths are mostly caused by hypertension, thrombosis or haemorrhage.
- A great proportion of maternity associated deaths still occur in the developing world. The commonest causes are haemorrhage, sepsis, unsafe abortion and hypertension.

REFERENCES

Al-Meshari A 1993 Maternal mortality in Saudi Arabia (1989–1992). Ministry of Health, Saudi Arabia

Association of Anaesthetists 1987 Anaesthetic services for obstetrics—a plan for the future. Association of Anaesthetists of Great Britain and Ireland/Obstetric Anaesthetists' Association, London

Bickerton TH 1936 A medical history of Liverpool from the earliest days to the year 1920. John Murray, London

Colebrooke L, Kenny M 1936 Treatment with prontosil of puerperal infections due to haemolytic streptococci. Lancet ii:1319–1322

Confidential Enquiries into Maternal Deaths in England and Wales. Fifteen triennial reports from 1952–1954 to 1993–1996, inclusive. HMSO and NSO, London

Högberg U 1985 Maternal mortality in Sweden. Umea University Medical Dissertation (new series) 156

Kaunitz AM, Spence C, Davidson TS, Rochat RW, Grieves DA 1984 Perinatal and maternal mortality in a religious group avoiding obstetric care. Am J Obstet Gynecol 150:826–831

Loudon I 1986 Deaths in child bed from the 18th century to 1935. Med Hist 30:1–41

Loudon I 1987 Puerperal fever, the streptococcus and the sulphonamides. Br J Med 295:485–490

Loudon I 1992 Maternal mortality. Clarendon Press, Oxford

Oxley WHF, Philips MH, Young J 1935 Maternal mortality in Rochdale. An achievement in a black area. BMJ 1:304–307

Urquhart DR, Fisk NM 1988 Transvaginal ultrasound in suspected ectopic pregnancy. BMJ 296:465–466

Walker G 1986 Family planning, maternal mortality and literacy. Lancet ii: 162

WHO 1967 Manual of the international classification of diseases, injuries and causes of death. 8th revision, vol 1. WHO, Geneva

WHO 1975 Manual of the international classification of diseases, injuries and causes of death. 9th revision, vol 1. WHO, Geneva

WHO 1992 Manual of the international classification of diseases, injuries and causes of death. 10th revision, vol 1. WHO, Geneva

Section 9
LEGAL PROBLEMS

49

Medico–legal aspects

Roger Clements

INTRODUCTION

The law governing the practice of medicine is complex and diffuse. In contrast to most other European countries, the law of England and Wales is not found in a single Code. While parliament has enacted a number of statutes governing medical practice, the regulation of that practice and the disciplining of doctors is delegated by parliament in the Medical Act 1983 to the General Medical Council. There are numerous differences both in organisation and statute in Scotland and in Northern Ireland; attention is drawn in the text to some of the important differences.

The European Community increasingly influences the law in the United Kingdom either within the provisions of the Treaty of Rome or through the European Convention of Human Rights, recently implemented in the Human Rights Act (Havers 2000). It is the civil law and particularly the tort of negligence that most concerns obstetricians because of the disproportionate contribution obstetrics makes to malpractice costs. The auditor general's NHS summarised accounts (England) 1997–1998 showed a total of £144 m charged to expenditure for clinical negligence in that year. The total provision for the cost of medical negligence in the summarised accounts as at

The diversity of legislation affecting the obstetrician includes:

1. criminal law

   - common law
   - statute law

2. NHS law
3. the laws controlling medical records
4. the registration of births and deaths
5. employment law
6. health and safety regulations
7. public health law
8. civil law

   - tort
   - judicial review
   - declaration

9. the coroner
10. the General Medical Council.

31st March 1998 was £394 m. This sum represents health organisations' best estimate of their share of future payments relating to certain or probable clinical negligence claims where costs can be reasonably estimated. A further £733 m is disclosed in the summarised accounts as contingent liabilities, where the outcome of cases is less certain, and provision for further costs is not required. In total the accounts show potential liabilities of some £1.8 billion, excluding the additional liabilities relating to incidents incurred but not yet reported, which could amount to another £1 billion.

National Health Service Litigation Authority (NHSLA) claims statistics (for England) as of 31st October 1999 show that obstetrics and gynaecology account for 32% of all claims by number but 63% of all claims by cost. There were 1212 outstanding cerebral palsy claims estimated to be worth £2000 m. A further 172 claims for Erb's palsy are estimated as costing £30 m.

THE CRIMINAL LAW

Much of English law is made by judges—the common law. Most criminal law is now codified and incorporated into Acts of parliament. Obstetricians are occasionally charged with murder, manslaughter, fraud and indecent assault but the criminal laws with which obstetricians most commonly find difficulty are:

> the Offences Against the Persons Act 1861
> the Infant Life (Preservation) Act 1929
> the Abortion Act 1967
> the Prohibition of Female Circumcision Act 1985
> the Human Fertilization and Embryology Act 1990

Abortion and assisted reproduction

> Confusion of thought, induced largely by turbulence of emotion, surrounds abortion more than any other medical subject (Puxon 1996).

The Offences Against the Persons Act 1861 made it an offence punishable by life imprisonment for any pregnant woman unlawfully to procure or attempt to procure her own miscarriage, and for any other person, whether a doctor or not, unlawfully to procure or attempt to procure a woman's miscarriage, whether she be with child or not.

The Infant Life (Preservation) Act 1929 made it an offence punishable by life imprisonment for any person to destroy the life of a child 'capable of being born alive'. It contained a rebuttable presumption of viability at 28 weeks.

The 1967 Abortion Act provided a defence to the offence of procuring a miscarriage under the 1861 Act but specifically did not provide protection under the Infant Life (Preservation) Act of 1929.

The 1967 Act effectively provided abortion on demand for the provision in section 1 'if two registered medical practitioners are of the opinion formed in good faith that the continuance of the pregnancy would involve risk to the life . . . or of injury . . . to the physical or mental health of the pregnant woman . . . greater than if the pregnancy were terminated . . .' can obviously be applied to any pregnancy since statistically delivery at term is more hazardous than early termination, other things being equal. The Act effectively allows abortion to be performed liberally within the NHS but imposes important restrictions in the private sector, aimed at preventing abuses, which were common in the 1960s before the legislation.

The Human Fertilization and Embryology Act 1990 provides a comprehensive and complex code of law controlling all procedures connected with human gametes and embryos. It is broadly based on the recommendations of the Warnock Committee. Its most important provision is the setting up of a licensing body, the Human Fertilization and Embryology Authority, with wide powers to license, inspect and control the operation of all persons carrying out any of the following activities:

> the creation or keeping of an embryo
> the storage of gametes
> the placing of sperm or eggs in a woman
> research on embryos.

Without a licence, any relevant operation is illegal and punishable on conviction by a fine or imprisonment of up to two years. The proper conduct of these activities is set out in a code of practice.

The law relating to termination of pregnancy was also amended by the Act. The 1967 Act specified no limit to the gestation of the pregnancy which might legally be terminated but specifically did not protect the doctor against the Infant Life (Preservation) Act 1929. Thus, abortion could not be performed legally after the age of viability, whatever that might be. The Human Fertilization and Embryology Act (S37) limits abortion to pregnancies that have not exceeded the 24th week, when abortion is to be performed on the grounds of the risks to the physical or mental health of the mother or any existing children in the family. However, the Act allows termination without any time limit where:

- the termination is immediately necessary to save the life or to protect the health of the woman from grave permanent injury, or
- there is a substantial risk that the child will be seriously handicapped.

The words *substantial* and *seriously* have yet to be defined by the courts.

In practice, most very late abortions are a consequence of the late diagnosis of serious fetal abnormality. Once the decision to perform a late abortion has been made, it is important to ensure that the fetus dies before the woman is delivered. The aim is to avoid the birth of a disabled child, not to add gross prematurity to already existing handicap. The Abortion Act (1967) states that:

> no person shall be under any duty . . . to participate in any treatment authorized by the Act to which he has a conscientious objection.

The only exception to this is when the abortion is necessary to save the mother's life or to prevent grave permanent injury to health. The doctor may subsequently have to establish his conscientious objection if the patient suffers thereby, and he should make clear from the beginning of the consultation that she is entitled to further opinions from doctors who are willing to recommend and perform termination of pregnancy.

The Abortion Act 1967 does not apply in Northern Ireland.

Genital mutilation

> Although it seems very likely that those who performed FGM (female genital mutilation) could, in any case, have been successfully prosecuted under sections 18 and 20 of the Offences Against the Persons Act, 1861, it was felt that a specific statute was needed . . . (Sheldon 1998).

Under the Prohibition of Female Circumcision Act no offence is committed by the woman but it is illegal to:

1. excise, infibulate or otherwise mutilate the whole or any part of the labia majora or labia minora, or clitoris of any person, or
2. aid, abet, counsel or procure the performance by another person of any of those acts on that other person's own body.

The Act presents serious difficulties to the obstetrician, particularly in the case of the woman who requests reinfibulation at the time of childbirth:

> . . . this seems to pose a particularly stark conflict between the duty of the medical practitioners to do no harm, and their duty to respect the patient's autonomy (Sheldon 1998).

THE CIVIL LAW

The commonest legal threat to the practising obstetrician is an action for the recovery of damages through the civil courts. An action for breach of contract may occasionally be brought against a private practitioner but it is more usual, when pursuing a doctor for defective care, to do so under the law of tort. A tort is a civil wrong, a breach of legal duty (excluding contract) with liability to damages. Examples of tort are negligence, assault, battery and trespass. Occasional actions for assault and battery (Puxon 1995) have succeeded but it is more common, even when defective consent is alleged, for the action to be brought in negligence. There are important differences:

> There are two fundamental distinctions between the two torts: first . . . intention is a necessary ingredient of assault and battery, whereas no intention is necessary in negligence; secondly, a trespass against a person (assault or battery) is actionable without any proof of damage and damages are at large. Where no damage is proved, nominal damages may be awarded for assault or battery. Aggravated damages may be awarded for any tort where the patient has suffered injury to [her] feelings as a result of the special circumstances of the case . . .
>
> In contrast, to establish negligence the plaintiff must prove that she has suffered actual loss and damage as a result of the negligent act. This distinction is vital in medical malpractice where causation of the damage suffered by the patient is often difficult to establish (Puxon 1995).

Medical malpractice litigation

Legal liability to pay compensation to a patient who has suffered some injury as a result of a medical action or omission usually only arises when some fault is established. As Lord Denning said in Hatcher v. Black (1954):

> Every surgical operation involves risks. It would be wrong, and indeed, bad law to say that simply because a misadventure or mishap occurred, the hospital and the doctors are thereby liable.

In most cases, fault will have to be established by the patient proving negligence. The law of negligence is made up of three elements:

1. the existence of a duty of care owed by the defendant to the claimant
2. a breach of that duty
3. damage caused to the claimant by that breach.

The duty of care

It is axiomatic that a doctor owes his patient a duty to exercise reasonable skill and care in relation to medical treatment. It is seldom that the existence or extent of that duty is a cause of dispute.

Health Authorities and Trusts have vicarious responsibility, for the errors of their clinical staff, whom they normally select. In addition to this vicarious responsibility, health service and other public hospitals also owe a direct duty to their patients. This distinction, while of considerable interest to lawyers, is not important in practice. Since the introduction of Crown Indemnity in 1990, doctors are no longer named in civil actions for negligence in the context of their health service work. Only in private and in general practice, where National Health Service indemnity does not apply, is a doctor's name likely to appear as a defendant.

The doctor's duty begins at the moment he undertakes to care for his patient.

Duty to the unborn child. Special arrangements have been necessary to define the duty owed to the unborn child, and these are of particular relevance in the context of obstetrics. The starting point is that the unborn child is not endowed with a legal personality and therefore has no rights, other than those which have been created piecemeal, usually by statute. The right of a child, after birth, to sue for damages inflicted in intrauterine life remained uncertain until, following the thalidomide tragedy, parliament enacted the Congenital Disabilities (Civil Liability) Act in 1976. This clarified the law but probably did not create it, for in two subsequent cases brought to the Court of Appeal of children born before 22nd July 1976 (the date on which the Act took effect) (Burton v. Islington Health Authority 1991) the court found that a child born alive could recover damages at common law for prenatal injury:

Damage to a fetus was within the foreseeable risk of harm that could arise from the defendants' negligence, and the cause of action arose when the fetus was born injured, at which point the plaintiff acquires the legal personality to sue (Jones 1996).

The Congenital Disability (Civil Liability) Act 1976 confers a right of action on a child who was born alive but disabled on or after 22nd July 1976, if the disability was caused by an occurrence which affected either parent's ability to have a normal healthy child or affected the mother during pregnancy, or affected the mother or child in the course of its birth. The Act only confers rights on children who are born alive, and does not apply in cases where the defendant's negligence causes the death of the fetus in utero although in such circumstances either or both parents may have an action that is independent of the Act. It is important to bear in mind that the child's rights under the Act derive from a duty owed to the mother and that the Act does not go so far as to create duties owed independently to the unborn child. If such a legislative enterprise were ever attempted it would have to define the stage of pregnancy at which fetal rights would accrue and reconcile them with termination of pregnancy, which is perhaps the ultimate compromise of any rights the unborn child might have. As it is, the possibility of a claim by the child against the mother is expressly excluded unless the mother was driving a motor vehicle, in which case she owes her unborn child the same duty of care as she owes to any other person. This exception is permitted on public policy grounds, because in most cases the true defendant in such a claim will not be the mother but the company who insures her while she is driving.

Once born, the fetus has legal rights which, before its majority, may be exercised through a litigation friend. The Limitation Act 1980 gives a child the right to bring an action at least until the age of 21 years. The limitation period within which an action for personal injury has to be brought (subject to the overriding discretion of a court to bring an action outside the time) is three years from the date of knowledge. Thus the age limit of 21 may be extended where the requisite knowledge is not acquired until after the age of 18 years; when the intellectual impairment is sufficient to prevent the child ever achieving legal competence, an action may be brought at any time on the child's behalf until three years after his death.

Wrongful life and wrongful birth. There is no cause of action in United Kingdom law for *wrongful life*. The Congenital Disabilities (Civil Liability) Act 1976 precludes an action by the child on the basis that he should never have been born. In McKay v. Essex Health Authority (1982) the plaintiff had been infected with rubella in utero and had been born with various handicaps as a consequence. She alleged negligence on the part of the doctor who treated her mother antenatally in that he knew, or should have known, of the infection and should therefore have advised the mother to terminate the pregnancy and thus prevent the birth of a handicapped child. There were various other claims in the action which resulted in the payment of some compensation, but the Court of Appeal rejected the claim. Not only could the judges not accept that anyone could have a duty towards a person, whether or not in utero, to terminate his life but, if there was any such right, it was impossible to say what should be the basis for the assessment of damages for a breach of it. The handicap was the result of the rubella, not of the doctor's failure to advise the mother to terminate the pregnancy, so compensation could not be paid for the pain and suffering of handicap compared to a healthy person. The difference that followed the omission to terminate was between not existing at all and existing in a disabled state, a distinction which defied quantification in money terms.

Where a child is born as the result of negligence on the part of a doctor, the parents may have a claim for *wrongful birth*. Since the mid 1980s, parents of children born as a result of negligent sterilisation or botched termination (Emeh v. Kensington and Chelsea and Westminster Health Authority 1995) have successfully claimed for the upbringing of the child. A recent decision in the House of Lords (McFarlane v. Tayside Health Board 1999), has effectively ended such claims. In this case the parents of a child conceived after the husband had had a vasectomy brought an action for negligence and the claim for damages included the cost of bringing up the child. The House of Lords allowed the mother's claim for pain, suffering and inconvenience of pregnancy and for the special damages of extra medical expenses, clothing and loss of earnings. Their Lordships however disallowed a claim for caring for a healthy normal child on the grounds that this did not satisfy the requirement of being fair, just and reasonable. Their Lordships took the view that the birth of a normal healthy baby outweighed any economic loss and therefore ruled that the parents were not entitled to recover the costs of caring for and bringing up the child. The child in this case was normal and it is as yet uncertain what view their Lordships will take if the child born as a consequence of wrongful birth is in some way handicapped.

Breach of duty

To establish negligence the claimant must prove that there was a breach of the duty of care:

> The duty of care is not absolute. The duty is discharged by doing what is reasonable in all of the circumstances of the case. Reasonableness is the standard set by law. What then is reasonable? How is it determined? The court needs to hear expert evidence on what is and is not acceptable practice. In medical negligence cases the court is assisted by application of the Bolam test (Powers & Barton 1995).

The case of Bolam v. Friern Hospital Management Committee (1957) enunciated a principle previously stated in the Scottish courts in Hunter v. Hanley (1955). In that case the test to be examined by the court, with the assistance of expert evidence, was set out by the court (Lockhart 1999):

1. Was there a usual and normal practice that any reasonably competent doctor using ordinary care would have followed?
2. Did the defendant depart from that practice?
3. Was the course that the doctor adopted one that no

4. Did that departure cause or materially contribute to the injury? (This is strictly causation rather than negligence.)

professional person of ordinary skill would have taken if they had been acting with ordinary care? (Lord Clyde said this is of *crucial* importance).

Two years later, J McNair enunciated the principle for the English Courts (Watt 1995). Reasonableness is normally approached by the courts by referring to the model of the reasonable man, one who is neither excessively foresighted nor particularly unable to judge the likelihood of future occurrences. Such a fictional character is often referred to as the man on the Clapham omnibus. But here, as the judge explained, the situation is different:

But where you get a situation which involves the use of some special skill or competence, then the test whether there has been negligence or not is not the test of the man on the Clapham omnibus, because he has not got this special skill. The test is the standard of the ordinary skilled man exercising and professing to have that special skill. A man need not possess the highest expert skill at the risk of being found negligent . . . it is sufficient if he exercises the ordinary skill of an ordinary competent man exercising that particular art.

But what if there are two views as to what constitutes reasonable care? The judge went on:

A doctor is not guilty of negligence if he has acted in accordance with a practice accepted as proper by a responsible body of medical men skilled in that particular art. Putting it the other way round, a doctor is not negligent, if he is acting in accordance with such a practice, merely because there is a body of opinion that takes a contrary view.

Thus a general practitioner is not expected to possess the skills of a consultant surgeon but a specialist is expected to exercise the ordinary skill of that specialty. If the threshold of skill is raised for the specialist, the question arises whether it is lowered for the junior doctor. Trainee doctors must exercise the level of skill appropriate to their posts, so a junior house officer will be expected to perform to the standards of a reasonably competent junior house officer. The level of skill must include the ability to know when he is outside this limit of skill and training and when more senior help is needed.

The position is that junior doctors and non-specialists are expected to know their limitations and to summon help when they get out of their depth. It is the consultant's responsibility to decide what he can reasonably delegate, according to post, qualifications and experience of his junior staff. It is the consultant's responsibility to ensure that junior doctors are aware of the limits of their skill and experience so as to know when to seek help; it is also the consultant's responsibility to make himself available to give that assistance. If help is sought but there is not enough consultant cover or other resources to provide the level of skill and care required in the circumstances, either at all or in time to prevent injury, the matter is then a resource issue for which the hospital is directly responsible.

The Bolam test was approved by the House of Lords in Whitehouse v. Jordan (1981) and further developed in Maynard v. West Midland Regional Health Authority (1984). In cases in which there are differences of medical opinion and practice, doctors will not be found negligent if a body of competent professional opinion supports their judgement and practice, even if another equally competent body of opinion considers that what they did was wrong.

A further matter that has been considered by the courts in dealing with the standards of care is the time at which the prevailing standards should be assessed. In many medical negligence cases the incident that is the subject of the claim will have taken place many years before the case comes to trial. In the interval, medical practice in the area may have moved on considerably, but the medical treatment will be judged by the prevailing standards at the date of treatment. While this may impose practical problems in identifying whether a practice accorded with a responsible body of opinion at the time in question, any other approach would be inequitable.

In December 1997 the House of Lords considered the Bolam test for the first time in nine years (Bolitho v. City and Hackney HA 1993). While sustaining the principle upon which expert evidence is assessed by the courts, the House of Lords added an important reservation, Lord Browne-Wilkinson expressing the view that a court is not bound to hold that a defendant doctor escapes liability for negligent treatment and diagnosis just because he submits evidence from a number of medical experts genuinely of the opinion that the defendant's treatment or diagnosis accords with sound medical practice. The court must be satisfied that the exponents of a body of opinion relied upon can demonstrate that such an opinion has a logical basis and that in forming those views the experts had directed their minds to the questions of comparative risks and benefits and reached a defensible conclusion. A judge might be entitled to the view that professional opinion was not capable of withstanding logical analysis and that the body of opinion relied upon was not reasonable or responsible (Watt 1999).

McNair J stated that the defendant had to have acted in accordance with a practice accepted as proper by a '*responsible* body of medical men'. Later he referred to 'a standard of practice recognized as proper by a competent *reasonable* body of opinion'. Again, (in *Maynard*) Lord Scarman refers to a *respectable* body of professional opinion. The use of these adjectives—responsible, reasonable and respectable—all show that the court has to be satisfied that the exponents of the body of opinion relied on can demonstrate that such opinion has a logical basis. In particular, in cases involving, as they so often do, the weighing of risks against benefits the judge before accepting a body of opinion as being responsible, reasonable or respectable, will need to be satisfied that, in forming their views, the experts have directed their minds to the question of comparative risks and benefits and have reached a defensible conclusion in the matter.

The role of the expert in assisting the court to understand the standards of care and the extent to which that standard has been complied with is explained below.

Adequacy of resources. In obstetric practice a lack of resources may be reflected in a number of ways: whether, for example, there is sufficient consultant cover to support junior staff with the interpretation of difficult cardiotocograms (CTG); whether, if a decision is made to intervene surgically, there is an unreasonable delay in doing so because facilities or anaesthetic cover are inadequate. These are resource issues, and consultants and hospital managers need to identify the point at which lack of resources exposes the patients (and thus indirectly the hospital and the doctors) to unacceptable risks.

Once a hospital has undertaken to provide treatment, lack of resources will not be accepted as an excuse for an inadequate standard of care. In the leading case (Bull v. Devon Area Health Authority 1993) the allocation of resources had led to a split site for the hospital's obstetric and gynaecological activities. In these circumstances, there was an inherent risk that an experienced obstetrician would not be able to attend within a reasonable time when required to do so. Despite the fact that the administrative arrangements were determined by the availability of resources, the court held that the delay in arrival of a qualified obstetrician (in this case to deliver a second twin) was unreasonable and the cover arrangements negligent.

The implications of the courts' decisions are that a hospital may decline to provide a service but, if the service is provided, it must be to a reasonable standard. Lack of funds is not an excuse for insufficient experienced cover to meet the needs of all patients on the labour ward, although the law does permit the number of beds to be limited so as to reflect the availability of resources. Similarly, the provision of emergency theatres needs to be reviewed since it may not be sufficient for a hospital to contend that delay in carrying out a caesarean section was a result of all theatres already being in use. It would be open to the court to find that administrative arrangements that had led to the situation were negligent and award damages accordingly.

Causation

It is not sufficient for the claimant to prove that there was a breach of duty on the part of the treating doctor or midwife; it is also necessary to prove that the breach of duty caused, or materially contributed to, her loss or injury. Proving causation is often much more difficult for the claimant than proving breach of duty. One of the difficulties in discussing causation is the very different approach taken by doctors and scientists on the one hand towards aetiology and by the courts on the other hand towards causation. The claimant must prove that the injury was caused by the defendant's breach of duty but the standard of proof is the same as for any other matter in the civil courts; it must be more likely than not. In other words it must be more than 50%. It does not have to be more than that. Once the court has decided the matter on the balance of probabilities (more than 50% likely) the court then goes on to regard that as fact and certain. While lawyers require proof on the balance of probabil-

ities, epidemiologists do not refer to proof, only to the probability of chance:

> The assertions of epidemiologists are *probabilistic* and *bio-statistical*, those of lawyers are *deterministic* and *individual*; it could be said that epidemiological assertions express the uncertainty of truth, while legal determinations express the fiction of certainty. The epidemiologist can only answer the question 'can X cause this condition?', not 'did X cause this condition?' (Puxon 1994).

In its simplest form, causation can be understood by the 'but for' test. In these circumstances the claimant demonstrates to the court that 'but for' the negligence of the defendant the damage would not have occurred:

> It is for the claimant to prove, on the balance of probabilities, that the defendant's breach of duty caused the damage. So where there are conflicting explanations for the claimant's condition, neither of which are wholly satisfactory, the defendant does not have to prove that his explanation is the correct one, though failure to prove it may be a factor in deciding whether the claimant's explanation of the cause should be accepted (Jones 2000).

Nevertheless the test is often applied in reverse, to consider whether, even if the defendant had not been negligent, the damage would have occurred in any event (Barnett v. Chelsea and Kensington Hospital Management Committee 1969). Where a number of factors may have contributed to the claimant's injury, the courts have (Bonnington Castings v. Wardlaw 1956, McGee v. National Coal Board 1972) a somewhat easier test for the claimant, one of 'material contribution'. Where there are such multiple possible causes of a claimant's injury, the claimant must demonstrate that the negligent cause made a material contribution to the damage and that his condition would have been very much better without that contribution. Merely increasing the risk of injury may not be sufficient to prove causation. In Wilsher (Wilsher v. Essex Area Health Authority 1980, Watt 1997) the House of Lords took the view that the retinopathy from which the infant claimant suffered could have been caused by the negligent administration of excess oxygen, but could also have occurred as a result of a number of other conditions in premature babies, all of which had afflicted the claimant. At the trial, the medical evidence was inconclusive as to whether the excess oxygen had caused the condition.

The House of Lords decided that, in cases where a claimant's injury was attributable to a number of possible causes and only one of those was the defendant's negligence, the combination of a breach of duty and the claimant's injury did not give rise to a presumption that the defendant had caused or materially contributed to the injury. The burden of proof remained on the claimant to prove a causative link between the defendant's negligence and his injury. In Wilsher, the retinopathy could have been caused by any one of a number of different agents and it had not been proved that it was caused by the failure to prevent excess oxygen being given, the burden of proof as to causation had not been discharged and the claim therefore failed. The House of Lords referred the case of Wilsher back for a retrial, in order to determine whether, as a matter of fact, the amount of oxygen administered through the negligence of the doctors was capable of having caused or materially contributed to the injury. The case subsequently settled.

Another difficult area, related to causation, is the *loss of a chance*:

> An alternative to the 'all or nothing' approach to causation (by which the claimant succeeds in full if the probabilities are greater than 50:50 but loses if the probabilities are lower than this) is to treat the claimant's damage as the 'loss of a chance'. This is best illustrated by Hotson v. East Berkshire Area Health Authority [1987] in which the plaintiff suffered an accidental injury to his hip in a fall which created a 75% risk that he would develop a permanent disability. Due to negligent diagnosis the hip was not treated for five days, and the delay made the disability inevitable. The plaintiff contended that the doctor's negligence had deprived him of a 25% chance of making a good recovery, whereas the defendant argued that the plaintiff had failed to prove, on the balance of probabilities, that the negligence caused the disability. The trial judge held that where a 'substantial chance' of a better medical result had been lost it was not necessary to prove that the adverse medical result was directly attributable to the breach of duty because the issue was the proper quantum of damage rather than causation. The plaintiff could prove causation of the lost chance and accordingly he was entitled to damages on the basis of 25% of the value of the claim for the full disability. In the House of Lords, however, the decision was overturned on the basis that the judge's finding that there was a high probability, put at 75%, that even with correct diagnosis and treatment the plaintiff's disability would have occurred, amounted to a finding of fact that the accident (not the error in diagnosis) was the sole cause of the disability. In other words this was not a 'lost chance' case, it was an all or nothing case—either the fall or the misdiagnosis caused the disability, and on the balance of probabilities (75/25) it was the fall (Jones 2000).

That remains the position in medical negligence actions but contrasts curiously with other professional negligence claims. It has long been the practice to allow in actions against solicitors damages based upon loss of chance. In a gynaecological case (Gascoine v. Ian Sherridan & Co and Latham 1994) the claimant's action against the gynaecologist and the radiotherapist for negligent treatment of cervical cancer was struck out for want of prosecution. In a subsequent action against her legal advisers the trial judge found that there was a 60% prospect of the claimant having succeeded against the doctors and the hospital and accordingly the claimant was awarded 60% of the full value of the claim.

Finally, Bolitho (Bolitho v. City and Hackney HA 1993, Watt 1999) illustrates the principle of negligent omission in which the court first has to determine what hypothetically would have occurred but for the negligent omission. If that finding results in establishing causation, the claimant succeeds. If, however, the finding indicates that the defendants would not have acted to avoid the damage, a new question arises. The court will then determine whether the defendants *should* have acted to avoid the damage and will do so on the basis of expert evidence, applying the Bolam test.

Quantum

Once a patient has shown that negligence led to loss, the remaining issue is the *quantum* or amount of damages. Damages are intended to restore the successful claimant to the position she would have been in but for the negligence. In personal injury cases, this is often a somewhat artificial exercise but the principle of English Law that damages are compensatory and not punitive has avoided the excessive awards that are sometimes said to exist in other jurisdictions.

The various categories by references to which damages are assessed are called *heads of damage*:

HEADS OF DAMAGE

A. General damages (non-pecuniary loss)

    1. damages for pain, suffering and loss of amenity
    2. interest on damages for pain, suffering and loss of amenity

B. Special damages (pecuniary loss, past [and interest on past losses up to the date of trial] and future), past and future losses and expenses:

    1. care
    2. accommodation/housing
    3. adaptation
    4. appliances
    5. extra clothing and household expenses
    6. speech therapy
    7. physiotherapy
    8. occupational therapy
    9. travel/transport
    10. medical expenses
    11. loss of earnings.

Damages that attempt to compensate in money for pain, suffering and loss of amenity are also called *general damages* and are calculated by reference to a judge-made tariff. In April 2000, The Court of Appeal, reviewing eight test cases, increased the level of such damages. At the top end of the scale the previous maximum of £150 000 was raised to £200 000. Below the maximum the percentage increase is tapered so that by £10 000 there is no increase.

The other heads of damage are known collectively as *special damages* and are particular to the circumstances of each case, with the result that each side in a case that cannot be successfully defended will expend substantial effort in order to strike as good a bargain on the quantum of damages as circumstances permit. There is an element of horse trading but, in large claims at least, it is not uncommon nowadays for the claimant's case on quantum to run to several hundreds of pages of close arguments, often prepared by accountants with the help of experts in the various regimens of therapy that are available. Bargaining down the quantum of claims is an equally complex activity, where skill counts as much as in many disputes about liability, and where a competent defence team can save large amounts of money. Some comment is appropriate about certain heads of special damages.

Nursing care. A plaintiff is entitled to medical treatment and nursing care to such extent as the court finds reasonable. Inevitably, the court will look sympathetically on the needs of a brain-damaged child who may need continuous nursing care for the rest of his life. Increasingly sophisticated medical and nursing care not only adds directly to these costs, but has led to increased life expectancy for even the most severely handicapped, which in turn leads to increasing awards to cover the cost of future care. There may be argument as to whether future care is provided privately or by the NHS.

Housing costs. This head covers the cost of purchasing and/or converting a property to fit the needs of a brain-damaged child, and his later needs as an adult. The accommodation must also be large enough to include parents and other carers. Damages are awarded for the cost of modifying existing accommodation or for the cost of borrowing to buy new property.

Loss of earnings. This covers the loss of future earning capacity in the brain-damaged child. The courts try to speculate as to the career path that the claimant might have had but for his disability. This exercise involves looking at the rest of the family before deciding such issues as whether the child would have gone to Eton and had a career at the bar, or else would have enjoyed a less prosperous life. A sum is awarded after a substantial discount to allow for the acceleration of earnings that the claimant would not normally have received until many years after the trial.

Discount. The House of Lords decision in Wells v. Wells (Wells v. Wells, Thomas v. Brighton Health Authority and Page v. Sheerness Steel plc 1999, Gumbel 1999a) has had a significant influence on the quantum of damage recovered by successful litigants. The judgement has had its most dramatic affects upon the damages awarded to cerebral palsy victims. The result of this judgement was to reduce the discount rate (the rate at which the successful litigant could be expected to receive interest on his lump sum award) from 4.5% to 3%. This had the effect of increasing the damages in one cerebral palsy claim from £1.85 m to £2.57 m (Young 1999).

The indication of the damages likely to be awarded in obstetric negligence cases has provided a series of reviews in *Clinical Risk* by Elizabeth Anne Gumbel QC (1997a,b, 1998, 1999a,b).

THE CIVIL PROCEDURE

In his report on the Civil Justice System in England and Wales *Access to Justice* (1996) Lord Woolf suggested wide-ranging reform of the system and proposed a new set of rules to bring those reforms into force. On the 26th April 1999 the Civil Procedure Rules 1998 (CPR) came into effect in England and Wales. The purpose of the rules (Gumbel 1999c) was not only to effect the substantive reforms proposed but to reduce the size of the rules, simplifying the language and eliminating

Latin. Part 1 of the new rules states the overriding objective 'of enabling the courts to deal with cases justly' ensuring that the parties are on an equal footing, saving expense and dealing with cases in ways which are proportionate to the amount of money involved, the importance of the case, the complexity of the issues and the financial position of each party. The rules impose upon the courts a duty to manage cases, a radical reform, taking the pace and control of litigation out of the hands of the parties.

The language of the rules is simplified; amongst other things the instigator of a civil action is no longer called a plaintiff but a claimant. There are two principal effects upon the conduct of medical negligence litigation. The pace of litigation is determined by the courts rather than by the parties, and the interminable delays under the old system should be avoided. Although medical negligence cases will seldom be suitable for the fast track there will nevertheless be a strict timetable imposed by the courts and penalties for default. The second effect is a requirement for greater openness between the parties and from the very beginning fuller statements of each party's case. It will no longer be possible for the statements of case (no longer called pleadings) to avoid the issues. This means that a defendant, in seeking to defend a clinical negligence action, will not be permitted simply to make a bland denial of the allegations but will be required to produced a reasoned argument and an alternative account.

In part 35 the rules spell out the duty of the expert witness (Clements 1999) to help the court, a duty that overrides any obligation of the expert to those instructing or paying him. Furthermore the expert, in the report for the court, must state that he or she both understands this duty and has complied with it. Such a declaration, recommended by the Expert Witness Institute, is set out in Figure 49.1.

The role of the expert is further defined by a Code of Guidance currently under review by the vice-chancellor (Draft Code of Guidance for Experts 1999). The Code distinguishes between *advice* by the expert in preparation of litigation and *report*, the document produced by the expert for the court which must be addressed to the court. The expert may be required to answer questions for clarification of the report. Failure to answer the questions may mean that the expert cannot be called to give evidence.

Experts are encouraged to meet so as to discuss their differences, and guidelines have recently been issued for consultation (Guidelines on Experts' Discussions in the Context of Clinical Disputes 2000).

THE CLINICAL DISPUTES FORUM

Before the Woolf Inquiry there was little communication between the professionals representing patients on the one hand and defendant health authorities and Trusts on the other. During the course of his inquiry Lord Woolf consulted many people, both lay and professional, with every possible connection with medical litigation. Several hundred people were drawn into working parties to develop ideas for reform. People who had never sat round a table together became working colleagues—judges and nurses, senior doctors and

Expert Witness Institute

Expert's Declaration

1. I understand that my overriding duty is to the court, both in preparing reports and in giving oral evidence.
2. I have set out in my report what I understand from those instructing me to be the questions in respect of which my opinion as an expert are required[1]
3. I have done my best, in preparing this report, to be accurate and complete. I have mentioned all matters which I regard as relevant to the opinions I have expressed. All of the matters on which I have expressed an opinion lie within my field of expertise.
4. I have drawn to the attention of the court all matters, of which I am aware, which might adversely affect my opinion.
5. Wherever I have no personal knowledge, I have indicated the source of factual information.
6. I have not included anything in this report which has been suggested to me by anyone, including the lawyers instructing me, without forming my own independent view of the matter.
7. Where, in my view, there is a range of reasonable opinion, I have indicated the extent of that range in the report.
8. At the time of signing the report I consider it to be complete and accurate. I will notify those instructing me if, for any reason, I subsequently consider that the report requires any correction or qualification.
9. I understand that this report will be the evidence that I will give under oath, subject to any correction or qualification I may make before swearing to its veracity.
10. I have attached to this report a summary of my instructions.

I believe that the facts I have stated in this report are true and that the opinions I have expressed are correct.

Signed   Date

Note

1. The point of this is to ensure that the expert is directing his/her opinion to the relevant issues. Experience shows that unless this is done, much time can be wasted on the wrong question.

Guidance notes

1. The declaration should be considered carefully by the expert. Signing it is not a routine matter. If any part of it requires modification for an individual case, it should be modified accordingly. Thus in some cases, an expert's instructions may limit the scope of the report and paragraph 2 may require modification accordingly.
2. The declaration is appropriate for only *civil* cases.
3. The declaration is not about ethics, but about responsibilities.
4. The declaration is only appropriately associated with the *final report* for exchange.
5. The declaration should be served as an appendix to the final report.

4th February 1999

Fig. 49.1 The Expert Witness Institute's Expert's Declaration.

plaintiff solicitors, plaintiff organisations (such as Action for the Victims of Medical Accidents), hospital staff and claims managers; all developed ways of working together. Early in the inquiry, in July 1995, Lord Woolf made a speech to a conference of health care providers at the Royal Society of Medicine. He called for the foundation of an umbrella organisation of people who would normally never talk to each other but who, as the inquiry had proved, could work together for the benefit of patients and health professionals alike. As a result the Clinical Disputes Forum (www.clinical-disputes-forum.org.uk) was founded in January 1996.

The Forum consists of representatives of every group involved in clinical negligence. There are client groups, those representing patients and consumers on the one hand and the health service managers, doctors and dentists on the other; the operators and funders of the system, solicitors on both sides, barristers and experts, the NHS Litigation Authority and the Legal Services Commission; then there are those who are neutral but central to the process, the Lord Chancellor's Department, the General Medical Council, the Law Society and the UKCC (regulating the nursing professions). Almost every point of view is represented so the Forum has a unique view of the problems within litigation and how best to solve them. The Forum has set itself a number of tasks, the first of which was to design a pre-action protocol for the resolution of clinical disputes. After extensive consultation the protocol was published in September 1998 (Pre-Action Protocol for the Resolution of Clinical Disputes 1998) and came into force on the 26th April 1999, at the same time as the CPR. Failure to comply with the protocol carries cost penalties. The main requirement of the protocol is that the claimant writes a letter of claim detailing the basis of the complaint *before* issuing proceedings. The defendant then has 14 days to acknowledge the letter of claim and a further three months in which to provide a *reasoned answer*. The experience of claims managers is that this exercise results in many of the more straightforward and smaller claims being resolved without recourse to litigation.

The Forum's next task was to provide the guidelines for experts' discussions referred to above (Guidelines on Experts' Discussions in the Context of Clinical Disputes 2000).

CLINICAL RISK MANAGEMENT

Clinical risk management may be defined as:

A particular approach to improving the quality of care, which places special emphasis on occasions on which patients are disturbed or harmed by their treatment (Vincent 1995).

The essential ingredients of a successful clinical risk management system are:

- the identification of adverse outcome
- analysis of the data base
- control and quality improvement
- funding.

The aims of clinical risk management:

To reduce and as far as possible eliminate harm to the patient

To deal with the injured patient

    continuity of care

    swift compensation for the justified claimant

To safeguard the assets of the organisation

    financial

    reputation

    staff morale

To improve the quality of care.

There is no denying that the impetus for risk management in the National Health Service has come from the escalating costs of malpractice litigation. The need has been increased by the recent procedural changes outlined above which make it essential for health care providers to identify adverse outcome and to investigate it at an early stage. However, responding only to those incidents that lead to litigation is to miss most of the problems. The Harvard Study (Brennan et al 1991), repeated elsewhere and shortly to be repeated in the United Kingdom, has demonstrated that only a tiny proportion (1 in 14 in the Harvard Study) of identified negligent events resulted in litigation. If clinical risk management is to achieve its aim of preventing harm to patients the aim must be to capture *all* adverse events, not only those resulting in litigation.

In the practice of obstetrics there are a number of problem areas that give rise to complaint and often to litigation:

- cerebral palsy
- shoulder dystocia
- vaginal birth after caesarean section (VBAC)
- anal sphincter injury
- consent.

Cerebral palsy

The cost of cerebral palsy claims dwarfs all other categories of litigation (Gumbel 1998, 1999a). The acknowledgement that only 10–15% of cerebral palsy can, on present medical knowledge and understanding, be linked to birth events is of little comfort to the defendants for the question before the court will be whether *in this particular case* the cerebral palsy relates to substandard care. More than a decade ago the criteria for linking intrapartum asphyxia with cerebral palsy were set out by Freeman & Nelson (1988).

---

1. Was there evidence of marked and prolonged intrapartum asphyxia?
2. Did the infant, as a newborn, exhibit signs of moderate or severe hypoxic-ischaemic encephalopathy during the newborn period, with evidence also of asphyxial injury to other organ systems?
3. Is the child's neurologic condition one that intrapartum asphyxia could explain?
4. Has the work-up been sufficient to rule out other conditions?

But of course the court does not require 'anything approaching a reasonable medical certainty'. The claimant must prove to the court that *on the balance of probabilities* causation of cerebral palsy flowed from the breach of care.

A concerted effort has recently been made by a group of paediatricians and obstetricians, chiefly from Australia and New Zealand (McLennan 1999), to define the prerequisites for proving a causal relation between acute intrapartum events and cerebral palsy. The consensus statement has not met with universal approval and appears to have some fundamental flaws (Dear et al 2000). The authors, for instance, insist that one of the essential criteria to define an acute intrapartum hypoxic event is 'evidence of a metabolic acidosis in intrapartum fetal umbilical artery cord, or very early neonatal blood sample (pH <7.00 and base deficit ≥ 12 mmol/l)'. Nowhere do they say where the evidence lies to support these figures and they appear to be unaware that in the majority of cerebral palsy cases coming before the courts there are no cord (or early neonatal) blood samples. Although the authors purport to give advice on how expert witnesses should behave they appear not to understand the burden of proof which is that *on the balance of probabilities* cerebral palsy is linked with birth events. The judgement will be made, more likely than not, on the available evidence before the court. Blood gases showing that there was no acidaemia at birth would of course be compelling evidence. The absence of blood gases is merely neutral. If it were not so, the message to all obstetricians and paediatricians would be clear—under no circumstances should blood gases be performed! That presumably was not the authors' intention.

For that minority of babies whose cerebral palsy is acquired during labour the commonest mechanism is asphyxia. In litigation, attention focuses on detection of intrapartum asphyxia and its prevention. Traditionally, the condition of the fetus has been assessed by auscultation of the fetal heart and examination of the amniotic fluid. Meconium in the liquor is a poor predictor of fetal asphyxia, particularly in the term baby, and so attention has focused on the fetal heart:

> . . . there is no evidence that intermittent auscultation using a Pinard stethoscope is of any value in intrapartum care. Emergency delivery of infants with a tachycardia (>160 beats/min) or a bradycardia (<120 beats/min) or with an irregularity of rhythm (another traditional sign of distress) detected using intermittent auscultation often resulted in infants showing every sign of perfect health, whereas others died unexpectedly in utero without any warning signs (Steer & Danielan 1999).

Historically, the first attempt to improve fetal monitoring was by fetal blood scalp sampling but the method is 'time consuming and inconvenient to perform, and uncomfortable for the mother' (Steer & Danielan 1999), not to mention the poor quality control and the often paradoxical results. In a medico-legal context there is often criticism of the defendants for relying on fetal scalp samples that were self-evidently wrong or were relied upon despite continuing abnormalities on the CTG. It must be clearly understood that the information about fetal pH is only valid at the time of the sample and has little predictive quality (i.e. a normal pH does not rule out the development of acidosis in the near future). In circumstances such as breech delivery where a period of hypoxia is inevitable during birth, it is doubtful whether fetal blood sampling has any place at all.

> Breech presentation presents special risks and in view of these there is little or no place for fetal blood sampling in a breech labour. The blood is more difficult to obtain from the tissues of the breech and it may be different from that obtained from scalp skin. If, having understood the normal mechanisms of CTG changes in a breech, there is a good indication for pH measurement then there is a good indication for caesarean section (Gibb & Arulkumaran 1997).

The enthusiasts for fetal blood sampling argue that its proper use reduces unnecessary operative delivery if the diagnosis of fetal distress relies only upon observations of the fetal heart rate. However meta-analysis (Steer & Danielan 1999) fails to show any clear advantage and at present the method is employed in a minority of district general hospitals.

The best opportunity to study the health of the fetus in labour is at present provided by electronic fetal monitoring. There is at present no consensus within the profession that electronic fetal monitoring is mandatory in all labours. The Dublin Study (McDonald et al 1985) in the mid 1980s led to the widespread acceptance of the improbable notion that listening to the baby some of the time is as good as listening to the baby all of the time. More recent studies (Thacker et al 1995, Vintzileos et al 1995) have shown a significant reduction in the deaths attributed to hypoxia with electronic fetal heart monitoring and a substantial and highly significant reduction in the incidence of neonatal seizures. Failure to understand, interpret and react to an abnormal CTG is the commonest accusation of the claimant in cerebral palsy cases. The CTG monitor confers no protection on the baby. To be effective, the monitor must be interpreted by adequately trained staff. In the context of clinical risk management, the single most important challenge to the maternity services is the 24-hour provision of midwifery and obstetric staff capable of interpreting the CTG and reacting appropriately to the abnormal trace. It is often argued that experts differ on the interpretation of CTGs: indeed they do, but that has little to do with the realities of litigation where so often barn door abnormalities are ignored, making it impossible to defend the claim.

Shoulder dystocia

The large number of claims for Erb's palsy are a cause of concern to the Litigation Authority. While obstetric brachial plexus palsy is the commonest injury to follow shoulder dystocia, it is not the most severe. Asphyxial damage to the baby, intrapartum death and soft tissue damage to the mother are also occasionally subjects of litigation. The problem is not a new one and was recognised by William Smellie in the 18th century who first described the typical lesion of the upper trunk of the brachial plexus (C5,6), subsequently associated with the name of Erb. Woods (1943) described the mechanics of shoulder dystocia in the 1940s and since then a number of other manoeuvres have been suggested for the relief of the impacted anterior shoulder. Until the publication of a specialist textbook on the subject (O'Leary 1992), general obstetric and midwifery texts were not always coherent in their advice to obstetricians and midwives confronted with this most terrifying of all obstetric dilemmas.

It is often claimed that shoulder dystocia is unpredictable and indeed much of it is. Nevertheless the predictors of a big baby and of shoulder dystocia are clearly documented in the literature:

THE PREDICTORS OF SHOULDER DYSTOCIA BEFORE LABOUR

- Excessive maternal birthweight
- Maternal obesity
- Diabetes mellitus
- Gestational age of greater than 41 weeks
- Previous shoulder dystocia
- Previous macrosomia
- Recognised macrosomia in the present pregnancy.

The prediction of birthweight is difficult, particularly towards the upper end of the weight range. Nevertheless, with improving ultrasound techniques, large babies are increasingly identified. Birthweight takes on a particular significance in diabetes where the shape of the baby favours shoulder dystocia. About half of all shoulder dystocia occurs in babies of normal birthweight (below 4 kilos) and it is difficult to devise a sensible programme for prevention of this complication. Nevertheless there is an evolving consensus (Roberts 1994) that caesarean section should be seriously considered for a diabetic where estimated birthweight is in excess of 4.5 kilos and for any baby whose predicted birthweight is above 5 kilos.

Shoulder dystocia is a rare complication in the labour ward and a shoulder dystocia drill should be taught to all midwives and junior obstetric staff. There is no time to consult the labour ward procedure book or protocol collection when the head is already born. Although the American College of Gynecologists (1997) comes to the unhelpful conclusion that 'there is no evidence that any one maneuver is superior to another in releasing an impacted shoulder or reducing the chance of injury', it reluctantly concedes that the McRoberts manoeuvre is easily facilitated and has a high success rate. The recommended sequence of manoeuvres in the current literature for the relief of this emergency is

---

- Change the position of the mother
  - McRoberts
  - all fours
- suprapubic pressure
- rotation of the shoulder (Woods–Rubin screw)
- delivery of the posterior arm.

The Zavenelli manoeuvre (cephalic replacement) deserves a mention but there are no convincing reports of its successful use in the UK literature.

Vaginal birth after caesarean section (VBAC)

Labour following a caesarean section differs only in one respect from other labours: it carries the risk of rupture of the caesarean section scar. The incidence of rupture is widely quoted as less than 1% (Dickinson 1999) but in fact incidences of 0.3–2% (American College of Gynecologists 1997) can be found in the literature. It seems likely that the true incidence is underreported. The consequences of scar rupture may be severe for both mother and baby; the principal issues arising in such circumstances are usually:

- consent
- the abuse of Syntocinon.

Before setting out on a trial of vaginal delivery with a caesarean section scar it is essential that the mother is informed of the risk. Since rupture of the scar is the *only* increased risk, that information must be specifically provided:

> I am not aware of any credible VBAC study that did not report adverse outcomes. Nor am I aware of any proponent of VBAC who would not advise patients of the risk of uterine rupture during labour (Gleicher 1991).

In retrospect, in cases where the scar has ruptured with an adverse outcome, it is likely that the parents will say that had the risks been put to them they would have chosen elective caesarean section. That argument can only be met by proper discussion beforehand and a full annotation of both the discussion and the decision. In advising the mother of the risks it is reasonable to stress the dangers inherent in delivery by caesarean section provided only that the risks of *elective* caesarean section are given for that is the true comparison. The risk of elective caesarean section to the baby is negligible; there are no reliable figures for risk to the mother of serious morbidity but the mortality is of the order of 1:10 000, a similar order of risk to that involved in driving a motor car.

Meta-analysis has not shown convincing evidence that Syntocinon used appropriately increases the risk of scar rupture. That is very different from the conclusion that Syntocinon is entirely safe in vaginal birth after caesarean section. The use of Syntocinon figures prominently in litigation following scar rupture and if the drug is to be used at all it must be employed with extreme caution. One of the myths surrounding scar rupture is that there are warning signs that presage the disaster. In many cases coming before the courts the tocograph suggests, by the frequency and elision of contractions, evidence of hyperstimulation in the period leading up to scar rupture.

Anal sphincter injury

There are no reliable figures for the incidence of anal sphincter injury following vaginal birth. Figures of 0.3–2% are quoted. The protective effect of episiotomy has never been demonstrated in a clinical trial and the literature on this subject is bedevilled by the lack of proper definition. Episiotomy, for instance, tends to be treated as one operation as if mediolateral episiotomy were the same as midline. It is seldom possible for the claimant to discharge the burden of proof that a third degree tear occurred through lack of skill or care. The accusation is usually that, an anal sphincter injury having occurred, the repair of it was defective. Sphincter injuries are missed because women are not properly examined in the third stage of labour. The injury goes unrecognised and is only subsequently repaired when the patient, weeks or months after the event, complains of anal incontinence. The results of such secondary repair are often disappointing. The claimant, in order to succeed in the courts, has to be able to demonstrate that primary repair would, on the balance of probabilities, have restored her continence. In the last decade, the follow-up of women after primary repair has revealed a disappointingly high incidence of imperfect continence. Until recently it was difficult for the claimant in such circumstances to discharge the burden of proof that, had the sphincter been repaired at the time of the injury, she would on the balance of probabilities have had her continence restored. A recent meta-analysis (Schofield & Grace 1999) has demonstrated that 66% of women regained full continence after primary repair but only 49% after secondary repair.

Consent

All treatment requires consent, for every woman has an absolute right to decide what should be done to her body:

> Every human being of adult years and sound mind has a right to determine what should be done with his body, and a surgeon who performs an operation without his patient's consent commits an assault for which he is liable in damages (Cardozo 1914).

For consent to be valid in law, three elements are required:

1. voluntariness
2. competence
3. knowledge (Clements 1995).

In expressing the relationship between the health care professional and the patient consent is a somewhat negative concept; the positive expression of that relationship is choice. In particular, for the obstetrician and the midwife dealing predominantly with normal women having uncomplicated pregnancies, the emphasis should be upon facilitating patient choice, providing sufficient information for the woman to decide which method of management is most acceptable to her. In obstetrics, as elsewhere, the obsession with the consent form and the need to have it signed often proves a distraction from the real business of informing the patient and allowing her to make the choice. In any event, in the context of labour ward treatment the consent form is of little assistance.

When an obstetrician obtains consent for an elective procedure the process is no different from that in any other branch of surgery. The patient must be given sufficient understanding to enable her to make a choice in circumstances where she is free to exercise choice. The introduction of the term informed consent is unhelpful in this regard. If the phrase means anything at all (what is uninformed consent?) it is a term of art relating to the standard applied by the courts in other developed countries. That standard, the standard of the prudent patient, applies throughout the developed world except in the British Isles. In these islands the courts still apply the test of the responsible doctor, in other words the amount of information required to be given is that which any reasonable doctor would give in the circumstances – the same test as for treatment (Bolam v. Friern Hospital Management Committee 1957, Watt 1995). At least that was the case before Bolitho (Bolitho v. City and Hackney HA 1993, Watt 1999). It remains to be seen to what extent the courts will apply the risk–benefit analysis to the question of information in the context of consent. It might, for instance, apply in the case of vaginal birth after caesarean section where the court might take the view that, even if other doctors did not warn of the risk of rupture of the uterus, a risk–benefit analysis would show that such practice would fail to measure up to a reasonable standard.

The circumstances in the labour ward prevent the imparting of critical information in sufficient quantity within a reasonable timescale to meet any objective analysis. In circumstances such as prolapsed cord or severe antepartum haemorrhage there is simply neither time nor opportunity to explain the treatment options in detail to a terrified woman. It may be argued (and has been so argued in the courts) that a woman in labour, in severe pain and under the influence of drugs is in any event not competent to give consent (Puxon 1997). Consent for obstetric procedures presents special difficulties to both doctor and patient. Some of it can be overcome by antenatal education and the imparting of information at a time when there is no crisis. Many emergency situations can be foreseen and good management should aim to create the circumstances in which, because complications have been anticipated, when the need to intervene does arise the tension associated with the emergency is reduced. It is unrealistic, however, to suppose that all emergencies can be foreseen. The obstetrician and the midwife should seek to build up a degree of trust in a patient such that she will be able to accept emergency advice given in her best interest.

On several recent occasions the courts have been asked to intervene in circumstances involving the refusal of treatment by a pregnant woman, refusal which might have threatened the life and well-being of her fetus and herself. In every case at first instance (and in the only case to come before the Court of Appeal in advance of the event) the courts have ruled in favour of intervention and have declared lawful caesarean section notwithstanding the refusal of the mother. In Re: MB (1997), Lady Justice Butler-Sloss, giving the leading judgement:

> rejected the submission that the rights of the unborn child should be weighed in the balance and upheld the principle that the competent mother has the unqualified right to decide whether or not to accept surgical intervention in childbirth. However on the facts the courts upheld the decision of the first instance judge who had held that the mother's phobia of the injection

needle rendered her incompetent (Lord Justice Thorpe 1999a).

The only occasion on which the courts have taken a different view was in the case of St. George's Healthcare NHS Trust ex Parte S (1999) in which, long after the event, the Court of Appeal was able to say that the autonomy of the woman is sacrosanct and must be preserved in future cases. In that case the Court of Appeal laid down guidelines for the future conduct of cases both by doctors and by lawyers, where maternal consent to intervention in pregnancy is refused. These matters, the absolute right of any adult to choose, to accept or refuse treatment and the rights of the fetus in law are discussed in detail elsewhere (Grace 1999, Lord Justice Thorpe 1999a,b).

CONCLUSION

In obstetric malpractice litigation three themes predominate:

- communication
- delay
- the cascade of events.

Consent issues are of course about communication and failure to communicate adequately with the patient to understand her wishes and to provide her with sufficient information to understand. But there are also communication issues between staff, handover of patients and communications, both vertical and horizontal, within the labour ward setting. It is essential in this context that if a midwife does not obtain a satisfactory clinical response from a junior doctor she should be empowered (and feel empowered) to go above the head of the junior doctor to someone more senior and if necessary to the consultant, so as to make sure that a proper clinical decision is made. Delay is ubiquitous in obstetric malpractice: delay in making observations and delay in interpreting those observations, delay in making decisions to intervene and delay in implementing those decisions. Birth asphyxia litigation is usually about delay above all else.

But obstetric disasters are not achieved by one end-player. They are usually the result of a cascade of events, a series of indecisions or wrong decisions starting in the antenatal period, usually with the absence of any decision at all continuing in the labour ward. Complicated (or high-risk) obstetrics involving twins, vaginal breech delivery, vaginal birth after caesarean section, or delivery of the macrosomic baby require planning, beginning in the antenatal clinic. On admission there is a further opportunity to assess risk factors but it may be more difficult later in labour when events move fast. The junior doctor or midwife left with a complex vaginal delivery ending in disaster is not usually the only person to have made a mistake, indeed he may not have made a mistake at all but is simply collecting the cumulative errors and omissions of more senior colleagues who had, and missed, the opportunity to intervene.

KEY POINTS

- Recent changes in the civil procedure rules have clarified the status of the expert, emphasising the expert's duty to the court. The reforms simplified the language and procedure of litigation, imposed upon the court the duty of managing cases and encouraged, by Pre-Action Protocols, a degree of openness and exchange of view before an action is started.
- Recent decisions in the courts have significantly increased the quantum of damage, partly by the increase in general damages and partly by reducing the discount rate from 4.5% to 3%.
- The Clinical Disputes Forum provides an opportunity for all the parties involved in clinical negligence litigation to contribute to debate and to further reform.

REFERENCES

Access to Justice 1996 Final Report to the Lord Chancellor on the Civil Justice System of England and Wales. HMSO, London

American College of Gynecologists 1994 ACOG committee opinion if vaginal delivery after a previous caesarean birth. Int J Obstet Gynaecol 48:127–129. 1995

American College of Gynecologists 1997 ACOG practice patterns: shoulder dystocia. Int J Gynaecol Obstet 60:306–313 1998

Barnett v. Chelsea and Kensington Hospital Management Committee [1969] 1QB 428, [1968] 2WLR422, [1969] 1A11 ER 1068

Bolam v. Friern Hospital Management Committee [1957] 2 A11 ER 118, [1957] 1 WLR 582, 1 BMLR 1

Bolitho v. City and Hackney HA [1993] 4 Med LR 381, [1993] 13 BMLR 111, [1998] AC232, [1997] 4A11 ER 771, [1997] 3WLR 1151, 39 BMLR I, [1998] PNLR 1, [1998] Lloyd's Rep Med 26

Bonnington Castings v. Wardlaw [1956] AC613, HL

Brennan TA, Leape LL, Laird NM, Herbert L, Localio AT, Lawthers AG 1991 Incidence of Adverse Events and Negligence in Hospitalized Patients. New England Journal of Medicine 324:370–6

Bull v. Devon Area Health Authority [1993] 4Med LR 117, CA

Burton v. Islington Health Authority [1991] 1A11 ER 825 and De Martell v. Merton and Sutton Health Authority [1992] 3A11 ER 8230; [1991] 2 Med LR 209

Cardozo J 1914 Schloendorff v. Society of New York Hospital. 105 NE 92

Clements RV 1995 Consent 1: the consultant's view. The Diplomate 2(2):139–143

Clements RV 1999 The new Procedure Rules: Part 35. Clinical Risk 5(3):90–98

Dear P, Rennie J, Newell S, Rosenbloom L 2000 Response to the proposal of a template for defining a causal relation between acute intrapartum events and cerebral palsy. Clinical Risk 6(4):137–142

Dickinson JE 1999 Previous caesarean section. In: James DK, Steer PJ, Weiner CP, Gonik B (eds) High risk pregnancy: management options, 2nd edn. WB Saunders, London, ch 67

Draft Code of Guidance for Experts 1999 Clinical Risk 5(5):168–172

Emeh v. Kensington and Chelsea and Westminster Health Authority [1995] QB 1012, [1984] 3A11 ER 1044

Gascoine v. Ian Sherridan & Co and Latham [1994] 5Med LR 437

Gibb DMF, Arulkumaran S 1997 Cardiotocographic interpretations: clinical scenarios. In: Fetal monitoring in practice, 2nd edn. Butterworth Heinemann, Oxford, ch 8

Gleicher N 1991 Mandatory trial of labour after caesarean delivery: an alternative viewpoint. Letter. Obstet Gynaecol 78(4):727

Grace J 1999 Should the foetus have rights in law? Med Leg J 67:57–67

Guidelines on Experts' Discussions in the Context of Clinical Disputes 2000 Clinical Risk 6(4):149–152

Gumbel EA 1997a Damages in obstetric negligence cases: part I—the calculation of damages. Clinical Risk 3:159–164

Gumbel EA 1997b Damages in obstetric negligence cases: part II—stillborn babies and badly injured babies who die. Clinical Risk 3:198–201

Gumbel EA 1998 Damages in obstetric negligence cases: part III—severely damaged babies who survive. Clinical Risk 4:110–115

Gumbel EA 1999a Damages in obstetric negligence cases: part IV—calculation of damages following the House of Lords' decision in Wells v. Wells. Clinical Risk 5:14–16

Gumbel EA 1999b Damages in obstetric negligence cases: part V—injuries to the mother, unplanned babies and loss of fertility. Clinical Risk 5:55–58

Gumbel EA 1999c The new Civil Procedure Rules: a first impression. Clinical Risk 53:86–89

Hatcher v. Black 1954 Times, 2nd July (QBD)

Havers M 2000 The impact of The European Convention on Human Rights on clinical negligence and medical law. Clinical Risk 6:51–55

Hotson [1987] AC750, [1987] 3WLR 232, [1987] 2A11 ER 909

Hunter v. Hanley [1955] SC200, [1955] SLT 213

Jones MA 1996 Medical negligence, 2nd edn. Sweet and Maxwell, London 1996, ch 2, para 037

Jones MA 2000 Causation and aetiology. Clinical Risk 6(3):106–112

Lockhart KB 1999 But you have not addressed the questions . . . Clinical Risk 5:59–60

Lord Justice Thorpe 1999a Consent for caesarean section, part 1—development of the law. Clinical Risk 5:173–196

Lord Justice Thorpe 1999b Consent for caesarean section, part 2—autonomy, capacity, best interests, reasonable force and procedural guidelines. Clinical Risk 5:209–213

McDonald D, Grant A, Sheridan-Pereira M, Boylan P, Chalmers I 1985 The Dublin randomized controlled trial of intrapartum fetal heartrate monitoring. Am J Obstet Gynecol 152:524–539

McFarlane v. Tayside Health Board [1999] 3WLR 1301

McGee v. National Coal Board [1972] 3A11 ER 1008, HL

McKay v. Essex Area Health Authority [1982] QB 1166, [1982] 2A11 ER 771

McLennan A 1999 A template for defining a causal relation between acute intrapartum events and cerebral palsy; international consensus statement. BMJ 319:1054–1059

Maynard v. West Midland Regional Health Authority [1984] 1WLR 634, [1985] 1A11 ER 635

O'Leary JA 1992 Shoulder dystocia and birth injury. McGraw Hill, New York

Powers M, Barton A 1995 Introduction to medical negligence law. Clinical Risk 1:37–39

Pre-Action Protocol for the Resolution of Clinical Disputes 1998 Clinical Risk 4:137–161

Puxon M 1994 Commentary on Reay v. British Nuclear Fuels [1994] 5Med LR 1 at 54

Puxon M 1995 The doctor and the criminal law: assault and battery. Clinical Risk 1:189–191

Puxon M 1996 The doctor and the criminal law: abortion. Clinical Risk 2:135–138

Puxon M 1997 The incompetent parturient. Clinical Risk 3:27

Re:MB [1997] 2FCR 541 AC. 38 BMLR 175–194

Roberts L 1994 Shoulder dystocia. In: Studd J (ed) Progress in obstetrics and gynaecology, vol 11. Churchill Livingstone, Edinburgh

Schofield PF, Grace R 1999 Faecal incontinence after childbirth. Clinical Risk 5:201–204

Sheldon S 1998 The doctor and the criminal law: female genital mutilation. Clinical Risk 4:189–192

St. George's Healthcare NHS Trust v. S, R v. Collins, x pS [1999] Fam 26 CA [1998] 3 WLR 936. 44 BMLR 160–196

Steer PJ, Danielian P 1999 Fetal distress in labour. In: James DK, Steers PJ, Weiner CP, Gonik B (eds) High risk pregnancy: management options, 2nd edn. WB Saunders, London, ch 64

Thacker SB, Stroup DF, Peterson HB 1995 Efficacy and safety of intrapartum electronic fetal monitoring: an update. Obstet Gynaecol 86:613–620

Vincent C 1995 Clinical risk management. BMJ Publications, London

Vintzileos AM, Nochimson DJ, Guzman ER et al 1995 Intrapartum electronic fetal heart monitoring versus intermittent auscultation: a meta-analysis. Obstet Gynaecol 85:149–155

Watt J 1995 Leading cases in medical negligence: Bolam v. Friern HMC. Clinical Risk 1:84–85

Watt J 1997 Leading cases in medical negligence: Wilsher v. Essex AHA. Clinical Risk 3:67–68

Watt J 1999 Leading cases in medical negligence: Bolitho v. City and Hackney HA. Clinical Risk 5:17–20

Wells v. Wells, Thomas v. Brighton Health Authority and Page v. Sheerness Steel plc [1999] 1 AC 345 HL [1998] 3 WLR 329. 43 BMLR 99–142

Whitehouse v. Jordan [1981] 1WLR246, [1981] 1 A11 ER 267, LH

Wilsher v. Essex Area Health Authority [1980] 2 WLR 557; [1988] 1 A11 ER 871

Woods CE 1943 A principle of physics as applicable to shoulder dystocia. Am J Obstet Gynecol 45:796–812

Young M 1999 Practical implications of the House of Lords' decision in Wells v. Wells, Thomas v. Brighton Health Authority and Page v. Sheerness Steel plc. Clinical Risk 5:23–24

50

Research in obstetrics and gynaecology

William Dunlop

INTRODUCTION

The quinquennial Research Assessment Exercise undertaken by all UK universities has done a great deal to impress upon the academic community the importance of research activity for the continuing success, both intellectual and financial, of university departments. Difficult choices have been made and, as a result, there has been substantial unease in certain departments. Reservations have been expressed about the competitiveness of obstetrics and gynaecology in this new hard-nosed environment. What evidence is there that the discipline has suffered? How can obstetrics and gynaecology compete successfully in the future? What are the constraints affecting academic development in the specialty? This chapter attempts to answer questions such as these.

INTERNATIONAL PERSPECTIVE

First, however, it is important to appreciate research endeavours in the United Kingdom from a global viewpoint. There is no doubt about the considerable health needs of women and children throughout the world. The World Health Organization (WHO) estimates that there are 120 million couples worldwide with unmet family planning needs, that 1600 women die each day in the course of pregnancy and childbirth and that at least 55 000 per day have a major complication, that more than 900 000 curable sexually transmitted diseases are contracted each day, that 30–40 million people have contracted HIV and that 60–80 million couples are infertile.

The World Health Organization described its Special Programme of Research, Development and Research Training in Human Reproduction in its Biennial Report for 1986–1987. The four cornerstones of reproductive health policy were identified as:

- family planning
- maternal care
- infant and child care
- control of sexually transmitted diseases.

The mandate of the Programme is outlined as follows:

"The Special Programme is a global programme of international research cooperation initiated by WHO to promote, coordinate, support, conduct and evaluate research in human reproduction with particular reference to the needs of developing countries by:

(i) promoting and supporting research aimed at finding and developing safe and effective methods of fertility regulation as well as identifying and eliminating obstacles to such research and development;

(ii) identifying and evaluating health and safety problems associated with fertility regulation technology, analysing the behavioural and social determinants of fertility regulation, and testing cost-effective interventions to develop improved approaches to fertility regulation within the context of reproductive health services;

(iii) strengthening the training and research capability of developing countries to conduct research in the field of human reproduction;

(iv) establishing a basis for collaboration with other programmes engaged in research and development in human reproduction, including the identification of priorities across the field and the coordination of activities in the light of such priorities."

Research priorities recently identified by WHO include:

- the development of new methods of fertility regulation for both women and men
- the introduction of new methods into family planning programmes
- study of the long-term safety of methods already in use and other aspects of epidemiological research in reproductive health
- study of social and behavioural aspects of reproductive health
- development of methods for controlling the spread of sexually transmitted disease which can cause infertility (HRP Online 2000).

NHS RESEARCH

The UK National Health Service Research and Development (NHS R&D) Programme was established in 1991 in order to improve the research base for the NHS. Approximately £65 million is currently spent on this programme. In addition, R&D support is available for NHS providers (£384 million) and the Department of Health commissions research through its own, separately funded, Policy Research Programme (£30 million) designed to inform ministerial policy and priorities.

The following priority programmes were previously identified and almost all of these have now completed commissioning work:

- cancer
- people with physical and complex disabilities
- asthma management

- evaluation of methods to promote the implementation of research findings
- mother and child health
- primary/secondary health care interface
- primary dental care
- mental health
- cardiovascular disease and stroke
- forensic mental health.

The programme for mother and child health was established in 1994, ratifying the 23 priorities recommended by an *ad hoc* advisory group. These priorities are set out in Table 50.1. Commissioning of research in these areas, totalling £6.5 million over 5 years, was carried out by a group of 18 members, none of whom was at that time a practising obstetrician or gynaecologist. Only 2 of the 50 listed projects have members of the Royal College of Obstetricians and Gynaecologists as principal investigators.

The organisation of NHS priority programmes in R&D is changing. The NHS Executive is moving towards a system which contains the following main programmes:

- health technology assessment
- service development and organisation
- new and emerging applications of technology
- national primary care development programme
- research methodology
- consumer involvement in R&D.

The total number of projects in each of these groups is set out in Table 50.2, together with an estimate of those topics which appear to be immediately relevant to obstetrics and gynaecology. The final column identifies grants held by members of the RCOG. Thus it can be seen that 6.7% of topics are relevant to obstetrics and gynaecology; of these, about one-third (2.4% of the total projects) were commissioned from members of the RCOG.

The Department of Health also produces the National Research Register (http://193.32.28.83/research/nrr.htm) of ongoing and recently completed research projects funded by, or of interest to, the United Kingdom's National Health Service. Ongoing projects currently number 18 250. A cursory analysis of the first 2 500 listed projects reveals that 225 (9%) are relevant to obstetrics and gynaecology, and of these 57 (25%, or 2.3% of the total) have members of the RCOG listed as lead researcher.

THE MEDICAL RESEARCH COUNCIL

The United Kingdom Medical Research Council (MRC; http://www.mrc.ac.uk) states that its purpose is:

- to encourage and support high-quality research with the aim of maintaining and improving human health
- to train skilled people, and to advance and disseminate knowledge and technology with the aim of meeting national needs in terms of health, quality of life and economic competitiveness
- to promote public engagement with medical research.

Table 50.1 Priority areas defined by the NHS R&D Advisory Group on Mother and Child Health

1. Evaluation of different models of maternity care.
2. Interventions during labour: short- and long-term outcomes.
3. Mental and physical health of mother after birth and impact on the family.
4. Evaluation of genetic services, to include access to, and delivery of, services; methods of education of professional staff and families; and evaluation of counselling and support for bereaved families.
5. Examination of causes, prevention, management and long-term outcome of babies born too early or too small.
6. Evaluation of the reasons for variation in outcome of the management of 'high-risk' neonates.
7. Impact of maternal and infant nutrition (including breast feeding) on health and development.
8. Identifying interventions, including development of parenting skills, to reduce harmful effects of social and physical environment on health and development of mother and child.
9. Investigation and management of common infant problems (e.g. night waking, crying, etc.).
10. Evaluation of the effectiveness and cost intervention to prevent injury, including an evaluation of the impact of such interventions on the quality of life of children, adolescents and their families.
11. Evaluation of the effectiveness and cost of the services provided for acutely injured children and adolescents.
12. Development of routine methods for the measurement of the age-related prevalence of disability and the development of appropriate outcome measures for evaluation of the services provided for infants, children, adolescents and their families with serious and/or disabling conditions.
13. Development and evaluation of methods to identify, correctly diagnose and provide for the needs of children and adolescents with complex disabilities and their families—with reference to models for the coordination of services within and between the health, social services and education sectors
14. Development and evaluation of methods of providing information to parents, children and adolescents with complex disabilities to allow effective use of services.
15. Development and evaluation of guidelines for the appropriate skill mix and settings for the treatment of important common chronic illnesses in childhood and adolescence, e.g. diabetes, recurrent acute lower respiratory tract illnesses (including asthma), epilepsy, orthopaedic problems, mental health problems.
16. Development and evaluation of methods to inform and empower parents, children, adolescents and school teachers to undertake the everyday management of important chronic childhood illnesses, e.g. asthma, diabetes.
17. Evaluation of the cost and effectiveness of the current different models of service delivery for children and adolescents with emotional, behavioural and learning disorders.
18. Evaluation of strategies to change health behaviours in children and adolescents, e.g. smoking, drugs, unwanted pregnancies.
19. Identifying the needs and views of young people on the appropriate delivery of adolescent services, especially primary health care services.
20. Population-based evaluation of the ease of access to and the use of health care services by children in need, in particular those from materially disadvantaged families and minority ethnic groups.
21. Paediatric pharmacology: the safety and efficacy of drugs and the evaluation of drug use for infants.

Table 50.2 NHS R&D Health Technology Assessment Programme

Topic group	Commissioned projects		
	Total	Relevant topic	O&G[a] grantholder
Acute care sector	45	4	3
Primary and community care	35	3	0
Pharmaceutical	38	1	0
Population screening	30	7	2
Diagnostics and imaging	36	2	1
Methodology	54	0	0
Projects commissioned for NICE	16	0	0
Totals	254	17	6

[a] Name in RCOG Register of Fellows and Members

During 1997, the MRC spent £308 million on research and training (Fig. 50.1). Eight core objectives were outlined in the MRC's Corporate Plan for 1996–1999:

1. to stimulate and strengthen research relevant to human health
2. to promote training and career development
3. to create and nurture productive environments for research
4. to encourage others to exploit the fruits of MRC research
5. to publicise research and its achievements as part of a strategy of promoting public understanding of science
6. to continue to maintain and develop professional standards and effective business management in all activities
7. to take account of the research needs of user communities—notably in the health service and public health, in industry and government—in developing and implementing scientific strategy
8. to develop partnerships with others providing, purchasing or sponsoring research—within and outwith the UK.

The MRC supports medical research in three main ways: through its research establishments, by awarding grants to individual scientists, and by providing support for postgraduate students. Research establishments include Interdisciplinary Research Centres, none of which currently has a focus directly related to clinical obstetrics and gynaecology, and MRC Units. There are currently 51 MRC Units. Only one, the MRC Human Reproductive Sciences Unit (formerly

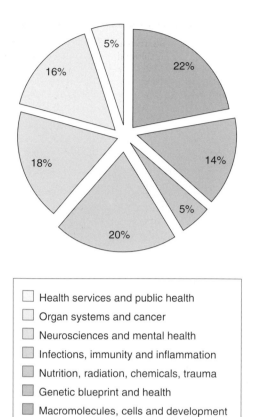

Fig. 50.1   MRC research expenditure 1997.

Legend:
- ☐ Health services and public health
- ☐ Organ systems and cancer
- ☐ Neurosciences and mental health
- ☐ Infections, immunity and inflammation
- ☐ Nutrition, radiation, chemicals, trauma
- ☐ Genetic blueprint and health
- ☐ Macromolecules, cells and development

Table 50.3   Summary of MRC research grant schemes

Centre Grants
To support a multidisciplinary research-centred environment, in partnership with a university, and having full-time, focused scientific leadership and management.

Programme Grants
To support long-term programmes of work, normally where the aim is to answer an interrelated set of questions.

Cooperative Group Grants
To establish or bring together critical research mass, predominantly within single universities, in ways which add value to individual projects and improve the productivity of research environments.

Development Grants
To help universities reach the point where they meet eligibility criteria for making applications for funding under the Co-operative Group Grants scheme.

Career Establishment Grants
To provide support for a fixed period for scientists recently appointed to university academic posts (within the last three years) to help them to establish themselves as independent principal investigators.

Innovation Grants
To provide short-term funding for high-risk, speculative and innovative research awarded on the basis of the applicant's achievement from previous MRC funding.

Strategic Project Grants
To support work which makes a specific contribution to implementing the aims of the Council's scientific strategy.

Trials Grants
To provide support for trials to provide high-quality evidence on the efficacy and effectiveness of interventions in medicine and the health services.

Reproductive Biology Unit) in Edinburgh, has a remit that is of direct relevance to clinical obstetrics and gynaecology. It is noteworthy, however, that the MRC Environmental Epidemiology Unit in Southampton has had a major interest in the fetal and childhood antecedents of adult disease.

The grant awarding process of the MRC has undergone radical reform in the past 5 years. A more strategic view has been taken in order that research strengths may be developed jointly with institutions of higher education. In consequence, the previous elaborate and relatively cost-ineffective scheme of project grants has effectively been disbanded. Current MRC research grant schemes are outlined in Table 50.3.

Obstetricians and gynaecologists previously appeared to have a creditable share of MRC research grant awards. In 1997, it was estimated that 21 of 31 academic units in obstetrics and gynaecology had some degree of MRC funding. Review of the MRC database at that time suggested that MRC support for research into human reproduction was even more widespread than this: in all but three of the UK universities with medical schools a relevant project or programme of research could be identified. With the reduction in project grant support, however, MRC funding will inevitably have reduced. Up to date information is not available.

MRC support for clinical trials in obstetrics and gynaecology has been reasonably substantial in the recent past. In 1997–1998, £1.3 million out of a total budget of £17.6 million was dedicated to 11 (out of a total of 144) clinical trials in obstetrics and gynaecology. In 1998–1999, spending in

relation to obstetrics and gynaecology had increased to £2.6 million out of a total budget of £17.9 million. It is noteworthy, however, that the number of trials supported had reduced to 8 (out of a total of 133).

By supporting postgraduate students, the MRC has contributed to the career development of individual research workers, both clinical and non-clinical, and has thereby helped to strengthen the research workforce in the UK. The MRC's personal award schemes are illustrated in Figure 50.2.

Training priorities have also been defined by the MRC. Areas specifically identified as of strategic importance include:

- bioinformatics
- quantitative biology
- primary care
- clinical neuroscience
- health of the public.

The MRC also organises a series of Health Services Research Training Fellowships (jointly with the NHS) as well as training for individuals from nursing and professions allied to medicine. A significant recent initiative has been a collaboration with the Royal College of Obstetricians and

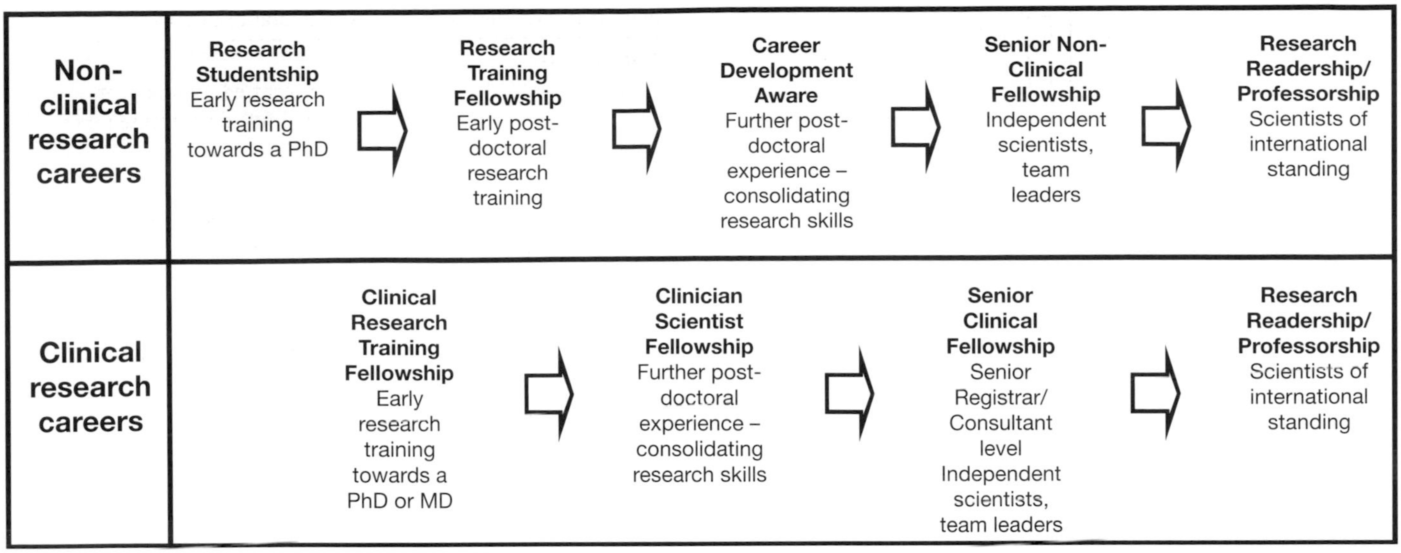

| Non-clinical research careers | Research Studentship
Early research training towards a PhD | → | Research Training Fellowship
Early post-doctoral research training | → | Career Development Aware
Further post-doctoral experience – consolidating research skills | → | Senior Non-Clinical Fellowship
Independent scientists, team leaders | → | Research Readership/ Professorship
Scientists of international standing |
| Clinical research careers | | | Clinical Research Training Fellowship
Early research training towards a PhD or MD | → | Clinician Scientist Fellowship
Further post-doctoral experience – consolidating research skills | → | Senior Clinical Fellowship
Senior Registrar/ Consultant level Independent scientists, team leaders | → | Research Readership/ Professorship
Scientists of international standing |

Fig. 50.2   MRC personal award schemes.

Gynaecologists in funding a number of joint training fellowships. These prestigious fellowships provide opportunities for training in the biomedical sciences in the UK. They are expected to lead to the award of a higher degree (PhD or MD) and applicants are judged in direct competition with those from other clinical disciplines by members of the MRC Clinical Training and Career Development Panel, supplemented by a member nominated by the College. Assessment criteria may include the issues listed in Table 50.4.

The MRC has defined research planning priorities. Those agreed for 1999 are listed in Table 50.5. It will be observed that relatively few of these relate directly to clinical obstetrics and gynaecology. Clinical priorities appear to relate predominantly to Government health initiatives. There is clearly a need to try to influence this process centrally.

It is difficult to ascertain with any certainty the extent of current MRC support for clinical obstetrics and gynaecology. Of the 2162 terms listed on the MRC Funded Projects Database, only 243 appeared to relate to the specialty. In order to obtain a clearer picture of research activity, a specialty-specific search strategy needs to be devised (see below).

CHARITIES SUPPORTING RESEARCH

Apart from the national sources of research funding, there is considerable potential for funding from medical research charities (Association of Medical Research Charities Handbook 2000). Those which are of particular relevance to research in obstetrics and gynaecology and which have an annual research expenditure of more than £1 million are outlined in Table 50.6.

Table 50.4   Issues relevant to the appointment to a training fellowship

Applicant
  Potential to be an excellent doctoral student
  Ability to carry out proposed work
  Commitment to a career in medical research
Project
  Clear objectives and hypotheses
  Technically feasible
  Achievable within timescale
  Intellectually challenging
  Useful for training
Training programme
  Research skills: subject-specific, generic, transferable
  Level and quality of supervision
  Monitoring
Centre
  Standing
  Appropriate for project
  Access to relevant facilities
  Suitable training environment

Table 50.5   MRC planning priorities 1999

The challenge of post-genome research
  Human and comparative genome research and gene identification
  Macromolecular structure, and functional analysis of gene products in health and disease
  Bioinformatics
  Technology development
  Social and ethical research relevant to human genetics
  MRC is also expanding its function for training in informatics
The health of the public
  Inequalities in health
  Behavioural interventions in health
  Early origins of disease
  Antibiotic resistance
Inflammation and immunobiological manipulation
Cardiovascular disease
Primary care

Table 50.6 Selected information about relevant UK medical research charities

Name	Approx. annual spend (£M)	Types of grant			
		Project	Programme	Clinical Research Fellowships	Other
Wellcome Trust	400.0	✓	✓	✓	✓
Cancer Research Campaign	56.0	✓	✓	✓	✓
Action Research	4.6	✓	✓	✓	
Tommy's Campaign	1.3	✓			✓
WellBeing	1.0	✓		✓	✓

The Wellcome Trust (http://www.wellcome.ac.uk)

The Wellcome Trust is the world's largest medical research charity, with assets of £13 billion. It is constituted so as to function independently of commercial and political pressures and has a mission 'to foster and promote research with the aim of improving human and animal health'. With an annual expenditure of over £400 million (more than the MRC), the Wellcome Trust is a major contributor to UK bio-medical research. Recently, there has been a noteworthy initiative involving the Trust and government agencies. In 1998, a Joint Infrastructure Fund (JIF) was established, with a total budget of £750 million, comprising £300 million each from the Wellcome Trust and the Department of Trade and Industry (DTI) and £150 million from the Higher Education Funding Council for England (HEFCE). This represents the largest investment in university research facilities for more than 40 years.

In addition to this major initiative, the Trust provides support by means of project and programme grants and career development grants. There is also an important emphasis upon funding to underpin international research collaboration, with a unique funding scheme for projects and workers in tropical countries. The Trust also provides funding for smaller infrastructure schemes (less than £750 000) and can earmark funds to take advantage of emerging scientific opportunities or to foster the development of particular scientific disciplines. Noteworthy in this respect was the Trust's investment, with other important charitable and governmental partners, in the development of research in cardiology (see below).

The Cancer Research Campaign
(http://www.crc.org.uk)

The Cancer Research Campaign (CRC) was founded in 1923 and has a mission 'to attack and defeat the disease of cancer in all its forms, to investigate its treatment, and to promote its cure'. It is by far the largest British cancer charity, with an annual expenditure in excess of £50 million. While the CRC has a wide range of interests, encompassing all aspects of cancer, there has been important support for women's cancers. In relation to gynaecology, there are currently interests

in familial susceptibility (notably breast and ovarian cancers), prevention of cancers (including cervical) caused by viruses, screening programmes, cancer treatment (including vaccine treatment for cervical cancer), the psychological needs of women with cancer, and cancer in women from minority ethnic groups.

Action Research (http://www.actionresearch.co.uk)

Action Research supports a broad spectrum of research with the objectives of preventing disease and disability (regardless of cause or age group) and of alleviating physical handicap. Programme and project grant support is available and there is a small number of prestigious research training fellowships for young clinicians and scientists. The annual expenditure on research is approximately £4.5 million.

Tommy's Campaign

Tommy's Campaign funds research into fetal health, the causes of premature birth, miscarriage and stillbirth. Awards are predominantly project grants and there is long-term support for research groups and individual research workers. The annual expenditure on research is currently about £1.3 million.

WellBeing (http://www.wellbeing.demon.co.uk)

WellBeing is the research arm of the Royal College of Obstetricians and Gynaecologists. It funds research into all aspects of women's health and the health of newborn babies. The major areas of interest are pregnancy, women's cancers and quality of life issues. Project grants of up to £80 000 are available and there is a small number of clinical research training fellowships. The annual expenditure on research is currently about £1 million.

RESEARCH STRATEGY

It is difficult to quantify the amount of research funding currently held by academic departments of obstetrics and gynaecology. It is unlikely that the forthcoming Research Assessment Exercise will clarify matters, since obstetrics and gynaecology will not be identified separately from the other clinical disciplines that constitute Unit of Assessment 03 (Hospital-Based Clinical Subjects). It seems likely that obstetrics and gynaecology has performed reasonably well in comparison with such disciplines as surgery and child health but relatively poorly in comparison with medical specialties, notably neurosciences. It is noteworthy that a concerted effort involving government agencies and major charitable bodies has substantially improved the research profile of cardiology within the last decade, and this discipline has been identified by both the government and MRC as a priority area for investment. No such priority is currently awarded to women's health. There is a need for a coordinated strategic approach to the development of research in this field.

In order to coordinate research activity and improve funding in obstetrics and gynaecology, it would be helpful to identify areas that are considered currently to be of importance by those carrying out research. In 1996, letters were sent to the heads of the 32 university departments of obstetrics and gynaecology, to the 23 RCOG regional advisers, and to the RCOG Scientific Advisory and Audit Committees. A preliminary list was presented to the Association of Professors of Obstetrics and Gynaecology and a small group was set up to edit the responses in 1997. The final list is presented in Table 50.7.

In order to focus research effort further, it will be necessary to prioritise research objectives, taking into account such factors as the clinical relevance of the topic in question, its scientific importance, and the likelihood of significant advance from research carried out at this time. One technique that can be used for this purpose is a Foresight Project, such as was carried out for cardiology. The process is outlined in Figure 50.3 and is further described here. The numbers in the following list refer to those in the figure:

1. It is first necessary to establish a robust database, defining the scope of the discipline, the resources currently committed to research, and the output in terms of research publications.
2. Further interviews with research workers and selected

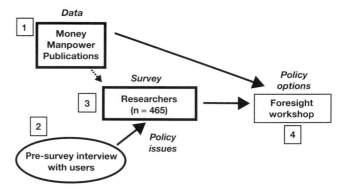

Fig. 50.3 Outline of the Cardiovascular Foresight Project. See text for explanation.

clinicians should be carried out when complete information is available. The model previously used may be considered appropriate.
3. A detailed survey of research workers should then be planned and executed in order to determine in a preliminary fashion the relative values which they would attribute to the topics identified.
4. A workshop involving research workers, clinical and non-clinical, as well as representatives of the profession and of the major providers of research funding can then be held, so that the final strategy can be drawn up. Appropriate representation is important so that the research community will develop a sense of ownership of the proposals.

Table 50.7 Research priorities in obstetrics and gynaecology, 1997

Clinical and laboratory research
Pre-implantation studies
Molecular genetics
Fetal abnormality
Fetal nutrition
Fetal behaviour
Human fertilisation
Implantation
Fertility regulation
Gametogenesis:
 • sperm count
 • oocyte culture
Climacteric:
 • psychology
 • patient selection
Cancer screening
Vaccines and cancer

Epidemiological and health services research
Menorrhagia trials
Rates of fetal growth
Infection:
 • pelvic inflammation
 • premature labour
 • cervical cancer
Hormone replacement therapy:
 • acceptability
 • uptake
 • continuity of treatment
 • rates of cancers
Translation of research into practice

ACADEMIC RECRUITMENT

There is increasing concern that good clinical scientists may be dissuaded from pursuing a career in obstetrics and gynaecology (Symonds & Arulkumaran 1999). This may be a generic problem affecting many academic disciplines (Richards 1997), but there is currently no evidence of a decline in numbers of academic posts within obstetrics and gynaecology (Rodeck 1999). On the other hand, a survey by the Academic Committee of the RCOG (Rodeck 1999) recorded a 23% reduction in MD and PhD students between 1997 and 1999. Of particular concern was the marked decrease (from 26 to 8) in postgraduate studentships funded by the MRC. Concerns of this sort in the United States of America have led to the introduction of innovative training programmes (Longo 1999). Similar initiatives are needed in the UK.

The past decade has seen major changes in postgraduate clinical training (Department of Health 1993). There is now great emphasis on structured training programmes leading to the award of a Certificate of Completion of Specialist Training which signifies the acquisition of a minimum standard of clinical competence. Such a move is in general to be welcomed but it carries the risk of encouraging all trainees to follow virtually identical career pathways, thus reducing the flexibility required for those who wish to have a less conventional career. Solutions to this problem have been suggested by working parties of the Royal College of Physicians of London (Arthur & Alberti 1999) and of the Academy of Medical Sciences (Savill 2000). Essentially, these groups have suggested an interdigitating package of training, with substantial periods of time spent away from clinical practice in order to complete research degrees and to learn the skills required to lead a research team. Such a solution may create problems for those who need to develop and maintain technical skills in order to function as a safe clinician. Thus it seems likely that somewhat different patterns of training will have to be devised for academic obstetricians and gynaecologists. What is important is to maintain the maximum possible degree of flexibility compatible with the delivery of effective training. It is to the advantage of trainees in obstetrics and gynaecology that the training programme attempts to assess competence rather than simply insisting upon the performance of a predetermined number of cases of certain types. Furthermore, it has already been possible to devise flexible programmes of training for subspecialists with the minimum of disruption to core specialist training. Nevertheless, it is important for the RCOG to clarify these issues. At the time of writing, reports from working parties auditing *structured training* and addressing the needs of *training for clinical academics* are being prepared. It is likely that significant changes will be proposed in the near future.

CONCLUSION

There is no room for complacency in relation to research in obstetrics and gynaecology. Funding of quality is becoming more difficult to secure and there are fewer research students, the seedcorn for our academic establishment in the future. The training needs of junior clinical research workers must be addressed with vigour and ways must be found to make an academic career a more attractive proposition than it appears to be at present. One important way of doing this is to show that research in obstetrics and gynaecology is held in high esteem. The development of a research strategy supported by the profession, by research workers and by government agencies is a vital part of this process.

Guidance for those wishing to embark upon a research project is set out below. Consultation is of paramount importance. Planning must be rigorous, feasibility and probity must be transparent, and funding must be secure. The recent increase in bureaucracy associated with research planning is frustrating for those eager to pursue new ideas but in the current climate of public accountability cannot be avoided.

KEY POINTS: GUIDANCE FOR RESEARCH WORKERS

- Identify an area of interest and define it clearly.
- Review literature using such resources as MEDLINE and the Cochrane Database.
- Make a working plan of the project.
- Ensure appropriate clinical, scientific and statistical advice.
- Review feasibility within the current working environment.
- Draw up a detailed research protocol taking further specialised advice.
- Obtain approval from local research and ethics committees.
- Submit approved protocol for peer review and funding.
- Inform colleagues of plans.
- Construct a database so that information can be easily processed later.
- Review progress regularly and compensate for any slippage.
- Analyse data with all relevant team members.
- Draft potential publications and target relevant journals.
- Write systematically in appropriate format for journal, delegating where necessary.
- Arrange local peer review of publication.
- Submit final version.
- Accept editorial amendments whenever possible.
- Consider submission to another journal if necessary.
- Review progress with colleagues and plan further research.

REFERENCES

Arthur MJP, Alberti KGMM 1999 Training in academic medicine: a way forward for the new millenium. J Roy Coll Physicians Lond 33:1–7

Association of Medical Research Charities Handbook 2000. Chartwell Press, Wigston, Leicestershire

Department of Health 1993 Hospital doctors—training for the future. The report of the working group on Specialist Medical Training (Calman Report). Department of Health, London

HRP Online 2000 http://www.who.int/hrp/about/index.html

Longo LD 1999 Training of academic staff in obstetrics and gynaecology in the USA. Baillieres Clin Obstet Gynaecol 13:403–421

Richards RE 1997 Clinical academic careers. Report commissioned by the Committee of Vice-Chancellors and Principals

Rodeck CH 1999 The second biennial survey of academic departments of obstetrics and gynaecology in the United Kingdom. RCOG, London

Savill J 2000 More in expectation than in hope: a new attitude to training in clinical academic medicine. BMJ 320:630–633

Symonds EM, Arulkumaran S 1999 Recruitment and training of academic staff in obstetrics and gynaecology. Baillière's Best Practice and Research. Baillière Tindall, London

WHO Special Programme of Research, Development and Research Training in Human Reproduction 1988 Research in Human Reproduction. Biennial Report 1986–87. World Health Organization, Geneva

Index